EDITED BY

ROBISON D. HARLEY, M.D., Ph.D., F.A.C.S.

Professor and Chairman, Department of Ophthalmology,
Temple University Health Sciences Center;
Director of Pediatric Ophthalmology Department, Wills Eye Hospital;
Chief Attending Surgeon, Saint Christopher's Hospital for Children

WITH CONTRIBUTIONS BY 46 AUTHORITIES

1975

PEDIATRIC OPHTHALMOLOGY

W. B. SAUNDERS COMPANY   PHILADELPHIA
LONDON
TORONTO

W. B. Saunders Company: West Washington Square
Philadelphia, PA 19105

12 Dyott Street
London, WC1A 1DB

833 Oxford Street
Toronto, Ontario M8Z 5T9, Canada

Pediatric Ophthalmology   ISBN 0-7216-4525-9

Print No.:   9   8   7   6   5   4   3   2   1

Dedicated To:
Loyde
Robison, Jr.
Ardee
Heather
Halvor II
William II
Robert B.
J. William D.
Larson L.
J. William, Jr.

For Their
Love
Patience
Loyalty
and
Understanding

Contributors

VICTOR H. AUERBACH, Ph.D.

Research Professor in Pediatrics (Biochemistry), Temple University School of Medicine; Director of the Enzyme Laboratory and Director of Research Chemistry, St. Christopher's Hospital for Children, Philadelphia, Pennsylvania.

Inborn Errors of Metabolism

CARROLL F. BURGOON, Jr., M.D.

Professor of Dermatology, Temple University Health Sciences Center, Philadelphia, Pennsylvania.

Ocular Changes in Skin Disorders

JOSEPH H. CALHOUN, M.D.

Senior Assistant Surgeon, Wills Eye Hospital; Clinical Affiliate of Children's Hospital, Philadelphia, Pennsylvania.

Disorders of Blood, Blood Vessels, Heart and Lungs: Histiocytosis Syndromes

MARIE A. CAPITANIO, M.D.

Professor of Radiology, Temple University School of Medicine; Chief of the Department of Radiology, St. Christopher's Hospital for Children, Philadelphia, Pennsylvania.

Radiologic Diagnosis and Therapy

GUY H. CHAN, Jr., M.D.

Associate Professor, Temple University School of Medicine; Assistant Surgeon, Department of Pediatrics and Motility, Wills Eye Hospital, Philadelphia, Pennsylvania.

Systemic Bacterial Diseases; Nutritional Deficiency Disorders; Drug Toxicity

FRANKLIN E. CIGNETTI, M.D.

Assistant Professor of Ophthalmology and Pathology, Eye and Ear Hospital of Pittsburgh, Pittsburgh, Pennsylvania.

Systemic Viral Diseases

JEAN-PIERRE COLLINS, M.D., F.R.C.P.(C.), C.S.P.Q.

Clinical Professor of Dermatology, University of Montreal; Attending Staff Dermatologist, Hotel-Dieu Hospital and Lakeshore General Hospital, Montreal, Canada.

Ocular Changes in Skin Disorders

MARTHA HAYDEN DANIS, M.D.

Formerly Associate Professor of Anesthesiology and Associate Professor of Pediatrics, Temple University School of Medicine; Chairman, Department of Anesthesiology, St. Christopher's Hospital for Children, Philadelphia, Pennsylvania. Present Appointment: Anesthesiologist, Emerson Hospital, Concord, Massachusetts.

Anesthesiology for Surgery of the Eye

JAY L. FEDERMAN, M.D.

Assistant Professor of Ophthalmology, Department of Pathology, Temple University Health Sciences Center; Assistant Professor, Department of Ophthalmology, Jefferson Medical College of Thomas Jefferson University; Senior Assistant Surgeon and Clinical Assistant in Pathology, Retina Service, Wills Eye Hospital; Assistant in Department of Ophthalmology, Lankenau Hospital, Philadelphia, Pennsylvania.

Fluorescein Angiography

JOSEPH C. FLANAGAN, M.D.

Assistant Professor, Jefferson Medical College of Thomas Jefferson University; Senior Assistant Surgeon, Oculoplastic Service, Wills Eye Hospital; Assistant in Ophthalmology, Lankenau Hospital; Associate Attending Surgeon, Fitzgerald Mercy Hospital, Philadelphia, Pennsylvania.

Diseases of the Lacrimal Apparatus; Disorders of the Lids

ROGER D. FREEMAN, M.D.

Associate Professor and Director, Services

for Handicapped Children, Department of Psychiatry, University of British Columbia; Active Staff, Vancouver General Hospital; Courtesy Staff, Children's Hospital and Sunny Hill Hospital for Children, Vancouver, Canada.

Emotional Components in Pediatric Ophthalmology

FRANCIS P. FURGIUELE, M.D.

Clinical Associate Professor of Ophthalmology, University of Pennsylvania School of Medicine and Scheie Eye Institute; Chief of Ophthalmology, Chestnut Hill Hospital; Attending Surgeon, Wills Eye Hospital, Philadelphia, Pennsylvania.

Disorders of the Conjunctiva

GLEN G. GIBSON, M.D.

Professor of Ophthalmology, Temple University Health Sciences Center; Senior Consultant for Wills Eye Hospital, Philadelphia, Pennsylvania.

Ophthalmic Examination of Infants and Children

LEONARD S. GIRSH, M.D.

Assistant Professor of Internal Medicine (Allergy Specialist), Temple University School of Medicine and Health Sciences Center; Pediatric Allergist, St. Christopher's Hospital for Children and Temple University School of Medicine and Health Sciences Center; Allergist, Holy Redeemer Hospital, Philadelphia, Pennsylvania.

Allergic States

W. RICHARD GREEN, M.D.

Associate Professor of Ophthalmology and Assistant Professor of Pathology, Johns Hopkins University School of Medicine; Ophthalmologist and Pathologist, Johns Hopkins Hospital, Baltimore, Maryland.

Tumors of the Eye, Lids, and Orbit

ALAN B. GRUSKIN, M.D.

Associate Professor of Pediatrics, Temple University School of Medicine; Director of Pediatric Nephrology, St. Christopher's Hospital for Children, Philadelphia, Pennsylvania.

Ocular-Genitourinary Manifestations of Diseases

JOSEPH W. HALLETT, A.B., M.D.

Clinical Professor of Ophthalmology, Jefferson Medical College of Thomas Jefferson University; Lecturer in Ophthalmology, University of Pennsylvania School of Medicine; Attending Surgeon and Chief of Uveitis Department, Wills Eye Hospital; Attending Ophthalmologist, Einstein Medical Center (Daroff Division), Philadelphia, Pennsylvania.

Disorders of the Uveal Tract

ROBISON D. HARLEY, M.D., Ph.D., F.A.C.S.

Professor and Chairman, Department of Ophthalmology, Temple University Health Sciences Center; Director of Pediatric Ophthalmology Department, Wills Eye Hospital; Chief Attending Surgeon, St. Christopher's Hospital for Children, Philadelphia, Pennsylvania.

Genetics; Diseases of the Orbit; Glaucoma; Collagen Diseases; Connective Tissue Disorders; Mycotic Infections; Ocular Parasitosis

LOUIS S. HEYMAN

Technical Consultant to Corneal Service and to Contact Lens Division, Department of Visual Physiology, Wills Eye Hospital, Philadelphia, Pennsylvania.

Corneal and Scleral Contact Lenses in Children

DAVID A. HILES, M.D.

Clinical Assistant Professor of Ophthalmology, University of Pittsburgh School of Medicine; Chief of Ophthalmology, Children's Hospital of Pittsburgh; Director, Fight for Sight Children's Eye Clinic, Eye and Ear Hospital of Pittsburgh, Pittsburgh, Pennsylvania.

Systemic Viral Diseases

ARTHUR H. KEENEY, M.D., D.Sc.

Dean of the School of Medicine and Professor and Acting Chairman, Department of Ophthalmology, University of Louisville School of Medicine, Louisville, Kentucky.

Growth and Development of the Eye; Trauma of Globe, Adnexa, and Orbital Walls

VIRGINIA T. KEENEY, M.D.

Associate Professor, Department of Family Practice, University of Louisville School of Medicine, Louisville, Kentucky.

Reading Disabilities in Children

JOHN A. KIRKPATRICK, M.D.

Professor of Radiology, Harvard Medical School; Radiologist-in-Chief, The Children's Hospital Medical Center, Boston, Massachusetts.

Radiologic Diagnosis and Therapy

PETER R. LAIBSON, M.D.

Professor of Ophthalmology, Jefferson Medical College of Thomas Jefferson University; Director, Cornea Service, and Attending Surgeon, Wills Eye Hospital, Philadelphia, Pennsylvania.

Diseases of the Cornea

REGINA LITTLE LESTER, B.A.

Blind Services Specialist, Pennsylvania Department of Public Welfare; Consultant to public and private agencies, low vision centers, and schools on visual functioning problems. Member of Advisory Committee, Regional Center for Deaf-Blind Children, Harrisburg, Pennsylvania.

The Visually Handicapped Child

DONELSON R. MANLEY, M.D.

Associate Professor of Ophthalmology, Temple University Health Sciences Center; Attending Ophthalmologist, St. Christopher's Hospital for Children; Associate Director of Department of Pediatrics and Motility, Wills Eye Hospital; Consulting Ophthalmologist, Overbrook School for the Blind; Consulting Ophthalmologist for Easter Seal Society of Greater Philadelphia, Philadelphia, Pennsylvania.

Strabismus; Glaucoma

LOIS J. MARTYN, M.D.

Assistant Professor in Pediatrics (Ophthalmology) and Instructor of Ophthalmology, Temple University School of Medicine; Assistant Attending Ophthalmologist, St. Christopher's Hospital for Children; Assistant Surgeon, Department of Pediatrics and Motility, Wills Eye Hospital, Philadelphia, Pennsylvania.

Pediatric Neuro-Ophthalmology; Mucopolysaccharidoses

P. ROBB McDONALD, B.S., M.D.

Professor of Ophthalmology, Jefferson Medical College of Thomas Jefferson University; Senior Consultant, Lankenau Hospital; Consulting Surgeon, Wills Eye Hospital, Philadelphia, Pennsylvania.

Disorders of the Lens

ADA MOFFITT, B.S.

Former Director, Orthoptics and Pleoptics, Department of Pediatric Ophthalmology, Wills Eye Hospital; Fight for Sight Children's Clinic, Philadelphia, Pennsylvania.

Orthoptics and Pleoptics

EVERETT MOODY, M.D.

Clinical Assistant Professor, University of Texas Southwestern Medical School; Director of Ophthalmology Division, Scottish Rite Hospital, Dallas, Texas.

Ophthalmic Examination of Infants and Children; Amblyopia

DON H. NICHOLSON, M.D.

Assistant Professor of Ophthalmology, University of Miami School of Medicine and Bascom Palmer Eye Institute, Miami, Florida.

Tumors of the Eye, Lids, and Orbit

ARNOLD B. POPKIN, M.D.

Instructor, Rutgers Medical School; Assistant Surgeon, Wills Eye Hospital, Philadelphia; Attending Ophthalmologist, Medical Center at Princeton, New Jersey, and Freehold Area Hospital, Freehold, New Jersey.

Electroretinography

HOPE H. PUNNETT, Ph.D.

Professor in Pediatrics, Temple University School of Medicine; Chief, Genetics Section, and Director, Cytogenetics Laboratory, St. Christopher's Hospital for Children, Philadelphia, Pennsylvania.

Genetics

HARRY SALEM, Ph.D.

Assistant Professor of Pharmacology, University of Pennsylvania School of Medicine, Philadelphia, Pennsylvania.

Allergic States

ROBERT A. SARGENT, M.D.

Clinical Instructor of Ophthalmology, University of Colorado Medical Center; Pediatric Ophthalmologist, The Children's Hospital, Denver, Colorado.

Ocular Manifestations of Skeletal Disorders

LOV K. SARIN, M.D.

Attending Surgeon, Wills Eye Hospital; Department of Ophthalmology, Lankenau Hospital, Philadelphia, Pennsylvania.

Fluorescein Angiography; Ultrasonography; Differential Diagnosis of Leukocoria

GERARD M. SHANNON, M.D., M.Sc.

Professor of Ophthalmology, Jefferson Medical College of Thomas Jefferson University; Attending Surgeon and Director of Oculoplastic Department, Wills Eye Hospital; Senior Attending Ophthalmologist, Nazareth Hospital and Holy Redeemer Hospital, Philadelphia, Pennsylvania.

Disorders of the Lids

JERRY A. SHIELDS, M.D.

Assistant Professor, Temple University School of Medicine; Assistant Surgeon, Retina Service, Wills Eye Hospital, Philadelphia, Pennsylvania.

Ultrasonography; Differential Diagnosis of Leukocoria

EDMUND B. SPAETH, M.D.

Emeritus Professor of Ophthalmology, University of Pennsylvania School of Medicine; Consultant, Wills Eye Hospital; Consultant, Graduate Hospital, University of Pennsylvania; Consultant, U.S. Naval Hospital, Philadelphia, Pennsylvania.

Diseases of the Orbit

GEORGE L. SPAETH, M.D.

Professor of Ophthalmology, Jefferson Medical College of Thomas Jefferson University; Director, Glaucoma Service, Wills Eye Hospital, Philadelphia, Pennsylvania.

Inborn Errors of Metabolism; Endocrine Disorders

PHILIP G. SPAETH, M.D.

Clinical Professor, Jefferson Medical College of Thomas Jefferson University; Associate Ophthalmologist, University of Pennsylvania School of Medicine; Attending Surgeon, Wills Eye Hospital, Philadelphia, Pennsylvania.

Corneal and Scleral Contact Lenses in Children

EDWIN C. TAIT, M.D., M.S.

Clinical Associate Professor of Ophthalmology, Temple University Health Sciences Center, Philadelphia; Chief of Ophthalmology, Montgomery Hospital, Norristown, Pennsylvania.

Refraction and Heterophoria

WILLIAM TASMAN, M.D.

Clinical Professor of Ophthalmology, Jefferson Medical College of Thomas Jefferson University; Attending Surgeon, Retina Service, Wills Eye Hospital, Philadelphia, Pennsylvania.

Diseases of the Retina and Vitreous

KENNETH C. TROUTMAN, D.D.S.

Associate Professor and Chairman, Department of Pediatric Dentistry, M.C.V.-V.C.U. School of Dentistry; Attending Pedodontist, M.C.V.-V.C.U. Hospital and Richmond Crippled Children's Hospital, Richmond, Virginia.

Ocular and Associated Dental Changes in Pediatric Syndromes

GEORGE O. WARING, M.D.

Assistant Professor of Ophthalmology, School of Medicine, University of California at Davis, California.

Diseases of the Cornea

SIDNEY WEISS, M.D.

Clinical Assistant Professor of Ophthalmology, University of Pennsylvania School of Medicine; Consultant in Ophthalmology, Wills Eye Hospital; Medical Director, Low Vision Center, Center for the Blind, Philadelphia, Pennsylvania.

Optical Aids for Children With Subnormal Vision

Foreword

Many years ago, when I first met Frank Costenbader, now the Dean of American Pediatric Ophthalmology, he told me he was limiting his practice to the care of children. I remember thinking at the time that practice in Washington, D.C., must be quite different from what I was accustomed to in Philadelphia. I knew that if I tried to limit my practice to youngsters under thirteen, my office would be empty many days of the week. Very few consultations would come my way from colleagues just because I espoused that particular portion of the ophthalmic garden to cultivate. All of my colleagues appeared to be quite happy with every case of strabismus or congenital cataracts that came their way for operation. There might be grandeur in being a pediatric ophthalmologist, but not much more. I would be faced with starvation, not stardom.

Today, things are quite different. The number of ophthalmologists limiting their practices to children has increased enormously, and rightly so. More and more reports of congenital and inherited pediatric syndromes having ocular complications are filling our journals. Research in the genetics and biochemistry of these conditions is occupying the attention of laboratory workers. A new society has been formed to create a proper forum where these problems can be discussed in depth by those concerned, saving time and compressing into one session what would otherwise be distributed over many sessions and conferences in the meetings of our general ophthalmological societies. The new American Association for Pediatric Ophthalmology now has several hundred members.

The knowledge demanded to meet the needs of the pediatric ophthalmologist calls for an authoritative textbook covering all phases of the subject, which this book does. In addition to the problems of strabismus and congenital cataracts, a text is needed in such a rapidly advancing discipline with particular emphasis on the latest developments in genetics, inborn errors of metabolism, newly recognized syndromes, pediatric neuro-ophthalmology and other ocular disorders peculiar to children.

The ophthalmologist who does not limit his practice to one age group needs a ready source of information to consult, for example, when a child is brought to his office with gross bodily deformities and clouding of the corneas. Recognizing that connective tissue disorders present themselves in young children in various types, the question arises, which one does this child represent? It is impossible to consult the literature during office hours, and some compact, ready reference must be found before one can proceed intelligently with the examination. The chapter on the Mucopolysaccharidoses in this book supplies this in table form together with a comprehensive description of each type of MPS. This is just one example of the usefulness of this book to the general ophthalmologist.

Pediatric ophthalmology seems to have come of age, and it is noteworthy that at the approximate first birthday of the American Association for Pediatric Ophthalmology, an excellent and authoritative textbook is published to supply this specialized knowledge to students and practicing ophthalmologists.

FRANCIS HEED ADLER, M.D.

The IV Stumbling Blocks to Truth

Invented by the Anglican Mage Br. Roger Bacon, O.F.M.

    I.   The Influence of Fragile or Unworthy Authority.

    II. Custom.

    III. The Imperfection of Undisciplined Senses.

    IV. Concealment of Ignorance by Ostentation of Seeming Wisdom.

—Don Tarquinio
Baron Corvo

Preface

Recent developments in ophthalmology have been especially apparent in the pediatric area. The mass of accumulated information in inborn errors of metabolism, genetics, congenital abnormalities, newly recognized syndromes, diagnostic techniques and therapy has become enormous in just a few years and alone justifies a review.

Inherent in the organization of data relating to basic and clinical sciences is the factor of obsolescence, a process involving the relentless sifting out of errors and misconceptions as new and more accurate information becomes available. Many portions of this text will soon be outdated, and we recognize this as a mark of progress. It will be the task of those who follow to continue to correct errors, identify misconceptions, reassemble data and insert basic new facts and information.

This volume was originally conceived as a teaching manual for residents, fellows and practitioners. A group of experts was invited to contribute essential information and material covering many special areas of ophthalmology as they relate to pediatrics.

In the effort to produce a text for instruction, and as happened, a reasonably definitive reference, the editor attempted to gather material with particular clinical value — material useful for residency training in ophthalmology, for practicing ophthalmologists and for pediatricians, with minimal emphasis on controversial subjects or untested research data.

The special consideration given certain subjects reflects the composite opinion of the authors and editor concerning their important relevance to particular aspects of pediatric ophthalmology. Generous use of illustrations and tables has been allowed.

It has been most stimulating to serve as both editor of and contributor to this book, but the major credit must be assigned to the many other individual contributors who took the time to create exceptional chapters in their particular fields of work. To them and to all who collaborated herein, the editor wishes to express his most sincere appreciation and gratitude.

Wills Eye Hospital and St. Christopher's Hospital for Children are rich storehouses of clinical material. They have provided the major background for this book. The two institutions complement each other uniquely in the cases most prevalently seen, St. Christopher's having many children with ocular manifestations of systemic disease, whereas at Wills one sees a wide spectrum of the most bizarre, often subtle, ocular abnormalities.

Two foundations and several individuals deserve special mention because of valuable contributions of equipment and personnel that have made possible the study of patients, the collection of data, and the utilization of research tools not readily available at many institutions. Fight for Sight, Incorporated, in New York, has operated and maintained the Children's Eye Center at Wills Eye Hospital, which averages 40 to 50 children daily and provides an opportunity for the study of an extremely wide variety of pediatric ocular disorders. The Pennsylvania Lions Eye Research and Sight Conservation Foundation has sponsored research development for many metabolic and degenerative diseases involving the eye that are included in this volume. Mr. and Mrs. Samuel Edelstein have been generous contributors to the eye research funds of both hospitals, enabling us to acquire special instruments not otherwise available.

I am especially appreciative of the members of the photographic department at Wills Eye Hospital, David Silva, Karen Albert and Laurel Weeney, and my secretaries, Bobi Perloff, Jessica Smith and Angela Agosto, who have worked countless hours in helping me to prepare manuscripts and illustrations.

Anyone may reasonably ask, "What are the compelling forces that drive an individual to compile such a mass of information on so specialized a subject?" I believe I responded both to a clear need for a current and reliable reference in pediatric ophthalmology and to a magnificent opportunity to collect and present the material for such a reference.

Perhaps all physicians in some way recognize an indebtedness to the profession of medicine and to influential teachers. Four individuals are prominent in my memory and deserve special citation. I wish to mention my ophthalmologist father, Halvor L. Harley, M.D., who awakened my first interest in medicine. Also, my professor of biology at Rutgers, Thurlow Nelson, Ph.D., who stimulated me to think; W. James Kennedy, M.D., of the Joseph Price Hospital, who taught me the art of patient care; and William L. Benedict, M.D., former head of Ophthalmology at the Mayo Clinic, who provided the wealth of clinical experiences that enriched the professional lives of so many of his former students.

It can be said of all who collaborated in this effort that we in no way consider this volume as the ultimate work on the subject of pediatric ophthalmology. On the contrary, we present it with the fervent hope that it will be corrected, improved, and supplemented by other colleagues who continue to be fascinated by this most interesting sub-speciality.

ROBISON D. HARLEY

Contents

Chapter 7

Everett A. Moody

Chapter 8

Edmund B. Spaeth and Robison D. Harley

Chapter 9

Joseph Flanagan

Chapter 10

DISORDERS OF THE LIDS.. 238

Gerard M. Shannon and Joseph Flanagan

Chapter 11

DISORDERS OF THE CONJUNCTIVA...................................... 256

Francis P. Furgiuele

Chapter 12

DISEASES OF THE CORNEA 273

Peter R. Laibson and George O. Waring

Chapter 13

DISORDERS OF THE UVEAL TRACT 326

Joseph W. Hallett

Chapter 14

DISEASES OF THE RETINA AND VITREOUS 347

William Tasman

Chapter 15

DISORDERS OF THE LENS 370

P. Robb McDonald

Chapter 16

GLAUCOMA IN INFANTS AND CHILDREN 390

Robison D. Harley and Donelson R. Manley

Chapter 17

TRAUMA OF THE GLOBE, ADNEXA, AND ORBITAL WALLS: PROPHYLAXIS AND IMMEDIATE THERAPY 413

Arthur H. Keeney

Chapter 20

OCULAR CHANGES IN PEDIATRIC SYSTEMIC DISORDERS 622

A. Ocular Manifestations in Endocrine Disorders.................... 622

George L. Spaeth

B. Ocular Manifestations in Disorders of the Blood, Blood Vessels, Heart, and Lungs, and in the Histiocytosis Syndromes 648

Joseph Calhoun

Chapter 29

ANESTHESIA IN THE PEDIATRIC PATIENT FOR SURGERY OF THE EYE...... 852
Martha Hayden Danis

Chapter 30

OCULAR CHANGES IN SKIN DISORDERS................................. 861
Carroll F. Burgoon, Jr., and Jean-Pierre Collins

Chapter 31

OCULAR MANIFESTATIONS OF SKELETAL DISORDERS............................ 885
Robert A. Sargent

Chapter 32

OPTICAL AIDS FOR CHILDREN WITH SUBNORMAL VISION.................... 900
Sidney Weiss

CONTENTS

CHAPTER 1

GROWTH AND DEVELOPMENT OF THE EYE

ARTHUR H. KEENEY, M.D., D.Sc.

INTRODUCTION

Optimal understanding of pediatric ophthalmology, and particularly the area of normal variation versus abnormal development, requires a working knowledge of embryology. The field of morphologic embryology has a long history of accuracy, beginning with Aristotle's *De generatione animalium* more than 300 years B.C. Many centuries of dormancy followed, however, until Hieronymus Fabricius prepared his beautifully illustrated *De Formato Foetus* in Venice in 1600, republished in 1967 in a facsimile edition by Cornell University Press. The next major advance, primarily in comparative embryology, came in 1651 from the splendid English physician William Harvey, who wrote *Exercitationes de Generatione*. The introduction of light microscopy or histology into embryology is properly a function of Marcello Malpighi of Italy in the 1670s. Many documentalists of specific components helpfully exploited the insight of microscopy, but it was not until German Nobel Prize laureate Hans

Spemann identified the "organizer concept" (1912–1936) that substantial advance was made in understanding *mechanisms* in embryology.

Though few Herculean figures rise in ocular embryology, Miss Ida Mann, first woman to be appointed ocular surgeon at Moorfields, produced more classic data than any other worker in detailed morphology of ocular development. The three editions of her book, *Development of the Human Eye* (1928, 1949, and 1964), bring the extensive bibliography of the field up to 1958.

The research reports offering the greatest contribution during the past two decades have been in the field of immunologic factors, amino acid formation, and protein synthesis in the ocular (and other embryologic) primordia. This is a logical outgrowth of the earlier decades that has developed from an understanding of embryologic biochemistry and has led to the identification of some 17 different crystallines in the embryonic lens. Of nearly equal fascination in the same decades has been the more detailed visualization of embryologic changes through the electron microscope. This has brought clarity to the previous controversy concerning anterior chamber angle development by showing tissue rarefaction and intercellular fenestration rather than simple atrophy or absorption.

The high linear accuracy and the non-destructive characteristics of ultrasonic measurements have further added to critical understanding of specific growth rates in development of each ocular component. These increasingly precise measurements have clarified much of the differential growth of various components which affect final interrelationships. A commonly recognized unit of embryologic development is the 5 mm. stage (crown-rump length) achieved early in the fourth week of gestation. At this time, the optic cups have formed by invagination from the optic vesicles, and the lens pit is morphologically distinct in the surface ectoderm. Still, the entire embryo and its membranes could nestle comfortably within a teaspoon. With far more precision, it is now easy to understand that the diameter of the eyes at approximately 10 weeks of gestation is 1 mm. Growth proceeds rapidly so that at the end of the fetal period, or the end of the twelfth week, the globes have reached a diameter of 3 mm., and by the end of the fourth lunar month the diameters have more than doubled to 6 or 8 mm. At the end of the sixth lunar month, the diameters are nearly doubled again to 12 mm. This rapid pace continues to birth, at which time the anterior-posterior diameter of the globes is approximately 15 mm., with a vitreous length of approximately 10.4 mm. in boys and 10.2 mm. in girls. In the first year of postnatal life, the vitreous length increases approximately 3.1 mm. in males and 3.0 mm. in females, and then in both sexes the increase is approximately 1.3 mm. a year from the second to the seventh year (Larsen, 1971). Prior to the use of ultrasound, it was not possible to derive measurements such as these that can be critically related to optical measurements. D. J. Coleman at Columbia Presbyterian Hospital has refined the accuracy of his M-scan ultrasound to 0.02 mm., which will assess growth and accommodative changes in axial diameter of the lens as well as thickness and even vascular pulsations in the choroid.

The complex narrative concerning development of individual tissues of the globe can easily be found well recorded in extensive detail in the classic textbook of Ida Mann (1964), in programed instruction format in the 1967 monograph of the American Academy of Ophthalmology and Otolaryngology (Pearson, 1967), in gatefold chronologic tables (Keeney, 1951), or in telegraphic outline (Keeney, 1966). It is vital, however, to be aware of certain neurologic and functional correlates which are often missed in step by step descriptions of ocular development. It is also essential to be aware of revised and new concepts which the past few years have added to understanding in this field.

The several types of RNA, the messengers from genetic DNA which carry developmental formulas for the templates of protein synthesis, are established in appropriate cells long before morphologic specialization can be visualized. Actual positioning of the eye is established in oogenesis, and by the time fertilization has occurred, the position of the lens is fairly well demarcated. The RNA-directed formation of intracellular amino acids, early polypeptide chains, and first stage proteins takes place before specialization of cells is seen in light microscopy. With the development of complex chemical molecular biology, there is also a concomitant mechanical molecular biology producing the structural changes or elongations of specialized visual cells. From the ocular point of view, both these components increase so rapidly that by early in the fourth week of gestation, or the approximately 4.5 mm. stage, the optic anlage constitutes the greatest mass of forebrain material.

The fetal or choroidal fissure which permits transient access of nutrient vessels into the optic cup begins to close in the fifth week and is completely closed in the sixth week or at the 16 mm. stage. Irregularities or failures in this closure produce the striking congenital anomalies seen as colobomas of the iris, zonule, lens, choroid, retina, or optic nerve. These may be of only casual significance in the appearance of the iris or may result in sight-devastating defects of vision involving the optic nerve.

VASCULAR DEVELOPMENT

Development of both arterial and venous passages is subject to considerable variation throughout the body, but traditionally this is held to be more common in the venous than in the arterial system. Vascular variations develop so commonly within the fundus that they have even been proposed by French criminologists as a method for personal identification. The presence of cilioretinal arteries, supplying the macular areas and posterior poles, is documented in 20 or 25 per cent of eyes. The vortex veins, collecting choroidal blood and serving as essential landmarks to the retinal surgeon, may at times appear as double the usual number of four or in large eyes may appear as posterior or choriovaginal veins. Such vascular components are generally finalized in their distribution well before the end of the period of the embryo. However, in the years since 1961, radiographic contrast studies of the superior ophthalmic vein through frontal vein injection have shown this single venous system to be highly consistent and free of developmental variations (Hanafee, 1972).

RETINA

Both improved chemical embryology and electron microscopy have identified the development of melanin in premelanosomes by the fifth week in the protoplasm of the cells of the pigment epithelium. By the ninth week, the microglial cells of mesenchymal origin begin the elaboration of identifiable mucopolysaccharides along the inner surface of the retina. About this time, the two layers of the optic cup, or the inner and outer layers of the retina, appear in physiologic apposition, though the potential cleavage plane between them persists throughout life as the embryologic source of retinal separation. This is commonly, though less aptly, referred to as "retinal detachment." Various hypoplasias of the macula have

been clinically recognized in association with poor central vision, but only in the last decade has the correlation of serous elevation in the macula with congenital pits of the optic nerve been established. These developmental defects seen in the nerve head were previously considered a curiosity of embryonic development and explained away on the basis of a minimal colobomatous defect. The use of fluorescein angiography has intimately coupled this defect with associated serous detachment of the macula even in mid adult life.

STRUCTURAL DEVELOPMENT OF THE GLOBE AND ITS RELATIONS TO REFRACTION

Growth and development of the human eye, particularly in relation to its overall or total refractive state (Kempf et al., 1928), has produced two major areas of continuing conflict in ophthalmic studies. First is the failure of earlier literature to subdivide the individual components of refraction when seeking to establish the hereditary modes of ametropia. The second has been more than a century of fragmentary findings and conjectural conclusions as to the degree and the methods by which environmental factors may modify inherited components of the globe. Early in the twentieth century, many biologists felt that hereditary and environmental modifications of structure were mutually exclusive alternatives. Recent decades, however, have clearly shown some interrelation between environmental factors and modifications in the genetic code.

In the final weeks of normal gestation, the lens is usually spherical, and the refractive index of the media is greater than in adult life. Thus, the refraction in premature birth (Fletcher and Brandon, 1955) and often at term (Gleiss and Pau, 1952) tends to be myopic by several diopters. However, the pupil at this stage in development is quite small, and of itself affords a compensatory source of better visual function. Atropine retinoscopy at birth generally reveals a scatter of refractive values conforming to the normal

Gaussian distribution and ranging from −3 to +8 diopters, but with a modal distribution of 1 to 3 diopters of hypermetropia (Wibaut, 1926).

Objective estimates of visual acuity in both the premature infant and the full-term newborn have indicated by elicited optokinetic nystagmus far better acuity (resolving power) than had been realized prior to the early 1960s (Dayton et al., 1964). Alternative evidence from EEG leads over the occipital cortex has shown on and off responses at birth, but never when the child was in natural sleep, prior to the age of one year. Photic driving of the usual occipital rhythm (2 to 7 per second) becomes frequent at the age of 5 months and almost constant at the age of 7 months. Apparently it is less marked and less frequent up to the age of one year. Absence of response to intermittent light stimulation does not indicate absence of useful vision, whereas the presence of occipital responses associated with apparent blindness suggests a potential improving prognosis or delayed myelinization (Stofft, 1961).

Actual development of total refraction and its components has shifted with growth and other developmental characteristics of populations, particularly in better documented and more intensively educated nations (Brown, 1938; Kempf et al., 1928; Slataper, 1950; Sorsby et al., 1961). Separate studies of more primitive populations, as in the Amazon basin and the Australian interior, have consistently shown an absence of myopia which has been related to visual requirements for survival in a hostile environment. The distribution of refractive errors in the more complex cultural nations has been a source of perplexity and changing values, particularly in recent decades.

The advent of ultrasound as an objective and simple instrument for measurement of ocular length, anterior chamber depth, and lens thickness has added much accuracy to this vital understanding of growth (Gernet and Olbrich, 1969; Leary et al., 1963). Without question, a correlative relationship of the components of refraction commonly maintains the limits of ametropia within the confines of plus to minus 4 diopters or so (Kettesy, 1949). The primary identified components are

(1) axial length; (2) anterior chamber depth; (3) corneal curvature (pars optica); (4) lens dimensions (thickness, anterior curvature, and posterior curvature); and (5) possible index factors. Of these, one of the most consistent is depth of the anterior chamber. Thus, literature a few decades ago (Kettesy, 1949; Wibaut, 1926) emphasized the "emmetropization of Straub" which in more current terminology is to be considered the nonpathologic or correlation ametropia within the range of plus or minus 3 or 4 diopters (Sorsby et al., 1962; van Alphen, 1961).

Contrariwise, the ametropia associated with specific pathologic conditions in refractive components of the eye or subsequent involutional changes in the retina may be considered as "miscorrelation" or a noncancellation by a combination of errors which generally exceeds the range of 5 or 6 diopters. Such conditions include spherophakia, staphyloma, megaloglobus, megalocornea, cornea plana, and excessive anterior chamber depth. Each of these components may constitute a separate genetic element. Statistically, the most common structural miscorrelation is that of axial myopia or what the environmental researcher would consider as "environmental myopic adaptation of axial length" (Young, 1963).

Environmental factors (Young, 1963) or isolated genetic patterns have been sought in anthropologic studies (Cass, 1966; Skeller, 1954), most of which have come under variously dissenting criticism. Similar studies have also been made among primates (Holm, 1937). Additional evidence from primates has been elicited in the primate research centers of this nation, particularly as championed by Francis A. Young, Ph.D., at the Primate Research Center of Washington State University in Pullman, Washington (Young, 1963; Young and Leary, 1967).

Colloquially designated *school myopia* or *study myopia* has been indeed associated with greater reading facility but seems to have eluded secure evidence of causal association between reading hours and axial length (Newman, 1929; Stansbury, 1948). The change in components other than axial lengths, however, has been documented by refractive analysis in the previous decade (Sorsby and Sheridan,

1953). Such a remote tissue as the retina apparently exercises a governing influence not only on the lens as seen grossly in its presence or absence in the salamander eye after experimental surgical excision of the embryonic retina, but also on correlated structural changes holding in balance the factors which could produce ametropia.

The potential environmental causes of myopia have been variously ascribed to not only excessive reading but poor light, poor diet, and poor print (Cass, 1966). An even more unusual approach has been that of gravity when the face is directed downward over the print, and this has been verified by three subsequent studies in monkeys (Levinsohn, 1929).

Even though consistent cause has not been demonstrated for the increasing myopic population (Otsuka, 1967; Sato, 1957) and sale of myopic spectacle lenses in the United States, therapeutic measures have been advanced (Bedrossian, 1966; Gostin, 1962). In general, these espoused treatments consist of mydriatic and cycloplegic drugs instilled one day to several days a week and fitting the growing child with an optimal distance correction plus an appropriate bifocal add to overcome the cycloplegic impairment of near vision. Such children may complain of light sensitivity and bifocal encumbrance. Better posture, diet, and lighting have been helpfully established as facilitating the speed and efficiency of the reading task, though these factors are questionably linked to developmental changes in the anatomy of the globes. A simple alternative seems to be that of encouraging the modestly myopic child to read and perform near tasks without spectacle correction.

Mechanisms postulated for axial elongation myopia subsequent to excessive near work generally relate to (1) tonically increased ciliary muscle contracture and (2) pressures of the long tendons of the lateral recti against the globes as held in convergence. Both these mechanisms potentially cause subtle increase in intraocular pressure and thereby produce pathologic elongation of the globe as related to the small percentage of children going on to high structural abnormalities.

DEVELOPMENT OF THE ANTERIOR CHAMBER AND STRUCTURAL PATHOLOGIC CONDITIONS UNDERLYING CONGENITAL GLAUCOMA

Analysis of anterior segment structural detail in fetal specimens (fourth lunar month through term) prior to the mid 1950s was plagued with some fixation artifacts and the concept of tissue absorption as a mechanism in creating the chamber angle. Initial observations of infants by clinical gonioscopy with low magnification did not clarify the actual mechanism and to some extent perpetuated the concept of mesodermal tissue filling the angle because of failure of resorption in the congenitally glaucomatous eye.

Development of the anterior chamber angle is now recognized (Smelser and Ozanics, 1971) to be primarily the product of (1) differential or excessive growth rates of the anterior segment as compared to the rest of the globe, particularly after the fifth lunar month; and (2) cleavage of tissue planes (Allen et al., 1955).

The components of the angle actually begin with a single layer of corneal endothelium which is established by the 12 mm. stage at the end of the fifth week. Embryologic purity would require that this be called *mesothelium* because of its mesodermal derivation. The use of the term endothelium, however, is firmly entrenched owing to its geographic position of ultimately lining the inner surface of the cornea. Simultaneously with this change, surface neuroectoderm, reunited over the lens vesicle, differentiates into corneal epithelium. By the end of the sixth week or the 16 mm. stage, future corneal stroma begins to form peripherally and extends over the entire dimensions of the cornea by the end of the seventh week or at 24 to 25 mm. At 17 mm., buds arise from the annular vessels and carry additional mesodermal tissue toward the anterior lens surface. This establishes, by the 22 mm. stage, a pupillary membrane in its peripheral portion, and at the same time, early iris stroma can be identified. By 24 mm., a very diaphanous but intact pupillary membrane is completed, and a relatively deep anterior chamber is present with its limiting apparent angles far anterior to their final position. Chamber depth is transiently reduced at the 25 to 30 mm. stage by pupillary membrane thickening and simultaneous thickening of the corneal stroma. The latter now develops collagenous staining.

At the 45 to 50 mm. stage (tenth week), 70 to 75 radial anlagen of the ciliary processes are formed by anterior growth of the optic cup margins. Simultaneously, there develops a condensation of cells with darkly staining, spindle-shaped nuclei arranged radially between the periphery of the corneal endothelium and the early scleral condensations. This forward extension is the early trabeculum and its posterior demarcation is the scleral spur, which becomes visible at the 48 to 50 mm. stage. Between the 50 and 65 mm. stages, the meridional ciliary muscle fibers condense. This is immediately followed by mesodermal iris thickening with concomitant vascular arcades. At the 76 to 85 mm. stage, the line of impending cleavage between the trabecular fibers and the ciliary body first is visible. Rapid growth, now in the anterior segment, causes apparent pupillary dilatation and pulls the ciliary processes peripherally from the lens. In the seventh month, the central vascular arcades shrink, the pupillary membrane opens, and Fuch's cleft appears between the true pupil and the absorbing pupillary membrane.

The angle of the anterior chamber deepens and enlarges peripherally by progressive cleavage, particularly in the last months and weeks of gestation. The continuing rapid growth of the anterior segment brings Schlemm's canal anterior to the scleral spur in the fifth month and anterior to the depth of the angle by the end of the eighth month. At birth, the usual relationships of scleral spur to Schlemm's canal and chamber angle are established, but the angle continues to be more narrow or acute for several years than it is in adult life. Circular fibers of the ciliary muscle do not appear until well into the first year of postpartum life.

Impairment of this cleavage between iris and ciliary body is a fundamental defect in the pathogenesis of congenital glaucoma. Associated with such cleavage is anterior insertion of the longitudinal and meridional ciliary muscle fibers. Contracture of such fibers compresses the trabeculum and Schlemm's canal rather than opening these structures as with normal or more posterior insertion. Scanning electron microscopy also reveals the development of intercellular pores in the continuous monolayer of polyhedral endothelial cells which smoothly cover the angle until the eighth month of gestation. Pore development is dramatically facilitated by the last weeks of rapidly differential growth and stretching of this layer.

Surgical goniotomy is successful in more than half these eyes by incising the anomalous trabeculum covering Schlemm's canal just posterior to the line of Schwalbe. Successful incision of the anomalous trabeculum (membrane or abnormal insertion) permits exposure of Schlemm's canal for adequate anterior chamber drainage. This permits access of aqueous to the trabeculum and allows posterior displacement of the ciliary muscles, which can then contract to facilitate trabecular opening.

GROWTH AND DEVELOPMENT OF THE LENS

For many decades it has been realized that the tip of the optic vesicle induces development of the lens placode in the overlying, single cell layer of surface ectoderm, which is originally cuboidal but eventually becomes columnar (Zwaan, 1972). This has been vaguely understood chronologically as to when it begins and when it ends. It has been only within the last decade that immunologic studies within the lens epithelium have identified the actual formation of crystallines, the various proteins of the lens, in the surface cells before morphologic elongations of the cells take place. Defects can occur here even before there is a morphologically specialized cell type.

In the differentiation of lens proteins and amino acids in the elongating cell of the lens placode, there have been at least 17 different forms of crystallines identified by immunofluorescence. These crystallines break down into three major groups which have some immunologic homogeneity and clearly give rise to the substance of the lens prior to elongation of the lens fibers.

The lens pit itself appears in the surface ectoderm at 6 to 7 mm., and this stage is morphologically understood. The lens pit then proceeds to formation of the lens vesicle by 8 or 9 mm. In early specimens, as pictured in older texts, there are "protoplasmic bridges" that go from the lens vesicle when it closes at 8 or 9 mm. to the reestablished surface ectoderm. By electron microscopy these protoplasmic bridges really do not exist. They appear to be coagulation defects which plagued light microscopists in earlier years. Present refined information is a result of better resolution and better understanding. These bridges are primarily artifacts.

The induction process itself continues for a long period of time and no one knows exactly when it ends. The factors responsible for lens induction are not exclusively in the tip of the optic cup but may also be as far back as the retinal anlage. Apparently, those bulbar components that come subsequently do not have any bearing on the development of the lens, cornea, or iris except as a complication. Elements present in the cup or even the retina anlage, in antecedent time, have a real bearing on lens formation.

As the lens epithelium differentiates at about 12 to 18 mm., pre-equatorial components may be identified as a germinal center. This delicate area gives rise to growing lens fibers. In the central portion of the epithelium, the cuboidal cells remain fairly stable or static, with a low mitotic rate throughout life. Nearer the lens equator, susceptibility to small insults increases, so that low doses of beta irradiation, even in adult life, cause peripheral punctate opacities. From the equatorial region, lens cells elongate to form irreversible fibers. These cells have complex potential in their seemingly simple development. They form acidophilic cytoplasm and also form an increasing complex array of gamma crystallines within these cells as they elongate from the anterior to the posterior poles of the lens. By electron microscopy, minute fibrils as small as 35 Ångstroms appear to be contractile elements extending the whole length of the cytoplasm of these cells. These seem to bend their cells mechanically so that they come into the suture network that arborizes anteriorly and posteriorly.

In general, the central epithelial cells are inactive, the pre-equatorial cells are germinal and commonly show mitosis, and the equatorial cells are the ones which elongate.

Cells in the nuclear area constitute the primary lens fibers which bridge the optic vesicle and by 18 mm. fill this cavity. After the 18 mm. stage, the equatorial cells begin to elongate and form the secondary lens fibers. Again, this growing area is where any sort of insult is much more likely to disturb the lens and its transparency than would similar trauma in the central area. As these cells elongate, the simple proteins in the cytoplasm are replaced by progressively more complex crystallines. A unique series of biochemical changes parallel rather precisely the morphologic changes which have been known for many years (Zwaan, 1968). Marie Jakus (1964) has shown by electron microscopy that the elongating fibers form a striking picture of uniform and homogeneous cells. In cross section, she has also shown the highly regular mosaic pattern of interdigitation of these elongating secondary fibers. From the standpoint of both optics and structural mechanics the lens presents a uniquely exquisite uniformity.

Differentiation of the primary or embryonal lens fibers closely parallels the periods of gestation, which are divided into (1) the embryonal period before three months gestational age and (2) the fetal period, from 3 months to term. Also, corresponding to this is the development of the vitreous and the hyaloid system. The primary vitreous and the hyaloid system reach their maximum development coincident with the embryonic period, but in the fetal period the hyaloid system atrophies and secondary vitreous is elaborated. The milestone of 3 months is pivotal in the development of the lens fibers, the vitreous, and the nutritive or hyaloid system that supplies the lens.

The lens, among all structures in the body, has the most elegantly concentrated and differentiated series of proteins. The lens is 30 per cent protein, and no other system in the body has such a high concentration. Therefore, the lens in its early stages of rapid growth and chemical differentiation has high nutritional requirements. These are met in part by the vitreous and in part by the hyaloid system which elaborates and then atrophies in correspondence with the metabolic needs. The lens is at all times avascular, so that its peculiar diffusional demands set it apart from almost every other structure in the body.

The capsule of the lens would seem to seal off the access of diffusional nutrition, which of course it does not. However, the capsule does appear concurrently with reduced metabolic requirements of the growing lens. The capsule is completed from two sources: (1) the lens epithelium secretes or develops a cuticular layer; and (2) much later in lens embryogenesis, as the 160 mm. stage is approached, the zonular layer and fibers are elaborated by the edge of the optic cup. Thus a double layering is achieved by a combination of cuticular (glass) membrane upon which is later superimposed a zonular layer.

The most important clinical factor here is the development of the capsulohyaloid ligament, the firm band that unites the anterior hyaloid and the posterior lens capsule. This is sometimes called the ligamentum hyaloideo-capsulare of Wieger (1883), a very old and very appropriate name. In recent literature this is referred to sometimes, perhaps incorrectly, as Egger's line (1924). The real importance of this attachment was accentuated by the introduction of alpha-chymotrypsin. This enzyme does indeed lyse the zonular attachments around the equator as an aid to lens removal but seems to have no effect on the capsulohyaloid ligament. In early life, not only in animals but also in humans, one may lift the lens forward along with the entire vitreous body as a result of the firm attachment of this ligament. Thus, a better approach to the division of the capsulohyaloid ligament or else a different approach to the removal of the lens is required in young patients in whom this ligament shows its greatest strength.

The lens development prior to birth produces essentially a spherical lens with an erect Y suture on the front and an inverted Y suture on the back. As life goes on, these suture lines ramify dichotomously and become exceedingly complex. The lens affords its well-known ability to demarcate the chronology of life or the time of insults by the continuing concentric annulations of lens fibers proceeding from the equator.

The lens itself reaches the adult nuclear thickness at about the age of 30, but the capsule does not reach its full adult thickness until about 50 years of age. Even so, there still continues the process of new fiber layering that compresses the nucleus, increases the refractive index, and makes the lens a constant mobile challenge to those of us who approach the problem of cataracts at any time of life.

REFERENCES

Allen, L., Burian, H. M., and Brailey, A. E.: A new concept of the development of the anterior chamber angle. Arch. Ophthal., 53:783, 1955.

Bedrossian, R.: Treatment of progressive myopia with atropine. Munich, Proc. XX Internat. Congress Ophthal. Excerpta Medica 1966, Part II pp. 612–617.

Brown, E. V. L.: Net average changes in refraction of atropinized eyes from birth to beyond middle life. Arch. Ophthal., 19:719, 1938.

Cass, E.: Ocular conditions amongst the Canadian western arctic Eskimo. In Weigelin, E. (ed.): Munich, Proc. XX Internat. Congress Ophthal., Excerpta Medica, 1966, Part II, pp. 1041–1053.

Dayton, G. O., Jones, M. H., Steele, B., and Rose, M.: Developmental study of coordinated eye movements in the human infant. Arch. Ophthal., 71: 871, June, 1964.

Fletcher, M. C., and Brandon, S.: Myopia of prematurity. Amer. J. Ophthal., 40:474, October, 1955.

Gernet, H., and Olbrich, E.: Excess of the human refraction curve and its cause. In Gitter, K. A., et al. (eds.). Ophthalmic Ultrasound Proceedings 1968. St. Louis, The C. V. Mosby Co., 1969, pp. 142–148.

Gleiss, J., and Pau, H.: Development of the refraction of the eye before birth. Klin. Mbl. Augenheilk., 121:446, 1952.

Gostin, S. B.: Prophylactic management of progressive myopia. Southern Med. J., 55:916, 1962.

Hanafee, W. N.: Orbital venography. Radiol. Clin. N. Amer., 10:63, 1972.

Hansson, H. A., and Jerndal, T.: Scanning electronic microscopic studies on the development of the iridocorneal angle of the human eye. Invest. Ophthal., 10:252, 1971.

Holm, S.: Ocular refraction among the Palenegrides of Gaboon in French equatorial Africa. Acta Ophthal., (Suppl. 13) 15:1, 1937.

Jakus, M. A.: Ocular Fine Structure. Boston, Little, Brown & Co., 1964.

Keeney, A. H.: Chronology of Ophthalmic Development. Springfield, Illinois, Charles C Thomas, 1951.

Keeney, A. H.: Development of vision. *In* Falkner, F. (ed.): Human Development. Philadelphia, W. B. Saunders Co., 1966, pp. 459–464.

Kempf, G. A., Collins, S. D., and Jarman, B. L.: Refractive errors in the eyes of children as determined by retinoscopic examination with a cycloplegic. U.S. Public Health Bulletin #182, Washington, D.C., U.S. Government Printing Office, 1928.

Kettesy, A.: The stabilization of the refraction and its role in the formation of ametropia. Brit. J. Ophthal., *33*:39, 1949.

Larsen, J. S.: Sagittal growth of the eye. III. Ultrasonic measurement of the posterior segment from birth to puberty. Acta Ophthal., 49:441, 1971.

Leary, G. A., Sorsby, A., Richards, M. J., and Chaston, J.: Ultrasonographic measurements of the components of ocular refraction in life. Vision Res., *3*:487, 1963.

Levinsohn, F. G.: Zur anatomie des kurzsichtig gemachten. Arch. f. Augenheilk. *100*:138, 1929.

Mann, I.: Development of the Human Eye. New York, Grune and Stratton. 3rd ed. 1964.

Maumenee, A. E.: The pathogenesis of congenital glaucoma—a new theory. Trans Amer. Ophthal. Soc., *56*:507, 1958.

Needham, J.: Biochemistry and Morphogenesis. Cambridge, The University Press, 1942.

Newman, F. A.: Acquired axial myopia. Amer. J. Ophthal., *12*:714, 1929.

Otsuka, J.: Research on the etiology and treatment of myopia. Acta Soc. Ophthal. Jap., *71*:1(Suppl.), 1967.

Pearson, A. A.: Development of the Eye: A Manual. Rochester, Minnesota, American Academy of Ophthalmology and Otolaryngology.

Pendse, G. S., Bhave, L. S., and Dandekar, V. M.: Refraction relation to age and sex. Arch. Ophthal., *52*:404, September, 1954.

Sato, T.: The Cause and Prevention of Acquired Myopia. Tokyo, Kanehara Shuppan Co., Ltd., 1957.

Skeller, E.: Anthropological and Ophthalmological Studies on the Angmagssalik Eskimos. Copenhagen, C. A. Reitzels Forlag, 1954.

Slataper, F. J.: Age norms of refractions and vision. Arch. Ophthal., *43*:466, 1950.

Smelser, G. K., and Ozanics, V.: The development of the trabecular meshwork in primate eyes. Amer. J. Ophthal., *71*:366, 1971.

Sorsby, A., Benjamin, B., and Sheridan, M.: Refraction and Its Components During the Growth of the Eye from the Age of Three. London, Her Majesty's Stationery Office, 1961 (Medical Research Council, Special Report Series #301).

Sorsby, A., Leary, G. A., and Richards, M. J.: Correlation ametropia and component ametropia. Vision Res., *2*:309, 1962.

Sorsby, A., and Sheridan, M.: Changes in the refractive power of the cornea during growth. Brit. J. Ophthal., *37*:555, September, 1953.

Stansbury, F. C.: Pathogenesis of myopia. Arch. Ophthal., *39*:273, 1948.

Stofft, P.: Development of visual function in infants. Ann. Oculist., *194*:133, 1961.

van Alphen, G. W. H. M.: On emmetropia and ametropia. Ophthalmologica Suppl., Vol. 142, Basel, S. Karger, 1961.

Wibaut, F.: Emmetropization and origin of spherical anomalies of refraction. Graefe's Arch., *116*:596, 1926.

Young, F. A.: The effect of restricted visual space on the refractive error of the young monkey eye. Invest. Ophthal., *2*:571, 1963.

Young, F. A., and Leary, G. A.: Comparison of the optical characteristics of the human, ape and monkey eye. Proc. Amer. Psych. Assoc. (75th Annual Convention), Washington, D.C., American Psychological Association, Inc., 1967, pp. 89–90.

Zwaan, J.: Immunochemical analysis of the eye lens during development. Thesis, University of Amsterdam, pp. XVII + 103. Rototype, Amsterdam, 1963.

Zwaan, J.: Lens specific antigens and cytodifferentiation in the developing lens. J. Cell Physiol., *72*:47 (Suppl. 1), 1968.

Zwaan, J.: Induction of the eye lens: facts and fancies. *In* Moscona, A. A., and Monroy, A. (eds.): Current Topics in Developmental Biology. New York, Academic Press, 1972.

CHAPTER 2

GENETICS IN PEDIATRIC OPHTHALMOLOGY

HOPE H. PUNNETT, Ph.D.
and ROBISON D. HARLEY, M.D., Ph.D.

The eye is uniquely suited for genetic studies. Observable abnormalities may be isolated phenomena limited to that tissue or clues to the presence of systemic disease or associated malformations. They may be due to single gene (mendelian) mutations, chromosomal abnormalities, teratogens, or multiple interacting genes, or the etiology may be unknown. In this chapter chromosomal disorders will be described in some detail and the basic genetic mechanisms outlined. Table 2–1, pediatric syndromes with their major ocular and systemic manifestations, and Table 2–2, ocular abnormalities and characteristics, indicate the extent of ocular involvement in congenital and/or genetic disorders.

MOLECULAR GENETICS

The phenotype or appearance of the individual is determined by his genotype,

his genetic constitution. The gene is definable in several ways. The most useful is that of function. The gene is that portion of the deoxyribonucleic acid (DNA) molecule which transmits the genetic information for the composition of a single polypeptide chain. Each molecule of DNA is composed of two intertwined strands, the double helix, held together by hydrogen bonds between the purine and pyrimidine bases. There are two purines, adenine and guanine, and two pyrimidines, cytosine and thymine. Whenever adenine occurs in one strand, it is paired with thymine in the other; the same is true for guanine with cytosine. The code is based on triplets of these bases; each triplet of bases codes for one of the 20 amino acids in human proteins. There are four bases, giving 65 possible combinations. Some redundancy exists, with 2 to 6 combinations coding for most amino acids, with the exception of methionine and tryptophan, each of which is coded for by only one combination. The three triplets which do not code for amino acids may serve as punctuation, marking the beginning and end of a chain.

The chromosomal DNA is in the nucleus. The protein synthesis for which it codes takes place in the cytoplasm, on ribosomes. The link between the gene and its product is RNA, which differs from DNA in that ribose replaces deoxyribose as the sugar, the base uracil replaces thymine, and it is single stranded. When a particular gene locus is active, that functional region of DNA attracts a complementary length of messenger RNA, which then migrates out of the nucleus to the ribosomes, where the polypeptide is synthesized. There it may combine with other polypeptides (specified by other genes) to form biologically active proteins and enzymes. Other genes may regulate, enhance, or repress these structural genes.

Each gene occurs at a particular position (its locus) on a specific chromosome. Since man is a diploid organism, with two sets of chromosomes, one inherited from each parent, his genes also occur in pairs, one member of each pair inherited from each parent. An individual is homozygous for a gene pair if the information specified by each member is identical. He is heterozygous if the two members code for different polypeptides. The alternate forms of a gene are called alleles and usually differ from the normal or "wild type" by a single base substitution in one base triplet, thereby changing the DNA code for that protein. These changes are called mutations. For example, the genes coding for hemoglobin A (normal) and hemoglobin S (sickle) and hemoglobin C are alleles. The end products differ from each other by one amino acid in a chain of 146. Hemoglobin A has glutamic acid in the position in which valine is found in hemoglobin S, and lysine in hemoglobin C. Although genes may exist in a number of allelic states, only two will be found in any one individual. With an increasing number of alleles many different combinations may occur in a population. Multiple allelism is an important source of genetic variation in man.

When in place of a single "normal" gene two (or more) alleles coexist in a population, there is a state of genetic polymorphism, defined by E. B. Ford (1940) as "the occurrence together in the same habitat of two or more discontinuous forms of a species in such proportions that the rarest of them cannot be maintained merely by recurrent mutation." Color blindness was probably the first genetic polymorphism to be recognized.

DOMINANT INHERITANCE

A gene is said to be dominant in its effect when it is manifest in a single dose, such that the mutant member of the gene pair interferes with or prevents expression of the normal allele. When a dominant gene occurs infrequently in the population, most individuals manifesting the gene will be heterozygous and the phenotype will indicate the presence or absence of the dominant allele directly. If the dominant gene is common, then both homozygous and heterozygous individuals will be present in the population and the phenotype will not be an accurate indicator of the genotype.

An individual with a dominantly inherited disease often has a family history of affected individuals in more than one generation (vertical transmission) (Fig. 2–1). In the case of the rare autosomal dominant disorder, an individual who manifests the disorder, mated to a normal partner, will pass the gene on to half of his children, regardless of sex. The other half of the children will receive the normal allele. Thus, the expectation for a normal child from each pregnancy will be 50 per cent and the expectation for an affected child will be 50 per cent also. This holds for each pregnancy, regardless of what the outcome of preceding pregnancies has been. "Chance has no memory."

If a child with a disorder which is usually inherited in a dominant manner is born to normal parents, he may represent a new mutation. The recurrence risk for other pregnancies is close to zero, because most detectable mutations occur in a single parental cell, a gamete. If the mutation were in a tissue sector which included germ cells, more than one affected child could be born. Although a rare occur-

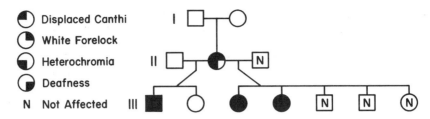

Figure 2–1 Pedigree illustrating the autosomal dominant transmission of Waardenburg's syndrome. (Adapted from DiGeorge, A. M., Olmsted, R. W., and Harley, R. D.: J. Pediat., 57:650, 1960.)

rence, such an event has recently been described. Two of six children born to normal parents had classic achondroplasia. One has married and borne two children, one of whom is also achondroplastic, thus demonstrating the dominantly inherited nature of the disorder in this family. Until the birth of an affected individual in the second generation, the possibility that the two achondroplastics represented a new, autosomal recessive form of achondroplasia could not be ruled out (Bowen, 1972).

Dominantly inherited disorders appear to skip a generation when an affected child is born to normal parents but has an affected grandparent. Careful examination of the presumed carrier parent may reveal minor stigmata of the disease or the parent may, indeed, be normal. In the latter case, the gene is said to lack penetrance. Penetrance is expressed quantitatively as the percentage of all those known to carry the gene (by virtue of affected progeny) who manifest the trait. Thus, a dominant gene, which is actually expressed in every individual who carries it, would have 100 per cent penetrance. If four family members descended from the same affected ancestor had affected progeny, but one was free of the disease, the gene would be 75 per cent penetrant in that family.

Some genes affect more than one organ. A gene which has multiple effects is pleiotropic. The complete expression of Waardenburg's syndrome (a dominantly inherited disorder) includes displaced canthi, heterochromia of the irides, white forelock, broad nasal root, and deafness. The gene is fully penetrant, since carriers always manifest displaced canthi. The other findings may vary in severity of effect among family members, providing an example of the variable expressivity of the gene (Fig. 2–1).

In summary, in autosomal dominant inheritance, there is usually a positive family history, with affected individuals in successive generations. In the absence of a family history, an affected individual may represent a new mutation or the parent may be a carrier in whom the gene is not penetrant. Males and females are affected equally. Statistically, 50 per cent of children born to an affected individual will also be affected unless there is incomplete penetrance.

RECESSIVE INHERITANCE

A disorder is recessively inherited when both mutant alleles are required for the effects of the genes to be manifest. A single recessive allele has no clinical effect in disorders inherited as autosomal recessive, although it may be possible to differentiate the heterozygous carrier state. A child with galactosemia is homozygous for the mutant allele, having received one mutant allele from each parent. The parents are obligate heterozygotes (carriers) who have one normal allele as well as the mutant and are phenotypically normal.

In a mating of two carriers, for every pregnancy the probability is equal that each parent will contribute either a normal or abnormal allele to the zygote. There are four possible genetic combinations: the homozygous normal child receives a normal allele from each parent; the heterozygote receives a normal allele from his mother and a mutant from his father, or vice versa; the affected child receives the abnormal gene from both parents. The expected ratio is 1 homozygous normal: 2 heterozygous normal: 1 affected (homozygous abnormal) offspring. Therefore, the probability is 3:1 that the embryo will have received at least one normal allele and be phenotypically normal.

When the enzyme defect is known in a recessively inherited metabolic disorder, it becomes possible to identify those relatives of an affected child who are carriers. The affected individual usually has little or no measurable enzyme activity, while the heterozygote has approximately half that of the normal homozygous individual. For example, the clinical manifestations of galactosemia are due to lack of activity of the enzyme galactose 1-phosphate-uridyl transferase. Heterozygotes for galactosemia have approximately half the enzyme activity (as measured in white cells and tissue culture fibroblasts) of individuals with two normal alleles. It is also possible to diagnose galactosemia and many other metabolic disorders in utero by measuring the enzyme level in tissue cultures of fetal cells obtained from amniocentesis.

In the case of rare recessive disorders, there is an increased incidence of consanguinity among the parents of affected individuals, both parents having received the mutant gene from the same common ancestor (Fig. 2–2). A gene may be relatively rare in one population, common in another. For example, the incidence of albinism in the United States is about 1 in 20,000. Among the San Blas Indians of Panama, it is 1 in 132. The genes for Tay-Sachs disease and familial dysautonomia are extremely rare except among Jews who trace their ancestry to Eastern Europe. This same population has a very low frequency of the gene for phenylketonuria (PKU). Cystic fibrosis is almost exclusively a Caucasian disease. The high frequency of some recessive genes is attributed to genetic drift within an isolated population (as in San Blas). For other genes, heterozygosity has conveyed a selective advantage. The selective survival of sickle cell heterozygotes in a malarial environment is the best known example of a balanced polymorphism. It has recently been suggested that heterozygosity for Tay-Sachs disease conveys resistance to pulmonary tuberculosis (Myrianthopoulos, 1972).

To summarize, in autosomal recessive inheritance there is usually no family history. The parents are clinically normal heterozygous carriers, with an increased incidence of consanguinity. Males and females are equally affected. There is a 25 per cent risk of an affected child with each pregnancy. Affected individuals will have affected children *only* if mated to an individual who is homozygous or heterozygous for the same gene.

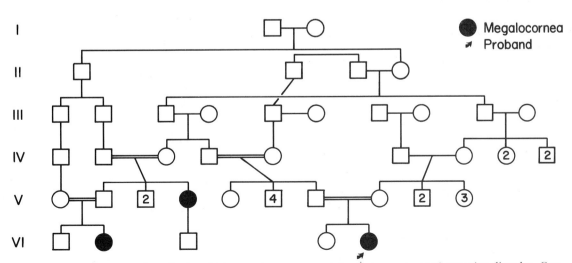

Figure 2–2 Pedigree of family in which megalocornea was inherited as autosomal recessive disorder. Consanguineous matings are indicated by double lines (═══).

X-LINKAGE

X-linked genes may be recessive or (less frequently) dominant. X-linkage refers to the location of the gene on the X chromosome. Females have two X chromosomes; males, one X and one Y. In the case of the X-linked recessive disorder, females are fully affected only when homozygous, carrying the abnormal gene on both X chromosomes. The female who is a heterozygous carrier transmits the abnormal gene to half of her daughters (who are carriers) and to half of her sons who manifest the disease because they have only one X chromosome (Fig. 2–3).

If the gene is dominant, a heterozygous female carrier would manifest the mutant phenotype. Males, being hemizygous for the X, are affected whenever their single X carries the mutated gene, recessive or dominant. Affected males transmit their single X chromosome to all their daughters who are obligate carriers for the X-linked recessive gene, affected for the X-linked dominant. Male-to-male transmission of an X-linked gene never occurs, since the male transmits his Y chromosome to his son.

The female carrier, heterozygous for an X-linked recessive disorder, may show similar but less severe manifestations than the affected hemizygous male. X-linked disorders of the eye for which phenotypic evidence of the carrier state is present in females include choroideremia, ocular albinism, and retinitis pigmentosa. The partial expression of the single recessive gene has been explained by the X inactivation theory of Mary Lyon (1961) (Lyon hypothesis). During the second to third week of embryonic life, one of the two X chromosomes in each cell of the female fetus differentiates as the inactive X. It becomes condensed during interphase and appears as a darkly staining mass at the nuclear membrane (Barr body or sex chromatin) (Fig. 2–5). Either the maternally contributed X or the paternally contributed X is inactivated at random in each cell. Most, if not all, of the genes on the inactive X are also inactive. Once this differentiation occurs, that same chromosome continues to be the inactive X during interphase in all the linear descendents of that cell. Therefore, the female is a mosaic of two cell types, those in which the genes on the X derived from her mother are active and those in which the X-linked genes from her father are active. The Lyon hypothesis is invoked to explain the splotchy fundus observed in the female carrier of ocular albinism, or the tapetal reflex in the carrier of X-linked retinitis pigmentosa.

In summary, in the case of an X-linked recessive disorder, half the sons of carrier females will be affected; half the daughters will be carriers like their mothers. The other 50 per cent of sons and daughters will be normal. In the case of an X-linked dominant disorder, half the children of an affected female will be affected, males and females equally. If there is a positive

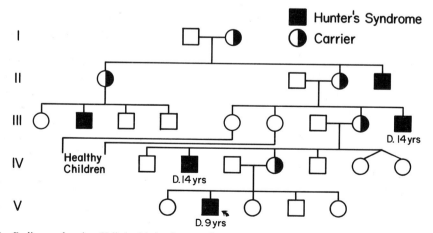

Figure 2–3 Pedigree showing X-linked inheritance of Hunter's syndrome. Note that affected males are related through their mothers.

PEDIGREE IN LOWE'S SYNDROME

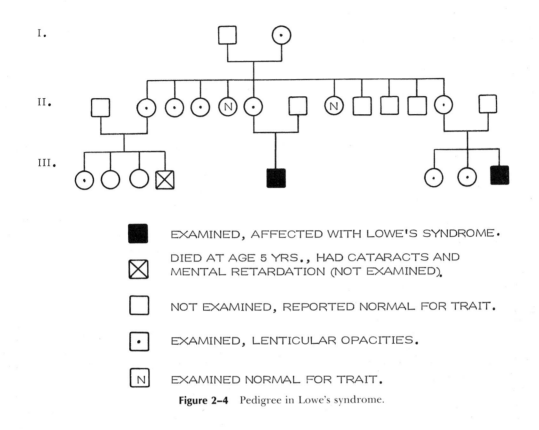

EXAMINED, AFFECTED WITH LOWE'S SYNDROME.

DIED AT AGE 5 YRS., HAD CATARACTS AND
MENTAL RETARDATION (NOT EXAMINED).

NOT EXAMINED, REPORTED NORMAL FOR TRAIT.

EXAMINED, LENTICULAR OPACITIES.

EXAMINED NORMAL FOR TRAIT.

Figure 2–4   Pedigree in Lowe's syndrome.

family history, it will be on the maternal side, with affected grandfathers having affected grandsons.

Since a male transmits his Y chromosome to his sons and his X to his daughters, male-to-male transmission of an X-linked disorder does not occur (except in those rare cases in which the son has Klinefelter's syndrome, the extra X chromosome being inherited from his father). All the daughters of a male with an X-linked recessive disorder will be obligate carriers; all the daughters of a male with an X-linked dominant disorder will be affected.

POLYGENIC AND MULTIFACTORIAL INHERITANCE

Polygenic and multifactorial inheritance afford an explanation of conditions in which there may be a familial component but which do not conform to single gene mendelian inheritance. The expression of the particular character or disease (i.e., strabismus, diabetes, cleft lip, spina bifida, anencephaly) may be dependent upon the presence of a critical number of genes with similar quantitative effect and which are inherited independently and act in an additive manner. Interaction with the environment also is implied in the term "multifactorial," as used by some genet-

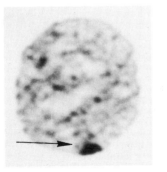

Figure 2–5   Barr body (sex chromatin) at the nuclear membrane in a cell from buccal mucosa of a normal female.

icists. A certain (unknown) threshold number of genes must be exceeded before the condition is expressed. The threshold value may differ for the two sexes as reflected in the differing incidence of pyloric stenosis and congenitally dislocated hip in males and females. Since pyloric stenosis occurs more frequently in males than females, a greater number of interacting genes is required for the female to express the anomaly. Therefore, the risk of an affected female having affected children is higher than that for an affected male. Those sex relationships would be reversed for congenitally dislocated hips, which is more common in females.

Multiple gene inheritance is undoubtedly important in determining quantitative ocular abnormalities. It has been suggested that refractive errors are polygenic and that heterophoria and binocular vision are among other quantitatable components of the visual system. The ratio of the diameter of the optic cup to that of the optic disc may also be controlled by multiple factors with additive effects (Armaly, 1967). Richter (1967) found evidence for multifactorial inheritance with threshold effect in the pedigrees of nearly a thousand children with concomitant strabismus. She suggested that inherited slight sensory and motor anomalies might be combined in different and continuously varying quantities to constitute the disorder.

The pattern of polygenic inheritance may resemble that due to autosomal dominance with low penetrance. However, in the former, affective individuals are usually first-degree relatives. In the case of dominance with low penetrance, affected individuals are found in many generations.

GENETIC HETEROGENEITY

Frequently, the same clinical entity (or phenotype) occurs with different modes of inheritance. This is genetic heterogeneity. The autosomally inherited Hurler syndrome and the X-linked recessive Hunter syndrome may be difficult to differentiate on the basis of physical findings in a young male child with the typical findings of mucopolysaccharidosis and no family history. Retinitis pigmentosa may be inherited as a dominant, recessive, or X-linked disorder within a given family. A complete family history and careful examination of unaffected family members who may be carriers are needed to determine the mode of inheritance for any individual family. In the absence of a revealing pedigree and demonstrated carrier state in parents, a female with retinitis pigmentosa may be either a new dominant mutation, or the homozygous recessive offspring of two heterozygous parents. The prognosis for her parents would be better if she were a new mutation, since there should be no other affected children. However, half of her children could be expected to inherit the deleterious mutant gene. If she were homozygous for the recessive form, her parents would face the 25 per cent risk of other affected children. If she were homozygous for the X-linked form, her mother would have to be a carrier and her father affected.

A striking example of genetic heterogeneity is exemplified by the case of the normally pigmented child born to albino Negro parents (Witkop et al., 1970). The parents had been told that if they had children, all would be albino. When a normally pigmented daughter was born, the father, concluding that the experts do not always have the answers, stated, "It is obvious that she [my wife] is a different kind of albino than I am." He was right. Each parent was homozygous at a different locus for albinism. The normal child was heterozygous at both loci. A similar family of albino parents with four normal children was reported by Trevor-Roper in 1952. In both families, hair bulb incubation in tyrosine differentiated the two types of albinos, one parent's hair bulb showing no pigment formation, the other developing intense pigment formation.

It is important to recognize the existence of genetic heterogeneity and to remember that every case of a clinical disease usually accepted as genetic may not be inherited, or, if inherited, may represent a different allele or a different gene at a different locus from the usual one.

GENES IN POPULATION

If a gene exists in only 2 allelic forms, *A* and *a*, each person in the population is either *AA*, *Aa*, or *aa*. If we designate the frequency of the gene *A* as *p*, then *p* would equal the frequency of all the *AA* individuals and half the *Aa* individuals. Similarly, the frequency, *q*, of *a* would be the frequency of *aa* and half the *Aa* individuals. Since the sum of the three frequencies (*AA*, *Aa*, and *aa*) equals 1.00, *p* plus *q* also must equal 1.00.

If all matings within the population occur at random in regard to genes *A* and *a*, the chance that a sperm carrying *A* will fertilize an *A* egg will be determined by the relative frequency, *p*, of *A*. The following table accounts for the genotypic origins of all individuals in the population.

Sperm	Egg	Zygote	Frequency
A	A	AA	$p \times p$ or p^2
A	a	Aa	$p \times q$
a	A	aA	$q \times p$ } or $2pq$
a	a	aa	$q \times q$ or q^2

The frequencies of *AA*, *Aa*, and *aa* individuals following random mating are p^2, $2pq$, and q^2, respectively, and will remain as such in all successive generations. This relationship is known as the Hardy-Weinberg law for the English mathematician and German physician who published it independently in 1908.

This formula may be used to estimate proportions of homozygotes and heterozygotes given the condition of random mating. For example, the incidence of oculocutaneous albinism is approximately one in 20,000 births. The frequency *q* of the albino allele may be calculated from the known frequency q^2 of the recessive homozygote: 1/20,000. We take the square root of 1/20,000 and arrive at $q = 1/141$. Since $p + q = 1$, the frequency of the normal allele $p = 1 - q = 1 - 1/141 = 140/141$. The carrier frequency, $2pq$, is $2 \times 1/140 \times 140/141$ or approximately 1/70. This means that one in every 70 people in the population is heterozygous for albinism. It is not surprising, therefore, that albino individuals married to normal spouses occasionally have albino offspring. One in every 70 albino:normal matings would be expected to be between an albino and a carrier, and half their children would then be albino.

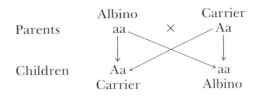

Parents: Albino aa × Carrier Aa

Children: Aa Carrier, aa Albino

It is important to understand the relationship between the frequencies for homozygous recessive individuals and for heterozygous carriers when consideration is being given to reducing the incidence of deleterious genes in a population. It has been estimated that each person is heterozygous for 5 to 7 such genes. The probability of an unrealted couple having a homozygous affected child is a function of the frequency of the specific gene in question. The risk of having a child with recessive albinism is the product of the probabilities of each parent being a carrier (1/70 × 1/70) × the 1/4 probability that any given pregnancy will result in an affected child. This equals 1/19,600, the approximate incidence of recessive albinsim with which we started.

CHROMOSOMAL ABERRATIONS

In 1956, Tjio and Levan established the chromosome number of man as 46. The chromosomal basis of Turner's (Ford et al., 1959), Klinefelter's (Jacobs and Strong, 1959), and Down's (Lejeune et al., 1959) syndromes were established shortly thereafter and other chromosomal diseases have since been delineated. Chromosome studies are now a major diagnostic tool in evaluation of children with congenital malformations and mental retardation or ambiguity of external genitalia. Approximately 1 in every 200 liveborn children and 20 to 70 per cent of spontaneous abortions carry a chromosome abnormality.

The normal human chromosome complement consists of 22 pairs of autosomes, and one pair of sex chromosomes (X and Y), divided into 7 groups on the basis of length and centromere position. Chromosomes 1, 2, and 3 constitute group A; 4 and 5, group B; 6 to 12 and X, group C; 13 to 15, group D; 16 to 18, group E; 19 and 20, group F; and 21, 22, and Y, group G (Fig. 2–6). Chromosome abnormalities may be numerical (extra or missing chro-

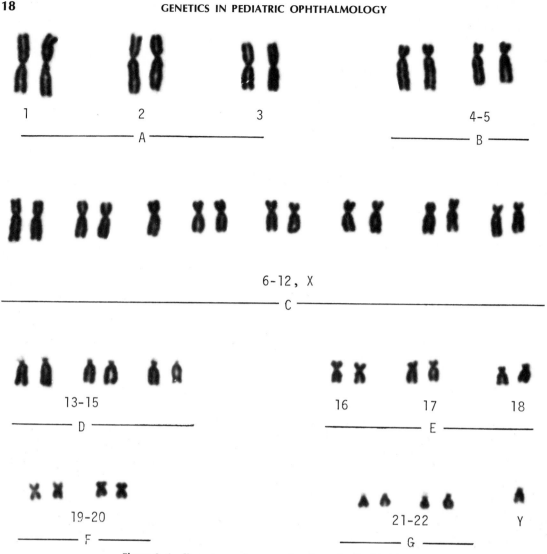

Figure 2–6   Karyotype of a normal male, stained with Giemsa.

mosomes) or structural (deletions, rings, translocations). A nomenclature system has been adopted to describe the human chromosome complement and indicate departures from normal. An extra chromosome is indicated by a plus (+), and a missing one by a minus (−), so that 47,XX+21 is a female with trisomy 21. The short arm of a chromosome is "p" and the long arm is "q"; therefore, 46,XY,5p− describes a male with a deletion in the short arm of one chromosome 5. A ring is indicated as "r" and translocation as "t." Quinacrine fluorescence (Caspersson et al., 1970) and Giemsa banding (Seabright, 1971) are special techniques which make it possible to identify each chromosome of

the complement (Figs. 2–7 to 2–9). Autoradiography has been used in the past to distinguish the inactive, late-labeling X from the remainder of the C group as well as to identify certain autosomes, but it is less useful than the newer methods.

Numerical Abnormalities

Most numerical chromosomal anomalies originate during gametogenesis in a parent and are due to nondisjunction or anaphase lag. Normally, homologous chromosomes pair and then segregate during the first meiotic division, members of each pair migrating to opposite poles,

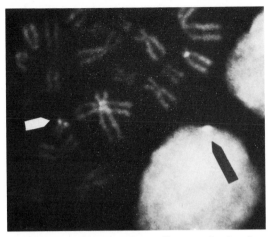

Figure 2–7 Portions of two adjacent cells, showing prominent fluorescence of distal portion of Y chromosome (white arrow) in dividing cell and fluorescent Y body in interphase nucleus (black arrow).

independently of their parental origin. Two cells, each with 23 chromosomes, result. This is followed by a second division. The primary gonocyte (spermatocyte and oocyte) thus produce 4 haploid germ cells, each with 23 chromosomes: 4 sperm in males, 1 egg and 3 polar bodies in females. Failure of separation of homologous chromosomes may occur in the first division, failure of chromatid separation in the second (Fig. 2–10). In either case, complementary gametes with 24 chromosomes (one present in duplicate) and 22 chromosomes (one missing) result. If the former is fertilized by a normal gamete (23 chromosomes), the zygote would have 47 chromosomes, one being present in triplicate (trisomy). If the latter, the zygote would have 45 chromosomes with one missing (monosomy). The autosomal trisomies compatible with term gestation are those of chromosomes 13, 18, 21, and 22. Trisomies of other chromosomes are usually lethal in utero and are identified in spontaneous abortions. Partial trisomies are produced by unbalanced translocation. Autosomal monosomy is also usually lethal, although monosomy 21 has been reported. It is impossible to rule out translocations or mosaicism in these cases.

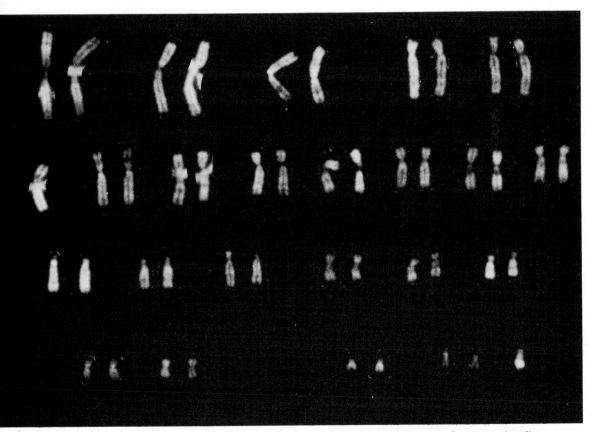

Figure 2–8 Karyotype of a normal male, stained with quinacrine mustard, showing fluorescent banding.

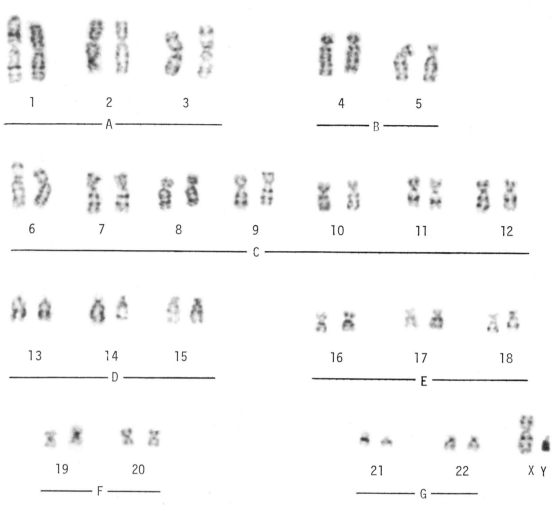

Figure 2–9 Karyotype of normal male, showing banding produced by trypsin treatment of Seabright (1972).

MEIOTIC DISJUNCTION - NON DISJUNCTION

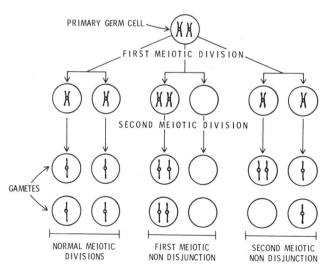

Figure 2–10 Diagram of meiosis for one pair of homologous chromosomes. Trisomy and monosomy resulting from nondisjunction in the first and second divisions are shown. (From Nelson, W. E., Vaughn, V. C., and McKay, R. J.: Textbook of Pediatrics. 9th ed. Philadelphia, W. B. Saunders Co., 1969.)

Nondisjunction of sex chromosomes has less severe consequences. Monosomy X is the cause of Turner's syndrome, and females with XXX and XXXX have been ascertained. Males with XXY (Klinefelter's syndrome) and XYY are not uncommon and increasing numbers of X and Y to XXXXY or XXYY are known.

If nondisjunction occurs after fertilization in an early division of the embryo, mosaicism results. Cell lines with trisomies and/or monosomies may persist in addition to normal cells. Cells with autosomal monosomies are nonviable, but monosomic X cells survive. Three cell types, 45X, 46XX, and 47XXX, may coexist in females who presumably began life as XX zygotes, a single mitotic nondisjunction producing the X and XXX cells.

The first identified human translocations were centric fusions between two acrocentric chromosomes (G/G, D/D, or D/G) which reduced the chromosome count by one, since the nonessential short arms were lost. Most of the translocations causing Down's syndrome and trisomy 13 are due to centric fusions (Fig. 2–11). Reciprocal translocations between biarmed chromosomes alter arm ratios without changing the chromosome number. Reciprocal translocations are usually detected through a child with multiple anomalies who inherited an unbalanced translocation from a normal balanced carrier parent. Deletion syndromes may also be inherited in this manner, although most deletions, rings, and the like are not inherited.

Case reports of familial translocations, unusual deletions, duplications, and so on abound in the literature. Most are of such limited occurrence that the clinical findings will not be described here. However, the ophthalmologist should be aware that there are many more chromosome abnormalities, in addition to the common syndromes, in which congenital abnormalities of the eye occur. We have seen pallor of the optic disc, heterochromia, Brush-

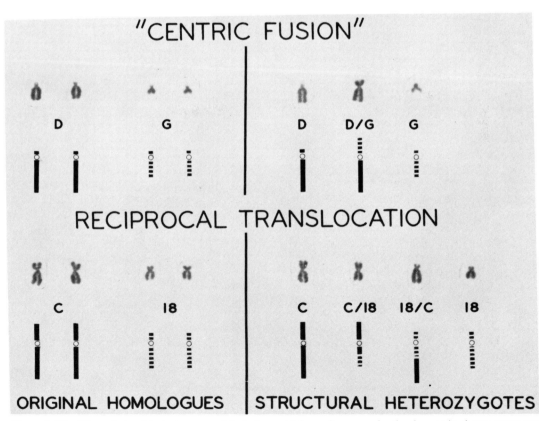

Figure 2–11 The relationship between centric fusion, which produces a reduction by one in chromosome number, and reciprocal translocation, which results in altered morphology, unchanged number. (From Gardner, L.: Endocrine and Genetic Diseases of Childhood. Philadelphia, W. B. Saunders Co., 1969.)

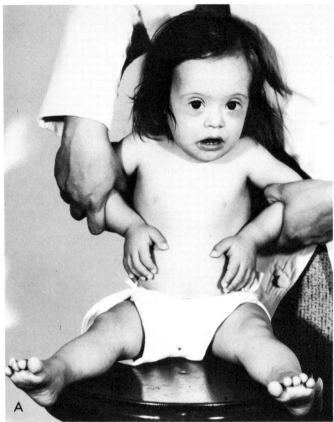

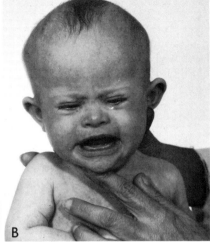

Figure 2–12 Down's syndrome. *A*, An 11-month-old boy with typical facies, stubby hands, and prominent sandal gap of the feet. *B*, Ectropion of all four eyelids in an infant with Down's syndrome.

field spots, epicanthal folds, ptosis, strabismus, colobomas and exophthalmos in children, each of whom carried a unique chromosomal abnormality.

TRISOMY 21 (DOWN'S SYNDROME). The most common autosomal abnormality is Down's syndrome, deriving its eponym from Langdon Down who first described the condition in 1866 (Fig. 2–12). Most children with Down's syndrome have 47 chromosomes with an extra chromosome 21 (Lejeune et al., 1959). Their parents have normal chromosomes and the trisomy is considered sporadic. About 6 per cent of children with Down's syndrome have 46 chromosomes, one of which represents the centric fusion of 21 and a D or G group chromosome. The translocation may have been inherited from a normal parent who has 45 chromosomes (the translocation replacing one 21 and one D or G) or have arisen de novo. There is no clinical difference between a child with trisomy and one with translocation. The incidence of Down's syndrome is 1 in 600 live births but is age dependent and climbs

with increasing maternal age to 1 in 40 for women over age 40. The risk of having a second child with Down's syndrome (47,+21) if both parents are chromosomally normal is only slightly higher (about 1 per cent) than that for all women of the mother's age. In the case of a parental translocation, the risk may be as low as 10 or as high as 100 per cent, depending on the translocation (Fig. 2–13).

Mosaicism for trisomy 21 is not uncommon. The clinical manifestations may vary from a normal phenotype to that of a typical Down's syndrome. Physically normal individuals with mosaicism are usually detected after the birth of a child with trisomy 21, when chromosomal investigation reveals an abnormal 47,+21 cell line in one parent. The risk of having further children with trisomy 21 may be as high as 50 per cent but cannot be calculated with any precision, since it depends upon knowing the proportion of trisomic cells in the gonad.

Systemic findings of Down's syndrome

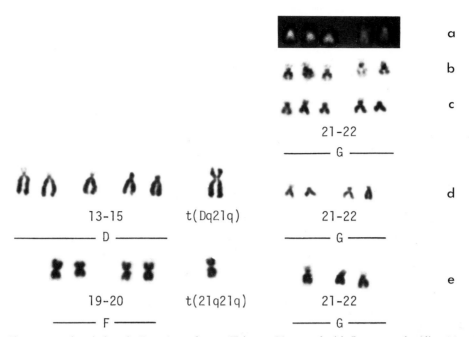

Figure 2–13 Chromosomal variations in Down's syndrome. Trisomy 21 proved with fluorescent banding (*a*) and trypsin banding (*b*). Centric fusion translocations involving the D and 21 (*d*), and two chromosomes 21 (*e*). In each case, the genetic information of chromosome 21 is present in triplicate. (*d* and *e* from Rodriguez, M. M., Valdes-Dapena, M., and Kistenmacher, M.: J. Pediat. Ophthal., *10*:54, 1973. Reproduced from the Journal of Pediatric Ophthalmology by permission of the publisher, Charles B. Slack, Inc.)

are hypotonia; mental retardation; brachycephaly; large protruding tongue; small nose with low, small bridge; small, often poorly defined ears; short, thick neck, stubby hands with a single palmar crease; clinodactyly of fifth digit with hypoplasia of middigital phalanges; short, stubby feet with wide gap between first and second toes; and congenital heart disease. Males are usually sterile; females may be fertile. Of the 21 reported children born to women with Down's syndrome, 13 were normal and 8 had trisomy 21 (Reiss, Lovrien, and Hecht, 1971).

The characteristic ocular findings in Down's syndrome are epicanthal folds, mongoloid slant of the eye, hypoplasia of the iris, Brushfield spots, myopia, keratoconus, esotropia, cataracts, and blepharitis. Ectropion of all four eyelids has been reported in Down's syndrome, and we have seen one case at St. Christopher's Hospital for Children.

TRISOMY 18 (EDWARDS' SYNDROME). The clinical findings of this trisomy are due to the presence of an extra chromosome 18 (Edwards, 1960). Rarely, an unbalanced translocation involving 18 may cause the syndrome. There is a marked preponderance of incidence among females. Most males with trisomy 18 probably die in utero. In a series of 40 cases of trisomy 18 diagnosed during a 10-year period in this laboratory, only 5 were males, and, of these, one was a 26-week spontaneous abortion and one had XY/XXY mosaicism. Two of the 40 had mosaicism for chromosome 18 (46,XX/47, XX,+18) but were clinically indistinguishable from full trisomies.

Those features which help to differentiate trisomy 18 clinically are microcephaly, characteristic facies (Fig. 2–14), low birthweight for gestational age, hypertonicity with limbs in flexion, limited hip abduction, apneic spells, and marked failure to thrive. The facial characteristics include a prominent occiput, with narrow bifrontal diameter; receding chin, micrognathia, and high arch palate; and low-set, large, malformed ears with poor helix development. The hand is usually flexed, with overlapping of second and fifth fingers and failure of development of interphalangeal creases. Rocker-bottom heels, webbing of toes, and dorsiflexion of a short great toe are common. Arch dermatoglyphic patterns are seen on most

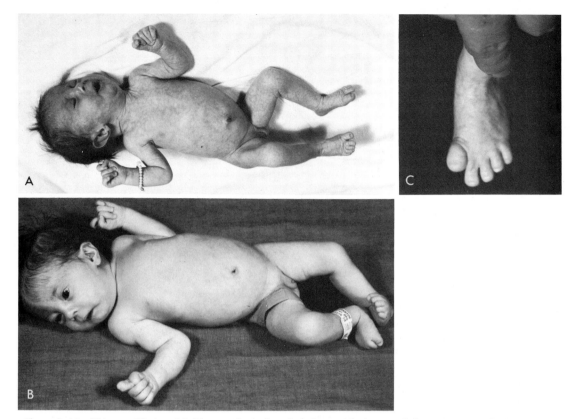

Figure 2–14 Trisomy 18. *A* and *B*, Two newborn female infants with characteristic appearance of micrognathia, low set ears, hypoplastic helix, and flexion deformity of fingers. Note slightly enlarged clitoris and club feet in *B*. *C*, Dorsiflexion of short great toe.

Figure 2–14 continued on opposite page.

finger tips. Lack of any arches may be taken as a contraindication for the diagnosis of trisomy 18. These babies have hypoplasia of adipose tissue and poor muscle development.

Renal anomalies and congenital heart disease occur in more than 65 per cent of cases. Pyloric stenosis, eventration of the diaphragm, and Meckel's diverticulum are found in 25 to 50 per cent of cases. In our series of 40 patients, 5 have had tracheoesophageal fistulas, a high proportion compared to other series. The oldest of our patients died at age 6. She was severely retarded and had reached no developmental milestones. The majority died before 1 year of age.

Eye anomalies in trisomy 18 are primarily orbital and palpebral, including hypertelorism and hypoplastic supraorbital ridges. However, ocular paralysis; coloboma of iris, choroid, or disc; corneal opacities; cataract; anisocoria; microcornea; keratitis; persistent hyaloid artery; areas of retinal depigmentation; and congenital glaucoma with optic atrophy have been described.

Microphthalmos, hypertelorism, blepharophimosis, small palpebral fissures, ptosis, mongoloid slant, and epicanthal folds were seen frequently in 26 out of 40 of the cases in our series. Seen at least once, in addition, were poor upper lid development preventing closure of eyes, exophthalmos (unilateral), dysconjugate movement, nystagmus, cataracts, lack of pupillary response, lid adhesions, and blindness. One of our male patients with trisomy 18 also had arhinencephaly, but his facies was that of the typical 18 trisomy. Small palpebral fissures and small optic nerves were the only ocular anomalies noted in that infant.

Pathologic studies of the eye in trisomy 18 are limited. In the 2 cases reported by Ginsberg et al. (1968) the most significant abnormalities affected the cornea, uveal tract, lens, and retina. Corneal opacities

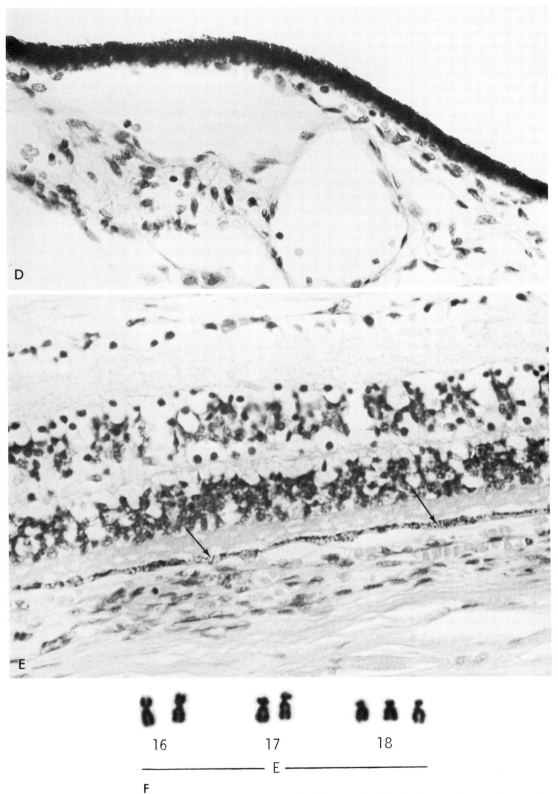

Figure 2–14 *Continued.* *D,* Retinal pigment epithelium displaying marked thickening and hyperpigmentation at the periphery (hematoxylin and eosin, ×256). *E,* Hypopigmentation of the retinal pigmentation (arrows) at the posterior pole (hematoxylin and eosin, ×256). *F,* E group chromosomes, with trisomy 18. (*E* and *F* from Rodriguez, M. M., Punnett, H. H., Valdes-Dapena, M., and Martyn, L. J.: Amer. J. Ophthal., 76:265, 1973.)

reflected retrograde changes (lamellar disorganization and fibrosis) of stroma. Anomalies of the ciliary process, breaks in the iris sphincter, posterior subcapsular cataract, and muscular abnormalities were described. Rodrigues et al. (1973) have observed abnormalities of the retinal pigment epithelium in the eye of our patient with trisomy 18 and XY/XXY mosaicism (Fig. 2–14D and E). No abnormalities were seen in the eyes of one other case (46,XX/47,XX,+18) studied by Green (1970).

TRISOMY 13 (PATAU'S SYNDROME). Infants with trisomy 13 (Patau et al., 1960) usually have normal birthweights and are hypotonic. About half have a cleft lip and/or palate (Fig. 2–15A). Those without clefts have a characteristic face with sloping forehead and bulbous nose (Fig. 2–15B).

Other anomalies include cardiovascular malformations, polycystic renal cortex, biseptate uterus in females, undescended testes and abnormal insertion of phallus in males, polydactyly of hands and feet, hyperconvex nails, capillary cutaneous defects, and cutaneous scalp defects. The central nervous system is markedly affected, with degrees of defects ranging from cyclopia (Fig. 2–15C) with absence of rhinencephalon, union of ventricles and thalami, and defects of corpus callosum, falx, and commissures to simple arhinencephaly with absence of olfactory nerves and lobes.

Ocular abnormalities are a cardinal feature of trisomy 13. Microphthalmia and anophthalmia are common. Uveal tract colobomas, cataracts, corneal opacities, glaucomas, hyperplastic vitreous bodies, intraocular or epibulbar cartilage, retinal dysplasia with tendency to herniate into adjacent tissue, optic atrophy, and defective angle development have been reported. Figure 2–15F and G, illustrating the eye of one of our patients, shows many of these anomalies (Rodrigues et al., 1973).

Most children with trisomy 13 have 47 chromosomes. However, a small number have 46 chromosomes, with D/D translocation, which usually occurs de novo but occasionally is inherited from a carrier parent. Males and females are equally affected. Of the 16 cases studied in this laboratory, 6 were females, 10 male; 12 were 47,+13, 3 were 46,−D,+t(DqDq). None of the children with a translocation had inherited it. One child was a mosaic 46,XY/47,XY,+13). Two of the children, still living at ages 5 and 7 years, respectively, are deaf and blind and have reached no developmental landmarks. Most children with trisomy 13 die before their first birthday.

TRISOMY 22. Trisomy 22 has been suggested as the cause of anomalies in children with 47 chromosomes and an extra G but lacking stigmata of Down's syndrome. With quinacrine fluorescence and differential staining, chromosomes 21 and 22 can now be distinguished, and we have reported the first case of trisomy 22 so diagnosed (Punnett et al., 1971). Until other previously described cases have been proved to be trisomy 22, the syndrome can not be adequately characterized. The eye abnormalities seen in the proved cases are limited to epicanthal folds and antimongoloid slant. In view of mental and physical retardation, low-set, large, abnormal ears, cleft palate, micrognathia, microcephaly, preauricular skin tags and/ or sinus, congenital heart disease, and anomalies of the external genitalia, it would be surprising if other eye defects are not reported.

Structural Abnormalities

The second group of clinically recognizable chromosomal syndromes is due to deletions resulting from breaks in a chromosome with loss usually of a terminal portion. If the deletion is limited to an egg or sperm, only a single child in a family will be affected. Deletions may also be inherited as the unbalanced form of a translocation for which a normal parent is a balanced carrier. Partial deletions of the short arms of 4, 5, and 18 and of the long arms of D group members and 18 occur frequently enough for each to be considered a syndrome. Children with ring chromosomes, which result from two breaks, with loss of chromatin from both ends, may resemble those with simple deletions of the same chromosome.

DELETION OF THE SHORT ARM OF CHROMOSOME 4. The physical findings in partial deletion of the short arm of 4 (46,4p−) are severe mental retardation, seizures, prominent glabella, midline scalp defect, preauricular dimple, cleft lip and palate or high arched palate, deformed nose, hemangiomas of the forehead, internal hydrocephalus, and undescended testes and hypospadias in males (Wolf et al., 1965). The eye anomalies include colobomas and unusually coarse structure of the iris, ocular hypertelorism, exophthalmos, and strabismus. No pathologic studies have been reported. The chromosomal anomaly may be either a de novo deletion or due to unbalanced segregation in the gamete of a carrier parent (Fig. 2–16).

DELETION OF SHORT ARM OF CHROMOSOME 5 (CRI DU CHAT). The syndrome due to the partial deletion of the short arm of chromosome 5 (46,5p–) was described by Lejeune in 1963. Children with this syndrome usually have a low birthweight and a slow growth rate, neonatally. They are hypotonic. The cat-like cry, which gives the syndrome its name, is attributed to an abnormality in structure of the larynx. It is striking in infancy but usually disappears with age. There is severe mental deficiency. Physical findings include microcephaly with a very round face in infancy, micrognathia, low-set ears, and congenital heart disease (Fig. 2–17). Ocular findings are antimongoloid slant, hypertelorism, epicanthal folds, exotropia, myopia, coloboma of iris, and optic atrophy. Like the syndrome of 4p–, the 5p– may represent a new event or be inherited from a carrier parent.

DELETED D. Over 30 children with deleted D or ring D chromosomes have been reported. Many of these children have similar physical findings, which include microcephaly, with trigonocephaly; prominent bridge of the nose; small chin; large, low-set, malformed ears; and facial asymmetry (Fig. 2–18). They are severely retarded. Males have shown hypospadias and undescended testes. Absent or hypoplastic thumbs are frequent.

Ocular findings include hypertelorism, narrow palpebral fissures, epicanthal folds, ptosis, microphthalmos, colobomas of the iris, and cataracts. Retinoblastoma has been reported in 7 children with Dq–, (5 bilateral, 2 unilateral) and 1 child with D ring.

It is not certain whether all the long arm deletions and the rings are derived from the same D chromosome. Identification, when made, was based on autoradiographic identification of the abnormal D. The D deletions and rings must now be restudied with quinacrine fluorescence and the new banding techniques. Until precise identification is made, we prefer to use the D group designation.

DELETED 18. Deletions of chromosome 18 may occur in either the short (18p–) or long (18q–) arm or in both, through ring formation (r18), following fusion of broken chromosome ends with the loss of terminal portions of both arms. Therefore, physical findings of r18 may overlap both the short arm and long arm deletion syndromes and will not be described separately (Fig. 2–19).

CHROMOSOME 18, DELETION OF SHORT ARM (46,18p–). The physical findings associated with the deletion (total or partial) of the short arm of chromosome 18 show a wide range. The mildest expression encompasses microcephaly, mental retardation, short stature, webbed neck, and immunoglobulin abnormalities (Fig. 2–20).

In its most severe form, the syndrome mimics trisomy 13, with the median facial dysplasia of cebocephaly or cyclopia and incomplete morphogenesis of the brain. Cardiac, renal, and gastrointestinal abnormalities are rarely seen in the 18q– syndrome.

The eye anomalies of the mildly affected children are hypertelorism, epicanthal folds, ptosis, and strabismus. Microphthalmia has been reported in the cebocephalics and the typical fused eyes are seen in cyclopia.

The only histopathologic study of the eye in an 18 deletion was reported by Yanoff, Rorke, and Niederer (1970) in a case of cebocephaly with a ring 18. Bilateral microphthalmia with cyst, intrascleral cartilage, intrachoroidal smooth muscle, and other anomalies were seen. No recognizable components of the optic system could be identified.

CHROMOSOME 18, DELETION OF LONG ARM (18q–). Partial deletion of long arm of 18 (deGrouchy et al., 1964) produces a syndrome marked by growth and developmental failure. The facies is striking, with microcephaly, midface hypoplasia,

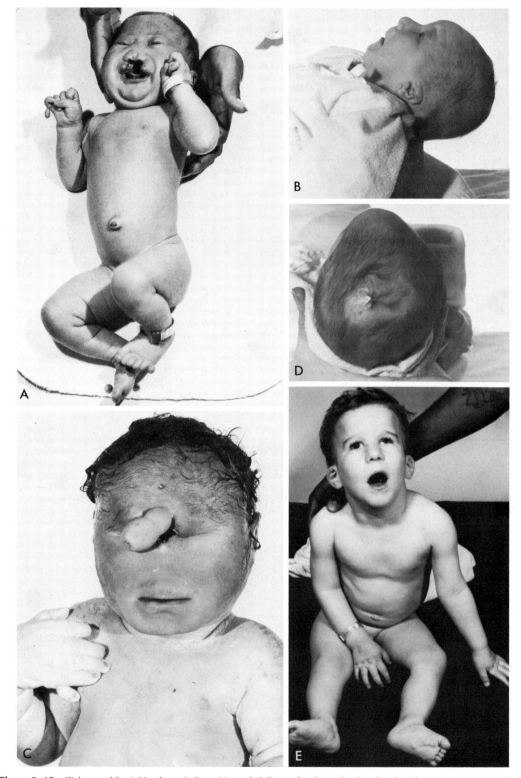

Figure 2–15   Trisomy 13. *A*, Newborn infant. Note cleft lip and palate, sloping forehead, supernumerary digit on all four extremities. *B*, Characteristic profile in infant without clefts, showing bulbous nose, sloping forehead, anomalies of external ear, and micrognathia. *C*, Cyclopia with extra digit. *D*, Scalp defect. *E*, Two and a half-year-old, severely retarded boy with mosaicism for trisomy 13. Characteristic face, with small eye on left; low set, abnormal ears; and tapering fingers with hyperconvex fingernails.

Figure 2–15 continued on opposite page.

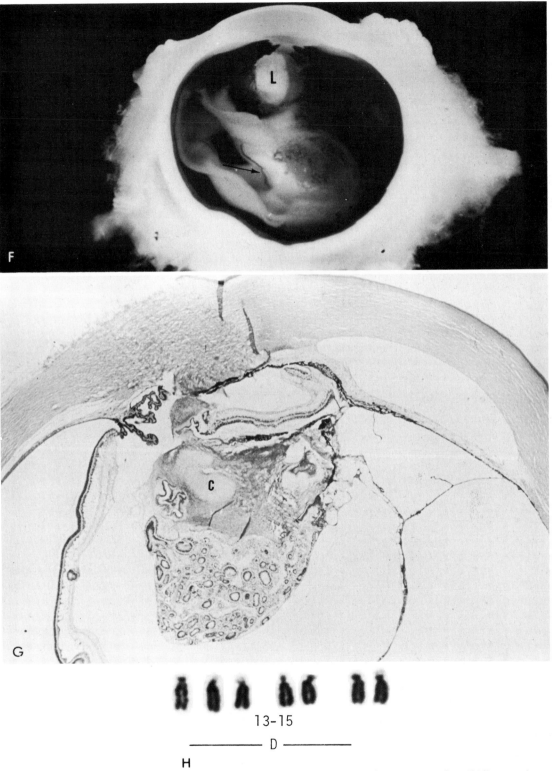

Figure 2–15 *Continued.* *F*, Microphthalmic left globe with microcornea. The cataractous lens (L) lies anterior to detached retina. The persistent hyaloid artery (arrow) is surrounded by persistent hyperplastic primary vitreous. *G*, The island of intraocular hyaline cartilage (C) lies in the plane of a uveal coloboma and is surrounded by persistent hyperplastic primary vitreous. Centrally, the embryonal retina shows numerous dysplastic rosettes (hematoxylin and eosin, ×4). (Rodrigues, M. M., Valdes-Dapena, M., and Kistenmacher, M.: J. Pediat. Ophthal., 1973. Reproduced from the Journal of Pediatric Ophthalmology by permission of the publisher, Charles B. Slack, Inc.) *H*, The D group chromosomes, with trisomy 13.

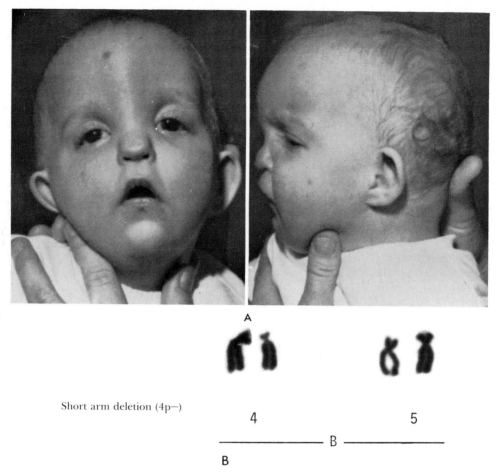

Short arm deletion (4p−)

A

4   5

B

B

Figure 2–16 *A*, One-year-old male with deletion of short arm of chromosome 4 (4p−). (Courtesy of Dr. O. J. Miller and Dr. Roy Breg. From Nelson, W. E., Vaughn, V. C., and McKay, R. J.: Textbook of Pediatrics. 9th ed. Philadelphia, W. B. Saunders Co., 1969.) *B*, Chromosomes of B group with deletion of part of short arm of 4.

and a carplike mouth. Ears have a prominent antihelix and/or antitragus. There is a narrow or atretic ear canal and hearing loss.

The fingers taper markedly, with a high frequency of whorl patterns. Single palmar creases are seen. Toes have abnormal placement, with the third toe placed above the second and fourth. Unusual fat pads occur on the dorsa of the feet. Dimples are prominent on knuckles, knees, elbows, and shoulders (Fig. 2–21).

Eye abnormalities include inner epicanthal folds, slanted palpebral fissures, nystagmus, ocular hypertelorism, microphthalmia, corneal abnormalities, cataracts, retinal defects, and abnormal optic discs.

Most individuals represent sporadic cases of partial deletion of the long arm of chromosome 18, but occasionally a parent may carry a balanced translocation.

"CAT'S EYE" SYNDROME. The "cat's eye" syndrome is a rare chromosomal syndrome. It is included in this chapter because one of the two associated anomalies is coloboma of iris and choroid. The other is imperforate anus or anal atresia with rectovesical or rectovaginal fistula. The facies are unusual, with hypertelorism, antimongoloid slant of the palpebral fissures, preauricular fistulas with skin tags, and a small chin. Most children have had psychomotor retardation.

The colobomas of the iris and choroid may be unilateral or bilateral. The shape of the iris resembles the cat's vertical pupil, thus the appellation "cat's eye." Cataracts, in addition to bilateral iris colobomas, were found in one mother with the same chromosome anomaly.

The 3 patients initially described (Schachenmann et al., 1965) each had an extra

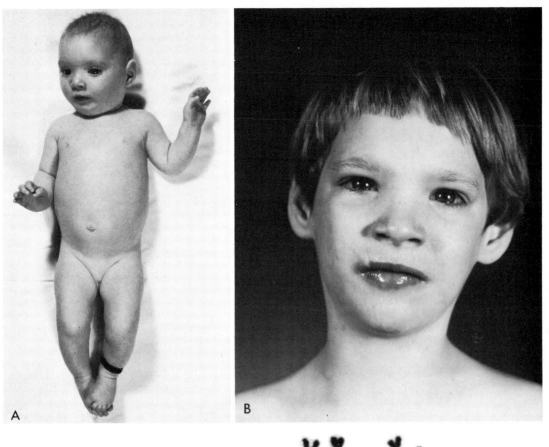

Short arm deletion (5p—)

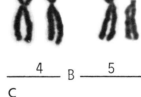

Figure 2–17 Child with deletion of short arm of chromosome 5 (5p—). *A*, At age 3 months. *B*, At 4 years of age. She has microcephaly, hypertelorism, epicanthal folds, and severe mental retardation. *C*, Chromosomes of B group with deletion of most of the short arm of 5.

acrocentric chromosome, smaller than either the 21 or 22. In those families in which more than one member has the extra chromosome, there has not been a correspondence of the full syndrome with the presence of the extra chromosome. The origin of the extra chromosome is not known.

Sex Chromosomes

The syndromes now known to be due to aneuploidy of the sex chromosomes were described before the development of modern cytogenetic techniques.

TURNER'S SYNDROME. Turner, in 1938, described several patients with infantilism, webbed neck, and cubitus valgus, establishing as a clinical syndrome a previously described endocrinologic disorder. The absence of sex chromatin in most Turner's syndrome patients was reported independently by three groups in 1954 (Decourt et al.; Polani et al.; Wilkins et al.). The first published 45,X karyotype (Ford et al., 1959) was confirmed by many laboratories within the same year. Approximately

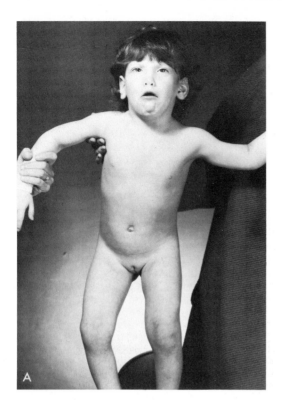

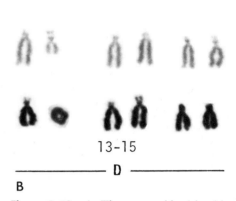

Figure 2-18 *A*, Three-year-old girl with ring chromosome 13, micrognathia, hypertelorism, internal strabismus of the right eye, bilateral colobomas of irides, epicanthal folds, and mongoloid slant of the eyes. (From Kistenmacher, M., and Punnett, H. H.: Amer. J. Human Genet., *22*:304, 1970.) *B*, Chromosomes of the D group, showing long arm deletion (13q−) and ring (13r) chromosome 13.

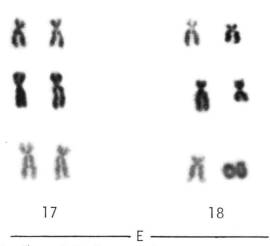

Figure 2-19 E group chromosomes, showing chromosome 18 with short arm deletion (18 p−), long arm deletion (18q−), and ring (18r).

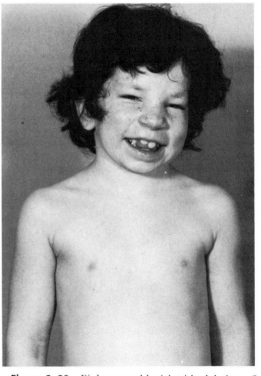

Figure 2-20 Eight-year-old girl with deletion of the short arm of chromosome 18, bilateral congenital ptosis, diabetes, and thyroiditis.

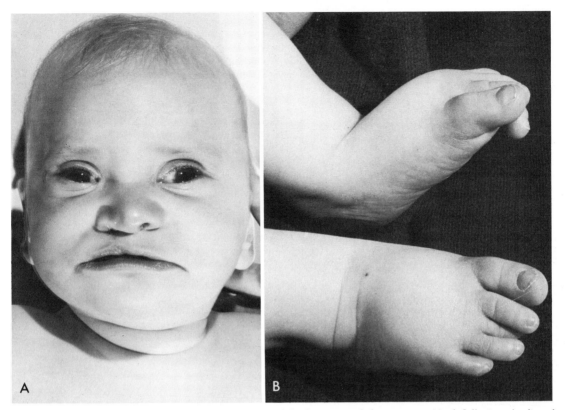

Figure 2–21 *A*, Ten-month-old infant with deletion of the long arm of chromosome 18, cleft lip (repaired) and palate, horizontal nystagmus, divergent strabismus, bilateral optic atrophy and macular anomalies. *B*, Abnormal insertion of third toe and fat pads on the dorsal aspect of feet.

80 per cent of girls with Turner's syndrome have 45 chromosomes, a single X, and no sex chromatin (Barr bodies). The remaining 20 per cent have other chromosomal variants. The unifying cytogenetic characteristic is the presence of a cell line which does not have two normal X chromosomes. It may lack the second X completely or have an abnormal second X (ring, fragment, deletion). The few who have Barr bodies are mosaics (45,X/46,XX) or have a long arm isochromosome (46,X,i[Xq]) (Fig. 2–22). Of the 44 girls with Turner's syndrome studied in this laboratory, 29 have 45,X karyotypes. The other 15 represent 7 different mosaic karyotypes, 5 of which include a normal 46,XX cell line.

The typical findings in Turner's syndrome are sexual infantilism, short stature, webbed neck, broad shield chest with widely spaced nipples, increased carrying angle, small uterus, and multiple pigmented nevi (Fig. 2–23). Recurrent ear infections are common. The ovaries consist of fibrous streaks with few or no follicles,

and failure to feminize may be the presenting problem in the older girl with few of the physical stigmata. Coarctation of the aorta is common and may account for some of the early childhood deaths. Autoimmune diseases, particularly Hashimoto's thyroiditis and diabetes, have been associated with the syndrome. Turner's syndrome in some newborn infants is characterized by lymphedema of the hands and feet which may persist into adulthood.

Ptosis and strabismus are the most common ocular lesions encountered. Congenital cataracts may occur, as well as those of later onset, particularly in association with diabetes. Refractive errors, corneal nebulae, blue sclera, and a variety of other anomalies have been reported. (In our laboratory chromosomal studies of a girl with 45,X/46,XX/47,XXX were initiated on the basis of optic disc pallor noted prior to surgery for strabismus at age 2.)

The incidence of color blindness in females with 45,X Turner's syndrome

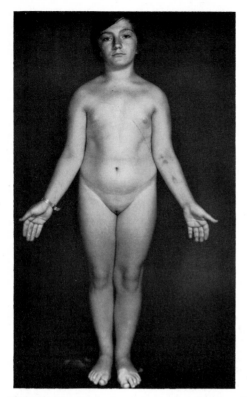

Figure 2–22   Turner's syndrome in a 15-year-old girl with short stature, cubitus valgus, and a goiter. Her karyotype is 45,X/46,XX. (From Nelson, W. E., Vaughn, V. C., and McKay, R. J.: Textbook of Pediatrics. 9th ed. Philadelphia, W. B. Saunders Co., 1969.)

a unilateral streak gonad is found with an abdominal testis on the other side.

KLINEFELTER'S SYNDROME. Klinefelter et al. in 1952 described a syndrome of gynecomastia, small testes with hyalinization of seminiferous tubules, absent spermatogenesis but normal Leydig cell complement, and elevated urinary gonadotropins. Patients with this clinical syndrome were shown to be chromatin positive by Plunkett and Barr in 1956, and to have 47,XXY sex chromosomes complement by Jacobs and Strong in 1959. Boys with more severe forms of Klinefelter's syndrome may have XXXY sex chromosomes and 2 Barr bodies, or XXXXY and 3 Barr bodies. Increasing numbers of X chromosomes cause greater physical and mental impairment. Males with XXXY are mentally retarded, may have radial-ulnar synostosis, scoliosis, microcephaly,

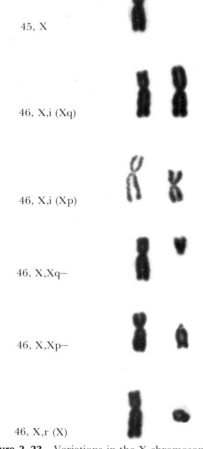

45, X

46, X,i (Xq)

46, X,i (Xp)

46, X,Xq–

46, X,Xp–

46, X,r (X)

Figure 2–23   Variations in the X chromosomes of Turner's syndrome, showing isochromosomes for the long arm (Xqi) and short arm (Xpi), deletions of the long arm (Xq–) and short arm (Xp–), and ring (Xr).

equals that seen in normal males, since only one X chromosome is present. In informative families, this easily recognized defect may identify the origin of the single X. If the girl with Turner's and her father are discordant (the child is color blind and the father normal, or the child normal and father color blind), the single X must have come from the mother. If both child and father are color blind and the mother is normal, the X may be assumed to be from the father.

Ambiguity of the external genitalia is not a feature of Turner's syndrome, but it is seen in children with 45,X/46,XY mosaicism in whom the physical findings of Turner's may be combined with varying degrees of pseudohermaphroditism. Some may resemble typical Turner's; others are phenotypic males. The Y chromosome usually induces some testicular development and subsequent masculinization (often incomplete) of genitalia. Frequently congenital heart disease, and prognathism (Fig. 2–24). The ocular findings are inner epicanthal folds, hypertelorism, upward slant of palpebral fissures, strabismus, Brushfield spots, and myopia.

The extra X may be either maternal or paternal in origin. Mosaicism (46,XY/47,XXY/48,XXXY or 48,XXXY/49,XXXXY) is common and may be explained by two successive nondisjunctions, the initial one in parental gametogenesis, the second in the zygote.

Considerable overlap with Klinefelter's syndrome has been seen in boys with 48,XXYY karyotypes who are unusually tall, with eunuchoid proportions and some degree of mental retardation. Some males have also exhibited the aggressive or bizarre behavior attributed to men with 47,XYY karyotypes. No phenotypic characteristics other than tall stature have been reported with the latter. The physical or

behavioral characteristics attributed to XYY males depends in large part upon how they were ascertained. The majority of XYY males were identified during surveys of British maximum-security hospitals, and their aggressive personalities have received inordinate publicity. Other XYY males have been identified owing to hypogonadism or infertility and are otherwise normal. The full range of phenotypic expression is not yet known.

Eye anomalies are not usually seen in the XYY syndrome, although myopia, dislocation of the lens, and bilateral retinal detachments have been reported.

CYTOPLASMIC INHERITANCE

The discussion thus far has dealt only with genetic factors within the nucleus. Are there non-nuclear determinants of heredity and can they be demonstrated in man?

For proof of non-nuclear (cytoplasmic) inheritance, the trait in question must be maternally transmitted. Most of the cytoplasm contributed to the zygote resulting from gametic fusion is contributed by the egg. The sperm's contribution is negligible. Therefore, if non-nuclear elements determine the inheritance of a trait, the progeny should resemble the mother.

There is evidence for cytoplasmic inheritance in protozoa, algae, fungi, insects, and higher plants. In some cases, although the particulate elements are transmitted through the egg cytoplasm, they require the presence of a specific genotype for activation or duplication of the particle. Mitochondria, viruses, and chloroplasts are inherited through the cytoplasm.

Is there evidence for cytoplasmic inheritance in man? Discrepancies in the inheritance of anencephaly and spina bifida (the same recurrence risk of 4 to 5 per cent for maternal half-siblings, and full siblings, and the lack of concordance in identical twins) led Nance (1969) to suggest cytoplasmic inheritance as a possible explanation. The case for Leber's optic atrophy, as another example, has been reopened by Erickson (1972) who also points out the difficulty in distinguishing between transplacental infection and cytoplasmic inheritance.

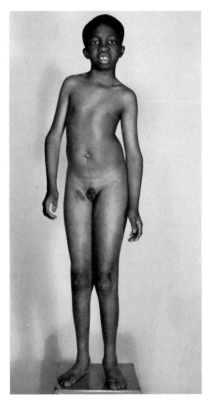

Figure 2–24 A 12-year-old boy with 48,XXXY/49,-XXXXY mosaicism. He has prognathism, epicanthal folds, scoliosis, hypogonadism, severe mental retardation, clinodactyly, and radial-ulnar synostosis. (From Nelson, W. E., Vaughn, V. C., and McKay, R. J.: Textbook of Pediatrics. 9th ed. Philadelphia, W. B. Saunders Co., 1969.)

TABLE 2–1 OCULAR CHANGES IN PEDIATRIC SYNDROMES

Disease	Ocular Manifestations	Systemic Manifestations	Inheritance
A-Beta-Lipoproteinemia Acanthocytosis (Bassen-Kornzweig)	Pigmentary degeneration of retina.	Spinocerebellar degeneration with ataxia. Spiny deformity of erythrocytes (acanthocytes). A-beta-lipoproteinemia. In homozygote, poor absorption of carotene and vitamin A. Dark adaptation restored with high levels of vitamin A.	a.r.
Achromatopsia (See Table 2–2)	Amblyopia, nystagmus, and photosensitivity. Visual acuity often 20/200. Total absence of color discrimination. Failure with Sloan achromatopsia test. Absent photopic ERG.		a.r.
Acrocephalosyndactyly (Apert's)	Exophthalmos, exotropia, optic atrophy, partial ophthalmoplegia, and cataracts.	Hypertelorism, hypoplastic maxilla, acrocephaly, syndactyly, abnormality of sutures.	a.d.
Aicardi Syndrome	Large, discrete areas of chorioretinopathy; microphthalmos	Spasms and toxic seizures in female infants, defects of corpus callosum, cortical heterotopia, dorsal vertebral anomalies, characteristic EEG, and mental retardation.	a.d. Lethal in the male
Albers-Schönberg (Osteopetrosis)	Cranial nerve palsies and blindness from marrow compression of foramina.	Thick, dense, fragile bones; pancytopenia from marrow obliteration. Serum calcium low, phosphorus elevated.	a.r.
Albinism (Oculocutaneous) 1. Complete Albinism	Iris is thin, pale blue. A characteristic orange reflex from the pupil occurs when light rays penetrating the pigment-deficient membranes of the eye are reflected back to the observer's eye. Prominent choroidal vessels with poorly defined fovea. Nystagmus, head-nodding, and frequently myopic astigmatism and strabismus. Marked photophobia. The eyelashes and eyebrows are white.	White hair and brows. Two distinct genotypes, depending on presence or absence of tyrosinase. Tyrosinase absent in complete albinism.	a.r.
2. Modified Complete Albinism	Slight pigmentation, some yellow pigment flecks at pupillary border. Minimal to absent red reflex. May be nystagmus, photophobia, and myopia. Choroidal vessels prominent.	Tyrosinase positive. In Caucasians, no phenotypic difference between tyrosinase positive and negative. In Negroes, slight pigmentation, golden hair, with tendency to hyperkeratoses and freckling in exposed areas of skin.	a.r.
3. Ocular Albinism	Marked deficiency of pigment in iris and choroid. Nystagmus and myopic astigmatism. Iris of female carrier is frequently translucent.	Normal pigmentation elsewhere.	X-r.
4. Amish Albinism	At birth, complete albinism with blue translucent irides and albinotic fundal reflex. Nystagmus and photophobia. Increasing pigmentation with age.	White hair and skin at birth. Increasing pigmentation with yellow hair and normal skin which tans. Biochemically, gives intermediate reaction between tyrosinase positive and negative.	a.r.

TABLE 2–1 OCULAR CHANGES IN PEDIATRIC SYNDROMES (*Continued*)

Disease	Ocular Manifestations	Systemic Manifestations	Inheritance
5. Albinism With Deafness	Typical ocular changes	Typical albinism with nerve deafness.	X-r.
Albright's Disease (Polyostotic Fibrocystic Dysplasia)	Unilateral proptosis, visual field defects, papilledema, optic atrophy.	Osteitis fibrosa cystica, pigmented areas of skin, and endocrine dysfunction and sexual precocity.	a.d.? Most cases sporadic
Alkaptonuria and Ochronosis	Scleral pigmentation most marked at recti muscle insertions.	Black colored urine on standing, osteoarthritis, valvular heart disease, atherosclerosis (homogentisic acid oxidase deficiency).	a.r.
Alpers' Diffuse Cerebral Degeneration	Cortical blindness.	Hyperkinesis, seizures, rigidity, opisthotonos.	a.r.
Alport's Syndrome	Cataracts, anterior and posterior lenticonus, spherophakia.	Nerve deafness, hemorrhagic nephritis.	a.d. with anomalous segregation
Alström's Disease	Retinitis pigmentosa and cataract.	Nerve deafness, diabetes mellitus in childhood, and obesity.	a.r.
Amaurotic Family Idiocy 1. Tay-Sachs Disease (GM$_2$ Ganglioside Storage Disease)	Cherry-red spot in macula, optic atrophy, gradual onset of ophthalmoplegia, visual loss to blindness.	Infants normal at birth but fail to thrive after 4 to 8 months, hypotonia, generalized CNS deterioration to spastic paraplegia, demented, frequent seizures, and death. Hyperacusis is a special sign. Occurs in Jewish children primarily. Biochemical heterogeneity. Absence of hexosaminadase A most common (type I); absence of hexosaminidase A and B in Sandhoff's variant (type II).	a.r.
2. Late Infantile Form of Amaurotic Family (Batten-Bielschowsky)	Dark-red spot on macula, optic atrophy.	Onset age 2 to 4, seizures, generalized CNS deterioration, visual loss, death, accumulation of ceroidlipofuscin.	a.r.
3. Juvenile Amaurotic Family Idiocy (Batten-Mayou-Vogt-Spielmeyer)	Reddish-brown spot in macula. Peripheral retinal degeneration, nystagmus, gradual visual loss to blindness.	Onset 5 to 7 years, mental deterioration, spasticity, seizures, hypertonus, death from intercurrent infection.	a.r.
4. Late Juvenile or Adult Form of Amaurotic Family Idiocy (Kufs')	No visual loss and fundi may be normal or show mild retinal pigmentary changes.	Onset age 5 to 25 years, rigidity and awkward gait, ataxia, dysarthria, epilepsy, and muscular rigidity. Storage of pigmented lipid.	a.r.
5. Generalized Gangliosidosis (GM$_1$)	Cherry-red spot in half of cases.	Low birthweight and failure to thrive, poor development, coarse features, joint limitation, kyphosis, and hepatomegaly. β-galactosidase deficiency.	a.r.

TABLE 2–1   OCULAR CHANGES IN PEDIATRIC SYNDROMES (*Continued*)

Disease	Ocular Manifestations	Systemic Manifestations	Inheritance
Aminopterin-Induced Syndrome	Shallow orbital ridge from severe hypoplasia of frontal bone. Broad nasal bridge and epicanthus. Prominent eyes.	Generalized congenital hypoplasia, cleft palate, and low-set ears. Partial syndactyly and hypotonia. Aminopterin, a folic acid antagonist, and methotrexate, the methyl derivative of aminopterin, have been used as abortifacient during first trimester.	Teratogen
Amyloidoses, Hereditary	Sheetlike hyaline vitreous opacities, visual loss, exophthalmos, ophthalmoplegia, corneal dystrophy from amyloid, conjunctival amyloidosis, pupils small and irregular.	Peripheral neuropathy, chronic gastrointestinal symptoms, hoarseness, autonomic dysfunction, occurs with high frequency in Portuguese. Genetic heterogeneity.	a.d.
Aniridia	Complete or partial absence of iris. Associated with coloboma in family. Nystagmus, hypoplasia of macula, glaucoma, cataract.	Cerebellar ataxia and oligophrenia reported. Increased incidence of Wilms' tumor associated with sporadic aniridia; rarely with familial.	a.d. Sporadic
Anophthalmos or Microphthalmos	Small rudimentary globe deep in orbit.	Polydactyly, craniofacial and brain malformations.	a.d. a.r. X-r.
Ataxia-Telangiectasia (Louis-Bar Syndrome)	Telangiectasia, bulbar conjunctiva in medial and lateral canthi, nystagmus, ocular motor apraxic movement, frequent loss OKN response, strabismus, and poor convergence.	Cutaneous telangiectasia of ears, cheeks, and antecubital space. Cerebellar ataxia, deficiency of IgA, lymphoreticular malignancy, recurrent sinopulmonary infections, and mental retardation.	a.d.
Basal Cell Nevus Syndrome	Strabismus, cataract, iris coloboma, hypertelorism. Synophrys.	Basal cell nevi over upper torso prone to carcinoma, mental deficiency, odontogenic cysts of mandible, misshapen teeth, bifid ribs.	a.d.
Behr's Syndrome (Cerebellar Ataxia with Optic Atrophy)	Optic atrophy, significant reduction of vision, nystagmus.	Ataxia, loss of coordination, pyramidal tract signs (including increased tendon reflexes, positive Babinski), mental deficiency, vesicle sphincter weakness.	a.r.
Carpenter's Syndrome (Acrocephalopolysyndactyly)	Lateral displacement of inner canthi and/or inner canthal folds.	Mental retardation, obesity, acrocephaly, polydactyly and syndactyly of feet, hypogenitalism, cardiac and other skeletal defects.	a.r.
Cataract, Congenital	Cataracts of all forms.	See Chapter 15 for diseases associated with cataract.	Depends on specific entity
Cerebral Sclerosis Group 1. Pelizaeus-Merzbacher Disease (Diffuse Cerebral Sclerosis)	Nystagmus, optic atrophy.	Symptoms similar to disseminated sclerosis and Friedreich's ataxia, mental deterioration, spasticity, athetosis. Similar to Schilder's disease.	X-r. (infancy) a.d. (late form)
2. Krabbe's (Globoid Cell Sclerosis)	Optic atrophy, nystagmus.	Demyelination, leukodystrophy and lipid storage, muscular rigidity, tonic spasms, early death. β-galactosidase deficiency.	a.r.

TABLE 2–1 OCULAR CHANGES IN PEDIATRIC SYNDROMES (*Continued*)

Disease	Ocular Manifestations	Systemic Manifestations	Inheritance
3. Scholz's (Subacute Diffuse Cerebral Sclerosis)	Cortical blindness, nystagmus.	Generalized CNS deterioration beginning at age 8 to 10, paralysis, deafness, early death. Intermediate between Pelizaeus-Merzbacher and Krabbe diseases.	X-r.
4. Spongy Degeneration of White Matter (Canavan's Disease)	Optic atrophy, nystagmus.	Macrocephaly, hypotonia early, spasticity later with decerebration, seizures, early death. Seen mostly in Jews.	a.r.
5. Metachromatic Leukodystrophy (Sulfatide Lipidosis)	Nystagmus, strabismus, cherry-red spot in macula, optic disc pallor.	Ataxia, hypotonia, seizures, CNS deterioration, dementia, death. Deficiency of aryl sulfatase A most commonly. Genetic heterogeneity.	a.r.
Cerebrohepatorenal Syndrome (Zellweger's Syndrome)	Bilateral congenital glaucoma, partial cataracts, and epicanthal folds.	Deficient growth, hepatomegaly with dysgenesis, albuminuria, polycystic kidney, patent ductus arteriosus, hypotonia, hypospadias, and camptodactyly. Calcific deposits in epiphyseal region of long bones. Mentral retardation. Early death.	a.r.
Charcot-Marie-Tooth (Progressive Neuritic Muscular Atrophy)	Reduced vision, nystagmus, and optic atrophy.	Atrophy of small muscles of hands and feet and then proximal arm and leg.	a.r. a.d. X-r.
Chédiak-Higashi Syndrome	Partial albinism, diminished uveal and retinal pigmentation with photophobia and nystagmus. Histologic examination of eyes has shown papilledema, lymphocytic infiltration of the optic nerve, leukocytes containing the typical metachromatic inclusion granules in the limbal area, iris, and choroid.	Neutropenia with tendency toward lymphocytosis, anemia, and thrombocytopenia. Hepatosplenomegaly, lymphadenopathy, and early death from recurrent infections, leukemia, lymphoma.	a.r.
Cockayne Syndrome	Cataract, pigmentary degeneration, and optic atrophy.	Dwarfism, precocious senile appearance, deafness, photophobia, and mental retardation.	a.r.
Congenital Alopecia	Bilateral cataracts.	Congenital absence or extremely poor development of hair of the scalp, trunk, pubic region, and eyebrows. Friedreich's ataxia, obesity, hyperhidrosis, and syndactyly.	a.d.
Conradi's Disease (Chondrodystrophia Calcificans Congenita)	Bilateral cataract, optic atrophy, and hypertelorism.	Punctate, calcific deposits in infantile, cartilaginous skeleton including epiphysis and joint capsules. Limbs are short, especially in their proximal segments. Joint contractures and calcification of tracheal cartilages may occur.	a.r.
Chromosomal Abnormality Syndromes 1. Deletion Syndromes			Usually sporadic but may be inherited as familial translocation.

TABLE 2–1   OCULAR CHANGES IN PEDIATRIC SYNDROMES (*Continued*)

Disease	Ocular Manifestations	Systemic Manifestations	Inheritance
a. Cri du chat. Partial deletion of short arm of chromosome 5 (5p−)	Hypertelorism, epicanthus, strabismus.	Slow growth, cat-like cry, mental retardation, hypotonia, microcephaly, simian crease, and congenital heart defect in 30%	
b. Partial deletion of short arm of 4 (4p−)	Iris coloboma.	Cleft palate, hypospadias.	Sporadic
c. Partial deletion of long arm of 18 (18q−)	Optic disc pallor, nystagmus, tapetoretinal degeneration.	Psychomotor retardation with microcephaly, prominent chin.	Sporadic or familial translocation
d. Partial deletion of short arm of 18 (18p−)	Hypertelorism, epicanthal fold, ptosis, strabismus.	Short stature, webbed neck, mental retardation.	Sporadic or familial translocation
e. Partial deletion of D long arm (Dq−) and ring D(Dr)	Epicanthal folds, ptosis, hypertelorism, microphthalmos, iris coloboma, retinoblastomas.	Mental retardation microcephaly, small chin, facial asymmetry.	Sporadic
2. Duplication Syndromes			
a. Cat's Eye Syndrome	Microphthalmos, coloboma, partial irideremia, absent macular areas, pale discs.	Anal atresia, preauricular skin tags, and umbilical hernia.	Extra small chromosome; sporadic or familial
b. Trisomy 13	Microphthalmos, enophthalmos, corneal opacity, cataract, retinal dysplasia with cartilage, hypoplasia optic nerve, and iris coloboma.	Low-set ears, cleft palate, flexion contracture of fingers, congenital heart defect, failure to thrive, severe CNS defects.	Usually sporadic, rarely inherited as translocation
c. Trisomy 18	Blepharoptosis, corneal opacity, short palpebral fissures, and epicanthal folds.	Micrognathia, congenital heart defect, "rocker-bottom" feet, low-set malformed ears, mental deficiency, and failure to thrive.	Usually sporadic, rarely inherited as translocation
d. Trisomy 21 (Down's Syndrome, Mongolism)	Mongoloid slant to palpebral fissures, epicanthus, cataract, Brushfield spots, strabismus and acute keratoconus with corneal hydrops.	Mongoloid facies, large tongue, obesity, hyperflexibility of joints, short 5th finger, hypotonia, simian crease, and mental retardation. Congenital heart disease.	Usually sporadic, 5 per cent due to familial translocation
3. Sex Chromosomes			
a. Turner's Syndrome (45 X) Mosaic Variants	Ptosis, color blindness, cataracts, strabismus, epicanthus, blue sclera, nystagmus.	Webbed neck, coarctation of aorta, lymphangioedema of hands and feet, small stature, and ovarian dysgenesis.	Sporadic
b. Klinefelter's Syndrome XXY, XXXY, XXXXY)	Hypertelorism, epicanthus, strabismus, Brushfield spots, myopia.	Mental deficiency, hypotonia, limited elbow pronation, low dermal ridge count on fingertips. Hypogenitalism with increasing X's.	Sporadic
Cornelia de Lange Syndrome	Long curly eyelashes, bushy eyebrows and synophrys, strabismus, myopia, optic atrophy, ptosis.	Short stature, mental retardation, low-pitched weak cry, microcephaly, hirsutism (esp. on back), reduction malformations of extremities.	Unknown

TABLE 2–1 OCULAR CHANGES IN PEDIATRIC SYNDROMES (*Continued*)

Disease	Ocular Manifestations	Systemic Manifestations	Inheritance
Crouzon's Disease (Craniofacial Dysostosis)	Exophthalmos, exotropia, optic atrophy, hypertelorism, and cataracts.	Craniofacial dysostosis, deafness, mental retardation, beak nose, and hypoplastic maxilla.	a.d.
Cryptophthalmos	Fusion of eyelids, unilateral or bilateral; microphthalmos.	Deformity of pinnae, atresia of auditory canal, malformed teeth, spina bifida, syndactyly, abnormal hairline.	a.r.
Cystic Fibrosis	Dilated dark, tortuous retinal veins; retinal hemorrhages.	Chronic pulmonary disease, intestinal malabsorption, excessive electrolytes in sweat (esp. NaCl), cirrhosis.	a.r.
Cystinosis (Fanconi Syndrome with Renal Tubular Defects)	Cystine crystals seen in cornea and conjunctiva with corneal microscope. Retinal pigmentary degeneration in periphery.	Small stature, aminoaciduria and renal failure. Renal tubular acidosis.	a.r.
Diabetes Mellitus	Rapid change in refractive error, cataract, retinal microaneurysms, retinopathy, retinitis proliferans, retinal detachment.	Hyperglycemia, glycosuria, with long-term effect on kidney, cardiovascular system, and eyes.	Familial but varying modes of inheritance
Dyskeratosis Congenita Syndrome	Blepharitis, ectropion, nasolacrimal obstruction or atresia of lacrimal ducts.	Hyperpigmentation of the skin, leukoplakia, nail dystrophy, sparse hair, pancytopenia and, testicular atrophy.	X-r.
Ectodermal Dysplasia (Marshall's Type)	Congenital or juvenile cataracts which may spontaneously absorb, myopia.	Midfacial hypoplasia, deafness, teeth deformity, low nasal bridge with short depressed nose. Mild hypohidrosis (25%).	a.d.
Ectodermal Hypohidrotic Dysplasia (Anhidrotic)	Tear deficiency leading to keratitis and photophobia, cataracts.	Hypohidrosis, episodes of hyperthermia, hypoplasia of sweat glands, scanty hair, hypodontia, finger nail dystrophy, and hypoplasia of mucous membranes. Chronic lung disease.	X-r. Rarely a.r.
Ehlers-Danlos Syndrome	Epicanthal folds, blue sclera, keratoconus, subluxation of lens, and retinal detachment.	Small stature, kyphoscoliosis, hyperextensibility of joints, dissecting aneurysm, intracranial aneurysm, hyperextensibility of skin and extreme fragility.	a.d.
Fabry's Disease (Angiokeratoma Corporis Diffusum)	Whorl-like corneal opacities are characteristic, corkscrew tortuosity of veins in posterior pole, spokelike lens opacities in 50%. Dilated, sausage-shaped conjunctival vessels, and periorbital edema.	Ceramide trihexoside lipidosis. Begins in childhood with burning pain in extremities and maculopapular eruption. Dark purple papules (angiokeratoma) common in males in bathing suit area. Edema of legs and face. Progressive renal failure, hypertension, and death. Deficiency in ceramidetrihexosidase.	X-r.

TABLE 2–1   OCULAR CHANGES IN PEDIATRIC SYNDROMES (*Continued*)

Disease	Ocular Manifestations	Systemic Manifestations	Inheritance
Falls-Kertesz Syndrome	Distichiasis of all four lids and partial ectropion of lower lids.	Chronic lymphedema of both lower extremities (Milroy's type) and pterygium colli.	a.d.
Familial Blepharophimosis	Epicanthus inversus, lateral displacement of inner canthi with short palpebral fissures and bilateral ptosis. Strabismus and nystagmus may occur.	Possible generalized hypotonia.	a.d.
Familial Dysautonomia (Riley-Day Syndrome)	Tear deficiency, corneal anesthesia, ulceration and corneal scarring.	Swallowing difficulties in infancy; emotional lability, insensitivity to pain, muscular hypotonia, hyperhidrosis, and skin blotching. Associated primarily with Jewish ancestry.	a.r.
Fanconi's Syndrome with Pancytopenia	Strabismus, ptosis, nystagmus, microphthalmos.	Pigmentation of skin, short stature, microcephaly, mental retardation, pancytopenia, abnormal ears and thumbs, and genital defects.	a.r.
Farber's Disease (Disseminated Lipogranulomatosis)	Grayish area posterior pole, with cherry-red spot and diffuse pigmentary mottling. Granulomas in and around eye.	Hoarse cry, subcutaneous swellings of extremities, irritability, progressive cachexia, and death (glycolipid infiltration). Deficiency in ceramidase.	a.r.
Flynn-Aird Syndrome	Severe myopia, bilateral cataracts, retinitis pigmentosa.	Bilateral nerve deafness, dental caries, kyphoscoliosis, skin atrophy, baldness, muscle wasting, mental retardation, ataxia, and seizures.	a.d.
Franceschetti's Syndrome (Treacher Collins', Mandibulofacial Dysostosis)	Lid coloboma, microphthalmos, antimongoloid slanting of lids.	Malar hypoplasia, malformation of auricles, conductive deafness, and mandibular hypoplasia.	a.d.
Freeman-Sheldon Syndrome (Whistling Face or Craniocarpotarsal Dystrophy)	Deep-set eyes, blepharophimosis, ptosis, strabismus, and epicanthus.	Masklike facies with small mouth presenting a "whistling" appearance. H-shaped dimple on chin, high palate, nasal speech, and club feet.	a.d.
Galactokinase deficiency	Juvenile cataracts	Galactosuria, galactosemia	a.r.
Galactosemia	Cataract, bilateral	Galactosemia, vomiting, galactosuria, failure to thrive, hepatosplenomegaly. (Deficiency in galactose 1-phosphate uridyl transferase.)	a.r.
Gaucher's Disease Type I – Noncerebral, juvenile	Wedge-shaped pinguecula, conjunctival pigmentation.	Splenomegaly, abnormal bruising, pathologic fractures.	a.r.
Type II – Cerebral, juvenile	Paralytic strabismus	Onset first few months of life. Hepatomegaly and splenomegaly, spasticity, failure to thrive, decerebrate rigidity, death in infancy.	a.r.
Type III – Cerebral, juvenile and adult	Paralytic strabismus	Onset 5 to 12 yrs., convulsions, tremors, emotional disturbances and progressive dementia (genetic heterogeneity). In all 3 types, defect is in β-glucosidase, and ceramide glucoside accumulates.	a.r.

TABLE 2–1   OCULAR CHANGES IN PEDIATRIC SYNDROMES (*Continued*)

Disease	Ocular Manifestations	Systemic Manifestations	Inheritance
Goldenhar's Syndrome (Oculoauriculo-vertebral Dysplasia)	Epibulbar dermoid involving conjunctiva and cornea, coloboma of lid.	External ear deformity or absence which may be associated with deafness. Preauricular cutaneous appendages. Mandibular hypoplasia, occipitalization of atlas hemivertebrae.	Not known
Goltz's Syndrome (Focal Dermal Hypoplasia)	Strabismus, coloboma, and/or microphthalmos.	Areas of hypoplasia and altered pigmentation of skin. Dystrophic nails, enamel hypoplasia, and syndactyly. Only females affected, presumed lethal in male.	a.d. or X-r ? (lethal in male)
Granulomatous Disease (Chronic) of Childhood	Pleomorphic, atrophic chorioretinal lesions, blepharitis, conjunctivitis, and keratitis.	Chronic suppurative lymphadenitis, eczematoid dermatitis, osteomyelitis, hepatosplenomegaly, pulmonary infiltrates and soft tissue abscesses and granulomas. Leukocytes ingest but cannot kill certain bacteria. Probable defect in cytoplasmic NADH oxidase and production of H_2O_2. Pigmented lipid histiocytosis.	x-r
Hallermann-Streiff (Dyscephalia Mandibulo-oculofacialis)	Bilateral microphthalmos and bilateral congenital cataracts which may resorb spontaneously, blue sclera, nystagmus.	Small stature, brachycephaly, malar hypoplasia, micrognathia. Small parrot-beak nose, skin atrophy over nose and scalp, sparse hair, hypoplasia of teeth, and hypotrichosis.	a.d.?
Hamartoses (Phakomatoses) 1. Sturge-Weber Syndrome	Congenital glaucoma, angiomatous formation in choroid, retinal detachment.	Flat facial hemangiomas, meningeal hemangiomas, seizures, mental deficiency.	Unknown
2. von Hippel-Lindau Syndrome	Angiomatous lesion in peripheral retina associated with dilated, tortuous vessels.	Cerebellar, spinal hemangiomas; adrenal, pancreatic cysts; hypernephroma of kidney; pheochromocytoma.	a.d.
3. Tuberous Sclerosis (Bourneville's Disease)	Retinal hamartomas.	Adenoma sebaceum, epilepsy, rhabdomyomas of kidney and heart, intracranial calcification.	a.d.?
4. Neurofibromatosis (von Recklinghausen)	Neurofibromatous lesion of retina, iris, or lids.	Café-au-lait spots on skin, skeletal changes, neurofibromas in skin and meninges.	a.d.
5. Wyburn-Mason's Syndrome (Angiomatosis of Midbrain and Retina)	Markedly enlarged retinal vessels. May involve orbit and optic nerve.	Angiomatous lesions of midbrain.	?
Hartnup's Disease	Nystagmus, photophobia, strabismus.	Aminoaciduria, pellagra-like skin rash, ataxia, mental deterioration, excess urinary indole excretion. Improves with nicotinamide.	a.r.
Hemophilia A	Oribtal, subconjunctival hemorrhage.	Prolonged bleeding and delayed clotting. Hemorrhages from mucous membranes, nose joints, gastrointestinal and genitourinary tracts, and intracranially. AHG factor VIII deficiency.	X-r.

TABLE 2–1   OCULAR CHANGES IN PEDIATRIC SYNDROMES (*Continued*)

Disease	Ocular Manifestations	Systemic Manifestations	Inheritance
Hemophilia B (Christmas Disease)	15% show ocular changes similar to Hemophilia B.	PTC factor IX deficiency.	X-r.
Hereditary Benign Intraepithelial Dyskeratosis (Witkop-Von Sallmann Syndrome)	Foamy gelatinous plaques on a hyperemic bulbar conjunctiva at nasal and temporal limbus may be noted by age 1. Corneal dyskeratosis can lead to severe visual loss.	Soft white folds and plaques involving mucosal surface of mouth, tongue, tonsils, and palate.	a.d. with high degree of penetrance
Homocystinuria	Dislocated lenses, cataract, secondary glaucoma, peripheral cystic degeneration of retina.	Osteoporosis, fractures, thrombosis, malar flush, mental retardation, fine fair hair (cystathionine synthetase deficiency).	a.r.
Hooft's disease (Hypolipidemia Syndrome)	Tapetoretinal degeneration resembling retinitis pigmentosa. Extinguished ERG.	Onset age 2. Red skin lesions on face and limbs. White nails, abnormal teeth, and mental retardation.	a.r.
Hyperlysinemia	Subluxation of lens, spherophakia, and strabismus.	Lax ligaments, hypotonic muscles, convulsions, and mental retardation. Hyperlysinemia and lysinuria. Genetic heterogeneity. Lysine ketaglutarate reductase deficiency in one form.	a.r.
Hyperphosphatasia, Hereditary (Juvenile Paget's Disease)	Optic atrophy and angioid streaks with macular changes. Blue sclera may be observed.	Onset prior to age 4. Symmetrical thickening of skull, bowing of long bones with osteoporosis, kyphoscoliosis, dwarfism, and deafness. High serum alkaline and acid phosphatase.	a.r.
Hypoparathyroidism	Zonular cataracts, phlyctenular keratoconjunctivitis, photophobia, blepharospasm, papilledema.	Tetany, hyperreflexia, metastatic calcifications, ectodermal changes. Neonatal onset. As above, plus moniliasis, idiopathic, later onset.	X-r. ?
Hypophosphatasia	Band-shaped keratopathy and calcific deposits in conjunctiva.	Onset early in life, with anorexia and vomiting. Similar to rickets clinically. Demineralization of bones and diminished alkaline phosphatase activity.	a.r.
Ichthyosis 1. Congenital Ichthyosis	Ectropion and keratopathy. Congenital cataracts may occur.	Hyperkeratosis involving especially articular folds, palms, and soles with generalized thick, scaly skin and hyperhidrosis.	a.r.
2. Lamellar Ichthyosis	Ectropion.	Dry, shining membrane envelops infant at birth. Skin membrane cracks and peels but reforms.	a.r.
3. Ichthyosis and Cataracts	Cortical cataracts.	Same as Congenital.	a.r.
4. Ichthyosis Vulgaris	Ichthyosis of lids, scales on lashes, punctate keratitis, corneal erosions, and stromal opacities, Lens changes.	Skin changes appear after 3 months of life. Mildest form.	a.d. X-r.

TABLE 2–1 OCULAR CHANGES IN PEDIATRIC SYNDROMES (*Continued*)

Disease	Ocular Manifestations	Systemic Manifestations	Inheritance
5. Bullous Ichthyosiform Erythroderma	Scales on lashes.	Similar to Congenital form but exhibiting bullae.	a.d.
6. X-linked Ichthyosis	Ocular changes as in ichthyosis vulgaris.	Similar to Vulgaris form but palms and soles normal.	X-r.
Infantile Subacute Necrotizing Encephalomyelopathy (Leigh's Syndrome)	Optic atrophy, nystagmus, intermittent ptosis, miosis.	Failure to thrive, vomiting, episodes of hypotonia, weakness, ataxia, dysarthria, convulsions, mental retardation, and death in early childhood. Subacute cases survive 10 to 15 yrs. Deficiency of pyruvate carboxylase activity resulting in impaired gluconeogenesis. Hyperpyruvicemia with hyper-alpha-alaninemia.	a.r.
Incontinentia Pigmenti (Bloch-Sulzberger)	Proliferative retinopathy, optic atrophy, strabismus, corneal opacities, cataract, PHPV.	Swirling patterns of skin pigmentation, hypodontia, skeletal defects, mental deficiency, patchy alopecia, microcephaly.	X-d. Lethal in male
Jeune's Syndrome (Thoracic Asphyxiating Dysplasia)	Loss of visual acuity and peripheral field, retinal degeneration with diminishing ERG.	Small stature, skeletal abnormalities (esp. small, fixed thoracic cage), respiratory failure in infancy, renal failure in later childhood.	a.r.
Kearn's Syndrome (External Ophthalmoplegia, Pigmentary Degeneration, and Cardiomyopathy)	Chronic progressive external ophthalmoplegia, pigmentary degeneration of the retina with abnormal ERG.	Cardiomyopathy, conduction defects, heart block, weakness of facial and laryngeal muscles, weakness of trunk and extremity musculature, deafness, small stature, EEG changes, and high CSF protein.	a.d.
Keratosis Palmoplantaris with Corneal Lesions (Richner-Hanhart)	Herpetiform lesions of the cornea and photophobia.	Painful, punctate keratoses of palms and soles, mental retardation, and hypotrichosis.	a.r.
Klippel-Feil Syndrome	Congenital strabismus. Bilateral Duane's retraction syndrome.	Congenital fusion of cervical vertebrae (esp. synostosis of atlas and axis). Short neck, immobile, often torticollis; spastic paraplegia, deafness, and mental deficiency. May be associated with platybasia.	a.r. a.d. irreg. Genetic heterogeneity
Laurence-Moon-Biedl Syndrome	Retinitis pigmentosa, optic atrophy, strabismus.	Obesity, polydactyly, hypogenitalism, mental retardation.	a.r.
Leber's Congenital Amaurosis	Blindness with normal fundi. May develop retinitis pigmentosa appearance later.	Mental retardation, epilepsy or neurologic disorders, rarely.	a.r. Probably more than a single genetic entity
Leber's Hereditary Optic Atrophy	Central scotoma, bilateral, not concurrent with eventual disc pallor (esp. papillomacular bundle).	Rarely, neurologic disturbances.	X-r., a.r. Genetic heterogeneity
Lenz's syndrome	Colobomatous microphthalmos, blepharoptosis, nystagmus, esotropia.	Microcephaly, short stature, mental retardation, dental diastema.	X-r.

TABLE 2–1   OCULAR CHANGES IN PEDIATRIC SYNDROMES (*Continued*)

Disease	Ocular Manifestations	Systemic Manifestations	Inheritance
Lipoid Proteinosis (Urbach-Wiethe)	Yellowish-white beadlike lesions on eyelid margins.	Hoarseness; yellow, confluent small papules on lips, tongue, extensor surface of elbows, and knees; intracranial calcification. Lesions PAS positive.	a.r.
Lowe's Syndrome (Oculocerebrorenal)	Congenital cataracts and glaucoma.	Aminoaciduria, renal rickets, retarded psychomotor development, muscular hypotonia, and mental retardation. Carrier state in female noted by diffuse, punctate lens changes.	X-r.
Macular Dystrophy (See Table 2–2)			
Mannosidosis	Small cloudy opacities beneath anterior lens capsule, optic discs pale with blurred margins.	Psychomotor retardation, gargoyle-like facies, cachexia, elevated sweat chlorides, susceptibility to infection, early death, α-mannosidase deficiency.	a.r.
Marfan's Syndrome	Dislocated lens, spherophakia, nystagmus, exotropia, myopia, retinal detachment.	Arachnodactyly, poor musculature, loose jointedness, pectus excavatum, kyphoscoliosis, cardiovascular defects.	a.d.
Marinesco-Sjögren Syndrome	Bilateral congenital cataract. Horizontal or rotary nystagmus, aniridia.	Oligophrenia and spinocerebellar ataxia. Similar to Sjögren's syndrome.	a.r.
Meckel's Syndrome	Microphthalmos, anophthalmos, cataract, partial aniridia, sclerocornea, cryptophthalmos, retinal dysplasia, and hypoplasia of the optic disc.	Occipital encephalocele, polycystic kidneys, polydactyly, congenital heart disease, abnormal genitalia, normal chromosomes.	a.r.
Menkes' Syndrome (Kinky Hair Disease)	Partial optic atrophy. Microcysta in pigment epithelium of iris	Cerebellar and focal cerebral degeneration. Failure to thrive. Kinky hair.	
Microphthalmos, Corneal Dystrophy, Mental Retardation, and Spasticity	Microphthalmos, corneal dystrophy (lattice), and pupillary changes.	Mental retardation, spasticity, and seizures.	a.d.?
Mieten's Syndrome	Corneal opacities, nystagmus, and strabismus.	Mental dullness, small stature, narrow nose with alae nasi, hypoplasia, short forearms, dislocation of proximal radius with flexion contracture of elbow.	a.r.
Moebius Syndrome	Bilateral, unequal involvement of 6th and 7th nerves, with frequent contracture of medial recti.	Deafness, syndactyly, polydactyly, absence of fingers or hand, and muscular weakness of tongue, neck, and chest. Mental retardation.	a.d. Variable expressivity
Mucopolysaccharidoses 1. Hurler's Syndrome (Gargoylism) MPS I H	Corneal clouding, ptosis, strabismus, thickened eyelids, glaucoma. Pigmentary degeration of retina occurs.	Large head, coarse features, short neck, protuberant abdomen, kyphosis, large tongue, stubby fingers, mental retardation. Hepatosplenomegaly. α-L-iduronidase deficiency. Excess urinary MPS.	a.r.
Scheie's Syndrome MPS I S	Corneal clouding but central central area less severely affected.	Dwarfism with large head, hands, broad abdomen protruding, deafness, (? mental retardation), stiff joints, similar appearance to Hurler's. May be allelic to Hurler's.	a.r.

TABLE 2–1 OCULAR CHANGES IN PEDIATRIC SYNDROMES (*Continued*)

Disease	Ocular Manifestations	Systemic Manifestations	Inheritance
2. Hunter's Syndrome MPS II	Cornea usually clear but mild clouding may be seen on slit lamp exam. Pigmentary degeneration of retina often seen.	Similar to Hurler's. Two forms, mild or severe physical and mental changes. Sulfoiduronate sulfatase deficiency.	X-r.
3. Sanfilippo's Syndrome MPS III	No specific eye change.	Mental retardation severe. Gargoyle features minimal. Type A—Heparitin sulfatase deficiency. Type B—N-acetyl-D glucosaminadase deficiency.	a.r.
4. Morquio's Disease MPS IV	Corneal clouding may occur but cornea usually grossly clear. Retinal pigmentary changes may be observed.	Osseous dystrophy of entire skeleton except head, thinning of vertebrae. N-acetylhexosamine sulfatase deficiency.	a.r.
5. MPS V (no syndrome assigned)			
6. Maroteaux-Lamy Syndrome MPS VI	Corneal clouding begins in early life.	Similar to MPS I but less marked. Mentality normal. Aryl sulfatase B deficiency suggested.	a.r.
7. β-glucuronidase Deficiency	Corneal clouding.	Similar to Hurler's. Ascites. β-glucuronidase deficiency.	a.r.
Muscular Dystrophy with External Ophthalmoplegia	Bilateral ptosis and extraocular muscle paresis progressing to immobility.	Progressive involvement of other muscle group including facial muscles, muscles of mastication, and muscles of neck, shoulder, and girdle. No response to Tensilon or Prostigmin.	a.d.
Myotonia Congenita (Thomsen's Disease)	Sudden closure of eyelids re-results in inability to open lids for several seconds. Esotropia rare.	Myotonia with inability to voluntarily relax contracted muscles. Muscular hypertrophy of arms, legs, and trunk and muscle weakness.	a.d.
Myotonic Dystrophy (Steinert's Disease)	Bilateral cataracts beginning as subcapsular opacities, pro-progressing to total opacities; ptosis and pigmentary retinopathy.	Myotonia, muscular wasting, mental deficiency, cardiac changes, and hypogonadism.	a.d. Variable expressivity
Nail-Patella Syndrome (Hereditary Osteo-onychodysplasia)	Dark, "clover-leaf" pigmentation of iris, cataract, ptosis, keratoconus, microcornea, and microphakia.	Hypoplasia and splitting of nails (esp. thumbnail), hypoplasia or absence of patella, spur in midposterior ileum, hypoplasia of scapula, and proteinuria, renal insufficiency.	a.d.
Niemann-Pick Disease		Usually among Jews, failure to thrive, rapid, progressive neuro-logic deterioration, blindness,	
1. Acute Neuronopathic "Crocker"	Macular cherry-red spot	hepatosplenomegaly, foam cells in bone marrow. Sphingomyelinase deficiency.	a.r.
2. Chronic Visceral without Nervous System Involvement	None	Hepatomegaly, pulmonary infiltration. Less severe deficiency of sphingomyelinase.	a.r.
3. Subacute or Juvenile	Macular cherry-red spot	As in 1, but more prolonged course, seizures. Sphingomyelinase activity normal or near normal.	a.r.
4. Nova Scotian	Undetermined	Neonatal jaundice, hepatosplenomegaly, ataxia, athetosis, seizures. Enzyme activity normal. Further genetic heterogeneity undoubtedly exists.	a.r.

TABLE 2–1   OCULAR CHANGES IN PEDIATRIC SYNDROMES (*Continued*)

Disease	Ocular Manifestations	Systemic Manifestations	Inheritance
Norrie's Disease	Blindness shortly after birth. PHPV, corneal opacity, cataract, phthisis bulbi, congenital retinal pseudoglioma.	Mental retardation, deafness, CNS degenerative changes.	X-r.
Oculocerebral Syndrome with Hypopigmentation	Microcornea, myopia, optic atrophy, cloudy vascularized corneas, and nystagmus.	Hypopigmentation, spasticity, athetosis, and mental retardation.	a.r.
Oculodentodigital Dysplasia (Meyer-Schwickerath)	Microphthalmos, microcornea, congenital glaucoma, and iris anomalies.	Typical facies presenting thin nose, hypoplastic alae, narrow nostrils, syndactyly, camptodactyly of 4th and 5th digits, enamel hypoplasia.	a.d.
Osteogenesis Imperfecta (van der Hoeve's Syndrome)	Blue sclera, anterior segment defects, and keratoconus. Cataract and ectopia lentis are rare.	Bones fracture easily, deafness 60%, dental defects, hyperflexibility of ligaments, skull anomalies, and scoliosis.	a.d. a.r.? Genetic heterogeneity
Osteopetrosis, Infantile form Mild form	Pigmentary degeneration of the retina, optic atrophy.	Generalized increase in bone density, large head, frequent fractures, anemia, and cranial nerve palsies.	a.r. a.d.
Oxycephaly	Exophthalmos, zonular cataracts, nystagmus, and optic atrophy.	Tower skull, convulsions, mental retardation, polydactyly, syndactyly, and deafness.	a.d.
Pachyonychia Congenita	Corneal thickening and cataracts.	Progressive thickening of anterior half of nail. Patchy to complete hyperkeratosis of palms and soles. Leukokeratosis of mouth and tongue. Teeth erupted at birth lost by 6 months.	a.d.
Peter's Syndrome	Central corneal leukoma, central defect of Descemet's membrane, and a shallow anterior synechia with peripheral anterior synechia. Cataract.	Skeletal anomalies and developmental defects of the gastrointestinal tract and central nervous system. Hydrocephalus and mental retardation.	a.r.
Pierre Robin Syndrome	Congenital glaucoma, retinal detachment, esotropia.	Micrognathia, cleft palate, glossoptosis.	No known genetic etiology: rarely X-r.
Porphyria, Acute Intermittent	Optic neuritis, bilateral ptosis, partial third nerve paralysis, and visual disturbances, retinal artery spasm.	Abdominal pain, mental depression, confusion, polyneuritis, transient hypertension, and seizures may be precipitated by drugs. Urine turns to burgundy red color on standing owing to increased porphobilinogen excretion.	a.d.
Prader-Willi Syndrome	Strabismus.	Small, obese stature, mental deficiency, hypotonus, small hands and feet, small penis and cryptorchism. Dental caries and diabetes mellitus of abnormal glucose tolerance response.	No known genetic etiology
Pseudoxanthoma Elasticum	Angioid streaks, hemorrhage in macula.	Thick, grooved, lax, yellowish skin involving neck, axillae, and orbital areas. Arterial medial thickening with secondary vascular insufficiency.	a.r.

TABLE 2-1   OCULAR CHANGES IN PEDIATRIC SYNDROMES (*Continued*)

Disease	Ocular Manifestations	Systemic Manifestations	Inheritance
Radial Aplasia— Thrombocytopenia (Absent Radius Syndrome)	Strabismus.	Thrombocytopenia, eosinophilia in 53%, absence or hypoplasia of radius, congenital heart defect in 25%.	a.r.
Refsum's Syndrome (Heredopathia Atactica Polyneuritiformis)	Atypical pigmentary retinal degeneration, night blindness, and diminished vision. Cataracts.	Polyneuropathy, ataxia, baldness, deafness, ichthyosis, muscular weakness, and increased spinal fluid protein. Defect in phytanic acid alpha-hydroxylase.	a.r.
Renal-Retinal Dystrophy	Progressive pigmentary retinal dystrophy leading to blindness, night blindness, attenuation of retinal vessels, optic atrophy, absence of ERG.	Interstitial nephritis.	a.r.
Retinitis Pigmentosa	Night blindness, narrowed arterioles, bone corpuscle-shaped pigment deposits, optic atrophy, ring scotoma.	Deafness, mutism, mental retardation, high arched palate.	a.d. X-r. a.r.
Retinitis Punctate Albescens	Related to retinitis pigmentosa. Numerous small yellow dots scattered over retina. May also contain pigment.	Deaf-mutism described.	a.r. X-r.
Rieger's Syndrome	Hypoplasia of anterior stromal leaf of iris with iridotrabecular adhesions inserted in corneal periphery. Microcornea, corneal opacity, and pupillary anomalies occur. Glaucoma is common.	Hypodontia, myotonic dystrophy, and mental deficiency. Hypertelorism 25%.	a.d. Variable expressivity
Rothmund's Syndrome (Poikiloderma Atrophicans Vasculare)	Bilateral cataracts developing in 3rd to 5th year. Corneal dystrophy	Telangiectases and hypogenitalism. Vascular skin lesions characterized by tightly stretched skin with patches of hypo- and hyperpigmentation.	a.r.
Rubinstein-Taybi Syndrome (Broad Thumb and Toe Syndrome)	Epicanthus, strabismus, refractive error, cataract, coloboma, ptosis, long eyelashes, and hypertrichosis.	Short stature, mental retardation, cryptorchism, fingers and toes broad (esp. the great toe), and low-set ears. Vertebral, cardiac, and renal anomalies may occur.	No known genetic etiology
Schwartz's Syndrome	Blepharophimosis, myopia, long eyelashes in irregular rows, microcornea.	Small stature, myotonia with sad, expressionless facies, joint limitation in hips; dystrophy of epiphyseal cartilage, wrist, fingers, toes, and spine. Vertical shortness of vertebrae, short neck, and low hairline.	a.r.
Sickle Cell Disease— Hemoglobin S	Venous tortuosity, arteriolar and venous occlusion, chorioretinal scars, comma-shaped conjunctival capillaries.	Normochromic anemia, joint, bone and abdominal pain during crises, death from intercurrent infection.	a.r.
Sickle cell Disease— Hemoglobin C	Arteriovenous abnormality extending into vitreous (sea fan), vascular occlusion, and chorioretinal scars.	Systemic symptoms milder but CNS signs may be present.	a.r.

TABLE 2–1   OCULAR CHANGES IN PEDIATRIC SYNDROMES (*Continued*)

Disease	Ocular Manifestations	Systemic Manifestations	Inheritance
Siemen's Syndrome	Congenital cataracts.	Hypoplasia, atrophy of skin.	a.r.
Sjögren-Larsson Syndrome	Pigmentary retinal degeneration (30%).	Icthyosis, spasticity, short stature, mental retardation, speech defects, short fingers and toes.	a.r.
Sjögren's Syndrome	Bilateral congenital cataracts, nystagmus, microphthalmos, and detached retina.	Oligophrenia.	?
Smith-Lemli-Opitz Syndrome	Bilateral ptosis, epicanthus, strabismus.	Mental deficiency, microcephaly, anteverted nostrils, syndactyly of 2nd and 3rd toes, hypospadias and cryptorchism in male.	a.r.
Spondyloepiphyseal Dysplasia, Congenital	Myopia, retinal detachment, cataracts, buphthalmos.	Short trunk and limbs, deformity of sternum, normal hands and feet, skeletal abnormalities of vertebral column and hips, absent femoral head. Deafness.	a.d.
Stickler's Syndrome (Progressive Arthro-Ophthalmyopathy)	Progressive myopia, retinal detachment, secondary glaucoma.	Pain and stiffness of joints with bony enlargement. Deafness and kyphosis.	a.d.
Sulfite Oxidase Deficiency	Bilateral dislocated lenses.	Severe neurologic impairment, mental retardation, and death in infancy. Deficiency of sulfite oxidase.	a.r.
Tangier Disease	Fine, dotted, stromal opacities in cornea.	Hepatosplenomegaly, peripheral neuropathy, dissociated loss of pain and temperature, and muscular wasting. Absence of alpha-lipoprotein.	a.r.
Turner's Phenotype (Pseudo-Turner's Syndrome)	Cataract and ptosis. Varying sexual development, normal chromosomes, and genetic heterogeneity. Occurs in both males and females.	Webbed neck, low-set ears, and typical facies. Pulmonary stenosis most common cardiac lesion.	a.d.
Unverricht-Lafora Disease (Progressive Familial Myoclonic Epilepsy)	Visual loss. Lafora bodies (inclusion bodies) reported in retina.	Seizures followed by myoclonic jerks. Mental retardation, dementia, ataxia, and death. Lafora bodies in brain, spinal nerves, liver, muscle.	a.r.
Usher's Syndrome	Retinitis pigmentosa, cataracts.	Nerve deafness, mental retardation, psychosis, and epilepsy.	a.r.
Von Gierke's Disease	Retinal changes consisting of discrete, nonelevated, round yellow flecks in macular area. No visual impairment.	Glycogen storage disease Type I characterized by absence of glucose-6-phosphatase. Short stature, hepatosplenomegaly, hypoglycemia, lactic acidosis, and hyperlipemia.	a.r.
Waardenburg's Syndrome	Lateral displacement of lower puncta and inner canthus, blepharophimosis, heterochromia, and hyperplasia of eyebrows medially.	Deafness, white forelock, and a broad nasal root.	a.d. Varying expressivity

TABLE 2–1 OCULAR CHANGES IN PEDIATRIC SYNDROMES (*Continued*)

Disease	Ocular Manifestations	Systemic Manifestations	Inheritance
Weil-Marchesani's Syndrome	Spherophakia, ectopic lens, myopia, possible glaucoma.	Short stature, brachycephaly, stubby fingers and toes, teeth malformed, and diminishing joint flexibility.	a.r.
Wildervanck's Syndrome (Cervico-oculo-acoustic)	Bilateral Duane's syndrome.	Congenital ipsilateral aplasia of auditory and facial nerve. Associated with Klippel-Feil syndrome.	X-d.? Lethal in male
Wilson's Disease (Hepatolenticular Degeneration)	Kayser-Fleischer ring, sunflower cataract.	Degeneration of lenticular nucleus and basal ganglia, cirrhosis of the liver, and jaundice. Malabsorption syndrome. Proximal tubular damage and renal aminoaciduria. Ceruloplasmin deficiency; copper accumulation in liver, brain, kidney, and cornea.	a.r.
Xeroderma Pigmentosa	Eyelids exposed to direct sunlight develop large freckles, followed by telangiectases and atrophic areas which become warty and undergo malignant degeneration. Photophobia and conjunctivitis.	Skin of face exposed to direct sunlight undergoes similar change. Tumors may be sarcomas, squamous cell or basal cell carcinomas. Death occurs during adolescence. Deficiency of DNA repair enzyme in some cases.	a.r.

The assistance of Mildred L. Kistenmacher, M.D., in the preparation of this table is gratefully acknowledged.
Key:
a.r. = autosomal recessive
a.d. = autosomal dominant
X-r. = X-linked recessive
X-d. = X-linked dominant

TABLE 2–2 OCULAR ABNORMALITIES AND CHARACTERISTICS

Hereditary and Developmental Ocular Abnormalities	Ocular Characteristics	Inheritance
A. *Complete Eyeball*		
1. Cyclopia	Associated with severe cranial and systemic abnormalities such as found in trisomy 13 and 18 and other chromosomal disorders.	a.r. or a variety of chromosomal abnormalities
2. Anophthalmos	Total anophthalmos rare. Small globe often found in deep socket. Usually associated multiple abnormalities such as trisomy 13. Can be drug-induced with thalidomide.	a.d., varying expressivity
3. Congenital Cystic Eyeball	Arrest in development of optic vesicle.	Not known
4. Microphthalmos	May be associated with ocular abnormalities, such as corneal opacities, cataract, microphakia, spherophakia, and hyperopia, and also systemic abnormalities, such as maternal rubella, toxoplasmosis, and many syndromes. Usually unilateral. Seen in trisomy 13.	a.d. or a.r., X-r.
5. Microphthalmos with Coloboma	May involve iris, choroid, or optic nerve; often associated with other systemic defects including trisomy 13.	a.d.
6. Microphthalmos with Cyst	Cyst extends inferiorly through fetal fissure consisting of abnormal sclera and retina. Differentiate from meningocele.	?
7. Coloboma	Represents closure failure of fetal fissure which may involve iris, ciliary body, choroid, retina, or optic nerve. Multiple structures may be involved, and associated findings include decreased visual acuity, strabismus, and nystagmus. Coloboma of the disc exists as an isolated finding in which the entire disc area is markedly enlarged with vessels appearing only at the margins. The colobomatous defect may involve just the inferior aspect of the disc and visual acuity is often severely reduced.	a.d., varying expressivity

TABLE 2–2   OCULAR ABNORMALITIES AND CHARACTERISTICS (*Continued*)

Hereditary and Developmental Ocular Abnormalities	Ocular Characteristics	Inheritance
8. Cryptophthalmos	A congenital abnormality in which skin of the forehead covers the eyeballs completely. It occurs unilaterally or bilaterally and may be associated with multiple anomalies including syndactyly, dental and urogenital abnormalities, and cleft palate.	a.r.?
9. Buphthalmos (Congenital Glaucoma)	Congenital infantile glaucoma characterized by epiphoria, photophobia, cloudy corneas, enlarged corneas, ruptures in Descemet's membrane, elevated tension, and glaucomatous cupping. Typical signs are present in 80 to 90 per cent during first year (see Chapter 16).	a.r.
10. Ocular Albinism	Marked deficiency in iris and choroid. Nystagmus and myopic astigmatism. Hypoplasia of macula. Female carrier frequently shows iris translucence. See systemic manifestations in Table 2–1.	X-r.
11. Congenital Melanosis	Spotted pigmentation of conjunctiva and sclera which may also involve lids, parts of face, and fundi.	a.d. a.r.
B. *Lid and Lacrimal Apparatus Abnormalities*		
1. Alacrima	Rare absence of tear secretion associated with corneal irritative symptoms. Also seen in Riley-Day syndrome.	a.r. or a.d.
2. Congenital Atresia of Nasolacrimal Duct	Common cause of tearing in infants. Rule out congenital glaucoma.	
3. Congenital Absence of Lacrimal Puncta	Unilateral most common.	a.d.
4. Lateral Displacement of Lower Lacrimal Puncta	See Waardenburg's Syndrome in Table 2–1.	a.d.
5. Coloboma of the Lid	Colobomas of the upper lid occur at junction of inner and middle third of lid. In the lower lid they occur chiefly toward outer third. Corneal opacities, microphthalmos, and iris and pupillary defects may be associated. Corneal dermoid and lid colobomas occur in Goldenhar's Syndrome.	?
6. Epicanthus	May be associated with ptosis. Common in Down's syndrome.	a.d.
7. Congenital Entropion and Ectropion	Entropion is more common in lower lid, while ectropion is more common in upper lids. Ectropion may occur secondary to skin disorder involving lids.	a.d.
8. Blepharochalasis	May occur congenitally from weak orbital septum and fat protrusion in upper lids.	a.d.
9. Ankyloblepharon	Inadequate separation of lid margins especially temporally.	a.d.
10. Epiblepharon	Horizontal fold of skin parallel to margin in upper but especially lower lid.	a.d.
11. Blepharoptosis	Commonly unilateral but may be bilateral. May have associated superior rectus paresis and strabismus. Must consider myasthenia gravis.	
12. Marcus Gunn Jaw-Winking Phenomenon	Elevation of lid with open mouth or with lateral jaw movement. Usually associated with ptosis.	a.d.
13. Distichiasis	Abnormal second row of lashes. May be associated with chronic lymphedema of lower extremities (Falls-Kertesz syndrome).	a.d.
C. *Corneal Abnormalities*		
1. Microcornea	Frequently associated with other defects including colobomas, cataract, nystagmus, glaucoma, strabismus, and other anterior segment changes.	a.d.
2. Megalocornea	Cornea diameter 12 to 15 mm. without glaucoma. May be observed in Marfan's syndrome.	X-r. rarely a.r. or a.d.
3. Keratoconus	A corneal ectasia commencing about age 10 with irregular astigmatism and irregular central shadow. It is usually bilateral, more common in females, and occurs with Down's syndrome.	a.d. or a.r.

TABLE 2-2 OCULAR ABNORMALITIES AND CHARACTERISTICS *(Continued)*

Hereditary and Developmental Ocular Abnormalities	Ocular Characteristics	Inheritance
4. Cornea Plana	Characterized by a flattened cornea, shallow anterior chamber, and a stromal opacity.	a.d. or a.r.
5. Corneal Dystrophies		
a. Granular Dystrophy (Groenouw Type I)	Granular opacities lying beneath Bowman's membrane in the axial region of cornea. Progressive visual loss. Onset during first decade.	a.d.
b. Macular Dystrophy (Groenouw Type II)	Fine diffuse clouding of superficial layers of central cornea. Significant visual loss by age 40. Onset during first decade.	a.r.
c. Lattice Dystrophy (Haab-Dimmer)	Characterized by presence of lines situated in anterior layers of central corneal stroma with periphery clear. Recurrent pain from epithelial erosions. Central corneal sensation decreased. Onset during first decade.	a.d.
d. Epithelial Dystrophy of Meesmann	Myriad punctate epithelial opacities, especially in area of palpebral fissure. Repeated attacks of corneal inflammation may lead to scarring. Visual loss rarely marked. Appears during infancy.	a.d.
6. Anterior Embryotoxon (Arcus Juvenilis)	A white circular ring parallel but separate from limbus by small margin of clear cornea. Appears during early life and may be observed with aniridia, blue sclera or megalocornea.	a.r.
7. Posterior Embryotoxon (Axenfeld's Syndrome)	A white, glassy ring localized peripherally in Descemet's membrane near the limbus is characteristic of the anterior displacement of Schwalbe's line — processes extend from the iris collarette to this ring across the anterior chamber angle. Often associated with glaucoma.	a.d./or a.r.
8. Mesodermal Dysgenesis of Rieger	See Table 2-1.	
D. *Hereditary Disorders of the Iris*		
1. Coloboma	Usually situated in inferior iris and may be associated with choroidal coloboma. Occurs unilaterally and bilaterally.	a.d.
2. Anisocoria	Rule out neurologic disorders.	a.d.
3. Congenital Miosis	Can occur in Horner's syndrome or as congenital absence of dilator pupillae fibers. May be associated with spasm of accommodation.	a.d.
4. Polycoria	In true polycoria, each pupil is surrounded by a sphincter. Isolated holes occur in iris without sphincter in iris dysplasia.	a.d.
5. Corectopia	Eccentric position of pupil.	a.d.
6. Persistent Pupillary Membrane	May be associated with anterior polar cataract. Has been reported associated with macrocornea and congenital cataracts.	a.d.
7. Aniridia (Irideremia)	Complete absence of iris does not occur. Often associated with cataracts, macular aplasia, nystagmus, strabismus, ectopia lentis, and diminished vision. (Occurs with Wilms' tumor, one in every 73 cases. Usually sporadic but aniridia on familial basis has been reported associated with Wilms' tumor.)	a.d.
8. Adie's Syndrome (Tonic Pupil)	Marked limitation in pupillary response to light and accommodation. Unilateral in 85 per cent. Frequent absence of knee or ankle jerks or both. Sensitive to Mecholyl, 2.5 per cent, causing intense miosis.	a.d.
9. Congenital Aplasia of the Iris	Mesodermal aplasia usually limited to one sector.	a.d.
10. Iris Heterochromia	May be hypo- or hyperpigmentation. May be unilateral or bilateral and can be associated with Marfan's or Sturge-Weber syndromes, Waardenburg's syndrome, and rubella embryopathy.	a.d.

TABLE 2–2 OCULAR ABNORMALITIES AND CHARACTERISTICS (*Continued*)

Hereditary and Developmental Ocular Abnormalities	Ocular Characteristics	Inheritance
E. *Hereditary Disorders of the Lens*		
1. Microphakia (Spherophakia)	May be associated with subluxation of the lens and secondary glaucoma.	a.r.
2. Coloboma of lens	Lens colobomas are situated inferonasally and occur alone or in conjunction with coloboma of the ciliary body. The lens border appears flat or notched, often with an absence of zonular fibers in the colobomatous area.	a.d. irreg.
3. Lenticonus	Characterized by a congenital conical protrusion of the anterior or posterior surface. May be associated with microphthalmos and iris abnormalities including pupillary membrane, iris coloboma, and iris angle changes.	a.d. or a.r.
4. Congenital Cataracts	See Chapter 15.	a.d., a.r., or X-r.
5. Ectopia Lentis (Dislocated Lens)	May occur as isolated finding but usually associated with syndromes:	
	Marfan's	a.d.
	Weil-Marchesani	a.r.
	Homocystinuria	a.r.
	Hyperlysinemia	a.r.
	Osteogenesis Imperfecta	a.d.
	Ehlers-Danlos syndrome	a.r.
	Sulfite oxidase deficiency	a.r.
F. *Disorders of the Vitreous and Hyaloid System*		
1. Mittendorf Dot	Remnant of hyaloid system attached to posterior lens capsule.	?
2. Persistent Hyaloid Artery	Persistent strand or vessel from posterior capsule to lens to optic disc. Bergmeister's papilla consists of absorbing hyaloid system anterior to the disc.	
3. Persistent Hyperplastic Primary Vitreous	Failure of hyaloid system regression. Unilateral in 90 per cent.	?
G. *Hereditary Functional Disorders of Retina and Choroid*		
1. Congenital Stationary Night Blindness (Essential Nyctalopia)	Occurs without ophthalmoscopic lesions. Myopia found in sex-linked recessive form. Amblyopia common. ERG response varies from mild reduction to complete absence of scotopic ERG. Photopic response usually normal.	a.d., a.r., or X-r.
2. Oguchi's Disease	Grayish-white metallic appearance of retina in light which regains normal appearance in the dark (Mizuo's phenomenon). A rare type of night blindness exhibiting slow dark adaptation. See Chapter 14.	a.r.
3. Day Blindness	Rare disorder in which vision is improved in dim illumination. Congenital day blindness may be accompanied by color blindness, amblyopia, and mental retardation.	a.r.
4. Color Blindness	Two types (Achromatopsia and Dyschromatopsia)	
a. Congenital Color Vision Dysfunction Syndrome or Achromatopsia	1. Cone—Monochromatism: rare; visual function good 2. Rod—Monochromatism: bilateral amblyopia (varying degree), nystagmus, photophobia, and total absence of color discrimination. Night vision is normal and high refractive errors are common. Cone ERG is absent. Failure with Sloan achromatopsia test. Complete achromatopsia is most common form but incomplete achromatopsia exists.	a.r.
b. Dyschromatopsia or Incomplete Color Blindness	Protonopic types confuse reds and greens and are insensitive to red light. Deuteranopic types confuse reds and greens but are sensitive to red light. Failure with pseudoisochromatic plates, Ishihara and Atlas of Hardy, Rand, and Rittler (H-R-R). Incomplete color blindness occurs	X-r.

TABLE 2–2 OCULAR ABNORMALITIES AND CHARACTERISTICS (*Continued*)

Hereditary and Developmental Ocular Abnormalities	Ocular Characteristics	Inheritance
	in about 8 per cent of males and less than 1 per cent of females. Men carrying one gene are affected since they are hemizygotes for the X chromosomes. Women carrying one pathologic gene are phenotypically normal and are not color blind. Women with two pathologic genes may exhibit the defect. Tritanopic types do not confuse reds and greens but are insensitive to blue and yellow.	a.d.
H. *Abnormalities of the Retina and Choroid*		
1. Hereditary Detachment of the Retina	May be associated with cystic degeneration and retinoschisis. Slow development with ultimate visual loss.	a.r.
2. Juvenile Retinoschisis	Progressive, degenerative retinal disorder which is usually bilateral. Frequently found inferior temporally, with cystic changes producing effect of retinal splitting. Massive vitreous bleeding occurs.	X-r.
3. Congenital Falciform Fold of the Retina	Folds may extend from disc to periphery, principally inferior temporal quadrant. Resembles retrolental fibroplasia.	a.r.
4. Retinal Dysplasia	Often associated with trisomy 13 in which dysplastic retina contains cartilage.	X-r.
5. Heredodegenerative	A large group of retinal disorders including typical and atypical pigmentary degeneration of the retina, occurring with systemic manifestations or alone, of varying genetic patterns. Macular degenerations may be classed in this group but will be considered separately. See chapter on Retina and Table 2–1.	a.r., a.d., or X-r.
a. Retinitis Pigmentosa Primary Pigmentary Degeneration)	Bilateral "bone corpuscular type" pigmentary accumulations usually noted in early childhood. Night blindness often first symptom, followed by visual field loss and progressive extinction of vision. ERG absent.	a.r. or a.d.
b. Retinitis Sine Pigmento	Retinal vessel narrowing and optic disc pallor. Similar to r.p. disorder without prominent pigmentary changes.	a.r.
c. Retinitis Punctata Albescens	Similar to r.p. except for numerous scattered white dots throughout retina.	a.r.
d. Fundus Albi Punctatus	Congenital night blindness with grayish-white mottling of the fundi. Vessels and optic disc normal. ERG normal.	a.r.
e. Retinoblastoma	Malignant neoplasm of the retina arising from the nuclear layer. Involvement is bilateral in 25 per cent of cases.	a.d.
f. Fundus Flavimaculatus (Flecked Retina)	Yellowish-white discrete lesions, particularly in posterior pole, especially peripheral, appearing in second decade. Macula may be involved. Gradual visual loss and abnormal ERG.	a.r.
g. Retinal Pigmentary Degeneration and Systemic Disorders	Typical and atypical retinal pigmentary changes have been recorded with Bassen-Kornzweig syndrome, cystinosis, Friedreich's ataxia, Hurler's disease, Leber's congenital amaurosis, Laurence-Moon-Biedl syndrome, myotonic dystrophy, Refsum's disease, Usher's syndrome, Cockayne's syndrome, and Pelizaeus-Merzbacher disease. Pigmentary retinopathy has also been observed in association with mental retardation, cataracts, myopia, nystagmus, deafness, and mutism.	
h. Choroideremia	Deficiency in color discrimination with pigmentary changes developing through the unmasking of choroidal vessels to final disappearance of the choroid. May represent an atypical r.p. Night blindness, visual field loss, progressive visual loss often to fifth decade, and absent ERG.	X-r.
i. Gyrate Atrophy of Choroid	Possibly atypical r.p. as above. Night blindness, with progressive loss of visual fields. Pigmentary changes with pale fundi, but retina appears normal about macula and disc.	a.d., a.r.
j. Choroidal Sclerosis	Scattered pigment clumps amidst prominent pale yellow choroidal vessels. Field defects with central vision loss.	a.r. or a.d.

TABLE 2–2 OCULAR ABNORMALITIES AND CHARACTERISTICS (*Continued*)

Hereditary and Developmental Ocular Abnormalities	Ocular Characteristics	Inheritance
I. *Macular Degenerations*		
1. Vitelliform Degeneration (Best's Disease)	Well-defined, round yolklike lesion in the macula with good vision is first sign. Pigmentary changes and visual loss follow. Usually affects children up to age 7.	a.d.
2. Juvenile Dystrophy (Stargardt's Disease)	Rapid loss of central vision followed by gradual fine pigmentary changes. Occurs between ages 8 and 18, with late development of peripheral lesions.	a.r. or a.d.
3. Late Form of Macular Degeneration	Senile type of macular degeneration include Kuhnt-Junius degeneration and macular degeneration of Haab. Dayne's honeycomb choroiditis and Tay's choroiditis represent the adult form.	a.r. or a.d.
J. *Disorders of the Optic Nerve*		
1. Myelinated Nerve Fibers	Usually unilateral. May be associated with myopia, coloboma oxycephaly, or neurofibromatosis.	a.d.?
2. Congenital Optic Atrophy	Marked visual loss and nystagmus. ERG normal.	a.r. or a.d.
3. Aplasia or Hypoplasia of Optic Nerve	Aplasia associated with gross malformations of globe (microphthalmos or cyclopia). Hypoplasia associated with marked visual loss or complete absence occurs as an isolated finding or with microphthalmos.	?
4. Coloboma of Nerve	Associated with diminished vision.	?
5. Congenital Crescents or Conus	Myopic crescent common at temporal margin. Arcuate scotomas associated with inferior crescents.	
6. Situs Inversus	Reversed vascular pattern in fundi.	
K. *Disorders of the Ocular Muscles*		
1. Congenital Ptosis	Usually unilateral. May be associated with superior rectus palsy.	a.d.
2. Duane's Syndrome	Usually unilateral and commonly involves left eye. Limitation of abduction and narrowing of palpebral fissure on adduction.	a.d.
3. Marcus Gunn Syndrome	Unilateral ptosis associated with lid elevation when mouth is opened. See also under Lid Disorders.	a.d.
4. Congenital Nystagmus	Often associated with other CNS defects. Rule out achromatopsia.	a.d. or a.r.
5. Congenital Esotropia	Marked alternating esotropia associated with insignificant refractive error with onset at birth or shortly thereafter.	a.d. irreg.
6. Accommodative Esotropia	Marked hyperopic refractive error. Onset at 2 or 3 years of age.	a.d. irreg.
7. Exotropia	May be intermittent or manifest.	irreg.
8. Tendon Sheath Disorder of Brown	Short anterior tendon sheath of superior oblique. Resembles inferior oblique paresis. Usually unilateral. Forced ductions indicated.	?
9. Progressive Muscular Dystrophy (Chronic Progressive External Ophthalmoplegia)	Onset in childhood with bilateral ptosis and progressive external ophthalmoplegia. Facial muscles often affected. Pigmentary degeneration of retina, cardiac abnormalities, and acanthocytosis may be present.	a.d.
10. Strabismus Fixus	Both eyes convergent. Difficulty to abduct eyes with forced ductions; medial recti replaced by fibrous bands.	?
11. Moebius' Syndrome	See Table 2–1.	
12. Ocular Motor Apraxia	Onset in infancy. Defective horizontal voluntary and attraction movements. Jerky overshooting head movements to fixate eyes in new position.	Varying expressivity
L. *Hereditary Refractive Error*		a.d.
1. High Hyperopia	Typical familial characteristics.	a.d. and a.r.
2. Myopia (High or Mild)	With or without strabismus and amblyopia.	
3. Astigmatism		a.d., a.r., or X-r.

Key:
a.r. = autosomal recessive
a.d. = autosomal dominant
X-r. = X-linked recessive

Literature Cited

Armaly, M. F.: Genetic determination of cup/disc ratio of the optic nerve. Arch. Ophthal., 78:35, 1967.

Bowen, P.: Two achondroplasts from normal parents. Reported at Fifth Conference on Clinical Delineation of Birth Defects, Baltimore, June 14, 1972.

Caspersson, T., Zech, L., and Johansson, C.: Differential binding of alkylating fluorochromes in human chromosomes. Exp. Cell Res., 60:315, 1970.

Decourt, L., Sasso, W. Da S., Chiorboli, E., and Fernandes, J. M.: Sobre o sexo genetico nas pacientes com sindrome de Turner. Rev. Assoc. Med. Brasil, 1:203, 1954.

de Grouchy, J., Royer, P., Salmon, C., and Lamy, M.: Deletion partielle des bras longs du chromosome 18. Path. Biol., 12:579, 1964.

Down, J. L. H.: Observations on an ethnic classification of idiots. Clin. Lect. Rep. Lond. Hosp., 3:259, 1866.

Edwards, J. H., Harnden, D. G., Cameron, A. H., Crosse, V. M., and Wolff, O. H.: A new trisomic syndrome. Lancet, 1:787, 1960.

Erickson, R. P.: Leber's optic atrophy, a possible example of maternal inheritance. Amer. J. Hum. Genet., 24:348, 1972.

Ford, E. D.: Polymorphism and taxonomy. In Huxley, J. S. (Ed.): The New Systematics. Oxford, Clarendon Press, 1940, p. 493.

Ford, C. E., Jones, K. W., Polani, P. E., deAlmeida, J. C., and Briggs, J. H.: A sex-chromosome anomaly in a case of gonadal dysgenesis (Turner's syndrome). Lancet, 1:711, 1959.

Ginsburg, J., Perrin, E. V., and Sueoka, W. T.: Ocular manifestations of trisomy 18. Amer. J. Ophthal., 66:59, 1968.

Green, W. R.: Personal communication, 1970.

Jacobs, P. A., and Strong, J. A.: A case of human intersexuality having a possible XXY sex determining mechanism. Nature, 183:302, 1959.

Klinefelter, H. F., Jr., Reifenstein, E. C., Jr., and Albright, F.: Syndrome characterized by gynecomastia, aspermatogenesis without A-Leydigism, and increased excretion of follicle-stimulating hormone. J. Clin. Endocr., 2:615, 1942.

Lejeune, J., Gautier, M., and Turpin, R.: Les chromosomes humains en cultur de tissues. C. R. Acad. Sci. (Paris), 248:602, 1959.

Lejeune, J., Lafourcade, J., Berger, R., Vilatte, J., Boeswillwald, M., Seringe, P., and Turpin, R.: Trois cas de deletion partielle du bras court d'un chromosome 5. C.R. Acad. Sci. (Paris), 257:3098, 1963.

Lyon, M. F.: Gene action in the X-chromosome of the mouse (Mus musculus L.) Nature (London), 190:372, 1961.

Myrianthopoulos, N. C., and Aronson, S. M.: Population dynamics of Tay-Sachs disease. II. What confers the selective advantage upon the Jewish heterozygote? Proceedings of fourth International Symposium on Sphingolipidoses, New York. Plenum Press, 1972. pp. 561–570.

Nance, W.: Anencephaly and spina bifida: a possible example of cytoplasmic inheritance in man. Nature (London), 224:373, 1969.

Patau, K., Smith, D. W., Therman, E., Inhorn, S. L., and Wagner, H. P.: Multiple congenital anomaly caused by an extra autosome. Lancet, 1:790, 1960.

Plunkett, E. R., and Barr, M. L.: Testicular dysgenesis affecting the seminiferous tubules principally, with chromatin-positive nuclei. Lancet, 2:853, 1956.

Polani, P. E., Hunter, W. F., and Lennox, B.: Chromosomal sex in Turner's syndrome with coarctation of the aorta. Lancet, 2:120, 1954.

Punnett, H. H., Kistenmacher, M. L., and ToroSola, M. A.: Diagnosis of trisomy 22 with quinacrine fluorescence. Pediat. Res., 5:654, 1971.

Reiss, J. A., Lovrien, E. W., and Hecht, F.: A mother with Down's syndrome and her chromosomally normal infant. Ann. Génét., 14:225, 1971.

Richter, S.: Zur Heredität des Strabismus concomitans. Humangenetik, 3:235, 1967.

Rodrigues, M. M., Punnett, H. H., Valdes-Dapena, M., and Martyn, L. J.: Retinal pigment epithelium in a case of 18 trisomy. Amer. J. Ophthal., 76:265, 1973.

Rodrigues, M. M., Valdes-Dapena, M., and Kistenmacher, M.: Ocular pathology in a case of 13 trisomy. J. Pediat. Ophthal., 10:54, 1973.

Schachenmann, G., Schmid, W., Fraccaro, M., Mannini, A., Tiepolo, L., Perona, G. P. and Sartori, E.: Chromosomes in coloboma and anal atresia. Lancet, 2:290, 1965.

Seabright, M.: A rapid banding technique for human chromosomes. Lancet, 2:971, 1971.

Tjio, J. H., and Levan, A.: The chromosome number of man. Hereditas, 42:1, 1956.

Trevor-Roper, P. D.: Marriage of two complete albinos with normally pigmented offspring. Brit. J. Ophthal., 36:107, 1952.

Turner, H. H.: A syndrome of infantilism, congenital webbed neck and cubitus valgus. Endocrinology, 23:566, 1938.

Wilkins, L., Grumbach, M. M., and vanWyk, J. J.: Chromosomal sex in "ovarian agenesis." J. Clin. Endocr., 14:1270, 1954.

Witkop, C. J., Nance, W. E., Rawls, R. F., and White, J. G.: Autosomal recessive oculocutaneous albinism in man: Evidence of genetic heterogeneity. Amer. J. Hum. Genet., 22:55, 1970.

Wolf, U., Reinwein, H., Porsch, R., Schroter, R., and Baitsch, H.: Defizienz an den kurzen Armen eines Chromosoms Nr. 4. Humangenetik, 1:397, 1965.

Yanoff, M., Rorke, L. B., and Niederer, B. S.: Ocular and cerebral abnormalities in chromosome 18 deletion defect. Amer. J. Ophthal., 70:391, 1970.

General References

Bergsma, D. (Ed.): Birth Defects, Atlas and Compendium. Baltimore, Williams and Wilkins, 1973.

Carter, C. O.: The inheritance of common congenital malformations. Progr. Med. Genet., 4:59, 1965.

Court Brown, W. M.: Males with an XYY sex chromosome complement. J. Med. Genet., 5:341, 1968.

Ford, C. E., and Clegg, H. M.: Reciprocal translocations. Brit. Med. Bull., 25:110, 1969.

Francois, J.: Genetic Aspects of Ophthalmology. Boston, Little, Brown and Co., 1968.

Goodman, G.: Clinical diagnosis of sex-linked ocular disorders. Symposium on Surgical and Medical Management of Congenital Anomalies of the Eye. Trans. New Orleans Acad. Ophthal. St. Louis, The C. V. Mosby Co., 1968.

Hamerton, J. L.: Human Cytogenetics. Vol. 1. General Human Cytogenetics, and Vol. 2. Clinical Cytogenetics. New York, Academic Press, 1970, 1971.

Holmes, L. B., Moser, H. W., Halldórsson, S., Mack, C., Pant, S. S., and Matzilevich, B.: Mental Retardation. An Atlas of Diseases with Associated Physical Abnormalities. New York, Macmillan Co., 1972.

Jacobs, P. A.: Structural abnormalities of the sex chromosomes. Brit. Med. Bull., 25:94, 1969.

Krill, A. E.: Hereditary Retinal and Choroidal Diseases. New York, Harper and Row, 1972.

Lejeune, J.: The 21 trisomy-current stage of chromosomal research. Progr. Med. Genet., 3:144, 1964.

McKusick, V. A.: Mendelian inheritance in man. 3rd ed. Baltimore, Johns Hopkins Press, 1972.

Punnett, H. H., and Mellman, W. J.: Familial chromosome translocations. In Gardner, L. (Ed.): Endocrine and Genetic Diseases of Childhood. Philadelphia, W. B. Saunders Co., 1969, pp. 668–681.

Roberts, J. A. F.: Multifactorial inheritance and human disease. Progr. Med. Genet., 3:178, 1964.

Roberts, J. A. F.: An Introduction to Medical Genetics. 5th ed. London, Oxford University Press, 1970.

Smith, D. W.: Recognizable Patterns of Human Malformation. Philadelphia, W. B. Saunders Co., 1970.

Stanbury, J. B., Wyngaarden, J. B., and Fredrickson, D. S.: The Metabolic Basis of Inherited Disease. 3rd ed. New York, McGraw-Hill Book Co., 1972.

Stern, C.: Principles of Human Genetics. 3rd ed. San Francisco, W. H. Freeman Co., 1973.

Strauss, B. S.: An Outline of Chemical Genetics. Philadelphia, W. B. Saunders Co., 1960.

Taylor, A. I.: Autosomal trisomy syndromes: A detailed study of 27 cases of Edward's syndrome and 27 cases of Patau's syndrome. J. Med. Genet., 5:227, 1968.

Thompson, J. A., and Thompson, M. W.: Genetics in Medicine. Philadelphia, W. B. Saunders Co., 1973.

Warkany, J.: Congenital Malformations. Chicago, Year Book Medical Publishers, 1971.

CHAPTER 3

OPHTHALMIC EXAMINATION OF INFANTS AND CHILDREN

EVERETT MOODY, M.D., and
GLEN GIBSON, M.D.

INTRODUCTION

Newcomers to the field of ophthalmology may be unaware of how rapidly our knowledge and abilities have changed in the very recent past in regard to the examination of very young patients. Twenty years ago this chapter might not have even been written and certainly would have been very different. The reasons are several. (1) It was taken for granted that most information was beyond our reach because adult tests did not work on children. (2) The importance of sensory maturation during the first years of life was underestimated. (3) Therapeutic measures applicable to infants were few, and therefore precise early examination was not so vital. Thus, elaborate examination of infants was thought to be not only impossible but unnecessary. Recounting a few specifics

will underscore the importance of mastering modern techniques.

Very few ophthalmologists attempted retinoscopy of infants 20 years ago. The indirect ophthalmoscope was not available and direct ophthalmoscopy was a heroic and special procedure and even then was usually futile. Children who could not read illiterate charts had written on their vision record "too young to determine." The slit lamp was for school-age children and the tonometer was for adults.

Clinicians accustomed to elaborate diagnostic regimens for strabismic school-age children were often frustrated at the thought of planning surgery for a 2-year-old. Infant surgery for congenital strabismus, now practiced in many medical centers, was beyond conception. Who could even dream of determining the vision, measuring the refractive error and angle of deviation, and defining the sensory anomalies in an infant 5 or 6 months of age?

Even if examination was possible, anesthesia hazards precluded surgical intervention. Cataract and glaucoma surgery techniques were not as sophisticated as they are today. The operating microscope was unavailable. Contact lenses were controversial for adult use and unthinkable for use on infants. Infant surgery was confined to heroic attempts at "blind" goniotomy for glaucoma and enucleation for retinoblastoma.

Modern concepts about sensory maturation occurring in the preschool years were incomplete and not widely disseminated. It was known that amblyopia developed only as a result of conditions present during the preschool years and was for the most part amenable to therapy before 6 to 9 years of age. However, the potential for binocularity in patients with congenital strabismus was unrealized until the early sixties (Taylor, 1963). Evidence is only now accumulating to statistically document the declining binocular potential which occurs between the sixth and thirty-sixth month in these patients (Ing et al., 1966).

Congenital cataracts and other causes of vision deprivation amblyopia have been neglected because of the poor visual results of therapy in the 3- to 6-year-old age group. It is becoming increasingly apparent that vision deprivation, strabismic, and anisometropic amblyopia (in order of decreasing severity) do not have equivalent prognoses. Evaluation of the results of current attempts at *earlier therapy* await accumulation of significant numbers of cases and maturation of the patients to the age when they can be tested with sophisticated techniques.

In light of these modern developments and knowledge, it is hoped and anticipated that a current treatise on this subject will interest and be useful to the practicing clinician as well as to the resident.

It will be assumed that the reader has already had some experience in the examination of adults. Differences, adaptations, and elaborations of adult versus pediatric examination will be emphasized in addition to personal prejudices as to examination technique. No effort has been made to exclude these, for these preju-

dices, borrowed heavily from many experienced examiners, probably represent the greatest value of the text.

COURTING THE CHILD

Good rapport is the key to examination of the child. Although many clinicians "seem to have natural talent" to this end, it is something that can be learned and cultivated.

Rapport starts in the outer office, where furnishings should include some things to make the youngster feel at home. A few carefully chosen, unbreakable, quiet, safe toys, a small table and chairs, storybooks, and perhaps even a specific children's area. Some thoughtful practitioners choose sturdy, cleanable furnishings, high door knobs, and doors which swing toward the examiner or nurse rather than into the area where a toddler might be standing. Street clothes or at least colored smocks are worn by many practitioners and their staff to avoid the fearful implications of white.

Choosing and training the personnel who will work with the children is as important as the physician's own personal talent for this special kind of sociability. Each professional will develop his own specific elaborations on the following general principles (Fig. 3–1):

1. CALL THE PATIENT BY HIS FIRST NAME.
2. AVOID NEGATIVE SUGGESTION.
   Assuming that the child fears the examiner is a mistake. If the examiner volunteers that he *will not hurt the child*, he is likely making a *fearful* rather than a reassuring suggestion. Also, avoid saying—"I just want to examine your eyes." This focuses the attention of the patient on himself. He will likely show his eyes widely or hide them; either way he is more difficult to examine.
3. OFFER A POSITIVE NEUTRAL SUGGESTION.
   Say "I want to show you something." He will be ready to look, which is the first and main thing he will be doing during the examination. His attention is distracted away from himself and away from the examiner. Children know that "show you" doesn't hurt and this serves as a positive substitute for the negative suggestion.

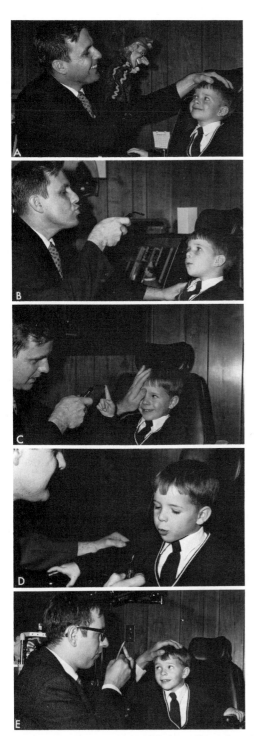

Figure 3–1 Courting the child (from above down). *A*, A puppet with story content; *B*, "coos" and noises; *C*, touching the light; *D*, "blowing it out"; and *E*, touching a specific place on a small picture—all enhance interest in the fixation target.

4. MAKE PHYSICAL CONTACT WITH SOME FRIENDLY GESTURE.

Children seem to fear what the examiner may do when he touches them even though the examiner "talks nicely." A gentle hand on the head, handgrasp crossing the room, assist into chair, handshake or other natural gentle physical gesture can bring the telltale smile that the child is reassured. A convenient trick is to ask him to hold something which you plan to use during the examination (like the occluder).

5. MAKE VERBAL CONTACT. INDUCE THE PATIENT TO SPEAK.

Ask him how old he is (or how "many" he is). Ask his teacher's name. Ask him to count something on the fixation target. Frequently a flood of words will flow once the first leak has sprung.

6. CULTIVATE A SPECIAL VOCABULARY. Red/green lenses are "Christmas glasses." Polaroid lenses are "magic glasses." If the top of a ball-point pen is called a "mirror," a child may be encouraged to see himself in it. Dr. Costenbader calls his remote cover test "peep-eye."

7. COLLECT INTERESTING FIXATION TARGETS WITH "ACCOMMODATIVE" DETAIL.

Small pictures pasted on tongue blades are handy for near fixation. Targets may be mounted on paper clips and hung on the examiner's glasses or held in his mouth to leave both hands free for the examination.

Animated, noisy battery-operated toys can be set up to be foot-activated. The best attention is in the first few seconds and manual control loses the best look. Foot activation also allows for seemingly "magical" operation. Multiple toys provide multiple looks, and a series of cubby holes in a cabinet at the end of the room permits each to light up and work in turn. If the toy has no light in its mechanism, a low-watt Christmas tree bulb or flashlight bulb can be included in the circuit. These toys are the best known devices for distant fixation in the very difficult under-2 age group (Friendly, 1970).

At the Wills Eye Hospital a continually run movie projector, placed at the end of the room, projects its films onto a screen positioned immediately above the projector. The whir of the projector comes from the same region as the screen which helps keep attention there. It also is "magically" operated by a foot pedal and a first-year resident found he could enhance the effect by pressing the child's nose as though it were the control button to turn it on. An appropriately placed mirror allows the doctor to follow the action on the screen and narrate if he desires. This device works best for the 2-year-old and up.

Although targets containing sufficient detail to require appropriate accommodation to be seen clearly are preferred, there are times when a light, especially one which can be "blinked" on and off, is the only target which will work. The light can be made red with a red lens, and if that lens is a Maddox rod, sound can be added by raking the light across the striations. Having the child blow the light out as though it were a match, or having him touch it with his finger, intensifies interest. A finger puppet may be placed over the light and the face illuminated from within; "winking" the light can be added.

8. GIVE FIXATION TARGETS "STORY CONTENT."

The interest potential of *any* device is multiplied many times if it has *story content.* "What are they doing on the boat? Mother is at the table; who else is there? He has blue eyes, and what color is his nose? What is he going to do with the tomahawk?" With a little imagination, story content can be given to *every part* of the examination.

9. SMILE.

A falsetto voice and homey sweetness is no short-cut to communication with children. Not only does it not fool them, but it may increase their anxiety as they wait to see what is hiding behind the sham.

Once the child has touched the examiner and spoken a few words to him, he is generally reassured and ready to see what the examiner has to show him.

HISTORY

The time-honored technique of allowing the parent to state the chief concern in her own words and recording it that way has unimpeachable merit. At the end of the examination, the chief concern should be reviewed to be certain it has received due attention.

Questioning conducted by the front office should not include "direct questioning" and "review of ocular symptoms." Questions like "Does he complain of burning eyes?" or "Does he sit too close to the T.V.?" obviously contaminate the thoughts of the historian. Spontaneous complaints of this nature have some merit but as a reply to direct questioning, most such items are entirely worthless.

The ability to skillfully conduct direct questioning depends on the examiner's knowledge of the syndromes which affect children.

Conditions which appear in childhood frequently involve material contained in the *birth, developmental,* and *family* histories. The tendency of congenital diseases to be multisystem makes the *past* history and *general health* of the patient of great importance also. The following questions are submitted to illustrate how a brief, complete review can be conducted.

Was his birth complicated? How much did he weigh?

Did he feed and breathe well right from the start?

Did he develop like the other children — walk and talk when he should?

Does he have unusual trouble keeping up with his classmates (playmates) of the same age?

Has he ever been hospitalized?

Does he take any medication?

Has the family doctor ever diagnosed or suspected any major illness?

Do any diseases run in the family?

Any eye diseases?

Anything not corrected by glasses?

Any crossed or lazy eye?

Any birth defects or neurological disease?

Do you or your husband wear glasses or have any eye trouble? His brothers? (No. and age) Sisters? (No. and age) Grandparents? Aunts and uncles?

History of previous eye care?

Age of first glasses?

EXAMINATION

Visual Acuity

Pediatric ophthalmologists, virtually without exception, take visual acuity themselves. If an occasional child peeks around the occluder, amblyopia might be missed. The child who sees poorly out of one eye is the very one who is most likely to try to peek. Latent nystagmus could easily be missed by an assistant. The ability to encourage a maximum effort is an art; it is important that the examiner know that a maximum effort has been achieved. Finally, taking the visual acuity is a wonderful opportunity to establish rapport, since it involves physical and verbal contact and the child who has performed successfully is "anxious to please" on the next test.

No part of the examination provides so much important information reliably or offers greater opportunity for the development of rapport in so short a time as the physician-executed visual acuity.

If full-line Snellen letters cannot be read, the illiterate tests (E game or figure charts) should be used in a full-line presentation, if possible. Otto Lippmann has found the stycar to be the best illiterate test (Lippmann, 1969). The "crowding phenomenon," present to a small degree in normals, is usually marked (2 or 3 lines difference) in amblyopes. Glasses should be worn if the patient has them and this should be noted on the chart. A near vision test has obvious value in the partially sighted patient but is of dubious value in the complete routine examination. Sustained near vision, advocated by some for school screening programs, clearly has no place in the office examination, since cycloplegic refraction will more clearly reveal the presence of hyperopia.

Occluder rejection is a common problem below age 3. Allowing the patient to hold the occluder while the history is being taken offers reassurance. He may prefer to hold it himself for the vision examination but he will need to be carefully watched. If the patient uses his hand for an occluder, the palm and not the fingers should be in front of the eye. In "peekers," a strip of 2-inch Micropore tape or an Elastoplast Occlusor will provide insurance and will more likely be accepted if called a "pirate's patch" (Fig. 3–2).

A prepared area of the record form will encourage more complete record keeping and make this information easier to find on review (Fig 3–3).

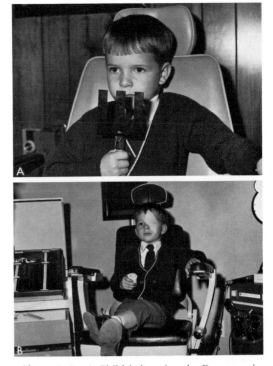

Figure 3–2 *A*, Child is learning the E game prior to the occlusion for the examination. Anxiety is allayed by the sense of accomplishment. *B*, Two-inch Micropore tape is used for occlusion while measuring the visual acuity in this "peeker."

Infant Visual Acuity

Although infants are illiterate, clinically useful estimates of the vision can be made. Ability to fix and follow a light is generally present by 2 months of age and well established by 3 months. Fixation of each eye, in turn, can be evaluated as good (if not unsteady), central (if not eccentric), and maintained (if fixation does not im-

V	OD 20/	FLP	SnL	c Rx
			E	
	OS 20/	SLP	Fig	s Rx

FLP – Full Line Presentation
SLP – Single Letter Presentation
SnL – Snellen Letters
Fig – Figures (pictures of objects)

Figure 3–3

mediately revert to the fellow eye in strabismus patients)...abbreviated GCM (Parks, 1966). "Maintained" indicates that there is not strong preference for one eye, suggesting equal or nearly equal vision. One eye is covered and it is noted that the infants look *steadily* at a light or fixation target and that the direction of gaze is roughly in the direction of the target (exact observation would require visuscopy, which is unreliable at this age). The eye is then uncovered. A strabismic patient who strongly prefers the eye just uncovered will switch fixation to that eye. This is good evidence of amblyopia in the fellow eye and is enough information to plan which eye to patch. Likewise, occlusion therapy can be followed until fixation can be held by either eye. This is an excellent example of how indirect evidence substitutes for an adult method with sufficient dependability to plan therapy and follow its course.

Covering the eye of a child who has *deep* amblyopia in the fellow eye will precipitate striking anxiety and avoidance maneuvers, since he is rendered severely handicapped by occlusion of the better eye.

"Crossed fixation," common in congenital esotropes with their large angles of strabismus, is an indication of nearly equal vision confirmed by those patients who have reached the age of literacy without surgical intervention. Their angle of deviation is so large (96 per cent being 40 prism diopters or more) (Ing, 1966) that it is more convenient to regard objects to their right with the left eye and *vice versa* than to turn their head. This phenomenon also probably contributes to the pseudoparesis of the lateral recti so characteristic of these children, since their condition makes abduction unnecessary.

The vision in an infant might be recorded thus:

OD:GCM	*OD*:GCM
OS:GC not M	*OS*:cries when OS covered

The history and observation of a child at play, with one or the other eye patched, allows some conclusions (recorded, "Picks up small objects with OD covered"). Optokinetic nystagmus is evidence of at least gross vision. Although the size of the stripes and the speed of the drum have been correlated to more specific visual acuity, the relationship is not yet clinically applicable. The optokinetic drum or tape test is an extremely valuable tool in which the examiner is interested in the presence or absence of the ocular response when the stripes are viewed both horizontally and vertically in either direction.

Head Posture

Note the position of the head of the child, especially as he tries to read the vision chart. Head position is described in three parameters: head up or down, face turned right or left, and chin up or down. Any one of these or a combination of two or three is possible (Fig. 3–4).

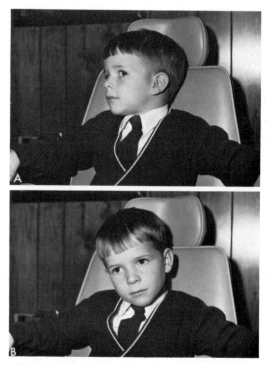

Figure 3–4 Abnormal head position is often accentuated when patient starts to regard detailed (accommodative) fixation target. *A*, Right face turn suggests right lateral rectus paresis (simulated). *B*, Right head tilt, left face turn, and chin down suggests isolated paresis of right inferior oblique (simulated).

Cover Testing

Extra attention will be given this phase of the examination because (1) there is little available detail in print, (2) the tests are of utmost importance, (3) recently acquired knowledge about small angle deviations has modified the classic regimen.

Prerequisite to cover testing is the ability of each eye in turn to be capable of central (foveal) fixation when the fellow eye is covered. If organic disease (cataracts, cloudy media, etc.) or functional conditions (eccentric fixation) prevent central fixation with either eye, then cover testing is *invalid* (Fig. 3–5).

Occluder technique emphasizes the prevention of fear. The traditional black paddle is handy, but if rejected, the examiner's hand or a thumb dropped from above may provide a more familiar, less threatening cover (Fig. 3–6). For very resistant infants, Dr. Costenbader advocates the remote cover test. A prescription pad or other handy cover is held about 18 inches from the infant's face, while a pen light is flashed at about 3 feet. The pad is placed so as to cast a shadow, first on one eye and then the other.

Prism technique includes the use of single prisms, a prism bar, split prisms (one over each eye, both base in or both base out), and stacked prisms (horizontal and vertical over the same eye) (Fig. 3–7).

Fixation targets should provide an *accommodative* stimulus if at all possible for *all types of strabismus* (Fig. 3–8). Unfor-

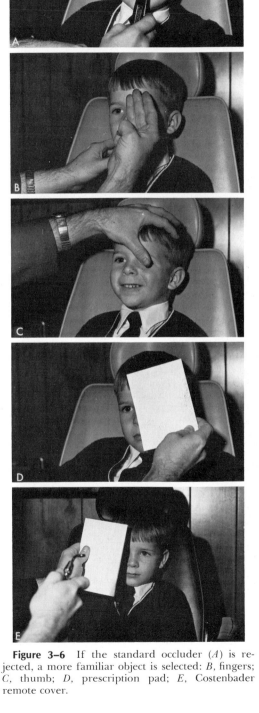

Figure 3–6 If the standard occluder (*A*) is rejected, a more familiar object is selected: *B*, fingers; *C*, thumb; *D*, prescription pad; *E*, Costenbader remote cover.

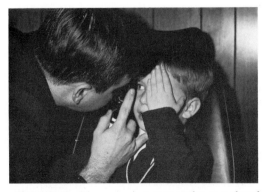

Figure 3–5 Visuscopy is a monocular test (hand covers the other eye) for a monocular condition (eccentric fixation).

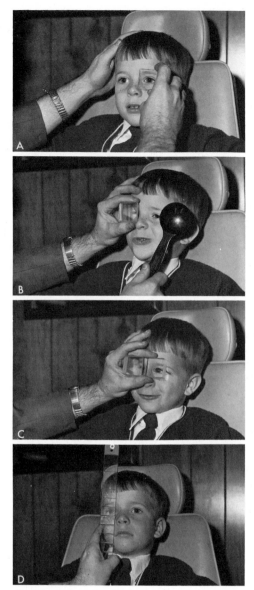

Figure 3–7 Prisms may be loose (*A*), stacked (horizontal and vertical over the same eye) (*B*), split (*C*), or on a bar (*D*). Use of the latter is encouraged when practicable.

tunately, nonaccommodative (muscle light) targets have been recommended by some for exotropes. The thought was that a couple of diopters of uncorrected hyperopia could be relaxed on a nonaccommodative target, bringing out the full extent of the exodeviation. What happens, however, is over-accommodation in order to get the two images together. In this manner a frank exotrope may appear to be only phoric. Using a target which

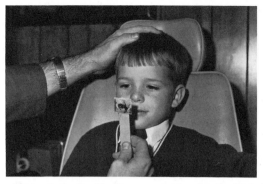

Figure 3–8 Small picture provides detail which, in order to be seen clearly, requires the patient to accommodate for the appropriate distance.

has detail on it offers a stimulus to a patient who under- or over-accommodates and simulates casual everyday seeing.

Vision charts at 20 feet and at 13 inches (1/3 meter) work well in older preschool and school-age children. The Costenbader accommodometer is ideal for near fixation (Fig. 3–9). Younger preschool children can be offered toys, movies, and the like with accommodative detail and story content to enhance interest.

Measurements are routinely made in the following six positions:

At 20 feet (6 M) (Fig. 3–10)
$\begin{cases} \text{(1) primary position} \\ \text{(2) up gaze center} \\ \quad \text{(c. 25°)} \\ \text{(3) down gaze center} \\ \quad \text{(c. 25 to 35°)} \\ \text{(4) right gaze (c. 25°)} \\ \text{(5) left gaze (c. 25°)} \end{cases}$

At 13 inches (1/3 M) { (6) primary position

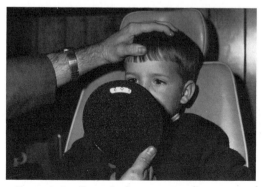

Figure 3–9 Costenbader accommodometer used as a near fixation target held at 13 inches.

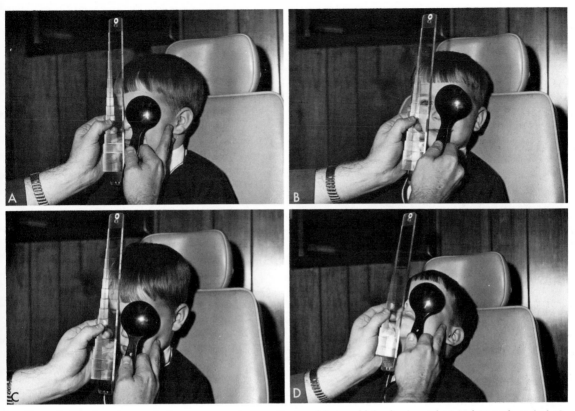

Figure 3–10 In prism and alternate cover testing, the head is turned for horizontal (*A* and *B*) and vertical (*C* and *D*) measurements, so that they may be taken with distant fixation targets.

Measurements in these positions give information about:

(1) A or V patterns
(2) lateral comitance
(3) accommodation-convergence relationship

Measurements as such are not routinely recommended for the oblique positions (see Versions).

Ocular deviations may be *diagnosed* as to their presence and type (heterophoria or heterotropia) by three maneuvers: the cover test, the uncover test, and the alternate cover test (Figs. 3–11, 3–12, 3–13). Once diagnosed, the deviation may be *measured* by addition of a prism of correctly chosen strength to neutralize movement of the eyes during various cover maneuvers (Figs. 3–14, 3–15, 3–16).

The Cover Test (Fig. 3–11)

The *cover test* is performed by having the patient look at an accommodative target with both eyes viewing. (It is a binocular test, even though one eye may be suppressing.) The examiner places an occluder over one eye while watching the fellow eye for a shift in fixation. A shift is evidence that the eye (the one not covered) was not regarding the target with its fovea while both eyes were viewing. The eye which is covered, then, was the only eye fixating the target while its fellow was deviated. The deviation is called *heterotropia* or, if the direction is specified, *esotropia, exotropia,* or *hypertropia.* A heterotropia is a *manifest deviation* because it exists (is manifest) under normal or casual seeing circumstances, i.e., with both eyes viewing. Notice that the patient enters the test with both eyes viewing: the cover test examines a *binocular* circumstance.

If no shift occurs, a heterotropia may still exist. If the occluder was placed before the deviating eye, the fellow eye would already be fixed on the target and no shift would be expected. Obviously in most cases the examiner already knows which eye is deviating because one eye is directed at the object of regard and the

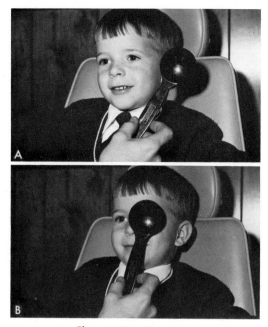

Figure 3–11 Cover test.

other is not. However, in small angle deviations, this is often not obvious and with very young children, it is sometimes hard to be sure that they are regarding the object intended.

To complete the test, the patient must be returned to binocular viewing for at least a couple of seconds so that fusion can be accomplished if there is that potential. The second eye is covered in the same manner as the first. The sequence is (1) cover one eye, observing the fellow; (2) uncover that eye for a few seconds; and (3) cover the second eye while observing the first eye. The sequence should be repeated to make sure that a subtle, rapid switch in fixation did not take place unnoticed during the binocular interval. Many strabismus patients can readily alternate fixation and if a switch occurs during the test, the examiner might be placing the occluder before the deviating eye each time. If this switch does occur, no shift would be present with maneuvers before either eye, leading to the false *conclusion* that both foveas were simultaneously regarding the target and that a manifest deviation does not exist. Close observation for this possibility and routinely repeating the sequence once or more makes this mistake unlikely.

The Uncover Test (Fig. 3–12)

During this sequence, each eye was not only covered but each was also uncovered. If the eye being uncovered is also observed for a shift, the *uncover test* is performed. The uncover test will now be treated separately only for didactic purposes. Obviously, the examiner has the opportunity to accomplish one as he does the other.

In the *uncover test*, the eye being uncovered is the *principal* object of the examiner's attention. Actually, both eyes must be observed simultaneously, making this a difficult test from the examiner's viewpoint. It is also difficult from the patient's viewpoint, because he is going from a monocular circumstance to a binocular one. Thus, he may suddenly be confronted with a diplopic world. His response to this situation may be (1) a *fusion response*, involving a shift of *one eye* (the deviating eye) so that both may regard the target with their foveas simultaneously; (2) a *switch in fixation response*, in which *both eyes* move in the same direction; or (3) no movement. In the last case, diplopia is handled by sensory adaptation, making motor adaptation unnecessary, or exact orthophoria exists.

Although the motor response to the cover test is immediate, this is often not

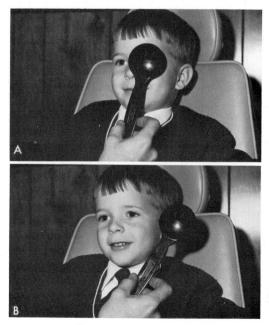

Figure 3–12 Uncover test.

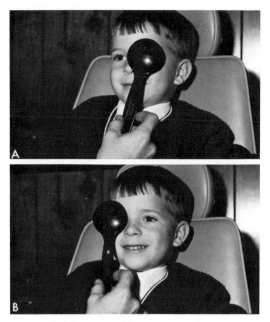

Figure 3–13 Alternate cover test.

true with the uncover test. Even more confusing, the patient may switch fixation and then fuse, resulting in a shift of both eyes followed by shift of the deviating eye in the opposite direction as it recovers.

The Alternate Cover Test (Fig. 3–13)

The *alternate cover* test is performed by moving the occluder directly from one eye to the other without allowing an interval for binocular viewing. Fusion is suspended throughout the test, since the patient is always viewing under *monocular* conditions. The position of the eyes with one eye occluded is called "the fusion free position," as emphasized by Walter B. Lancaster.

If no ocular shift occurs as the occluder is moved directly from one eye to the other, then the eyes are truly aligned. Even with fusion suspended, the foveas are in position to regard the target without having to shift.

However, if a shift does occur, a deviation exists. If that deviation is corrected by fusion—i.e., if the deviating eye moves into alignment under binocular conditions—then the deviation is said to be *latent* and is called a heterophoria (phoria, for short).

It should be apparent that the alternate cover test does not diagnose a phoria by

itself but depends on the findings of the cover test. The alternate cover test demonstrates that a deviation exists under monocular conditions. If the deviation persists under binocular conditions, it is a *manifest* deviation called a *tropia*. If it is present under monocular but not binocular conditions, it is a *latent* deviation brought out only by the suspension of fusion and is called a *phoria*.

A misconception has been fostered by the unfortunate wording, "the occluder is moved swiftly from one eye to the other," leading to the widely held notion that a rapid fanning back and forth of the occluder helps break up fusion. Actually, the occluder need not be moved very fast, since the following edge uncovers one eye about the same time as the leading edge covers the fellow eye. A brief moment should be allowed for fixation to be accomplished by the uncovered eye before reversing the direction of the occluder (Fig. 3–17).

The Prism and Alternate Cover Test (Figs. 3–14 and 3–15)

To this point *diagnosis* of deviations has been discussed. Addition of a prism allows for *measurement* of deviations. The test used clinically is the *prism and alternate cover test*. A prism is held before *either* eye

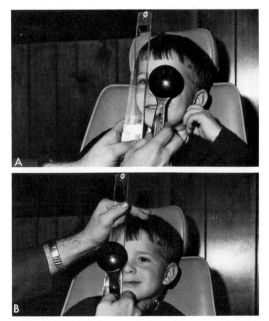

Figure 3–14 Prism and alternate cover test (OD fixing).

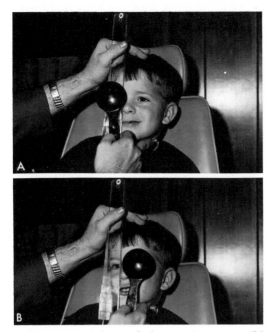

Figure 3–15 Prism and alternate cover test (OS fixing).

with the apex in the direction of the deviation. (Unfortunately, the position of the prism is classically described according to its base: base in, base out, base up, base down.) The alternate cover maneuver is then performed and if an ocular shift is present, another prism is chosen. The correctly chosen prism deflects light from the target onto the fovea of the deviating eye making an ocular shift unnecessary. The strength of the neutralizing prism is the measurement of the deviation.

The use of a *prism bar is strongly recommended,* since *rapid* selection of the correct prism is important in dealing with the short attention span of children.

The neophyte may be amazed that when the occluder is moved from left to right the effect of the neutralizing prism may be different from when it is moved from right to left. In this case, both measurements are recorded and noted as "OD fixing" and "OS fixing" (Figs. 3–14 and 3–15). "OD fixing" means the patient entered the test with the OD viewing (the occluder passes from OS to OD) and *vice versa.* This difference immediately suggests a paretic strabismus.

Clinically, the prism is not used with the other maneuvers: cover and uncover. In

the former case, the prism would be introduced to binocular seeing, artificially altering any natural disparity in the images presented to the two eyes, invalidating the test. A prism and uncover test still has all the disadvantages of the uncover maneuver previously described.

The *classic diagnostic regimen* includes these tests. (1) A *cover test* reveals the presence or absence of a manifest deviation (tropia). If there is no manifest deviation, (2) the *alternate cover test* is done to reveal the presence or absence of a latent deviation (phoria). *Either* deviation is then measured by (3) the *prism and alternate cover test.*

According to the "classic" regimen, it is *assumed* that the "angle of deviation in the fusion free position" measured by the prism and alternate cover test is equal to *either* type of deviation and no allowance is made for the simultaneous existence of a phoria and a tropia.

However, it has been appreciated in the last decade that in certain small angle deviations, this situation does exist. The angle of deviation in the fusion free position (one eye covered) is partially reduced (the phoric component), but a small manifest deviation (tropia) persists under bin-

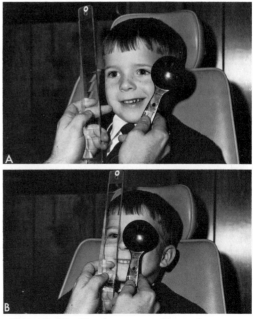

Figure 3–16 Simultaneous prism and cover test (OD is deviating eye).

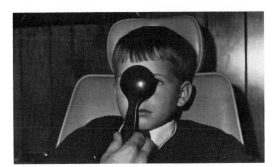

Figure 3–17 Since the trailing edge of the occluder leaves one eye about the same time as the leading edge covers the fellow, there is no need for speed or jerky movements (fanning) in performing the alternate cover maneuver.

ocular conditions. (This complex thought is illustrated in Figure 3–18). Classic concepts so thoroughly exclude this possibility that a long and slow re-education process is predicted. This fascinating story is beyond the scope of this chapter but the motor test involved shall be described here (Parks, 1961).

The Simultaneous Prism and Cover Test (Fig. 3–16)

It has already been stated that the prism and alternate cover test measures the angle of deviation in the fusion free position. This can be thought of as the whole angle of which the phoric and tropic components constitute the parts (Fig. 3–18). If either part can be measured, the difference between the part and the whole is the remaining part. It is convenient to measure the tropic component with the *simultaneous prism and cover test*. This test is performed by introducing the occluder before the fixating eye and introducing the correctly chosen prism before the deviating eye *simultaneously*. A correctly chosen prism neutralizes the shift of the deviating eye.

The test is not without its difficulties. First, the ocular shift must be studied behind a prism immediately after it has been moved into place. However, with a little practice, the apparent displacement of the eye due to the prism is easily distinguished from the actual shift of the eye.

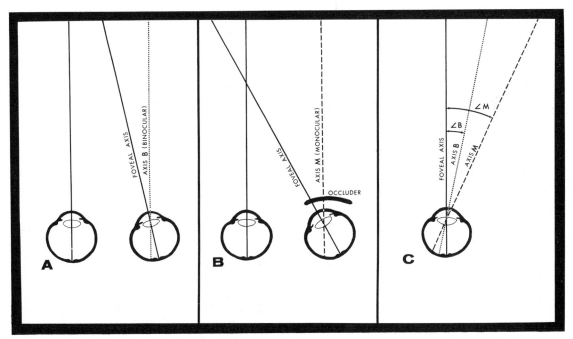

Figure 3–18 *A,* Under binocular conditions, axis B makes an angle (up to 8 prism diopters) with the foveal axis (the tropic component).

B, Under monocular conditions, axis M projected through the occluder into the eye makes an angle (up to 20 prism diopters) with the foveal axis (the total angle or the fusion free position).

C, Composite diagram of the deviating eye shows angle B, the tropic component (measured by the simultaneous prism and cover test); angle M, the total angle (measured by the prism and alternate cover test); and angle M minus angle B, the phoric component.

Another problem is that the test does not work unless *the occluder is placed before the fixating eye and the prism before the deviating eye.* The phenomenon is characteristic of small angle deviations, and gross observation as to which is the deviating eye is necessarily more difficult. Also, many of these patients can rapidly alternate their fixation. *The correct performance of the test the first time sets up circumstances for incorrect performance with the next prism choice in a patient who alternates easily.* When the occluder goes before one eye, fixation is switched to the fellow and unless there is strong preference for the first eye (which there frequently is not) it will remain there. The examiner then must change the prism and occluder to opposite hands or, more easily, he can occlude the other eye for a moment, switching fixation back to the original eye.

When should the simultaneous prism and cover test be employed?

(1) When the deviation is less than 20Δ on prism and alternate cover test.

(2) When stereoacuity is 67 seconds or worse.

(3) On all postoperative strabismus patients.

It need not be used if the cover test indicates orthophoria.

The importance of this test should be well understood. The tropic components of these deviations have been observed to be only up to 8 prism diopters in amount. This is the angle of deviation with which the patient does his everyday casual binocular seeing. In a routine workup done along classic lines, the patient would have a tropia on the cover test. The amount of shift would only be 8 prism diopters or 4° but measurements are not taken on the cover test. The examiner would then do the usual prism and alternate cover test, measure 20 prism diopters deviation, and assume that this is the measure of his tropic deviation. He might be prejudiced by this large measurement to recommend surgery, whereas the actual tropic component which this patient has to walk around with is a mere 8 prism diopters, hardly a cosmetic problem in most patients.

It is an interesting observation that several experienced clinicians have been faced with this problem frequently enough in postoperative patients to view the ac-

curacy of routine measurements (prism and alternate cover) as invalid or at least misleading in postoperative patients. The particulars of the reason for their skepticism have now come to light, vindicating their clinical judgment. Now, however, we have a test to actually measure the discrepancy.

Measuring the Deviation by Other Than Cover Testing

When cover testing is impossible because of organic disease, eccentric fixation, or lack of cooperation, very good estimates of ocular deviations can be made. Probably the best method is the reverse Krimsky test. In this test, a prism is held before the fixating eye (the prism bar is the best) and the patient fixates a light bright and large enough to be seen as a corneal reflex (ordinary muscle light). The prism is changed until the corneal reflexes are symmetrically centered, but not necessarily geometrically centered, since adequate allowance should be made for angle *kappa.* Most infants beyond 4 months can cooperate sufficiently for this test (Fig. 3–19).

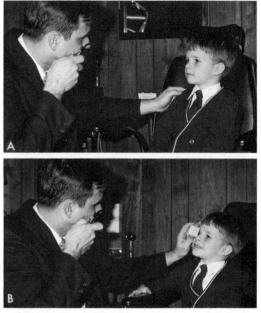

Figure 3–19 *A,* Hirschberg estimates of deviation (1 mm. asymmetry = 7° or 14 prism diopters). *B,* Reverse Krimsky: increasing prism placed before the fixating eye until corneal reflexes are symmetrical. The fixation light is held adjacent to the visual axis of the examiner's viewing eye.

In an exceptionally uncooperative patient, Hirschberg estimates may have to be done. Although Hirschberg recommended specific landmarks — e.g., pupillary margin — as having certain values, it is probably more accurate to estimate the decentration of the reflex in millimeters, using a point symmetrical to the reflex in the fixating eye. This can be multiplied by 15 prism diopters and be very close to a measured deviation.

In making estimates by either method, it is imperative to have the light in the same line as the *examiner's viewing eye*. In fact, it is a good idea to hold the muscle light touching the examiner's cheek as a reminder.

Versions (Range of Motion of the Eyes Together)

Versions should be checked in the nine diagnostic positions of gaze. This has already been accomplished during cover testing in five of these nine positions. Examination of the *oblique positions* can be done by gross observation as the patient follows a near target into these positions (Fig. 3–20). The rationale for this somewhat controversial short cut is as follows: Clinically, the examination need only be gross because any surgical plans based on these observations (recession or myotomy of the inferior obliques in almost every case) is gross, maximum, and standard. Also, unnecessary examination should be omitted to conserve the child's limited attention span.

The findings may be graded as small, medium, or large. It is simple and convenient to limit reference to the findings as an *underaction* or *overaction of an oblique*. Notice that the *underaction of any oblique could be expressed as overaction of the yoke* (always a vertical rectus — see Fig. 3–21). "Underaction" and "overaction" are simply descriptions of the position of the eyes. They do not imply the etiology of the deviation (paresis, hypertrophy, contracture, and so forth).

There is a need to simplify our recording of the examination. For example, overaction of the superior oblique muscles in

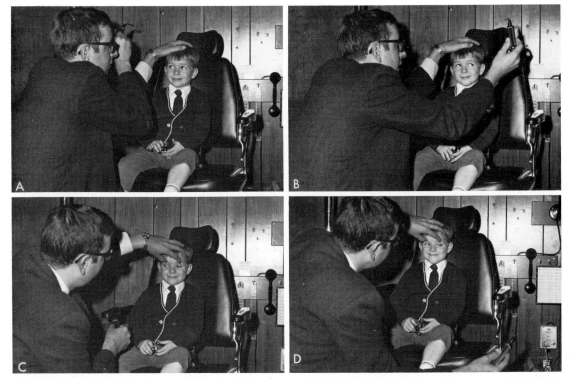

Figure 3–20   Versions are done at near (*A* and *B*). Right and left inferior oblique muscles are tested (*C* and *D*). Estimates of the amount of underaction or overaction are graded (none, slight, moderate, severe).

OVERACTION OF THE		UNDERACTION OF THE OPPOSITE	
superior oblique	IS	inferior rectus	
inferior oblique	THE	superior rectus	
superior rectus	SAME	inferior oblique	
inferior rectus	AS	superior oblique	

Figure 3–21

both eyes may be written O.A.S.O.O.U. Similarly, bilateral underaction of the inferior oblique muscles may be recorded as U.A.I.O.O.U.

Ductions (Range of Motion of One Eye at a Time)

If versions are full, testing each eye separately is superfluous. If versions are not full, ductions need only be done in the field of action of the suspected limitation; versions having proved the full range of the other ductions.

It is not uncommon for congenital esotropes to have limited abduction. Non-ophthalmologists frequently interpret this as sixth-nerve paralysis, even to the point of doing neuroradiological procedures. Patching of one and then the other eye usually results in improvement of ductions within hours or days at most. Even without patching, ductions improve with age in these patients.

If the child does not allow manual covering of each eye, 2-inch Micropore tape will frequently work.

A chair that swivels is of great help in observing ductions and versions. To check right gaze (medial rectus OS or lateral rectus OD) have the infant sit on the mother's lap with his legs extending to the left and turn the chair to the left, holding the target to the far right. The

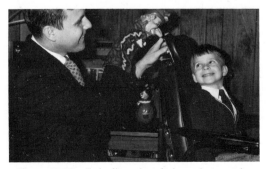

Figure 3–22 Swiveling the chair makes versions possible without restraining the head manually.

child will dextrovert the head maximally to the right, but then must use a maximum dextroversion of the eyes (Fig. 3–22). Attempts to hold the child's head straight manually are invariably frustrated with resistive movements and prompt lack of interest in the target. Noisy targets (like jangling keys) held at close range work best.

Maddox Rod

Small vertical deviations can contribute to dissociation, making an otherwise latent deviation manifest. Furthermore, these small vertical deviations may be masked by more sizeable, but perhaps less significant, horizontal deviations. The sensitivity of this test, to pick up an important small deviation which by other methods could be easily overlooked, has earned a well justified place for this test in the routine examination.

A red Maddox rod offers more dissociation, which is desirable in this test. The striations of the Maddox rod are held vertically before one eye while the patient fixates a distant (20 feet away) muscle light. The patient sees a "red horizontal line" with this eye and a "white dot" with the fellow eye. He is quizzed as to their relative position. The patient sometimes requires a little time before observing the red line, unless the room is sufficiently darkened.

The wording of the question is problematic with children. If the examiner asks, "Is the dot on the line?", many children will think of a ball on a table and respond "No" when the line goes right through the dot. Preferred phraseology would be "Does the dot touch the line?"

If the dot does not touch the line, ask whether it is above the line or below it. Interpreting the answer is important and it is well to have a routine for thinking this through. If the dot appears above the line, the image is striking inferior retina and this eye must be relatively hypodeviated.

(If the dot appears *high*, that eye is *low*.)

The amount of the hyperdeviation can quickly be assessed by placing the appropriate vertical prism in front of either eye until the "dot touches the line."

An interesting frustration of this test is that the Maddox rod may act as a partial occluder and manifest a small dissociated hyperdeviation. The eye behind the Maddox rod will be higher, usually by a prism diopter or two. This can be quickly checked by placing the Maddox rod before the other eye. If the fellow is now the higher, the deviation is that of a dissociated hyperphoria. If the original eye is still higher, the vertical is of the ordinary, so-called "true" hyperdeviation.

Use of the Maddox rod for *horizontal* deviations is frustrated by spurious data because of the fusion capability of dissimilar images which many patients possess and the lack of accommodation control. (A fixation light is not an accommodative target.) The Maddox rod should be used routinely *only* for *vertical* deviations (Fig. 3–23).

Color Vision

Color vision should be routinely tested. The H-R-R pseudoisochromatic plates are an excellent test series, since they examine for yellow-blue as well as red-green defects and there is a rough quantitation capability. The directions enclosed with the test are explicit, but a few commonly overlooked features will be mentioned here. The first four plates both teach the test and screen for malingerers; they are seen by all color defectives. The next six plates

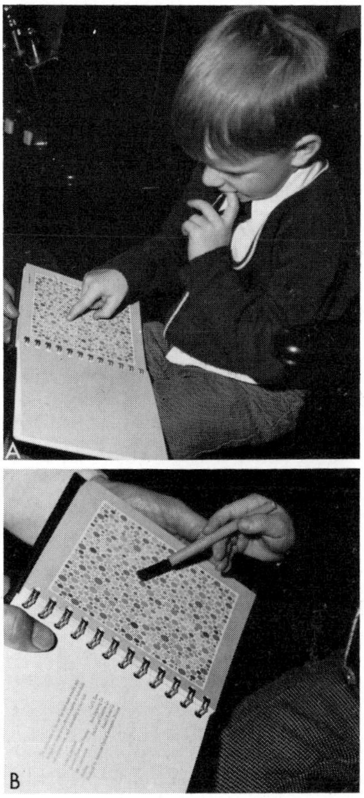

Figure 3–24 Testing color vision with the H-R-R plates. Illiterate child tracing figure with fingers will soil plates. Dry paintbrush recommended.

are called screening plates, since they test mild defects with desaturated figures. Testing beyond the sixth "screening plate" is a waste of time if the patient has identified these correctly. Use of the Macbeth-Easel Lamp (for illumination) and dry paintbrush (to prevent discoloration of the plates) is frequently neglected. (Fig. 3–24). This test can be done by medical assistants.

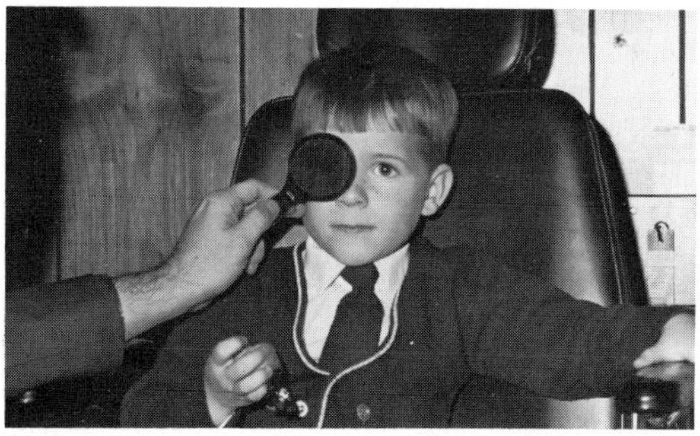

The Farnsworth D-15 color chips may be used on those patients who fail the H-R-R. According to experts, only functionally significant defectives fail the former test, whereas the latter is a very rigid screener. Neither of these tests discriminates anopes (total color defectives) from anomalies (partial defectives). This requires testing with an anomaloscope, which is well beyond the range of routine examination (Linksz, 1964).

The Ishihara test is an exacting one which no individual with a color vision defect can read without making any mistakes.

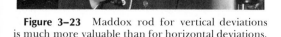

Figure 3–23 Maddox rod for vertical deviations is much more valuable than for horizontal deviations.

Near Point of Accommodation

This test not only measures accommodation, but also ensures elucidation of strabismus at near (Fig. 3–25).

Stereoacuity — The Titmus Test

Since the Edgar Wirt test is out of print, the Titmus test is the best available. Check the plates to be sure that it is correctly made; the two images should be exactly side by side (not vertically displaced).

Stereoacuity is graded in arc seconds disparity. The button card is best performed by children if they are asked to push the high button back down on the page. It wears the card out to have the plates scratched with the pressing, but the game is much more fun that way and cooperation is infinitely better.

The first button or two is eccentrically placed to the monocular child. (Try it yourself with one eye closed.) Regard correct answers at this level only with suspicion. Some children who will not see stereoscopically will guess the button by this clue.

There is obviously a big cooperation factor, but children who are able to read letters can generally perform to *better than 70 seconds*. A score below 67 seconds virtually proves bifoveal fusion (Parks, 1968).

Showing the House Fly test picture to a 3- to 6-year-old child will frequently produce a giggly or frightened response, especially since he has been told he is wearing "magic glasses" (Fig. 3–26). This can be taken as evidence that the fly ap-

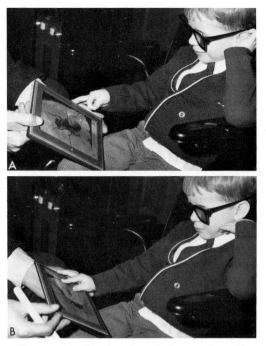

Figure 3–26 Stereoacuity: *A*, Stereopsis, evident from appropriate grasp of the wing image. *B*, Test turned 90°; even normals see wings as flat.

pears as three-dimensional. If the response is doubtful, ask him to pick up the wings. Some children who are experiencing binocular stereopsis will advance their hand from the front until it strikes something. The examiner frequently cannot tell whether the child anticipated striking the wing or if he was just going for a flat image. Encourage him to bring his hand in from the side. To be quite certain, the examiner may turn the plate sideways; in this position the fly will not be seen stereoscopically by anyone (the disparity is now vertical). Ask if it now appears different.

A number of prominent pediatric ophthalmologists use this test on every patient 3 years of age or older to assure peripheral binocularity (3000 to 67 seconds of arc) or excellent bifoveal binocularity (less than 67 seconds of arc). For those scoring 67 seconds or worse, it is wise to search for central suppression in one eye with the Worth 4 dots test, Bagolini lenses, red-green perimetry, Polaroid vectograph, or 4-diopter prism test. This recommendation is based on the observation of Marshall Parks that he has never seen a patient

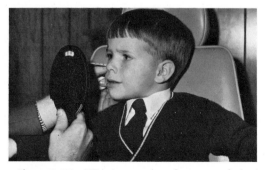

Figure 3–25 NPA (near point of accommodation) is measured with 20/40 symbol of the Costenbader accommodometer.

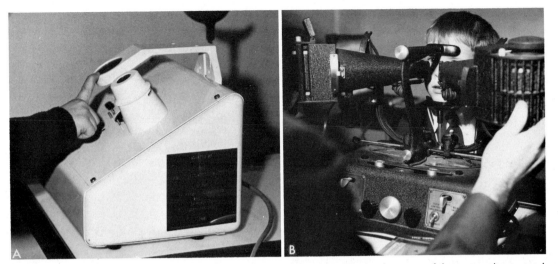

Figure 3–27 Haidinger's brushes (*A*) and the major amblyoscope (*B*) require more elaborate equipment, take longer to use, and generally are operated by specially trained orthoptists.

with central suppression of one eye score better than 67 seconds on the Wirt stereoacuity card (similar to the Titmus) (Parks, 1968).

Although *not routinely performed on every case*, other sensory tests will be discussed here. Notice that all these tests are inexpensive, fast (1 to 2 minutes), and done in full room illumination and with minimal dissociation to preserve the casual seeing condition. Children are not placed close to instruments which might induce near reflexes (Fig. 3–27).

Tests for Central Suppression

Worth 4 Dots

Worth 4 dots test has been traditionally performed at distance and near and discrepancies have been blamed entirely on variations in the deviation at the two distances. More recently, it became apparent that the main difference is the angle subtended by the dots. At a standard distance (6 meters), the 4 dots subtend 1.25 degrees, whereas they subtend 6 degrees at 33 cm. If a patient has a central suppression zone in the deviating eye (usually 3 to 5 degrees), he would give a monocular response to the 1.25-degree test and a fusion response to the 6-degree test, simply because the latter falls outside the scotoma (Fig. 3–28). The angle subtended by the

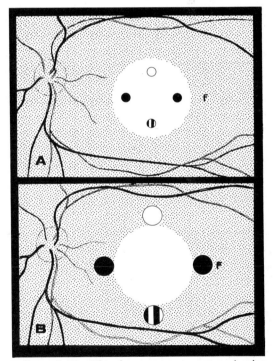

Figure 3–28 The clear area represents a circular scotoma on the nasal retina of the deviating eye (F = fovea).

A, From 10 feet away the hand-held 4 dots fall within the scotoma and are not seen by this eye. *B,* The same eye viewing the 4 dots at closer range, which now subtend an angle great enough to fall on seeing retina. The patient gives a fusion response at this distance. The illustration diagrams all 4 dots; of course, only 2 or 3 would be seen by this eye, depending on the particular filter worn before it.

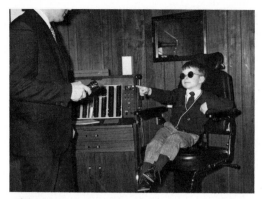

Figure 3–29 Examiner approaches patient from 10 feet up to his nose and records the distance at which 4 dots are first recognized.

fusion response is given and measure the distance to the patient (Fig. 3–29). The angle subtended on the retina can be calculated from the chart (Fig. 3–30) and reflects the size of the central suppression scotoma. Beyond 10 feet, normal patients have retinal rivalry and a fusion response cannot be expected with targets that small (Stager and Phelps, unpublished data). Obviously, there is need for a variable size 4 dot test that can be placed at a standard distance.

Bagolini Lenses

A Bagolini lens can be made by streaking an oily thumb across a plano lens. In fact, the streaking of oncoming headlights at night is caused by road film that has been streaked on the windshield by the wipers. Fine striations behave like a micro-Maddox rod, rendering a spot of light into a streak perpendicular to the striations. Commercially available Bagolini lenses

dots can be varied by changing the distance of the near test.

A good routine is to approach the patient from about 10 feet with the standard "flashlight testing instrument" until a

WORTH 4 DOT CONVERSION TABLE
WORTH 4 DOT FLASH LIGHT

DISTANCE FROM PATIENT		DEGREES (APPROX.)
METERS	FEET - INCHES	
6 M.	20	.33°
4 M.	13	.50°
3 M.	9.5	.67°
2 M.	6.5	1°
1 M.	3'3"	2°
67 cm.	2'2"	3°
50 cm.	20"	4°
33 cm.	13"	6°
25 cm.	10"	8°
20 cm.	8"	10°
17 cm.	7"	11°
15 cm.	6"	13°
12.5 cm.	5"	16°
10 cm.	4"	20°
8 cm.	3"	26°
DISTANT WORTH 4 DOT		1.25°
A.O. VECTOGRAPH SLIDE		.48°

Figure 3–30 (After Stager.)

can be placed in a trial frame (over the distance correction, if any) so that the striations are at right angles to each other. The examiner does not have to remember the position of the striations because he can see the reflected streaks as the patient sees them when he positions himself exactly in front of the patient. A hand-held muscle light is used and the child is asked to draw the lines with his finger in the air just as he sees them (Fig. 3–31). Children with bifoveal fusion see a perfect cross (×). If central suppression is present, the central scotoma in the deviating eye appears as a break in the line corresponding to that eye (╳). Usually the examiner must call the attention of the patient to the break. He can receive some reassurance that he is not talking the patient into something not seen by eliciting that the break is in the line corresponding to the deviating eye. A child with rapid alternation readily switches his suppression from eye to eye as fast as he switches fixation. If total suppression of the deviating eye occurs, the patient will see only one line or the other [／] or [＼].

This test requires a more sophisticated patient than does the stereoacuity and Worth 4 dots. It has the advantage, however, that it simulates casual seeing best of all sensory tests, since the dissociation is minimal.

A sophistication of the test is to dim the light in an effort to see if one of the lines extinguishes before the other in subtle sensory adaptations.

Red-Green Perimetry

Red-green perimetry can be performed with red-green glasses in a fully illumin-

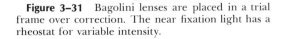

Figure 3–31 Bagolini lenses are placed in a trial frame over correction. The near fixation light has a rheostat for variable intensity.

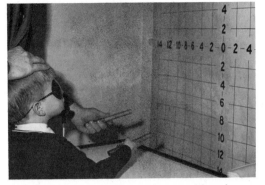

Figure 3–32 Binocular perimetry with red-green glasses in full room illumination. Patient holds projector corresponding to the deviating eye and places spot of light on examiner's spot (color corresponds to the preferred or fixating eye).

ated room with any of several available red and green projection pointers. The patient is placed 1 meter from the wall and graduated charts (Lancaster, Hess, and others) can be used if desired (Fig. 3–32).

A color spot is projected on the wall corresponding to the fixating eye. The patient is handed the pointer of the color corresponding to the deviating eye and asked to place his "spot" of light on the other spot. He may head directly for the central spot, but if there is a central suppression scotoma, he will become uncertain and wander around in the central vicinity. Upon questioning, he will report that the light disappears just as he is about to reach the other spot. (It moves within his scotoma.)

A child who has no binocularity will see only one dot at a time, whereas one who has fusion will accomplish the task.

The test does not work well for rapid alternators, since they will alternately lose one spot, then the other. It is sometimes difficult to tell a total suppressor from one who has central suppression only. However, the test can be performed at age 4 and above, as long as the child has a strong preference for one eye.

The test is not analogous to ordinary Lancaster red-green techniques which are done in the dark without peripheral stimuli available.

Polaroid Vectograph

Children with central or total suppression of one eye will delete letters on the AO Polaroid vectograph. The patient wears special Polaroid glasses (polarized vertically in one eye and horizontally in the other). The slide is projected also in a polarized fashion, so that some of the letters on the vision chart are presented to the OD only, some to the OS only, and some to both. Illiterate children who can count can also perform the test by counting the letters seen. The test is exquisitely sensitive and is being investigated for school screening as well as office use.

The 4-Diopter Prism Test

This test should be mentioned as a quick and inexpensive sensory test which can be performed by the physician (Fig. 3–33). Its mechanism and its numerous pitfalls have been outlined well and at length in recent literature (Romano, 1969). It is by far the least reliable of the group for identifying total or regional suppression but has some merit.

Notice that the sensory testing described herein is directed toward proving (1) total suppression, (2) central suppression, or (3) no suppression of the deviating eye. This represents an assay of whether the child has (1) no binocularity, (2) peripheral binocularity only, or (3) bifoveal binocularity. It is felt that the first has a poor prognosis for maintaining alignment while the second and third have excellent prognoses. These decisions can be reached before the third birthday in most all cases and often before the second birthday.

Notice also that determining ARC and NRC is generally ignored. This represents a prejudice of the clinician whose practice deals with prompt management of strabismus as soon as it is detected. In these practices, it is a rare thing to do a sensory examination on a child who has a large enough angle, who is (1) old enough to test for retinal correspondence and (2) also has an angle of deviation large enough to make such observations reliable. (It is very difficult to test NRC, ARC, and no RC reliably in small angle deviations.)

Fusional Vergences

The ability of a child to converge or diverge behind a changing prism in order to maintain fusion is a valuable test but not done routinely. If good vergences are

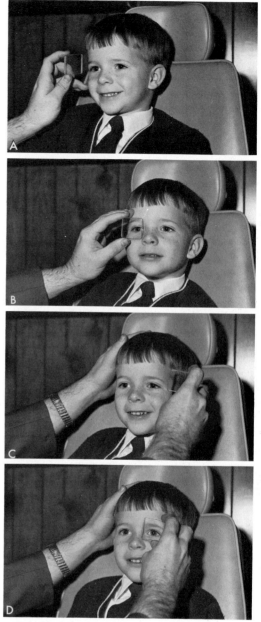

Figure 3–33 Four diopter prism test. *A* and *B*, Four diopter prism placed over OD with central scotoma; no movement OU. *C* and *D*, Prism placed over OS, the fixating eye; both eyes move to right. When prism is removed, both eyes make simultaneous movement to left, the primary position.

demonstrated, it indicates binocularity and both a capability and desire to maintain it. Prism power is increased until fusion cannot be maintained and one eye swings back to a neutral and more comfortable position (Fig. 3–34). This can be grossly observed; therefore, this test can be done

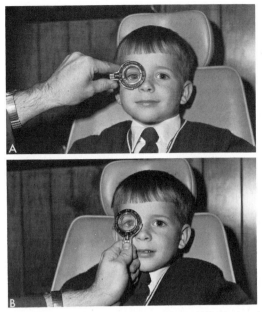

Figure 3–34 Horizontal and vertical fusional vergences.

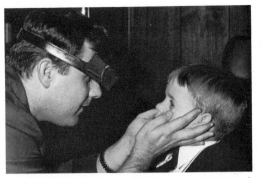

Figure 3–35 External examination may be made with loupe before mydriasis, which may cause some irritation.

in infants as early as the fourth month of life. Accommodative targets are used. A "make" figure can also be obtained if the child is old enough (6 years or so) to report accomplishment of fusion as the prism strength is reduced.

A rotary prism is usually used. However, a prism bar can be substituted (horizontally or vertically), but apparent displacement of images is jerky. The speed with which the examiner advances a rotary prism or a bar affects the end point, making reproducible results vary somewhat.

EXTERNAL EXAMINATION

This may require manipulation of the child, at least manual retraction of the lower lids. It should be delayed until *just before* dilatation in case rapport is spoiled (Fig. 3–35). It should be done *before* dilatation in order to place medicinal reactions in their proper perspective. The lid margins, follicular hypertrophy in the conjunctiva, and preauricular nodes are routinely given special attention.

Refraction

Since refraction techniques are discussed elsewhere, only a few comments

will be made here. Cycloplegic refraction is essential in children. The presence of strabismus, the youth of the child, and the darkness of the iris increase the indication for atropine. However, Cyclogyl (2%) is felt to be adequate in most cases by an increasing number of clinicians. Atropine ointment (1%), instilled for 2 days prior to the refraction, is the best cycloplegic for children. Atropine sulfate (0.5%) ointment is preferred for children under age 1.

A good routine is to dilate and do retinoscopy on each child the first time he is seen in the office, even if he has had a refraction elsewhere. On subsequent visits, most alert children in the latter grade school years can be manifested, starting from the last objective data (Fig. 3–36). Hesitant responses or large changes should clue the examiner to repeat objective refraction (retinoscopy) and repeat cycloplegia.

The authors' personal prejudice is to employ streak retinoscopy with plus cylinders (after Copeland). Children are capable of either dial or cross-cylinder refraction.

Retinoscopy of infants in their mothers' laps without physical restraint and with hand-held lenses is possible in the overwhelming majority of children over 3 months of age. Cultivation of this art is well worth maximum effort. A final resort, after all whistling and cooing has failed, is to turn out all lights except that of the retinoscope (after Evans). With the retinoscope being the only light in the room, only the rarest child will not look at it. During retinoscopy, children are asked to look directly at the light of the retinoscope (Fig. 3–37).

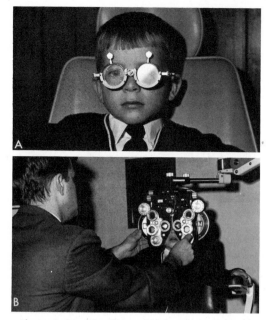

Figure 3–36   Manifest refraction is done only on follow-up visits. Trial frame technique (*A*) is generally superior to the phoropter (*B*) in the pediatric age group. In the very cooperative patient, however, the phoropter saves time.

Loose lenses must be used in very young children, and the thin-rimmed type is preferred. The Oculus trial frame for children is a good one (Fig. 3–38).

Children tolerate objective prescriptions and large changes far more readily than adults.

Slit Lamp and Aplanation Tension

As with many other aspects of examination, clinicians have surprised themselves at how much can be accomplished by simply *trying harder* with very young children at the slit lamp. Infants can usually be supported by the parent with one arm under the buttocks and the other hand on the back of the head (Fig. 3–39). Examination follows along adult lines except for the greater speed and patience required.

The examiner should be especially alert to routine examination of the retrolental space. Vitreous basitis (pars planitis) presents even more silently in childhood than in young adulthood.

Aplanation tonometry can be accomplished at this time. Since angle closure is

ever so rare in children, it is convenient to examine with the slit lamp and take the tension after dilatation.

Fundus Examination

Indirect ophthalmoscopy at one of the two lowest settings (2.5 or 4.0 V), with the child in the sitting position, is by far the best screening method. The ophthalmoscope can be called a "moon hat" and the child is told that if he looks hard enough, he can see the moon. Restraining children under two is often necessary but should be done only after an unrestrained attempt.

If the child is turned upside down in

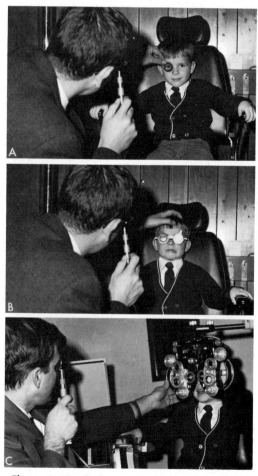

Figure 3–37   Retinoscopy with: (*A*) Hand-held spheres and cylinders, (*B*) trial frame, (*C*) phoropter. An increasing ability to cooperate is required from top to bottom.

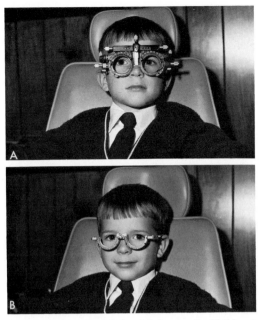

Figure 3–38 *A*, Adult trial frame; *B*, Children's trial frame (Oculus).

the parent's lap with his legs straddling the parent's waist, the head can be grasped between the parent's knees. The hands can be held by the parent across the chest and

the examiner has one hand free to support the lid (Fig. 3–40).

Older children will allow examination to and past the equator but far peripheral examination is justifiably omitted from the *routine* examination.

A record format will serve to summarize the routine children's examination described so far. It also will emphasize how much information can be gained by a well organized clinician in a brief 15 to 20 minutes (excluding waiting time for mydriasis).

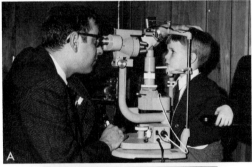

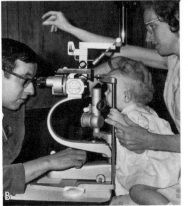

Figure 3–39 Slit lamp: *A*, Child; *B*, Infant.

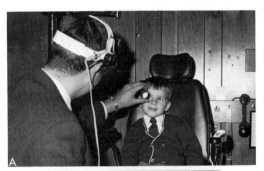

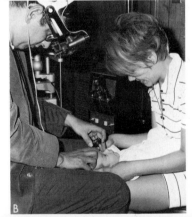

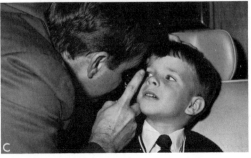

Figure 3–40 Ophthalmoscopy: *A*, preferred routine; *B*, uncooperative patient; *C*, undilated pupil on follow-up exams only, when manifest refraction alone is used.

Patient Record

Johnny Child (C.R. Child, 240 Post Oak, Phila.)
Age 4 (BD 6-26-67)
Birth weight
Birth and development
Past history
Family history
Previous eye care
Chief concern: Intermittently crossed eyes
Dir. questioning: Onset 6 mo. age, getting more freq. & longer dur.
Posture and demeanor: No head tilt, not hyperactive

OD 20/40	c−s Rx	← ───────With and without glasses
	FL−SL	← ───────Full Line, Single Letter presentation
OS 20/40	Sn−E−Fig	← ───────Snellen Letters−E game−Picture Figures

Wearing (date)

OS
OS

Cover testing:

ET 20

ET 25   ET 25 ET 25
            ET′ 40

ET 25

Versions: Slight OA SO OU (overaction of superior oblique, bilaterally)

Color vision: Normal
Stereo: Fly
Vert. Maddox rod: no hyper.

Cycloplegic: Cyclogyl 1% × 2 (blue irides)
Retinoscopy:

OD +3.25 +0.50 × 95	OD 20/40
OS +3.00 +0.50 × 85	OS 20/40

Slit lamp: Neg.
Tension: Attempted
Fundus: Neg.

Diagnosis: Esotropia, probably accommodative
Therapy: Full Rx given
Plan: Return in 3 weeks to re-evaluate deviation, repeat
     stereo, W4, give prognostication then.

Notice that conclusions, therapy, and plan are clearly outlined.

There is some danger that the contents of this paper may be misunderstood to imply that examination of the infant is so complex as to be accomplished only by a few. Quite to the contrary. It is felt that the overwhelming majority of clinicians can cultivate these abilities.

To be successful in the examination of children, the accomplished ophthalmologist should be

1. Convinced of the need for it.
2. Convinced that he can do it.

3. Sensitive to communications with children.
4. Flexible, adapting to the ability and willingness of children to cooperate.
5. Persistent in trying techniques, even though they frequently fail at a given age.

ADDENDUM

Examination Under Anesthesia

Keratometry can be done under anesthesia by removing the usual head brace and pushing the keratometer table up to the patient, with his head turned to the side. Pressure on the lids must obviously be avoided. The same warning applies to retinoscopy.

Aplanation tonometry can be done with the Draeger unit. Since all sedatives reduce the intraocular pressure, premedication, except for atropine, should be avoided. Anesthetic agents themselves lower the pressure, the least offender being Ketamine, an intramuscular or intravenous agent recently released by the FDA (Bryan, 1967). Tension should be measured immediately after induction.

Indirect and direct fundoscopy, gonioscopy, and slit lamp examination are also possible under anesthesia.

ACKNOWLEDGMENTS

Credit is given to several clinicians visited in 1969 (by the junior author) whose ideas and methods have been unblushingly borrowed. Chief credit goes to Marshall M. Parks. Other pediatric ophthalmologists visited include: Frank Costenbader (the world's first such subspecialist), Dan G. Albert, David Friendly, John O'Neill, David R. Stager, and Wills' own Robison D. Harley and Donelson R. Manley. Other ophthalmologists who do not limit their practice to children but who have special interest in strabismus and other problems of children were also visited, including Gunter von Noorden, Paul Romano Otto Lippmann, and William Phelps.

Special thanks to William Stenstrom for the art work and to David Silva for photography.

REFERENCES

Bryan, B.: Symposium on Intraocular Pressure Determination With General Anesthesia: A Review of the Literature. University of Texas Southwestern Medical School, Dallas, Texas. March, 1967.

Friendly, D.: Presentation to the Costenbader Club, April, 1970.

Ing, M., Costenbader, F. D., Parks, M. M., and Albert, D. G.: Early surgery for congenital esotropia. Amer. J. Ophthal., *61*:1419, 1966.

Lancaster, W. B.: Strabismus Symposium of the New Orleans Academy of Ophthalmology. St. Louis, The C. V. Mosby Co., 1958.

Linksz, A.: An Essay on Color Vision and Clinical Color Vision Tests. New York, Grune & Stratton, 1964.

Lippmann, Otto.: Vision of young children. Arch. Ophthal., *81*:763, June, 1969.

Parks, M. M.: Growth of the eye and development of vision. *In* Liebman and Gellis (eds.): The Pediatrician's Ophthalmology. St. Louis, The C. V. Mosby Co., 1966, pp. 15–25.

Parks, M. M.: Stereoacuity as an indicator of bifixation. International Strabismus Symposium, Basel, S. Karger, 1968.

Parks, M. M., and Eustis, A.: Monofixational esophoria. Amer. Orthopt. J., 1961.

Romano, P. E., and von Noorden, G.: Atypical responses to the four-diopter prism test. Amer. J. Ophthal., *67*:935–941, June, 1969.

Taylor, D. M.: How early is early in the management of strabismus. Arch. Ophthal., *70*:752, 1963.

CHAPTER 4

DIAGNOSTIC TECHNIQUES

FLUORESCEIN ANGIOGRAPHY

Jay L. Federman, M.D., and Lov K. Sarin, M.D.

Fluorescein has been used by the medical profession since it was first synthesized by von Baeyer in 1871. This unique dye was introduced to investigative ophthalmology by Paul Ehrlich in 1881. Its importance in the development of fundus angiography and as a clinical diagnostic test has only been exploited since the report of Novotny and Alvis in 1961. This to a large extent is the result of modern advances in technology. The sophisticated photographic equipment available to document fluorescein angiography has helped us to understand clinically the relationship of the retinal and choroidal circulation in normal and pathologic states of the fundus. Although this important study has been confined to large clinical centers, it can be used in the office as a diagnostic aid. A knowledge of a few basic properties of fluorescein, important related anatomic concepts, and normal fluorescein patterns is necessary to carry out and understand the fluorescein angiographic study.

CHEMICAL AND PHARMACOLOGIC PROPERTIES

Sodium fluorescein is a brown crystalline substance with a molecular weight of 376.27. It is highly water soluble and in aqueous solution is yellow-red in color. When excited, it fluoresces, emitting a yellow-green color. In vitro it is excited when radiant energy of 490 nm. is absorbed. This momentarily changes its electron vibrational state, and radiant energy of 520 nm. is emitted. The degree of fluorescence is dependent upon many factors, including pH, concentration, light intensity, and temperature.

In whole blood (in vivo) fluorescein is excited by radiant energy of 465 nm. and emits radiant energy of 524 nm.; 40 to 85 per cent of the dye is absorbed by plasma proteins (predominantly albumin), while 15 to 17 per cent is bound to erythrocytes. A small portion remains free as a negatively charged ion. Fluorescein is rapidly eliminated from the bloodstream by the kidneys and metabolized to a lesser extent by the liver. Most of it is excreted within an hour and is usually completely gone within 24 hours. Occasionally traces may be found 4 to 5 days after injection. The excretion of fluorescein in the urine will cause a positive Benedict's test, but will not show positive with Clinistix or test tapes.

Toxicity is rare, reactions ranging from mild itching, erythema, hives, nausea, and vomiting to anaphylactic type reactions. The incidence of all types of reactions is thought to be less than 1 per cent. An emergency tray, airway, oxygen, and emesis basin should be available when intravenous fluorescein is being administered. The emergency tray might include epinephrine, Benadryl, aramine, and steroids.

OFFICE TECHNIQUE

Although it is important to be able to document fluorescein angiography photographically, this test should by no means be confined only to large hospital centers. This test can easily be performed without the help of an assistant as an office procedure and should be used.

The area used for the study should be dark and the observer should be in a state of at least partial dark adaptation. It is important for the patient to be comfortable and prepositioned. One arm of the patient is extended for injection of the dye into the antecubital vein. A butterfly extension needle on a syringe with 5 cc. of 10 per cent fluorescein is placed in the vein. A slit lamp with a Goldmann or Hruby lens and a direct or indirect ophthalmoscope can be used to observe the study. We prefer the Haag-Streit slit lamp with a 3-mirror Goldmann lens. The indirect ophthalmoscope with a Nikon 20 D lens gives a better overall view than does the direct ophthalmoscope. When using a slit lamp, the cobalt blue filter is used. With the indirect or direct ophthalmoscope a Kodak 47 Wratten gelatin filter is placed over the light source. While observing the area of interest, the study is initiated by rapidly injecting the fluorescein over a 2- to 3-second period. The area should be carefully studied for approximately the first 30 seconds, at 3 to 5 minutes and at 20 to 60 minutes from the time of injection. The presence or absence of fluorescence should be documented. A simple chart (Table 4–1) filled in during the study may be helpful for interpretation later.

ANATOMIC CONSIDERATIONS

The normal retina has essentially no extracellular space and is completely transparent. In the macular area the inner

TABLE 4–1 FLUORESCENCE OF TISSUE ACCORDING TO PHASE

Tissue Observed	Filling Phase 6 to 30 sec.	Recirculation Phase 3 to 5 min.	Late Phase 20 to 60 min.
Disc	+	+	0,+
Retinal tissue	0	0	0
Retinal vasculature	++	+	0
Retinal pigment epithelium	0	0	0
Choroidal tissue	+	++	+
Choroidal vasculature	++	+	0
Lesion to be studied	?	?	?

0 = Negative fluorescence
+ = Weak to moderate fluorescence
++ = Marked fluorescence
? = Unknown

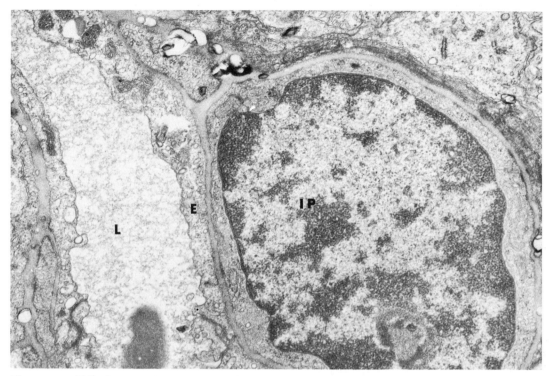

Figure 4–1 This electron micrograph shows a portion of a retinal capillary in cross section. The capillary endothelial cell (*E*) and intramural pericyte (*IP*) form the wall of the vessel. The endothelium shows a relatively constant thickness of cytoplasm limited on both sides by cell membrane with no apparent structures to allow a passive transfer of material from within the lumen (*L*) of the capillary to the surrounding retinal tissue. Human retina (uranyl acetate and lead citrate, ×28,100). (Courtesy of Dr. J. L. Federman.)

layers of the retina are pushed aside, these layers being absent in the fovea. Since the vasculature of the retina is confined to the inner layers, there are no retinal capillaries in the foveal area (Fig. 4–5B). The retinal vasculature can be considered as a completely closed system (Fig. 4–1). Under normal circumstances no fluorescein escapes from these vessels into the surrounding tissue. Therefore, during the normal angiographic study, the entire retinal vascular system is sharply defined as fluorescein-filled vessels surrounded by the transparent retinal tissue against the dark background of the retinal pigment epithelium (Fig. 4–5B).

The retinal pigment epithelium (Fig. 4–2) is a single layer of cells each of which is filled with approximately the same number of melanin granules. In the periphery these cells are flat and wide; they become more cuboid in shape in the posterior pole and columnar in the fovea. Therefore, as one approaches the fovea from the peripheral retina the layers of pigment

granules become much thicker. Depending upon the degree of pigmentation of the fundus, the view of the underlying choroidal circulation is markedly obscured in the macula as compared to the surrounding retina (Figs. 4–4 and 4–5A, B, and D). For this reason, the capillary network around the fovea and in the posterior pole is enhanced when filled with fluorescein (Fig. 4–5B). In addition to this optical effect, the retinal pigment epithelium is important physiologically in acting as a barrier to the passage of fluorescein from the choroid into the retina. Normally fluorescein is not thought to be taken into the pigment epithelium cells.

The choroid is a highly vascularized tissue supplying and draining the choriocapillaris, which is separated from the retinal pigment epithelium by Bruch's membrane. The capillary system in the choroid is fenestrated (Fig. 4–3) and there is a rapid, passive transport of fluorescein into Bruch's membrane and the surrounding extravascular space of the choroid.

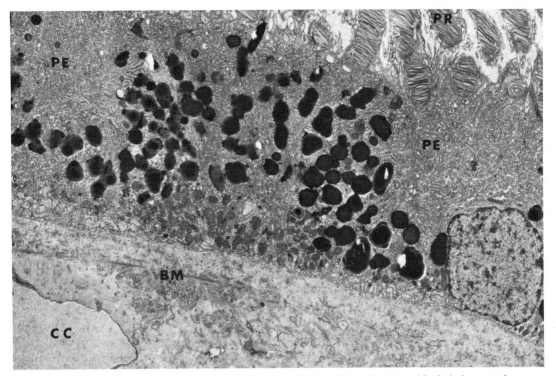

Figure 4–2 Electron micrograph showing retinal pigment epithelial cells (*PE*) with their large melanosomes separating the photo receptors (*PR*) of the retina from Bruch's membrane (*BM*) and the choriocapillaris (*CC*). Human retinal pigment epithelium (uranyl acetate and lead citrate, ×6000). (Courtesy of Dr. J. L. Federman.)

The vascular system of the choroid can thus be thought of as an open system as opposed to the closed vascular system of the retina.

The disc, anterior to the lamina cribosa, is composed of capillaries, nerve fibers, and glial supporting tissue. These capillaries, similar to the retina, show filling with no leakage into the surrounding tissue (Figs. 4–5*A*, *B*, and *C*). Because this tissue is transparent the structures behind are visualized. The lamina cribosa and the myelinated nerve fiber bundles of the optic nerve, permeated by connective tissue septa, both appear to fluoresce. The fluorescence of these structures is exaggerated because of their normal white color. The fluorescence of the disc is sharply demarcated by the surrounding retinal pigment epithelium (Figs. 4–5*A*, *B*, and *C*).

A basic knowledge of these anatomic concepts is necessary for a clear appreciation of the sequence of events in the normal fundus during fluorescein angiog-

raphy. Fluorescein patterns indicative of disease result from a breakdown of these anatomic and physiologic relationships. Thus, fluorescein angiography is an important aid in diagnosing and understanding the pathophysiology of many diseases.

NORMAL ANGIOGRAPHIC STUDY

The average arm to retina circulation time is approximately 10 to 13 seconds. The initial background choroidal fluorescence represents the filling of the choriocapillaris (Fig. 4–4) and is seen just prior to the appearance of fluorescein in the main retinal arteries. If a cilioretinal artery is present, it fills at the same time as the choriocapillaris (Fig. 4–4). The patchy filling of the choriocapillaris is first seen in the posterior pole and then spreads toward the periphery. Fluorescein is first seen in the main retinal arteries as the

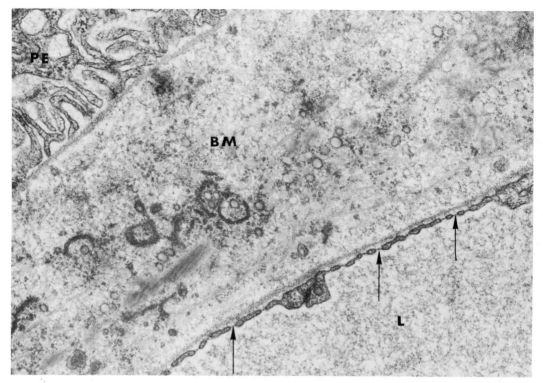

Figure 4–3   This electron micrograph shows in cross section the fenestrations (arrows) in the wall of a capillary of the choriocapillaris. These pores may act as openings to allow a passive transfer of material from within the lumen (*L*) of the capillary into Bruch's membrane (*BM*) and the surrounding extravascular tissue of the choroid. The basal infoldings of the retinal pigment epithelial cells (*PE*) are seen. Human choroid (uranyl acetate and lead citrate, ×36,000). (Courtesy of Dr. J. L. Federman.)

choriocapillaris in the midperiphery fills. This represents the arterial inflow phase (Fig. 4–5*A*) and occurs most rapidly in the peripapillary and macular areas. The venous outflow phase (Figs. 4–5*B* and *C*) preceded by the capillary transition phase

also occurs first in the peripapillary and macular areas.

After the initial filling of the choriocapillaris, fluorescein rapidly leaks out of the vessels into the extravascular choroidal tissue. Shortly, the concentration

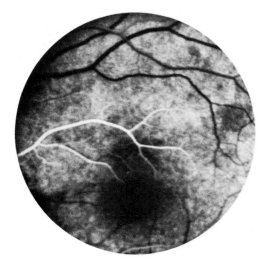

Figure 4–4   Normal fluorescein angiogram of the left eye of a 14-year-old white male clearly showing filling of the choriocapillaris (choroidal flush or choroidal filling phase) and cilioretinal artery before the retinal arteries fill with fluorescein. (Retinal Service, Lankenau Hospital.) (Courtesy of Dr. J. L. Federman.)

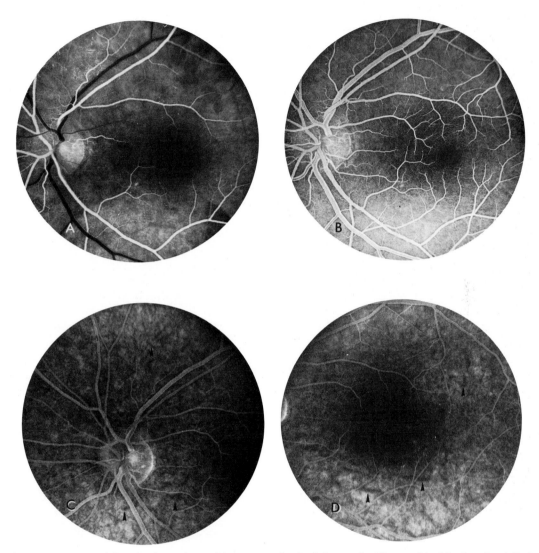

Figure 4–5 Normal fluorescein angiographic sequence in the left eye of a 12-year-old white female. *A*, Retinal arteries filled with fluorescein. The arterial phase and the capillary transition phase are complete. There is very early laminar filling of veins (early venous filling phase). The background choroidal flush is obscured by pigment at level of retinal pigment epithelium in the macula. Capillaries on the disc are filling with fluorescein. *B*. Venous phase showing fluorescein filling all retinal vessels. The fovea is free of retinal vessels. Retinal capillaries surrounding the fovea stand out against the high concentration of pigment at the level of the retinal pigment epithelium which is obscuring background choroidal fluorescence. Capillaries on disc are seen. *C*, Late venous phase showing fluorescence of disc, its borders sharply outlined by pigment at the level of the retinal pigment epithelium. The fluorescence of the lamina cribosa and nerve fiber bundles of the optic nerve is more pronounced through the small central optic cup. In the surrounding choroidal tissue the large choroidal vessels (arrows) are seen in dark relief against the more concentrated fluorescein-filled extravascular tissue. *D*, Recirculation phase showing fluorescein equally distributed throughout retinal vessels, but less concentrated than in Fig. 4–5*B*. The concentration of fluorescein is greater in the extravascular tissue compared to the intravascular space of the choroid. For this reason the large choroidal vessels (arrows) appear dark. (Retinal Service, Lankenau Hospital.) (Courtesy of Dr. J. L. Federman.)

Time After Injection	Phase
8–10 seconds	Choroidal vascular filling
10–12 seconds	Retinal arterial filling
11–13 seconds	Retinal capillary transition
12–14 seconds	Retinal venous drainage or filling
10–13 seconds	Choroidal extravascular filling
3–5 minutes	Recirculation
5–20 minutes	Removal fluorescein from vascular system
10–60 minutes	Removal fluorescein from choroidal extravascular tissue

in both intra- and extravascular spaces becomes equal. During the recirculation phase, when the intravascular concentration is less, one can see the choroidal vessels standing out against the surrounding fluorescein-filled tissue (Figs. 4–5C and D).

The important times and phases during the angiographic test to study or document are given in the accompanying chart. It is important to remember that these times vary from patient to patient, but normally the sequence remains unchanged.

ABNORMAL FLUORESCEIN ANGIOGRAPHY

Any disturbance to the normal physiology and normal anatomic relationships of the fundus will cause specific fluorescein angiographic patterns. Such patterns can be classified according to changes seen in the disc, retina, retinal pigment epithelium, and choroid.

Disc

The presence of fluid in the nerve fiber layer and subretinal fluid surrounding the disc margins seen in papilledema will cause fluorescence of the disc with indistinct margins (Fig. 4–6). It is difficult to differentiate pseudo from true papilledema with fluorescein. However, drusen (Fig. 4–7), choroidal hemangiomas, and capillary hamartomas are easily differentiated. Congenital variations of vessels, the presence of Bergmeister's papilla, optic pits, and coloboma will influence the normal angiographic pattern.

Retina

The presence of fluid within the retinal tissue due to trauma, inflammation (Figs.

4–6, 4–10, 4–22A and B), and vascular abnormalities (Figs. 4–16, 4–17A and B, and 4–18) will cause fluorescence of that tissue. The typical fluorescein pattern of cystoid macular edema (Figs. 4–22B and C) is seen secondary to inflammation and retinal tears. Hemorrhages (Figs. 4–6, 4–8, 4–9, and 4–19), whether preretinal or retinal, will obscure the background choroidal fluorescence and the retinal vasculature depending on the location in depth. Inflammatory tissue (Fig. 4–10) with or without fibrosis involving both choroid and retina will fluoresce. Inflam-

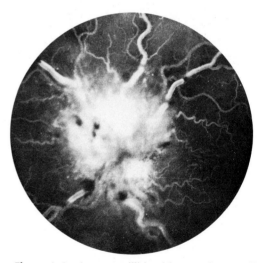

Figure 4–6 Acute papillitis with secondary papilledema seen in the left eye of a 15-year-old white male. There is a history of malaise and a diagnosis of cat scratch fever with positive lymph node biopsy. There is leakage of dye into the vitreous and the edematous tissue extending along the nerve fibers beyond the borders of the optic disc. Engorgement of the veins with blockage of the surrounding fluorescence by hemorrhages is seen. (Retina Service, Wills Eye Hospital. Terrance Tomer, photographer.)

Figure 4–7 Drusen of the optic disc seen in the right eye of an 18-year-old white male. These structures of a hyaline-like material will fluoresce, clearly differentiating this entity from true papilledema. (Retina Service, Wills Eye Hospital. Terrance Tomer, photographer.)

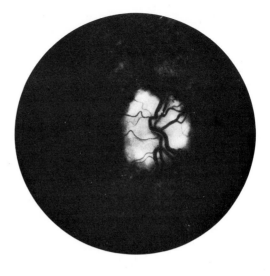

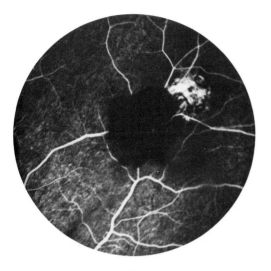

Figure 4–8 This 16-year-old white male with trauma to the left eye shows a superficial retinal hemorrhage extending into the vitreous which obscures the surrounding fluorescence. Adjacent to the hemorrhage is an area of chorioretinal inflammation which shows fluorescence. (Retina Service, Wills Eye Hospital. Terrance Tomer, photographer.)

Figure 4–9 This 18-year-old white female with angioid streaks received a traumatic blow to the right eye. Hemorrhages obscuring the surrounding fluorescence are seen along the course of all the angioid streaks. The left eye showed angioid streaks with no hemorrhages. (Courtesy of Dr. John McGavic, Retina Service, Wills Eye Hospital. Johnny Justice, photographer.)

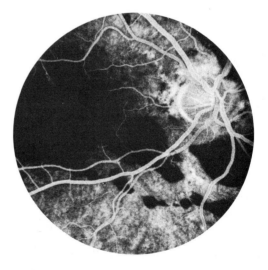

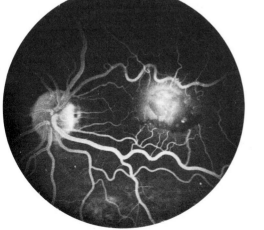

Figure 4–10 The right eye of an 8-year-old Negro male with a chorioretinal scar involving the macula. Hyperplasia of the retinal pigment epithelium obscures the surrounding fluorescence of the fibrous connective tissue. The differential diagnosis is traumatic chorioretinitis, congenital toxoplasmosis, and nematode endophthalmitis. (Retina Service, Wills Eye Hospital. Terrance Tomer, photographer.)

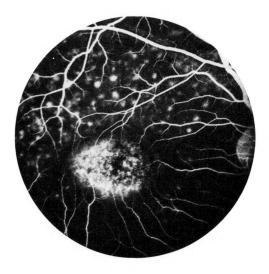

Figure 4–11 This 8-year-old white female with central heredodegeneration of the pigment epithelium (Stargardt's disease or Behr's disease) shows transmission of the choroidal fluorescence through small pigmented areas scattered around the macula. In the macula, in addition to transmission of the choroidal fluorescence, there is staining of intraretinal fibrous tissue. Here there is loss of central vision first. (Retina Service, Wills Eye Hospital. Terrance Tomer, photographer.)

mation of retinal vessels (Figs. 4–22A and B) will cause staining of the vessel wall and leakage of fluorescein into the surrounding retinal tissue. Various conditions which lead to aneurysmal and neovascular formations of the retinal vessels show leakage of fluorescein (Figs. 4–16, 4–17A and B, 4–18, and 4–19) due to abnormal permeability.

Retinal Pigment Epithelium

Changes in the distribution and concentration of the melanosomes at the level of the retinal pigment epithelium will influence the amount of transmission (Figs. 4–11 to 4–14), or obscuration (Figs. 4–10 and 4–12), of the background choroidal fluorescence. Collection of fluorescein within or just below the retinal pigment epithelial cells (Figs. 4–15A and B) will cause specific fluorescein patterns. Hemorrhage (Fig. 4–9) at the level of the retinal pigment epithelium will obscure the background choroidal fluorescence.

Choroid

Hemorrhages below the retinal pigment epithelial cells will obscure the background and surrounding fluorescence but may stain late, whereas a serous detachment stains early. Areas of inflammation may caused hyperfluorescence early and retention of dye late, whereas choroidal hemangiomas (Fig. 4–21) will show filling and hyperfluorescence early with little

(*Text continued on page 98.*)

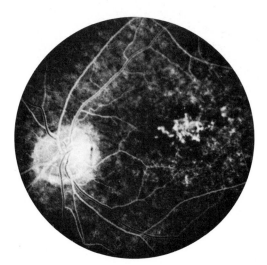

Figure 4–12 Seventeen-year-old white male with diffuse heredodegeneration of the pigment epithelium, probably a variant of the central type (Fig. 4–11) but may also be a type of retinitis pigmentosa. This patient complained of night blindness for the past 8 years before he noticed a decrease in central vision. Here there is transmission of the choroidal fluorescence through many small depigmented areas scattered throughout the fundus and in the macula. There is also obscuration of the choroidal fluorescence by pigment clumping in the macula. (Courtesy of Dr. P. Robb McDonald, Retinal Service, Lankenau Hospital, and Dr. J. L. Federman.)

Figure 4–13 The salt and pepper mottled appearance of the pigment epithelium in a patient with rubella retinitis. There is transmission of the background choroidal fluorescence through many small pigment epithelial defects. (Courtesy of Dr. Alfred Lucier, Retina Service, Wills Eye Hospital. Terrance Tomer, photographer.)

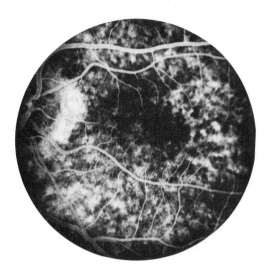

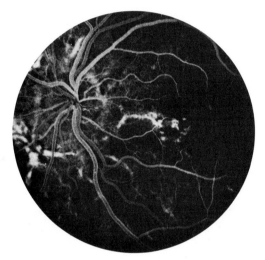

Figure 4–14 Angioid streaks seen in the right eye of this 16-year-old white male show transmission of the background choroidal fluorescence through the breaks in Bruch's membrane. These usually radiate from the optic disc and clinically may be confused with blood vessels. (Retina Service, Wills Eye Hospital. Terrance Tomer, photography.)

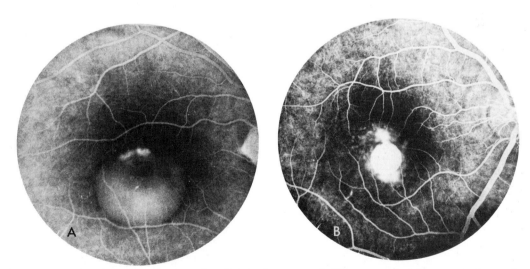

Figure 4–15 Heredomacular degeneration (Best's disease or vitelliform macular degeneration) seen in two brothers. *A*, Right eye of a 7-year-old white male showing pseudofluorescence of the typical egg yolk lesion at the level of the pigment epithelium. At this stage the visual acuity is still normal. *B*, Right eye of the 8-year-old brother showing true fluorescence of the egg yolk lesion centrally with adjacent small areas of fluorescence, indicating the beginning of the disruptive stage. Here the visual acuity is slightly less than normal. (Courtesy of Dr. Kenneth Nase, Retina Service, Wills Eye Hospital. Terrance Tomer, photographer.)

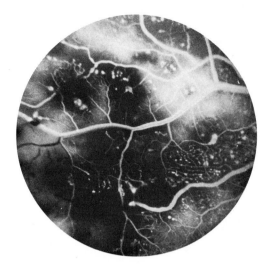

Figure 4–16 Fluorescein clearly shows the tel-angiectatic and aneurysmal beaded vessels in the right eye of this young male with Coats's disease. There is leakage of fluorescein with staining of the subretinal exudation. The left eye shows no changes. (Retina Service, Wills Eye Hospital. Terrance Tomer, photographer.)

Figure 4–17 Angiomatosis retinae (von Hippel's disease) seen in the right eye of an 18-year-old white female. *A*, The arterial phase shows the filling of the retinal capillary hamartoma with its large feeder arteriole. *B*, The venous phase shows the lesion completely filled with fluorescein, drained by a large tortuous venule. (Courtesy of Dr. William Annesley, Retina Service, Wills Eye Hospital. Terrance Tomer, photographer.)

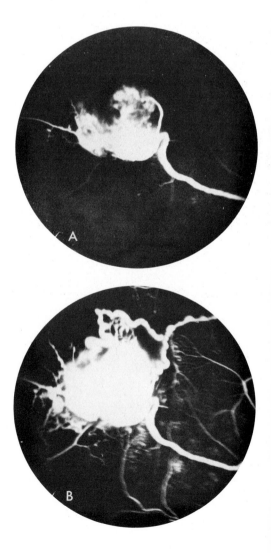

Figure 4–18 Right eye of a young Negro male with SC sickle cell disease showing leakage of fluorescein into the vitreous from the neovascular arteriovenous anastomoses. Note the retinal zone of avascularity peripheral to these formations. (Retina Service, Wills Eye Hospital. Terrance Tomer, photographer.)

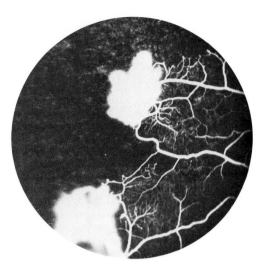

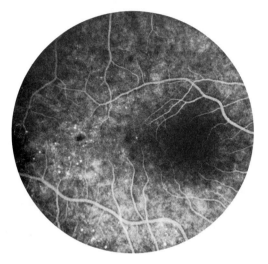

Figure 4–19 The posterior pole of the right eye of a young diabetic showing the retention of fluorescein by the microaneurysms and obscuration of the background choroidal fluorescence by small deep retinal hemorrhages. These early changes, not seen clinically, are clearly shown with fluorescein. (Retinal Service, Lankenau Hospital.) (Courtesy of Dr. J. L. Federman.)

Figure 4–20 Obscuration of the background choroidal fluorescence by a choroidal nevus (arrows) seen in the right eye of this young white male. (Retina Service, Wills Eye Hospital. Terrance Tomer, photographer.)

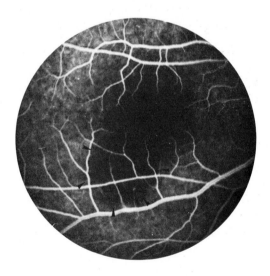

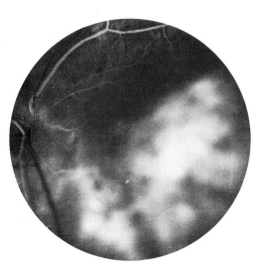

Figure 4–21 A large elevated choroidal hemangioma (Sturge-Weber disease) is seen in the left eye of this young white male. Marked filling of the vascular spaces within the choroidal hemangioma, with leakage, is already seen during the capillary transition phase of the retinal circulation. (Courtesy of Dr. William Annesley, Retina Service, Wills Eye Hospital. Terrance Tomer, photographer.)

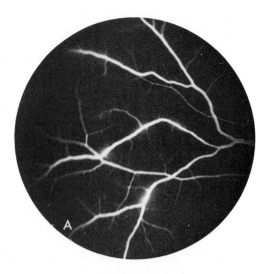

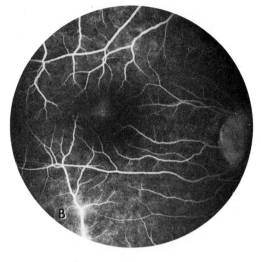

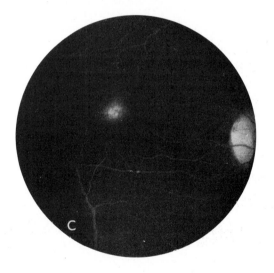

Figure 4–22 The right eye of a 17-year-old female with sarcoid uveitis. *A,* Fluorescein leaks from focal areas of periphlebitis along the course of retinal vessels in the midperiphery. *B,* Recirculation phase showing focal areas of periphlebitis in the posterior pole. Fluorescein is beginning to accumulate in the retinal tissue in the macular area. *C,* Late phase angiogram shows increased fluorescence of the macula in a typical pattern of cystoid macular edema. (Retina Service, Wills Eye Hospital. Terrance Tomer, photographer.)

late fluorescence. A choroidal nevus (Fig. 4–20) will often block out the surrounding choroidal fluorescence and does not stain, whereas a malignant melanoma or metastatic tumor may show an abnormal circulation and stains both early and late.

REFERENCES

Amalric, P., Bessou, P., and Biau, C.: Aspects of fluoresceiniques de la papille et de la région peri-papilaire. Bull. Soc. Franc. Ophthal., *80*:334, 1967.

Archer, D, Krill, A. E., and Newell, F. W.: Fluorescein studies of normal choroidal circulation. Amer. J. Ophthal., *69*:543, 1970.

Cunha-Vaz, J. G., and Maurice, D. M.: The active transport of fluorescein by the retinal vessels and the retina. Physiol. J., *191*:465, 1967.

Curry, H. F., Jr., and Moorman, L. T.: Fluorescein photography of vitelliform macular degeneration. Arch. Ophthal., *79*:705, 1968.

Dollery, C. T., Hodge, J. V., and Engel, M.: Studies of the retinal circulation with fluorescein. Brit. Med. J., *2*:1210, 1962.

Dollery, C. T., Mailer, C. M., and Hodge, J. V.: Studies of fluorescence photography of papilloedema in malignant hypertension. J. Neurol. Neurosurg. Psychiat., *28*:241, 1965.

Ernest, J. T., and Krill, A. E.: Fluorescein studies in fundus flavimaculatus and drusen. Amer. J. Ophthal. *62*:1, 1966.

Gass, J. D. M.: Stereoscopic Atlas of Macular Diseases, A Funduscopic and Angiographic Presentation. St. Louis, The C. V. Mosby Co., 1970.

Gebler, P., and Shah, A.: Fluorescein study of

albipunctate dystrophy. Arch. Ophthal, *81*:164, 1969.

Krill, A. E.: The retinal disease of rubella. Arch. Ophthal., 77:445, 1967.

Krill, A. E., and Chishti, M. I.: Fluorescein studies in diseases affecting the pigment epithelium. Trans. Amer. Opthal. Soc., 66:269, 1968.

Krill, A. E., Morse, P. A., Potts, A., and Klein, B.: Hereditary vitelliruptive macular degeneration. Amer. J. Ophthal., *61*:1405, 1966.

Krill, A. E., Newell, F., and Chishti, M. I.: Fluorescein studies ,in diseases affecting the pigment epithelium. Amer. J. Ophthal., 66:470, 1968.

Maeda, H., Ishida, N., Kawauchi, H., and Tuzimura, K.: Reactions of fluorescein-isothiocyanate with proteins and amino acids. Biochem. J., 65:777, 1968.

Miller, S. J. H., Sander, M. D., and Feytche, T. J.: Fluorescein fundus photography in the detection of early papilloedema and its differentiation from pseudo-papilloedema. Lancet, 2:651, 1965.

Morse, P. H., and MacLean, A.: Fluorescein fundus studies in hereditary vitelliruptive macular degeneration. Amer. J. Ophthal., 66:485, 1968.

Novotny, H., and Alvis, D. L.: A method of photographing fluorescence in circulating blood in the human retina. Circ., *124*:82, 1961.

O'Day, D., Crock, G., Galbraith, J. E. K., Parel, J. M., and Wigley, A.: Fluorescein angiography of normal and atrophic optic disc. Lancet, 2:224, 1967.

Rubin, M. L., Kaufman, H. E., Tierney, J. P., and Lucas, H. C.: Intraretinal nematode. Trans. Amer. Acad. Ophthal. Otolaryng., 72:885, 1968.

Sanders, M. D., and Ffutche, T. J.: Fluorescein angiography in the diagnosis of drusen of the disc. Trans. Ophthal. Soc. U.K., 87:861, 1967.

Stein, M. R., and Parker, C. W.: Reactions following intravenous fluorescein. Amer. J. Ophthal., 72: 861, 1971.

Welch, R., Maumenee, E., and Wahlen, H. E.: Peripheral posterior segment inflammation, vitreous opacities, and edema of the posterior pole. Arch. Ophthal., 64:540, 1960.

Wessing, A., and VanNoorden, G. K.: Fluorescein Angiography of the Retina. Textbook and Atlas. St. Louis, The C. V. Mosby Co., 1969.

Zweng, H. C., Little, H. L., and Peabody, R. R.: Laser photocoagulation and retina angiography. St. Louis, The C. V. Mosby Co., 1969.

ULTRASONOGRAPHY IN PEDIATRIC OPHTHALMOLOGY

Jerry A. Shields, M.D., and Lov K. Sarin, M.D.

INTRODUCTION

Ultrasonography is an important diagnostic technique in several fields of modern medicine. In recent years it has become popular in ophthalmology, and it is used extensively in many eye centers. It is particularly important as a diagnostic adjunct in the evaluation of eyes with opaque media, but it has other applications as well. This chapter will deal with the practical use of diagnostic ultrasonography in pediatric ophthalmology.

PRINCIPLES AND EQUIPMENT

The basic physics of ultrasonography as applied to ophthalmic diagnosis are discussed in detail in textbooks on this subject. Briefly, when a transmitted wave of ultrasound meets an interface of different acoustic impedance, one portion is reflected as an echo and another portion passes through the tissue until it meets another interface of different acoustic impedance. The portion that is reflected forms an echo pattern which may be displayed on an oscilloscope and photographed (Fig. 4–23).

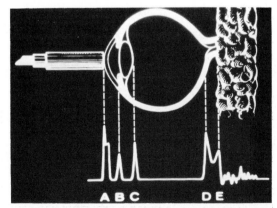

Figure 4–23 Diagram showing relationship between normal ultrasonogram and ocular tissues. (*A*) Opening echo from the cornea. (*B*) Anterior lens surface. (*C*) Posterior lens surface. (*D*) Posterior wall of globe. (*E*) Orbital fat.

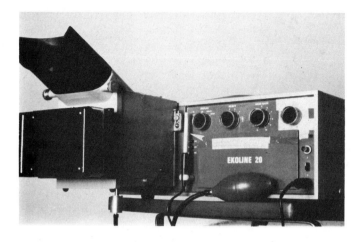

Figure 4–24   Ekoline 20′ A-scan unit. On the left is a camera over the oscilloscope for immediate polaroid photographs. The white arrow indicates the transducer. (Courtesy of Smith-Kline Instrument Co.)

Two types of diagnostic ultrasound are widely used in ophthalmology. The A-scan (time amplitude) provides a linear pattern with an echo or "spike" representing each change in acoustic impedance within the eye. The B-scan technique yields an acoustic cross section of the eye that resembles a histological slide of the globe and consequently is easier to interpret. In our clinic we have used the Ekoline 20′ A-scan unit from the Smith Kline Instrument Company (Fig. 4–24), the Bronson-Turner B-scan unit (Fig. 4–25), and the Sonometrics Ophthalmoscan unit which incorporates both the A-scan and B-scan techniques (Fig. 4–26A). The Ophthalmoscan utilizes a water bath placed around the eye as a coupling medium (Fig. 4–26B). Most of this chapter will discuss B-scan ultrasonography which is more widely used today.

TECHNIQUE

In the case of the Ekoline unit, topical anesthesia is utilized, and the ultrasound transducer is placed directly on the cornea or sclera with the use of a coupling medium such as methylcellulose. In uncooperative children, the transducer may be placed on the closed eyelid rather than on the cornea, although this decreases the accuracy of measuring ocular dimensions.

With the Bronson-Turner unit, the transducer, again with the use of a coupling medium such as methylcellulose, is placed directly on the closed eyelid. Consequently, this test can easily be performed on uncooperative or crying children and satisfactory readings obtained.

The Sonometrics Ophthalmoscan unit is very precise. Because of the necessity of the water bath around the eye being

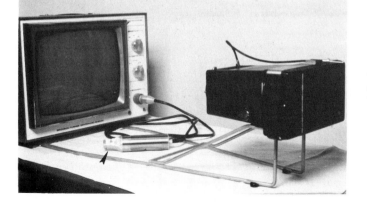

Figure 4–25   Bronson-Turner B-scan unit. The echoes detected with the transducer (arrow) may be displayed on the television screen and photographed. (Courtesy of Storz Instrument Co., St. Louis.)

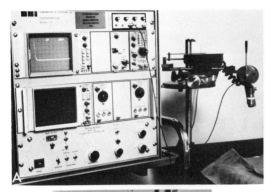

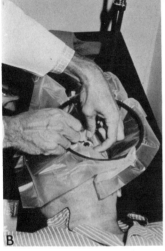

Figure 4–26 *A*, Sonometrics ophthalmoscan unit. The screen above displays the A-scan and the one below displays the B-scan. The hand-operated transducer is shown on the right. *B*, Application of the water bath. A water-tight plastic drape holds the water over the eye during the test. (Purchased through Medical Instruments Research Associates, Boston.)

tested, however, it is difficult to utilize this unit with infants and uncooperative children unless general anesthesia is employed.

THE NORMAL ULTRASONOGRAM

A normal A-scan pattern is shown in Figure 4–27. Distinct spikes can be obtained at the cornea, anterior lens, posterior lens, and posterior bulbar complex. Diffuse echoes occur from the orbital tissues.

A normal B-scan ultrasonogram done with the Bronson-Turner unit is shown in Figure 4–28. Details of the anterior segment cannot be resolved, but the pos-

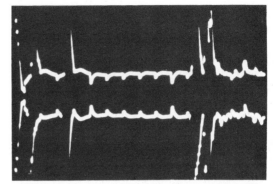

Figure 4–27 Normal A-scan ultrasonogram. The echoes correspond with those seen in Figure 4–23, with the cornea to the left and the orbit to the right. By convention, the upper pattern represents the right eye and the lower pattern, the left.

teriorly located structures can be adequately evaluated.

A normal B-scan pattern with the Sonometrics Ophthalmoscan unit is shown in Figure 4–29. The resolution of the an-

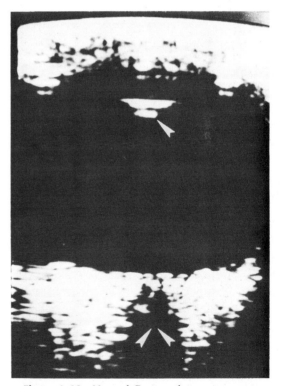

Figure 4–28 Normal B-scan ultrasonogram performed with the Bronson-Turner unit. The cornea is above and the orbit below. The top arrow demonstrates the posterior lens echo and the bottom arrow shows the optic nerve shadow. The large black area in the center represents normal vitreous.

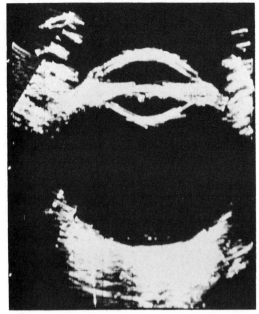

Figure 4–29 Normal B-scan ultrasonogram as seen with the Sonometrics ophthalmoscan unit. Note that the cornea, iris, and lens are clearly delineated and that the picture is similar to a histologic section of a globe.

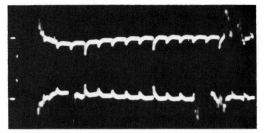

Figure 4–30 Abnormally long globes in high myopia. The right eye (*above*) measures 30 mm. in anteroposterior diameter, and the left eye (*below*) measures 26 mm.

terior segment is quite distinct, and the cornea, iris, and lens, as well as the posterior portion of the globe and orbit can be well delineated.

THE ABNORMAL ULTRASONOGRAM

Ultrasonography can provide useful clinical information in the following conditions:
1. abnormal size of the eye;
2. certain congenital abnormalities;
3. cataracts and subluxated lenses;
4. vitreous alterations;
5. retinal detachments;
6. intraocular tumors;
7. ocular trauma such as penetrating injuries or intraocular foreign bodies;
8. orbital tumors, foreign bodies, and inflammation.
It is most useful in eyes with opaque media such as corneal opacities, cataracts, or vitreous hemorrhage. In such instances, important clinical information can often be obtained.

Any currently available ultrasound unit may be employed to evaluate the size of the globe. If the ultrasound measurements indicate a large eye, one might suspect congenital glaucoma or myopia (Fig. 4–30). If the eye is smaller than normal, one may consider phthisis bulbi, persistent hyperplastic primary vitreous, or other causes of microphthalmos (Fig. 4–31).

Ultrasound may be helpful in the evaluation of certain congenital abnormalities within the eye. It can be utilized to detect the extent of the hyaloid remnants and retinal detachment in cases of persistent hyperplastic primary vitreous (Fig. 4–32). In such cases the scans should be taken through several planes, because it is often difficult to illustrate the entire hyaloid system in one section.

Certain abnormalities of the lens may be detected and evaluated with ultrasound. For example, in the case of cataracts, we see increased echoes from the posterior lens which outline the configuration of the lens better than in the normal state (Fig. 4–33). This is useful to the corneal surgeon

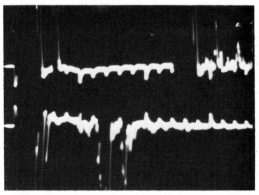

Figure 4–31 Microphthalmia of the left eye. The right eye (*above*) measures 24 mm. in anteroposterior diameter, whereas the left eye (*below*) is only 12 mm. in length.

Figure 4–32   B-scan ultrasonogram of posterior hyperplastic primary vitreous. The mound posteriorly represents a focal mass of tissue over the optic disc (arrows). The linear echo in the vitreous represents persistent hyaloid vessels.

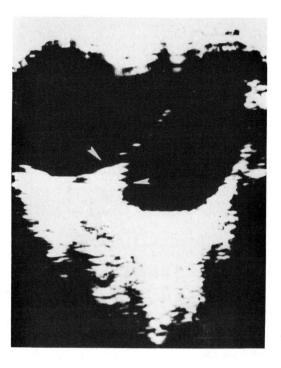

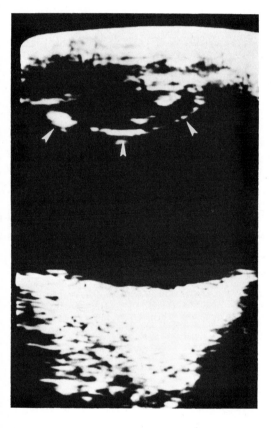

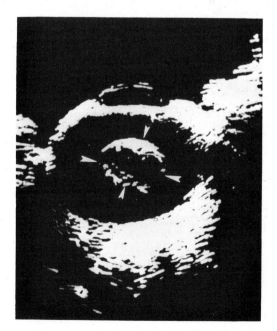

Figure 4–33   Dense cataract. Note that the lens can be outlined better than in the normal ultrasonogram (arrows).

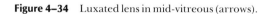

Figure 4–34   Luxated lens in mid-vitreous (arrows).

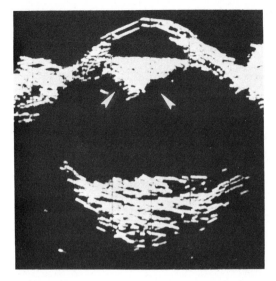

Figure 4–35 Dense cyclitic membrane (arrows).

Figure 4–36 Diffuse echoes in the vitreous representing vitreous hemorrhage (arrows). These echoes disappear when the sensitivity is decreased slightly.

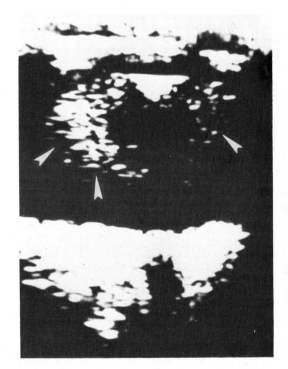

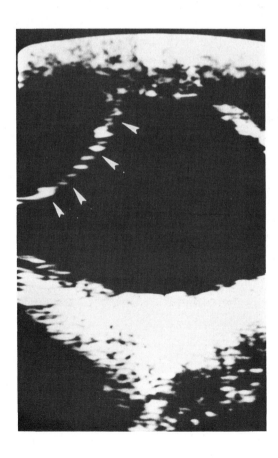

Figure 4–37 Choroidal detachment, showing a linear echo passing from the region of pars plana to the equator (arrows).

who may want to know whether a cataract is present when he is planning a corneal transplant. Subluxated or totally luxated lenses may be demonstrated with ultrasound as well (Fig. 4–34).

In eyes which have experienced inflammation or trauma, one can sometimes demonstrate a cyclitic membrane in the retrolental area (Fig. 4–35). It is clinically important to the surgeon planning a cataract extraction to know that such a dense membrane exists behind the cataractous lens.

The degree and extent of a vitreous hemorrhage may also be demonstrated with ultrasound. Hemorrhage appears as diffuse echoes in the vitreous cavity which tend to disappear when the sensitivity of the machine is lowered (Fig. 4–36).

In eyes that have hypotony secondary to surgical or nonsurgical trauma, ultrasound may demonstrate the presence and size of a detachment of the choroid (Fig. 4–37). In such cases, a linear echo within the globe extends from the pars plana region to the equator. Ultrasound can localize the best site for surgical drainage of fluid in such instances.

Ultrasound is most useful in detecting the presence of a retinal detachment in eyes with opaque media. In the case of a total retinal detachment, a typical linear echo extends from the optic nervehead to the region of the ora serrata (Fig. 4–38). This configuration differs from the choroidal detachment mentioned above. The lack of echoes posterior to this linear pattern indicates that the detachment is probably a serous rather than a solid type. It is particularly important to do ultrasound on children with traumatic cataracts prior to performing cataract surgery (Fig. 4–39). In some instances, ultrasound may be useful in determining the pathogenesis of a retinal detachment. For example, ultrasound can occasionally demonstrate a retinal dialysis, which is highly suggestive of previous trauma (Fig. 4–40). Consequently, ultrasound may have medicolegal as well as clinical importance.

The evaluation of intraocular tumors in children may be facilitated with the use of ultrasound. In contrast to the serous detachment of the retina, tumors usually demonstrate a solid pattern (Fig. 4–41). The ultrasound technique is particularly

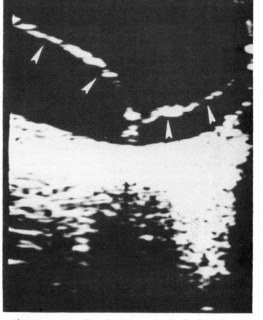

Figure 4–38 Total serous retinal detachment. Note the linear echoes passing from the optic disc to the ora serrata (arrows).

useful in those instances where a retinoblastoma presents in an atypical clinical manner such as vitreous hemorrhage (Fig. 4–42). Ultrasound is also useful in the diagnosis of other intraocular tumors in children. Malignant melanomas, although rare in children, may be easily diagnosed with this technique (Fig. 4–43).

Ultrasound may be useful in the diagnosis and evaluation of inflammatory detachments. In these cases, a small, solid mass may be seen in association with a total retinal detachment (Fig. 4–44). This may be similar to a tumor with an adjacent retinal detachment, and in such cases the clinical history may be important in arriving at the proper diagnosis.

In children with ocular trauma, ultrasonography may be a very useful diagnostic adjunct. After a penetrating injury to the globe, one can often demonstrate echoes along the course of the penetrating object. These are due to organizing hemorrhage along the penetrating tract

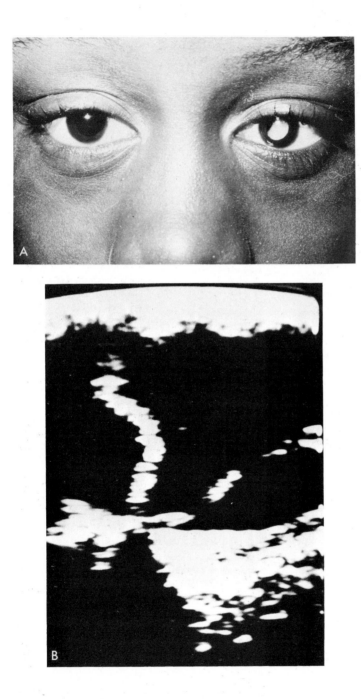

Figure 4–39 *A,* Child with opaque traumatic cataract in the left eye. *B,* Ultrasound shows a total serous retinal detachment.

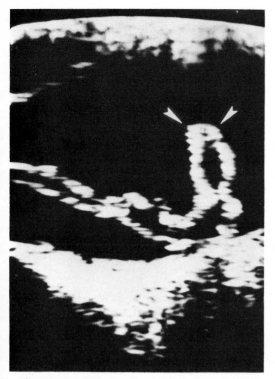

Figure 4–40 Giant retinal dialysis. Note that the linear echo does not extend to the ora serrata, but rather folds back upon itself in the mid-vitreous (arrows). Child had ocular trauma from parental abuse.

(Fig. 4–45). Such a pattern helps the clinician determine the extent of the injury and tells the surgeon where to look for a possible posterior rupture of the globe.

The use of ultrasound in the diagnosis and evaluation of intraocular foreign bodies is well established. With the use of ultrasound, the foreign body can be demonstrated as a dense echo in the vitreous, although at high sensitivities it may be difficult to differentiate the presence of a foreign body from a hemorrhage within the vitreous (Fig. 4–46A). When the sensitivity is lowered, however, the echo from the foreign body will persist, whereas that from the hemorrhage will disappear (Fig. 4–46B). Ultrasound can be further used to evaluate foreign bodies in conjunction with a magnet. If an intraocular foreign body is magnetic, it will move abruptly toward a magnet placed against the adjacent sclera. This movement can be visualized on the oscilloscope, enabling the surgeon to evaluate whether or not a foreign body is magnetic prior to taking the patient to the operating room for its removal. Ultrasound may also be used to

check the accuracy of x-ray localization of a foreign body. In contrast to x-ray, ultrasound permits precise localization of the wall of the globe, and thus with ultrasound, a foreign body lying immediately in front of the retina will not be falsely localized in the retrobulbar area. It is not uncommon for x-ray to show a foreign body localized in the anterior portion of the orbit, whereas ultrasound will verify that it is actually in the globe.

The role of ultrasound in the diagnosis of various conditions of the orbit is increasing. It is utilized to localize and sometimes to differentiate a number of orbital tumors, orbital cysts, orbital foreign bodies, and, in some cases, inflammatory processes within the orbit.

In patients with proptosis, one can often demonstrate the location, size, and sometimes the diagnosis of an orbital tumor (Fig. 4–47). An orbital cyst will show an acoustically empty area, although at times it may be difficult to differentiate such cysts from a tumor.

Orbital foreign bodies within the retrobulbar areas can be demonstrated with ultrasound and documented by lowering the sensitivity of the machine as we have in-

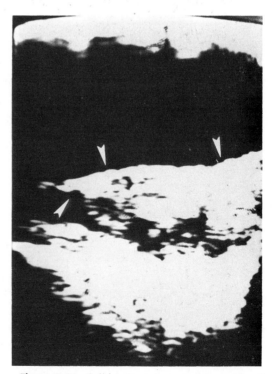

Figure 4–41 Solid pattern in posterior portion of globe, compatible with intraocular tumor (arrows). Diagnosis was retinoblastoma.

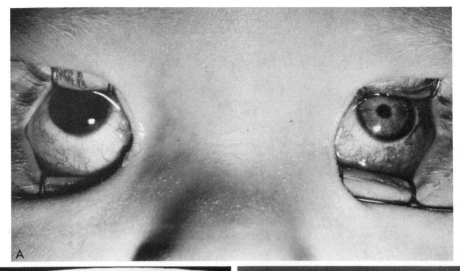

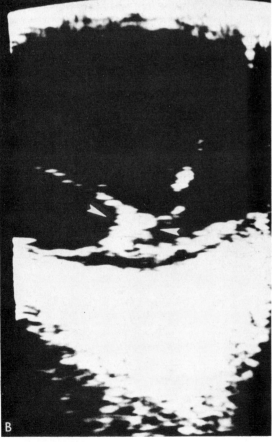

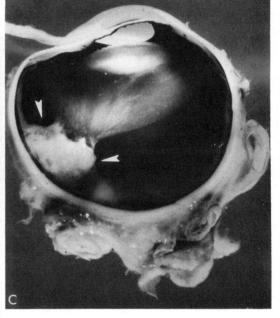

Figure 4–42 *A*, Clinical photograph of one-year-old child with spontaneous vitreous hemorrhage OD. *B*, Ultrasound showing solid mass in posterior pole with linear echoes into vitreous (arrows). *C*, Section of the gross globe showing retinoblastoma corresponding to the solid echo seen with ultrasound (arrows). The linear echoes were due to hemorrhage along the posterior surface of a totally detached vitreous.

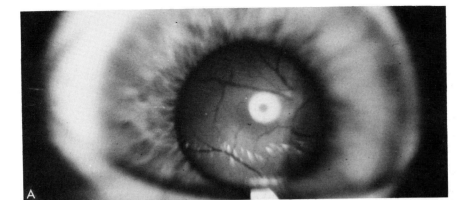

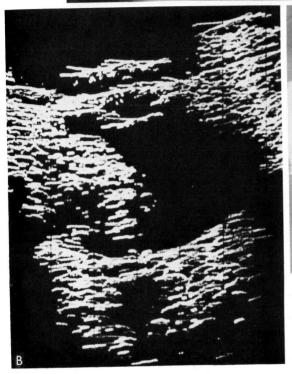

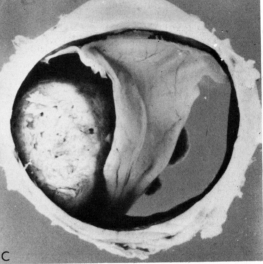

Figure 4–43 *A*, Clinical photograph of a total retinal detachment in a 15-year-old patient. A clear view of the posterior segment could not be obtained. *B*, Ultrasound showing dome-shaped tumor pattern on nasal side. *C*, Section of gross globe showing large malignant melanoma of choroid corresponding to the tumor pattern noted with ultrasound.

dicated with intraocular foreign bodies. Inflammatory processes within the orbit can be diagnosed by the absence of a space-occupying lesion, and sometimes by thickened rectus muscles characteristically seen in thyroid ophthalmopathy.

SUMMARY

Diagnostic ultrasound has many practical applications in pediatric ophthalmology. It is useful in the evaluation of patients with abnormal eye size, as seen in congenital glaucoma or microphthalmia. It is helpful in detecting cyclitic membranes, vitreous hemorrhage, retinal detachments, tumors, and other such conditions when opaque media preclude visualization of the fundus. In eyes that have experienced trauma, ultrasound is useful in delineating the extent of penetrating injuries or the presence of intraocular or orbital foreign bodies. In addition, it may be utilized to localize and diagnose orbital tumors, cysts, foreign bodies, and inflammatory conditions. It is an important diagnostic adjunct in pediatric ophthalmology.

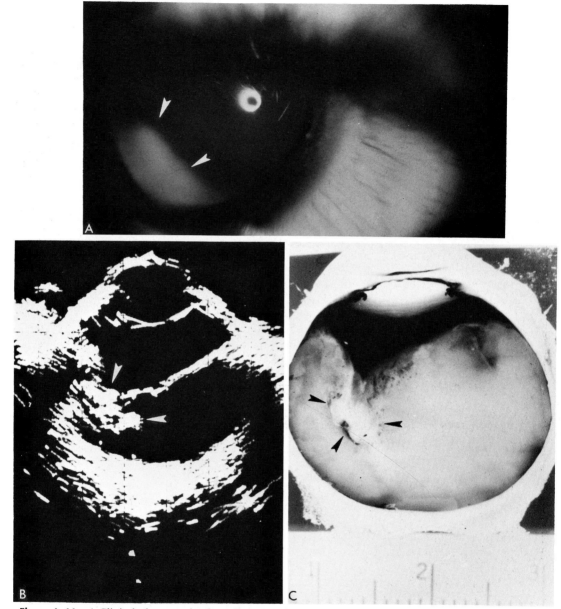

Figure 4–44 *A*, Clinical photograph of a yellow mass in the vitreous of a ten-year-old child (arrows). *B*, Ultrasound showing a semi-solid mass (arrows) with a total retinal detachment. *C*, Section of gross globe showing inflammatory mass (arrows). Diagnosis was presumed nematode endophthalmitis.

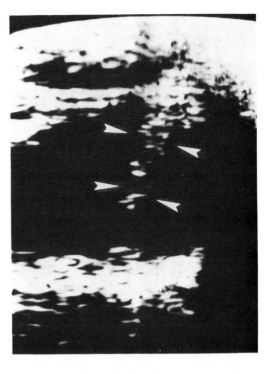

Figure 4–45   Focal echoes in vitreous due to hemorrhage along tract of penetrating injury (arrows).

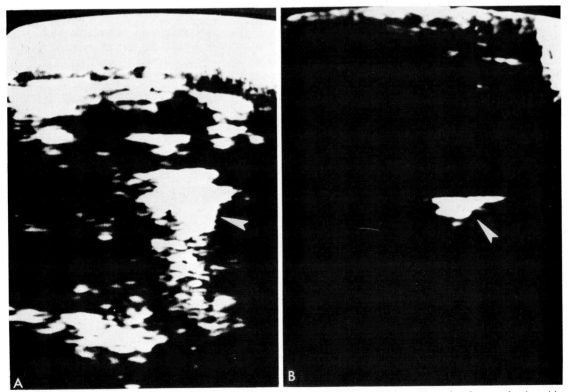

Figure 4–46   *A*, Diffuse echoes throughout vitreous representing hemorrhage. Note the dense echo in midvitreous (arrow). *B*, By lowering the sensitivity, all of the hemorrhage and soft tissue echoes disappear, but the dense echo persists (arrow). This is diagnostic of an intraocular foreign body.

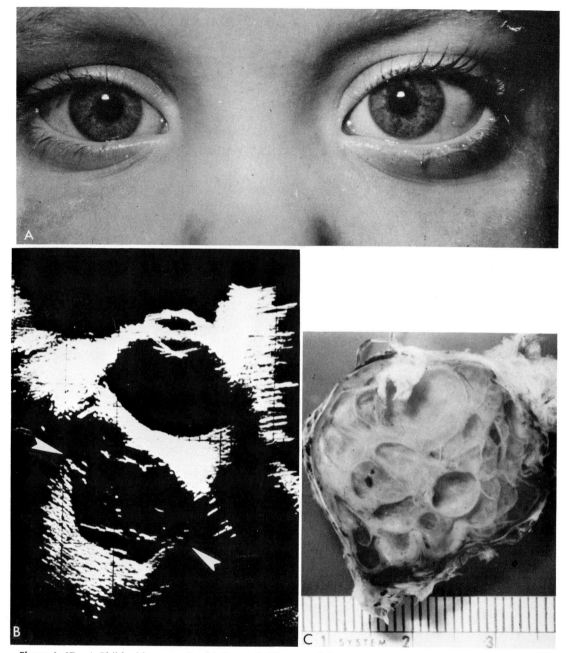

Figure 4–47 *A,* Child with proptosis of left eye. *B,* Ultrasound demonstrated a large orbital mass (arrows). The ultrasound diagnosis was probable orbital hemangioma. *C,* Surgically removed specimen showing cavernous hemangioma of orbit.

REFERENCES

Bronson, N. R., Jr.: A simple B-scan ultrasonoscope. Arch. Ophthal. *90*:237, 1973.

Coleman, D. J., Konig, W. F., and Katz, L.: A hand operated ultrasound scan system for ophthalmic evaluation. Amer. J. Ophthal. *68*:256, 1969.

Gitter, K. A., Meyer, D., and Sarin, L. K.: The use of ultrasound in the diagnosis of eyes with opaque media. Amer. J. Ophthal. *64*:100, 1967.

Gitter, K. A., Meyer, D., White, R. H., Jr., Ortolan, G., and Sarin, L. K.: Ultrasonic aid in the evaluation of leukocoria. Amer. J. Ophthal. *65*:190, 1968.

Gitter, K. A., Keeney, A. H., Sarin, L. K., and Myer, D. (eds.): Ophthalmic Ultrasound: Proceedings of the 1968 International Congress of Ultrasonography in Ophthalmology. St. Louis, The C. V. Mosby Co., 1969.

Goldberg, R. E., and Sarin, L. K. (eds.): Ultrasonics in Ophthalmology. Philadelphia, W. B. Saunders Co., 1967.

CHAPTER 5

REFRACTION AND HETEROPHORIA

EDWIN C. TAIT, M.D.

REFRACTION

BASIC CONCEPTS

The refractive procedure for children does not differ greatly from that for adults except in two major areas. First, there is an age limit below which no subjective confirmation of the objective findings can be accomplished, and second, the examiner must be inventive and be able to adjust his thinking and performance to meet the level of understanding and cooperation of the child. It is unusual for a child of 4 years or younger to give any meaningful answers to the usual refractive question of whether a lens makes the vision better or worse. In most instances, the final refractive error must be determined from the objective means of retinoscopy. After the child has learned to respond to a visual acuity chart, it is often more meaningful to have him try to read successively smaller letters as lenses are varied rather than ask him to compare clarity until a maximum visual acuity is obtained.

Some 5-year-old and often 7-year-old children can give a fairly reliable subjective answer to the question of better or worse and children above this age group can be refracted much the same as the adult group.

TECHNIQUE OF PEDIATRIC REFRACTION

The physician must genuinely enjoy children and young people and create an atmosphere of unhurried efficiency. Any show of impatience is quickly detected by the child and no more playful cooperation may be expected.

Small children always behave better sitting on a parent's lap and infants will require a nursing bottle or pacifier to remain still. Sudden movements are to be avoided. Playing with the retinoscope light about the child's hands or legs or examining the mother first are reassuring measures for the child.

The refractionist must be expert with adults before attempting an examination on a child. One must depend on objective measurements to a large degree and frequently the observation must be performed during a short interval. Holding the child's head should be done only as a last resort.

Children are easier to examine and less fearful if other children are nearby but not distracting. The room should be partially lighted, except in the case of infants who will look at a light best in total darkness.

Retinoscopy of a child's eye can be best performed with loose lenses. The regular trial frame cannot be used before age 3, although there are some child's frames which can be tolerated. The phoropter cannot be used well on small children be-

cause they do not hold their heads still nor do they fixate for more than a few seconds at a time.

Fixation can be maintained on the refractionist's forehead for brief intervals if the child's attention can be directed toward some imaginary object.

Visual Acuity

In order to have a useful notation of *visual acuity*, it is necessary to have some vision testing systems which can be used for preschool children and adjustable for youngsters of school age. Figure 5–1

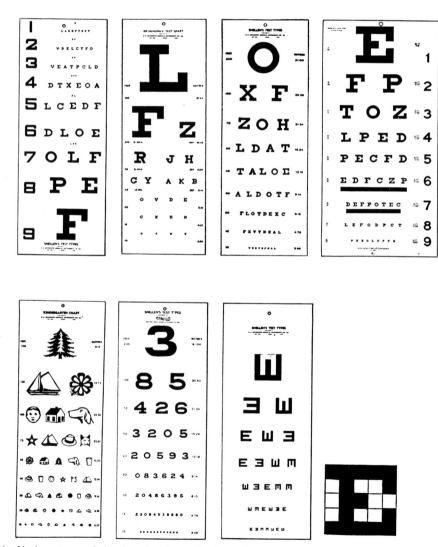

Figure 5–1   Various types of visual acuity charts (Snellen), designed so that the objects will subtend a 5-minute angle at the given distance. Their details subtend a 1-minute angle as far as possible. The **E** at lower right illustrates this principle in its construction.

shows a sampling of the charts which have been devised.

The two most useable are the outlines of familiar objects and the E chart. These charts are adaptable to projection type instruments. One of the poor features with the outline chart is that the exposure of children to outlines varies considerably and not all are familiar with the objects, especially those in the disadvantaged groups. The E chart is useful from about the age of 3, and in many instances if the examiner or an assistant will first demonstrate with his or her fingers regarding the chart, the patient will be able to learn in one short session. If necessary, the mother can be instructed to teach the child at home. The E chart has been successful in the preschool screening tests. In the very young child, a notation of the fixation may be the only visual notation possible.

It must be remembered that the average child does not respond to 6/6 vision until about 5 years of age and before this age 6/9 may be normal. Also, at any age not all eyes resolve to 6/6 even though no pathologic condition or excessive refraction can be observed. In the presence of a marked refractive error, especially a high astigmatic error, the immediate result from a cycloplegic refraction may be less than 6/6 (Fig. 5–2).

Wearing of the proper correction for several months often results in an im-

TABLE 5–1 CENTRAL VISUAL ACUITY: DISTRIBUTION OF MAXIMAL CORRECTED VISUAL ACUITY FOR 2000 INDIVIDUAL HEALTHY EYES (TAIT)

Visual Acuity at 6 Meters	Number of Eyes
6/3	16
6/4	84
6/5	808
6/6	792
6/7.5	168
6/10	107
6/12	25

proved central visual acuity response and presumably a stimulated foveal function (Table 5–1).

Unequal vision is a finding which should alert the refractionist and an extra effort must be made to account for the difference. Anisometropia is frequently associated with amblyopia.

Refraction Method

In performing the actual refractive procedure, the most useful instrument will be the retinoscope followed by the keratometer (in children old enough for keratometric measurements). The prescription given is usually entirely dependent on the findings of retinoscopy with an allowance made for the normal ciliary tonus paralyzed by adequate cycloplegia. The use of cycloplegia in children, even up to their early teens, is necessary because they will not maintain fixation for any given period of time and this change of fixation, together with a change of accommodation at frequent intervals, makes it impossible to arrive at a satisfactory answer without the use of cycloplegic agents. There are two major effects from all cycloplegic agents which are vitally important in pediatric refraction procedures. The first of these is a paralysis of the active accommodation to a sufficient degree so that changes in fixation by the child will not cause sudden changes in the accommodation. The cycloplegia is considered adequate if the residual accommodation is less than 2 diopters. The second result of the cycloplegia is a temporary paralysis of the tonus of the ciliary muscle. This effect on the ciliary muscle is recognized

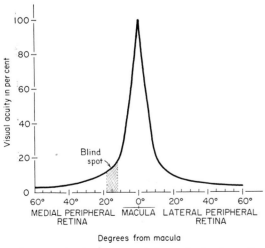

Figure 5–2 Average variation of visual acuity over retina, in terms of percentage and according to Snellen notation.

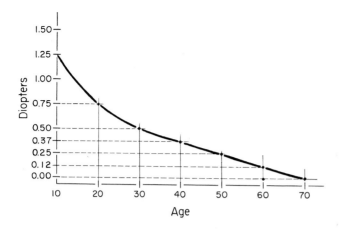

Figure 5–3 Maximum value of normal ciliary muscle tonus in seven age groups.

by a difference in the cycloplegic and post-cycloplegic refractive figures and is often called latent hyperopia in the farsighted group.

The basic tonus of the ciliary muscle in children is relatively higher than that of adults and in the very young can be as much as 1.75 diopters and as much as 1.00 diopter at the age of 10 (Fig. 5–3; Table 5–2).

It is important to remember this second effect of the cycloplegia, so that in making a final correction for hyperopia in children an adequate allowance is made for this ciliary tonus in order that the child will not be over-corrected for his distance vision. For example, if a 5-year-old child were found to have a moderate farsighted astigmatism with a basic sphere of 4.5 diopters under adequate cycloplegia, the actual prescription for the spherical part would be approximately 1.00 to 1.25 diopters less than that found under cycloplegia. If this allowance were not made the child would be over-corrected for dis-

tance and his distance vision would be blurred. This small reduction in the spherical correction is particularly applicable for the child with normal muscle balance. The approximate allowance figures for different ages can be seen in Table 5–2.

However, for the esotropic or esophorotropic child, a full atropine correction is essential. If the child wears the glasses before the atropine effect has disappeared, the adjustment to the glasses is facilitated. Most small children with accommodative esotropia seem to accept the blur for the brief time it takes to clear. When the mother states that the child wears the glasses all day or reaches for them in the morning, one can be reasonably sure they are correct. On the other hand, if he repeatedly hides them in the sandbox or under a chair, it might be well to recheck your retinoscopic findings.

Accommodation and Accommodative Amplitude

Accommodation is the ocular process in which the eye keeps the object of regard in focus on the retina as the object approaches the eye. This is accomplished by interaction of the ciliary muscle and the crystalline lens. By relaxing the accommodation, the eye can see objects clearly as they recede from the eye. Essentially, the eyes keep the object and the macula in conjugate focus. The mechanism of just how contraction of the ciliary body increases the curvature of the lens is not fully understood. Young and Helmholtz

TABLE 5–2 USUAL DIFFERENCE IN DIOPTERS BETWEEN LENS FINDINGS UNDER 1 PER CENT ATROPINE CYCLOPLEGIA AND THE FINAL LENS CORRECTION IN VARIOUS AGE GROUPS

Age (years)	Difference in Diopters
6	1.25
10	1.00
15	0.87
20	0.50
30	0.25
40	0–0.25

asserted that the lens in its capsule assumed a more spherical form with an increased convexity of the anterior surface when circular fibers of the ciliary body contracted and relaxed the zonular fibers.

Uncorrected refractive errors will change the accommodation needed, increasing it in hyperopia and decreasing it in myopia, and tests for accommodation must be made with full correction if they are to be meaningful. Accommodation can be tested by the approach method until blurring of print occurs or by adding concave lens power until blur occurs either at distance or at 13 inches (monocularly adjusting for the 3 diopters already in use). The amplitude of accommodation is approximately 14 diopters according to any of these tests in children 8 to 10 years of age.

Except for instances in which the accommodation is paralyzed by trauma, infection, or intracranial disease, it is extremely rare to find a reduced range of accommodation in children. This may be explained by the fact that the amplitude greatly exceeds the amount used by children in everyday ocular use.

Theoretically, *emmetropia* exists when there is no refractive error under cycloplegia, with the ciliary muscle relaxed and the light rays focused on the retina uninfluenced by the ciliary muscle action. Practical emmetropia exists when the refractive error is near zero with the normal ciliary muscle-tonus present but with distance fixation, so that no accommodational action is stimulated. Because of the greater tonus of the ciliary muscle in children, it is necessary to use a stronger cycloplegic agent for the young child and therefore atropine is used, starting 2 days before the refraction is scheduled (Fig. 5–3).

Cycloplegics and Mydriatics

The most commonly used cycloplegic in children up to the age of 6 is atropine sulfate. It is preferable to prescribe 1/2 per cent atropine ointment for children under 2 years of age, especially if they are lightly pigmented. One per cent atropine ointment is satisfactory for darkly pigmented children at a younger age and all children above the age of 2. Atropine in oil suspension may be equally satisfactory. Atropine solution is to be avoided, since it may be absorbed by the nasal mucous membranes following rapid passage down the lacrimal canaliculi. Digital pressure over the puncta will minimize absorption.

Many children are sensitive to atropine and react with flushing, dryness, elevated temperature, and irritability. Atropine ointment should be instilled 3 times a day for 2 days prior to the examination. The additional advantage of this technique is that the medicine is instilled at home instead of the office, which permits the physician a better opportunity for relating to a more cooperative child.

If atropine cannot be used, homatropine hydrobromide solution 2 per cent instilled every 10 minutes for 5 times may be substituted. Cyclopentolate hydrochloride (Cyclogyl) 1 or 2 per cent has the advantage that one drop instilled twice in each eye, 5 minutes apart, prepares the child for refraction in 45 minutes. Cyclogyl is regarded as a close substitute for atropine as a cycloplegic in the refraction of the strabismic child. However, the refraction must be performed 40 to 50 minutes after the last drop or the results are not accurate.

Systemic reactions with Cyclogyl include visual and space disorientation. The strange behavior of the child may be disturbing to the parent unless explained.

When refractions are being performed under anesthesia it is essential to prepare the patient just as one would for an office visit. This is especially true when short-acting anesthetics such as ketamine are used.

In accommodative esotropia, a repeated cycloplegic refraction may often reveal additional hyperopic correction 6 months or one year later.

Medical students and pediatricians frequently ask what the best method is for pupillary dilatation prior to a fundus examination. Tropicamide (Mydriacyl) 1/2 to 1 per cent combined with 10 per cent phenylephrine (Neo-Synephrine) is effective and quick-acting.

Newborn and premature children must have adequate mydriasis for an effective examination with the indirect or direct ophthalmoscope.

REFRACTIVE ERRORS

Refractive errors in children are genetically determined, but since there are so many variables concerning the final refractive error the actual hereditary patterns are difficult to evaluate. Generally, the larger refractive errors are recessive and the simple refractive states are dominant. However, the corneal curves, anterior chamber depth, and curvatures of the anterior and posterior surfaces of the lens are all components in the production of the refractive error and are factors which may compensate for the change in axial length during growth.

The eye may increase its axial length from 17 mm. at birth to 24 mm. at the age of 8 and would theoretically change the refraction about 30 diopters. However, these marked changes usually do not occur, therefore some variation in other factors must compensate for the growth changes.

Whether due to axial or curvature factors or both, a simplified diagram will demonstrate the focus of the parallel light rays on the retinal plane in emmetropia (on the retinal plane), hyperopia

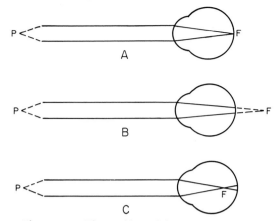

Figure 5–4 The position of the posterior principal focus (*F*) of the eye with relation to the retinal plane: *A*, in emmetropia; *B*, in hyperopia; *C*, in myopia. Parallel incident light rays originate at a single point (*P*) at infinity. A normal amount of ciliary muscle tone (tonic accommodation) is assumed to be present.

(behind the retinal plane), and myopia (in front of the retinal plane) (Figs. 5–4 and 5–5).

Hyperopia

Most children are *hyperopic* at birth, with refractive errors of 2 to 3 diopters fre-

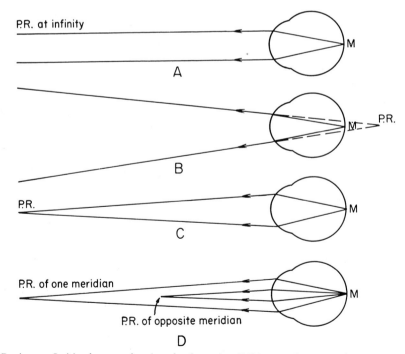

Figure 5–5 Conjugate foci in the eye, showing the far point (*P.R.*) as conjugate to the retina (*M*): *A*, in emmetropia; *B*, in hyperopia; *C*, in myopia; and *D*, in astigmia (with far points of the two major meridians).

quently found. From this stage to 3 years of age there is an apparent increase in hyperopia even though conceivably there must be an increase in eye size due to growth during this period. From 7 to 14 years of age there is a rapid decrease in the hyperopia. However, it has been my experience that if the hyperopia in this age group is associated with esotropia, the loss of hyperopia is much slower and may not happen at all in some instances. Hyperopic errors of 5 diopters or more are often associated with partial amblyopia and ocular muscle imbalance, notably internal strabismus. The partial amblyopia may be binocular but it is more often associated with a unilateral high hyperopia and it may be impossible to improve the visual acuity with any refractive measures, occlusion, or orthoptic techniques.

Very often in young people with low degrees of hyperopia the visual acuity for distance seems better without correcting lenses, possibly because the slight absorption and reflection of light by the lenses results in a retinal image less bright and sharp than that formed without them. Occasionally, there also seems to be some pupillary constriction as the result of the accommodation used for distance when no convex lenses are worn, and such a lessening of the diameter of the pupils will, by reducing the size of the retinal diffusion circles, give better vision.

Young children who are actually hyperopic may simulate myopia by holding objects very close to the eyes. In these cases, the hyperopia is usually of considerable amount and the child avoids the use of accommodation by bringing the object in which he is interested so close that he can see it by means of the large retinal diffusion circles. This is a very inefficient process and, of course, results in very slow and labored reading together with extreme difficulty in other visual tasks. The parents and the school teacher usually mistakenly tell the refractionist that the child is nearsighted.

Correction of Hyperopia

The correction of hyperopia in children is usually unnecessary, since the accommodational range for them is adequate to overcome even relatively high errors with the necessary two-thirds diopter reserve of accommodation for comfort. Glasses for neutralization of hyperopia are important for associated sensorimotor anomalies or if there are asthenopic symptoms associated with school work. Glasses for unilateral hyperopia and amblyopia should be used together with patching of the better eye in an effort to attain the maximum vision possible in the hyperopic eye. It should be remembered that the final correction in hyperopia, not associated with strabismus, should be less than that found under cycloplegia for maximum distance visual acuity.

Myopia

Myopia in children, statistically a less frequent condition, results in the need for lens correction in a higher percentage of individuals than hyperopia. This occurs, however, not from symptoms of asthenopia (although frontal or nuchal headaches are possible with excessive squinting of the eyelids which the myopic individual may use to produce a pinhole effect) but from the inability to see clearly at distance fixation with minor amounts of myopia (>1.00D). The slight distance blur may be interpreted as normal and the individual may be unaware of any difficulty unless he compares himself with a normal sighted child. With the advent of school screening programs, myopia is being discovered earlier but sometimes in rather minor amounts.

The treatment of the ordinary myopic child is easy and consists of prescribing the least amount of correction which will result in 6/6 vision. Any amount over 0.75 diopters will be significant, especially in the average school classroom.

Myopia may also be excessive on a congenital basis and this type often does not increase with age but it is associated with varying degrees of amblyopia. Progressive or malignant myopia is associated with a rapidly progressing myopia as well as vitreous and fundus changes. Unilateral high myopia is commonly associated with amblyopia and presents a therapeutic problem. Occlusion of the better eye until vision improves to 20/40 is possible if commenced early. Contact lenses are now prescribed for such cases, regardless of age, at the Wills Eye Hospital.

Correction of Myopia

Various treatment methods have been advanced in an attempt to reduce the progression of both simple and progressive myopia. It has not yet been definitely proved that any method influences either type to any degree. Methods that have been explored include bifocals or reading glasses, contact lenses, and cycloplegic drops. Surgical correction has been advocated by José Barraquer. The method consists of trephining a corneal button, planing off the undersurface, and then resuturing the altered corneal button. Reduction in myopia is produced by flattening the corneal surface.

Bifocals or reading glasses may be used in an attempt to reduce the pull on the anterior choroid during ciliary muscle contraction and thereby lessen the amount of stretching of the choroid. If bifocals are used, the amount should not exceed 1.50 diopters and the bifocal segment must be one-half the height of the entire lens, so that looking over the top of the bifocal is discouraged for near work. Tait found that he was able to demonstrate the beneficial effect of bifocals in progressive myopia during a 20-year experience. Myopic children require yearly examinations and if their visual acuity is less than 20/20, another refraction is indicated.

Contact lenses are used and are credited with reducing the degree of progressive myopia. However, no definite prolonged studies with adequate controls have been carried out, so that whether the contact lens effect is real or apparent is not yet established. Contact lenses do present some problems in the case of very young children and require considerable cooperation by the parents.

Cycloplegic drops used at bedtime have been advocated in order to relieve ciliary muscle pull on the choroid and reduce ciliary muscle congestion. The cycloplegic used is metabolized overnight and does not interfere with close work the next day.

Although there is no definite indication that any one of these methods is usually effective, it is wise to try one or more methods in order to effect the best final result for the progressively myopic child. Attention to the general health, nutrition, and hygiene of the eyes is important and should be considered. Excessive near work in a poor light should be discouraged.

Astigmatism

Astigmatism presents one of the most difficult of all problems to the pediatric refractionist. It is often difficult to refine the axis or the amount of astigmatism in children up to 5 years of age, especially in amounts up to 2 diopters. Moderate amounts of astigmatism are tolerated by children without symptoms and yet the refractionist will wonder if this child's visual performance would be enhanced by correction of the condition. The retinoscope provides the basic answer and usually the prescription must be written from this single evaluation.

Correction of Astigmatism

It is sometimes better in moderate amounts of astigmatism to "rock" the cylinder (move the axis 10 degrees either way and have the child read the letters in each position) rather than to try to establish an equal blur with the crossed cylinder. The axis is used which gives the best visual acuity. Corneal astigmatism can be measured by keratometry in children about age 4 and above and gives an indication of the axis. Since children have not developed any degree of dynamic compensatory lenticular astigmia, a close approximation of the lens power can be ascertained if allowances are made for the lens effectiveness of the spherical component.

The keratometer also will indicate at once the presence of irregular astigmatism which cannot be treated by conventional optical means but will require contact lenses or surgical intervention.

An astigmatic correction should be given to those children with asthenopic complaints, regardless of the degree, and to those individuals with unilateral astigmatism and secondary amblyopia. Correction of significant amounts of astigmatism should be made for school work even when unaccompanied by symptoms.

Anisometropia

Anisometropia, or a refractive error which is different in each eye, produces the effect of having one eye always out of focus and images of different size in each eye. If the error is of any magnitude, either alternating vision or monocular preference with possible amblyopia in the non-fixing eye with or without a muscle imbalance may develop. The refraction problem can be solved with ordinary glasses but the image size disparity cannot.

Contact lenses are useful in selected cases of unilateral high refractive error, including those associated with aphakia. The corneal measurements in the very young require the use of general anesthesia and a special keratometer mounted for use in the operating room. The cooperation of the parents is essential for the success of this type of therapy.

Subnormal Vision

Subnormal vision occurs in children on either a congenital or acquired basis. In these individuals ordinary eyeglasses are of no benefit and some form of special help is necessary. If the visual handicap is beyond correction, a school specializing in teaching methods for partially sighted individuals is recommended. The handicap produced by low vision will vary from person to person and will depend to some extent on the individual's personal drive to do visually demanding work. It should be noted that in children there often may be a disparity between the distance and near visual acuity, and many children with 20/200 vision at distance may see fairly fine print at near by bringing the material very close to the face. For example, in spite of the nystagmus observed in albino children, it is not unusual for them to read small print quite well even with their distance vision handicap.

Bilateral aphakia following successful cataract surgery is another form of subnormal vision which deserves comment. For children under 3 years of age, it is often difficult to make them wear their aphakic correction, even after rechecking to make sure it is accurate. The small child will remove his glasses and proceed to run about the house and see well enough for his immediate needs to the amazement of all. As they become more interested in examining objects more in detail, they accept their aphakic correction. Contact lenses are indicated for aphakia under optimum circumstances.

TABLE 5-3 RELATION BETWEEN VISUAL ACUITY NOTATIONS AND PERCENTAGES OF MACULAR VISUAL EFFICIENCY (STERLING AND SNELL).

Snellen Notation Feet	Meters	Visual Angle in Minutes	Visual Efficiency in Per Cent	Percentage Loss of Vision
20/20	6/6	1	100.0	0.0
20/25	6/7.5	1.25	95.6	4.4
20/30	6/9	1.50	91.4	8.6
20/40	6/12	2	83.6	16.4
20/50	6/15	2.5	76.5	23.5
20/60	6/18	3	69.9	30.1
20/70	6/21	3.5	63.8	36.2
20/80	6/24	4	58.5	41.5
20/90	6/27	4.5	53.4	46.4
20/100	6/30	5	48.9	51.1
20/120	6/36	6	40.9	59.1
20/140	6/42	7	34.2	65.8
20/160	6/48	8	28.6	71.4
20/180	6/54	9	23.9	76.1
20/200	6/60	10	20.0	80.0
20/220	6/66	11	16.7	83.3
20/240	6/72	12	14.0	86.0
20/260	6/78	13	11.7	87.3
20/280	6/84	14	9.8	90.2
20/300	6/90	15	8.2	91.8
20/340	6/102	17	5.7	94.3
20/380	6/114	19	4.0	96.0
20/400	6/120	20	3.3	96.7
20/500	6/150	25	1.1	98.9
20/600	6/180	30	0.6	99.4
20/800	6/240	40	0.1	99.9

By utilizing the central vision notation, it is possible to estimate the visual efficiency (in per cent) and the percentage loss of vision.

Table 5–3 might be utilized for children with decreased vision to help guide them into occupations which would be possible with their degree of visual efficiency.

The methods used for subnormal vision correction are either to make the printed material large, as done with the elementary school material, or to enlarge the material by magnification. Basically, devices that are worn like spectacles are of two types: *telescopic lenses* for distance enlargements and *microscopic lenses* for enlargement of near work. These optional devices tend to set the child apart and thus will not be worn well in regular school but may be used at home. The microscopic lenses are available at most opticians and reach a maximum of 40D, giving a 10X magnification. The reading must be held at the tip of the nose and enlarges only a few letters at a time. (See Chapters 28 and 32.)

FUNCTIONAL DISTURBANCES

Children may indicate that they are unable to see better than 6/60 in one or both eyes. Yet, following a cycloplegic refraction, a minimal refractive error may be found which is disproportionate to the visual disability. If the remainder of the eye examination, including visual fields, is normal and a small correction results in 6/6 vision, one may suspect a functional element. If after subsequent visits plano lenses result in 6/6 vision, the pediatrician should be alerted to investigate for a psychological problem at home or at school.

HETEROPHORIA

Heterophoria is defined as a latent deviation of the visual axes of the eyes which is compensated for by the fusional vergence reflexes. While this is basically true, the sensorimotor reflexes operative in the formation of heterophoria are different for distance and near fixation. Therefore, it is difficult to have an all-encompassing definition, especially when the clinical significance, the adjustment, and the deficiencies in adjustment to heterophoria are considered.

The subject of heterophoria, therefore, will be considered from the standpoint of the reflexes concerned in the formation of the heterophoria and the necessary fusional correction first for distance fixation and then for near fixation.

For distance fixation, the reflexes concerned are the ones which produce the basic balance innervation (tonus) to all the ocular muscles. As defined by Best and Taylor, the tonus of any muscle is determined by the small amount of constant innervation which is reaching the muscle to keep it ready for action. In the event of a movable organ (without muscle loading), it is the balance between opposing muscle groups in the absence of cerebral innervation to move the organ which controls the postural characteristic of the organ. In reference to the eye, it has been noted that the extraocular muscles are more powerful than necessary so that muscle loading almost never occurs. When measuring heterophoria, the eyes are in the primary position and, therefore, there is no cerebral innervation to move the eyes (unless fixation wanders), so that the position of the visual axes under dissociation should reflect the basic balance innervation (tonus) of the opposing muscle groups.

Just what makes the balance of opposing muscle groups produce an eso-, exo-, hyper-, or cyclophoria usually cannot be determined in any given case. However, heredity plays an important part in distance fixation anomaly. An old compensated palsy could also produce a heterophoria at distance. Whatever the cause, it is sufficient to say that the actual position occurs because the balance of tone in the opposing group is such that the visual axes are directed apart.

Although most ocularly comfortable people are *orthophoric* at distance, there are individuals who have a latent deviation but who are still comfortable while others with the same measurement are ocularly uncomfortable. The difference between ocular comfort and a sensorimotor asthenopia is usually a reflection of the adequacy of the fusional vergence reflex in a direction opposite to the heterophoria. It was found empirically that if the fusional vergence measurement was twice the heterophoria (remembering that the vergence measurements start with the heterophoria already compensated to the zero reading on the prisms), the patient will not have symptoms referable to the heterophoria. If fusional vergence is less than twice the heterophoria reading, the heterophoria will have to be seriously considered as a factor in the production of ocular symptoms.

The symptoms of inadequately compensated distance heterophoria, in children old enough to complain, are referred to as panoramic *asthenopia*, i.e., symptoms of eye strain for all ocular activity, distance and near. In children too young to complain, there is often restlessness and inattention, with objective evidence of strain such as chronic hyperemia of lids and ocular congestion. One of the most frequently encountered problems may be observed with intermittent exotropia in which there is a heterotropia for distance and a heterophoria of varying degrees for near fixation. At first glance, this may appear as a heterotropia problem but actually represents a deficiency in fusional convergence for distance in which single binocular vision is possible for near but not for distance. A high *exophoria* for distance may give the same symptoms if associated with an inadequate fusional vergence. *Esophoria* too great for the fusional divergence will also give ocular discomfort. Since *esophoria* requires fusional divergence for correction, small degrees of esophoria deviation may be the cause of symptoms because fusional divergence is not developed to the degree of fusional convergence either at distance or at near fixation. For example, 10^Δ of esophoria would require 20^Δ of fusional divergence for comfort, a figure not reached by most individuals.

All patients should have a cycloplegic refraction and be evaluated with full correction. Orthoptic exercises may be tried but they are seldom successful in influencing the distance fusional vergence power.

If the objective or subjective symptoms are great enough to warrant treatment of a distance heterophoria problem, the correction, with few exceptions, is surgical, with the aim of placing the visual axes in such a position that the fusional vergence reflexes will then be adequate. For example, if an individual had a 15^Δ of esophoria and a prism divergence of 10^Δ, surgical correction to place the visual axes to 5^Δ of esophoria would place the heterophoria within correctable limits by fusional divergence.

Vertical deviations also have a vergence correction, but in amounts over 1^Δ the vertical vergence is almost universally inadequate, so that some correction is necessary if the patient is having symptoms. Except for infrequent cases in which the heterophoria can be corrected by weakening a yoke muscle, most corrections are effected by vertical prisms.

The reflexes governing the position of the visual axes for near fixation are different from those for distance. This can be appreciated best by considering the difference between orthophoria for distance and orthophoria for near. At distance, orthophoria represents parallelism of the visual axes under dissociation, whereas at near, orthophoria represents a convergent movement of the visual axes of from 15^Δ to 21^Δ for the visual axes to intersect at 1/3 meter. The actual amount of convergence movement required for 1/3 meter can be calculated by multiplying the interpupillary distance in centimeters by 3. The reflexes concerned in the convergence movement of the visual axis at near are *fusional convergence, tonic convergence, proximal convergence*, and *accommodative convergence. Tonic convergence* is the basic tonus of the medial rectus muscles with the eyes in the primary position free from any fusional impulses. *Proximal convergence* is the amount of convergence induced by a sense of nearness of an object. *Fusional convergence* is initiated reflexively by the stimulus to fuse objects approaching or receding from the eyes. *Accommodative convergence* is that portion of the total convergence mechanism which is initiated by the stimulus to accommodate.

If the accommodative convergence reflex develops normally, there will be a convergence movement of the visual axes to cross at a fixation of 1/3 of a meter for 3^Δ of accommodation, and orthophoria results. If the accommodative convergence reflex does not develop completely there will be a limited convergence movement of the visual axes for accommodation and high exophoria at the near point is found. The degree to which A-C reflex develops will determine the amount of exophoria found. It must be remembered that the A-C reflex does not develop fully in every individual and the resulting exophoria at near is not necessarily the cause of asthenopia. If near symptoms exist with exophoria, it is almost always the result of fusional convergence insufficiency (remote near point) and not the exophoria with near. This can be appreciated in light of the fact that the amount of convergent movement of the visual axes to converge from parallelism at a distance to intersect at 1/3 of a meter, assuming a constant pupillary distance, is the same, regardless of the amount of exophoria at near (Fig. 5–6).

Esophoria at near fixation, with the refractive error adequately corrected by proper lenses, results from an excessive convergent response to a normal accommodative stimulus. The symptoms are associated with asthenopia for close work, but in children the response may be to avoid reading and studying and the child is considered to have reading problems.

Treatment for esophoria at near is to lessen the accommodative stimulus by the use of convex lenses, a sufficient amount of lens power being used to reduce the esophoria to near orthophoria. It is rarely necessary to exceed +2.00D, since there is usually a 4^Δ to 6^Δ reduction of esophoria for 1D of lens power used.

The near heterophoria is a modification of the distance position by the accommodation convergence reflex, and when considering heterophoria, both distance and near reading must be utilized in the final analysis. For example, if an individual had 10^Δ of exophoria for distance and 10^Δ of exophoria for near, it would represent a basic balance anomaly (exophoria at distance) but a normal accommodation convergence reflex, since the near exophoria is just a reflection of the distance starting position.

The range of heterophoric measurements can be seen from Figure 5–7. It may be noted that most individuals are orthophoric at distance and have approximately 8^Δ of exophoria at near. However, these are not to be considered as normal values, since all the corrective reflexes determine the significance and possible symptoms related to the heterophoria.

Although the *near point* of convergence is not basically a part of the heterophoria problem, there is one aspect in which it is of vital importance. During the movement of the visual axes from parallelism at distance to near fixation with fusion (convergence), it should be remembered

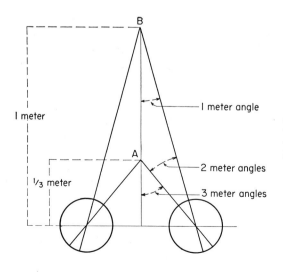

Figure 5–6 Relative convergence. When fixation is moved from the distal point *B* to the proximal point *A*, the convergence is *positive*, relative to the original fixation at point *B*, and is the value of 2 meter angles. When fixation is moved from the proximal point *A* to the distal point *B*, the convergence is *negative*, relative to the original fixation at point *A*, and is also equal to 2 meter angles.

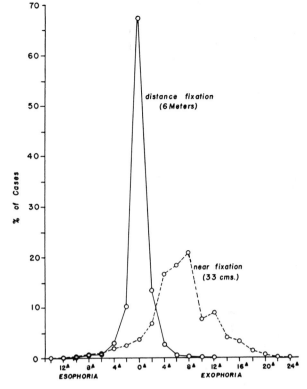

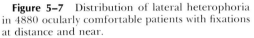

Figure 5–7 Distribution of lateral heterophoria in 4880 ocularly comfortable patients with fixations at distance and near.

that the visual axes start with parallelism, so that an exophoria at distance must be compensated before normal convergence occurs. Therefore, if an exophoria exists, it will require that much more additional convergence power to be adequate. For example: If a patient is orthophoric at distance, he will require 18$^\Delta$ of convergence to see singly at near (60-mm. P.D.) and require 18$^\Delta$ additional convergence power at near for comfort. If he has 10$^\Delta$ of exophoria at distance, he will use 10$^\Delta$ of convergence to get to parallelism at distance and then use 18$^\Delta$ to converge to near fixation, a total of 28$^\Delta$. He would then need 28$^\Delta$ of convergence reserve at near, which is outside the usual range. This explains why exophoria at distance produces symptoms at all fixation distances.

With the exception of the fixation targets and cover testing, all other tests for heterophoria are subjective and, therefore, will not be possible until school age in most individuals.

When using the fixation targets and alternate cover to neutralize the ocular movement, a series of prisms is held over one eye in increasing power until the refixation movement stops. The apex of the prism should be held in the direction of the deviation, since this method takes advantage of the fact that light rays are bent toward the base of the prism in known amounts until the prism diopters of the deviation are recorded (Figs. 5–8 and 5–9).

If the deviation is desired in degrees, a conversion can be made utilizing the table (Table 5–4). However, in most instances, it is easier to utilize prism diopters in dealing with heterophoria.

To summarize, the heterophoria measurements are done with an accurate lens correction in place and with subjective testing whenever possible, with a target for near which will stimulate accommodation. The distance heterophoria is determined and the amount of fusional vergence reserve is calculated in the direction opposite to the heterophoria.

The near heterophoria is determined and the figures are related to the distance reading. If nearly equal to the distance

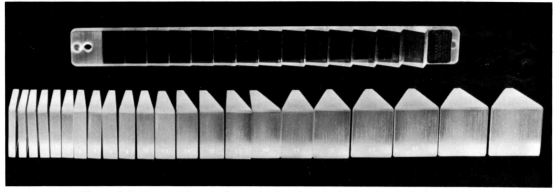

Figure 5-8   Loose prisms in foreground and vertical prism bar in background.

reading, then the problem is one of a distance difficulty with a normal accommodative convergence reflex. If the near reading is greater toward the esophoric side than distance (or less exophoric than at distance), the patient has an exaggerated accommodation convergence reflex in addition to the distance problem, if present. Exophoria at the near point is of no real significance and the patient generally will not have difficulties from this but will have symptoms only if he has a reduced fusional convergence at near fixation.

The following chart lists the heterophoric anomaly on the left side with the suggested treatment in the opposite column.

HETEROPHORIC ANOMALY	TREATMENT
Basic balance anomaly (heterophoria at distance too great for fusional vergence in opposite direction).	Surgical. Prisms used if surgery refused or if physical condition contraindicates.
Accommodative convergence excess (esophoria at near).	Convex lens power sufficient to reduce esophoria at near.
Combination of above A. Exophoria at distance with less at near or actual esophoria at near.	A. Surgery to correct distance problem and convex lens power for near fixation.
B. Exophoria at distance with more at near.	B. Surgery for distance problem. None for near.

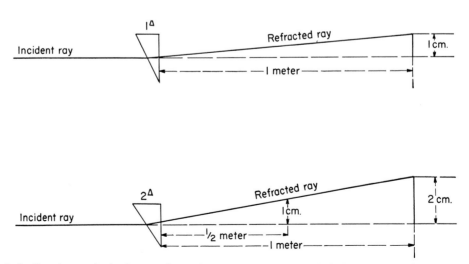

Figure 5-9   Prentice method of measuring prisms in terms of their deviating power (prism dioptrics), illustrating comparative deviations of 1^Δ and 2^Δ prisms.

TABLE 5–4 RELATIONSHIP BETWEEN PRISM DIOPTRIES (Δ) AND DEGREES (°) OF ARC IN CONVERGENCE AND DIVERGENCE (APPROXIMATELY 1° = 2 Δ).

Prism Dioptries (Δ)	Degrees (°) of Arc	Prism Dioptries (Δ)	Degrees (°) of Arc
1	35′	15	8° 32′
2	1° 9′	16	9° 5′
3	1° 43′	17	9° 39′
4	2° 18′	18	10° 12′
5	2° 52′	19	10° 46′
6	3° 26′	20	11° 19′
7	4°	25	14° 3′
8	4° 35′	30	16° 42′
9	5° 9′	35	19° 17′
10	5° 43′	40	21° 48′
11	6° 17′	45	24° 13′
12	6° 51′	50	26° 34′
13	7° 24′	55	28° 48′
14	7° 58′	60	30° 58′

DUANE-WHITE CLASSIFICATION OF ANOMALIES OF CONVERGENCE

Ever since 1896, when Duane presented a new classification of the motor anomalies of the eye, those who have used his system have divided convergence anomalies into four general groups. According to Duane, convergence anomalies can be described as either convergence insufficiency, convergence excess, divergence insufficiency, or divergence excess. This system of classification is still very popular and perhaps more widely used at this time than at any other. The diagnostic concepts have been developed and presented in detail by White and other of Duane's pupils, and adhered to, in turn, by their successors.

This system of classification is based almost entirely on the motor responses of convergence, and, except for accommodative influences, does not at all consider the stimuli which are responsible for the observed responses. In view of the widespread use and understanding of the Duane-White viewpoint, however, it is necessary to present and discuss its four major groups in terms of the stimulus-response mechanisms which have been described in preceding pages.

Following is a summary of the Duane-White classification of convergence anomalies, with the major points of differentiation:

A. *Convergence Insufficiency:*
  1. Lateral orthophoria or slight exophoria for distance
  2. Marked exophoria at 1/3 meter
  3. Pc (near point of convergence) 2 inches or more from nose
  4. May be accommodative or nonaccommodative
  5. May be secondary to divergence excess

B. *Convergence Excess:*
  1. Orthophoria or moderate esophoria for distance
  2. Marked esophoria at 1/3 meter
     Accommodative convergence excess due to
     (a) Uncorrected hyperopia
     (b) Myopia with excessive concave lens correction
     (c) Beginning presbyopia
     (d) Cycloplegia
  3. May be complicated with divergence insufficiency either as cause or effect

C. *Divergence Insufficiency:*
  1. Primary
     (a) Esophoria for distance (not over 8D)
     (b) Esophoria at 1/3 meter (small amount)
  2. Secondary
     (a) Esophoria for distance great
     (b) Esophoria for near greater than for distance
  3. May be secondary to a convergence excess

D. *Divergence Excess:*
  1. Exophoria for distance marked
  2. Exophoria at 1/3 meter less or equal
  3. Primary convergence normal (Pc normal)
  4. Secondary convergence less (Pc remote) (Fig. 5–10)

The first of these groups, that of *convergence insufficiency,* is marked by the pres-

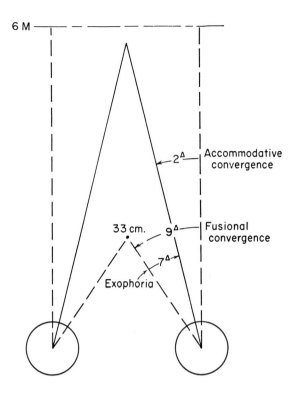

Figure 5–10 Convergence insufficiency; high exophoria (14△) for near, with orthophoria for distance (P.D. = 60).

ence of considerable exophoria at the near point. From the reflex standpoint, this means that the patient has only a small amount of accommodative convergence, but, as has been demonstrated previously, it matters little how much accommodative convergence is present in a given case as far as comfort is concerned, unless, of course, it is excessive. The amount of exophoria at near depends on the amplitude of the accommodative convergence reflex which is not in use under normal conditions of fixation. Duane early recognized the fact that many individuals with great exophoria for near fixation are comfortable, and the position of the near point of convergence was then introduced as a factor in diagnosis. The convergence near point in most individuals depends on the extent of the fusional convergence reflex, and it was properly recognized that in the presence of an adequate amount of fusional convergence, as manifested by a close near point, the individual would be comfortable. The case would still be classed, however, as one of convergence insufficiency on the basis of the marked exophoria at the near point, Occasionally, however, a close convergence near point may be the result of coexistence of a well-

developed accommodative convergence reflex and a poor fusional convergence reflex. A simple approach type of convergence test, therefore, may be quite misleading.

The nonaccommodative character of some of these cases has been recognized, for example, the case of a myope who does not accommodate very much or at all for the near point and who will, in consequence, usually have a marked exophoria. In this case, again, it was not realized that the increased exophoria at the near point, under dissociation, was caused by a lack in the accommodative convergence reflex.

Convergence insufficiency cases, therefore, can be much more accurately classed on the basis of their tonic vergence balance for distance and the presence or absence of an adequate fusional convergence amplitude.

The second group, that of *convergence excess*, is represented by those in which there is a normal or nearly normal tonic vergence balance for distance, but in which there is esophoria at the near point. These cases are further divided into those in which there is an actual accommodative convergence excess because of uncorrected hyperopia, those presenting a my-

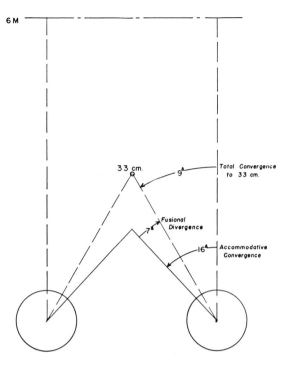

Figure 5–11   Convergence excess: marked esophoria (14ᐃ) for near, with orthophoria for distance (P.D. =60).

opia with excessive concave correction, those in which there is beginning presbyopia and the patient strains to see, and those showing the effects of the excessive ciliary innervation occasionally demonstrated by a patient under cycloplegia (Fig. 5–11).

All these last four groups, of course, would be eliminated if the tests were made with adequate lens corrections for the ametropia present, including an adequate lens addition for the artificial presbyopia in the cycloplegic case.

Those cases in which the marked esophoria at the near point persists despite adequate ametropic corrections are considered as the nonaccommodative convergence excess group. These cases constitute something of a problem when considered only from the standpoint of the motor manifestations. They can be recognized easily, however, by the binocular reflexes as representing cases of an exaggerated accommodative convergence reflex. They represent the patients in whom the normal exercise of accommodation results in an abnormally great associated reflex to convergence, apparently caused in most instances by a reduction in synaptical resistance or by the facilita-

tion of reflexes often resulting from a generally disturbed nervous system.

The third group, representing *divergence insufficiency*, is divided into two subgroups, *primary* and *secondary* (Fig. 5–12).

The *primary* group is composed of those cases in which there is considerable tonic convergence for distance, with a lesser amount of esophoria at 1/3 meter. The smaller amount of esophoria at the near point represents, of course, an amount of accommodative convergence well within the usual limits of distribution, and the anomaly therefore is due to a maldistribution of tonic reciprocal innervation which produces the esophoria for distance. If this can be compensated for by an adequate amplitude of fusional divergence, the patient will have comfortable and efficient vision. If the amplitude of fusional divergence is insufficient, discomfort always ensues and single binocular vision is threatened.

In the *secondary divergence insufficiency* group, the esophoria at the near point is greater than the amount at distance, thus representing, in addition to the tonic convergence innervational fault present in the primary variety, the effect of an excessive accommodative convergence re-

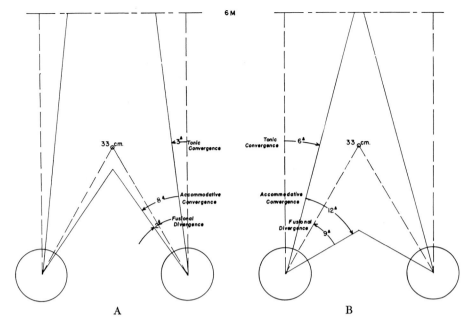

Figure 5–12 Divergence insufficiency, primary and secondary. *A*, Primary divergence insufficiency: moderate esophoria (6$^\Delta$) for distance, with less (4$^\Delta$) for near (P.D. = 60). *B*, Secondary divergence insufficiency: great esophoria (12$^\Delta$) for distance, with more (18$^\Delta$) for near (P.D. = 60).

flex. Such a patient would require fusional divergence not only for distance but also considerably more at the near point, and this, in many cases, is not available. Practically, of course, the excessive esophoria for near in these individuals could be relieved for the time being, although not eliminated, by the prescription of added convex lens power for use at the near point.

The fourth and last group, *divergence excess*, includes those cases in which the distribution of tonic reciprocal innervation to the extraocular muscles for distance results in considerable exophoria, with the exophoria at the near point being equal or less than that for distance (Fig. 5–13). Comfort in such cases would naturally depend on the amplitude of fusional convergence, and this is recognized in the Duane classification, in that individuals with a normal convergence near point are differentiated from those with a remote near point. The possibilities for comfort in a given case, of course, depend on the useable amplitudes of fusional convergence. On the basis of the foregoing discussion, it can be seen that the Duane classification does not present mutually

exclusive groups, because the manifest findings on which it is based may permit the individual to be placed into two or possibly more of the groups.

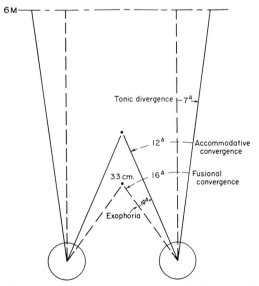

Figure 5–13 Divergence excess: marked exophoria (14$^\Delta$ for distance, with less (8$^\Delta$) for near (P.D. = 60).

REFERENCES FOR HETEROPHORIA

Adler, R. H.: Physiology of the Eye. St. Louis, The C. V. Mosby Co., 1965.

Boeder, P.: An Introduction to the Mathematics of Ophthalmic Optics. Rutland, Vermont, Charles E. Tuttle Co., Inc., 1937.

Duke-Elder, S.: Practice of Refraction. 5th Ed. St. Louis, The C. V. Mosby Co., 1949.

Linksz, A.: Physiology of the Eye. Vol. 1, Optics. New York, Grune and Stratton, Inc., 1950.

Mellick, A.: Convergence. Brit. J. Ophthal., 33: 755–763, 1949.

Mellick, A.: Convergence deficiency—An investigation into results of treatment. Brit. J. Ophthal., 34:41–46, 1950.

Parrish, R. K.: An Introduction to Visual Optics. A Manual of the Amer. Acad. Ophthal. and Otolaryngol., Rochester, Minnesota, 1967.

Scobee, R. G., and Green, E. L.: Relationships between lateral heterophoria, prism vergence, and near point of convergence. Amer. J. Ophthal., 31:427–441, 1948.

Tait, E. F.: Fusional vergence. Amer. J. Ophthal., 32:1223–1230, 1949.

Tait, E. F.: Stimulus-response mechanisms in binocular coordination. Amer. J. Ophthal., 33:1751–1762, 1950.

Tait, E. F.: Accommodative convergence. Amer. J. Ophthal., 34:1093–1107, 1951.

REFERENCES FOR REFRACTION

Blair, H. L., and Martens, T. G.: Refraction and visual physiology. Annual Review. Arch. Ophthal., 71:889, 1964.

Cowan, A.: Refraction of the Eye. Philadelphia, Lea and Febiger, 1948.

Fonda, G. E.: Refraction Problems. A Manual of the Amer. Acad. Ophthal. and Otolaryngol., Rochester, Minnesota, 1969.

Rubin, M. L.: Optics and visual physiology. Annual Review. Arch. Ophthal., 75:836, 1966.

Sloane, A. E.: Manual of Refraction. Boston, Little, Brown and Co., 1961.

Snydacker, D., and Newell, F. W.: Refraction. A Manual of the Amer. Acad. of Ophthal. and Otolaryngol., Rochester, Minnesota, 1952.

Tait, E. F.: Textbook of Refraction. Philadelphia, W. B. Saunders Co., 1951.

CHAPTER 6

STRABISMUS

DONELSON R. MANLEY, M.D.

ANATOMY

There are six extraocular muscles attached to each eye:

1. Medial rectus
2. Inferior rectus
3. Lateral rectus
4. Superior rectus
5. Inferior oblique
6. Superior oblique

The rectus muscles course from their origins in the apex of the orbit to their tendinous insertions in the sclera anterior to the equator of the globe. The oblique muscles, on the other hand, have an oblique course in the orbit and are inserted posterior to the equator.

Each eye is held in place within the orbit by a system of connective tissue structures which allow the eye to be easily moved in any direction. *Tenon's capsule* is that part of the orbital fascia lining the outside and inside of the muscle cone. The anterior portion of the capsule runs under the conjunctiva from the insertion of the rectus muscles to the limbus, at which point it is inseparably fused with the conjunctiva. The *check ligaments* are condensations of the orbital fascia, which run from the outer aspect of the rectus muscles to the orbital rim. These give added stability to the globe within the orbit.

A line connecting the midpoint of the in-

sertions of the rectus muscles reveals that a spiral, rather than a circumference, is formed. This spiral, known as the *spiral of Tillaux*, is of importance for two reasons: (1) During surgery, the surgeon remains properly oriented by knowing these insertional distances, and this provides the safeguard of operating the correct muscle; (2) In reoperations, measuring the insertional distance of a muscle from the limbus will provide some information as to the type and amount of previous surgery.

Medial Rectus
(Internal Rectus) (Table 6–1)

This muscle arises from the medial portion of the annulus of Zinn in the apex of the orbit and passes forward along the medial orbital wall. It is the largest of the extraocular muscles and is supplied by a branch of the inferior division of the third cranial nerve, which enters the muscle on its bulbar side approximately 15 mm. from the muscle's origin.

Inferior Rectus

The inferior rectus arises from the inferior portion of the annulus below the optic foramen. It passes downward and laterally along the floor of the orbit, forming an angle of 23° with the visual axis of the eye. A branch of the inferior division of the third cranial nerve enters its bulbar sur-

TABLE 6–1 EXTRAOCULAR MUSCLES: LENGTHS OF MUSCLE AND TENDON WITH INSERTIONAL DISTANCES FROM THE LIMBUS

	Distance from Insertion to Cornea (in mm.)	Length of Muscle and Tendon (in mm.)	Length of Tendon (in mm.)	Width of Tendon at Insertion (in mm.)
Medial rectus	5.5	40.8	3.7	10.3
Inferior rectus	6.5	40	5.5	9.8
Lateral rectus	6.9	40.6	8.8	9.2
Superior rectus	7.7	41.8	5.8	10.6
Superior oblique	14 to 18	60.0	30.0	variable; 11 is the average
Inferior oblique	16 to 25	38	1–2	variable; 9 to 10 is the average

face 13 to 15 mm. from the muscle's origin. The inferior rectus is attached to the lower lid by means of fascial connections of its sheath; these connections are important, as they may cause the position of the lower lid to be altered when large amounts of surgery are performed on the muscle.

Lateral Rectus (External Rectus)

The lateral rectus has two sites of origin. It arises from the portion of the annulus which spans the medial aspect of the superior orbital fissure and it also has an origin from the lateral ends of the superior and inferior orbital tendons. The sixth cranial nerve enters its bulbar side 15 mm. from the muscle's origin.

Superior Rectus

The superior rectus arises from the upper part of the annulus just below the origin of the levator muscle. It passes forward, upward, and laterally, forming an angle of 23° with the visual axis of the eye (Fig. 6–1). A branch of the superior division of the third cranial nerve enters the muscle on its bulbar side, approximately 15 mm. from the muscle's origin. Surgery on this muscle may also affect the

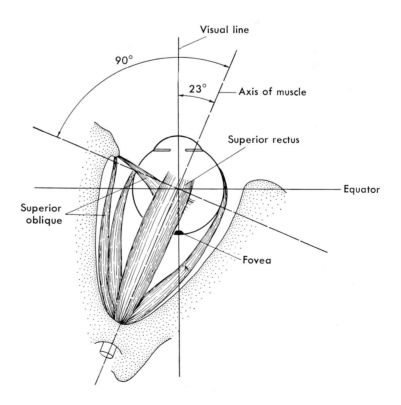

Figure 6–1 Diagram of muscles seen from above, showing origin and insertion of superior rectus. (From Moses, R. A.: Adler's Physiology of the Eye. 5th ed. St. Louis, The C. V. Mosby Co., 1970.)

width of the palpebral fissure by changing the position of the upper lid. As with the inferior rectus, a too-generous recession will widen the fissure, whereas a large resection will narrow it.

Inferior Oblique

The inferior oblique arises from the periosteum of the maxillary bone, a few millimeters posterior to the orbital rim and a few millimeters lateral to the bony orifice of the nasolacrimal duct. From its origin it passes laterally, upward, and posteriorly, making an angle of 51° with the visual axis of the eye. It passes beneath the inferior rectus, to which it is intimately attached by a fusion of their sheaths into the *ligament of Lockwood*. This ligament is of importance, for it gives support to the eye within the orbit, it may become entrapped by a fracture of the floor of the orbit, and at times it would appear to act as the physiological origin of the inferior oblique muscle. The muscle passes under the lateral rectus to insert in the posterior lateral quadrant of the eye, posterior to the equator. A branch of the inferior division of the third cranial nerve enters the muscle on its bulbar surface just lateral to the lateral border of the inferior rectus muscle.

Superior Oblique

The superior oblique originates in the apex of the orbit from the periosteum, covering the sphenoid bone just medial to and above the optic foramen. It is the longest extraocular muscle (60 mm.) and is divided into two parts:

1. *Direct part:* origin to trochlea is 40 mm. long.

2. *Reflected part:* trochlea to insertion is 20 mm. long.

From its origin, the muscle passes forward and upward along the medial wall of the orbit and becomes a rounded tendon 10 mm. posterior to the trochlea. After passing through the trochlea, it changes direction, running downward, backward, and laterally, forming an angle of 51° with the visual axis of the eye (Fig. 6–2). The tendon inserts in the posterior lateral quadrant behind the equator. The fourth cranial nerve enters the muscle on its orbital side, approximately 12 mm. from the origin of the muscle.

MOTOR PHYSIOLOGY

The primary position of the eyes is that natural position in which the head is erect

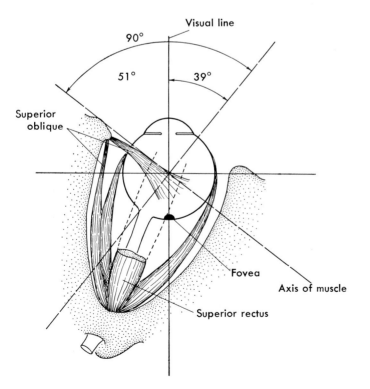

Figure 6–2 Diagram of origin and insertion of muscles from above, with superior rectus cut away. Physiologic origin of superior oblique at trochlea. (From Moses, R. A.: Adler's Physiology of the Eye. 5th ed. St. Louis, The C. V. Mosby Co., 1970.)

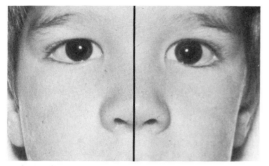

Figure 6–3 The primary position and the median plane.

upon an erect body and the gaze is directed exactly in advance toward the horizon (Fig. 6–3). It is felt that under these conditions the visual axes are exactly aligned in the normal individual, and a minimum of muscular innervation is present. For purposes of measurement, the eyes are directed toward an object located on a level with the eyes at a distance of 20 feet from them. Glasses are worn if necessary, and accommodation is controlled by using suitable targets for fixation. For purposes of terminology, the head is divided into two symmetrical parts by the median plane, which passes anterior to posterior. This plane is used as the reference for many of the terms describing eye movements.

Fick's Axes and Listing's Plane (Fig. 6–4)

These useful concepts are used to explain the movement of the eye around a theoretical center of rotation. The three axes are designated as X, Y, and Z. Voluntary rotations may be made horizontally around the Z axis and vertically around the X axis; involuntary torsional rotations occur around the Y axis. The Y axis runs through the center of rotation of the eye at right angles to Listing's equatorial plane.

The functions of the motor system of the eyes are:

1. to bring a sharp image of the object of regard on each fovea;

2. to enlarge the visual field, that is, to transform the visual field into the field of fixation;

3. to maintain the image of the object of regard on the fovea;

4. to insure at all times the proper relative position of the two eyes, so that binocular vision is made possible and maintained.

To achieve this requires an intricate system of voluntary and reflex eye movements. In addition, the resting position of the eyes must be normal. Abnormal orbital development may cause the positioning of the eyes to be such that normal alignment of the visual axes is impossible. The extraocular muscles and their fascial connections must be normal, and there must be a proper relationship between accommodation and convergence.

Eye movements may be classified (1) according to their nature or (2) by the direction of their movement (Table 6–2).

Eye Movements Classified by Their Nature

VOLUNTARY EYE MOVEMENTS

Voluntary eye movements originate in area 8 of Brodmann; corticobulbar fibers pass from the frontal cortex through the internal capsule to the brain stem nuclei of the nerves to the extraocular muscles. There are oculogyric centers for conjunctive and disjunctive voluntary eye movements. When the head is moved from the primary position, voluntary eye move-

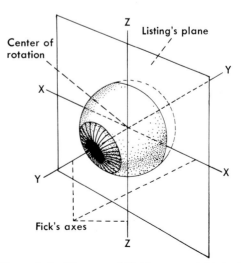

Figure 6–4 Diagram of Fick's axes and Listing's plane. (From Moses, R. A.: Adler's Physiology of the Eye. 5th ed. St. Louis, The C. V. Mosby Co., 1970.)

TABLE 6–2 CLASSIFICATION OF OCULAR MOVEMENTS

I. According to their nature
  A. Voluntary
  B. Reflex
    1. Optomotor (psycho-optic, optic fixation)
      a. following
      b. fixation
      c. fusional
      d. vergence
    2. Postural
      a. semicircular canals
      b. otoliths
      c. neck muscles
II. According to the direction of their movement
  A. Monocular (ductions)
    Adduction .... Abduction
    Sursumduction .... Deorsumduction
    Incycloduction............. Excycloduction
  B. Binocular (versions and vergences)
    1. Versions (conjugate movements)
      Dextroversion........... Levoversion
      Sursumversion .... Deorsumversion
      Dextrocycloversion ... Levocycloversion
    2. Vergences (disjunctive movements)
      Convergence .... Divergence
      Right   Right
        sursumvergence ... deorsum-
                          vergence
      Incyclovergence........Excyclovergence

---

ments must be modified according to the new position of the head in space in order to bring about the desired change in the position of the visual axes. For the most part, the vestibular apparatus brings about this desired influence.

REFLEX EYE MOVEMENTS

Optomotor Reflexes (Psycho-Optic, Optic Fixation)

Optomotor reflexes are so named because a visual stimulus results in a movement of the eyes to follow and fixate the object of regard. These reflexes begin to develop as soon as the newborn infant opens its eyes, and they are well developed by the third month. The visual information is received in area 17 of the occipital lobe and is relayed to areas 18 and 19. The optomotor reflexes are initiated from these latter two areas and pass to the brain stem and the nuclei of the nerves to the extraocular muscles. These reflexes require visual perception and interest, and are easily demonstrated in most infants after the third month. Defects such as cataracts and glaucoma can interfere with the normal development of these reflexes. Hence it is of importance that structural problems and refractive errors be identified and corrected, if possible, in early infancy.

FOLLOWING REFLEX. The following reflex maintains the image of the moving object of regard on the fovea. It is responsible for the response seen in optokinetic nystagmus. Whenever the image of the object of regard moves off the fovea, an increase in tonus occurs to those muscles which will turn the eyes reflexly to follow the object.

FIXATION REFLEX. After the following reflex has moved the eyes in the desired direction following the object of regard, the fixation reflex maintains the image of the object on the fovea. The powerful stimulus for this is brought about by the marked difference in the visual acuity between the fovea and the retina, just off the fovea. The normal development of this reflex is of great importance to the infant. A clear image of the object must be focused on the fovea. Hence, a high refractive error may prevent this and poor fixation will result. Any abnormality that interferes with the visual axis may result in the development of a poor fixation reflex. Before the child can tell us how well he sees, we use the fixation reflex clinically to evaluate visual acuity. An infant should have central fixation (foveal) in each eye and should be able to maintain it. Eccentric fixation (off the fovea) results in decreased visual acuity (amblyopia).

FUSIONAL REFLEXES. Fusional reflexes are concerned with the maintenance of bifixation (each fovea directed at the object of regard at the same time), and vergences are also important in this regard.

VERGENCE REFLEXES. These may be horizontal, vertical, or torsional and are stimulated by retinal image disparity occurring when the visual axes are not properly aligned. For example, exophoria produces temporal retinal image disparity and thus stimulates fusional convergence, which realigns the visual axes. The amplitudes of fusional vergences may be measured.

Postural Reflexes

Postural reflexes result from impulses originating in the inner ear, which contains the cochlea (hearing) and labyrinth (equilibrium). Hearing originates as impulses from the receptors in the organ of Corti; the impulses are transmitted by the auditory division of the eighth cranial nerve. Through the cochlear connections, the eyes may reflexly turn in any direction in response to an auditory stimulus.

SEMICIRCULAR CANALS. The labyrinth contains the three semicircular canals, the utricle, and the saccule. The canals contain endolymph, and each canal has a dilated end called the ampulla. The canals are continuous, with the utricle and saccule in a closed system. When the head is moved rapidly, the flow of endolymph within the canals is altered, and this alteration in flow stimulates the hair cells of the cristae located in each of the ampullae. This results in a reflex impulse from the three ampullary nerves to the vestibular portion of the eighth cranial nerve, and this reflex innervation produces compensatory contractions in the extraocular muscles and in the muscles of the neck, trunk, and extremities. Labyrinthine responses are studied clinically by rotating the individual in a chair (Bárány test) or by caloric testing using warm and cold water.

OTOLITHS. The utricle and saccule contain a sensory epithelium covered with hair cells that is overlayed with a gelatinous membrane in which are embedded small sandlike concretions called *otoliths*. Changes in the position of the head in respect to gravity cause the otoliths to pull on the hair cells, resulting in reflex innervation relayed by the vestibular nerves. Utricular reflexes function through the influence of gravity and are responsible in part for the following:

Doll's head phenomenon: When the chin is depressed, the eyes tonically deviate upward, and when the chin is elevated, the eyes deviate downward. This reflex is often used clinically in evaluating the extraocular movements of an infant.

Compensatory torsional reflex: When the head is tilted to either shoulder, the otoliths initiate reflex impulses that are sent to the extraocular muscles, and torsional movements of the eyes around the antero-posterior axis occur. This reflex is often used clinically in the evaluation of cyclovertical muscle weakness.

NECK MUSCLES. The influence of prioception from the neck muscles is unknown.

Eye Movements Classified by Direction

MONOCULAR MOVEMENTS

Ductions

Ductions are monocular rotations; they occur around the X, Y, and Z axes of Fick. For nomenclature the median plane is used for reference.

ADDUCTION—rotation of the eye toward the median plane. Rotation occurs around the Z axis.

ABDUCTION—rotation of the eye away from the median plane. Rotation occurs around the Z axis.

SURSUMDUCTION (ELEVATION)—upward rotation of the eye, occurring around the X axis.

DEORSUMDUCTION (DEPRESSION)—downward rotation of the eye, occurring around the X axis.

INCYCLODUCTION (INTORSION)—rotation of the upper end of the vertical meridian of the cornea nasally toward the median plane, occurring around the Y axis. Involuntary.

EXCYCLODUCTION (EXTORSION)—rotation of the upper end of the vertical corneal meridian away from the median plane, occurring around the Y axis. Involuntary.

BINOCULAR MOVEMENTS

Versions

Versions are rapid, synchronous, conjugate, and saccadic movements of the eyes. They allow the eyes to be moved quickly in any direction so that a visual stimulus can be fixated by the foveas (fixation reflex) and a moving stimulus can be followed (following reflex).

DEXTROVERSION — both eyes rotate to the right.

LEVOVERSION — both eyes rotate to the left.

SURSUMVERSION (ELEVATION) — both eyes rotate upward.

DEORSUMVERSION (DEPRESSION) — both eyes rotate downward.

DEXTROCYCLOVERSION — rotation of the eyes around their anteroposterior axis so that the upper end of the vertical meridian of the cornea rotates to the right.

LEVOCYCLOVERSION — rotation of the eyes around their anteroposterior axis so that the upper end of the vertical meridian of the cornea rotates to the left.

In the clinical sense the term *versions* is also used to describe binocular rotations in the diagnostic positions of gaze.

Vergences

Vergences are slower, synchronous and disjunctive movements of the eyes; that is, the visual axes of the eyes move in opposite directions. Vergences may occur concurrently with versions, but they respond to different stimuli, are controlled through different neuropathways, are slower in execution, involve different groupings of muscles, and serve a different purpose. For the most part, vergences are concerned with the maintenance of binocular vision, and they allow the visual axes to remain aligned on the object of regard at any viewing distance.

CONVERGENCE — both eyes rotate toward the median plane.

DIVERGENCE — both eyes rotate away from the median plane.

RIGHT SURSUMVERGENCE — the right eye rotates upward while the left eye rotates downward.

RIGHT DEORSUMVERGENCE — the left eye rotates upward while the right eye rotates downward.

INCYCLOVERGENCE — rotation of the eyes around their anteroposterior axis so that the upper end of the vertical corneal meridian of each cornea rotates toward the median plane.

EXCYCLOVERGENCE — rotation of the eyes around their anteroposterior axis so that the upper end of the vertical corneal meridian of each cornea rotates away from the median plane.

Actions of the Extraocular Muscles (Table 6-3)

The actions to be discussed are those that have proved to be clinically valid in humans.

The medial and lateral rectus muscles have horizontal actions, whereas the cyclovertical muscles have both a vertical and a torsional action. These actions of the cyclovertical muscles change as the eyes are rotated from the primary position to other directions of gaze.

Medial Rectus

The action is solely that of adduction to turn the eye inward toward the median plane.

TABLE 6-3 ACTIONS OF THE EXTRAOCULAR MUSCLES

Muscle	Primary Action	Secondary Action	Synergists
MR	Adduction	None	SR and IR
LR	Abduction	None	SO and IO
SR	Elevation		IO
		Adduction	MR and IR
		Intorsion	SO
IR	Depression		SO
		Adduction	MR and SR
		Extorsion	IO
SO	Intorsion		SR
		Depression	IR
		Abduction	LR and IO
IO	Extorsion		IR
		Elevation	SR
		Abduction	LR and SO

Lateral Rectus

The action is solely that of abduction to turn the eye outward, away from the median plane.

Superior Rectus

In the primary position the superior rectus is primarily an elevator and has little intorsion effect. As the eye is abducted, the elevating action increases and the intorsion effect decreases. When the eye is abducted 23°, elevation is the only action and there is no torsion effect. As the eye is adducted, intorsion increases and the elevating effect decreases. When the eye is adducted 67°, intorsion is its only action and there is no elevating effect. Adduction is a secondary action of the superior rectus and would be greatest in midline upgaze.

Inferior Rectus

In the primary position the inferior rectus is primarily a depressor and has little torsion effect. As the eye is abducted, the depressing effect increases and the torsion effect decreases. When the eye is abducted 23°, depression is the only action and there is no torsion effect. As the eye is adducted, extorsion increases and the depressing effect decreases. When the eye is adducted 67°, extorsion is its only action and there is no depressing effect. Adduction is a secondary action and would be greatest in midline downgaze.

Superior Oblique

In the primary position, intorsion is the main action, and there is little depressing effect. As the eye is abducted, the intorsion effect increases and the depressing effect decreases. When the eye is abducted 39°, intorsion is its only action and there is no depressing effect. As the eye is adducted, the intorsion effect decreases and the depressing effect increases. When the eye is adducted 51°, no intorsion effect is present, and the depressing effect is maximum. The secondary action of abduction is present to a limited extent in the primary position, and this increases in midline downgaze.

Inferior Oblique

In the primary position, extorsion is the main action and there is little elevating effect. As the eye is abducted, the extorsion effect increases and elevation decreases. When the eye is abducted 39°, extorsion is the only action and there is no elevating effect. As the eye is adducted, the extorsion effect decreases and the elevating effect increases. When the eye is adducted 51°, no extorsion is present and the elevating effect is maximal. The secondary action of abduction would be greatest in midline upgaze.

Yoke Muscles (Figure 6–5)

Each of the six extraocular muscles of each eye has a direction of gaze in which its action is maximum. The muscles have

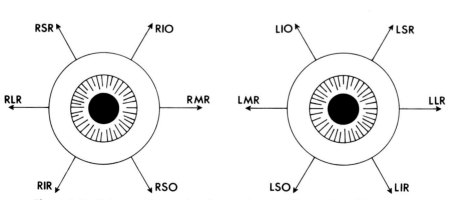

Figure 6–5 Yoke muscles moving the eyes into the diagnostic positions of gaze.

been grouped into pairs of yoke muscles, and each pair moves the eyes maximally in one direction.

```
Eyes right
  (dextroversion)..................RLR and LMR
Eyes up and right
  (dextrosursumversion)...........RSR and LIO
Eyes up and left
  (levosursumversion ..............LSR and RIO
Eyes left
  (levoversion).......................LLR and RMR
Eyes down and left
  (levodeorsumversion)............LIR and RSO
Eyes down and right
  (dextrodeorsumversion) ........RIR and LSO
```

Synergistic Muscles (Table 6–3)

Each of the extraocular muscles has a primary action, and this action is enhanced by the synergistic muscles, whose *secondary* actions are the same as the primary action of the muscle under consideration. For example, the primary action of the lateral rectus muscle is abduction. Both the superior and inferior obliques have a secondary abducting effect that enhances the abducting effect of the lateral rectus. Thus both of the obliques are synergists of the lateral rectus.

Hering's Law (Equal and Simultaneous Innervation)

This law has been stated as follows: In all voluntary movements of the eyes, equal and simultaneous innervation flows from the oculogyric centers to the muscles of both eyes concerned with the desired direction of gaze. For example, in looking up and to the right (dextrosursumversion), the right superior rectus elevates the right eye in abduction while the left inferior oblique elevates the left eye in adduction. Both of these muscles receive that amount of innervation (equal) at the same time (simultaneous) required to move both eyes up and to the right an equal amount. Hering's law applies in all movements involving muscle pairs concerned with movement, such as versions and vergences, and it also explains the difference between primary and secondary deviations. In primary deviation the normal eye is used for fixation, whereas in secondary deviation the eye with the paretic muscle is the fixating eye.

Sherrington's Law (Reciprocal Innervation)

Ths extraocular muscles are reciprocally innervated; that is, if one muscle contracts, its antagonist simultaneously relaxes. For example, in abduction of the right eye, the right lateral rectus contracts and the right medial rectus simultaneously relaxes.

FEATURES OF STRABISMUS

Strabismus has varied characteristics that are used singly or in combination for classification purposes. These include:

1. Age at onset—congenital, infantile, acquired.
2. Intermittency—phoria or tropia, cyclic.
3. Relationship to accommodation—accommodative and nonaccommodative.
4. Relationship to the AC/A ratio—the deviation at near is different from that at distance.
5. Comparison of up- and downgaze—A and V patterns.
6. Different measurements in various positions of gaze—comitant and noncomitant.
7. Size of the deviation—monofixation syndrome.

Overlapping may occur, and time or surgery may change one type of deviation into another.

The visual axis of an eye joins the fovea with the fixation point and passes through the nodal point of the eye. Strabismus exists when the visual axes are not properly aligned. For example, an esodeviation exists when the visual axes cross in front of the point of fixation, whereas an exodeviation is present when the visual axes diverge from one another.

Deviations of the Visual Axes

PHORIA—a misalignment of the visual axes that is kept latent by fusion.

PHORIA-TROPIA (INTERMITTENT TROPIA)—an intermittent misalignment of the visual axes that is both latent (phoria) and manifest (tropia). As long as fusion is sufficient to overcome the misalignment, a phoria exists. When the deviation exceeds this amplitude, a tropia occurs.

TROPIA—a manifest misalignment of the visual axes that is not controlled by fusion.

Fusion may be decreased (illness, fatigue) or absent (congenital esotropia).

MOTOR TESTING PROCEDURES

Motor testing determines the type (qualitative) and the amount (quantitative) of strabismus present. Determination of strabismus requires very careful observation of the child, for some children may only appear to have strabismus when their visual axes are aligned (pseudostrabismus), while others may appear to have straight eyes and yet have strabismus. This discrepancy is often explained by the *angle kappa*.

Angle Kappa

The angle kappa is formed by the pupillary line and the visual axis, assuming that the pupil is centered accurately in relation to the center of the cornea (Fig. 6–6). The corneal light reflection (CLR) is usually thought to be located superficially on the anterior surface of the cornea, but it actually lies approximately 4 mm. posterior to the cornea and is the first Purkinje image (Fig. 6–7). Clinically it appears to the ophthalmologist that the angle kappa is measured from the anterior surface of the cornea (Fig. 6–6).

Measurement of the Angle Kappa

In clinical practice the angle kappa is measured by observing the relation of the CLR to the center of the pupil. The angle is called positive when the CLR is nasal to the center of the pupil and negative when the CLR is temporal.

A perimeter or amblyoscope may be used to measure the angle, but the easiest way is to use a fixation light. A light is held approximately 1 foot in front of the patient's right eye while a cover is held in front of the left eye. The patient is asked to fixate the light with the right eye. If the CLR is centered (Fig. 6–8) there is no angle kappa. If the CLR is nasal to the pupillary line (Fig. 6–9) there is a positive angle kappa, and if the CLR is temporal to the pupillary line (Fig. 6–10) there is a negative angle kappa. As mentioned previously, eccentric fixation may be mistaken

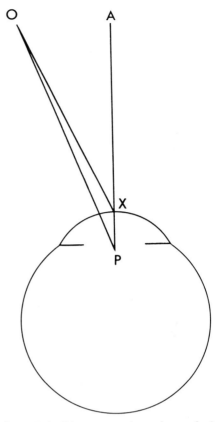

Figure 6–6 Diagram to show the angle kappa.
P = Center of the pupil
X = Point of the cornea which lies in the central pupillary line
O = Fixation point
AP = Central pupillary line
Angle OPA = Angle kappa
Angle OXA = Angle kappa, as measured clinically
(Redrawn from Lyle, T. K., and Wybar, K. C.: Lyle and Jackson's Practical Orthoptics in the Treatment of Squint. London, H. K. Lewis Co., 1967.)

for an angle kappa, and one should check the visual acuity and the fixation pattern with the Visuskop. True eccentric fixation should be associated with amblyopia, and the Visuskop will indicate whether or not fixation is by the fovea.

To insure accuracy, the examiner must keep his own eye directly behind the test light being held in front of the patient. This will avoid any error in interpreting the position of the CLR.

Positive Angle Kappa (Fig. 6–9)

1. The CLR is nasal to the pupillary line.

2. A small positive angle is a common finding in many normal eyes.

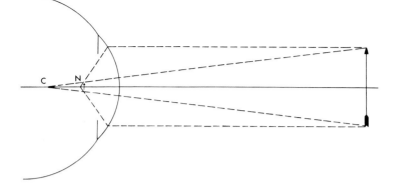

Figure 6–7 Relative size and position of images with convex mirror. This diagram serves to illustrate that the corneal light reflex is in reality a subcorneal light reflection of reduced size. (Redrawn from Krimsky, E.: The Management of Binocular Imbalance. Philadelphia, Lea and Febiger, 1948.)

3. Simulates an exotropia.

4. Causes an exotropia to appear greater than it is.

5. Causes an esotropia to appear less than it is.

6. Retinopathy of prematurity may cause retinal dragging (Fig. 6–11) so that the fovea is temporal to its usual location. An individual with this condition may appear to have an exotropia, although the visual axes are aligned. Ophthalmoscopic examination will reveal the retinal dragging.

Negative Angle Kappa (Fig. 6–10)

1. CLR is temporal to the pupillary line. This is not a common occurrence in an otherwise normal eye.

2. Simulates an esotropia.

3. Causes an esotropia to appear greater than it is.

4. Causes an exotropia to appear less than it is.

5. Eccentric fixation nasal to the fovea commonly occurs in esotropia and will appear similar to a negative angle kappa.

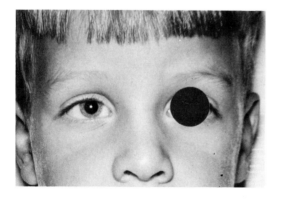

Figure 6–8 No angle kappa. Corneal light reflection is centered in right eye.

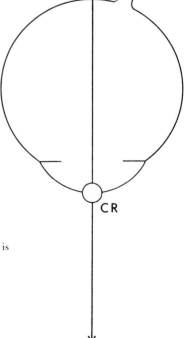

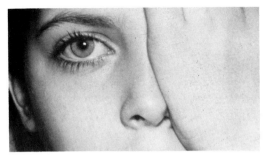

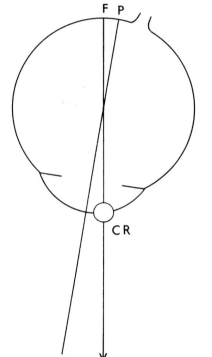

Figure 6–9 Positive angle kappa of the right eye. The corneal light reflection is nasal to the pupillary line.

6. The major anatomic cause of a negative angle kappa is high myopia. Occasionally in retinopathy of prematurity, the fovea may be dragged nasally rather than temporally.

Methods of Measurement of Strabismus

Once strabismus is known to be present, it must be measured. Three of the many clinical methods will be discussed in detail.

Hirschberg Test

This is a rapidly performed objective test that is useful in infants and uncooperative children and adults.

The cornea is approximately 12 mm. in diameter and has a radius of curvature of approximately 8 mm. Therefore each millimeter on its circumference equals 7° or 14Δ (1° = 2Δ). Clinically, it is convenient to use three locations for the estimation of the amount of strabismus present. Locations of the CLR (Fig. 6–12) are:

1. Pupillary margin = 15° (30Δ)
2. Midway between the

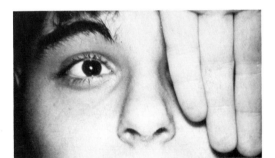

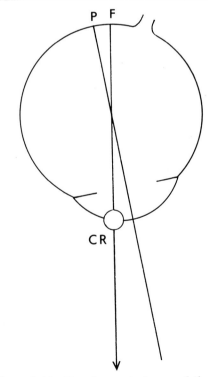

Figure 6–10 Negative angle kappa of the right eye. The corneal light reflection is nasal to the pupillary line.

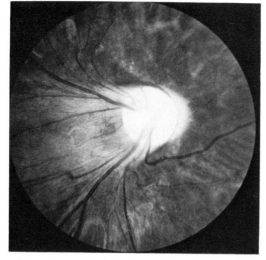

Figure 6–11 Retinal photograph of the right eye showing temporal dragging of the retina. This will cause the macula to be located temporal to its normal position, changing the relationship between the visual line and the pupillary line. A positive angle kappa is the result.

     pupillary margin and
     the limbus   = 30° (60Δ)
  3. At the limbus   = 45° (90Δ)

Initially, one should check the location of the CLR of each eye separately to determine if an angle kappa exists, for this must be taken into consideration in the estimation of the amount of strabismus present. Following this, a light is held directly in

front of the patient, and near measurements are easily made. As the patient looks directly at the light, the location of the CLR on the cornea of the deviating eye is evaluated. Distance measurements are more difficult to take and require a bright light and a dark room. Some of the additional limitations of this test are:

1. It does not control accommodation (Fig. 6–13).

2. As it is difficult to judge fractions of a millimeter, it is not possible to be more accurate than to the nearest 7° (14Δ).

3. The size of the pupil will affect the measurements (Fig. 6–14).

4. The amount of the displacement of the CLR depends on the position of the fixating eye, and if the fixating eye is not looking straight ahead, the position of the CLR on the deviating eye will be affected. (Fig. 6–15).

5. In individuals with dark irides, there may be little or no contrast between the pupil and the iris (Fig. 6–16), and this makes it difficult to measure the decentration of the CLR.

Krimsky Prism Reflex Test (Fig. 6–17)

This is a rapidly performed test and is more accurate than the Hirschberg test because it measures the strabismus in prism diopters. The Krimsky test requires greater patient cooperation and may be performed in one of two ways:

1. In a manifest strabismus the prism is

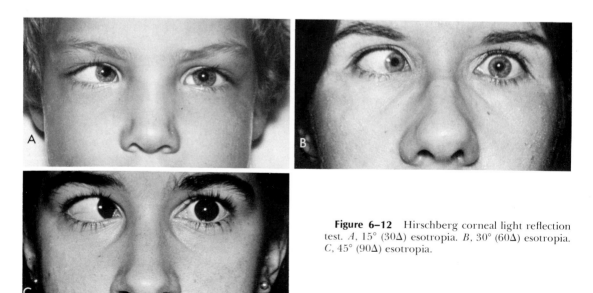

Figure 6–12 Hirschberg corneal light reflection test. *A*, 15° (30Δ) esotropia. *B*, 30° (60Δ) esotropia. *C*, 45° (90Δ) esotropia.

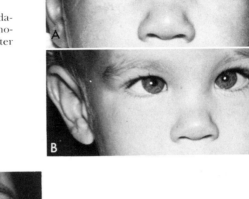

Figure 6–13 Eight-month-old child with accommodative esotropia. *A*, Eyes are straight without accommodative effort. *B*, Large esotropia is apparent after accommodation has been stimulated.

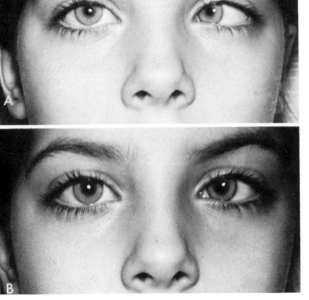

Figure 6–14 Individual with 35 prism diopters of left esotropia by cover test. In *A* the CLR is at the pupillary margin, indicating 15° of esotropia, while in *B* the CLR is nasal to the pupillary margin as a result of the pupil being larger than in *A*.

Figure 6–15 Esotropia of both eyes. As neither eye is centered it is difficult to have a reference point for the estimation of the decentration of the CLR.

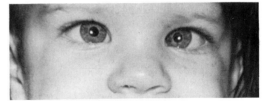

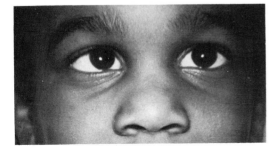

Figure 6–16 Dark irides make it difficult to see the pupil, so that the location of the CLR is difficult to determine.

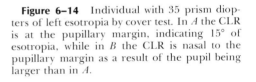

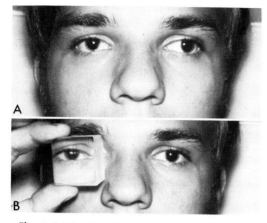

Figure 6–17 *A*, Subject has a large left exotropia and count fingers vision. A positive angle kappa in the right eye accentuates the appearance of the exotropia. *B*, Modified Krimsky test. Base-in prisms of increasing strength are placed before the fixating right eye. The end point has been reached when the left eye appears straight. It has almost been reached in this illustration. (From Manley, D. R. (ed.): Symposium on Horizontal Ocular Deviations, St. Louis, The C. V. Mosby Co., 1971.)

used to move the displaced CLR so that it becomes centered in the pupil. The strength of the prism necessary to accomplish this is a measure of the amount of strabismus present. In esotropia, the CLR is displaced temporally because the eye is turned inward. A prism will move ths position of the CLR in the direction of its apex. Therefore, in esotropia, the strength of the base-out prism necessary to center the CLR in the pupil is a measure of the amount of strabismus. Distance measurements are more difficult to take than those at near, and the angle kappa must also be taken into consideration. Frequently a prism is held before each eye so that both CLRs become centered. This method of testing is most useful in infants.

2. A second method is useful in older children and adults with good vision in one eye and poor vision in the other (Fig. 6–17). The prism is placed before the fixating eye, which then moves in the direction of the apex of the prism. The deviating eye will follow conjugately. The strength of the prism required to center the deviating eye is a measure of the strabismus. For example, if the left eye is esotropic, a base-out prism is placed before the right eye; the right eye will then move to the left and the left eye will follow. The end point has been

achieved when the prism before the right eye has moved the eyes to the left so that the left eye appears to be looking straight ahead. This is the *modified Krimsky test*, which allows distance and near measurements to be taken quickly. Accommodation in the fixating eye is controlled with this test.

Cover Testing (Figs. 6–18 and 6–19)

The cover test is the most accurate method available for measuring strabismus; it requires patient cooperation, good visual acuity (fixation) in each eye, and careful observation by the examiner. The test does not depend on the corneal light reflection, and the angle kappa does not need to be considered. The components of cover testing are:

1. Monocular cover-uncover
2. Alternate cover
3. Simultaneous prism-cover

MONOCULAR COVER-UNCOVER (Fig. 6–18). After carefully observing the patient, the examiner should perform this test first. This is a qualitative test and will determine the type (phoria, tropia) and direction (eso, exo, hyper) of the strabismus. If an individual has orthophoria, the visual axes will be aligned at the point of fixation; if orthophoria is not present, the visual axes will be misaligned. By covering and uncovering each eye separately, one can study the fixation behavior of each eye and thereby evaluate the type of misalignment.

The individual is asked to fixate a distant object with the head held in the primary position. The examiner covers one eye and carefully watches the fixation behavior of each eye; the cover is then removed. This test may be repeated several times. The other eye is then covered and uncovered in a similar manner. The following fixation patterns may be observed:

Orthophoria. Neither eye will move.

Heterophoria. The eye under cover will move in the direction of the phoria. (e. g., the eye will turn nasally if esophoria is present), as fusion is disrupted by the cover. When the cover is removed, the previously covered eye will move in the opposite direction to refixate. The three types of heterophoria are:

   esophoria—the eye under cover moves
       toward the nose and then
       moves temporally to refix-

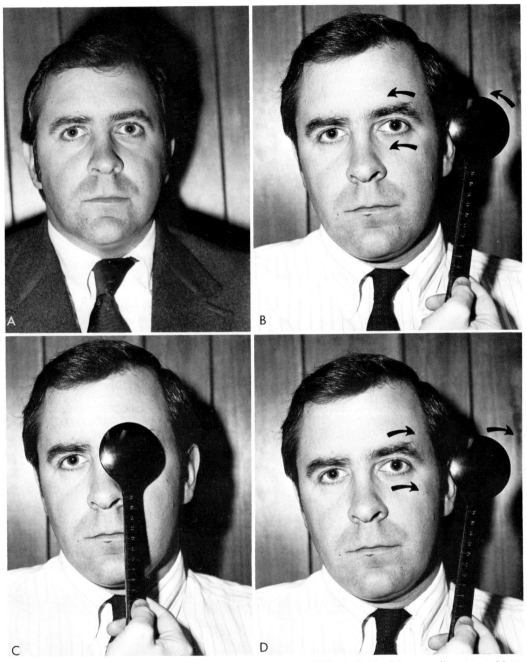

Figure 6–18 Techniques of monocular cover-uncover testing. *A*, The individual fixates a distant test object and is observed by the examiner for the presence of strabismus. *B*, The cover approaches the left eye while fixation is being maintained. *C*, The cover is placed in front of the left eye, and both eyes are carefully observed for any movement. None is observed. *D*, The cover is then removed from the left eye, and again both eyes are carefully observed for any movement. None is seen. These maneuvers are then repeated in front of the right eye. (From Manley, D. R. (ed.): Symposium on Horizontal Ocular Deviation. St. Louis, The C. V. Mosby Co., 1971.)

ate after the cover has been removed.

exophoria—the eye under cover moves away from the nose and then moves nasally after the cover has been removed.

hyperphoria—the eye under cover moves upward and then moves downward after the cover has been removed.

Since phorias are usually symmetrical, they are not commonly designated as right or left.

Heterotropia. In a tropia, the visual axes are not aligned at the point of fixation. Covering the deviating eye will result in no movement, since the other eye is already fixating the object of regard. However, covering the fixating eye will require the deviating eye to fixate the object of regard, and the examiner will observe this movement. Tropias are often designated as right or left if one eye is preferred for fixation. For example, if the right eye is the deviating eye, it is called a right tropia. If the eyes alternate and neither is preferred for fixation, it is called alternating tropia. There are four types of heterotropia:

esotropia—when the fixating eye is covered, the deviating eye moves temporally to fixate.

exotropia—when the fixating eye is covered, the deviating eye moves nasally to fixate.

hypertropia—when the fixating eye is covered, the deviating eye moves downward to fixate.

hypotropia—when the fixating eye is covered, the deviating eye moves upward to fixate.

Phoria-tropia. In some individuals the eye will deviate for a variable period and then refixate. These individuals have a phoria-tropia or intermittent tropia.

ALTERNATE COVER TEST (Fig. 6–19). Alternate cover testing is performed by placing the cover before one eye and then quickly moving it over to cover the other eye before fusion can be regained. This test is quantitative and uncovers the total deviation. When combined with prisms (alternate cover-prism test) the total deviation can be measured. As the cover is alternately placed before the eye(s), prisms of increasing strength are placed before the eye(s) until no shift is seen. When the prism placed before the eye(s) is of sufficient strength to neutralize the shift, the end-point has been reached. As an example, consider a right esotropia of 30 prism diopters. As the cover is moved back and forth, each eye will move temporally to refixate. Base-out prisms of increasing strength are placed before the eye(s) (the apex of the prism is placed in the direction of the tropia), and alternate covering is continued. No shift will be seen when a 30 diopter prism is placed before the eye. In larger deviations it is helpful to split the prisms between the eyes rather than to have one large prism before one eye.

SIMULTANEOUS PRISM-COVER TEST (Fig. 6–20). This test is less well known and does not have to be performed in every individual. It allows the examiner to determine how much of the total deviation is tropia and how much is phoria. If monocular cover-uncover reveals a small tropia shift, this shift may be measured by placing the prism before the deviating eye and simultaneously placing the cover before the fixating eye. Alternate cover testing will then reveal that a larger deviation is present; this represents the total deviation. The phoria component is the difference between the amount of tropia and the total deviation. For example, if an individual is found to have a right esotropia of 6 prism diopters and alternate cover testing reveals a total deviation of 20 prism diopters, there is an esophoria of 14 prism diopters.

ESODEVIATIONS

Definitions

Esophoria—a convergent alignment of the visual axes that is kept latent by fusion.

Esophoria-Tropia (intermittent estropia) —an intermittent convergent alignment of the visual axes that is both latent *(phoria)* and manifest *(tropia)*.

Esotropia—a manifest convergent alignment of the visual axes that is not controlled by fusion.

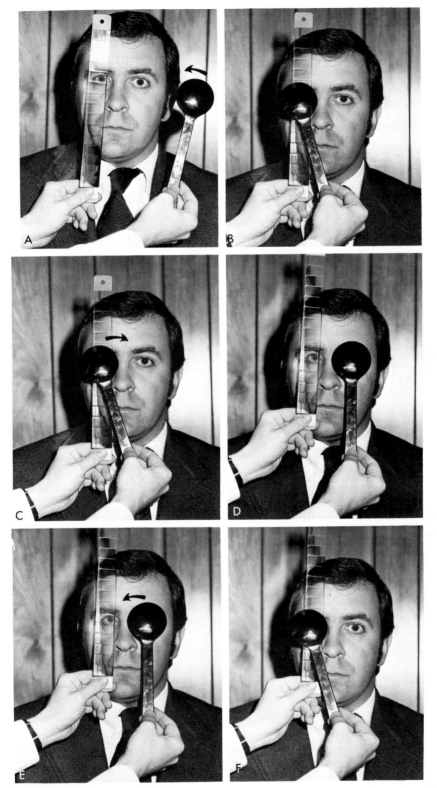

Figure 6–19 Techniques of prism alternate-cover test. This test disrupts fusion and measures the total deviation. The cover is rapidly moved back and forth before each eye to prevent the individual from regaining fusion. The prism is placed before one eye and increased in strength until no further shifting of the eyes occurs. When the shift has been neutralized, the measurement of the deviation will have been determined by the strength of the prism required. (From Manley, D. R. (ed.): Symposium on Horizontal Ocular Deviations. St. Louis, The C. V. Mosby Co., 1971.)

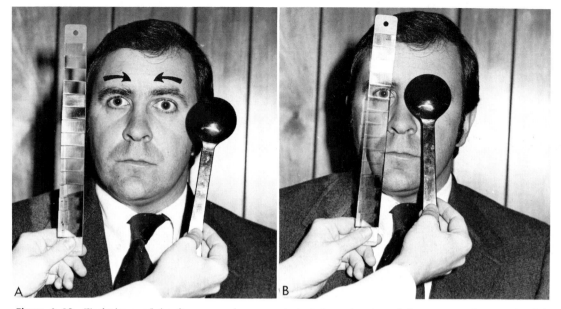

Figure 6–20 Techniques of simultaneous prism-cover test. *A,* An estimation of the amount of esotropia of the right eye is made. *B,* A prism of that strength is placed before the right eye, and at the same time, the cover is placed before the left eye. Covering the left eye causes the right eye to pick up fixation. When the prism placed before the right eye equals the amount of the tropia, no shift will be seen, and the end point will have been reached. If a stronger prism is necessary, both the prism and cover are removed, the prism bar moved upward, and then both the prism and cover are again placed before their respective eyes. This test measures the amount of tropia in a deviation that has a superimposed phoria. (From Manley, D. R.: Symposium on Horizontal Ocular Deviations. St. Louis, The C. V. Mosby Co., 1971.)

Convergence Excess—an esodeviation that is greater at near than at distance.

Divergence Insufficiency—an esodeviation that is greater at distance than at near.

Clinical Classification of Esodeviations

1. Congenital esotropia
   a. Pseudoesotropia
   b. Esotropia
   c. Strabismus fixus, Möbius syndrome, Duane's syndrome
2. Acquired esotropia
   a. Infantile esotropia
   b. Accommodative esotropia
      (1) Deterioration
   c. Primary nonaccommodative esotropia
   d. Mixed accommodative and nonaccommodative
   e. Secondary esotropia
      (1) Blind spot syndrome
3. Cyclic esotropia
4. Monofixation syndrome

Congenital Esotropia

Pseudoesotropia (Fig. 6–21)

This condition is probably the most common reason an ophthalmologist is asked to evaluate an infant. Pseudoesotropia is the appearance of having an esotropia when in fact no actual convergent alignment of the visual axes is present.

Usually the infant's parents or grandparents have noticed an intermittent crossing of the eyes when the infant gazes to the side. The epicanthal folds that cover the nasal bulbar conjunctiva are prominent, and a flat nasal bridge is usually present. Examination reveals that no strabismus is present, and an explanation is then given to the parents. It is helpful to demonstrate the epicanthal folds to them. The infant is then followed and re-evaluated every 6 months, as it is possible that a true esotropia may develop at a later date.

True Congenital Esotropia (Fig. 6–22)

The term congenital esotropia is usually applied to any esotropia that is known to

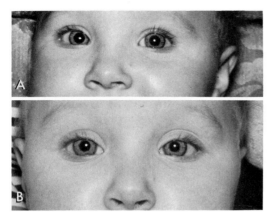

Figure 6–21 Pseudoesotropia. *A*, Epicanthal folds and a flat nasal bridge frequently give the appearance of esotropia when the infant looks to the side and the entire nasal bulbar conjunctiva is covered. *B*, Same infant, gazing slightly to the right. The nasal bulbar conjunctiva is covered by the prominent epicanthal folds more than the right eye, giving the appearance of a left esotropia.

have been present prior to 6 months of age. Unfortunately, many parents and physicians believe that it is not abnormal for an infant's eyes to be crossed, and thus they may let a considerable amount of time elapse before having an ophthalmological examination performed. This is unfortunate, as an undiagnosed retinoblastoma may be the cause and treatment may be delayed. Other defects, such as cataracts, may also be treated if they are detected early, and thus it is *imperative* that an examination be performed as soon as the strabismus has developed.

ETIOLOGY

The etiology of true congenital esotropia is largely unknown, although it is generally believed to result from an imbalance of tonic convergence and divergence. This is supported by the common clinical fact that when an infant or child develops strabismus as a result of sensory impairment in one eye (injury, cataract, retinoblastoma), it is usually an esotropia.

CLINICAL FINDINGS

. *Congenital.* The esotropia is present at birth or appears within the first few months of life. In most instances the term congenital is used if the esotropia is present prior to 6 months of age.

2. *Large deviations* are the rule. Although some are 30 to 40Δ, the majority are larger, measuring 50Δ or more.

3. *Good visual acuity in each eye.* Since the

actual acuity cannot be measured, the fixation reflex is evaluated in each eye. If fixation is central and maintained in each eye, the eyes will alternate their fixation, and this is the usual finding in congenital esotropia. Although most infants do not have amblyopia, it must be remembered that amblyopia *may* be present, in which case there will be no alternation of fixation. Amblyopia in an infant can be demonstrated (1) when the same eye is always chosen for fixation, (2) when the deviating eye demonstrates eccentric fixation associated with strabismus, and (3) by the unhappy attitude of the infant when the better eye is covered. Amblyopia at this age can be treated with a few weeks of occlusion therapy. Elimination of amblyopia will make it easier to subsequently evaluate such associated clinical findings as overaction of the inferior obliques and the A and V patterns. An infant's visual acuity is evaluated by presenting targets of decreasing size to the infant's eyes until the targets become too small to be fixated and optokinetic nystagmus is no longer elicited. It has been demonstrated that adult acuity is reached by 3 years of age.

4. *Crossfixation* is usually present as the infant looks across its nose with the esotropic eye rather than abducting the nonfixating eye. Clinically it may appear that there is a bilateral sixth nerve palsy, and this diagnosis is commonly made. Good abduction can usually be demonstrated.

a. In the office the mother covers the fixating eye, and a suitable object such as a milk bottle is moved into the diagnostic positions. The infant will

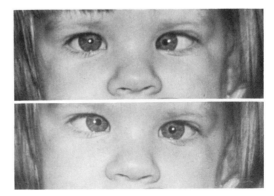

Figure 6–22 Congenital esotropia showing alternation of fixation. The esotropia measures approximately 15 degrees by the Hirschberg test.

usually follow the object, and abduction is noted.

b. Abduction may also be demonstrated by stimulating the vestibular apparatus. The examiner holds the infant face to face and quickly rotates 360° to his left (the infant's right) while standing in the same place. The infant's eyes will be seen to conjugately deviate to the infant's left, demonstrating abduction. The examiner then repeats the process, rotating in the opposite direction.

c. Another useful technique is to have the infant fixate straight ahead as it sits in the mother's lap. Again, an interesting object such as a milk bottle is held directly in front of the infant. While he is fixating, his head is quickly rotated to the right and left. Ths eyes will attempt to continue to fixate, and abduction is demonstrated.

d. If abduction cannot be demonstrated in the office, a few days of occlusion at home will usually prove that it is present.

5. *Heredity.* There is often a history of strabismus in the family.

6. *Similar distance-near measurements* are found.

7. *Refractive error.* Although any type of refractive error may be found, the majority are hypermetropic and less than +2.50 sphere in each eye.

8. *Nonaccommodative esotropia.* The esotropia usually does not improve when antiaccommodative therapy is used. After surgery, the residual esotropia may be partially accommodative, especially in those infants with hypermetropia of +4.00 sphere or more. Some infants may develop an accommodative component after 2 years of age.

9. *Absence of binocular function.* This can be demonstrated in older children with untreated congenital esotropia.

10. *Inferior oblique overaction, dissociated vertical deviations,* and *latent nystagmus* are often seen.

TREATMENT

The treatment of congenital esotropia is surgery, commonly performed around 6 months of age. Evidence is accumulating that better binocularity is achieved if the visual axes are aligned as early as possible.

Some ophthalmologists prefer to recede both medial rectus muscles initially and then resect both lateral rectus muscles at a later date for the residual esotropia that may be present. On the other hand, an equally satisfactory result may be obtained by initially performing a horizontal recess-resect on one eye and later performing a similar operation on the other eye. Satisfactory results are obtained with either method. Quite often the inferior obliques must also be weakened. Since the response to surgery is so variable, the parents should initially be told that more than one operation may be necessary. Often the horizontal alignment is quite good, and after 2 or 3 years of age a dissociated vertical deviation may appear that is occasionally noticed by the parents. If this becomes constant (tropia), additional surgery will have to be performed to correct it.

There is a gratifying psychological effect on the parents of infants whose eyes have been straightened. Of interest is the common report of parents that the infant's motor functions have improved after surgery. The infant begins to walk, is able to reach for objects with greater coordination, and in general appears to the parents to develop more rapidly.

Strabismus Fixus, Möbius Syndrome, Duane's Syndrome

In the evaluation of congenital esotropia one should remember several other entities that may appear similar. These are strabismus fixus, Möbius syndrome, and Duane's syndrome.

STRABISMUS FIXUS is a rare type of congenital esotropia in which the medial rectus muscles are tight and inelastic. Forced ductions will reveal that the eyes cannot be turned temporally past the midline. Surgical treatment is necessary, and the medial rectus muscles are receded 5 to 6 mm. This may correct the esotropia, but the lack of abduction persists.

MÖBIUS SYNDROME is extremely rare and consists of congenital bulbar paralysis including facial diplegia, pontine paralysis of lateral gaze, and paralysis of the tongue. Other congenital defects may be found in association. These include deafness, webbed fingers or toes, supernumerary digits, defects of the muscles of the chest, neck, or tongue, and even absence of hands, feet, fingers, or toes. The mouth is fixed open and the eyelids cannot be closed completely. Because of a bilateral abducens paralysis, the eyes will not abduct.

DUANE'S SYNDROME is discussed on pp. 179–180.

Acquired Esotropia

Infantile Esotropia

This is a more inclusive term than congenital esotropia and includes any esotropia that is present prior to 1 year of age. This group has a higher incidence of sensory defects, such as cataracts, retinal disorders, and optic nerve dysplasias. One should always remember than accommodative esotropia may appear in infants under 1 year of age.

Accommodative Esotropia (Fig. 6–23)

An accommodative esodeviation is one that results from the activation of accommodation.

ETIOLOGY. Etiologic factors involved are (1) hypermetropia, or (2) high AC/A ratio, or (3) a combination of the two. Most normal children have hypermetropia and do not have esotropia, whereas most of the children with esotropia have hypermetropia. It is believed that the esotropia may develop in part because of unstable

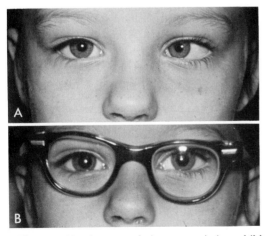

Figure 6–23 Accommodative esotropia in a child with similar distance-near measurements. *A*, Without glasses there is a left esotropia of approximately 15 degrees (Hirschberg). *B*, Same child wearing single vision lenses which have aligned the visual axes.

equilibrium resulting from a fusion defect. How this is transmitted to offspring remains unknown.

TECHNIQUES OF EXAMINATION

Accommodation must be stimulated and controlled. This requires the use of small detailed fixation targets for distance and near that are suitable for the age and interest of the child. (A light is not satisfactory.) During examination, the synkinetic near response is stimulated. This consists of the following triad:

1. Accommodation
2. Accommodative convergence
3. Pupillary constriction

A proper relationship between accommodation and accommodative convergence (AC/A ratio) helps to insure bifixation at any viewing distance.

Visual acuity testing requires that the target be suitable for the child's age and ability. Adult acuity is reached by 3 years of age, but it is usually difficult for a child under this age to verbalize what he sees. In these younger children, the fixation ability of each eye is evaluated. Fixation should be central and maintained in each eye, and alternation should be present. As soon as the child is able to respond to letters, the E game and letters should be used. The symbols should be presented in a horizontal line rather than singly; this insures that amblyopia will not be overlooked. A child may have 20/30 acuity with single symbols, whereas symbols presented linearly reveal that the acuity is actually 20/70.

To measure the deviation, proper spectacles should be worn, and the measurements should be made in the primary position at both distance and near. The comparison between the alternate cover and prism measurements at distance and near will determine the distance-near relationship for that individual, and this measurement will affect what form of treatment is used. Measurements should also be taken in straight up- and downgaze to determine whether an A or V pattern is present.

Cycloplegic refraction should be performed. Two per cent cyclopentolate hydrochloride (Cyclogyl) is a popular agent and in most instances provides adequate cycloplegia. If cycloplegia is incomplete, as occurs with dark irides, or if an unusual refractive error is present, atropine is preferred.

Ophthalmoscopic examination with the binocular indirect ophthalmoscope should be performed in all cases; this is the most important part of the examination. Abnormalities may be the cause of the strabismus or may prevent improvement of amblyopia.

CLINICAL FINDINGS

1. Age at onset is usually around 2½ years, with a range between 6 months and 7 or 8 years.

2. The size of the deviation is less than that seen in congenital esotropia. The usual range is between 20 and 45Δ.

3. Amblyopia is a common finding and requires vigorous treatment. Amblyopia is one of the sensory adjustments that occur. When the visual axes become misaligned there is visual confusion (each fovea being directed at a different object in space). This is not recognized by the child, as the brain will not integrate the dissimilar images resulting from one fovea looking at one object while the other fovea is directed at a completely different object. Visual confusion is eliminated by suppression of the deviating fovea by the brain, and amblyopia is the result. Occlusion of the better eye will force the fovea of the deviating eye to be used, and this is the better method of treatment of amblyopia. The younger the child at onset of the esotropia and the longer the duration of the esotropia prior to treatment, the more severe the amblyopia.

4. When the esotropia develops, diplopia (the same object in space seen twice) will result, as the image of the object of regard in space will be received by the fovea of the straight eye and also by the extrafoveal nasal retinal area of the esotropic eye. Another sensory adjustment made by the child is the elimination of diplopia by suppression of the peripheral retinal area of the deviating eye which received the image of the object of regard. For this reason, diplopia is usually absent in a child with accommodative esotropia.

5. Binocular function can be demonstrated with various tests, including the Worth 4 lights, Bagolini glasses, after images, and the synoptophore. Because the visual axes are no longer aligned and previously corresponding retinal areas cannot continue to enjoy their previous directional values, a third type of sensory

adjustment occurs. Anomalous retinal correspondence (ARC) develops, thus providing binocularity in the presence of a manifest deviation.

6. Heredity plays an important role in accommodative esotropia. It is not uncommon for one parent or a close relative to have a similar problem. All siblings should be completely evaluated, even though they may be thought to be normal.

7. The refractive error and the distance-near relationship are closely interrelated. As mentioned, there are two etiologic factors: (1) hypermetropia and (2) an abnormal distance-near relationship. Some children have a combination of the two.

Hypermetropia. Any type of refractive error may be present in accommodative esotropia, but the majority of cases have moderate hypermetropia. Parks found that the average hypermetropia was +4.75 sph. equivalent in the lesser of the two hypermetropic eyes. Children with high hypermetropia (+7 or +8 sph.) are less likely to develop accommodative esotropia.

Children with hypermetropia as the etiologic factor usually have similar distance-near measurements. In the past, this type of esotropia has been called pure accommodative or refractional accommodative esotropia.

Abnormal distance-near relationship. Children with this type have high AC/A ratios and would be expected to develop a large esotropia as a result of a small amount of accommodation. One would expect the refractive error to be smaller, and Parks' study showed that the average hypermetropia in this group was 2.25 sph. equivalent in the lesser of the two hypermetropic eyes. These children have an esotropia at near that is greater than that at distance. In the past, this type has been called hypoaccommodative, hyperkinetic, and convergence excess accommodative esotropia.

MANAGEMENT OF ACCOMMODATIVE ESOTROPIA

Early treatment of accommodative esodeviations is important if the sensory complications and the motor complication of nonaccommodative esotropia are to be avoided. Therapy is antiaccommodative in nature and may be of two types: (1) *optical* — single vision lenses or bifocals, and

(2) *medical*—miotics. In some children both may be used.

Optical therapy

Glasses provide emmetropia at distance and correct any astigmatism, so that accommodation is unnecessary. If the child also has a high AC/A ratio, further antiaccommodative therapy will be required at near in the form of bifocals. An add of +2.50 is usually used in the form of an executive bifocal. In deciding the type and strength of glasses, the refractive error, the AC/A ratio, the visual acuity, the age of the child, and the fusional divergence amplitude must be considered. The glasses should provide good visual acuity, alignment of the visual axes for distance and near, and visual comfort. One frequently asked question is, "What is the least amount of plus-sphere one would give a child with esotropia?" To answer this, one should determine what the distance-near relationship is. The more abnormal this relationship, the more important a small correction becomes and the more significant are small hypermetropic errors. In children under 4 years of age, full cycloplegic findings are given. After age 4, some children may not tolerate full correction, especially if they have not previously worn glasses. One should give as much plus-sphere as possible so as to align the visual axes and at the same time not blur the distance visual acuity.

As the child grows older, the distance-near abnormality tends to normalize. This allows the bifocal to be gradually reduced in strength, and frequently by the age of 9 or 10 years the bifocal can be eliminated. Similarly, single vision lenses may be reduced in strength if this reduction is consistent with good visual alignment of the visual axes. The child's fusional divergence amplitude can be expanded by purposefully reducing the strength of the glasses over a period of time. One must accept the fact, however, that there are some children who are committed to wearing glasses for life. In many older individuals, contact lenses work well.

Miotic therapy

Miotics are useful as a diagnostic test and as a method of treatment of accommodative esotropia. There is usually little additive effect when miotics are used in addition to glasses. Miotics are long-acting cholinesterase inhibitors for topical use, and they enhance the effect of endogenously liberated acetylcholine in the iris, ciliary muscle, and other parasympathetically innervated structures of the eye. Some of the ocular effects are miosis, potentiation of accommodation, and an increased facility of outflow of aqueous humor.

Miotics will depress both plasma and erythrocyte cholinesterase levels in patients after a few weeks of eyedrop therapy. If miotics are used, the parents are given the name and dosage so that they may notify an anesthesiologist if general anesthesia is contemplated. Succinylcholine (Anectine, Sucostrin) may be given prior to intubation; this relaxes skeletal muscle by persistent depolarization of the motor end-plate of the muscle. If a person has been on anticholinesterase drugs, less plasma cholinesterase will be available to hydrolyze the succinylcholine. As a result, more of it will arrive at the motor end-plate than is usual, causing an over-effect. There will be greater and more prolonged depolarization at the motor end-plate, and prolonged apnea may occur.

Prior to using these drugs, one should inquire about the child's history. Precautions for use include epilepsy, bronchial asthma, spastic gastrointestinal disorders, peptic ulcer, retinal detachment, and uveitis. Adverse reactions include stinging, burning, lacrimation, lid muscle twitching, conjunctival and ciliary redness, browache, induced myopia, iris cysts, conjunctival thickening, nasal lacrimal canal obstruction, and lens opacities. Iris cysts may be controlled by using 10% phenylephrine (Neo-Synephrine) in addition to the miotic.

Commonly used miotics. Echothiophate iodide (Phospholine iodide) is reconstituted to form 5 cc. of solution and is supplied in four strengths—0.03%, 0.06%, 0.125%, and 0.25%. It is stable at room temperature for 1 month and for a year if refrigerated.

For diagnostic purposes, 1 drop of 0.125% echothiophate iodide is instilled daily for 2 or 3 weeks. If a favorable response occurs, the strength should be reduced to 0.125% every other day or 0.06% every day. The 0.03% strength is successful in some cases.

Isoflurophate, diisopropyl flurophosphate, DFP (Floropryl) is hydrolyzed by water, and it is important that the tip of the tube or dropper not come into contact with the lids or a moist surface, because it is possible for the drug to become inactivated by tears. The drug is supplied in two dosage forms:

1. 0.1% anhydrous peanut oil solution, 5 ml.

2. 0.025% ointment, 3.5 g.

The ointment form is recommended for strabismus; 1 drop of ointment every night for 2 weeks is used diagnostically. If the esotropia responds, an accommodative component has been determined. For treatment, 1 drop is instilled daily for 2 weeks, then reduced to 1 drop every other day, and then 1 drop once a week for 2 months. If benefit cannot be maintained with a dosage of 1 drop every 48 hours, treatment should be discontinued.

Demecarium bromide (Humorsol) is supplied in two dosage strengths—0.125% and 0.25%. It does not have to be reconstituted, requires no refrigeration, and is stable at room temperatures for up to 3 years. For diagnosis, prescribe 1 drop daily for 2 weeks, than 1 drop every 2 days for 2 or 3 weeks. For treatment, prescribe 1 drop in each eye every day for 2 to 3 weeks, then reduce the dose to 1 drop every other day for 3 to 4 weeks. Reduce this to 1 drop twice a week, and if improvement continues, decrease to 1 drop every week. If, after 4 months, control still requires 1 drop every 2 days, the therapy should be stopped.

DETERIORATION. Some children whose eyes were initially straightened by antiaccommodative therapy will develop a nonaccommodative esotropia as they grow older. This frustrating development occurs more often in those children with abnormal distance-near relationships. When this nonaccommodative component appears, it is wise to re-evaluate the child. Amblyopia may have developed and should be treated, refraction may reveal that the hypermetropia has increased and the glasses must be strengthened, and occasionally uveitis or papilledema will have appeared. Careful ophthalmoscopic examination should be performed. If the nonaccommodative component cannot be eliminated, it may eventually require surgery.

Primary Nonaccommodative Esotropia

This type of esotropia develops between the ages of 1 and 3 years, and appears clinically similar to accommodative esotropia except that when antiaccommodative therapy is instituted the esotropia does not decrease. If amblyopia is present, it should be treated, and surgery is necessary to align the visual axes.

Mixed Accommodative and Nonaccommodative Esotropia

If a portion of the esotropia responds to antiaccommodative therapy, surgery is performed for that part of the deviation that is not corrected by glasses or miotics.

Secondary Esotropia

Secondary esotropia is an esotropia that develops following surgery for exotropia. A small esodeviation following surgery for exotropia is usually transient and desirable. However, if the esotropia persists, it must be re-evaluated and treated. Patching to prevent amblyopia may be necessary, and antiaccommodative therapy may reduce the deviation. If these measures fail, surgery will be necessary.

BLIND SPOT SYNDROME. If the secondary esotropia is between 25Δ and 35Δ, the blind spot (optic disc) will serve as a suppression scotoma. This is not a common occurrence.

Cyclic Esotropia

This is an uncommon type of esotropia that appears and disappears in a periodic manner. Usually the esotropia appears in a regular 48-hour cycle, although 72- and 96-hour cycles have also been reported. On the squinting day, the esotropia is large and associated with suppression and no diplopia. On the nonsquinting days, no deviation or only a small esophoria is present, and binocular function is good. Amblyopia is absent.

Abnormal EEG, epileptiform seizures, personality changes, excessive sleepiness, and increased frequency of micturition have been observed.

The mechanism of cyclic esotropia remains unknown, and glasses are of little help. Surgery has been reported as yielding good results.

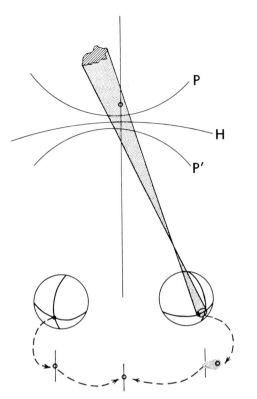

Figure 6–24 Right esotropia with a suppression scotoma encompassing the object of regard and the fovea. This adaptive mechanism overcomes visual confusion. H, horopter and P and P' outline the boundries of Panum's fusional space. (Dr. Manley Modified from Parks, M. M., and Eustis, A.: Amer. Orthopt. J., *11*:38–45, 1961.)

Monofixation Syndrome (Fig. 6–24)

The monofixation syndrome is a small angle tropia (up to 6 to 8Δ) associated with peripheral fusion. Although the type of tropia may be exo- or hyper-, the majority are estropia, so this entity is discussed here. A number of characteristic findings occur in regular association and identify this entity. Monofixation is a constant finding in that, under binocular viewing circumstances, the fovea of one eye is used for fixation while the fovea of the deviated eye is suppressed.

Clinical Findings

MONOFIXATION. Under binocular viewing circumstances, one eye fixates and there is a small tropia of the other eye with suppression of its fovea. The monofixation pattern can be diagnosed by using the monocular cover-uncover test as well as the 4Δ test (Fig. 6–25).

TROPIA. A small tropia of up to 6 to 8Δ may be seen. The 4Δ test does not determine the direction of the tropia, whereas the monocular cover-uncover test does. There may be an esotropia (majority), exotropia, or hypertropia, or any combination of these.

AMBLYOPIA. Amblyopia is usually present, although one may occasionally see a patient with equal visual acuity.

RETINAL CORRESPONDENCE. The retinal correspondence is usually thought to be anomalous and usually harmonious.

PERIPHERAL FUSION is present in monofixation syndrome and can be demonstrated using the Bagolini striated glasses, Worth 4 lights, and the major amblyoscope.

STEREOPSIS. Individuals with monofixation syndrome have less than perfect stereopsis, as detected by the Wirt stereotest. The stereoacuity is 67 seconds of arc or less.

SUPPRESSION OF FOVEA OF DEVIATING EYE. An absolute macular scotoma is present under binocular viewing circumstances and disappears when the vision is tested monocularly. The scotoma can easily be demonstrated using the Polaroid vectograph slide.

Practical Aspects of the Monofixation Syndrome

Many individuals with a small tropia have amblyopia and poor stereoacuity and yet seem to have straight eyes. The cause of the visual defect may therefore not be apparent. Unnecessary worry and evaluation will be prevented if the problem can be explained by finding a small tropia. The amblyopia is best treated by occlusion of the better eye.

EXODEVIATIONS

Proper alignment of the visual axes requires that the eyes be placed in proper position. In addition, there must be a normal balance between convergence and divergence mechanisms.

There are two factors in the pathogenesis of the exodeviations. First, mechanical causes may place the eyes in a position of divergence that cannot be overcome by convergence mechanisms. Crouzon's dis-

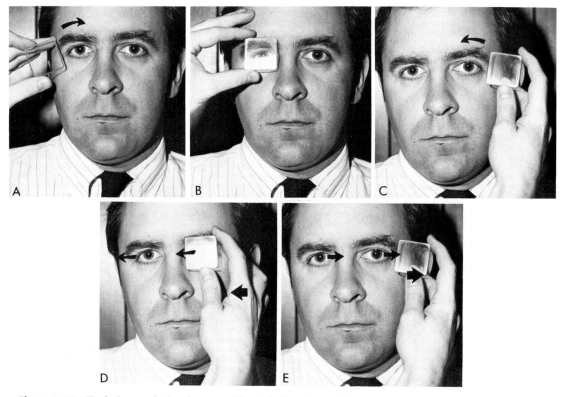

Figure 6–25 Techniques of 4Δ prism test. The individual has a 5Δ monofixational esotropia of the right eye. Under binocular circumstances a suppression scotoma is present around the right fovea. The individual is asked to fixate a small symbol at distance with both eyes uncovered. *A*, The prism base out approaches the right eye. *B*, The prism is before the right eye and deflects the image of the symbol temporally on the retina of that eye. This is unnoticed because this new location lies within the suppression scotoma; hence, no change in fixation of the right eye occurs. *C*, The prism base out approaches the left eye, and in *D* it is before the left eye. The prism deflects the image of the symbol so that the image falls temporal to the fovea of the left eye. The left eye will quickly shift its fixation toward the direction of the apex of the prism, moving the fovea temporally and refixating the image of the symbol. The right eye will conjugately move to the right at the same time. *E*, The prism is removed from the left eye, and both eyes shift conjugately to the left as the left eye again refixates to its original position prior to the test. (From Manley, D. R.: Symposium on Horizontal Ocular Deviations. St. Louis, The C. V. Mosby Co., 1971.)

ease with its abnormal orbital osteology is an example (Fig. 6–26).

The second factor is an abnormality in the relationship between convergence and divergence. Divergence is an active process, and when it is excessive an exodeviation develops which may then be modified by the convergence mechanisms. The centers and pathways of divergence are unknown.

Definitions

Exophoria—a divergent alignment of the visual axes that is kept latent by fusion.

Exophoria-Tropia (intermittent exotropia)—an intermittent divergent alignment of the visual axes that is partially latent (*phoria*) and partially manifest (*tropia*).

Exotropia—a manifest divergent align-

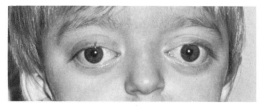

Figure 6–26 Craniofacial dysostosis (Crouzon's disease). Ocular findings include exophthalmos, hypertelorism, downward slanting palpebral fissures and exotropia. Optic atrophy may be present.

ment of the visual axes. It occurs (1) when the magnitude of the deviation exceeds the compensatory abilities of fusion or (2) when the compensatory abilities of fusion are decreased (illness, fatigue) or absent entirely (injury, cataract).

Divergence Excess—an exodeviation greater at distance than at near. This occurs when excessive divergence impulses occur.

Pseudodivergence Excess—an exodeviation that initially seems to be greater at distance than at near. When the near measurement is remeasured with a +3.00 sphere before each eye, the near deviation increases, and approximates or equals the distance deviation. Why some near deviations respond in this manner while others do not remains unclear.

Basic Exotropia—an exodeviation that measures the same at both distance and near. In this instance there is a secondary failure of convergence at near.

Convergence Insufficiency—an exodeviation that is greater at near than at distance. In this instance there are inadequate accommodative and fusional convergence impulses.

Secondary Exotropia—an exotropia that occurs following surgery for esotropia. (Also called consecutive exotropia by some ophthalmologists.)

Consecutive Exotropia—an exotropia that spontaneously develops from an esotropia.

Usually the esotropia has significant hypermetropia and amblyopia present. (Also called secondary exotropia by some ophthalmologists.)

Classification of Exodeviations

Exodeviations may be classified according to fusion (exophoria, intermittent exotropia, or constant exotropia) or by the distance-near relationship (divergence excess, basic, and convergence insufficiency). (See Table 6–4.) One classification that has been found clinically useful is the following:

1. Pseudoexotropia
2. Congenital exotropia
3. Acquired exodeviations
   a. Exophoria
   b. Intermittent exotropia
   c. Secondary exotropia
   d. Consecutive exotropia

Pseudoexotropia

Pseudoexotropia may be present as a result of a positive angle kappa or a wide interpupillary distance. Some normal children may appear to have an exotropia when they look to the side (Fig. 6–27). One should remember that retinopathy of prematurity may cause a positive angle kappa as a result of temporal dragging of the macula.

TABLE 6–4 CLASSIFICATION OF EXODEVIATIONS*

Duane	AC/A ratio	Abbreviation	
Divergence excess	High	XT	= 30Δ
		X′	= 4Δ
		X′ (+3.00) =	4Δ
Pseudodivergence excess	High	XT	= 30Δ
		X′	= 4Δ
		XT′ (+3.00) =	30Δ
Basic	Normal	XT	= 30Δ
		XT′	= 30Δ
		XT	= 10Δ
Convergence insufficiency	Low	XT′	= 20Δ

*From Manley, D. R.: Classification of the exodeviations. *In* Manley, D. R. (ed.): Symposium on Horizontal Ocular Deviations. St. Louis, The C. V. Mosby Co., 1971, p. 132.

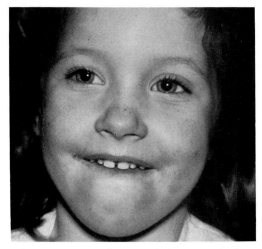

Figure 6–27 Pseudoexotropia in a normal 4-year-old child. A positive angle kappa in the right eye is accentuated when the eyes look to the right, giving the appearance of an exotropia.

Congenital Exotropia (Fig. 6–28)

True congenital exotropia does occur, although much less commonly than congenital esotropia. In many instances it is the result of an imbalance between divergence and convergence; the refractive error is normal, and there may be decreased adduction and increased abduction. Occlusion will usually demonstrate that good adduction is present. Surgery is usually necessary; as the angle of the exotropia is usually quite large, more than one operation may be required.

Acquired Exodeviations

Exophoria

A small exophoria is commonly seen in normal children who remain asymptomatic and require no treatment. As the deviation is latent, the parents do not notice it, and it usually is detected by the ophthalmologist on a routine examination. A large exophoria may be symptomatic, producing eyestrain and blurry vision. If glasses are worn, a hypermetropia may be undercorrected or a myopia overcorrected. Surgery is not usually necessary.

Intermittent Exotropia

This is the most common type of exodeviation seen in children and is usually first noticed by the parents after the child has reached the age of 2. The incidence is greater in older children than in younger children, and there is a strong hereditary influence. There are four types of intermittent exotropia, based on the distance-near relationship. These are:

1. Divergence excess
2. Pseudodivergence excess
3. Basic
4. Convergence insufficiency

DIAGNOSIS

As already mentioned, the parents will usually notice that one eye turns out; this is more pronounced when the child is looking off at the distance, toward the end of the day when tired, or when ill. The child will usually realign the visual axes to regain fusion, and the deviation remains intermittent. A notable characteristic of intermittent exotropia is the child's closure of one eye when out-of-doors on a sunny day. Thus a seasonal improvement may be noticed during the winter. There are two common explanations for this. One is that out-of-doors there are fewer near clues to stimulate convergence; the second is that the bright light dazzles the retinas and disrupts fusion.

SENSORY FINDINGS

Children with exodeviations develop suppression quite easily, which explains the lack of symptoms and the absence of diplopia in most instances. Amblyopia, anomalous retinal correspondence, and eccentric fixation are unusual.

CLINICAL FINDINGS (Fig. 6–29)

1. *Divergence excess*—the exotropia is greater when measured at distance than at near. If possible, it is wise to take the

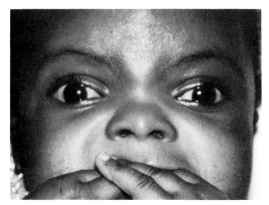

Figure 6–28 True congenital exotropia noticed at birth.

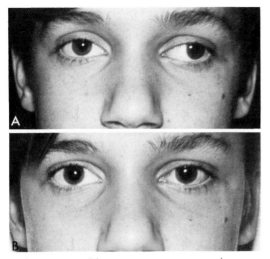

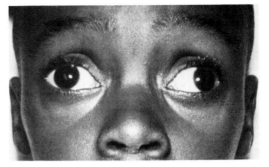

Figure 6–30 Basic type of exotropia with similar distance-near measurements. Adduction was full in each eye.

Figure 6–29 Divergence excess exotropia occurring in a 7-year-old boy. *A,* A left exotropia at distance of 35 prism diopters. *B,* An exophoria at near of 8 prism diopters.

measurement at extreme distances, to uncover as much of the exotropia as possible. This deviation is noticed more when the child is looking off in the distance, or when he is tired or ill. At near, the deviation is much smaller and may only be a small exophoria. When the near measurement is retaken with +3.00 sphere before each eye, the near deviation does not increase appreciably.

2. *Pseudodivergence excess.* Clinically this is exactly similar to divergence excess, with one exception. When the near measurement is repeated with +3.00 sphere, it increases and may be as great (or in some children, greater) as the distance exotropia. Why some near deviations increase in this manner remains unclear.

3. *Basic*—the distance and near measurements are similar (Fig. 6–30).

4. *Convergence insufficiency*—the near exodeviation is greater than that at distance. These children have poor con-

vergence amplitude, a poorly sustained or remote near point of convergence, and blurring of vision at near; they may also complain of diplopia.

TREATMENT (Table 6–5)

1. *Divergence excess.* If the deviation is less than 15Δ and fusion is good, it may be possible to help this condition by optical methods. Correction of any refractive error is important. If hypermetropic spectacles are being worn, reducing their strength will stimulate accommodative convergence. If myopic spectacles are being worn, increasing their strength will accomplish the same thing. These optical methods may be employed, but it must be realized that accommodative convergence is being stimulated when the primary problem is a lack of sufficient fusional convergence. Orthoptic excercises may be helpful in some children.

In deviations over 15Δ, surgery may be necessary. When the exotropia at distance is 20Δ or more, surgery is almost always required to correct the deviation. This type of exotropia does not necessarily worsen as the child get older, and it is helpful to repeat the measurements at 3- to 4-month intervals. In this way the ophthal-

TABLE 6–5 SURGICAL TREATMENT OF EXODEVIATIONS*

Exotropia	Recommended Surgery
Divergence excess	Recess LR of OU
Pseudodivergence excess	Recess LR of OU, or resect MR and recess LR—same eye
Basic	Resect MR and recess LR—same eye
Convergence insufficiency	Resect MR of OU

*From Manley, D. R.: Classification of the exodeviations. *In* Manley, D. R. (ed.): Symposium on Horizontal Ocular Deviations. St. Louis, The C. V. Mosby Co., 1971, p. 135.

mologist is able to determine the clinical course, and the parents are able to report their impressions as well. Surgery is performed to eliminate the distance exotropia (see Table 6–5). This may be in the form of a recession of both lateral rectus muscles or a monocular recession-resection. There is no evidence that better results are obtained using the latter procedure on the fixating eye as opposed to the nonfixating eye. Surgery may be performed as early as possible, provided the surgeon has been able to measure the deviation. If an undercorrection occurs in the immediate postoperative period, the deviation will probably recur. A small overcorrection of less than 20Δ occurring in the first 2 weeks following surgery is desirable, as it is usually temporary and ultimately will provide the better result. If the overcorrection persists, one should wait patiently for it to decrease. It is important to follow the child closely, to prevent sensory adaptation to the esotropia. If the esotropia is 25Δ or 30Δ, the blind spot may be used by the child to eliminate diplopia. Alternate patching may be necessary to prevent suppression, amblyopia, and the development of anomalous retinal correspondence. Antiaccommodative therapy in the form of glasses or miotics may be necessary. In a small number of children, the secondary esotropia is permanent and persists for many months or even years. It should be re-evaluated and treated as a new case of esotropia. Surgery for this is usually quite successful.

2. *Pseudodivergence excess.* Surgery is planned to eliminate the distance exotropia; this may be accomplished by a recession of both lateral rectus muscles or by a monocular recession-resection. The choice remains that of the surgeon. Postoperative evaluation and results are similar to those noted for divergence excess, in the preceding paragraph.

3. *Basic.* The treatment is usually a recession of the lateral rectus and a resection of the medial rectus of the deviating eye. Postoperative evaluation and results are similar to those for divergence excess. It has not been proved that an overcorrection is as desirable in this type.

4. *Convergence insufficiency.* Orthoptic exercises are quite helpful in this type of exotropia, and an attempt is made to increase the fusional convergence amplitude. Base-in prisms for near work may be helpful.

Surgery may be performed, and although the distance exotropia is eliminated, there may be a residual near exotropia. If surgery is performed for the near deviation, there may be a postoperative esotropia at distance with diplopia.

Secondary Exotropia (Fig. 6–31)

This type of exotropia follows surgery performed for esotropia. Quite often the esotropia was variable or partially accommodative, or significant hypermetropia and amblyopia were present. This type of deviation is commonly seen in adults who had surgery for esotropia as children.

A small secondary exotropia may be treated conservatively by weakening the hypermetropic spectacles, thereby stimulating accommodative convergence. If glasses are not being worn, the deviation should be evaluated completely, and surgery performed as necessary.

Consecutive Exotropia

This type of exotropia develops spontaneously from an esotropia. Quite often the esotropia was accommodative, and significant hypermetropia and amblyopia are common findings. Treatment is similar to that for secondary exotropia.

A AND V PATTERNS

The A and V patterns are esotropias and exotropias in which there is a significant difference in the horizontal deviation in straight upward gaze when compared with straight downward gaze. There are four types:

1. *V-ET (V-esotropia)* has a greater esotropia in downgaze than in upgaze.

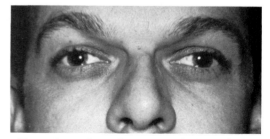

Figure 6–31 Secondary exotropia in a 27-year-old male. Onset of esotropia at age 2 years which was partially accommodative. Surgery performed at age 7 years. Exotropia appeared around 9 years of age and slowly increased during the teen-age years.

2. *A-ET (A-esotropia)* has a greater esotropia in upgaze than in downgaze.
3. *V-XT (V-exotropia)* has a greater exotropia in upgaze than in downgaze.
4. *A-XT (A-exotropia)* has a greater exotropia in downgaze than in upgaze.

The terminology of A and V is intended to be descriptive of the position of the eyes when the deviation is the greatest. Surgical principles take into account two factors. The first is the abducting effect of the oblique muscles in midline up- and downgaze. The inferior obliques have an abducting effect of up to 15Δ in straight upgaze and negligible effect in the primary position. The superior obliques have as much as 45Δ of abducting effect in straight downgaze and approximately 15Δ abducting effect in the primary position. Therefore, weakening the inferior obliques can increase an esotropia or decrease an exotropia in upgaze. The superior obliques have a similar, although greater, effect in straight downgaze and to a lesser extent in the primary position.

The second clinical factor is that when the insertions of the horizontal rectus muscles are moved up or down, their pulling power is altered. The principle of placement direction is: *Move the muscle in the direction where the greatest weakening is desired.* For example, in V-esotropia the deviation is greater in downgaze than in the primary position. Since a greater effect is desired in downgaze, the medial rectus muscles should be lowered in addition to being receded. It is usually satisfactory to move the insertions of the muscles 5 mm.

The etiology of the A and V patterns is variable, and I would agree with Dunlap in favoring the combined school as to etiology: "The combined school considers the etiology of the A-V patterns to be variable, and further, that some patients have dysfunction of the horizontal muscles with no vertical component existent, let alone contributory, while others have a clear-cut demonstrable vertical dysfunction."

There are a number of surgical procedures that one might perform for these patterns. The procedures to be mentioned are those with which I have had experience and from which I have obtained satisfactory results.

V-ET (Fig. 6–32)

This is usually associated with overaction of the inferior obliques and underaction of

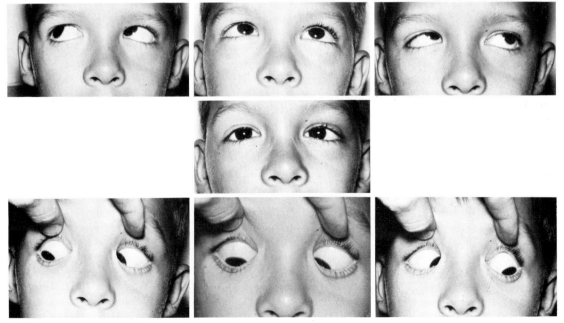

Figure 6–32 V pattern in esotropia. The esotropia increases in straight down gaze and decreases in straight up gaze. Overaction of both inferior oblique muscles causes greater abduction in up gaze. Underaction of both superior oblique muscles causes decreased abduction in down gaze. (From Harley, R. D.: *In* Manley, D. R.: Symposium on Horizontal Ocular Deviations. St. Louis, The C. V. Mosby Co., 1971.)

the superior obliques. Weakening the inferior obliques will decrease their abducting power in straight upgaze, which is desirable; at the same time, the hypertropia of the adducted eye in side gaze will be corrected. The medial rectus muscles are receded an appropriate amount for the esotropia in the primary position, and lowering their insertions will give the desired greater effect on the esotropia in downgaze.

A-ET (Fig. 6–33)

This is usually associated with underaction of both inferior obliques and overaction of both superior obliques. Usually the overaction of the latter is not as great as that seen in the A-XT, and it is usually not necessary to weaken these muscles. Satisfactory results may be obtained by receding both medial rectus muscles for the esotropia in the primary position and raising their insertions by 5 mm. Resecting and lowering the lateral rectus muscles may be performed later if necessary. When the overaction of the superior obliques is marked, they may be weakened at the same time that the medial rectus muscles are receded.

V-XT (Fig. 6–34)

This is usually associated with overaction of both inferior obliques; underaction of the superior obliques, when present, is usually not marked. Usually both lateral rectus muscles are receded and both inferior obliques weakened. In some instances it may be desirable to also raise the lateral rectus muscles if the V pattern is quite large.

A-XT (Fig. 6–35)

This is usually associated with underaction of both inferior obliques and marked overaction of both superior obliques. Usually the superior obliques are weakened to eliminate the marked difference that is present in the exotropia between the primary position and downgaze. Horizontal muscle surgery is also performed for the exotropia. Interestingly, this type of pattern often has an associated vertical strabismus of the dissociated type.

In some instances an exotropia may have overaction of all of the oblique muscles, resulting in an "X" pattern. It is usually sufficient to eliminate the exotropia by operating the horizontal rectus muscles

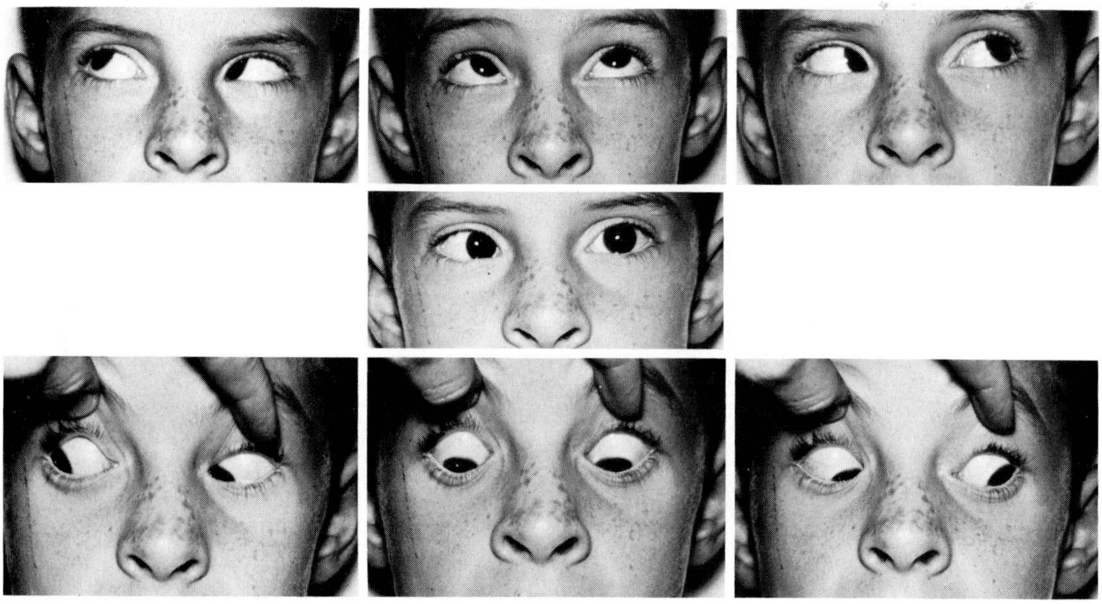

Figure 6–33 A pattern in esotropia. The esotropia increases in straight up gaze and decreases in straight down gaze. Underaction of both inferior oblique muscles causes decreased abduction in up gaze. Overaction of both superior obliques muscles causes increased abduction in down gaze. (From Harley, R. D.: *In* Manley, D. R.: Symposium on Horizontal Ocular Deviations. St. Louis, The C. V. Mosby Co., 1971.)

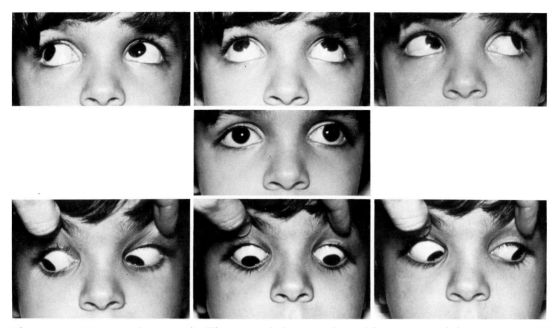

Figure 6–34 V pattern in exotropia. The exotropia increases in straight up gaze and decreases in straight down gaze. Overaction of both inferior oblique muscles causes increased abduction in up gaze. Underaction of both superior oblique muscles causes decreased abduction in down gaze.

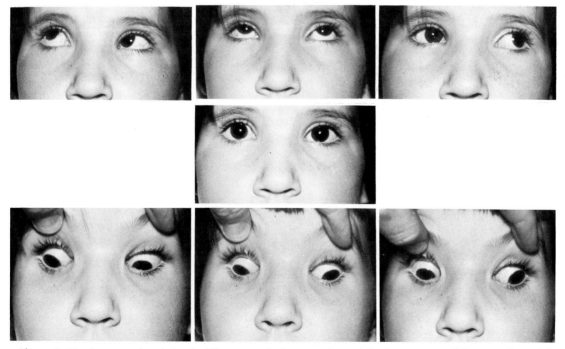

Figure 6–35 A pattern in exotropia. The exotropia increases in straight down gaze and decreases in straight up gaze. Overaction of both superior oblique muscles causes increased abduction in down gaze. Underaction of both inferior oblique muscles causes decreased abduction in up gaze.

rather than weakening all of the oblique muscles. When the exotropia has been eliminated, the overaction of the oblique muscles is usually less apparent.

Note: If the surgeon prefers the monocular recession-resection operation, the appropriate offsetting of the medial and lateral rectus for these patterns will produce a satisfactory result.

VERTICAL STRABISMUS

Although many of the horizontal deviations are accompanied by vertical deviations, there are a number of entities that are primarily vertical in nature; these will be discussed in this section.

Most of the horizontal deviations are nonparalytic and occur in otherwise healthy children. One must approach the vertical deviations with greater suspicion, as they are often caused by injury or disease that affects one or more of the vertically acting muscles. The history is important, and one should inquire about injury, previous surgery, general health, and fluctuations in the deviation. In the complete evaluation one must include monocular rotations (ductions), binocular rotations (versions), primary and secondary deviations, measurements in the diagnostic positions of gaze, including right and left head tilt, and forced ductions. Forced ductions should always be performed, and general anesthesia is usually necessary in a child. If the child is old enough, diplopia evaluation may be possible if suppression is not present.

If one suspects that a hypertropia is present, cover testing should be carefully performed. A pseudohypertropia will have no shift of the visual axes. If the hypertropia is of the dissociated type there will not be a corresponding hypotropia of the other eye when the eyes are alternately covered. Most hypertropias have a corresponding hypotropia of the other eye.

Classification of Vertical Strabismus

1. Pseudovertical strabismus
2. Dissociative vertical strabismus
3. Comitant vertical strabismus

4. Incomitant vertical strabismus
   a. Brown's syndrome
   b. Double elevator palsy
   c. Orbital injury, including blowout fracture of the floor of the orbit
   d. Isolated cyclovertical muscle palsy
      i. Superior oblique palsy
      ii. Superior rectus palsy
      iii. Inferior rectus palsy
      iv. Inferior oblique palsy
   e. Orbital tumors
   f. Endocrine myopathy
   g. Postoperative

Pseudovertical Strabismus (Fig. 6–36)

Some children "appear" to have a hypertropia even when cover testing reveals that there is no misalignment of the visual axes. Complete examination usually reveals the reason. Some of the more common explanations are: vertical angle kappa, vertically displaced macula, orbital asymmetry, lid retraction, displaced globe by a tumor, and

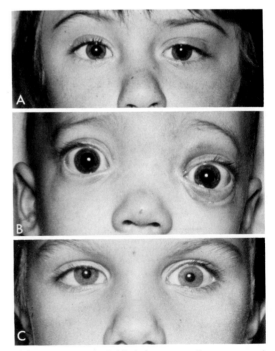

Figure 6–36 *A,* Orbital asymmetry is present and the left eye appears to be lower than the right. No misalignment of the visual axes is present. *B,* Orbital tumor has pushed the left eye downward. The visual axes remain aligned. *C,* Unilateral retraction of the left upper lid results in the left eye appearing to be lower (pseudohypotropia).

macular degeneration with eccentric fixation above or below the fovea.

Dissociative Vertical Strabismus (Fig. 6–37)

This is also called *alternating sursumduction, occlusion hyperphoria, double hypertropia,* and *double dissociative hypertropia.* The diagnosis is confirmed by the cover test. When the cover is placed before one eye, the eye will elevate, extort, and usually abduct. When the cover is removed, the eye will depress, intort, and adduct to the position it had prior to cover testing. The deviation may be a phoria, a phoria-tropia, or a tropia, and it may be unilateral or bilateral. One eye may be more affected than the other, and the magnitude of the deviation may be different in the various diagnostic positions of gaze. The main differentiating feature of this entity is the finding on alternate cover testing that there is no corresponding hypotropia of the other eye.

Because of suppression, there are usually no symptoms in dissociative vertical strabismus, but the affected child or his parent will complain of one eye being higher than the other. Most children with this devia-

tion will have had congenital esotropia or another type of strabismus with onset in infancy.

The cause remains unknown, but is thought to be innervational. Overaction of an inferior oblique may be seen in association with but does not cause dissociative vertical strabismus.

Resecting the inferior rectus of the involved eye will help anchor the eye so that it does not elevate as readily. Postoperatively there may be narrowing of the palpebral fissure with some restriction of upward gaze, and the parent should be told of this possibility. Weakening the inferior oblique or superior rectus has produced disappointing results.

Comitant Vertical Strabismus

The hypertropia is the same in the primary position as it is in gaze to the right and left. Evaluation reveals that no over- or underaction of any muscle is present. If the deviation is small (15Δ or less), one should lower the involved eye or raise the lower eye by operating an appropriate vertical rectus muscle. If the deviation is larger (20Δ or more), two vertical rectus muscles may be operated. It is preferable that one muscle of each eye should be operated. For example, if an individual had 20Δ of left hypertropia, one could recede the left superior rectus and the right inferior rectus. This would weaken a vertical muscle with a greater vertical effect in right gaze (RIR) and also weaken a vertical muscle with a greater vertical effect in left gaze (LSR). Such a procedure would be preferable to operating the LSR and LIR, which would be expected to have more effect in left gaze than right gaze.

Because the oblique muscles have less vertical action in the primary position than the vertical rectus muscles, it is preferable to operate on the latter to correct a hypertropia in the primary position.

Incomitant Vertical Strabismus

Brown's Syndrome (Fig. 6–38)

Under elevation of an eye in adduction has been observed clinically for many years and has usually been described as an iso-

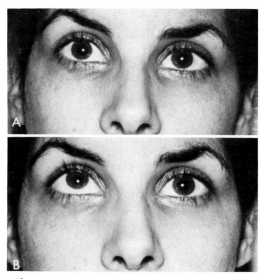

Figure 6–37 Dissociative vertical strabismus. *A,* No vertical deviation is present. *B,* Following occlusion of the right eye, a large dissociated right hypertropia is apparent. On alternate cover testing there is no corresponding hypotropia of the left eye.

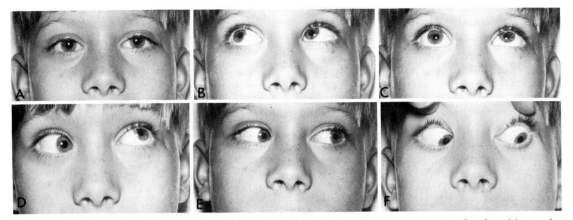

Figure 6–38 Brown's syndrome of the right eye (typical). *A*, There is no compensatory head position and a exophoria in the primary position of 6Δ. *B*, Slight overaction of the left inferior oblique. *C*, Limitation of the right eye in upward gaze. *D*, No elevation of the right eye in adduction and widening of the right palpebral fissure. This limitation remained the same on monocular rotations as well. *E*, Slight downshoot of the right eye in adduction (levoversion) and slight widening of the right palpebral fissure. *F*, No overaction of the right superior oblique.

lated paralysis or pseudoparalysis of the inferior oblique. In 1945 Brown found that a short sheath of the superior oblique tendon was present in this condition, and in 1950 he reported what has since been called the superior oblique tendon sheath syndrome of Brown. Since that time, other causes have also been found, and in some individuals no anatomic explanation is found at the time of surgery.

CLINICAL FEATURES

The clinical features of Brown's syndrome are as follows:

1. The main finding is restriction or absence of elevation in adduction, appearing clinically as a weakness of the inferior oblique. The degree of limitation of elevation is the same on version, duction, or passive rotation. As the eye gradually rotates from its position of adduction toward elevation in abduction, there will be a corresponding increase in elevation. The gradual increase in elevation will be a straight line from the midhorizontal plane in full adduction to full elevation near straight upgaze.

2. There is usually widening of the palpebral fissure on adduction.

3. There is little or no overaction of the homolateral superior oblique.

4. If any change in the horizontal alignment occurs in straight upgaze, it is always an exotropia which results in a V pattern.

5. Downshoot of the affected eye may be present in adduction.

6. There may be a compensatory head position.

7. There is usually normal or near normal muscle balance in the primary position.

8. Forced ductions are positive.

9. Although usually unilateral, the syndrome may be bilateral.

Brown has subdivided the entity into true and simulated tendon sheath syndromes, as in the following classification:

I. True sheath syndrome
   a. *Typical:* no underaction of the homolateral superior rectus.
   b. *Atypical:* significant underaction of the homolateral superior rectus.

II. Simulated sheath syndrome
   a. Spontaneous recovery cases have been reported, but none in an individual found to have a positive forced duction test.
   b. Intermittent cases: These have been related to rheumatoid arthritis, and to injury and inflammation in the region of the trochlea.
   c. Following orbital floor fracture.

ETIOLOGY

According to Brown, the true sheath syndrome is caused by a congenitally shortened anterior sheath of the superior oblique tendon. In most cases, however, one is unable to determine the cause of the restriction. The etiology is a spectrum of disorders, and a differential diagnosis based solely on the clinical features is impossible.

TREATMENT

Treatment is not necessary unless there is a compensatory head position and a downshoot of the involved eye with a vertical deviation. If the forced ductions are normal, surgery will probably not be helpful. If the forced ductions are positive, the restriction must be identified. In some instances it has been found that the fine attachments between the tendon and the anterior sheath restrict movement of the tendon within the sheath. After these attachments are lysed, the forced ductions may improve, and the eye is then sutured in a position of elevation in adduction for 5 to 6 days. This procedure has been helpful in some instances.

Double Elevator Palsy (Fig. 6–39)

Weakness of both elevators of the same eye (superior rectus and inferior oblique), usually congenital, is the major feature of this condition. Elevation is limited through the entire upper field: in the temporal field as a result of the superior rectus and in the nasal field from the inferior oblique.

There may be a true ptosis or pseudoptosis accompanying the muscle problem. The true ptosis is due to a weakness of the levator, whereas the pseudoptosis is brought about by the involved eye being lower. When the nonparetic eye is used for fixation, the paretic eye is lower and the lid follows the eye down. Three clinical varieties may be seen:

1. Binocularity is maintained by tilting the head backward so as to move the eyes into the field of the depressors. Vision is usually normal, and when the head is placed in the primary position, diplopia may be demonstrable. This is the most common type.

2. Fixation is with the nonparetic eye, and the paretic eye is hypotropic. It is in this type that ptosis is most noticeable. Vision in the paretic eye is often 20/200 or less.

3. Fixation is with the paretic eye. In this type the nonparetic eye has a pronounced secondary deviation which makes this the most disfiguring of the three types. Vision in the nonparetic eye is often reduced. This is the least common type.

TREATMENT

Double elevator palsy must be differentiated from those conditions causing a restriction in upward gaze. These include blowout fracture of the orbital floor, atypi-

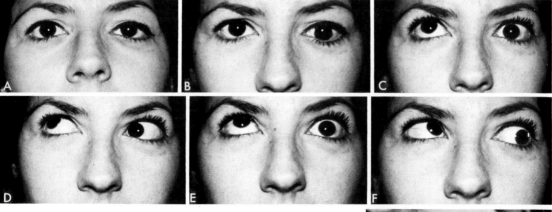
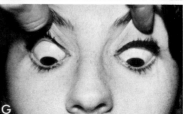

Figure 6–39 Double elevator palsy of the left eye. *A*, Fixation with right eye: eyes are in a slight down gaze position because of chin elevation. *B*, Fixation with nonparetic eye in primary position results in a left hypotropia and pseudoptosis. *C*, Fixation with paretic eye results in marked secondary deviation of the right eye. Note that the left upper lid has elevated to its normal position, indicating that this is a pseudoptosis. *D*, Inability to elevate the left eye in adduction (LIO). *E*, Inability to elevate the left eye in straight up gaze (LIO and LSR). *F*, Inability to elevate the left eye in abduction (LSR). *G*, Normal depression of both eyes.

cal Brown's syndrome, and endocrine myopathy with involvement of the inferior rectus. Forced ductions and x-rays are of great importance. If these are normal, surgery may be performed to help improve the compensatory chin elevation and the hypotropia in the primary position. Transposition of the medial and lateral rectus muscles of the paretic eye up to the superior rectus works quite well.

Orbital Injury: Fracture of the Floor of the Orbit (Fig. 6–40)

Following injury to the orbital region, the thin floor of the orbit may break, and some of the orbital contents, including the inferior rectus, may become entrapped. This may cause a vertical strabismus. If the inferior rectus is entrapped, there will be a restriction in upward gaze with good depression. Other associated signs are narrowing of the palpebral fissure caused by

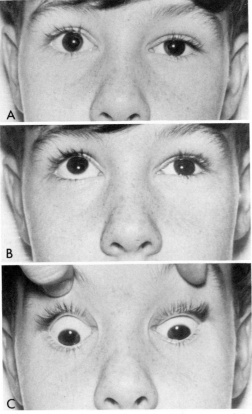

Figure 6–40 Blowout fracture of the floor of the left orbit. *A,* Enophthalmos and narrowing of the palpebral fissure of the left eye. *B,* Restriction of upward gaze of left eye. *C,* Normal depression.

enophthalmos, and decreased sensation in the area supplied by the infraorbital nerve. There is usually a history of trauma, with external evidence of injury to the orbital region. X-rays should be obtained to determine if a fracture is present. Forced ductions are important, and should be performed to determine whether a mechanical restriction is present.

TREATMENT

In the acute phase it may be necessary to repair the floor of the orbit with a synthetic material, after the inferior rectus has been freed and the forced ductions are normal. If the ocular motility is normal and enophthalmos is not present, it may not be necessary to insert a plate in the floor. Each patient must be carefully evaluated and treated accordingly.

In the chronic phase it may not be possible to free the inferior rectus, because of the healing that has occurred in the floor region. Under these circumstances it may be wiser to perform strabismus surgery on the basis of the type of hypertropia that is present. Forced ductions are of importance before, during, and following surgery.

Two other types of vertical strabismus may occur following orbital injury:

1. Injury to the inferior rectus or its nerve supply. This will cause a hypertropia that increases in downgaze and decreases in upgaze. This type of problem is usually not corrected by repair of the floor, and strabismus surgery is usually necessary after a period of 9 to 12 months if the inferior rectus weakness does not spontaneously improve.

2. Paresis of the superior oblique of either eye may occur as a result of the blunt head trauma. This type of vertical strabismus will not be improved by the repair of the floor of the orbit. If spontaneous improvement does not occur within 9 to 12 months, surgery will be necessary.

Isolated Cyclovertical Muscle Palsy

Any of the eight cyclovertical muscles (vertical rectus and oblique muscles) may be paretic, either singly or in combination, resulting in an incomitant hypertropia. The paresis may be congenital, or it may be acquired as the result of injury or disease.

In the primary position, the vertical

TABLE 6–6A THREE-STEP TEST FOR LEFT HYPERTROPIA

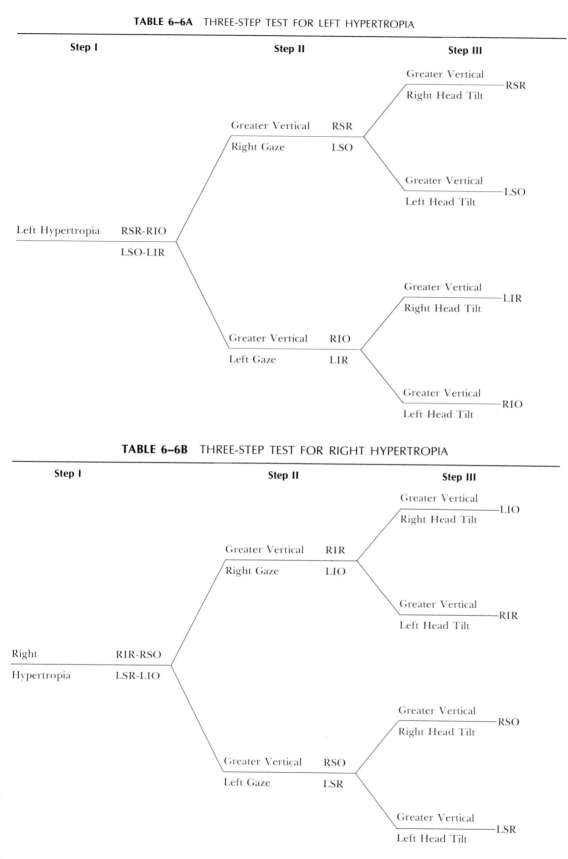

TABLE 6–6B THREE-STEP TEST FOR RIGHT HYPERTROPIA

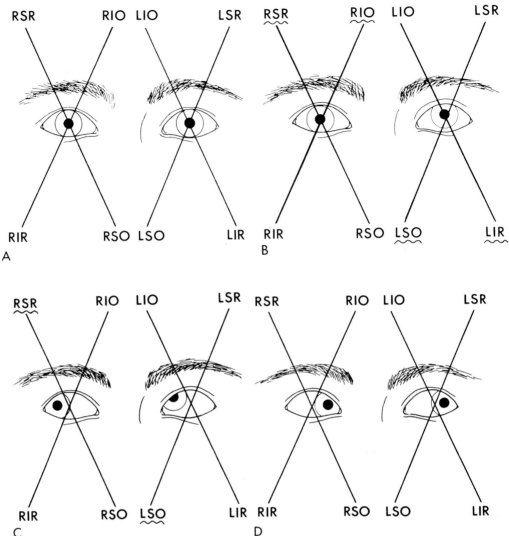

Figure 6–41 *A,* Primary position showing the positions of gaze in which the vertical actions of the cyclovertical muscles are maximal. *B,* Left hypertropia, which could be caused by a weakness of the LSO, LIR, RIO, or RSR. *C,* Left hypertropia greater in straight gaze (LSO-RSR). *D,* No hypertropia in straight left gaze.

Illustration continued on opposite page.

position of the eyes is controlled mainly by the vertical rectus muscles (VRM), while the obliques control mainly the torsional position. As the eye is abducted, the vertical action of the vertical rectus muscles increases and their torsional action decreases. In adduction, the vertical action of the obliques increases and their torsional action decreases. Torsional deficits are difficult to measure, and, although confirmatory, are usually not diagnostic. The correct diagnosis may be made by measuring the vertical position of the eyes in straight

right and left gaze, including head tilting to either shoulder (three step test).

Let us take as our example paresis of the left superior oblique muscle. The left superior oblique is a depressor of the left eye, and its vertical effect increases when the eye is adducted or turned to the right. When the left eye is abducted, the vertical action decreases. If the muscle is weak, there will be a left hypertropia that is greater in right gaze than in left gaze. In addition, the left hypertropia will be greater when the head is tilted to the left

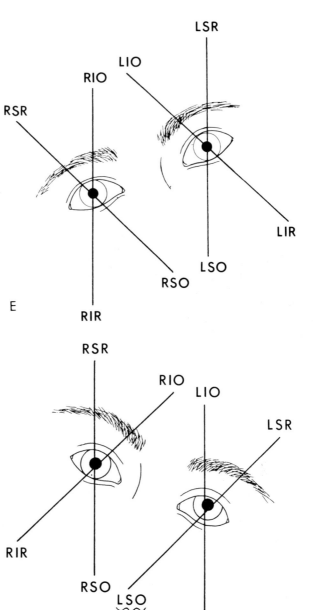

Figure 6–41 *Continued. E,* No hypertropia on right head tilt. *F,* Left hypertropia increases on left head tilt (LSO).

shoulder than to the right shoulder, as a result of the effect of gravity on the otolith apparatus.

The three step test is invaluable and should be mastered. It is valid when one is dealing with a paresis of an isolated cyclovertical muscle. Any individual with a hypertropia should be carefully evaluated with this test. However, it should be noted that this test is less helpful in individuals who have had surgery, injury, or endocrine (thyroid) disease.

THREE-STEP TEST (TABLE 6–6)

Figure 6–41*A* shows the field of greatest vertical action of the eight cyclovertical muscles as the patient faces the observer. Let us analyze a left hypertropia caused by weakness of the left superior oblique (Fig. 6–41*B*).

Step 1 (Fig. 6–41*B*). A left hypertropia is the same as a right hypotropia. Thus the cause of an LHT could be a weakness of a depressor of the left eye (LSO-LIR) or an elevator of the right eye (RSR-RIO). The fact that an LHT is present indicates that one of four muscles is weak (LSO, LIR, RSR, or RIO).

Step 2 (Fig. 6–41C and D). The left hypertropia is greater in straight right gaze than in left. The paretic muscle must be one whose vertical action is greater in right gaze. The two muscles are the RSR and the LSO. The RIO and the LIR are eliminated because their greatest vertical action is to the left.

Step 3 (Fig. 6–41, E and F). Both the LSO and the RSR are intorters, and the superior oblique is a depressor whereas the superior rectus is an elevator. When the head is tilted toward the right shoulder, the intorters of the right eye (RSR-RSO) intort, and their vertical actions are in balance (Fig. 6–41E). No hypertropia is present.

However, when the head is tilted to the left shoulder, the left hypertropia increases, confirming a diagnosis of weakness of the left superior oblique (Fig. 6–41 F). This occurs because when the head is tilted toward the left shoulder the intorters of the left eye (LSO-LSR) will attempt to intort the eye, and since the depressing power of the LSO is weak, the elevating power of the normal LSR will cause the eye to elevate.

The superior oblique is the most commonly affected muscle. Weakness of a superior rectus, inferior rectus, or inferior oblique is less common, and the three-step test is helpful in correctly diagnosing a paresis of one of these muscles. Prior to performing Step 3, it is helpful to remember that the final muscle pair will always be two superior muscles (SR-SO) that are intorters, or two inferior muscles (IR-IO) that are extorters. When the pair are *intorters*, the greater hypertropia occurs when the head is tilted *toward* the side of the eye having the paretic muscle. For example, if the LSO is paretic, the greater vertical would be found when the head is tilted to the left. When the final pair are extorters, the opposite is true: the greater hypertropia occurs when the head is tilted to the side *opposite* the eye having the paretic muscle. For example, if the right inferior oblique is paretic, the greater vertical would occur when the head is tilted toward the left shoulder.

ETIOLOGY

Many of these conditions appear to be congenital, and they occur in otherwise healthy children. Some are acquired as a result of injury, and many are idiopathic. One should always remember that myasthenia gravis or a brain stem glioma may present as a cyclovertical muscle palsy.

TREATMENT

After the patient has been completely evaluated, the strabismus may persist, and surgery is often necessary. Surgery should be performed on a vertically acting muscle whose greatest vertical action is in the field of greatest vertical action of the paretic muscle. For example, if the LSO is weak (Fig. 6–41C), the choices are: LSO, LIO, RSR, and RIR. A comparison of the vertical deviation in the three diagnostic positions of gaze to the side of the greatest vertical deviation will help the surgeon decide which muscle should be operated. These positions are: up-right, straight-right, and down-right. If the measurements are the same in these three positions, any of the four muscles would be correct. Usually, however, the LSO, LIO, or the RIR are operated. If the hypertropia is greatest in up-right gaze, the choice would be between the LIO and the RSR. (Usually the LIO is the preferred muscle.) If the hypertropia is greatest in down-right gaze, the choice would be between the LSO and the RIR. Some ophthalmologists prefer to tuck the paretic SO, while others prefer to weaken the yoke IR.

It is wise to operate on one muscle at a time, following which the strabismus is reevaluated. Any residual hypertropia is corrected as necessary. A second muscle may have to be operated 8 to 10 weeks later. It is unusual for a third muscle to be operated, and I have not yet seen a patient requiring surgery on all four muscles.

SUPERIOR OBLIQUE PALSY (FIG. 6–42)

This is the most common cyclovertical muscle palsy, and often appears to be on a congenital basis in an otherwise healthy child. The parents notice that one eye is higher than the other, and there may be a compensatory head position. Usually the face is turned into the field of action of the weak superior oblique. For example, in an LSO weakness, the head is tilted to the

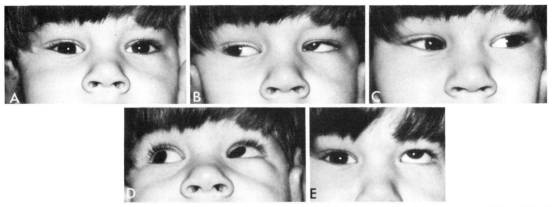

Figure 6–42 Left superior oblique palsy in a child. *A*, Small left hypertropia in the primary position. *B*, Left hypertropia increases in right gaze. *C*, No hypertropia in left gaze. *D*, Overaction of the left inferior oblique. *E*, Left hypertropia increases on left head tilt. Right head tilt not shown, as no hypertropia was present.

right shoulder, the face is turned to the right, and the chin is depressed. This position allows better alignment of the visual axes when the child is looking straight ahead.

The degree of head turn is not always proportional to the size of the hypertropia. The vertical fusional ability of the child may limit the deviation to a phoria or an intermittent tropia, and the parents may seldom notice a hypertropia. In some children the deviation becomes more evident as they grow older, and it is often difficult to determine the age of onset. Diplopia is seldom noticed, and surgery may be necessary when the hypertropia increases. In addition to correcting the strabismus, surgery will improve the head position.

Head trauma may cause a weakness of a superior oblique, although the trauma may not have been severe enough to have caused loss of consciousness. It is not always possible to prove that the palsy was the result of trauma, because the child may have had a pre-existing paresis.

Many superior oblique pareses appear to be idiopathic, as there is no history of head injury and the neurological evaluation is negative.

At first glance, skew deviation may appear to be similar to a superior oblique weakness, and one must make this differentiation.

Some surgeons prefer to tuck the superior oblique as the initial procedure, while others prefer either to weaken the inferior oblique of the eye with the paretic superior oblique or to weaken the inferior rectus of the nonparetic eye.

SUPERIOR RECTUS PALSY (FIG. 6–43)

Most superior rectus palsies appear to be congenital, and in the mild cases there is a pseudoptosis of the involved eye caused by the hypotropia. In the more severe cases there may be an associated levator muscle weakness, and in all probability this represents a partial third cranial nerve palsy. The family history is important, as other family members may have total external ophthalmoplegia or a third cranial nerve weakness.

A compensatory head position may be present, and the face is usually turned into the field of action of the paretic muscle, although in some cases the face is turned to the side of the paretic superior rectus.

The differential diagnosis includes blowout fracture of the orbit and double elevator palsy. X-rays and forced ductions are of importance preoperatively.

In mild cases, a recession of the inferior rectus of the paretic eye and resection of the paretic superior rectus will improve the hypotropia and the pseudoptosis. If the deviation is larger it may be necessary to weaken the inferior oblique of the nonparetic eye. Lid surgery may be necessary if a ptosis remains after the hypotropia has been corrected in the primary position.

INFERIOR RECTUS PALSY (FIG. 6–44)

Most inferior rectus palsies in children either are congenital or are acquired as a

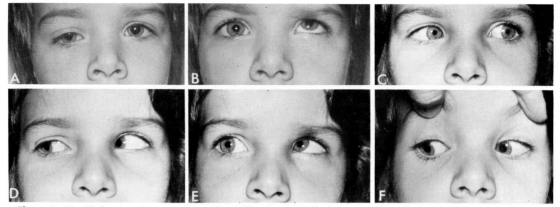

Figure 6–43   Right superior rectus paresis. *A,* Fixation with the left eye. There is a right hypotropia associated with a pseudoptosis. *B,* Fixation with paretic right eye resulting in marked secondary deviation of left eye. Note that the right upper lid has elevated to normal position, proving that a pseudoptosis was present. *C,* No hypertropia in straight left gaze. *D,* Left hypertropia increases in straight right gaze (fixation with left eye). *E,* Up-right gaze, showing underaction of right superior rectus (fixation with left eye). *F,* Down-right gaze, showing overaction of right inferior rectus (left eye fixating).

result of injury to the orbital region. There is a hypertropia of the eye with the paretic muscle. Widening of the palpebral fissure is usually present as a result of the upper lid's moving upward with the eye. The hypertropia increases in side gaze to the side of the paretic muscle and is usually greatest in the field of action of the inferior rectus.

In congenital pareses, the child is usually otherwise in good health and the family history is negative for a similar condition. Amblyopia may be present and should be treated in infancy.

Traumatic pareses may be difficult to diagnose correctly. The injury may be blunt or sharp. Blunt injuries may result in contusion to the orbital region, with swelling and vertical diplopia. Impaired depression with good elevation results and this must be differentiated from the poor elevation and good depression that result from blowout fracture of the floor of the orbit owing to entrapment of the inferior rectus. The inferior rectus may become paretic as a result of hemorrhage into the muscle, contusion of the muscle, or injury to the muscle nerve. It is not possible clinically to determine the exact mechanism. Sharp injuries often cause laceration of the inferior conjunctiva and lower eyelid. It is wise to explore the region of the

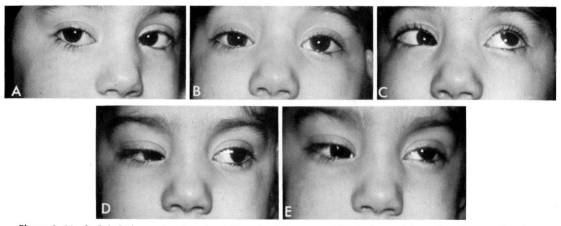

Figure 6–44   Left inferior rectus paresis. *A,* Eyes in right gaze, which is the position of comfort, and no hypertropia is present. *B,* Left hypertropia in the primary position. *C,* Up-left showing marked overaction of left superior rectus. *D,* straight left gaze showing left hypertropia. *E,* Down-left gaze showing underaction of the left inferior rectus.

inferior rectus to make sure that it has not been severed from the globe. Usually it has not, and the paresis must be assumed to be similar to that caused by blunt injury.

A compensatory head position is often present in inferior rectus paresis and is usually one of slight chin depression with the face turned to the side of the paretic muscle.

TREATMENT

Congenital paresis requires surgical correction, and forced ductions should always be performed to determine if any limitation is present. If forced ductions reveal that the eye cannot be rotated inferiorly, the ipsilateral superior rectus may be contracted and will have to be receded. If the forced ductions are normal, the inferior rectus is resected, as the hypertropia is usually greater in downgaze. In a severe paresis it may be necessary to operate both of these muscles.

INFERIOR OBLIQUE PALSY

True inferior oblique paresis does occur, but it is uncommon. It may be acquired following injury, and the hypertropia is usually not as large as that present with pareses of the other cyclovertical muscles. The underaction of the inferior oblique causes diplopia that may be present only in the field of action of the paretic muscle. On monocular rotations the eye usually elevates well in adduction. There is overaction of the ipsilateral superior oblique, and this helps to determine that the underaction of the inferior oblique is caused by weakness and not by an anatomical restriction as seen in Brown's syndrome. Forced ductions are normal. In upgaze the inferior oblique is an abductor, and a weakness of this muscle would produce an esotropia. If any pattern is present, one would expect it to be an A pattern.

DIFFERENTIAL DIAGNOSIS

Since Brown's syndrome is not uncommon, it must be differentiated from inferior oblique paresis. In most instances this is not difficult, because of the different clinical characteristics and positive forced ductions found in Brown's syndrome. In some cases of mild Brown's syndrome, the differentiation may be difficult to make, especially if the forced ductions are normal.

Bilateral paresis of the inferior obliques is extremely uncommon and has followed severe head injury in adults. Bilateral underaction of the inferior obliques may be seen in an A pattern esotropia or in a bilateral Brown's syndrome.

TREATMENT

If the paresis persists after 9 to 12 months, and the child is otherwise neurologically normal, a satisfactory result is usually obtained by receding the superior rectus of the nonparetic eye.

Vertical Strabismus Caused by Orbital Tumors (Fig. 6–45)

Any orbital tumor may cause a vertical strabismus by displacing the globe or affecting one of the extraocular muscles or their nerve supply. The type of strabismus is determined by the location and growth of the tumor. One should look for associated signs such as exophthalmos, hemorrhages of the retina, conjunctiva, and lids, anterior displacement of the posterior portion of the eye, and limitation of rotation of the eye.

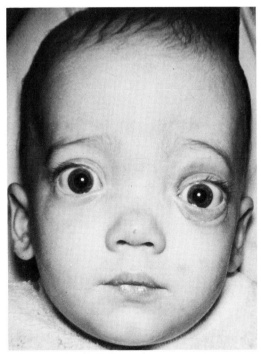

Figure 6–45 Left hypotropia occurring in a 6-month-old child caused by rhabdomyosarcoma. Tumor was growing in the superior part of the orbit and displaced the globe inferiorly.

Endocrine Myopathy

This is uncommon in children.

Postoperative Vertical Strabismus

This type of strabismus follows surgery on the extraocular muscles. No vertical strabismus is noted prior to surgery, but after surgery it is present. It usually results from operating the wrong muscle or is caused by the inadvertent weakening of a vertically acting muscle while operating on another muscle. A vertical rectus muscle may be mistaken for a horizontal rectus muscle. It is possible to weaken the inferior oblique while operating the lateral rectus muscle. These types of strabismus are preventable. The surgeon should be familiar with the anatomy of the extraocular muscles and use sound surgical techniques.

CONGENITAL MOTOR ANOMALIES

There are other entities that are present at birth and represent varying etiologies. Some of these are thought to result from structural anomalies of the extraocular muscles or their attachments, while others appear to result from innervational abnormalities. The etiologies of some remain unknown.

Congenital Familial External Ophthalmoplegia (Fig. 6–46)

This uncommon problem consists of bilateral ptosis and partial to complete external ophthalmoplegia of both eyes. The eyes are usually in a downgaze position and cannot be elevated to the primary position. As a result, the individual develops a compensatory chin elevation in order to see straight ahead. Congenital external ophthalmoplegia is inherited as a dominant trait; some affected members of the family may have a less complete form, such as a third nerve paralysis of one eye.

Surgical treatment for the complete form is not usually recommended.

Congenital Third Nerve Paralysis (Fig. 6–47)

This type of strabismus results from a paralysis of all the muscles supplied by the oculomotor nerve of one eye. It is usually unilateral. The individual has ptosis, hypotropia, and exotropia of the affected eye. Amblyopia is common and should be treated vigorously in infancy. Other family members should be examined for a similar condition; occasionally this entity may be seen in an individual whose family has con-

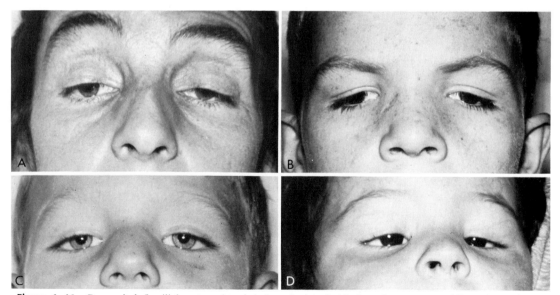

Figure 6–46 Congenital familial external ophthalmoplegia. *A*, Mother demonstrates bilateral ptosis; chin elevation and total inability to move the eyes were present. *B*, Eight-year-old son; *C*, Five-year-old son; *D*, Eighteen-month-old daughter all demonstrated similar findings as the mother.

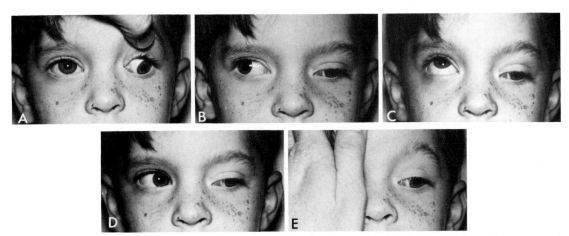

Figure 6–47   Congenital third nerve palsy of left eye. *A*, Primary position showing exotropia and hypotropia of left eye. Ptosis is also present and upper lid is held to show position of eye. *B*, Right gaze showing lack of adduction. *C*, Up gaze showing lack of elevation. *D*, Left gaze. *E*, Monocular rotations of left eye. Eye remained in this position during attempted adduction and elevation.

genital familial external ophthalmoplegia. Surgical correction is necessary and usually includes a recession of the inferior rectus of the affected eye for the hypotropia and a horizontal recession-resection for the exotropia. It may be necessary to utilize the superior oblique to hold the eye straight. Ptosis surgery is performed after the eye has been straightened.

Retraction Syndromes

These entities have in common varying degrees of retraction of the globe, narrowing and widening of the palpebral fissure, and limitation of extraocular movements. There are horizontal and vertical retraction syndromes, and some individuals have a combination of the two.

Horizontal Retraction Syndrome (Fig. 6–48)

The typical type is Duane's retraction syndrome (Stilling-Turk-Duane syndrome), which has the following characteristics:

1. Decreased abduction of one eye, usually the left.

2. Widening of the palpebral fissure on attempted abduction.

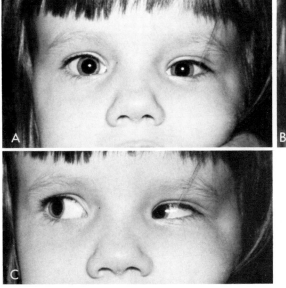

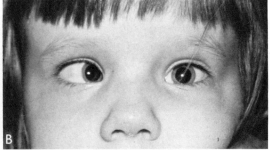

Figure 6–48   Duane's horizontal retraction syndrome of left eye. *A*, Left esotropia in primary position, with narrowing of left palpebral fissure; *B*, absence of abduction of left eye; *C*, full adduction of left eye with narrowing of fissure. Retraction of eye was also present.

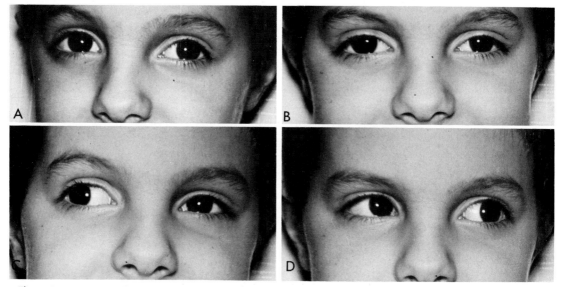

Figure 6–49   Duane's horizontal retraction syndrome of left eye with decreased adduction of the eye. *A*, Compensatory right face turn with eyes looking to the left. *B*, Primary position; there is a left exotropia of 18 prism diopters. *C*, Decreased adduction of left eye with narrowing of the fissure. *D*, Full abduction of left eye.

3. Full or decreased adduction.

4. Narrowing of the palpebral fissure on adduction.

5. Retraction of the eye on adduction.

6. Poor convergence wherein the affected eye does not converge fully, although the normal eye does.

7. The affected eye may upshoot or downshoot in adduction.

8. There may be a variable A or V pattern.

9. Amblyopia is not common, and there

may be a face turn toward the affected side to maintain binocularity.

10. A variable zone of binocular vision may be present.

Atypical types include those with decreased adduction (Fig. 6–49) and a combination of decreased abduction and adduction.

Vertical Retraction Syndrome

This type is less common and is characterized by an upshoot (Fig. 6–50) or a

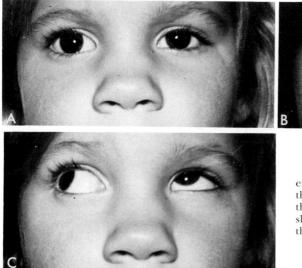

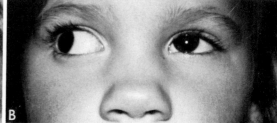

Figure 6–50   Vertical retraction syndrome of left eye. *A*, Primary position showing slight narrowing of the left palpebral fissure. *B*, On straight right gaze the left eye elevates slightly. *C*, Up and right gaze shows greater elevation of the left eye; retraction of the eye was also present.

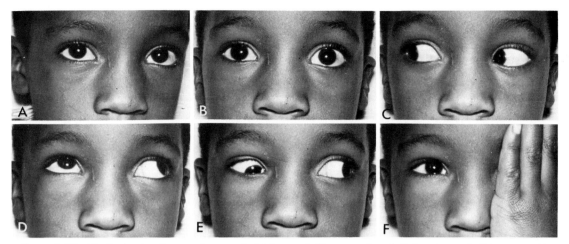

Figure 6–51 Vertical retraction syndrome of right eye. *A*, Compensatory left face turn. *B*, Primary position reveals small exotropia of right eye. *C*, Right gaze; no strabismus is present. *D*, Up-left gaze shows upshoot of right eye. *E*, Straight left gaze showing marked downshoot of right eye; retraction of eye and narrowing of fissure also present. *F*, Straight left gaze showing decreased adduction of right eye.

downshoot (Fig. 6–51) of the adducted eye. Narrowing of the fissure and retraction of the globe are usually present in adduction. Although a compensatory face turn may be present, most of these individuals have little strabismus in the primary position.

ETIOLOGY

1. *Myogenic theory.* Fibrosis of the lateral rectus has been reported, and retraction and fissure narrowing are thought to result from the medial rectus pulling against the tight and inelastic lateral rectus. In some individuals the poor abduction is the result of a tight medial rectus, as confirmed by forced ductions prior to and following severance of the medial rectus from the sclera. In some individuals the forced ductions are normal, as is the appearance of the extraocular muscles during surgery.

2. *Innervational theory.* Electromyography has revealed decreased firing of the lateral rectus during attempted abduction and increased firing of the lateral rectus on adduction. This paradoxical innervation presumes an abnormal innervation to the lateral rectus from the third nerve. Narrowing of the fissure and retraction are thought to result from co-contraction of the horizontal rectus muscles during adduction. In some individuals the upshoot in adduction has been shown to result from increased firing of the superior rectus and is not the result of overaction of the inferior oblique.

SURGERY

Forced ductions are important prior to surgery. Surgery is performed to eliminate the strabismus in the primary position and to straighten the head. If an individual has straight eyes in the straight-ahead position, surgery is not necessary. When strabismus is present in the primary position it is usually an esotropia (Fig. 6–48), and a generous recession of the medial rectus is often all that is necessary. A recession of the medial rectus of the other eye may also be performed if necessary. Resection of the involved lateral rectus is usually not indicated and may cause further narrowing and retraction. Less commonly an exotropia may be found in the primary position (Fig. 6–49), and a resection of the medial rectus may be necessary to improve adduction, especially if forced ductions are normal. If forced ductions indicate that the eye cannot be easily turned nasally, a recession of the lateral rectus may be necessary if this muscle is found to be causing the restriction. Surgery for the upshoot and downshoot is not usually necessary, as there is little or no strabismus in the primary position.

REFERENCES

Albert, D. G.: Small angle esotropia. Amer. Orthopt. J. *12*:39–44, 1962.
Allen, J. H. (ed.): Strabismus Ophthalmic Symposium II. St. Louis, The C. V. Mosby Co., 1958.

Alvaro, M.: Simultaneous surgical correction of vertical and horizontal deviations. Ophtalmologica, *120*:191, 1950.

Arruga, A.: Effect of occlusion of amblyopic eye in amblyopia and eccentric fixation. Trans. Ophthal. Soc. U. K., *82*:45, 1962.

Arruga, A.: Surgical overcorrections. J. Pediat. Ophthal., 2:15, April, 1965.

Asbury, T.: The role of orthoptics in the evaluation and treatment of intermittent exotropia. *In* Arruga, A. (ed.): International Strabismus Symposium, University of Giessen (1966). Basel, S. Karger, 1968.

Axelsson, U., and Holmberg, A.: The frequency of cataract after miotic therapy. Acta Ophthal., *44*:421–429, 1966.

Bagolini, B.: Post surgical treatment of convergent strabismus, with a critical evaluation of various tests. Int. Ophthal. Clin., *6*:633–667, Fall, 1966.

Bangerter, A.: Prophylaxis and therapy of amblyopia. *In* Arruga, A. (ed.): International Strabismus Symposium, University of Giessen (1966). Basel, S. Karger, 1968.

Bérard, P. V.: Prisms: their therapeutic use in strabismus. *In* Arruga, A. (ed.): International Strabismus Symposium, University of Giessen (1966). Basel, S. Karger, 1968.

Berke, R. N.: Surgical treatment of hypertropia. *In* Haik, G. M. (ed.): Strabismus. Symposium of the New Orleans Academy of Ophthalmology. St. Louis, The C. V. Mosby Co., 1962.

Bietti, G. B., and Bagolini, B.: Problems related to surgical overcorrection in strabismus surgery. J. Pediat. Ophthal., 2:11, April, 1965.

Blodi, F. C., Van Allen, M. W., and Yarbrough, J. C.: Duane's syndrome: A brain stem lesion. Arch. Ophthal., *72*:171, 1964.

Breinin, G.: The physiology of the "A" and "V" patterns. Trans. Amer. Acad. Ophthal. Otolaryng, *68*:363, 1964.

Brinker, W. R., and Katz, S. L.: New and practical treatment of eccentric fixation. Amer. J. Ophthal., *55*:1033, 1963.

Brown, H. W.: Congenital structural muscle anomalies. *In* Allen, J. H. (ed.): Strabismus Ophthalmic Symposium (I). St. Louis, The C. V. Mosby Co., 1950.

Brown, H. W.: True and simulated superior oblique tendon sheath syndrome. Docum. Ophthal., *34*:123, 1973.

Burian, H. M., and Spivey, B. E.: The surgical management of exodeviation. Trans. Amer. Ophthal. Soc., *62*:276, 1964.

Burian, H.: Symposium: The "A" and "V" patterns in strabismus; treatment. Trans. Amer. Acad. Ophthal. Otolaryng., *68*:375, 1964.

Burian, H. M.: Exodeviations: their classification, diagnosis and management. Amer. J. Ophthal., *62*:1161, 1966.

Burian, H. M.: Occlusion amblyopia and the development of eccentric fixation. Amer. J. Ophthal., *62*:853, 1966.

Burian, H. M., and Spivey, B. E.: The surgical management of exodeviations. Amer. J. Ophthal., *59*:603, 1965.

Callahan, A.: The arrangement of the conjunctiva in surgery for oculomotor paralysis and strabismus. Arch. Ophthal., *66*:241, 1961.

Chamberlain, W., and Caldwell, E.: The significance of monofixational phoria. Amer. Orthopt. J., *14*:152, 1964.

Cooper, E. L.: Surgical management of secondary exotropia. Trans. Amer. Acad. Ophthal. Otolaryng., *65*:595, 1961.

Cooper, E. L.: Purposeful overcorrection of exotropia. *In* Arruga, A. (ed.): International Strabismus Symposium, University of Giessen (1966). Basel, S. Karger, 1968.

Costenbader, F.: The management of convergent strabismus. *In* Allen, J. (ed.): Strabismus Ophthalmic Symposium. St. Louis, The C. V. Mosby Co., 1950.

Costenbader, F.: Infantile esotropia. Trans. Amer. Ophthal. Soc., *59*:397–429, 1961.

Crawford, J. S.: Congenital fibrosis syndrome. Canad. J. Ophthal., *5*:331–336, 1970.

Dayton, G. O., Jones, M. H., Aiu, P., Rawson, R. A., Steel, B., and Rose, M.: Developmental study of coordinated eye movements in the human infant. Arch. Ophthal. *71*:865, 1964.

Duane, A.: Congenital deficiency of abduction associated with impairment of abduction, retraction movements, contraction of the palpebral fissure and oblique movements of the eye. Arch. Ophthal., *34*:133, 1905.

Duke-Elder, S., and Wybar, K.: System of Ophthalmology. Vol. VI. Ocular Motility and Strabismus, St. Louis, The C. V. Mosby Co., 1973.

Dunlap, E. A.: Diagnosis and surgery of double elevator underaction. Mem. IV Congr. Panam. Oftal., *3*:1554, 1952.

Dunlap, E. A.: Surgical management of intermittent exotropia. Amer. Orthopt. J., *13*:20, 1963.

Dunlap, E. A.: Vertical displacement of the horizontal recti. J. Pediat. Ophthal., 2 (4): 37, 1965.

Dunlap, E. A.: Overcorrections in exotropia surgery. *In* Arruga, A. (ed.) International Strabismus Symposium, University of Giessen (1966). Basel, S. Karger, 1968.

Dunlap, E. A.: Vertical displacement of horizontal recti. *In* Symposium on Strabismus. Ed. by Publications Committee, New Orleans Academy of Ophthalmology. St. Louis, The C. V. Mosby Co., 1971. pp. 320–322.

Fink, W. H.: The A and V syndromes. Amer. Orthopt. J., *9*:105, 1959.

Fitton, M., and Jampolsky, A.: A case report of spontaneous consecutive exotropia. Amer. Orthopt. J., *14*:144, 1964.

Flynn, J. T., and Vereecken, E.: Amblyopia therapy. Results at the Giessen Clinic. Brit. J. Ophthal., *51*:804, 1967.

Friendly, D. S., Manson, R. A., and Albert, D. C.: Cyclic strabismus — a case study. Docum. Ophthal., *34*:189, 1973.

Goldstein, J. H.: The intra-operative forced duction test. Arch. Ophthal., *72*:647, 1964.

Goldstein, J. H.: Monocular vertical displacement of the horizontal rectus muscles in the A and V patterns. Amer. J. Ophthal., *64*:265, 1967.

Goldstein, J. H.: The role of miotics in strabismus. Survey Ophthal., *13*:31–46, 1968.

Gorman, J. J., Cogan, D. G., and Gellis, S. S.: An apparatus for grading the visual acuity of infants on the basis of optokinetic nystagmus. Pediatrics, *19*:1088, 1957.

Görtz, H.: The corrective treatment of amblyopia with eccentric fixation. Amer. J. Ophthal., *49*: 1315, 1960.

Haik, G. M. (ed.): Strabismus. Symposium of the New Orleans Academy of Ophthalmology. St. Louis, The C. V. Mosby Co., 1962.

Harcourt, R. B.: The objective assessment of visual function in young children. Brit. Orthop. J., *26*:1, 1969.

Hardesty, H.: Diagnosis of paretic vertical rotation. Amer. J. Ophthal., 56:811–816, 1963.

Hardesty, H.: Treatment of recurrent intermittent exotropia. Amer. J. Ophthal., *60*:1036, 1965.

Hardesty, H.: Overcorrected intermittent exotropia. Amer. J. Ophthal., *66*:80, 1968.

Hardesty, H.: Treatment of under and overcorrected intermittent exotropia with prism glasses. Amer. Orthopt. J., *19*:110, 1969.

Helveston, E. M., and von Noorden, G. K.: Microtropia. A newly defined entity. Arch. Ophthal., 78:272–281, 1967.

Helveston, E. M.: A two-step test for diagnosing paresis of a single vertically acting extraocular muscle. Amer. J. Ophthal., *64*:914–915, 1967.

Helveston, E. M.: Atlas of Strabismus Surgery. St. Louis, The C. V. Mosby Co., 1973.

Hiles, D. A., Davis, G. T., and Costenbader, F. D.: Long term observations on unoperated intermittent exotropia. Arch. Ophthal., *80*:436, 1968.

Hoyt, W. F., and Nachtigäller, H.: Anomalies of ocular motor nerves: neuroanatomic correlates of paradoxical innervation in Duane's syndrome and related congenital ocular motor disorders. Amer. J. Ophthal., *60*:443, 1965.

Hugonnier, R., and Clayette-Hugonnier, C.: Strabismus, Heterophoria, Ocular Motor Paralysis. 2nd ed. (translated by S. Véronneau-Troutman). St. Louis, The C. V. Mosby Co., 1967.

Ing, M., Costenbader, F. D., Parks, M. M., and Albert, D. G.: Early surgery for congenital esotropia. Amer. J. Ophthal., *61*:1419–1427, 1966.

Irvine, S.: A simple test for binocular fixation. Amer. J. Ophthal., *27*:740–746, 1944.

Jampolsky, A.: Management of exodeviations. *In* Haik, G. M. (ed.): Strabismus. Symposium of the New Orleans Academy of Ophthalmology. St. Louis, The C. V. Mosby Co., 1962.

Jampolsky, A.: The prism test for strabismus screening. J. Pediat. Ophthal., *1*(1):30–34, 1964.

Jampolsky, A.: Oblique muscle surgery of the A-V patterns. J. Pediat. Ophthal., *2*:31, 1965.

Jampolsky, A.: Overcorrections in strabismus. Highlights Ophthal., *8*:75, 1965.

Khawam, E., Scott, A. B., and Jampolsky, A.: Acquired superior oblique palsy. Arch. Ophthal., 77:761, 1967...

Knapp, P.: Treatment of divergent deviations. Allen, J. H. (ed.): Strabismus Ophthalmic Symposium, II. St. Louis, The C. V. Mosby Co., 1958.

Knapp, P.: Vertically incomitant horizontal strabismus: the so-called "A" and "V" syndromes. Trans. Amer. Ophthal. Soc., 57:666, 1959.

Knapp, P.: The surgical treatment of persistent horizontal strabismus. Trans. Amer. Ophthal. Soc., 63:75, 1965.

Knapp, P.: The surgical treatment of double elevator paralysis. Trans. Amer. Ophthal. Soc., 67:304–323, 1969.

Lang, J.: Evaluation in small angle strabismus or microtropia. *In* Arruga, A. (ed.): International Strabismus Symposium, University of Giessen (1966). Basel, S. Karger, 1968.

Lang, J.: Amblyopia of microtropia. *In* Strabismus '69, Transactions of the Consilium Europaeum Strabismi Studio Deditum Congress. St. Louis, The C. V. Mosby Co., 1970.

McDonald, R. J.: Secondary esotropia. Amer. Orthopt. J., *20*:91, 1970.

McGinnis, J. M.: Eye movements and optic nystagmus in early infancy. Genet. Psychol. Monogr., 8:321, 1930.

McNeer, K., Scott, A. B., and Jampolsky, A.: A technique for surgically weakening the inferior oblique muscle. Arch. Ophthal., 73:87, 1965.

McNeer, K., and Jampolsky, A.: An evaluation of underacting inferior oblique muscles. Amer. J. Ophthal., *60*:114, 1965.

Manley, D. R. (ed.): Symposium on Horizontal Ocular Deviations. St. Louis, The C. V. Mosby Co., 1971.

Metz, H. S., Scott, A. B., and O'Meara, D., et al.: Ocular saccades in lateral rectus palsy. Arch. Ophthal., *84*:453–460, 1970.

Moore, S.: Orthoptic treatment for intermittent exotropia. Amer. Orthopt. J., *13*:14, 1963.

Moore, S.: The prognostic value of lateral gaze measurements in intermittent exotropia. Amer. Orthopt. J., *19*:69, 1969.

Moses, R. A.: Adler's Physiology of the Eye. 5th ed. St. Louis, The C. V. Mosby Co., 1970.

Ogle, K. N.: Fixation disparity. Amer. Orthopt. J., *4*:35, 1954.

Ogle, K. N.: Fixation disparity and oculomotor imbalance. Amer. Orthopt. J., *8*:21, 1958.

Ordy, J. M., Latanick, A., Samorajski, T., and Massopust, L. C.: Visual acuity in newborn infants. Proc. Soc. Exp. Biol. Med., *115*:677, 1964.

Parks, M. M.: Abnormal accommodative convergence in squint. Arch. Ophthal., 59:364–380, 1958.

Parks, M. M.: Isolated cyclovertical muscle palsy. Arch. Ophthal., *60*:1027–1035, 1958.

Parks, M. M.: Comitant deviations in children. *In* Haik, G. M. (ed.): Strabismus, Symposium of the New Orleans Academy of Ophthalmology. St. Louis, The C. V. Mosby Co., 1962.

Parks, M. M.: Ocular motility. Lecture Notes, Lancaster Course, Colby College, Maine, 1965.

Parks, M. M.: and Friendly, D. S.: Treatment of eccentric fixation in children under four years of age. Amer. J. Ophthal., *61*:395–399, 1966.

Parks, M. M.: Symposium: Infantile esotropia, summary and conclusions, Amer. Orthopt. J., *18*:15, 1968.

Parks, M. M.: The monofixation syndrome. Trans. Amer. Ophthal. Soc., 67:607–657, 1969.

Raab, E. L., and Parks, M. M.: Recession of the lateral recti. Arch. Ophthal., 82:203, 1969.

Raskind, R. R., and Burian, H. M.: Bilateral resections. Amer. J. Ophthal., *64*:78, 1967.

Reinecke, R. D., and Cogan, D. G.: Standardization of objective visual acuity measurements. Arch. Ophthal., *60*:418, 1958.

Reinecke, R. D., and Miller, D.: Strabismus, A Programmed Text. New York, Appleton-Century-Crofts, 1966.

Romano, P. E., and von Noorden, G. K.: Atypical responses to the four-diopter prism test. Amer. J. Ophthal., *67*:935, 1969.

Ruskell, G. L.: Some aspects of vision in infants. Brit. Orthop. J., *24*:25, 1967.

Scott, A. B.: Active force tests in lateral rectus paralysis. Arch. Ophthal., *85*:397–404, 1971.

Scott, A. B., and Knapp, P.: Surgical treatment of superior oblique tendon sheath syndrome. Arch. Ophthal., *88*:282–286, 1972.

Stanworth, A.: The A and V phenomena. Brit. Orthopt. J., *25*:12, 1968.

Swan, K. C.: The blindspot mechanism. *In* Allen, J. H. (ed.): Strabismus Ophthalmic Symposium (II). St. Louis, The C. V. Mosby Co., 1958.

Symposium on Strabismus. Ed. by Publications Committee, New Orleans Academy of Ophthalmology. St. Louis, The C. V. Mosby Co., 1971.

Tamler, E.: Pure and impure A-V syndromes. Arch. Ophthal., *66*:524, 1961.

Taylor, D. M.: How early is early surgery in the management of strabismus? Arch. Ophthal., *70*:752, 1963.

Tour, R.: Surgical overcorrection in convergent strabismus. Amer. Orthopt. J., *8*:59, 1958.

Urist, M. J.: Horizontal squint with secondary vertical deviations. Arch. Ophthal., *46*:245, 1951.

Urist, M. J.: Recession and upward displacement of the medial rectus muscles in A-pattern esotropia. Amer. J. Ophthal., *65*:769, 1968.

Urist, M. J.: Surgical treatment of esotropia with bilateral depression in adduction. Arch. Ophthal., *55*:643, 1956.

Urrets-Zavalia, A., Jr., Solares-Zamora, J., and Olmos, H. P.: Anthropological studies on the nature of cyclovertical squint. Brit. J. Ophthal., *45*:578, 1961.

Verhoeff, F.: The so-called blindspot mechanism. Amer. J. Ophthal., *40*:802–808, 1955.

Voipio, H., and Hyvarinen, L.: Objective measurement of visual acuity by arrestovisography. Arch. Ophthal., *75*:799, 1966.

von Noorden, G. K.: Occlusion therapy in amblyopia with eccentric fixation. Arch. Ophthal., *78*:776, 1965.

von Noorden, G. K.: Etiology and pathogenesis of fixation anomalies in strabismus. Trans. Amer. Ophthal. Soc., *67*:668, 1969; Amer. J. Ophthal., *69*:210, 1970.

von Noorden, G. K., and Maumenee, A. E.: Atlas of Strabismus. 2nd ed. St. Louis, The C. V. Mosby Co., 1973.

Walsh, F. B., and Hoyt, W. F.: Clinical Neuro-Ophthalmology. Baltimore, Williams and Wilkins, 1969.

Watson, A. G.: A new operation for double elevator paralysis. Trans. Canad. Ophthal. Soc., *25*:182, 1962.

Windsor, C. E.: Surgically overcorrected esotropia: a study of its causes, sensory anomalies, fusional results, and management. Amer. Orthopt. J., *16*:8, 1966.

Wolin, L. R., and Dillman, A.: Objective measurement of visual acuity (using opto-kinetic nystagmus and electro-oculography). Arch. Ophthal., *71*:822, 1964.

Zauberman, H., Magora, A., and Chaco, J.: An electromyographic evaluation of the retraction syndrome. Amer. J. Ophthal., *64*:1103, 1967.

CHAPTER 7

AMBLYOPIA

EVERETT A. MOODY, M.D.

DEFINITION

Amblyopia signifies *reduced visual acuity* (measured under monocular conditions) *not correctable by refractive means and not attributable to obvious structural or pathological ocular anomalies* (Schapero et al., 1968). Although amblyopia may occur in both eyes, it is important to understand that the condition is revealed by a monocular test, the visual acuity being measured with only one eye viewing. It is possible for a patient to read well with either eye when the fellow is covered, but to have suppression of vision in one eye when both eyes are viewing. This, of course, would not be amblyopia but "suppression."

How much vision loss is required before the diagnosis of amblyopia is applied is subject to debate. Some clinicians would argue that 20/15 vision in one eye and 20/20 vision in the other represents amblyopia in the latter. This concept has merit, but general usage usually implies a vision of 20/30 or worse in the amblyopic eye.

CLASSIFICATION

Until recent years *amblyopia ex anopsia* has been used as a synonym for amblyopia as defined above. Gunter Von Noorden and others have restricted the use of the term *ex anopsia* to the so-called "disuse" amblyopia (Von Noorden, 1968), meaning the type which arises from interruption of the visual response by severe ptosis, cataract, or other pathological condition. Others prefer to discard the term *ex anopsia* altogether and refer to this type as disuse or occlusion amblyopia.

Amblyopia may be associated with (1) strabismus; (2) occlusion (disuse), i.e., cataract, retrolental mass, ptosis, cloudy media, corneal leukoma, inadvertent prolonged patching, and so on; (3) ametropia (both eyes having severe refractive error); or (4) anisometropia. Although the term "organic amblyopia" is used to include the organically caused condition, many authors feel that this particular form of amblyopia is excluded by the definition, since, if the organic cause is known, it is no longer called amblyopia. Cases in which amblyopia is suspected but not known to be organic would be more properly grouped as (5) *amblyopia of unknown etiology*. (6) Hysterical amblyopia would be a final classification.

Eccentric fixation, like amblyopia, is a monocular phenomenon, but it relates to direction rather than to visual acuity. Good visual acuity is associated with foveal fixation, whereas extrafoveal fixation or unsteady fixation is invariably associated with reduced visual acuity.

185

The factors leading to anomalies of fixation in strabismic amblyopia were investigated by Von Noorden. His study of the relationship between anomalies of relative subjective localization in binocular vision (anomalous retinal correspondence) and the monocularly determined fixation pattern indicated that the angle of anomaly is not usually quantitatively related to the monocular eccentric fixation.

Von Noorden indicates the presence of a wide spectrum of sensory and motor adaptations that contribute to eccentric fixation.

1. Some amblyopic patients fixate at the margin of an organic or functional central suppression scotoma to obtain better vision. In this phenomenon, the fovea remains the zero center of oculomotor orientation and the sensation of indirectness of viewing may or may not be appreciated by the patient. Paradoxical fixation and eccentric fixation in occlusion or stimulus deprivation amblyopia are examples of this group.

2. In amblyopic patients with the onset of strabismus within the first year of life, the adaptation is more complete and the motor component of the fixation reflex becomes associated with an eccentric area (foveal function reduced by suppression) which then acquires a foveal characteristic of becoming the zero point for oculomotor orientation.

3. In the third group (most advanced form of adaptation) the eccentric retinal area may be used for both binocular and monocular vision.

Additional factors probably influence the development of eccentric fixation, and the role of motor factors on fixational behavior in strabismic patients deserves investigation.

FUNCTIONAL VS. ORGANIC AMBLYOPIA

It is necessary to distinguish between functional and organic amblyopia. In functional amblyopia, no apparent cause can be found for the unilateral visual deficit, whereas in organic amblyopia a lesion is evident and accounts for the loss in vision. However, organic amblyopia may exist subclinically so that it may be difficult to clearly differentiate the two forms and may account for the limited success we may encounter in some patients.

Furthermore, functional amblyopia may be associated with active suppression or the amblyopia may have been acquired from disuse. Such a theory is further complicated by a report of Riesen, Kurk, and Mellinger (1953), who found that animals reared in the dark from birth have defective vision. Wiesel and Hubel (1963) have produced impressive evidence indicating a definite reduction in cellular response from the visual cortex in kittens occluded from birth. When the occlusion was removed, there was no functional improvement even after one year. Similar results were obtained when a newborn kitten was made surgically exotropic without occlusion. Such evidence suggests that organic changes were associated with visual deprivation in the newborn kitten. Atrophy of neurons in the lateral geniculate body of the kitten has been identified. In low luminances, the vision of the amblyopic eye approaches the vision of the normal eye. Isolated letters can be perceived better than letters in a line, a phenomenon known as "crowding."

The amblyopic eye is characterized by reduced foveal function, whereas the peripheral vision is usually normal.

Neutral Density Filter Test

This test attempts to differentiate functional from organic amblyopia. A filter which reduces the visual acuity of a normal eye to 20/30 (Kodak Wratten Gelatin Filter #96 N. D. 300) is placed before the eye. Through such a filter, a normal eye is reduced to 20/30 while the vision in the functionally amblyopic eye remains unchanged. However, in organic amblyopia reduced illumination reduces visual acuity.

Prognosis for Various Types of Amblyopia

It is of more than academic importance that amblyopia is classified. It is becoming increasingly apparent that the *prognosis for the various types of amblyopia differs greatly. Occlusion or "disuse" amblyopia* produces a very early and profound visual loss which is amenable to treatment probably only in the early years of life. *Strabismic amblyopia* is less profound, probably starts at a somewhat later date as the child begins to try to use his eyes together, and can generally be reversed to normal or near normal vision if treated prior to the age of 4. In addition, significant returns of vision can be made in the 5-, 6- and 7-year-old child. *Ametropic amblyopia* is rarely severe probably because the ametropia causes the child to perform visual tasks poorly enough to come to medical attention at an early age. The poor seeing eye goes undetected until a secondary strabismus appears or a school screening is performed. *Anisometropes have a better prognosis than strabismic amblyopes.* Reversal of 20/200 amblyopia in the early teen-ager is not uncommon in cases of anisometropia, whereas this is rare in cases of strabismic amblyopia. Data to support this observation are being gathered at Wills and other hospitals. Large series of cases have not been reported heretofore, chiefly because we have assumed that all types of amblyopia had equivalent prognoses and no effort was made to treat some of these older children with anisometropic amblyopia.

Medical and Surgical Correction

The aim of treatment of amblyopia is to provide opportunity for the amblyopic eye to see clearly at as early an age as possible. Medical and surgical therapy must be directed at occlusion amblyopia at the very earliest time, since the prognosis in these cases is so dependent on early therapy. In 1969, on the seventh day of his life, an infant with congenital cataracts was operated on (Paton, 1971). It will be years before we know if this aggressive therapy is rewarded by good vision but this exemplifies current concepts of aggressive therapy.

Early surgical therapy for strabismus, of course, helps prevent amblyopia. However, it should be made clear that the reason for operating on a child with congenital esotropia between 6 and 12 months of age is based, *not primarily on an effort to prevent amblyopia, but rather on an effort to provide binocularity.* Loss of fusion potential increases in patients allowed to remain strabismic somewhere in the interval from 9 months to approximately 3 years. Patients whose eyes have been straightened with surgery by age 9 months seem to have a fair chance for some form of fusion capability. By 3 years of age this chance is greatly reduced (Ing et al., 1966). The prognosis for continued visual alignment is heavily dependent on the child's ability to fuse, at least peripherally.* Fusion of any kind allows the child to practice using the eyes together daily (a sort of walking-around orthoptics) and this goal should not be undervalued.

Historically, the knowledge that strabismic amblyopia is reversible in most cases up to 4 years of age has led clinicians to procrastinate surgery to this age, feeling that amblyopia prevention is the chief goal of early surgery. By this time, hope for binocularity in congenital esotropes is virtually nonexistent.

Ametropic and anisometropic amblyopia demand prompt recognition and refractive correction. The value of contact lenses in anisometropia to minimize aniseikonia is generally appreciated. Contact lenses are also of benefit for correction of symmetrical high refractive errors. By simply trying harder it has been discovered that contact lenses are easily fitted as early as 4 months of age. In fact, it is easier to introduce them at this age than between 2 and 4 years because of behavioral problems. The mother inserts the lens up to about age 5; after that the child assumes the responsibility for insertion and removal. Success with contact lenses in the very young is directly proportional to the interest and abilities of the mother.

Special mention should be made of the anisometropia occurring with congenital glaucoma. Distention of the ocular coats frequently produces a myopia which may be only partially compensated by flattening of the cornea. Failure to correct the

---

*Peripheral fusion means that there is regional suppression centrally in the nonpreferred eye while the overlapping peripheral visual fields are fused.

refractive error before amblyopia becomes permanent only substitutes one disease for the other.

Patching

Even if surgical and medical means have provided the best opportunity for vision, there is still the problem of the patient preferring one eye over the fellow. Our basic therapeutic effort here is to patch the preferred eye.

There are so many devices and schemes for partial patching that it should be heavily underscored that *there is neither substitute nor peer for full-time patching* in the treatment of amblyopia. The experienced clinician can recall cases in which half-hearted occlusion attempts were practiced by a family for many months until finally some convincing "turnkey" is found to impress the parent or the child with the importance of this simple therapy. Then when total occlusion is accomplished, the immediate result is rapid recovery of vision after a long history of failure.

When the clinician has experienced a few of these cases for himself he is impressed not only with the value of total occlusion but also with the importance of an aggressive approach as he explains for the first time the patching regimen to the parents. *The parent who is convinced of the importance of winning the battle with the child the first day is rewarded on two accounts. First, as the vision improves, resistance to patching becomes less. Secondly, to avoid rewarding a child's manipulation is the best defense against it.*

It has been felt that giving small detailed visual tasks during the period of occlusion commensurate with the vision of the child speeds the visual recovery, although it does not seem to improve the final result. Expensive devices need not be employed for this, since coloring book exercises suffice for the initial ranges of vision. Filling in the loops of letters in small print is excellent for the better ranges of vision as therapy progresses.

Patching Problems

Patient acceptance of a patch in the reasonable child can be encouraged by

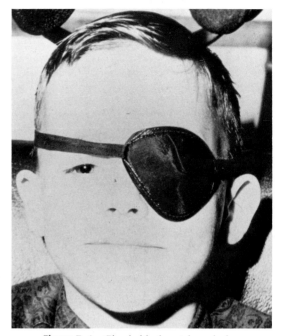

Figure 7–1 Classic black patch occluder.

propaganda. The Jolly Roger Club and Peanuts cartoons have helped make patching more socially acceptable in the younger set. Painting designs on the patches and making homemade patches of material matching the child's dress have been successful incentives. In most cases, children will peek from under any patch which is not taped to the skin (Elastoplast Occlusor and Opticlude patches), but placing a pirate's patch over the tape often makes a satisfactory solution for the child who insists upon authenticity (Figs. 7–1 and 7–2).

Summer patching is convenient from a schooling standpoint but sweating be-

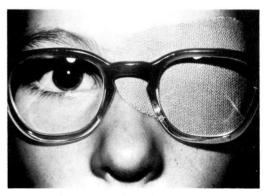

Figure 7–2 Elastoplast Occlusor.

neath the patch is often a problem. (Be warned about procrastinating until summer.) Tincture of benzoin applied to the skin around the lid will often improve adhesiveness. Skin breakdown can be combated with steroid skin creams and hypoallergenic tape.

Arm splints may have to be used but all have been incriminated at one time or another in causing skin breakdown or pressure pareses. Pinning long shirt sleeves at the wrist to the diaper is a good measure.

The author has never sutured the lids closed but it is conceivable that the need for this severe measure might arise. A case of corneal breakdown and abrasion with use of tissue glues is known and, at least for the present, glue is not recommended. An opaque or blurring contact lens may work and is convenient if the child has to be fitted with them anyway. The employment of soft contact lenses may be particularly useful as a technique for occlusion, but requires frequent observation.

This large bag of tricks should underscore the need for tenacious insistence of the physician that successful total occlusion be performed.

Partial Occlusion

Partial occlusion (part-time or patching a spectacle lens only) is not recommended as initial therapy but is a satisfactory holding technique to discourage recurrence. The AO occluder lens is a good cosmetic substitute for the frosted lens. These glasses can be worn part of every day or part of every week. Hair spray or magic

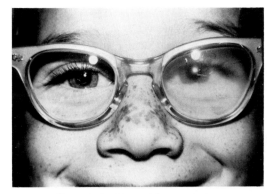

Figure 7–4 Frosted lens occluder.

mending tape is less expensive if cosmesis is not a major issue. Paste-on "mod" occluders for glasses are popular (Bausch & Lomb). (See Figures 7–3 through 7–7.)

Patching the Infant

Most amblyopes recognized in infancy have strabismus. The amblyopic eye can be identified as the nonpreferred eye. A cross-fixater (one who regards objects to the right with the left eye and objects to the left with the right eye) can be assumed not to have amblyopia. Eye preference not only identifies the amblyopic eye, but also provides the end point for amblyopia therapy, i.e., equal preference.

Strong preference is reversed within a week in almost all children less than a year of age if occlusion therapy has been accomplished as prescribed. Therefore, a return visit in *one week* is indicated, and perhaps a word of caution should be given to the parents should there be any reason for delay in returning. Amblyopia can

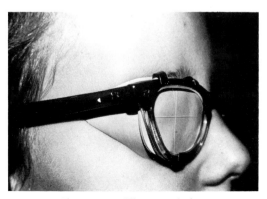

Figure 7–3 Clip-on occluder.

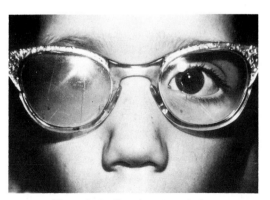

Figure 7–5 Scotch tape occluder.

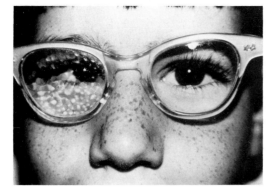

Figure 7–6   Nail polish occluder.

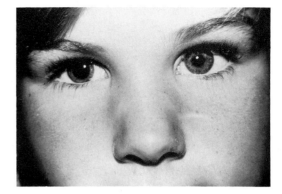

Figure 7–8   Atropine cycloplegia used as a mechanism for blurring vision in one eye.

occur very rapidly in the patched eye. Although this is readily reversible, it could be disastrous if a gross misunderstanding were to take place and the child were to go for months without being seen.

A problem arises when the first available operating time is a month away, and the amblyopia has been reversed in a week. A good solution is to have the mother strike a match in front of the child each morning when she first visits his crib. The child will regard the bright light with one eye or the other. This eye is patched for the remainder of the day and this regimen is followed until surgery. Atropine ointment 1 per cent may be instilled daily in the eye preferred for fixation. This technique may be useful if the amblyopia is mild (Fig. 7–8).

Pleoptic Therapy

Pleoptic therapy for amblyopia was initially received with great excitement but in controlled studies has failed to prove superior to simple patching (Fletcher, M.:

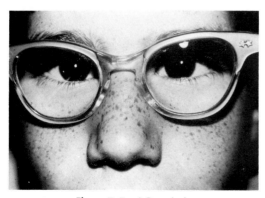

Figure 7–7   AO occluder.

Amer. Orthop. J., 1968.) The devices employed are, once again, to stimulate vision in the amblyopic eye, which can be done with more simple and inexpensive means.

In brief, pleoptic therapy for amblyopia consists of efforts to stimulate the macula of the amblyopic eye with flashing lights, moving targets, and other means. Following recognition of eccentric fixation by means of the visuscope, pleoptic therapy attempts to place a scotoma on the eccentrically fixating point with a bright flash. This encourages preference of the normal macula area for fixation. In addition, attention can be called to the macula area by stamping a ring scotoma around the macula of the eccentrically fixating eye with a specially devised pleoptiscope which is a modification of the visuscope. The patient is then instructed to look at the center of the scotoma circle.

There are times when hospitalization for amblyopia therapy is definitely justified, not so much for the pleoptic benefit, but to provide an opportunity for the child to be observed in a controlled environment to ensure that complete patching is being accomplished. *One does not like to give up on patching without full assurance that complete patching without improvement has been accomplished.* Pleoptics has been shown to be successful in some refractory cases of amblyopia but visual acuity will not remain good unless binocular vision can also be achieved.

RECURRENT AMBLYOPIA

Once patching has brought the vision up to normal, amblyopia may recur if treatment is not continued. Patients who have a central suppression scotoma in the deviating eye under binocular conditions will frequently have this progress to a frank amblyopia (under monocular conditions.) This has happened as late as age 9. All amblyopes should, therefore, have periodic rechecks at least through this age.

PRESCHOOL VISION SCREENING

Preschool vision screening is advisable to detect amblyopia in time for successful treatment. A simple visual acuity with illiterate tests performed on 3- and 4-year-old children is ideal. Strabismic amblyopia generally tips its hand to alert parents in time for amblyopia to be treated. Anisometropic amblyopia cannot be detected early by parents. In this case, we depend entirely on screening tests.

AVOIDING GRAVE ERRORS IN TREATMENT

A thorough funduscopic examination is absolutely imperative in all cases of suspected amblyopia. Unfortunately, there are cases in which the child presenting with strabismus has undergone amblyopia therapy for a time and subsequently has been found to have a lesion in the posterior pole capable of interfering with normal macular function.

It is likewise shocking to see a patient who has had strabismus surgery and is found to have severe amblyopia and gives the history that there has never been any attempt at amblyopia therapy.

A more common and equally tragic situation is one in which a strabismic child is given preoperative treatment for amblyopia but postoperatively is discharged without follow-up to detect and treat a recurrence.

SUMMARY

Amblyopia has several causes and the prognosis for vision varies greatly with the etiology. Notably, occlusion amblyopia must be treated in the early months of life to have a good prognosis. Anisometropic amblyopia can be treated even in the teenager with good results and one should not assume that the patient is beyond the age of good response but should engage in a trial of therapy. Although strabismic amblyopia has a good prognosis through age four, delaying therapy of the amblyopia and the squint may result in recovery of the amblyopia but loss of binocularity.

Full-time occlusion of the good eye with a patch applied to the skin provides the best and most secure way to treat amblyopia. The clinician should not abandon amblyopia therapy short of 20/20 unless he feels well assured that full-time patching has been accomplished for a substantial period of time (that amount depending on the age of the child). Emphasis is given to the importance and value of preparing the parents with sufficient encouragement and instruction so that they are able to accomplish full-time patching right from the outset.

In the care of infants, strong preference of one eye implies amblyopia of the fellow eye. Even without quantitative visual acuity, the amblyopia treatment can be conducted, since the preferred eye is the one to be patched and the endpoint of therapy is equal preference of the two eyes. Clinicians who are not used to patching infants for amblyopia are warned that this process may be reversed within one week and prolonged patching can cause amblyopia in the fellow eye. Following improvement in the amblyopic eye to 20/30 or 20/20, periodic patching of the good eye may be required until satisfactory binocular vision can be established.

The importance of screening preschool children with illiterate vision tests for detection of amblyopia in time for adequate therapy is emphasized.

Amblyopia treatment is basically simple, relatively inexpensive and unexciting enough to be neglected by both parents and physicians. However, the rewards of this simple treatment are enormous in terms of vision saved. The success rate is directly proportional to the following of three principles:

1. Early detection and treatment.
2. Aggressive insistence on *complete* patching.

3. Adequate follow-ups at least through age 9.

REFERENCES

Hubel, D. H., and Wiesel, T. N.: Binocular interaction in the cortex of kittens reared with artificial squint. J. Neurophysiol., 26:1041, 1965.

Ing, M., Costenbader, F. D., Parks, M. M., and Albert, D. G.: Early surgery for congenital esotropia. Amer. J. Ophthal., 61:1419, 1966.

Paton, D.: Personal communication, 1971.

Riesen, A. H., Kurk, M. I., and Mellinger, J. C.: Interocular transfer of habits learned monocularly in visually naïve and visually experienced cats. J. Comp. Physiol. Psychol., 46:166, 1953.

Schapero, Cline, Hofstetter, *Dictionary of Visual Science.* Philadelphia, Chilton Book Co., 1968.

Von Noorden, G. K., and Maumenee, A. E.: Stimulus-deprivation amblyopia. Amer. J. Ophthal., 65:220, February, 1968.

Von Noorden, G. K.: Etiology and pathogenesis of fixation anomalies in strabismus. I. Relationship between eccentric fixation and anomalous retinal correspondence. Amer. J. Ophthal., 69:210, 1970.

Von Noorden, G. K.: Etiology and pathogenesis of fixation anomalies in strabismus. II. Parodoxic fixation, occlusion amblyopia, and microstrabismus. Amer. J. Ophthal., 69:223, 1970.

Von Noorden, G. K.: Etiology and pathogenesis of fixation anomalies in strabismus. III. Subjective localization. Amer. J. Ophthal., 69:228, 1970.

Von Noorden, G. K.: Etiology and pathogenesis of fixation anomalies in strabismus. IV. Roles of suppression scotoma and motor factors. Amer. J. Ophthal., 69:236, 1970.

Wiesel, T. N., and Hubel, D. H.: Single-cell responses in striated cortex of kittens deprived of vision in one eye. J. Neurophysiol., 26:1003, 1963.

Wiesel, T. N., and Hubel, D. H.: Extent of recovery from effects of visual deprivation in kittens. J. Neurophysiol., 28:1060, 1965.

CHAPTER 8

DISEASES OF THE ORBIT

EDMUND B. SPAETH, M.D.,
and ROBISON D. HARLEY, M.D.

INTRODUCTION

The orbital cavities are situated on either side of the sagittal plane of the skull between the cranium and the facial structures. Superior to the orbits is the anterior cranial fossa, medially are the air sinuses and nasal cavity, inferiorly are the maxillary sinuses (fluid), laterally are the supporting zygomatic arches, and superolaterally are the temporal and middle cranial fossa.

The orbit has the approximate shape of a quadrilateral pyramid whose base is directed forward and laterally and whose apex contains the optic foramen and the superior orbit fissure. In the child the interorbital distance is generally small and the eyes appear close together. With the growth of the frontal and ethmoidal air cells the interorbital distance increases. This fact often explains the apparent improvement of the esotropic position with growth. The maxillary sinus is small at birth and the frontal sinus is usually not well developed before age 9. Ethmoid sinuses are present at birth.

Classification

Orbital structures may be altered by developmental, inflammatory, vascular, traumatic, metabolic and systemic disorders, or neoplastic diseases. Orbital involvement may be further considered under the following categories: primary, secondary, or metastatic.

Diagnostic Considerations

Since the orbital cavity is a closed space, exophthalmos or proptosis is a primary manifestation of orbital disease. The degree and rate of development of the protruding eye may vary considerably depending on various factors. The following diagnostic steps are important:

1. *History of proptosis and age of patient.* Has the proptosis developed slowly or rapidly? Do periodic exophthalmometer readings indicate growth (Fig. 8–1)? Does the eyeball protrusion vary with position or from day to day? Has there been a history of trauma? How is the general health of the child?

2. Does the exophthalmos involve both eyes or one eye?

3. Does the proptosis appear to be inflammatory or noninflammatory? Is there evidence of sinus disease or a recent upper respiratory infection?

4. *Palpation of mass.* Is proptosis compressible? Hard masses are more apt to be malignant, not inflammatory. Does eye-

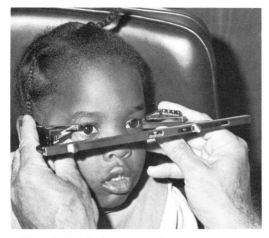

Figure 8–1   The Hertel exophthalmometer in use. For successive readings, the same lateral orbital distance is essential.

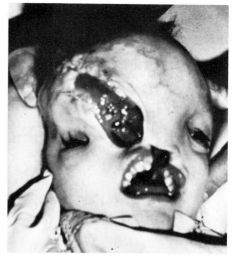

Figure 8–2   Failure of cleft closure. (Courtesy of Harold Falls, M.D.)

ball pulsate? Can auscultation detect a bruit? Vascular lesions or defects in the posterior orbit may transmit a pulsation. In which direction is the proptosis? The position of the mass is often of diagnostic aid.

5. *Ocular motility.* The presence of diplopia or restriction of movement can be affected by orbital disease and is significant concerning the nature of the lesion.

6. Has visual acuity been affected? Are visual fields normal? Tumors adjacent to the optic nerve or even intracranial tumors with orbital extension may produce characteristic field changes.

7. *Fundi changes.* Optic nerve pallor, papilledema, venous congestion, refractive changes, and retinal striae in the posterior pole are diagnostic aids in orbital diseases. Optic nerve glioma classically produces visual loss as a primary symptom.

8. Various x-ray techniques of the orbit reveal signs of bony erosion and invasion. Physical examination of the child may disclose the presence of metabolic diseases or other systemic disorders.

CONGENITAL DISORDERS OF THE ORBIT

Developmental abnormalities of the orbit concern the ophthalmologist because of the secondary effects which may occur

to the eye (Fig. 8–2). Orbital changes are usually accompanied by marked skull deformities. Shallowness of the orbits may produce proptosis to such a degree that the lids have difficulty closing (Fig. 8–3). Manipulation about the lids in shallow orbits has resulted in protrusion of the eyeball beyond the lids, a disturbing situation for the ophthalmologist and patient. In addition to proptosis, exotropia is often associated with widely separated eyes. Blepharoptosis, papilledema, and optic atrophy may be observed with orbital defects, especially the crainostenoses.

(See Plate I.)

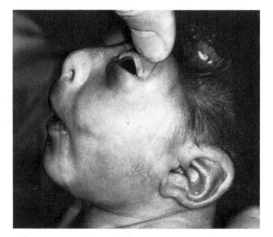

Figure 8–3   Ancephalic with bilateral exophthalmos.

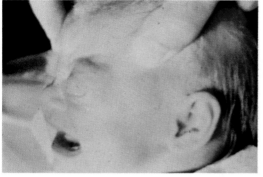

A

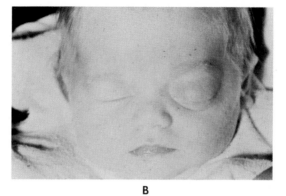

B

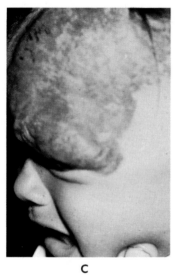

C

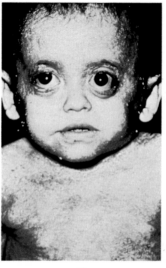

D

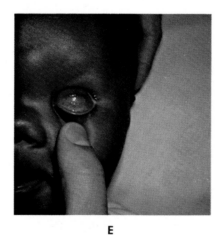

E

PLATE I

(*A*) and (*B*) Teratoma of orbit.

(*C*) Hemangioma involving orbit, lid, and forehead.

(*D*) Hand-Schüller-Christian disease. (Courtesy of Dr. Harold Falls.)

(*E*) Neuroectodermal dysplasia.

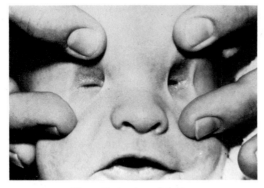

Figure 8–4   Anophthalmos.

When the eye is extremely microph-thalmic or apparently absent, the orbit may be only slightly smaller or much smaller than normal. Failure of ocular development apparently does prevent orbital development (Figs. 8–4 to 8–8).

According to Kennedy:

"Striking and characteristic bone changes occurring in the orbit following enucleation of one eye at an early age are described for the rabbit, cat and human. The previous experimental work on three rabbits reported by Thomson has been repeated and substantiated. The changes are represented by a decrease in the orbital measurements in the magnitude of 12.6 per cent for the rabbit and 26.8 per cent for the cat as determined from the dry skulls."

In the human these bony changes in the anophthalmic orbit were determined from the roentgenograms of a series of 42 patients in whom the enucleation has oc-curred between the first day and the 14th year. Cephalometric roentgenographic determinations showed a decrease in the orbital measurements up to 15 per cent when no orbital implant had been used, and up to 8 per cent when an implant had been inserted. The magnitude of change decreased the later the enucleation was performed.

The insertion of an orbital implant results in less contraction of the develop-ing anophthalmic orbit. This is suggested in the cat experimentally and is evident in the human, with its benefit being greater the earlier in life the enucleation occurs. This supports the findings of Pfeiffer.

The altered orbital volume cannot be determined satisfactorily from either the dried animal skull or the roentgenograms in humans. Empirically, however, the de-creased orbital volume in the human might be 20 to 30 per cent, and even as high as 50 per cent (Fig. 8–8). An orbital implant appeared to reduce the loss in volume.

Facial asymmetry, as evidenced by in-crease in the midline to lateral orbital margin measurement, can occur in two thirds of the patients. The interorbital region measurements show little variation.

The canal of the optic nerve is smaller on the enucleated side as reported by Luzsa and others. This was evident in all the cats and in 93 per cent of the humans. The average decrease in humans was approximately 17 per cent, but may be as high as 50 per cent."

Roentgen ray therapy to the orbital region may cause additional reduction in

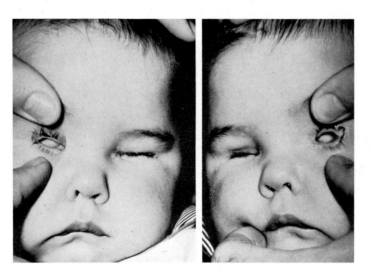

Figure 8–5 Clinical anophthalmos. Extremely small globes found in orbit.

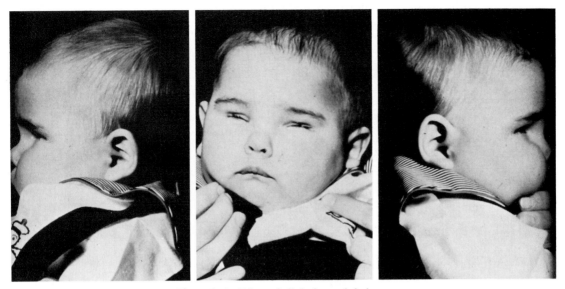

Figure 8–6 Bilateral clinical anophthalmos.

orbital measurements far greater than those resulting from simple enucleation. Enucleation in infancy is seldom recommended except in instances of retinoblastoma and gross ocular deformities.

While the orbit has been observed to be extremely shallow and small with apparent anophthalmos, absence of the orbit is rare. In cyclopia, the two orbits are united into a single median opening (Figs. 8–9, 8–10 and 8–11). Blodi has summarized the congenital anomalies of the skull affecting the eye.

(See Plate II.)

Microphthalmos with Cyst (Fig. 8–12).

When closure of the fetal cleft has been incomplete, neuroectodermal tissue may herniate into the orbit. The condition is almost invariably associated with microph-

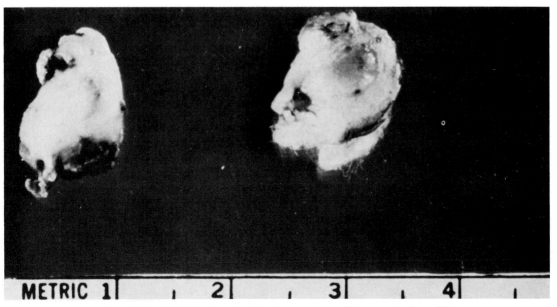

Figure 8–7 Marked microphthalmic eyes removed from posterior orbit.

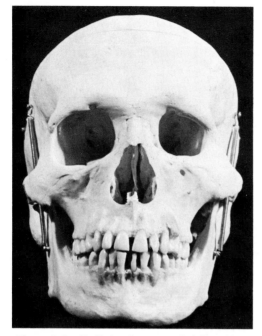

Figure 8–8 Skull showing normal right orbit and markedly underdeveloped abnormal left orbit, probably congenital anophthalmos. (Courtesy of Dr. R. E. Kennedy.)

thalmos which may be almost completely developed or rudimentary. Since the cyst occupies a large portion of the orbit, it must be differentiated from a primary tumor. The cyst contains neuroectodermal elements which are poorly differentiated, so the mass may be termed neuroectodermal dysplasia. Proliferated glial and fibrous connective tissue are frequent components giving the mass some firm consistency which can lead to a mistaken diagnosis.

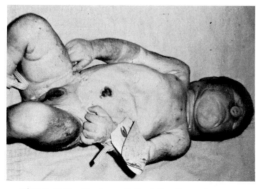

Figure 8–9 Cyclops. Infant lived one hour.

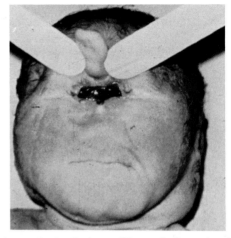

Figure 8–10 Cyclops. View of face showing fused orbit and proboscis.

Meningocele, Encephalocele or Hydroencephalocele

A herniation of cranial contents into the orbit may be classified as a meningocele, encephalocele or hydroencephalocele, depending on the composition of the herniated material.

Cranial contents may herniate through natural openings or bony defects. Anterior cephaloceles usually appear at the upper medial aspect and displace the globe temporally. The mass is fluctuant and reducible with firm pressure.

A congenital defect in the greater wing of the sphenoid has been observed to produce pulsating exophthalmos, espe-

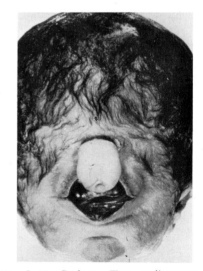

Figure 8–11 Cyclops. Two rudimentary eyes present in one orbit.

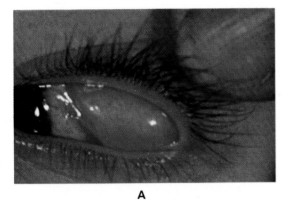

A

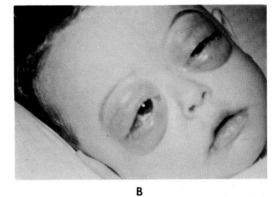

B

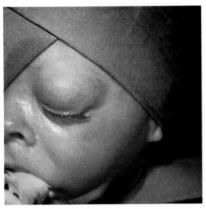

C

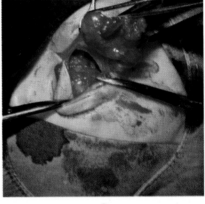

D

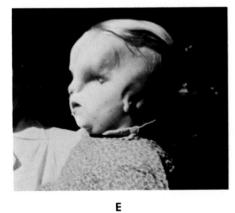

E

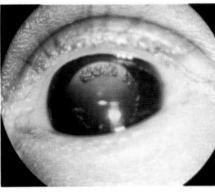

F

PLATE II

(*A*) Dermoid extending from orbit.

(*B*) Reticuloendotheliosis (Letterer-Siwe syndrome). (Courtesy of Dr. Harold Falls.)

(*C*) Capillary hemangioma of orbit and lid approached through a brow incision.

(*D*) Hemangioma dissected from posterior orbit (same case as *C*).

(*E*) Atypical rhinencephaly. Medial portion of orbital walls in contact, partially excluding the nose. (Courtesy of Dr. Harold Falls.)

(*F*) Cataract of prematurity. Birth weight: 2 pounds, 7 ounces. Infant was two months premature.

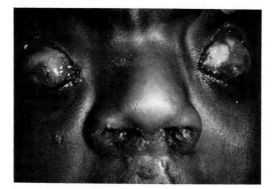

Figure 8–12   Bilateral microphthalmos with cyst.

cially when the head is in the dependent position.

Dysostoses of the Cranial Bones (Figs. 8–13 to 8–16)

Nager and DeReynier classify the deformities into five sections—craniostenosis, craniofacial dysostosis of Crouzon, mandibulofacial dysostosis of Franceschetti, hypertelorism and a group of rare entities.

Premature closure of one or more sutures of the skull results in a head deformity producing damaging effects to the brain and the eyes.

CONGENITAL CRANIOSYNOSTOSIS (CRANIOSTENOSIS). This condition originates during embryonic development and may be associated with other skeletal defects. Early recognition is important before deleterious effects have developed. Neurosurgical procedures for the relief of premature suture closure are available.

When the sagittal suture is closed prematurely, the head becomes long and narrow (*scaphocephaly*). A bony ridge often marks the closed suture. Male children are more frequently affected than females. Associated ocular or neurologic disorders rarely occur with these defects. *Plagiocephaly* is a slanted skull in which premature union of the sutures involves only half the head.

Closure of one coronal suture results in a severe deformity *oxycephaly* or *turricephalus* with involvement of the face and orbit on the same side. The roof of the orbit is depressed and exophthalmos, strabismus, nystagmus, papilledema, optic atrophy and visual disturbances may occur. Congenital cataract and oxycephaly may be associated defects.

ACROCEPHALOSYNDACTYLY (APERT'S SYNDROME) (FIG. 8–17). This is a disorder in which the head is pointed anteriorly (*acrocephaly*) and there are abnormalities of the sutures with syndactyly of the fingers and sometimes of the toes. It has been observed in several generations transmitted as an autosomal dominant. The eyes are widely spaced and prominent and exotropia is common. In *cleidocranial dysostosis* (absence of clavicle and delayed ossification of fontanelles) unilateral proptosis has been noted.

CRANIOFACIAL DYSOSTOSIS (CROUZON'S DISEASE). This is a syndrome characterized by acrocephaly, beak-shaped nose, hypoplastic maxilla, hypertelorism, exophthalmos, and exotropia. The orbits may be very shallow, and the disorder is transmitted as a dominant trait with varying expressivity. Absence of the superior rectus muscle bilaterally has been observed.

MANDIBULOFACIAL DYSOSTOSIS (FRANCESCHETTI'S SYNDROME) (FIGS. 8–18 AND 8–19). Mandibulofacial dysostosis is characterized by hypoplasia of the facial bones, especially in the malar bones, producing a characteristic "bird face." Malformations of the lid in the form of the antimongoloid slant, ectropion of the lower lid and at times colobomas are observed. There are also malformations of the ear, cleft palate and hair growth anomalies.

HYPERTELORISM (FIGS. 8–20 AND 8–21). Hypertelorism is characterized by an abnormally large distance between the eyes and an apparent broad nasal root. The lesser sphenoid wings are overdeveloped and the greater wings underdeveloped. Diagnosis is suspected by the wide interpupillary distance and exotropia. Mental deficiency is common and the condition appears genetically determined. Proptosis is not frequent but exotropia and optic atrophy occur with the pronounced cases.

TRIGONOCEPHALY (FIG. 8–22). This is a premature synostosis of the frontal bones. A keel-like ridge forms on the forehead and nasal root. The optic nerves may be damaged by pressure.

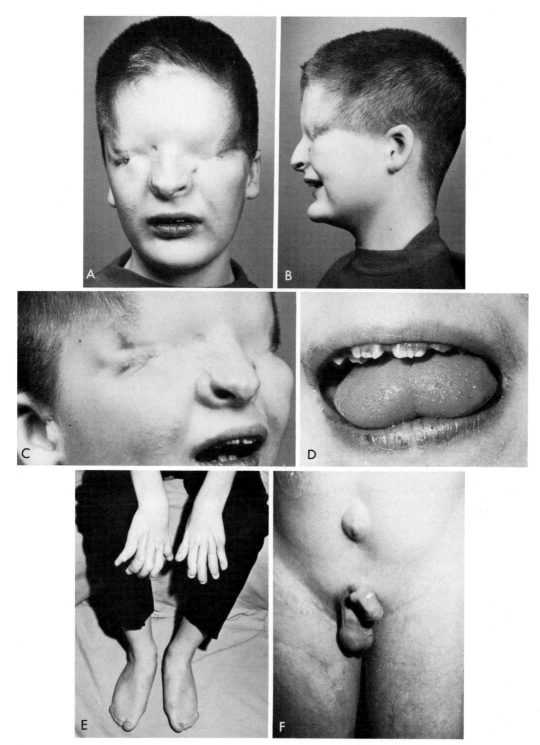

Figure 8–13 *A*, Cryptophthalmos associated with multiple congenital abnormalities. Complete covering of eyes by skin. Anterior segment usually deformed. Eye measurements by ultrasound. *B*, Side view. Hairline extending over entire temple area. *C*, Close up. Notching of right nostril and external ear deformity. *D*, Cryptophthalmos exhibiting malformation of teeth. *E*, Cryptophthalmos showing syndactyly of fingers and toes. Flexion deformity of fingers is postoperative. *F*, Cryptophthalmos associated with umbilical hernia and penis deformity. (Courtesy of Dr. Carl H. Ide and Dr. Paul B. Wollschlaeger.)

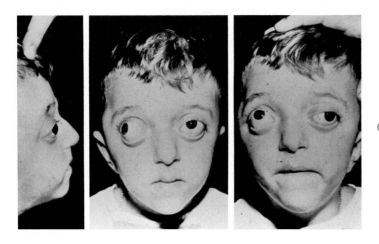

Figure 8–14 Craniofacial dysostosis (Crouzon's disease).

ACQUIRED DISORDERS OF THE ORBIT

Orbital Inflammation

Orbital inflammatory conditions, with the exception of direct trauma, develop secondary to inflammation or infection of adjacent structures such as the paranasal sinuses, nasopharyngeal cavity, surrounding skin and bones, fascial structures, orbital vessels, and the brain.

Inflammatory Edema of the Orbit

The eyelids may be intensely swollen and the eye may be partially proptosed as a result of reactive edema. Marked conjunctival chemosis and erythema are common signs in both. Orbital edema occurs most commonly in children in association with acute purulent ethmoiditis, acute antral disease, abscessed teeth or acute dacryocystitis. Orbital edema must be differentiated from orbital cellulitis.

Orbital Cellulitis and Abscess (Figs. 8–23, 8–24 and 8–25)

Orbital cellulitis is characterized by the signs of marked orbital edema together with limitation of ocular movement, a brawny induration of the lids, and systemic signs. Fever and lassitude are present. In the absence of penetrating trauma, acute purulent sinusitis is the most common cause. With the nasal tissues shrunken, purulent drainage can usually be identified. Although an abscess may develop, it is difficult to drain in the presence of marked edema. Treatment must be directed toward sinus drainage and large doses of antibiotics. Complications of orbital cellulitis are cavernous sinus thrombosis, meningitis, and brain abscess.

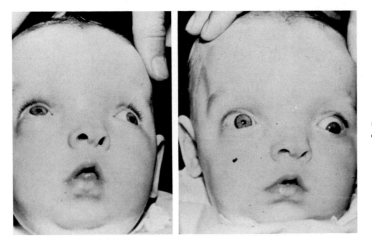

Figure 8–15 Craniofacial dysostosis (Crouzon's disease) illustrating hyperexodeviation.

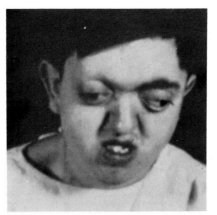

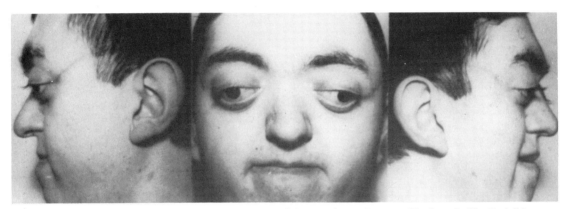

Figure 8–16   Case of craniofacial stenosis at age 12, and 20 years later. (Presented by Spaeth. The Bedell Lecture 1964.)

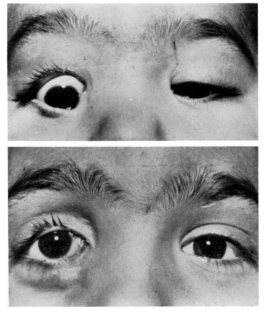

Figure 8–18   Unilateral case of lid coloboma and orbital margin defect simulating mandibulofacial dysostosis, complicated by lacrimal sac and lacrimal nasal duct deformity, before and after the surgery.

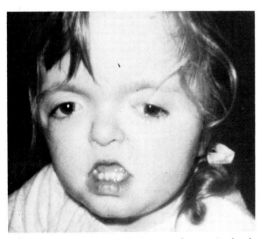

Figure 8–17   Hypertelorism and exotropia in Apert's syndrome.

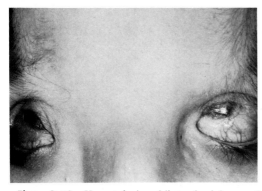

Figure 8–19 Hypertelorism, bilateral coloboma of lids associated with symblepharon xerophthalmia (Franceschetti's syndrome?).

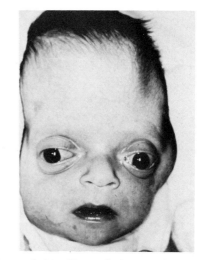

Figure 8–21 Hypertelorism and oxycephaly. (Courtesy of Harold Falls, M.D.)

Mucocele of the Paranasal Sinuses (Fig. 8–26)

Mucocele of the ethmoid sinuses is the most frequent mucocele encountered in children. Frontal sinus disease is not apt to occur before age nine or ten. Mucoceles protrude into the orbit through bony defects in the presence of chronic sinus disease. They have been seen frequently in cystic fibrosis patients. The mucocele usually involves the anterior ethmoidal cells and may present as a firm, fluctuant mass at the upper inner aspect of the orbital margin. The diagnosis can be confirmed by x-ray and sinus inspection (See Chapter 21, Figure 21–29A.) Surgery of the mucocele can be performed by incising the periosteum adjacent to the orbital margin, so that one is able to replace the trochlea in the normal functioning position.

Osteoperiostitis

Periostitis occurs most commonly as the result of trauma but may originate from the extension of an infection in adjacent structures. It frequently leads to the development of a staphylococcic osteomyelitis, resulting from accessory nasal sinusitis (chiefly maxillary sinus), infected tooth roots, or occasionally in association with childhood illnesses. There is intense lid swelling, proptosis, motility limitation, pain and tenderness on pressure. It is essentially an orbital abscess, and x-ray will disclose bone disease. Fistulas have been known to develop but are generally more common with chronic disease such as a retained foreign body or tuberculosis.

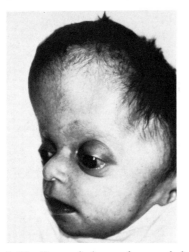

Figure 8–20 Hypertelorism and oxycephaly with associated exophthalmos. (Courtesy of Harold Falls, M.D.)

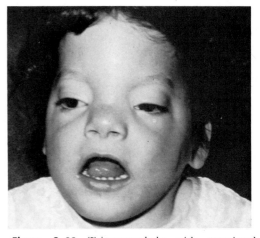

Figure 8–22 Trigonocephaly with associated residual exotropia and repaired choanal atresia. Child has had two operations for exotropia.

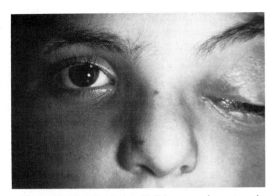

Figure 8–23 Orbital cellulitis secondary to ethmoid sinusitis (white female, age 8).

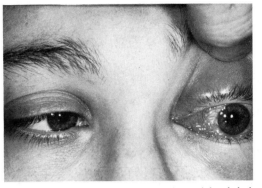

Figure 8–25 Orbital cellulitis with partial ophthalmoplegia.

Tenonitis

An uncommon entity associated with edema, chemosis of the conjunctiva, and exquisite pain on ocular movement, tenonitis has been observed postoperatively following trauma or childhood illnesses. During the migratory phase of Trichinella, when the parasite is invading the extraocular muscles, the symptoms suggest a tenonitis as well as myositis.

Cavernous Sinus Thrombosis

Infections about the face and nose require special handling, since the angular branch of the facial vein anastomoses with the ophthalmic veins in the orbit and these veins drain directly into the cavernous sinuses.

Prior to the development of antibiotics, this disease was usually fatal and still must be considered of grave consequence. Other foci of infection about the nose and throat have been observed.

The patient becomes acutely ill, exhibiting all the signs and symptoms of a fulminating septic process. At first the condition resembles a severe orbital cellulitis, but the pressure from behind becomes so severe that papilledema, venous engorgement, and visual loss develop. Bilateral involvement is a poor prognostic sign.

Severe headache and meningeal signs may occur and complete ophthalmoplegia is indicative of cavernous sinus disease rather than orbital cellulitis. Treatment consists of massive doses of an antibiotic and drainage of the infected area together with supportive care by the pediatrician, neurologist, and neurosurgeon.

Dacryoadenitis and Dacryocystitis

Dacryoadenitis is a rare occurrence in a child but may develop concurrently with mumps. Chronic dacryoadenitis is more apt to suggest sarcoid or tuberculosis. Characteristically, there is pain, swelling and displacement of the eye down and nasalward. Proptosis is not common. Acute purulent dacryocystitis is common secondary to obstruction of the nasolacrimal duct and must be differentiated from acute orbital cellulitis.

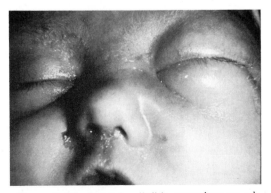

Figure 8–24 Orbital cellulitis secondary to ethmoiditis (white male, age 2).

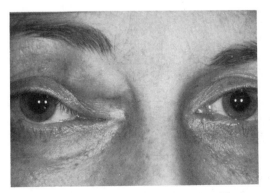

Figure 8–26 Mucocele of right ethmoid sinus (white female, age 16).

Chronic Orbital Inflammation

Chronic orbital inflammatory disease must be differentiated from orbital tumors. The inflammatory mass may be divided into nongranulomatous and granulomatous.

Nongranulomatous Lesions

Pseudotumor of the orbit falls into this category.

The etiology is often unknown. Even after biopsy the diagnosis may be reported as chronic round cell infiltration which invites some concern as to the true nature of the process. The clinical course is varied, since the onset may be sudden or slow. It is usually unilateral, with proptosis, some limitation of ocular movement, a palpable mass, and congestion. The condition has a tendency toward remission but can be improved with corticosteroid therapy. We have recently observed a 15-year-old boy with pseudotumor show 75 per cent improvement in 3 months following surgical exploration and without the administration of systemic cortisone. At times the second orbit becomes involved months later. It must be differentiated from malignant lymphoma and Hodgkin's disease.

Granulomatous Lesions

Granulomatous lesions of the orbit consist of tuberculosis, syphilis, sarcoid, mycoses and parasites.

TUBERCULOSIS. Tuberculosis of the orbit is rare and reaches the orbit by extension from adjacent structures or metastasis. Trauma may be a precipitating factor in cases of tuberculous periostitis. The formation of a sequestrum with sinuses opening near the eyebrow is a characteristic.

SARCOIDOSIS. Sarcoidosis involving the lacrimal glands or occurring deeper in the orbit usually involves older children or adults in our experience.

SYPHILIS. Syphilis of the orbit involves the periosteum near the anterior margin to form a painless swelling. Spaeth reported a gumma in which pain preceded the proptosis.

MYCOSES. The fungi which have been known to involve the orbit to produce a granulomatous lesion are Actinomyces, Aspergillus, Mucor and Sporotrichum. Acute mucormycosis involving the orbit was reported by Gregory and coworkers. There was proptosis, external ophthalmoplegia, and meningoencephalitis in an uncontrolled diabetic. The fungus infection may begin in the nasopharynx and spread to the orbit and central nervous system, resulting in death.

PARASITIC INFECTION. The following parasites have been discovered in the orbit: Trichinella, Cysticerca, Onchocerca and Echinococcus. Cysticerca larva, *Taenia solium* (pork tapeworm), are more commonly found to migrate intraocularly than within the orbit. Although the microfilaria found in onchocerciasis commonly invade the eye causing blindness, it was never observed in the orbit during a survey of a large endemic area in Guatemala. Echinococcus (hydatid cyst) of the orbit is frequently encountered in North Africa, South America, Central Europe and Australia, but rarely in North America. It occurs particularly where dogs are used for tending sheep and cattle. Hydatid cysts are especially common in young people and develop in the liver, lung, brain, or orbit. A large multilocular cyst with scolices was recently excised from the orbit of a 10-year-old Tunisian girl. The ophthalmologist stated that hydatid cyst was a common occurrence.

Toxocara canis and catis. According to Wills Eye Hospital records, *Toxocara canis* and *catis* have been observed within the eye but not in the orbit.

Trichinosis. Trichinosis often affects the extraocular muscles. During the period of larval encystment there is lid edema, marked chemosis, and pain on ocular movement.

WEGENER'S GRANULOMATOSIS. This condition may be a variant of periarteritis nodosa and is characterized by the following: necrotizing granulomatous lesions, especially in the respiratory tract; generalized and focal necrotizing vasculitis; and a necrotizing glomerulitis which eventuates in death. The orbit is involved by direct extension from the nasopharynx and sinuses.

LETHAL MIDLINE GRANULOMA. This condition begins with a gradual destructive process involving the center of the face. Edema about the nose is followed by

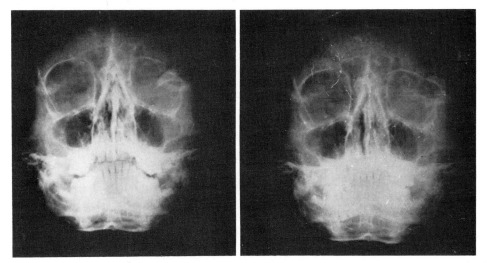

Figure 8–27   Orbital rim fracture following sledding collision accident, before and after open reduction.

ulceration of the septum and palate. The orbit is secondarily involved as the process extends to adjacent structures.

INJURIES TO THE ORBIT
(Figs. 8–27 and 8–28)

Penetrating injuries may be significant for three reasons:

1. Damage to orbital structures.
2. Orbital bleeding with or without retained foreign bodies.
3. Intracranial perforation of the posterior orbital wall.

Fractures about the orbit, particularly blowout fractures of the orbital floor or fractures of the orbital margins with deformity, are common. Damage or inclusion of the soft tissue must be of primary concern. (See Chapter 17 on ocular trauma.)

VASCULAR CONDITIONS OF THE ORBIT (Fig. 8–29)

Vascular lesions of the orbit are frequently secondary to inflammatory disease of the vessels and hematopoietic disorders. Primary vascular lesions consist of *hemangiomas, aneurysms, lymphangiomas, orbital varices,* and *carotid-cavernous fistulas.* Orbital thrombophlebitis may be associated with orbital cellulitis and cavernous sinus thrombosis. It most commonly originates from adjacent structures, from penetrating trauma, or as a metastasis from infected areas. Serious complications, including meningitis, may develop.

Hemangiomas (Fig. 8–30)

Cavernous hemangioma is the most frequently encountered primary tumor in

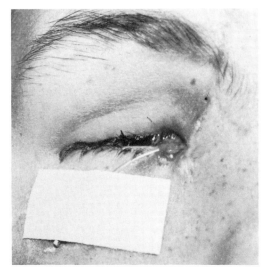

Figure 8–28   Traumatic fracture of floor and medial wall of orbit; partial exenteration of orbit; rupture of bony lacrimal nasal duct. First stage in therapy, restoration of lacrimal nasal duct by dacryocystorhinostomy and indwelling polyvinyl tube.

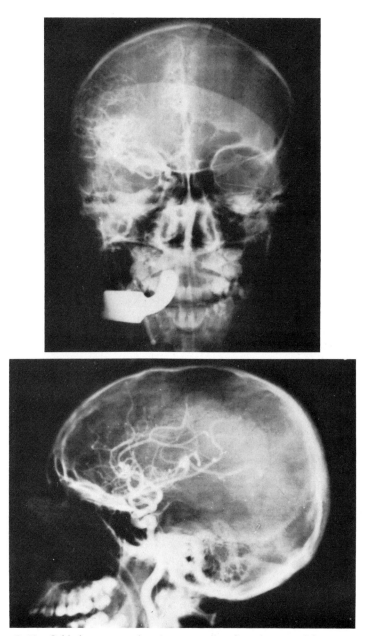

Figure 8–29   Orbital aneurysmal varices extending from intracranial venous origin.

the orbit. It is usually present at birth, although hemorrhage into the mass would make one consider it a growth of recent origin. It may be recognized as a lid swelling or proptosis and characteristically increases in size when the child cries or strains. Capillary hemangiomas present similar clinical findings but are less common.

Aneurysms

Aneurysms must be exceedingly uncommon but traumatic arteriovenous fistulas occur and are characteristically recognized by pulsating exophthalmos and a bruit heard through the closed eyelid. Nonpulsating aneurysm has been reported as a complication of orbital neurofibromatosis.

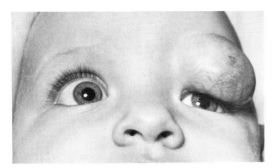

Figure 8–30 Hemangioma of lid, anterior to orbital rim.

Hemangio-endotheliomas and Lymphangiomas (Fig. 8–31)

Hemangio-endotheliomas are vascular tumors but are solid compared to cavernous hemangiomas and should be excised, although radiation has a beneficial effect. Lymphangiomas are congenital, benign, slowly progressive tumors of the lymph vascular system. Jones analyzed 62 cases involving the ocular adnexa, of which 47 per cent involved the orbit. The age of onset of this group of 29 patients was 6.2 years. Ten patients had lymphangiomas at birth, while 16 patients developed signs prior to age 15. Hemorrhage into lymphangiomas is common. Aspiration of the blood followed by the application of a pressure dressing may be effective. Excision is indicated, since these tumors are not radiosensitive.

Orbital Varices

Varices are unusual vascular formations characterized by variable and transient proptosis induced by crying, coughing, sneezing, or placing the head in a dependent position for 5 seconds. The proptosis may also be exaggerated with pressure on the jugular vein. Thromboses of elements within the varix produce episodes of swelling followed by shrinkage. The mass consists of numerous dilated, coiled vessels and may present some difficulty on attempted removal. X-ray may indicate the presence of calcified thrombi as a diagnostic aid, and contrast media studies of the orbital vessels may be most significant. When suspected, it is wise to be prepared for blood replacement prior to surgical excision of the mass.

Carotid-Cavernous Fistulas

This serious problem is characterized by pulsating exophthalmos and usually induced by trauma to the orbit or as a result of basilar skull fracture. The fistula consists of a rupture of the carotid artery into the cavernous sinus resulting from a crack in or displacement of the sphenoid bone which has ruptured the vessel wall. Characteristically the patient hears an intermittent roaring noise, a bruit, and there is a palpable thrill and variable involvement of ocular motility. Conjunctival vessels are commonly engorged and tortuous. Diagnosis can be established by

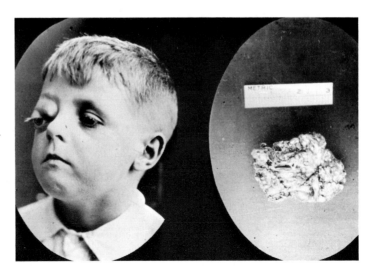

Figure 8–31 Hemangio-endothelioma (white male, age 6).

digital compression of the carotid. Treatment by homolateral carotid ligation is effective, although spontaneous cure by thrombosis has been observed.

Orbital Hemorrhage (Fig. 8–32)

Trauma is the most common cause of orbital hemorrhage. It may occur from blunt compression injuries or penetrating wounds into the retrobulbar structures. Proptosis is moderate but the lids may be tightly closed and there is a firm resistance on pressure such as follows hemorrhage from retrobulbar injection. Intraocular tension may be raised and pulsation of the central artery has been noted. Visual and motility disturbances occur but are temporary. Vomiting may be induced. Birth trauma and difficult forceps delivery may give rise to proptosis from orbital hemorrhage.

BLOOD DYSCRASIAS. Blood dyscrasias, especially *leukemia*, are the commonest nontraumatic causes of orbital hemorrhage. Ecchymosis usually accompanies the proptosis, and the child is obviously ill and exhibits a sickly pallor. Orbital hemorrhage has been seen in *scurvy*, in which case the bleeding is subperiosteal and the proptosed eye is displaced opposite to the collection. Other less common causes are *vitamin K deficiency*, causing newborn proptosis; *intracranial vascular tumors;* and *subdural hematoma*.

CHLOROMA. Chloroma is a green-colored tumor that may spread into the orbit in atypical forms of myelogenous leukemia. Tumor masses are found throughout the periosteum of the skull and meninges. The mass is firm and the green color results supposedly from an intermediate substance in the breakdown of hemoglobin. In a differential diagnosis of proptosis, the importance of history, physical examination, x-rays of skull or orbit, and white cell count with differential and sedimentation rate must be uniformly considered.

ORBITAL DISEASE SECONDARY TO METABOLIC OR SYSTEMIC DISORDERS (Fig. 8–33)

Orbital diseases secondary to metabolic or systemic disorders include hyperthyroidism, histiocytosis syndromes (eosinophilic granuloma of bone and Hand-Schüller-Christian and Letterer-

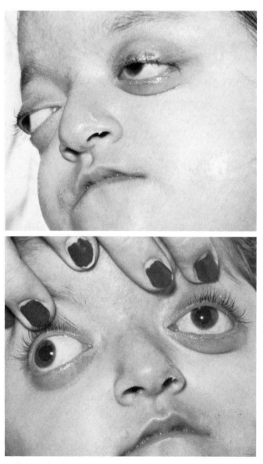

Figure 8–33 Eosinophilic granuloma. (Service of the late Dr. Howard Childs Carpenter, Graduate Hospital, University of Pennsylvania, Philadelphia.)

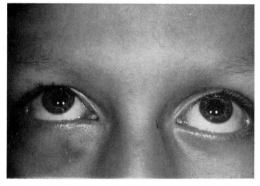

Figure 8–32 Organized hematoma, right lower orbital margin.

Siwe syndromes), neurofibromatosis, and bony diseases (osteoma, hyperostosis, infantile cortical hyperostosis [Caffey's disease], osteopetrosis (Albers-Schönberg disease), and fibrous dysplasia of bone).

Hyperthyroidism

Hyperthyroidism is much more common in adults than in children. They make up approximately 1 per cent of all patients with hyperthyroidism. Eighty per cent of the children involved are between ages 10 and 15 and girls are affected more often than boys in a ratio of 6 to 1. Congenital hyperthyroidism may be observed in infants, occurring secondary to a mother's hyperthyroidism. Exophthalmos is present in most cases but is rarely marked and may be unilateral.

Upper lid retraction is one of the earliest and most reliable signs. It may be quite subtle and noted at the beginning of attempted down gaze.

Irritability and hypermotor activity are characteristic. The clinical diagnosis can be confirmed with the aid of special laboratory tests such as the protein-bound iodine determination and the uptake of radioactive iodine (I^{131}).

Diplopia and corneal exposure rarely occur in children. If lid closure did become a problem, lateral wall decompression would be indicated. General therapy remains the function of the pediatrician. Hyperthyroidism occurs occasionally with *polyostotic fibrous dysplasia* and sexual precocity.

Histiocytosis Syndromes

Eosinophilic Granuloma of Bone (Histiocytosis X)

This condition occurs as a lesion involving the skeletal system with cystic areas of granulation tissue. Phagocytic histiocytes and eosinophils are characteristic. Cystic lesions involving the orbit produce proptosis. Painful swellings over other bony areas, which can be curetted and irradiated, provide a clue to the diagnosis.

Hand-Schüller-Christian Syndrome

This is a chronic systemic disorder of the histiocytosis group which has osseous lesions and additional involvement of the viscera. Characteristically, there is orbital infiltration with proptosis, defects of the membranous skull bones, and diabetes insipidus. The proptosis is usually bilateral but not symmetrical. Polydipsia and polyuria are classic symptoms. Antitumor chemotherapy promises the greatest hope for eventual control of the granulomatous process.

Letterer-Siwe Syndrome

This is the most serious clinical problem and occurs in those infants exhibiting major visceral involvement. It is generally fatal. The skin, liver, spleen, bone marrow, and skeleton become involved. Diagnosis is made from the biopsy of the skin lesions. Proptosis occurs but is not common in this condition.

Bony Diseases of the Orbit

Osteomas

Osteomas are seen occasionally in older children and generally arise from the paranasal sinuses. Sphenoidal osteomas may produce visual impairment. Papilledema and some ocular displacement may be present.

Hyperostosis

Hyperostosis is characterized by a diffuse thickening of the orbit, usually in association with a meningioma.

Infantile Cortical Hyperostosis (Caffey's Disease)

This condition manifests a hyperplasia of subperiosteal bone and thickening of the periosteum, according to Iliff and Ossofsky (1962). Symptoms begin in the early weeks of life and not later than 6 months. Fever, irritability, and pseudoparalysis are encountered. Anemia and elevated alkaline phosphatase are reported. Multiple bones are involved. Proptosis is not common.

Fibrous Dysplasia of Bone

This manifests itself as a filling of the bony medullary cavity with fibrous hyperplasia. When orbital bones are affected, the volume of the orbit is reduced. Proptosis and some swelling about the orbital margin are present. All bones may be involved. Diagnosis is confirmed by the roentgenologic appearance.

Osteopetrosis (Albers-Schönberg Disease)

This is known as the "marble bone disease." Sclerosis begins near the epiphyseal lines and affects the skull base and long bones. Orbital volume and the optic foramina are decreased, resulting in proptosis and optic atrophy.

NEOPLASMS OF THE ORBIT

A. *Primary*
　1. Benign
　　a. Hemangioma—cavernous and capillary
　　b. Hemiangio-endothelioma
　　c. Lymphangioma
　　d. Dermoid and epidermoid cyst (choristomas)
　　e. Neurofibroma
　　f. Neurilemoma
　　g. Benign lymphoma
　　h. Adamantinoma
　　i. Lipoma, fibroma, leiomyoma and chondroma
　　j. Benign mixed cell tumor of lacrimal gland.
　2. Malignant
　　a. Teratoma
　　b. Sarcoma
　　　1. Rhabdomyosarcoma
　　　2. Liposarcoma
　　　3. Lymphosarcoma and reticulum cell sarcoma
　　　4. Hemangio-endothelio-sarcoma
　　　5. Fibrosarcoma
　　c. Optic nerve glioma
　　d. Lacrimal gland tumors, malignant
　　e. Melanoma of orbit
B. *Secondary*
　1. Benign
　　a. Osteoma
　　b. Meningioma
　　c. Intracranial tumors involving the orbit
　2. Malignant
　　a. Neuroblastoma
　　b. Malignant nasopharyngeal tumors
　　c. Chloroma
　　d. Sarcoma of paranasal sinuses
　　e. Malignant lymphoma
　　　1. Hodgkin's disease
　　　2. Leukemia
　　f. Malignant melanoma of orbit
　　g. Retinoblastoma
　　h. Intracranial tumors invading the orbit

PRIMARY BENIGN TUMORS
(Figs. 8–34 and 8–35)

Hemangioma

Hemangioma is the most common orbital tumor and the most common cause of proptosis among primary orbital tumors. These tumors are often associated with vascular lesions of the skin and may be present at birth, with growth noted during the first years of life. A rapid

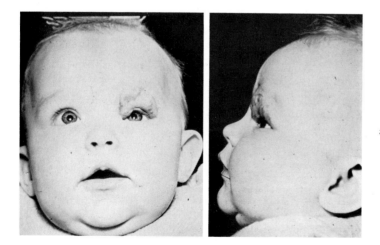

Figure 8–34 Hemangioma of lid and orbit.

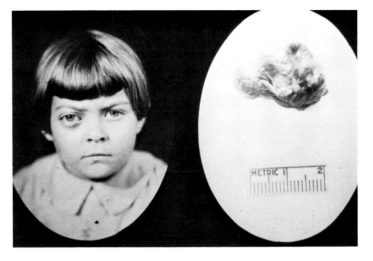

Figure 8–35 Hemangioma successfully removed from right orbit.

increase in size is generally associated with hemorrhage and thrombosis. For *benign hemangioendothelioma* and *lymphangioma*, the reader is referred to Vascular Conditions of the Orbit (p. 207).

Choristoma

Choristoma is a tumor composed of tissue elements which normally are not present at this location. Such tumors include *dermoid cysts, epidermoid cysts,* and *teratomas.*

Dermoid or Epidermoid Cysts (Fig. 8–36). These are congenital tumors composed of sebaceous material, hair follicles, and elastic fibers representing a "rest" of the primitive ectoderm in the area of a fetal cleft. They are frequently attached to bone in the upper temporal aspect of the orbital margin. They are firm to palpation with some bony erosion at the site of attachment. The majority of anteriorly situated dermoid cysts can be excised easily. Every effort should be made to remove the tumor in one piece, since the contents of the dermoid cyst are irritating. Deep orbital dermoid cysts extending into the orbital roof may requite neurosurgery to assist removal.

Neurofibromas

Neurofibromas are slow-growing congenital tumors of the peripheral nerves. Large plexiform neurofibromas may produce a slowly progressive proptosis and may also involve the lids. Pulsation indicates intracranial extension. Neurofibroma of the orbit may occur as an isolated lesion or represent a part of the generalized disease (von Recklinghausen's disease). The association between neurofibroma and optic nerve glioma is well known. Palpation of the mass in the lids has a typical "bag of worms" feel and excision of the tumor is often incomplete. Neurilemomas (Schwannomas) are slow-growing and derived from the sheath of Schwann. The growth is well encapsulated and composed of orderly patterned tumor cells. Complete excision is curative. Neurilemoma may undergo malignant change (Figs. 8–37 to 8–40).

Benign Lymphomas and Plasmomas

Benign lymphomas and plasmomas consist of infiltration of the tissues with

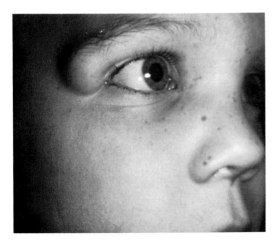

Figure 8–36 Dermoid cyst, orbital margin.

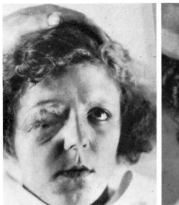

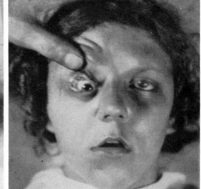

Figure 8–37 Skin and orbital neurofibromatosis, complicated by nonpulsating orbital aneurysm.

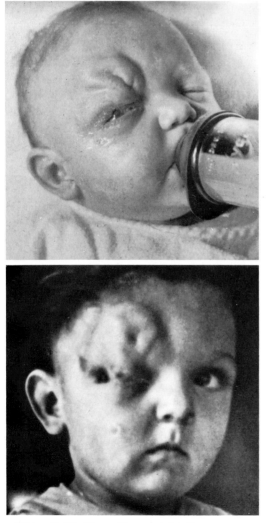

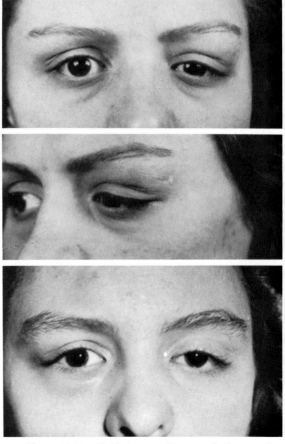

Figure 8–38 Neurofibroma in infancy, accompaned by a blind right eye because of optic nerve atrophy. Same case after bone flap to forehead.

Figure 8–39 Orbital neurofibroma, before and after orbitotomy.

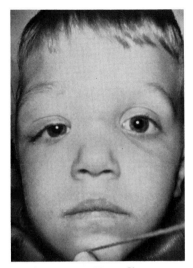

Figure 8–40 Neurofibroma.

lymphocytes and plasma cells respectively. The diagnosis is confirmed with biopsy and the growths are sensitive to radiation.

Adamantinomas (Fig. 8–41)

Adamantinomas are rare growths composed of epithelial cells originating from tooth buds. Although of low-degree malignancy, they exert their effect by direct extension into the orbit and displace the globe upward. They tend to spread by direct extension into the maxillary sinus and orbit.

Primary Malignant Tumors (Figs. 8–42 and 8–43)

Teratomas

Teratomas comprise tissue elements derived from the three primary embryonic cell layers. The tumors are noted at birth, grow rapidly, and are highly malignant. The proposed eye is dwarfed by the extent of the tumor mass. The tumor consists of skin, hair, sebaceous glands, cartilage and connective tissue, and epithelium of endodermal origin. Immediate excision of the mass offers the only hope for survival.

Rhabdomyosarcomas (Figs. 8–44 and 8–45)

Rhabdomyosarcoma is the most common malignant tumor of mesenchymal origin and also the commonest orbital malignancy in children. Tumors may be

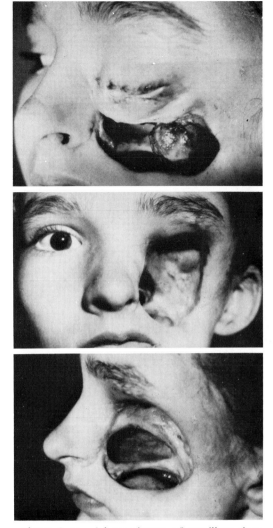

Figure 8–41 Adamantinoma of maxillary sinus, recurrent, invading the orbit. Front and lateral views after orbitotomy.

classified into three histological types which are found predominantly in Caucausian males under 10 years of age. Embryonal rhabdomyosarcoma is the most common histological type and characteristically develops in the upper nasal orbit, displacing the eye down and outward. Early exenteration seems to offer the best opportunity for care, although recent results indicate a favorable outcome with prompt massive x-ray therapy, as with cobalt-60. The brain and lungs are primary sites for metastases. Extension has occurred into the orbit from a primary tumor site on the surface of the upper lid, outer angle.

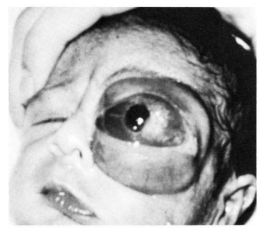

Figure 8–42 Teratoma in newborn.

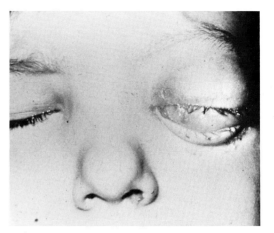

Figure 8–44 Rhabdomyosarcoma (white male, age 10).

Liposarcomas, Fibrosarcomas, and Hemangio-endotheliosarcomas (Figs. 8–46 and 8–47)

These, derived from their cell elements, have been reported from the orbit but must be rare.

Certain primary *malignant lymphomatous tumors* composed solely of lymphocytes are referred to as *lymphosarcomas* (Fig. 8–48). When the tumor originates from the reticulum cell, it is known as a *reticulum cell sarcoma*, which is closely related to a type of *Hodgkin's disease.* Proptosis may occur in Hodgkin's disease in children.

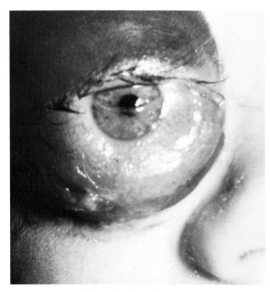

Figure 8–43 Teratoma.

Optic Nerve Gliomas (Figs. 8–49 and 8–50)

Optic nerve glioma is a slow-growing tumor derived from the interstitial cells, astroglia and oligodendroglia. As gliomas increase in size they produce enlargement of the bony optic canal, which is a prime diagnostic feature. Loss of vision is the first symptom, but since the tumors are usually present in the first decade, it is rare that the parent of the child is aware of it. Since the tumor grows in the muscle cone, the proptosis is directed straight outward. Optic atrophy is a common finding, although if the growth approximates the globe, papilledema may result. If the tumor is confined to the nerve, excision of the orbital position of the nerve and tumor is sufficient to result in a cure. Intracranial extension through the optic nerve foramen has occurred. If biopsy of the optic nerve resection suggests such extension, then a transfrontal neurosurgical approach is necessary as a secondary operation. Invasion of the globe by glioma, even when the tumor grows almost adjacent to the eyeball, rarely occurs. The relationship of von Recklinghausen's disease and optic nerve glioma has been mentioned.

Lacrimal Gland Tumors

These may be classified into benign and malignant mixed cell tumors and carcinomas. The majority of mixed cell tumors are benign and are composed of a blending of epithelial and connective tissue elements. The tumors are multi-

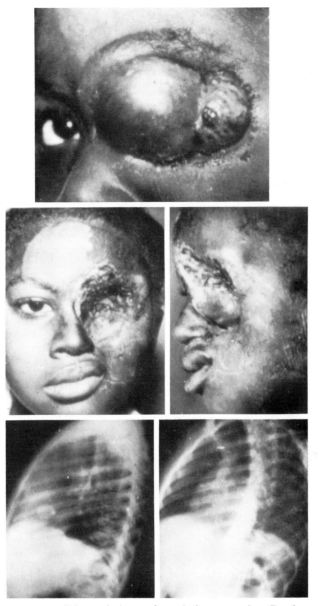

Figure 8–45 Rhabdomyosarcoma. Primary lesion and surgical exenteration. Death occurred from pulmonary extension. (J. Pediat. Ophthal., *1*:2, 1964.)

lobulated but are well encapsulated and adherent to the periosteum. They are locally invasive and tend to recur if not completely removed.

Nearly 50 per cent of all epithelial tumors of the lacrimal gland are *carcinomas* and the majority are of the adenoid cystic variety. This tumor spreads along nerves and vessels, penetrates bone, and offers a poor prognosis. As soon as the diagnosis

has been established, exenteration is required.

Melanomas of the Orbit (Fig. 8–51)

Melanoma of the orbit is derived from melanocytes which have extended beyond the scleral coat on the vessels. The juvenile melanoma is a junctional nevus and should be excised. *Malignant melanoma* is extremely rare in children.

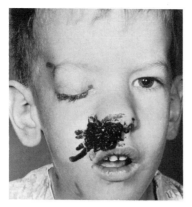

Figure 8–46 Hemangiosarcoma (white male, age 7).

SECONDARY BENIGN TUMORS

Osteomas

Osteomas may occur in the orbit or neighboring sinuses. They have the appearance of normal or sclerotic bone and are often exostoses. Bony growths may be associated with teratomas and particularly with the anterior ethmoidal cells. Osteomas should be excised before they produce symptoms caused by pressure.

Meningiomas

Meningiomas are tumors that usually develop in the skull but may be primary in the orbit. The tumors extend to the orbit by involving the bones or by extension through the optic foramen. Meningiomas are classified according to their clinical site and can be divided into three categories: suprasellar, presellar, and sphenoidal ridge meningiomas. Symptoms are related to pressure exerted on adjacent structures. Sphenoid ridge meningiomas may produce optic atrophy, field changes and proptosis x-ray changes are characteristic. The surgical management must be planned in conjunction with a neurosurgeon.

SECONDARY MALIGNANT TUMORS
(Figs. 8–52 and 8–53)

Neuroblastomas

Neuroblastoma arises from the adrenal medulla of infants and young children. When it metastasizes to the orbital bones, it produces periorbital hemorrhage, lid

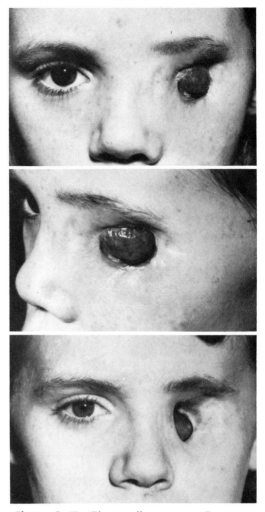

Figure 8–47 Giant cell sarcoma. Recurrence after primary exenteriation. Final cure after subsequent surgery.

ecchymosis, and marked proptosis. A recurrent ecchymosis of the lid is often the first sign of the disease. The patients then develop pallor, weight loss, and a palpable abdominal mass. An intravenous pyelogram will demonstrate a kidney displaced by a mass. Breakdown products of epinephrine and norepinephrine can be found in the urinary excretion.

Malignant Nasopharyngeal Tumors

Malignant nasopharyngeal tumors are more common in adults than in children but do occur in the latter. The tumors may be sarcomas or carcinomas and spread rapidly to the nasal sinuses and invade the orbit and cranial cavity. Lacri-

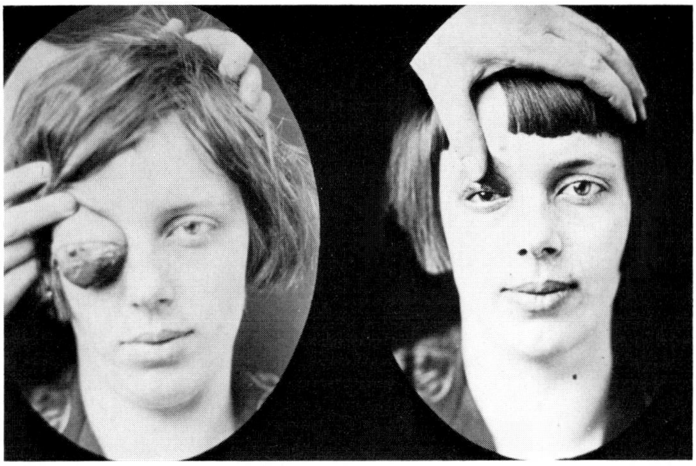

Figure 8–48 Orbital lymphosarcoma presented with proptosis, ecchymosis, and diplopia. Rapid growth in a few months (white female, age 16).

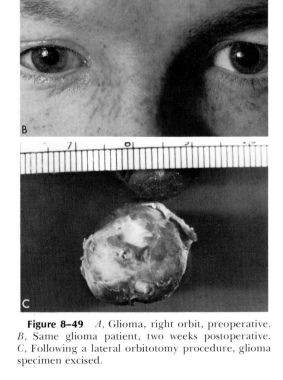

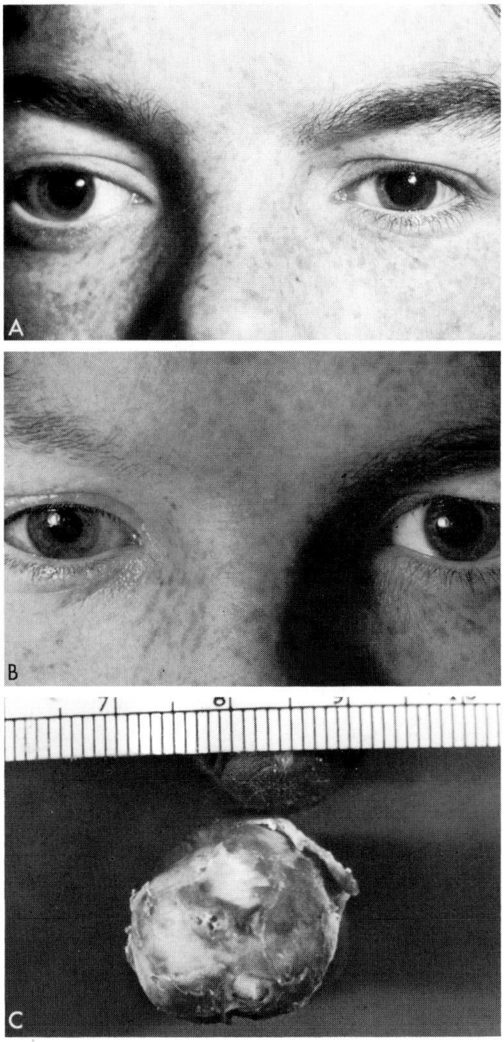

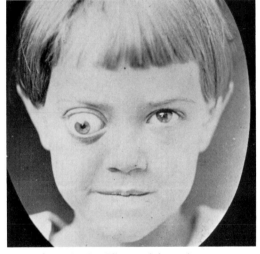

Figure 8–50 Glioma, right optic nerve.

Figure 8–49 *A*, Glioma, right orbit, preoperative. *B*, Same glioma patient, two weeks postoperative. *C*, Following a lateral orbitotomy procedure, glioma specimen excised.

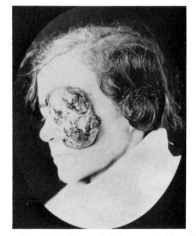

Figure 8–51 Melanoepithelioma (white female, age 19).

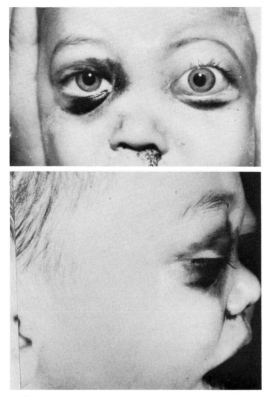

Figure 8–52 Hypernephroma with orbital metastases (renal cell carcinoma).

mation, lateral rectus muscle palsy, nasal obstruction, and pain are early signs. An 11-year-old boy was seen with lymphosarcoma in which mild epistaxis was the presenting sign prior to proptosis and orbital involvement. The prognosis is poor, although radiation brings temporary relief.

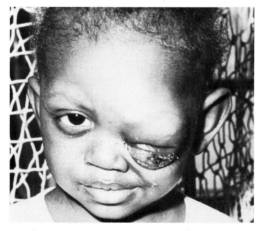

Figure 8–53 Neuroblastoma in 3-year-old.

Sarcoma of the Paranasal Sinuses

This tumor may occur but is rare in children. The usual type is a giant cell sarcoma.

Malignant Lymphoma

In children the development of an orbital tumor may be the first indication of *leukemia or malignant lymphoma* and may be next to rhabdomyosarcoma insofar as frequency of malignant orbital neoplasms is concerned. A biopsy specimen confirms the presence of a malignant lymphomatous process, so that a careful examination of the child is necessary to reveal the exact nature of the disease. The prognosis is poor, since acute leukemias and reticulum cell malignant lymphoma are likely diagnoses. Hodgkin's disease is a neoplasm involving the reticulum cells. Proptosis and ecchymosis about the lids is common.

Burkitt's undifferentiated lymphoma affects African children between ages 2 and 12. It frequently involves the orbit and maxillary bone, with a predilection for the jaw. It is a malignancy in which the virus etiology is considered convincing. A herpes type of virus designated as EB virus has been found with electron microscopy. Burkitt's lymphoma has been reported in the United States, Canada, and Japan.

Malignant Melanoma and Retinoblastoma

These may extend into the orbit and are considered in more detail in Chapter 30, Ocular Neoplasms in Childhood.

TREATMENT OF ORBITAL TUMORS IN CHILDREN

Medical

Rhabdomyosarcoma

Rhabdomyosarcoma may be treated by exenteration or radiation. This important tumor of children must first be identified by biopsy before a preferential decision can be made. Reese, and others, favor massive dose radiation at the present time, having used cobalt-60 in 17 cases, two of which had recurrent following exenteration.

Infantile Hemangiomas

Infantile hemangiomas in the anterior

portion of the orbit also respond satisfactorily to radiation given cautiously.

TREATMENT OF HEMANGIOMAS. Six principal methods of treatment have been described for orbital hemangiomas in infants and children: cryotherapy, surgical diathermy, sclerosing agents, radiotherapy, corticosteroids, and excision. Present day therapeutic methods favor the implantation of radon seeds, the use of steroids, or surgical excision.

Experience with the systemic administration of corticosteroids for the suppression of orbital hemangiomas has been limited. The usefulness of corticosteroids was discovered during attempts to control bleeding problems in children exhibiting large, diffuse hemangiomas and thrombocytopenia.

More favorable results have been reported following the systemic use of steroids for infantile hemangiomas of the ocular adnexa, but the inherent risk of such therapy for infants must be considered.

Final judgment on the efficacy of such treatment cannot be formed, and results remain inconclusive.

Lymphangiomas

Lymphangioma is characterized by hemorrhage into the large endothelial-lined spaces. Aspiration of the blood and a pressure dressing is often successful.

Radiation is indicated when the chiasm has become involved from a *optic nerve glioma* or when the resected nerve end shows tumor cells.

CHEMOTHERAPY

This form of therapy is becoming increasingly important in childhood oncology. It is no longer in the realm of experimentation, since specialists are available for assistance.

ORBITAL SURGERY

Surgical Approaches for Tumor Excision

There are two primary approaches to the orbit in children. The method selected depends upon the position of the mass and the displacement of the globe. The expo-

sure for lesions in the orbital roof is best performed by means of a brow incision, but care must be exercised not to interfere with lid innervation or trochlea function. Transconjunctival routes with the aid of a lateral canthotomy are frequently sufficient for a biopsy. An approach through the lower lid is rarely used except for abscess drainage or an orbital floor fracture. Most tumors deep in the orbit are best reached via a lateral wall orbitotomy.

Figure 8–54 *A, B,* and *C* from the *Atlas*

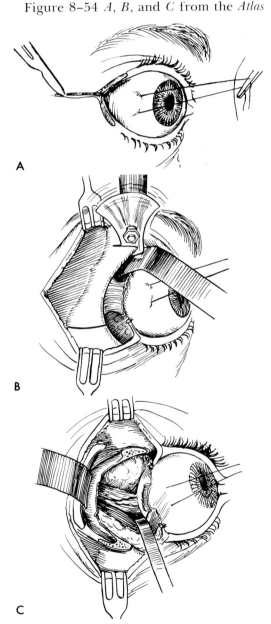

A

B

C

Figure 8–54 *A, B,* and *C* are line sketches from *Atlas of Eye Surgery* (see bibliography), illustrating the principal steps in the Krönlein technique.

of Eye Surgery by Paton, Smith, Katzin, and Stillwell illustrates the skin incision and orbitotomy, which is a modified Krönlein technique.

STEPS

1. A retraction suture is placed under the tendon of the lateral rectus muscle and the medial halves of the lids are sutured closed. The skin incision is made 35 mm. long down to temporal fascia, followed by a lateral canthotomy which is tagged by suture.

2. The periosteum of the lateral orbital wall is incised and freed with a periosteal elevator, especially at the superior and inferior bony cut sites.

3. The orbital contents are retracted away from the lateral margin and the bone is incised superiorly for a distance of 10 to 12 mm. by the Stryker saw, which is held at an angle of 45 degrees to the floor of the orbit.

4. The lateral wall is fractured outward with rongeur forceps and the periosteum and periorbita are incised horizontally, exposing the orbital contents. The lateral rectus muscle and tendon are to be identified. The tumor should be isolated by displacing adjacent orbital structures.

5. Following tumor removal, the orbital periosteum is sutured, and the bone flap is replaced and held in place by suturing the periosteum overlying the bone incisions. The canthal ligament must be carefully replaced at the lateral tubercle.

6. The skin is closed and the lids may remain sutured if much edema is anticipated. A pressure dressing for 48 hours is advisable.

EXENTERATION OF THE ORBIT

Exenteration may be performed with or without a split-thickness skin graft. The decision often depends on the need for postoperative radiation, since the amount of radiation may produce graft sloughing.

STEPS

1. The lids are firmly sutured. An incision is made just inside the orbital margin below the brow, without any attempt to preserve the lids. The incision goes to the periosteum entirely about the orbital margin.

2. The periosteum is incised and freed with a periosteal elevator. The periosteum is stripped, beginning at the upper temporal margin. The trochlea is detached and the canthal ligaments are severed.

3. Special care is required along the nasal wall, since the ethmoid bones are fragile. The periosteum can be freed as far as the apical stump, where heavy curved scissors are required to cut the nerve and other apical attachments as close to the bone as possible.

4. The orbital contents are removed, bleeding vessels are secured, and a split-thickness graft is cut from the thigh or abdomen, if this step is planned.

5. The graft is placed into the prepared dry socket and generalized pressure is exerted by means of a sterile sponge. The edges of the graft are trimmed and sutured to the incised skin margin, if possible. The graft must remain undisturbed for 10 days. This is possible with a properly placed pressure bandage dressing.

6. Temporal muscle transpositions can be fashioned by way of a trephined bony opening in the lateral wall to compensate for the cavity which is created, but this may interfere with the prosthesis, and is not recommended in pediatric patients.

7. The ocularist is able to tailor a prosthesis fitted to glasses that closely matches the fellow eye.

Socket reconstruction in older children may be required in cases of a contracted socket caused by the chronic irritating effect of a poorly fitting, roughened prosthesis; following trauma; or as the end result of a chemical burn. In mild or moderate contractions, the results can be good, provided surgical repair is begun soon.

The affected fornix is incised horizontally the entire length and the dissection is carried down to the periosteum of the orbital margin, which is generally the inferior. Healthy conjunctiva is saved but scar tissue is excised entirely. A mold of sufficient size is fashioned to provide a snug fit. Following complete hemostasis, a split-thickness graft is spread over the mold and then placed firmly in the socket.

Cleaning and irrigation of the socket must be attended to daily and with tender care. The mold should remain in place for adequate healing to take place over a period of 6 to 8 weeks.

If sufficient pressure cannot be maintained on the mold, stems connected to spectacles or head dressings may be required. After two months the patient should be ready for a permanent prosthesis.

More recently, expanding type conformers have been made available that can be adjusted in size by injecting some fluid into the conformer through the socket tissue.

The assistance of a well-trained ocularist adds measurably to the final successful result. Markedly contracted sockets are rarely seen in children. Several excellent texts on the plastic reconstruction of the orbit are available.

ACKNOWLEDGMENT

The authors would like to dedicate this chapter to two outstanding Philadelphia pediatricians, bridging two generations, Dr. Howard C. Carpenter and his associate, Dr. Joseph R. Ritter. They stimulated the interest of one author (E.B.S.) in pediatric ophthalmic lesions through many years of association.

REFERENCES

Albert, D. M., Rubenstein, R. A., and Scheie, H. G.: Tumor metastasis to the eye: Part II. Clinical study in infants and children. Amer. J. Ophthal., 63:727, 1962.

Apple, D. J.: Metastatic orbital neuroblastoma originating in the cervical sympathetic ganglionic chain. Amer. J. Ophthal., 68:1093, 1969.

Blodi, F. C.: Developmental anomalies of the skull affecting the eye. Arch. Ophthal., 57:593–609, 1957.

Duke-Elder, S.: Textbook of Ophthalmology. Vol. 5. St. Louis, The C. V. Mosby Co., 1952, p. 5427.

Gregory, J. E., Golden, A., and Haymoker, W.: Mucormycosis of the central nervous system. Bull. Johns Hopkins Hosp., 73:405, 1943.

Harley, R. D.: Exophthalmos in the newborn. Amer. J. Ophthal., 26:1314, 1943.

Heine, L.: Die Krankheiten des Auges, in Zusammenhang mit der inneren Medizin und der Kinderheilkunde. Berlin, Verlag Springer, 1921.

Henderson, J.: Orbital Tumors. Philadelphia, W. B. Saunders Co., 1973, p. 139.

Hiles, D. A., and Pilchard, W. A.: Corticosteroid control of neonatal hemangiomas of the orbit and ocular adnexa. Amer. J. Ophthal., 71:1003, 1971.

Hogan, M. J., and Zimmerman, L. E.: Ophthalmic Pathology. 2nd ed. Philadelphia, W. B. Saunders Co., 1968.

Iliff, C. E., and Ossofsky, H. J.: Tumors of the Eye and Adnexa in Infancy and Childhood. Springfield, Illinois, Charles C Thomas, 1962.

Jones, I. S.: Lymphoangiomas of the ocular adnexa; and analysis of 62 cases. Trans. Amer. Ophthal. Soc., 57:602, 1959.

Kennedy, R. E.: The effect of early enucleation on the orbit. Amer. J. Ophthal., 60:227, 1965.

Liebman, S. D., and Gellis, S. S.: The Pediatrician's Ophthalmology. St. Louis, The C. V. Mosby Co., 1966.

Nager, F. R., and DeReynier, J. P.: Pract. Oto-rhino-laryng., Supp. 2:1, 1948.

Nelson, W. E., Vaughan, V. C., and McKay, R. J.: Textbook of Pediatrics. 9th ed. Philadelphia, W. B. Saunders Co., 1969.

Paton, R. T., Smith, B., Katzin, H. M., and Stilwell, D. (Illustrator): Atlas of Eye Surgery. 2nd ed. New York, Blakiston Division, McGraw-Hill Book Co., 1962.

Reese, A. B.: The treatment of ocular and orbital tumors in children. Amer. J. Ophthal., 2:274, 1970.

Scheie, H. G., Hambrick, G. W., Jr., and Barness, L. A.: A newly recognized forme fruste of Hurler's disease (gargoylism). Amer. J. Ophthal., 53:753, 1962.

Spaeth, E. B.: The Bedell Lecture 1964. J. Pediat. Ophthal., 1:2, 1964.

Spaeth, E. B.: Principles and Practice of Ophthalmic Surgery. 4th ed. Philadelphia, Lea & Febiger, 1948.

Straatsma, B. R.: Ocular manifestations of Wegener's granulomatosis. Amer. J. Ophthal., 44:789, 1957.

Tasman, I. S.: Eye Manfestations of Internal Disease. 3rd ed. St. Louis, The C. V. Mosby Co., 1951.

The Ophthalmologic Staff of the Hospital for Sick Children in Toronto: The Eye in Childhood. Chicago, Year Book Medical Publishers, Inc., 1967.

Thomson, W. E.: The determination of the influence of the eyeball on the growth of the orbit by experimental enucleation of one eye in young animals. Trans. Ophthal. Soc. U.K., 21:258, 1901.

CHAPTER 9

DISEASES OF THE LACRIMAL APPARATUS

JOSEPH FLANAGAN, M.D.

GENERAL CONSIDERATIONS

Anatomy and Physiology

The lacrimal apparatus is composed of structures which produce tears (lacrimal gland, glands of Krause and Wolfring, meibomian glands, glands of Zeis and goblet cells) and structures responsible for the drainage of tears (upper and lower puncta, upper and lower canaliculi, common canaliculus, lacrimal sac, and nasolacrimal duct). The tear fluid is isotonic with blood plasma or slightly hypertonic, and its high protein content lowers the surface tension, which enhances the wetting of the corneal epithelial surface, thus improving the optics of the cornea. The only enzyme found in tears is lysozyme, which has antibacterial properties. The tears also protect the eye by washing away foreign matter. The pH of tears is approximately that of blood, i.e., 7.35. The accessory glands of Krause and Wolfring are the primary secretors under normal conditions, whereas the lacrimal gland provides the profuse tearing from corneal irritation or emotional states.

Approximately 1 cc. of tears is produced in 24 hours.

Embryology and Innervation

The lacrimal gland is derived embryologically from an ectodermal invagination from the conjunctiva and is composed of an orbital portion and a palpebral portion, separated by the fascia of the levator. The secretory innervational fibers are from the parasympathetic system. They originate in the pons above the superior salivary nucleus and reach the gland by way of the facial nerve, greater superficial petrosal nerve, sphenopalatine ganglion, and zygomatic branch of the maxillary division of the trigeminal nerve. The lacrimal nerve is a branch of the ophthalmic division of the trigeminal nerve. It has no secretory function but is an afferent pathway for the reflex arc. The lacrimal gland is also innervated by sympathetic fibers from the superior cervical ganglion which reach the gland by way of the carotid plexus and the lacrimal artery, while some fibers join the parasympathetic fibers and reach the gland via the lacrimal nerve.

Reflex lacrimation is easily produced by stimulation of the trigeminal, optic, or olfactory nerves. Approximately 12 ducts collect the tear fluid from the tubules of the gland and pass through the palpebral portion of the gland and empty the tears into the upper cul-de-sac temporally. The tears then travel nasally as a strip along the upper and lower lid to the lacrimal lake. An oily layer derived from meibomian glands and the accessory sebaceous glands of Zeis on the surface prevent wetting of the lid margin and spilling over of the tears onto the cheek.

The lacrimal drainage apparatus is derived embryologically from the nasooptic fissure. This becomes buried as a solid epithelial cord because of the growing together of the lateral nasal processes from above and the maxillary processes from below. The epithelial cord thickens and divides to form the nasal lacrimal duct, and the canaliculi develop as outbuddings from its upper end. Canalization of the passageways starts at the upper end and progresses downward. A thin membrane separating the nasolacrimal duct from the nasal mucosa usually persists up to the time of birth. Tears drain through this system by virtue of capillary attraction, gravity, and the lacrimal pump.

The concept of the lacrimal pump has been proposed by Dr. Lester Jones. It is composed of the superficial head of the pretarsal muscle, the deep head of the preseptal muscle, the lacrimal fascia, and the medial palpebral ligament. The lacrimal fascia converts the lacrimal fossa into a completely closed cavity, thereby forming a diaphragm which creates alternate positive and negative pressure brought about by contraction of the superficial and deep heads of the pretarsal muscle and deep head of the preseptal muscle. Winking creates a constant pumplike mechanism which draws the tears into the lacrimal sac and expresses them into the nose.

ANOMALIES OF LACRIMAL SECRETION

Anomalies of lacrimal secretion may range from decreased tearing to complete absence of tearing (alacrima) or the hypersecretion of tears. Decreased tearing may be diagnosed by the Schirmer test, utilizing a strip of #41 Whatman filter paper. Normally 10 to 15 mm. of the strip is moistened over a period of 5 minutes. If tearing is decreased, the cornea will also stain with rose bengal. If tear production is not excessive and epiphora is present there is an obstruction in the drainage system. The presence of total obstruction is diagnosed by irrigation and probing. Dye tests are of no value in the diagnosis of complete obstruction but are valuable in the differential diagnosis of partial obstruction. They indicate whether the epiphora is a result of canalicular or nasolacrimal duct obstruction or to hypersecretion. These tests have been described by Dr. Lester Jones as follows:

Diagnostic Methods

PRIMARY DYE TEST. One drop of 1 per cent fluorescein solution is instilled in the conjunctival sac. A small cotton-tipped metal applicator moistened with a mixture of 1:1000 epinephrine and 5 per cent cocaine solution is introduced into the inferior meatus in the nasal cavity at intervals of from 1 to 5 minutes. If the cotton comes out stained with the dye, it is a *positive* test. A positive primary dye test proves that there is no obstruction in the lacrimal passages and that the epiphora is due to hypersecretion. If after 3 to 5 minutes there is no dye on the cotton, it is a *negative* test.

SECONDARY DYE TEST. If the result of the primary dye test is negative, the dye is washed from the conjunctival sac and the patient's head is tipped forward far enough for fluid to run out from the anterior naris into a white basin. One mm. of normal saline solution is injected via a lacrimal cannula inserted in the canaliculus as far as the internal common punctum. If the fluid comes out of the nose stained with the dye, it is a *positive test*. A positive secondary dye test proves that there is no obstruction at the punctum nor in the canaliculus and that the lacrimal pump is functioning as far as the tear sac, which fills with the dye. The partial obstruction is in the nasolacrimal duct. If there is no dye in the fluid from the nose, it is a *negative* test. A negative secondary dye test demonstrates that no dye has reached the tear sac and proves that the primary cause of the epiphora lies in the canaliculi.

Alacrima

A congenital absence of the secretions of tears may be present because of the absence of the lacrimal gland in the anomaly of cryptophthalmos. A congenital absence of the secretion of tears in the presence of a lacrimal gland is rare. The condition is usually bilateral and tears are not shed from birth on, even in the presence of irritation of the cornea. The Schirmer test is negative, and on clinical examination the eye is seen to be irritated and photophobic with a positive reaction to rose bengal. Corneal scarring and vascularization usually result. Three etiologic factors have been suggested. They are (1) the persistence of the congenital condition of alacrima, (2) an absence or hypoplasia of the lacrimal gland, and (3) a neurogenic abnormality. The third is the most popular theory because of the common association of this disorder with other nervous anomalies, especially abnormalities of the cranial nerves.

Absence of lacrimation occurs also in two syndromes—*the anhidrotic type of ectodermal dysplasia* and *familial autonomic dysfunction.* This latter condition is also known as the *Riley-Day syndrome,* which is a syndrome inherited as an autosomal recessive trait and usually seen in children of Jewish extraction. The ocular findings are characteristic. There is decreased to complete absence of lacrimation, with a hyperemic conjunctiva and a stringy discharge. The cornea is hypoesthetic, which further complicates the picture. Corneal ulceration and scarring are prominent.

The treatment of alacrima primarily involves conservative measures such as the use of a demulcent, e.g., artificial tears; if this is not sufficient, occlusion of the lacrimal punctum with the Hyfrecator may be necessary. In cases of autonomic dysfunction, stimulation of the lacrimal gland may be brought about by the subcutaneous injection of Prostigmine (neostigmine) (0.25 mg.) or Mecholyl (3 mg.), or the local instillation of Eserine (physostigmine) ointment. The severe cases of the *Riley-Day syndrome* often require a partial tarsorrhaphy to protect the cornea. More radical treatment includes parotid duct transplant followed by a conjunctival-antrorhinostomy to drain the excessive amount of "tears" formed by the parotid gland.

Lacrimal Hypersecretion

A congenital tendency to excessive lacrimation is rare, but it has been reported occurring familially in association with hyperhidrosis, hypertrichosis, and diffuse cranial hyperostosis.

ABERRANT LACRIMAL GLAND

Aberrant lacrimal gland tissue may appear anywhere under the conjunctiva, particularly on the temporal side. Treatment is surgical excision if there is any cosmetic blemish; however, conservative nonsurgical treatment is usually indicated. The aberrant lacrimal gland tissue is identical histologically to normal lacrimal gland tissue. Lacrimal gland tissue rarely occurs intraocularly as a congenital anomaly.

CYSTS

Congenital cysts of the lacrimal gland are rare and must be differentiated from tumors. They occur in the orbital lobe of the lacrimal gland and may cause considerable proptosis. Surgical excision is the treatment of choice. A Krönlein approach may be necessary if it extends far back into the orbit.

DERMOID CYSTS

Dermoid cysts or dermolipomas of the lacrimal glands may occur and must be differentiated from malignancies. Treatment is surgical excision.

FISTULA

Congenital lacrimal fistulas are rare and, when present, they appear as a sinus tract above the tarsal plate in the lateral portion of the upper lid. Tears may drain from such a fistula and cause excoriation of the skin on the face. Lashes may be seen to grow out of such a fistula. Treatment consists of surgical excision of the fistula and closure of the defect in layers.

DACRYOADENITIS

Acute Dacryoadenitis

Acute dacryoadenitis is rare in children except when it occurs as a complication of mumps.

Chronic Dacryoadenitis

Chronic dacryoadenitis produces ptosis and a palpable lump. It may occur secondary to Boeck's sarcoid, Hodgkin's disease, tuberculosis, leukemia, or mononucleosis. The systemic nature of the disease must be investigated and a biopsy may be helpful.

ANOMALIES OF THE DRAINAGE SYSTEM

Ectasia

Ectasia of the lacrimal passageways is a rare anomaly which depends on the malunion of the nasal process, so that the facial fissure remains open with the site of the lacrimal passageway represented as a furrow on the cheek. The defect which may result can range from an inconspicuous fistula opening onto the cheek to a complete grotesque facial cleft. These anomalies can be explained on the basis of faulty embryological fusion, but the more grotesque anomalies with marked facial disfigurement probably result from the trauma of amniotic bands. The treatment of the fistula consists of excision of the fistula with closure in layers. The facial clefts require multiple surgical procedures for reconstruction.

ANOMALIES OF THE PUNCTA AND CANALICULI

As noted previously the upper and lower canaliculi arise embryologically as epithelial buds from the cord which forms the lacrimal sac and the nasolacrimal duct. The inferior canaliculus buds off from the lateral aspect of the epithelial cord and is involved more commonly with congenital abnormalities than the upper canaliculus. The overlying surface may fail to separate, which results in the absence of the punctum. As the result of faulty development or trauma of amniotic bands, various anomalies may result, including absence of the canaliculus or punctum, supernumerary puncta and canaliculi, and abnormalities of the shape or position of the puncta. When these conditions are hereditary the inheritance shows the characteristics of an autosomal dominant trait with variable penetrance and expression.

Congenital Obstruction of Lacrimal Drainage System

Nordlöw and Vennerholm analyzed 100 cases of congenital obstruction of the lacrimal passageways and found that the cause in 12 per cent lay in the punctum or canaliculus, 21 per cent in the duct and canaliculus, and 67 per cent in the nasolacrimal duct.

Nasolacrimal Duct Atresia

Atresia of the nasolacrimal duct is usually caused by failure of canalization. The most common site of blockage is at the lower ostium where failure of dehiscence results in atresia or the formation of a valvelike fold. Guerry and Kendig found some impatency in 6 per cent of unselected full-term infants. The membrane usually opens spontaneously before the onset of the secretion of obvious tears in the first few weeks of life. Occasionally, gross abnormalities of the nasolacrimal sac and duct are present, especially if there are associated anomalies of the nasal bones.

If obstruction of the lacrimal passageways is not relieved, dacryocystitis and development of a mucocele will invariably occur. In children, acute suppurative inflammation of the sac left unattended will commonly give rise to a fistula. The fistula drains below the medial canthal ligament on the lateral side of the nose, as shown in Figure 9–1. If there is failure of canalization at the upper end of the epithelial cord as well as the lower end of the cord, a congenital cystic sac will occur. A chronically tearing eye must be differentiated from the initial stages of congenital glaucoma, and tonometric deter-

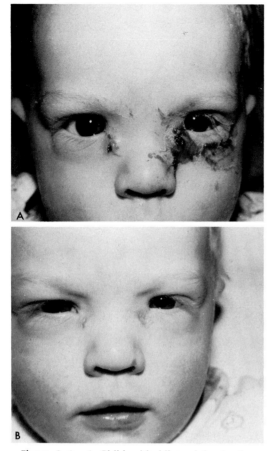

Figure 9–1 *A*, Child with bilateral lacrimal sac abscesses, with fistula formation inferior to the medial canthal ligament. *B*, Appearance 2 weeks after bilateral incision and drainage and treatment with local and systemic antibiotics. This child went on to have bilateral dacryocystorhinostomies performed one year apart.

minations are indicated. The presence of a discharge such as occurs in chronic dacryocystitis makes this possibility less likely.

TREATMENT. Treatment of the various anomalies is not necessary unless tearing is present or there is a possibility of a complication occurring such as dacryocystitis.

Atresia of the Lacrimal Punctum

When there is a pure failure of dehiscence of the overlying epithelium, the canaliculus remains separated from the lid margin by a fine membrane. This type of anomaly occurs more commonly in the lower lid. This membrane may be per-

forated by a fine needle, followed by dilatation with a punctum dilator. If this fails, a pigtail probe is inserted into the upper canaliculus and out through the lower punctum by way of the common punctum. At times it is necessary to cut down on the tip of the probe as it pouts at the site of the imperforate punctum. A 6–0 black silk or nylon suture is then passed in the reverse direction and tied on to the side of the nose. This suture is left in place for 4 weeks and is usually sufficient to maintain a patent punctum. Such a procedure may also be used if there is a limited area of atresia of the canaliculus; if the canaliculus is absent, a glass tube procedure, as described later in this chapter, is necessary.

Obstruction of the Nasolacrimal Duct

Obstruction of the nasolacrimal duct often opens spontaneously during the first few weeks of life. Massage over the lacrimal sac four times a day for at least 2 or 3 months is often successful. Chemotherapeutic agents or antibiotics are used locally if there is a secondary conjunctivitis. If the obstruction persists, as evidenced by continual tearing, probing of the nasolacrimal duct will be necessary. This procedure should be performed under general anesthesia to minimize the production of false passageways. The age at which this is done depends largely on the anesthesia department. For a child 6 months of age anesthetic risks are minimal and this is a good time to perform probing.

If probing is necessary, an attempt is first made to irrigate through the lower canaliculus with a fluorescein-stained saline solution, as shown in Figure 9–2*A*. The hydrostatic pressure may be sufficient to overcome a membranous valvelike obstruction. A soft rubber catheter is inserted into the nasal cavity to see if the irrigating solution reaches the inferior meatus. If this is unsuccessful, the next step is to occlude the upper punctum with a punctum dilator and again irrigate through the lower canaliculus, as shown in Figure 9–2*B*. This creates a closed system and again increases the hydrostatic pressure which may overcome the obstruction. If the fluorescein-stained solution still does not gain entrance to the inferior meatus when the upper punctum

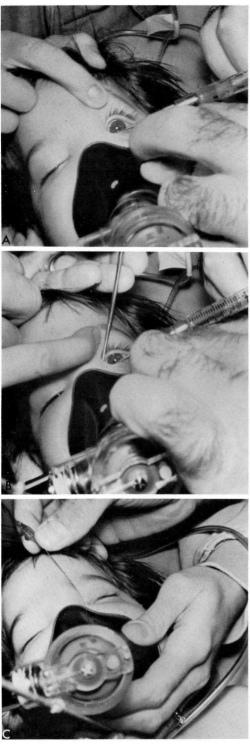

Figure 9-2 *A,* Irrigation through inferior canaliculus with fluorescein-stained saline solution. *B,* Same procedure as in *A,* performed while upper canaliculus is obstructed with a punctum dilator. *C,* Bowman probe passed delicately through nasolacrimal duct via the upper canaliculus.

is occluded, a single 0 Bowman probe is inserted into the upper punctum and passed vertically for approximately 2 mm. and is then rotated into the horizontal position and passed medially until it strikes the nasal bone. As contact is made with the nasal bone the end of the probe is rotated into a vertical position so that the lower end is directed toward the first molar tooth, as shown in Figure 9-2C. The probe is then delicately passed until it strikes the floor of the nose under the inferior turbinate. A second probe may be passed into the nose so that the surgeon can feel the metal-to-metal contact or, if preferred, a fluorescein-stained solution can be irrigated through the upper or lower canaliculus with the child on his side. If successful, the yellow-stained solution can be recognized in the nose or throat when aspirated by means of a soft rubber catheter. In the majority of cases, one probing is all that is necessary, but there are a few cases where the procedure will have to be repeated. If a secondary probing is necessary, impaction of the inferior turbinate must be ruled out by nasal examination.

DACRYOCYSTITIS

Acute Dacryocystitis

In the presence of acute dacryocystitis the initial treatment is medical, utilizing local and systemic antibiotics, especially penicillin. If this does not produce a prompt response, incision and drainage may be necessary. As soon as the acute infection is controlled, probing in an attempt to prevent cicatricial closure of the duct is performed.

Chronic Dacryocystitis

TUBERCULOUS INFECTIONS OF THE SAC. These occur secondary to affected adjacent structures such as bone, skin, nose, or conjunctiva. Fistula formation is characteristic.

GUMMATOUS FORMATIONS. These are rare but have been known to involve the sac, causing complete obstruction of lacrimal drainage. Dacryocystitis is common in *leprosy* secondary to nasal complications.

TRACHOMA OF THE SAC. These may occur secondary to the conjunctival disease. Coalescing follicles have been reported in the sac wall. Chronic inflammation leads inevitably to fibroblastic proliferation, shrinkage, and destruction of the sac.

MYCOTIC INFECTIONS OF THE SAC. These are common after nasolacrimal duct blockage. Actinomycosis, rhinosporidiosis, and other fungi may cause dacryocystitis. Streptothrix may proliferate in the sac and form large casts which can be expressed with pressure through the puncta. Recurrences are common. Diagnosis is confirmed by recognition of the hyphae of the fungus.

CANALICULITIS

Acute canaliculitis may follow traumatic probing, especially in the presence of bacterial infection.

Chronic canaliculitis and secondary stenosis are common in advanced trachoma.

Tearing may result from mycotic concretions obstructing the canaliculi. Diagnosis may often be suspected upon attempted probing, at which time concretions may be encountered and felt. The concretions may be expressed or may be removed with a fine curette, care being taken not to damage the endothelial lining. A lump may be palpated between two fingers.

If the canaliculus is opened, a complete cast may be observed. Simple mycotic filaments have been described as Leptothrix, while branching forms are labeled Streptothrix.

When probing is unsuccessful, the surgeon must perform a dacryocystorhinostomy. In children, the operation is performed under general anesthesia. The preferred procedure is the Kasper modification of the Moser-Toti operation. The procedure popularized by Dr. Kelvin Kasper, described in his technique manual, follows.

DACRYOCYSTORHINOSTOMY: DESCRIPTION OF OPERATION

Incision

The site of the incision is located by drawing a horizontal line through the orbit. This line will bisect the medial canthus. The fornix or dome of the sac lies slightly above or superior to this line. Our incision is a straight one, placed midway between the medial canthus and the bridge of the nose. This is medial to the angular vessels and should be 2 cm. or less in length. A beginner may make a longer incision, possibly 3 cm. in length. With continued practice one will learn to work through a smaller opening (Fig. 9–3).

Very firm pressure is made on the knife and the first cut carries down *through* the periosteum. If this is not done on the original incision, subsequent cuts might shred the periosteum and this we wish to keep intact.

The skin, subcutaneous tissue, angular vessels, and periosteum are all reflected in an unbroken layer. One does not see the medial palpebral ligament owing to the position of our incision. In this position the periosteal fibers have not thickened to form the medial palpebral ligament but are still fanned out as their fibers attach to the frontal process of the maxillary bone. However, as the periosteum is reflected lateralward and one gets closer to the medial canthus, the periosteal fibers thicken to form the medial palpebral ligament (tendo oculi) which gives origin to the orbicularis muscles.

Small rakes are held in the wound retracting the soft tissues—pressure from the rakes helps control any oozing. A fine suction tip at this stage is invaluable. It is placed deep in the incision, resting on the *upper* or *superior*

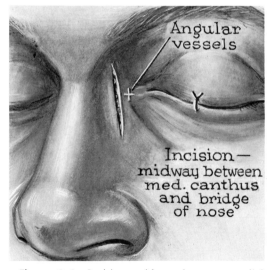

Figure 9–3 Incision midway between medial canthus and bridge of the nose—length about 2 cm., one third above medial canthus and two thirds below. This places angular vessels lateral to the incision. "X" marks site of angular vessels.

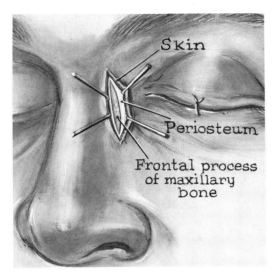

Figure 9–4 This drawing shows the early stages of reflected skin and periosteum. Exposed bone is frontal process of the maxillary bone. Later, when the bony window is formed, this bone will be ex-enterated almost up to the line of incision.

part of the *cut periosteum.* A Freer submucous knife is then used as a periosteal elevator and reflection started by working from the line of incision lateralward toward the medial canthus. The tissue medialward (toward bridge of nose) is *not* disturbed (Figs 9–4 and 9–5). The upper part of the periosteum is less adherent and it is expedient to work from above downward toward the anterior lacrimal crest. As the periosteal fibers directly over the anterior

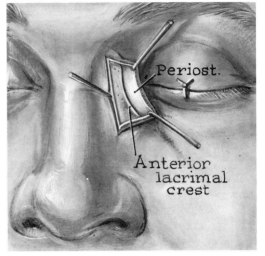

Figure 9–6 Anterior lacrimal crest has been reached in this drawing and immediately over the edge of the lacrimal sac will become visible.

lacrimal crest are approached one will find them very resistant, but when the crest is reached, and its edge passed over, practically all resistance disappears. At this stage the edge of the sac becomes visible and entrance into the anterior portion of the lacrimal fossa has been made (Figs. 9–6 and 9–7).

From now on the reflection of the periosteum becomes very easy, assuming of course that instructions were followed about starting above and working down. The sac at this stage can be reflected very readily out of the fossa with no effort at all. The attachment of the periosteum to the floor of the lacrimal fossa is so

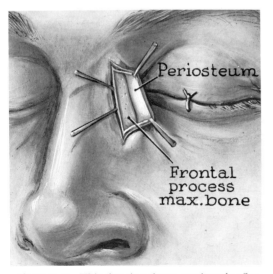

Figure 9–5 This drawing shows continued reflection of the periosteum off the frontal process of the maxillary and a closer approach to the anterior crest. The lacrimal sac is immediately visible when you pass over the *edge* of the anterior crest.

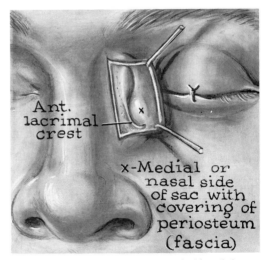

Figure 9–7 The medial or nasal side of the sac with its covering of periosteum (fascia). The superior and inferior portion of the fossa can also be observed.

loose, and the floor so thin, that one can easily poke a hole through the floor.

At this stage the operator should be able to identify a portion of the nasal process of the maxillary bone, the anterior lacrimal crest, the lacrimal fossa, the posterior lacrimal crest from its superior border to its inferior border, and the lacrimal sac dipping down into the bony nasolacrimal canal. The reflected periosteum should be intact from the line of incision posteriorward to the posterior lacrimal crest. There is no need to carry the reflection farther than the posterior lacrimal crest (Figs. 9–8 and 9–9).

If one should become a bit hazy about his anatomy after starting a dacryocystorhinostomy, try to remember the horizontal line bisecting the orbit and passing through the medial canthus. The sac fornix is always above this line but most of the body of the sac is below or inferior. Also, if you palpate the inferior orbital rim and move your finger medialward you will be resting on the anterior lacrimal crest. It is well to keep the above aids in mind.

After reflection of the periosteum has been completed back to the posterior lacrimal crest, all the structures clearly outlined, we are ready to make our window.

An initial opening (Fig. 9–10) (large enough to allow entrance of a small biting punch) is made *deeply* in the inferior portion of the lacrimal fossa just in front of the posterior lacrimal crest. No effort is made to preserve nasal mucous membrane. There is no later attempt to suture sac to nasal mucosa. This opening in the floor of the fossa is continued upward, running parallel to the edge of the

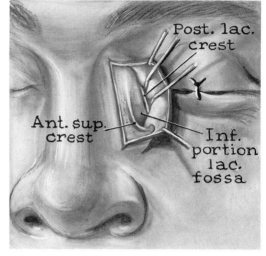

Figure 9–9 Entire floor of the lacrimal fossa has been exposed and the periosteum reflected to the posterior lacrimal crest.

posterior lacrimal crest and extending to the superior limit of the lacrimal fossa. The posterior boundary of the window is thus formed. Next, the remaining portion of the lacrimal fossa is exenterated (Fig. 9–11), followed by the very hard bone of the anterior lacrimal crest (Fig. 9–12). About 5 mm. of the anterior lacrimal crest is removed. The finished window likely measures about 1.5 cm. from superior to inferior border and about 1 cm. from the

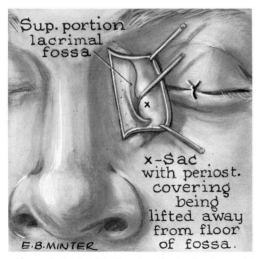

Figure 9–8 In this drawing the lacrimal sac with its periosteal covering has been retracted laterally and lifted away from the fossa floor.

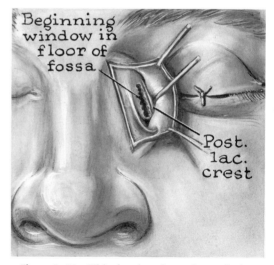

Figure 9–10 This drawing shows the preliminary opening in the lacrimal fossa. It is made in the inferior portion just anterior to or in front of the posterior lacrimal crest and then extended upward to the superior boundary of the fossa.

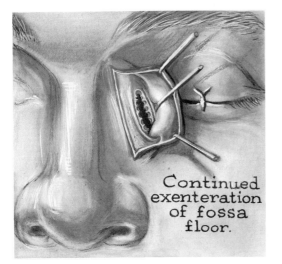

Figure 9–11 Continued exenteration of the fossa floor is illustrated. The anterior lacrimal crest is still intact.

posterior lacrimal crest to the anterior boundary.

We use biting instruments to exenterate the bone. Stryker saws supplemented with biting instruments can be employed or bone drills may be used.

After completion of the window, an 0 or 00 Bowman probe is passed through the lower canaliculus into the sac cavity—tenting out the medial (nasal) side of the lacrimal sac (Fig. 9–13). This gives us an idea of the size and boundaries of the sac.

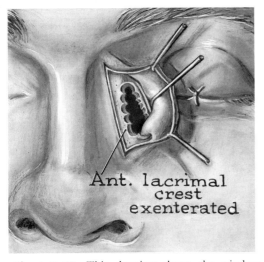

Figure 9–12 This drawing shows the window shaping up. The anterior lacrimal crest has been exenterated and all the bone (with nasal mucosa) between anterior and posterior lacrimal crests has been removed.

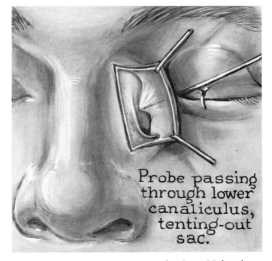

Figure 9–13 A Bowman probe 0 or 00 has been passed through the lower canaliculus into the sac cavity and is shown tenting-out the medial or nasal side of the sac. The inferior portion of the sac is seen just before it dips down into the bony nasolacrimal canal.

Formation of Flap

In Fig. 9–14, the broken line seen on the medial side of the sac indicates where the sac will be entered and incised. This broken line is placed along the anterior margin of the sac and meets a line above and below, at the superior margin and at the inferior margin of the sac. These last two lines extend posteriorward to the posterior lacrimal crest.

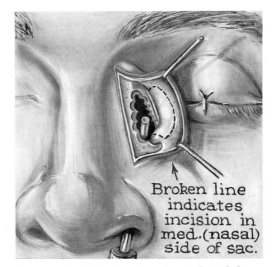

Figure 9–14 Broken line shows site of future incision in the medial (nasal) wall of the sac. Suction tip has been passed intranasally and merely indicates the clean open window.

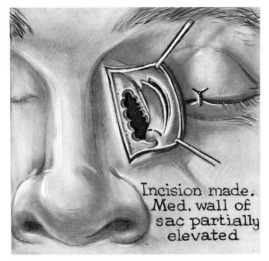

Figure 9–15 Incision has been made in the medial (nasal) side of the sac and our flap starts to take shape. As the incision is continued the medial side of the sac will fall away, exposing the interior of the sac, the lateral wall, and its common opening of the lacrimal duct.

In Fig. 9–15, the medial or nasal side of the sac has been incised and the wall partly turned back. When all the lines are connected (Fig. 9–16), we will have a free flap—hinged on a line running parallel to the posterior lacrimal crest (Fig. 9–17). The flap falls over the posterior boundary of our bony window—in this case the posterior lacrimal crest. If the flap is too wide it can be trimmed. No packing

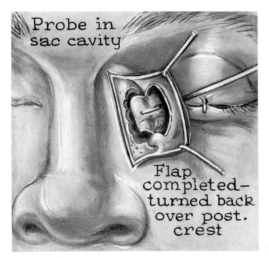

Figure 9–16 Probe has been passed through the lower canaliculus and presents itself in the sac cavity. The flap has been completed and is shown posterior to the probe. If the flap had been left standing the protruding probe would push it over into the position as we now see it.

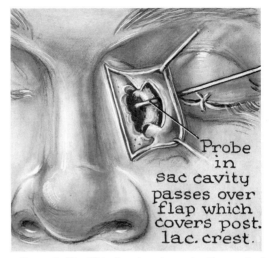

Figure 9–17 This drawing shows the flap pushed down and covering the entire posterior lacrimal crest.

is necessary to keep it in place. Our window will heal and almost one half the window perimeter will be covered by mucous membrane from the flap.

This flap was adapted from Dr. Lester Jones' intranasal operation and I call it the "Jones Flap." Considerable time and effort is saved performing the external dacryocystorhinostomy operation when the step of suturing nasal mucosa to sac wall is eliminated.

Wound Closure

In closing our wound we use Number 000 plain catgut and join periosteum to periosteum. If one studies the first few figures he will see that the periosteum lateral to the incision is reflected but that the periosteum medial to the incision is left attached to the bone, so that in reality we are suturing periosteum to soft tissue. The lateral and medial borders of periosteum are, however, approximated. Number 6 silk on an atraumatic needle is used for skin closure. Usually we pass a probe through the canaliculus and check its position intranasally in the newly formed indow. A simple dressing is placed over the eye. Routinely we have the patient lie with head turned on one side or the other so that any bleeding comes out the front of the nose and not down the back of the throat.

Postoperative Care

First three days postoperative the patient is not touched except to tidy up a dirty exterior.

No irrigations—no probing. An antibiotic eye-drop is used and an antibiotic may or may not be used systemically. Sutures are removed in 72 hours and at this time the interior of the nose is checked. One usually finds an accumulation of debris in the window area. This is gently cleaned out. If the healing area appears to be dry we may use light mineral oil drops for several days. During this first week postoperatively there is nothing particularly gained by irrigation and the healing tissues might be disturbed. One must admit, however, that there is a pleasant feeling of satisfaction in watching saline squirting through the new window.

Occasionally we find the septum and nasal lateral wall extremely close. In this case be careful not to allow adhesions to form and cause closure of the window.

CONJUNCTIVODACRYO-CYSTORHINOSTOMY

When a canalicular obstruction is present, one must use the Lester T. Jones glass tube technique. A dacryocystorhinostomy is performed as previously described and after this the caruncle is excised. A Graefe knife is used to create a tract for the tube. Initially a #200 polyethylene tube is sutured into the area where the caruncle was excised with three 6-0 black silk sutures. Before the tube is inserted, a flange is created on the proximal end of the tube by flaming it with a match. This tube is replaced by a glass tube in two weeks. Much attention must be given to the tube and therefore the parents must be instructed in the cleaning and care of the tube. It is best to leave the tube in for as long a time as possible, even permanently, if there is no irritation. The tube may be removed for short intervals daily after several months with periodic dilatation to ensure patency of the sinus tract.

DACRYOCYSTECTOMY

Dacryocystectomy is rarely if ever performed in children if there is any chance for promoting drainage into the nose. It is rarely necessary to be subjected to the lifetime annoyance of a chronically tearing eye.

TRAUMA

Trauma to the medial aspect of the lids often results in damage to the canaliculus. It is important to repair lacerations of the canaliculus as a primary procedure, especially when it involves the lower canaliculus. The cut ends of the canaliculus must be approximated and splinted with a suture to ensure re-epithelialization of the canaliculus. The various stages and the pigtail probe are shown in Figure 9–18. The probe is inserted into the upper punctum and passed into the sac. It is then gently passed into the proximal end of severed canaliculus, then through the distal end, and out through the punctum of the lower lid. A 6-0 black silk or nylon suture is then attached to the end of the probe and is withdrawn in the opposite direction. The ends of the suture are then tied and taped to the side of the nose. The lid is then repaired as shown in Chapter 10. The suture through the canaliculi is moved slightly when the patient is seen in the office and it is removed after 4 weeks. If lacerated canaliculi are not repaired primarily, the resultant lacrimal obstruction is often very difficult to correct and may require a *dacryocystorhinostomy* with a glass tube implant.

TUMORS OF THE LACRIMAL SYSTEM

Tumors of the canaliculus and lacrimal sac are rare and are usually nonmalignant. They result from *granulomatous inflammations* and *polyps* in the majority of cases (Fig. 9–19). Tumors of the sac do not necessarily present inferior to the medial canthal ligament as acute infections, but abscesses do, and this is an important diagnostic point. Treatment consists of excision and biopsy of these masses. If the tumor is benign, nothing more need be done if tearing and infection do not ensue. If obstruction results, it is treated as listed above, according to the location of the obstruction.

Tumors of the lacrimal gland must be exceedingly rare in children. Mixed tumor is the commonest lacrimal gland tumor in

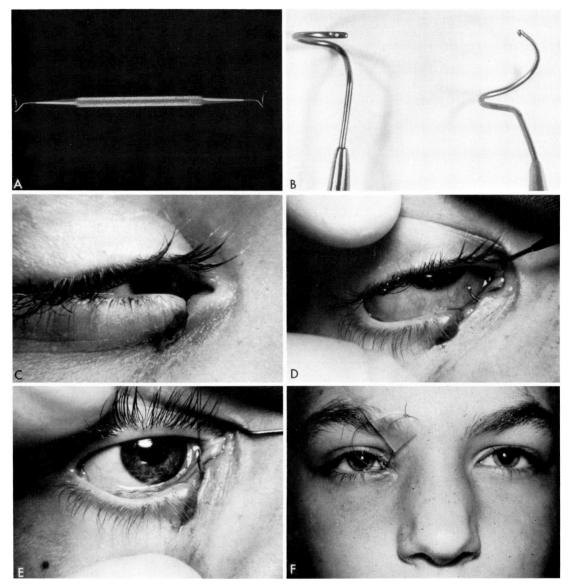

Figure 9–18   *A*, Pigtail probe. *B*, The probe with the perforation for the suture is less traumatic than the one with the barb on the end. *C*, Laceration of the right lower lid involving the canaliculus. *D*, Probe through proximal portion of the canaliculus. *E*, 6-0 black silk suture being withdrawn in the reverse direction. *F*, Silk suture taped to side of nose; it remains in place for 4 weeks.

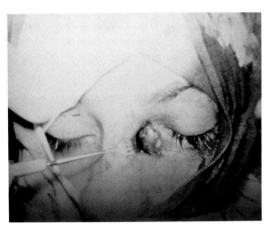

Figure 9–19 Granuloma of the sac in a 10-year-old boy.

adults but we have no record of this tumor in children at the Wills Eye Hospital.

ACKNOWLEDGMENT

I would like to thank the late Dr. Kelvin A. Kasper for his excellent guidance in teaching me how to treat problems of the lacrimal system and for his assistance in the preparation of the manuscript.

REFERENCES

Crawford, J. S.: The Eye in Childhood. Chicago, Year Book Medical Publishers, Inc., 1967, p. 139.

Duke-Elder, S.: System of Ophthalmology. Vol. 3: Normal and Abnormal Development. Part II: Congenital Deformities. St. Louis, The C. V. Mosby Co., 1963.

Guerry, D., and Kendig, E. L.: Congenital impatency of the nasolacrimal duct. Arch. Ophthal., 39:193, 1948.

Jadassohn, W., Grasset, N., and Brun, R.: Hyperhidrose, hypersécrétion lacrymale, hypertrichose, hyperostose de la calotte crânienne. Bibl. Ophtal., 47:591, 1957.

Jones, L. T.: Practical fundamentals of anatomy and physiology. Trans. Amer. Acad. Ophthal., 62:669, 1958.

Jones, L. T.: Lacrimal drainage reconstruction. In Smith, B., and Converse, J. M. (co-chairmen): Proceedings of the Second International Symposium on Plastic and Reconstructive Surgery of the Eye and Adnexa. St. Louis, The C. V. Mosby Co., 1967.

Kasper, K. A.: Dacryocystorhinostomy. Survey Ophthal., 6:95, 1961.

Kasper, K. A.: Illustrated Monograph of Dacryocystorhinostomy. Residents' Instruction Program, Wills Eye Hospital.

McDonald, P. R.: Personal communication.

Mishima, S., and Maurice, D.: The effect of normal evaporation on the eye. Exper. Eye Res., 1:46–52, 1961.

Nordlöw, W., and Vennerholm, I.: Congenital atresiae of the lacrimal passages: Their occurrence and treatment. Acta Ophthal. (Kobenhagen), 31:367, 1953.

Riley, C. M., Day, R. L., Greeley, D. McL., and Langford, W. S.: Central autonomic dysfunction with defective lacrimation. I. Report of five cases. Pediatrics, 3:468, 1949.

Silverman, S.: Microphthalmos with congenital defect of the lacrimal apparatus. Brit. J. Ophthal., 17:351, 1933.

CHAPTER 10

DISORDERS OF THE LIDS

GERARD M. SHANNON, M.D.,
and JOSEPH FLANAGAN, M.D.

The congenital anomalies of the eyelids were first classified systematically by August von Ammon in the 19th century, and were divided into three types by Sir Stewart Duke-Elder, approximately based on chronological development. First, there are anomalies dependent on abnormal formation of the lid folds, which are seen early in development and include cryptophthalmos, microphthalmos, and coloboma. Second, there can be anomalies in the differentiation of the lid margins, which occur between the fifth and sixth months of development. Differentiation begins in the nasal portion of the lid area and is usually complete at the time of lid separation in the sixth month; anomalies include ankyloblepharon, congenital ectropion, and congenital entropion. Finally, anomalies occur in the differentiation of the tissue of the lids, and produce a variety of conditions which may include the tarsus, the skin of the lids and its pigmentation, congenital tumors, and the motility of the lids through involvement of the palpebral musculature.

CRYPTOPHTHALMOS

Cryptophthalmos is a rare condition in which there is complete failure of the development of the lid folds (Fig. 10–1), so that epithelium which is normally differentiated into cornea and conjunctiva becomes part of the skin which passes continuously from the forehead to the cheek. It might also be noted that the left eye of this child (Fig. 10–1) presents a microblepharon as well as a microphthalmos. At surgery, this child had a very small conjunctival sac, with a disorganized globe; there is little that can be done surgically for this type of eye. The microblepharon present in the left eye creates an additional problem in that there is exposure and keratinization of the cornea due to lagophthalmos. In many cases, entropion also occurs.

CONGENITAL COLOBOMA

A coloboma of the lid is a defect affecting primarily the lid margin. One or all

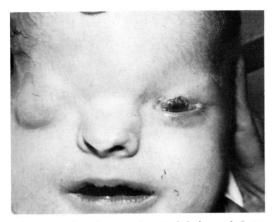

Figure 10–1 *Right eye:* Cryptophthalmos. *Left eye:* Microblepharon with congenital entropion of the upper lid, lagophthalmos, microphthalmos, and corneal keratinization.

four lids may be involved, and the defect may vary from small indentation of the lid border to nearly complete absence of the lids; these latter defects are uncommon. Colobomas are more common in the upper lid, where they usually occur nasally. When they occur in the lower lid, they are usually found laterally and may be associated with craniofacial dysostosis (Fig. 10–2). The entire thickness of the lid is frequently absent and the edges of the defect are rounded and covered with conjunctiva which unites the lid to the bulbar conjunctiva. Unusual cases may

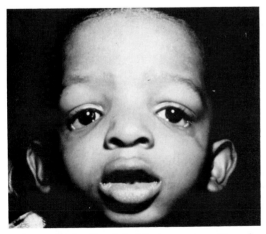

Figure 10–2 Craniofacial dysostosis with colobomas of the lower lids (Treacher-Collins syndrome).

show absence of the tarsus only. If the defect is large, corneal exposure and ulceration may occur. Colobomas of the lid are thought to be the result of trauma from amniotic bands, or of a localized failure of adhesion of the lid folds. Amniotic band constriction usually causes the gross defects associated with other anomalies such as facial fissures. The small lid defects unassociated with other anomalies probably arise from a failure of the adhesion of the lid folds, or a premature breaking of the adhesion, resulting in a lag of growth.

Treatment

Colobomas of the lids do not have to be treated immediately unless there is corneal exposure. The majority of cases can be handled at the age of 2 or 3 when the child is a better anesthetic risk, and there is also an increase in the laxity of the lid tissues. Most colobomas can be closed by an end-to-end anastomosis. The edges are freshened by excision of a very small amount of lid border tissue, and then approximated with three interrupted sutures of 6-0 black silk, one at the posterior border, one at the anterior lid border (lash line), and one in the area of the grey line. These sutures are tied and left long. While the assistant uses these sutures for traction, the remainder of the defect is closed in two layers. The pretarsal fascia is closed with interrupted 4-0 chromic catgut and the skin is closed with interrupted 6-0 black silk. The three sutures on the lid border are then incorporated into one of the skin sutures to prevent their rubbing on the cornea. Figure 10–3*A* to *C* shows a patient treated in this manner.

If additional tissue is necessary, relaxation may be obtained by performing a lateral cantholysis. A lateral canthotomy is followed by a tenotomy of the superior or inferior cruz of the lateral canthal tendon. The lateral portion of the lid may then be mobilized nasally and the margins approximated as previously described. If it is felt that this will not be sufficient, the defect may be closed by the methods proposed by Hughes, Beard and Cutler, or Mustardé, utilizing various flaps and skin grafts.

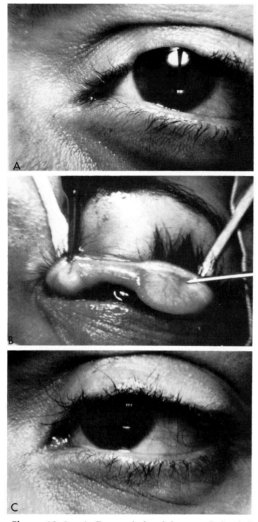

Figure 10–3 *A*, Congenital coloboma of the left upper lid. *B*, Lid everted to show absence of the tarsus in the area of the coloboma. *C*, Postoperative appearance.

ANKYLOBLEPHARON

Ankyloblepharon exists when the lid margins are fused together over some portion of their length, producing shortening of the palpebral fissure. The condition is divided into (a) external ankyloblepharon, in which the outer canthus is fused; and (b) internal ankyloblepharon, in which the inner canthus is fused. External ankyloblepharon is the more common type. Ankyloblepharon is an unusual condition which may be genetically determined, but the exact cause or mechanism is not clearly understood.

Treatment

The treatment of ankyloblepharon is entirely surgical; the plastic procedures are all based on the separation of the lids so that the interpalpebral fissure length is increased.

CONGENITAL ECTROPION

Congenital ectropion rarely occurs as a separate, primary entity. Eversion of the lid margins occurs most commonly in conjunction with congenital ptosis, epicanthus inversus, and blepharophimosis. It has also been reported to occur with microphthalmos, buphthalmos, and orbital cysts. The ectropion is usually more severe in the lateral portion of the lid than when it is found nasally.

Treatment

If the ectropion is minimal, surgery may not be required. If it involves only the lateral one-third of the lid, a temporal tarsorrhaphy may be sufficient to correct the cosmetic blemish. When the ectropion is extensive, and especially when there is a deficiency of skin in the lateral portion of the lid, a full thickness skin graft from the retroauricular area must be utilized to correct the defect. After the bed is prepared, a full-thickness skin graft is sutured into the bed with multiple interrupted 6–0 black silk sutures. The lower lid is then suspended from the brow by two 4-0 black silk sutures to keep the bed of the graft flat. The sutures which suspend the lid are removed after 48 hours; the skin sutures are removed after 10 days. The child should wear a transparent eye shield for two weeks to prevent trauma to the grafted area.

CONGENITAL ENTROPION

Congenital entropion, or the turning inward of the entire lid margin, rarely occurs as an isolated phenomenon. When it does present itself as a primary defect, it usually involves the lower lid, although involvement of the upper lid has been reported. Entropion in infants and children is more often a condition secondary to epicanthus or epiblepharon of the lower lid. It is frequently associated with microphthalmos and enophthalmos, i.e., conditions in which there is a lack of support to the posterior border of the lid.

Primary entropion results from a general absence of the tarsal plate or from a hypertrophy of the marginal portion of the orbicularis muscle. The congenital absence of the tarsal plate is the most common cause of congenital entropion of the upper lid. When hypertrophy of the marginal portion of the orbicularis is responsible, the resultant entropion is of the spastic type, similar to that seen in senile spastic entropion. Whether it is the result of absence of the tarsal plate or hypertrophy of the orbicularis muscle, entropion in children is often familial, with more than one instance occurring in the same sibship.

Treatment

When the entropion is secondary to an epicanthus, it will usually respond when the epicanthus is treated surgically. Those cases secondary to epiblepharon tend to disappear early in life before the lashes become stiff and consequently do not cause corneal problems. With the differential growth of the facial bones, the epiblepharon is usually corrected spontaneously and the secondary entropion resolves. When secondary corneal changes occur, surgical treatment of the entropion is a necessary and simple surgical procedure involving the skin and muscle of the lid. An incision is made along the lower lid approximately 3 mm. from the lid border. A horizontal strip of orbicularis muscle is excised, particularly the marginal bundles. The orbital septum may be shortened by the technique described by Jones et al. This tightening of the orbital septum prevents the tarsus from tipping in toward the globe and also prevents the preseptal portion of the orbicularis from sliding over the pretarsal portion, thereby preventing the inward rotation of the lid margin.

EPIBLEPHARON

Epiblepharon is a condition characterized by the presence of a horizontal fold of skin across either the upper or lower lid,

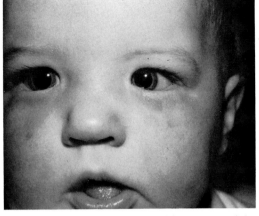

Figure 10–4 Epiblepharon with no corneal involvement; therefore no surgery is indicated.

which forces the lashes against the cornea. It often has a familial basis. The condition tends to correct itself by the differential growth of the facial bones; rarely does a keratitis occur, but when it does it is an indication for surgical intervention. That surgery is often not necessary, as shown by Figure 10–4.

EURYBLEPHARON

In this condition there is a generalized enlargement of the palpebral aperture which is greatest in the lateral aspect, with a localized outward displacement of the lateral canthus. The lateral canthus is displaced inferiorly, with a downward displacement of the lateral half of the lower lid. On superficial examination, children with this condition may be diagnosed as having congenital ectropion. This condition may be hereditary, having the characteristics of an autosomal dominant trait, and may be seen in several members of the same family in its milder forms. Figures 10–5A and B show a typical displacement downward and laterally of the lateral canthus, which increases the size of the palpebral aperture; this particular case is associated with a craniofacial dysostosis. A secondary enlargement of the palpebral aperture can occur due to other conditions such as buphthalmos, staphyloma, and proptosis. This, however, would be obvious because of the changes in the globe.

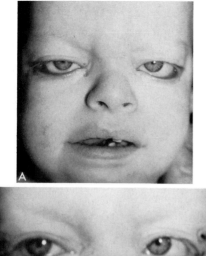

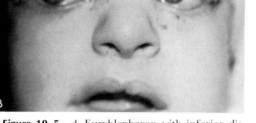

Figure 10–5 *A*, Euryblepharon with inferior displacement of the lateral canthus. *B*, Immediate postoperative appearance after a lateral canthoplasty.

Two other examples of this condition are shown in Figures 10–6*A* and *B* and 10–7*A* and *B*. These cases were treated differently because of the difference in degree of involvement. The young boy in Figure 10–6 has a generalized enlargement of the palpebral fissure; however, the dis-

placement of the lateral canthus is not prominent. When treated he was 16 years old; under local anesthesia a temporal tarsorrhaphy was performed on each eye, with the sutures remaining in place for 10 days. The bilateral temporal tarsorrhaphy was sufficient to decrease the dimension of the palpebral aperture and give the lids a normal appearance. The other case was a 3-year-old child (Figures 10–7*A* and *B*) with enlargement of the palpebral aperture and a downward displacement of the lower lid and lateral canthus. The defect was repaired in three stages: the first stage consisted of a free tarsal graft from the upper right lid to the lower right lid, creating an ectropion; second, a free skin graft from behind the right ear to the right lower lid was made to correct the ectropion, and at the same time a free tarsal graft from the left upper lid to the left lower lid was made. The final procedure was a free skin graft from behind the left ear to correct the surgically produced ectropion of the left lower lid. Figure 10–7*B* shows the postoperative appearance of the patient at 6 weeks. No further surgery was necessary in either of these children.

EPICANTHUS

Epicanthus consists of a semilunar fold of skin running downward at the side of the nose, with its concavity directed to the inner canthus (Figure 10–8). This condi-

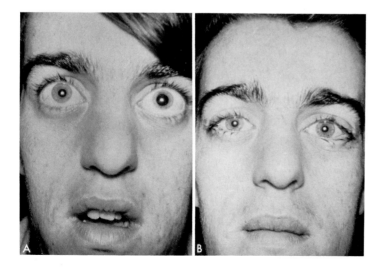

Figure 10–6 *A*, Preoperative appearance of euryblepharon in 16-year-old boy. *B*, Postoperative appearance after bilateral lateral tarsorrhaphy.

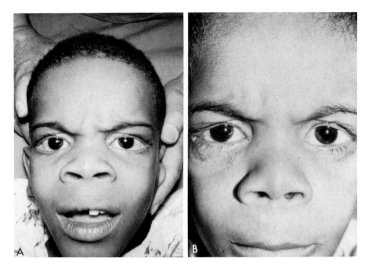

Figure 10–7 *A,* Congenital euryblepharon with downward displacement of the lateral canthus. *B,* Final appearance after three surgical procedures.

tion can occur as an isolated problem or combined with other defects and may appear as arising above or below the canthus. The type that arises inferiorly is usually associated with blepharophimosis and ptosis. In many instances a simple epicanthus may resolve spontaneously, therefore surgery is best deferred until after age 5. Investigation of other family members before surgery is decided upon is also helpful. However, when surgery is indicated, the Y-V is probably the simplest of all procedures (see Figures 10–9*A* to *D*). Procedures described by Spaeth and Mustardé, using rotating flaps, will give satisfactory results when properly performed, even in the most complicated blepharophimosis cases. It is necessary in

many cases to increase the horizontal length of the lids by doing a lateral canthotomy. In addition to performing the skin flaps or the double Z-plasties, it is important that the medial canthus be shifted nasally and reattached by means of transnasal wirings in order to get a satisfactory cosmetic canthal effect (see Figure 10–10*A* and *B*).

TELECANTHUS

Telecanthus indicates a wide intercanthal distance, with the interpupillary distance remaining normal. Although this is often associated with epicanthus and blepharophimosis, it can occur as a single, primary finding, or as a result of trauma. This condition should be repaired using the Mustardé or the Y-V type of procedure described previously. It is usually necessary to wire the medial canthus after correcting any bony deformity that might be present, using the same technique as that described for epicanthus.

Figures 10–11*A* and *B* show a patient in which only one side needed correction because the defect was caused by trauma. The canaliculus was intubated, the sac identified, a dacryocystorhinostomy performed, and the medial canthus was wired transnasally to a plastic plate on the opposite, normal side. The flaps were reconstructed in the Y-V manner. The transnasal wiring described by Troutman, Converse, and Smith, although effective,

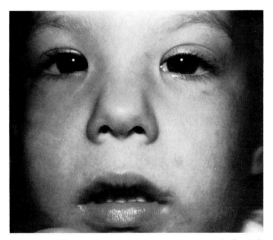

Figure 10–8 An example of congenital epicanthus.

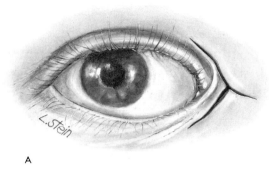

A

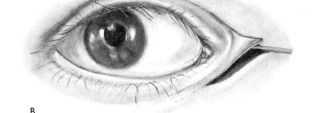

B

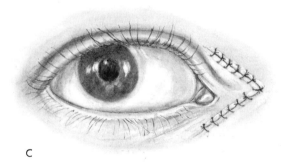

C

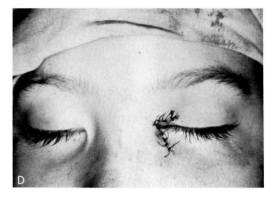

D

Figure 10–9 *A,* Incision for preparing skin flap. *B,* Undermining of skin to allow for movement of tip. *C,* Skin sutures in V-shape flattening epicanthal fold. The skin at the junction of the Y flap is rotated medially to apex of V, thus flattening the epicanthus. *D,* Unoperated right epicanthal fold; immediate postoperative appearance after Y-V procedure in *A, B,* and *C.*

does carry with it the possibility of exposed wires in the nasal cavity. For this reason, patients should have a careful postoperative follow-up.

BLEPHAROPTOSIS

Ptosis may be congenital or acquired, and since these are two entirely different conditions, the treatment is quite different in each case. The frequency of congenital ptosis as compared to the acquired condition varies between 9:1 (Berke and Fox) and 3:2. Although the term congenital ptosis would seem to indicate that the condition exists at birth, this is not always the case. In fact, the ptosis may not be observed until some time after birth. The basic cause of this condition is a dystrophy of the levator muscle—the muscle relaxes as well as contracts poorly. There is a definite relationship between the presence or absence of striated muscle and the amount of ptosis. Exceptions to this are the ptoses seen in blepharophimosis and in the jaw-winking syndrome.

Preoperative Evaluation

The evaluation should indicate the degree of ptosis, the amount of levator function, the condition of the lid fold, and

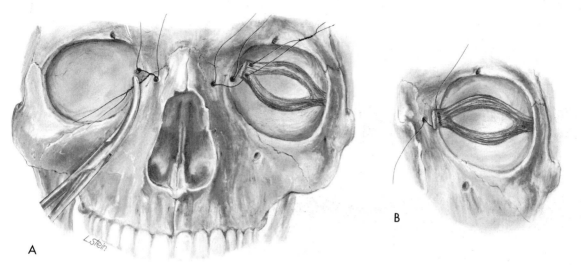

Figure 10–10 *A*, Transnasal wiring of the medial canthus on left, using double set of stainless steel wires. *B*, Position of canthus when drawn into place; free wires are used for skin traction.

the presence of associated anomalies. In apparently unilateral cases, the uninvolved eye should be carefully evaluated for a slight amount of ptosis. The degree of levator function is determined by measur-

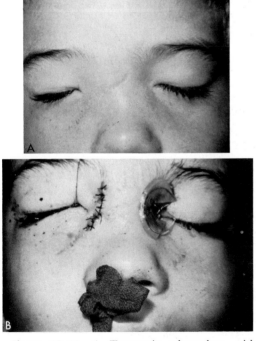

Figure 10–11 *A*, Traumatic telecanthus, with obstruction of the lacrimal sac on the right side. *B*, Immediate postoperative appearance, showing transnasal wire tied over plastic button. (See text for complete description.)

ing the excursions of the upper eyelid margin as the eyes travel from "eyes down" to "eyes up" position. It is important to fix the frontalis for this measurement. A movement of 2 mm. has been classified as absence of levator function. Eight mm. would be considered good, 5 to 7 fair, and 4 or less poor.

Surgery to Correct Congenital Ptosis

There are only two basic methods of correcting ptosis: one involves a shortening of the levator muscle to increase its efficiency; the other is a suspension of the lid to the brow, frontalis or superior rectus fascia. This last procedure is difficult and has possibilities for many complications. There are various techniques for the resection of the levator muscle, and they will be discussed in the order used, from correction of a slight amount of ptosis to correction of the more severe cases.

The Fasanella-Servat operation is a superior tarsectomy which includes the levator aponeurosis. This procedure will vary among operators, but basically the technique is the placement of two curved hemostats on the upper border of the tarsus, including the palpebral conjunctiva and Müller's muscle, to a depth of approximately 3 mm. Catgut sutures are placed above the hemostats while the tissue below is excised. The procedure next in complexity is that of levator resection through the conjunctiva. The original procedure by Blaskovics, and later modified by Iliff and Berke, has produced good results cosmetically.

Lastly, levator resection through the skin is used when there is a great amount of correction to be obtained. In this procedure, the resected levator can be advanced along the surface of the tarsus to give a more accurate method of approximating the opposite lid. This procedure produces a deep lid fold, therefore much care should be taken so that its location is not changed in reference to the other eye (Figs. 10–12A to G).

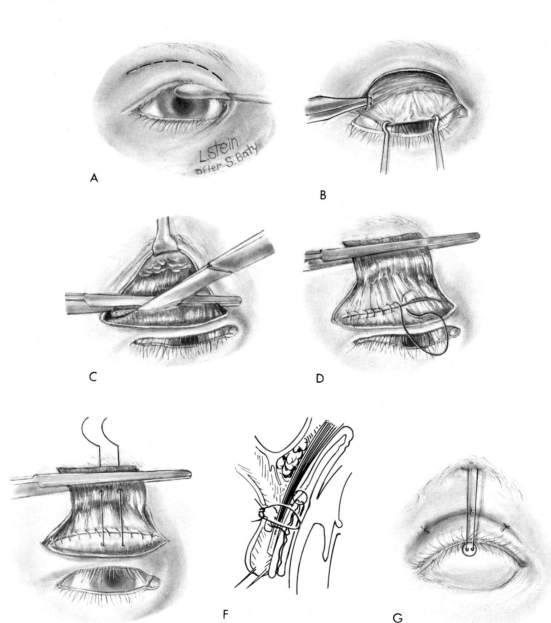

Figure 10–12 External levator resection (modified from Smith). *A*, Mark position of lid fold. *B*, Skin is pulled down, showing pretarsal orbicularis which has to be incised for exposure of the tarsal plate. *C*, Fibers of levator and Müller's muscle cut below clamp. *D*, Closure of conjunctiva and tarsus. *E*, Suture placed into tarsus securing levator. Position of sutures in levator determines around of correction. *F*, Cross section showing position of conjunctiva, tarsal plate, and levator muscle with sutures in place. *G*, Temporary suture for corneal protection under dressing.

In the operation for suspension many materials have been used, such as fascia lata, silk, and plastic suture materials and Silastic bands. All these materials will give good results if the sutures are placed in the proper position under proper tension.

The choice of operation will be determined by the amount of levator function present, the presence of the ptosis unilaterally or bilaterally, and other complicating factors such as extraocular muscle palsies. In Figure 10–13, the patient had a slight to moderate unilateral ptosis which was corrected by a levator resection using the external approach.

Complications of Ptosis Surgery

Under-Correction

The most obvious immediate complication is under-correction; however, in cases where the external route has been used, this problem has been at a minimum. Should the under-correction persist for several months, re-operation is indicated.

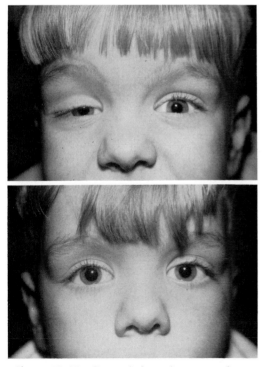

Figure 10–13 Congenital ptosis, pre- and postoperative appearance. Corrected by the external approach.

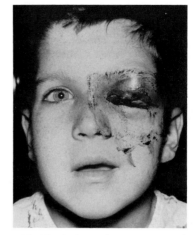

Figure 10–14 A large hematoma produced by injury following ptosis surgery.

This re-operation is then best handled by the external approach, although the resection can be repeated using the same technique originally performed. Should under-correction result where there is little levator function present, a suspension operation would be the procedure of choice, using fascia lata or alloplastic material. Injury in the immediate postoperative course can be a complication; an example is shown in Figure 10–14 in which a child who upon discharge from the hospital was struck by his sister's schoolbag. This produced a large hematoma which necessitated revising the wound, removing the hematoma, and re-attaching the levator stump.

Over-Correction

This can occur most often when the external route is used. Although overcorrection can occur in the procedures for congenital ptosis, it is most frequently seen in the correction of the secondary and traumatic types. Correction of this complication is imperative because of the possibility of corneal exposure. Although tenotomy has been recommended, complete revision of the wound with recession of the levator has given the best results for this condition.

Other Complications

Slight lid lag occurs in many operations which nevertheless have given a good cosmetic result. Careful exposure of the orbital septum during surgery will help to prevent lid lag. Lagophthalmos, with resultant corneal exposure and damage, is a very serious complication. Prompt surgical correction should be instituted; artificial tears and ointment may be used as a temporary corrective measure. Abnormal lid folds is a complication that is easily prevented by matching the lid fold on the opposite side as a secondary operation.

Ectropion, although it can occur, is rare and usually the result of too great an excision of the levator or tarsus. This can be prevented by suturing or fixing the lid skin to the tarsal plate so that the lashes are placed in the proper position; this is also the procedure of choice for correction of this complication. Entropion can occur when the lid is improperly placed; this can be prevented by attaching the skin of the lid to the anterior surface of the tarsal plate. Prolapse of the conjunctiva of the fornix can occur and can be easily treated by the use of a mattress suture placed in the fornix and brought out through the skin.

Infection is probably the most severe complication and should be treated vigorously immediately upon diagnosis. Scarring can occur as a reaction to the absorbable sutures and, because of this, care should be exercised in their use in any secondary operations for ptosis.

MARCUS GUNN OR JAW-WINKING SYNDROME

This condition occurs in approximately 5 per cent of patients with congenital ptosis. It is usually associated with some weakness of the superior rectus muscle. If the ptosis is the dominant feature, then correction of the ptosis is indicated. Care must be exercised, otherwise an overcorrection will be produced when the abnormal wink reflex occurs. However, if the wink reflex is dominant, with an increased size to the vertical measurement of the palpebral fissure, the operation of choice is detachment of the levator and a frontalis sling procedure. Correction of the extraocular muscle problem should be done prior to ptosis surgery. Figures 10–15A and B show a typical jaw-winking syndrome, epiblepharon, and congenital entropion.

ACQUIRED AND TRAUMATIC PTOSIS

The management of acquired ptosis, although similar to that for the congenital type, has several differences. In traumatic types of acquired ptosis, surgical correction is accomplished following a period of 6 to 12 months from the time of injury by resecting the scar with reapproxima-

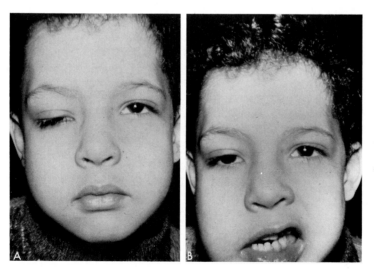

Figure 10–15 Typical jaw-winking syndrome involving right eye. *A,* Ptosis present when mouth is closed. *B,* Retraction of lid seen when jaw is moved.

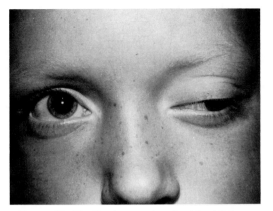

Figure 10–16 Ptosis associated with third-nerve paralysis.

CONGENITAL TUMORS

The most common congenital tumors affecting the lids are nevi, angiomas, and neurofibromas. Dermoid cysts may occur in the lids, but these are usually primary tumors of the orbit or orbital margin which may involve the lids secondarily.

Nevi are common benign congenital tumors which are relatively unpigmented at birth but which may enlarge and darken at puberty. A very common location for a nevus is along the lid border, as shown in Figure 10–17. Such nevi vary greatly in size and shape and may be sessile or pedunculated. They usually do not cause any concern until there is an increase in pigmentation and a resultant cosmetic blemish. Treatment depends on the location and size of the lesion. Treatment is not necessary if the lesion is stable in size and pigmentation. However, it is often wise to remove these tumors while they are small, in the hopes of preventing an increase in size and the necessity of major surgery at a later date. If the nevus involves the lid margin, it can often be shaved off flush with the lid margin by means of a razor blade knife. Suturing is not required and the anatomy and growth pattern of the lashes need not be disturbed. If the lesion does not involve the lid margin, simple excision and repair of the defect with accurate approximation of the skin margins will give a good cosmetic result.

Angiomatous tumors may occur in the lids as a single entity but are most commonly associated with other findings. For example, a nevus flammeus or port-wine

tion of the tissues and special concern for normal anatomic relationships. Care should be taken so that only a very small amount of levator is resected, as in this type of ptosis the effect of levator resection is much greater than that achieved in the congenital type. The acquired ptosis that is seen other than that due to trauma should also be treated with more conservatism than congenital ptosis, since the results of any levator resection in the presence of functioning levator muscle will produce a greater effect than in the congenital type. The Fasanella-Servat operation is an excellent procedure for minimal amounts of acquired ptosis. Should there be no levator function present, the procedure of choice is a suspension of the lid to the brow. This can be carried out using fascia lata, 4-0 Supramyd, or 3-0 Mersiline sutures. This procedure will give better results than those obtained by using a crutch applied to glasses, although this latter procedure has to be done to elevate the lid on those occasions when levator function is absent.

Ptosis associated with third-nerve paralysis should be treated with special care, giving first consideration to the eye muscle problem (Fig. 10–16). Then a suspension operation to bring the lid to the approximate height of the other eye can be done as a secondary procedure. Surgical treatment of a third-nerve paralysis should be carried out only after the patient has been thoroughly evaluated and the possibility of other neurologic diseases eliminated.

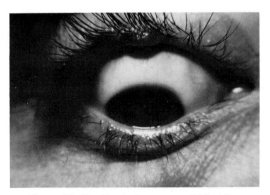

Figure 10–17 Dermal nevus on lid border.

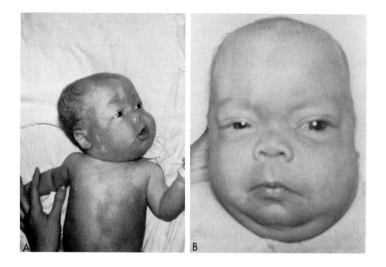

Figure 10–18 Sturge-Weber syndrome. *A*, Port-wine stain involving left side of body. *B*, Congenital buphthalmos, left eye.

stain, a telangiectasis of the deeper skin capillaries which often involves the area of the face innervated by the trigeminal nerve, is associated with the Sturge-Weber syndrome. Congenital glaucoma and choroidal hemangiomas may also accompany this hamartomatous syndrome. Figures 10–18*A* and *B* show a child with extensive cutaneous involvement and congenital glaucoma of the left eye. The recognition of these tumors is important because of their association with serious intraocular or intracranial problems. Congenital glaucoma occurs more commonly when the tumor involves the upper lid. When treatment is attempted by skin grafting or by tattooing the area, the cosmetic result is often more disfiguring than the original condition. Therefore these tumors are best left untreated.

Angioblastic hemangiomas (strawberry hemangiomas) usually occur as a single entity, unassociated with other ocular diseases. They are more common in premature infants and may cause quite a cosmetic blemish because of their discoloration (Fig. 10–19). These tumors usually increase in size during the first year of life; however, after this, spontaneous regression is common to the point at which they disappear, by the age of 5 or 6. It is important to explain the situation to the parents and to tell them that the tumor will increase in size and cause more of a cosmetic defect with time, but after this improvement may be expected. Several modes of therapy have been ad-

vanced, with surgical excision, cyrotherapy and the injection of a sclerosing agent being the most popular. We feel that these tumors should not be treated in the great majority of cases and that spontaneous regression gives the best cosmetic result. If surgery is necessary, cryotherapy is the treatment of choice. It is extremely important that these cases not be treated by radiation therapy. Figure 10–20 shows a 10-year-old girl who received radiation therapy for an angioblastic hemangioma. There is a poor cosmetic result, with visual function reduced to light perception from glaucoma and secondary cataract. After radiation therapy she also required several operative procedures to ameliorate the trichiasis secondary to the cicatricial

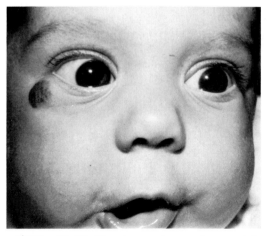

Figure 10–19 Strawberry hemangioma, right lower lid.

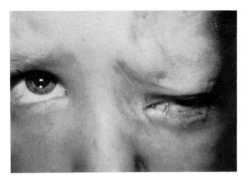

Figure 10–20   Hemangioma treated with radiation. Patient has trichiasis, glaucoma, cataract, and marked scarring.

changes. It is important that the parents be warned against shopping around in the hope that they will find someone to treat their child at an early age.

In neurofibromatosis the lid may be involved because of the presence of a plexiform neuroma. The diagnosis is not difficult if an adequate history is obtained and a thorough physical examination is performed to discover the telltale café au lait spots anywhere on the child's body. The plexiform neuroma may cause a mechanical ptosis or severe cosmetic defect. Surgical treatment is not indicated unless either the ptosis or blemish is prominent. Surgical removal of the tumor may also produce a traumatic ptosis which will then require subsequent repair.

The lids may be involved secondarily by any tumor of the orbit which may occur in childhood. There is a tendency for the lids to become involved in metastatic neuroblastoma and this diagnosis must be considered in young children, especially if ecchymosis of the lid is a prominent feature.

TRAUMATIC INJURIES

The most common traumatic injuries to the lids of young children are lacerations due to blunt trauma, dog bites, and sharp instruments. Before repairing lid lacerations it is extremely important to rule out serious ocular injury. If the laceration does not involve the lid margin, surgical repair involves apposition of the skin margin with multiple fine sutures.

The defect may have to be closed in layers if the deeper tissues are involved. It is extremely important to recognize involvement of the levator muscle, since functional results are best when this muscle is repaired as a primary procedure. A traumatic ptosis following laceration which does not resolve spontaneously over a period of approximately 6 months is difficult to correct.

If the laceration involves the lid margins, it is important to try to approximate them exactly, so that there will be no notching of the lid border. The repair of these lid lacerations is shown in Figures 10–21A to D. The lid margins are approximated with three 6-0 black silk sutures. The first suture is inserted into the posterior lid border of each side of the defect. This is followed by a similar suture into the anterior lid border in the area of the lash line. The assistant then pulls on these sutures to bring the lid margins into apposition. A third suture is then inserted into the area of the gray line. These three sutures are then tied and left long. The remainder of the defect is closed in two layers, with the pretarsal fascia being closed with interrupted 4-0 chromic catgut suture. The skin is closed with interrupted 6-0 black silk and the three sutures on the lid margin are incorporated into one of the skin sutures to prevent their inversion, with possible subsequent irritation to the cornea. The skin sutures are removed after 4 days, whereas those on the lid margin are left in place for 2 weeks. The age of the patient and his ability to cooperate determine whether these repairs can be performed under local or general anesthesia. The three sutures on the lid margin maintain approximation while the lid heals, prevent notching and trichiasis, and are easier to insert than either the "figure-of-eight" or "halving" type.

If a portion of the lid is missing, an attempt should be made to locate and suture it into the defect as soon as possible. The skin and structures of the lid are especially vascular and there is an excellent chance of the graft taking, with a minimal possibility of infection. Where missing tissue is grafted, it is wise to place the child on prophylactic antibiotics. A moderate pressure dressing is applied for

36 hours, and the sutures are removed in 10 days to 2 weeks.

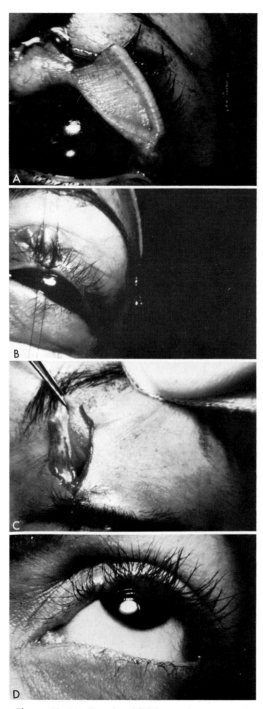

Figure 10–21 Repair of lid laceration. *A*, Vertical laceration through lid border. *B*, Sutures at anterior and posterior lid border, and one in area of the gray line. *C*, Remainder of defect is closed in two layers. *D*, Postoperative appearance.

BURN INJURIES

Burns may result from caustic materials coming into contact with the lids or from thermal injuries. Lye burns are more serious than acid burns because of continuing damage. Acid burns are self-limiting because of protein coagulation, which prevents further penetration of the acid; however, they can be very serious if a large amount in concentrated form comes into contact with the skin. Ocular complications resulting from such injuries can be devastating. When caustic material comes into contact with the lids, the immediate treatment consists of a very thorough lavage with water. After this, frequent applications of steroid ointments will help prevent cicatricial changes. If scarring is severe, lagophthalmos, entropion, or ectropion may result. Temporary tarsorrhaphies may prevent the contracture which causes these complications. If scarring and contracture are severe, surgical lysis of the adhesions, excision of the scar tissue, and full-thickness skin grafts may be necessary.

INJURIES CAUSED BY FOREIGN BODIES

Foreign bodies may enter the eyelids under many circumstances and should be removed whenever possible, especially if infection is present. Special attention should be given to the globe, and any injuries to it must be promptly and properly treated. Vegetable matter, either as the primary or secondary foreign body, often incites an intense reaction and may result in a chronic draining fistula until removed. Special x-rays, including bone-free dental films, may be necessary to localize such nonmetallic foreign bodies. In the pediatric age group, treatment consists of surgical removal under general anesthesia.

LID INVOLVEMENT WITH BACTERIAL LESIONS

Chalazion

A chalazion is a lipogranuloma of the meibomian gland which results from the obstruction of the gland duct and is usually located in the midportion of the tarsus, away from the lid border. It may occur on the lid margin if the opening of the duct is involved. Secondary infection of the surrounding tissues may develop, with subsequent swelling of the entire lid.

Chronic meibomitis may predispose a patient to recurrent chalazion formation and should be eradicated whenever possible. Chalazia can cause pressure on the globe, with subsequent alteration in the refractive error, and should therefore be eliminated before glasses are prescribed.

Small chalazia may resolve spontaneously; however, if they are large or if there is secondary infection, treatment is required. Initially this involves the use of warm compresses, followed by the instillation of antibiotic drops four times a day. For a small child, ointment may be preferred. It is important to stress continual use of the medication for several days after spontaneous rupture of a chalazion to prevent its recurrence. If the lesion does not respond to medical management, an incision with drainage and excision of the wall are necessary. In young children this is best done under general anesthesia on an outpatient basis. It is risky to try to perform such surgery under local anesthesia in a child because of the possibility of injuring the globe while injecting the local anesthetic agent or while performing the surgery.

Hordeolum

A hordeolum is a purulent staphylococcal infection of the glands of Zeis or the hair follicle. Initially there is diffuse swelling followed by localization on the lid margin. Treatment is the same as that given for a chalazion. Recurrences commonly result from autoinoculation and inattention to average hygienic care. General health measures and autogenous vaccine may be required in difficult situations.

Blepharitis

Chronic blepharitis is common in children and may result in secondary blepharoconjunctivitis, recurrent chalazia, loss of lashes (madarosis), and thickening of the lid margins (tylosis cialiaris).

The simple squamous variety is characterized by hypertrophy and desquamation of the epidermis near the lid margin, resulting in erythema and scaling of the lid border.

The ulcerative variety of blepharitis is the result of a secondary infection. Initially there is a purulent inflammation of the glands of the lid margin, which results in the formation of small ulcers.

Treatment consists of warm compresses, tarsal massage, removal of the scales and crusts with a moist cotton applicator, and instillation of an antibiotic ointment 3 or 4 times daily. The treatment must be continued for several weeks until the blepharitis is completely eradicated; otherwise, recurrence is most likely. The blepharitis may continue for several years despite treatment. Refraction will probably be necessary and glasses helpful, especially if astigmatism is present. Stubborn cases may respond to desensitization with a staphylococcus-streptococcus vaccine.

Impetigo Contagiosa

Impetigo contagiosa is a contagious pyoderma seen most often in the summer months. Characteristically, vesicles form and then erupt, resulting in the formation of a yellowish crust. This crusting is the result of local invasion of staphylococcus or streptococcus. Treatment consists of removal of the crusts and the local application of an antibiotic ointment.

LID INVOLVEMENT WITH VIRAL DISEASES

Vaccinia

Vaccinia of the lids usually results from autoinoculation during the first week after vaccination. The most frequent site of involvement is the inner aspect of the lower lid. Figure 10–22 shows a child with extensive involvement of both lids. If the lid alone is involved, the condition is not dangerous, but the possibility of con-

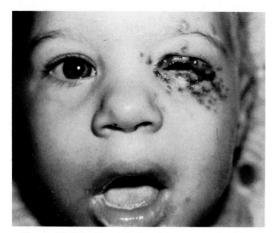

Figure 10–22 Vaccinia involving upper and lower lids on left side from autoinoculation.

junctival and corneal involvement makes prompt treatment necessary. Treatment consists of the application of idoxuridine (IDU) drops locally, and vaccinia hyperimmune gamma globulin administered systemically. The pustules resulting from such autoinoculation may produce scarring of the lid.

Herpes Simplex

Primary herpes simplex may occur in children aged 6 months to 5 years, and when it does, it is usually clinically asymptomatic. When the eye is involved in primary herpes simplex the initial lesion is usually on the lid or lid margin. This gives rise to the latent infection which may persist throughout life and be activated by many nonspecific stimuli. The most common ocular manifestation involves the cornea, but the lids may be affected in a recurrent infection. Herpetic blepharitis is characterized by the formation of vesicles which subsequently break down and ulcerate to form a yellowish crusted surface. These recurrent episodes usually clear completely within 10 to 14 days. IDU ointment may be helpful in early cases. Because recovery occurs spontaneously, treatment is supportive and prophylactic, utilizing antibiotic ointment to prevent secondary bacterial infection.

Herpes Zoster

Herpes zoster ophthalmicus is caused by the varicella-herpes zoster group of viruses. It is unusual in childhood, but the upper or lower lids may be involved if the first or second division of the trigeminal nerve is affected. Vesicles occur at the inner half of the upper lid when the supratrochlear branch of the first division is involved, and along the side and tip of the nose if the nasociliary branch is involved. In the latter instance, severe keratitis and uveitis may occur. With lid involvement only, treatment is mainly symptomatic, with emphasis on prevention of a secondary bacterial infection. Convalescent serum concentrated gamma globulin may be helpful.

Molluscum Contagiosum

Molluscum contagiosum is a viral skin disorder which may cause a secondary follicular conjunctivitis when the lid margins are involved. The typical skin lesion is a small nodule with an umbilicated center and minimal signs of inflammation. These lesions may be incised and curetted but simple expression or touching the lesion with electrocautery is sufficient.

LID INFECTIONS WITH FUNGI

Eyelid infections due to fungi are on the increase with the advent of antibiotics, steroids, and various antimetabolites used in cancer chemotherapy. There is often a history of trauma involving vegetable matter. Diagnosis requires a strong index of suspicion, proper culture utilizing Sabouraud's medium, and wet smears cleared with 10 per cent potassium hydroxide.

Actinomycosis

The organisms of the family Actinomycetaceae, which includes Actinomyces and Nocardia, enter the skin at the site of trauma. A nodular lesion results which may rupture through the skin and discharge "sulfur granules" containing the fungus. Diagnosis is made by finding branching filaments upon microscopic examination of these granules. Treatment consists of the administration of systemic penicillin.

Nocardia

Nocardia is considered an aerobic genus of the family Actinomycetaceae, which may cause a chronic suppurative process associated with granuloma and draining sinuses. Treatment consists of systemic penicillin and the removal of any foreign material.

Candida

Candida is a yeastlike fungus which may cause thrushlike infections, especially in the presence of pregnancy, alcoholism, vascular stress, and heavy sweating. In the eye it may cause a pseudomembranous conjunctivitis presenting as a shallow, indolent corneal ulcer. Diagnosis is made by direct examination of a scraping which has been treated with 10 per cent potassium hydroxide and demonstration of the chlamydospore after culture on Sabouraud's medium. Alkaline lotions are very helpful, and if the disease affects the skin, gentian violet is recommended. Nystatin is usually combined with the above treatment.

Blastomyces Dermatitidis

The eyelids may be involved in the cutaneous form of blastomycosis (Gilchrist's disease). Lid involvement produces multiple small abscesses around the lashes, scarring, and subsequent ectropion. The cornea and conjunctiva may be secondarily involved. Diagnosis is made by demonstrating thick-walled, double-contoured, budding yeasts in material taken from the affected tissue or exudate. If the lesion is localized it should be excised; if it is diffuse, iodides, stilbamidine or propamidine are recommended.

LID INVOLVEMENT WITH ARTHROPODS

Pediculosis

Louse infections of the lids result in severe itching and irritation. There is a predilection for the lids to become involved with the pubic louse. This type of infection has become more prevalent among adolescents within the last few years. Diagnosis is made easily on slit lamp examination when the ova and adult crab louse may be observed. Treatment consists of improving the patient's personal hygiene and the application of a 0.5 per cent eserine ointment.

Contact Dermatitis

The skin of the eyelids may resemble crepe paper and appear loose in its normal state, but it becomes markedly swollen with contact to noxious agents. The skin of the lids initially becomes red, itchy, and irritated. Common irritants include some local medications (atropine, for example), cosmetics, nail polish, soaps, poison ivy, sumac, and so on. Treatment consists of removal of the initiating substance when it can be identified. Symptomatic relief may be obtained by using systemic antihistamines and local steroid preparations.

REFERENCES

Beard, C.: The surgical treatment of blepharoptosis: a quantitative approach. Trans. Amer. Ophthal. Soc., 64:401, 1966.

Berke, R. N.: Congenital ptosis: a classification of two hundred cases. Arch. Ophthal., 41:188, 1949.

Berke, R. N.: A simplified Blaskovics operation for blepharoptosis. Arch. Ophthal., 48:460, 1952.

Blaskovics, L.: A new operation for ptosis with shortening of the levator and tarsus. Arch. Ophthal., 52:563, 1923.

Cutler, N. L., and Beard, C.: A method for partial and total upper lid reconstruction. Amer. J. Ophthal., 39:1, 1965.

Duke-Elder, S.: System of Ophthalmology. Vol. 3, Diseases of the Outer Eye. Part I: Conjunctiva. St. Louis, The C. V. Mosby Co., 1965, p. 310.

Duke-Elder, S.: System of Ophthalmology. Vol. 3, Normal and Abnormal Development. Part II: Congenital Deformities. St. Louis, The C. V. Mosby Co., 1963, p. 827.

Fox, S. A.: Correction of ptosis. In New Orleans Acad. Ophthal. Otolaryng. Symposium on Surgery of the Ocular Adnexa. St. Louis, The C. V. Mosby Co., 1966, pp. 41–57.

Hughes, W. L.: Ophthalmic Plastic Surgery. Rochester, Minnesota, Amer. Acad. Ophthal. Otolaryng., 1961. (A.A.O.O. Home Study Manual.)

Iliff, C. E.: A simplified ptosis operation. Amer. J. Ophthal., 37:529, 1954.

Jones, L. T., Reeh, M. J., and Tsujimura, J. K.: Senile entropion. Amer. J. Ophthal., 55:463, 1963.

Mustardé, J. C.: Repair and Reconstruction in the Orbital Region: A Practical Guide. London, E. & S. Livingstone, Ltd., 1966.

Mustardé, J. C.: The treatment of ptosis and epicanthal folds. Brit. J. Plast. Surg., 12:252, 1959.

Smith, B., and Cherubini, T. D.: Oculoplastic Surgery: A Compendium of Principles and Techniques. St. Louis, The C. V. Mosby Co., 1970.

Spaeth, E. B.: Further consideration on the surgical correction of blepharoptosis (epicanthus). Amer. J. Ophthal., 41:61, 1956.

Troutman, R. C., Converse, J. M., and Smith, B. (eds.): Plastic and Reconstructive Surgery of the Eye and Adnexa. Washington, D.C., Butterworths, 1962.

CHAPTER 11

DISORDERS OF THE CONJUNCTIVA

FRANCIS P. FURGIUELE, M.D., F.A.C.S.

INTRODUCTION

To many physicians, conjunctivitis as a disease does not seem as important as glaucoma or retinal detachment, probably because in most instances it represents a lesser threat to serious visual loss. Its broad scope of etiologies and easy accessibility for study make it no less interesting than other ophthalmic diseases. Moreover, in cases such as trachoma or gonorrheal ophthalmia, the blindness that often follows makes it important that one have a proper understanding of the problem of conjunctivitis so that early recognition and treatment may prevent serious sequelae. The material in this chapter covers the more common disorders of the conjunctiva. It is intended to offer a descriptive clinical approach, a differential diagnosis, and suggested laboratory studies which will help in the management of the patient presenting with conjunctivitis. For those who suffer from the disease, the ailment is an ocular discomfort of varying degree that may become chronic and disabling.

Certain conditions likely to be encountered such as "spots" on the conjunctiva, pigmentations, degenerations, or trauma will be covered only briefly in order to avoid overlap with other chapters in this text.

ANATOMY

The conjunctiva is a thin transparent lymphoid mucous membrane that covers the anterior surface of the globe and the posterior surface of the eyelids. These portions are known respectively as the bulbar and palpebral conjunctiva. They unite in a rather loose redundant part that forms a fold in the upper and lower portion. On the nasal side a fold of conjunctiva forms a crescent known as the plica semilunaris. Medial to the plica and lying in the canthus is a fleshy body known as the caruncle. The whole of the conjunctiva projected backward in the fornices forms a sac known as the cul-de-sac. Although anatomically the conjunctiva ends at the limbus, embryologically it is continuous with the cornea. The conjunctival sac has been likened to a lymph node which has been split and lined with a mucous epithelium. The conjunctiva therefore participates not only in epithelial diseases but also in those involving the reticuloendothelial and lymphatic systems. The conjunctiva secretes mucus, which is essential to the health of the cornea. Chronic diseases affecting the secretion provided by the conjunctiva may lead to serious visual impairment. Histologically the conjunctiva is divided into two layers: the superficial or epithelial layer and a subepithelial layer. The latter is made up of adenoid tissue and fibrous tissue. The blood supply of the conjunctiva comes from the palpebral branches of the nasal and lacrimal arteries of the eyelids and from the anterior ciliary vessels.

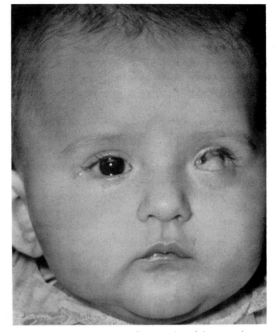

Figure 11–1 Dermatolipoma involving conjunctiva and cornea.

TUMORS OF THE CONJUNCTIVA (BENIGN)

The principal tumors occurring on the conjunctiva are the nevus, dermoid cyst, dermolipoma, and hemangioma.

Nevus

This is a very slightly elevated lesion, usually salmon in color but may be a deep brown, depending on the degree of pigmentation. These tumors are usually benign and rarely become malignant. They rarely require excision unless there is some question of possible malignancy because of tumor enlargement.

Dermoid Cyst and Dermolipoma

Dermoid cysts and dermolipomas have a similar clinical appearance. They are elevated, smooth, rounded in shape, and usually straddle the limbus, often in the upper outer quadrant. The dermolipoma (Fig. 11–1) is usually composed of connective and adipose tissue. Glandular tissue, hair follicles, and hair shafts occurring in the tumor are usually characteristic of the dermoid cyst.

Hemangioma

These tumors are comprised of dilated blood vessels and may or may not be elevated. They usually do not require treatment.

Pterygium

This is a triangular or winged-shaped connective tissue overgrowth of the conjunctiva. The thickened mass is usually located in the exposed portions of the bulbar conjunctiva, more commonly on the medial aspect, with the apex of advancing growth toward the cornea and at times intruding on or several millimeters into the cornea. Occupations in which exposure to wind, dust, and other irritants is common tend to aggravate the lesion. Treatment is usually indicated when the cornea is encroached upon and the eye is symptomatic. Excision followed by beta radiation or thio-tepa is usually satisfactory, although recurrence is common.

MALIGNANT MELANOMA AND LYMPHOMA

Malignant melanoma and lymphoma are uncommon malignant tumors of the conjunctiva (see Chapter 33, Ocular Tumors). Lymphoma as a primary ocular entity is rare and must be differentiated from benign lymphoid hyperplasia. These conditions are diagnosed by excision biopsy and pathologic evaluation. Disagreement may occur among pathologists, especially regarding lymphoma diagnosis on biopsy specimens.

SPOTS

Most commonly noted spots are nevi (pink to brown), pinguecula (yellowish-white), isolated collections of vessels (red), pterygium (yellow to red), and pigmentations from exogenous or systemic causes. They vary in color, size, number, and distribution. For example, small collections of capillaries, petechial spots, and nevi may occur singly or in number, but they usually appear on the bulbar portion of the conjunctiva. Isolated patchy spots of grey pigment often surround the exits of episcleral vessels. The increase of pigmentation and elevation of these lesions are often of concern to the parent. A simple excision of singular lesions often reveals them to be benign nevi. On rare occasions malignant melanoma may be found. In certain cases of deep scattered pigmentation of the conjunctiva, sclera, iris, and deeper ocular structures, the diagnosis of melanosis oculi should be considered. This lesion requires careful observation because of its increased potentiality to change to malignant melanoma.

Pingueculum

This is a benign lesion appearing as a yellowish white, slightly elevated mass involving the bulbar conjunctiva and representing an elastic and hyaline degenerative change of the conjunctiva. No treatment is required unless for cosmetic reasons, in which case a simple excision will suffice.

Pigmentations

Continued use of epinephrine or silver solutions such as argyrol produce black discoloration of the conjunctiva. The conjunctival palor of anemia or the scleral icterus related to hyperbilirubinemia should be considered as an integral part of the examination of the conjunctiva.

Lithiasis (Conjunctival Concretions)

These are yellow-appearing spots on the palpebral conjunctiva caused by degenerative changes in the conjunctiva (glands of Henle). They usually are asymptomatic but occasionally behave like a foreign body when they erode through the surface and scratch the globe. Removal with a sharp curette or knife is required under these circumstances.

CONJUNCTIVITIS

Peculiarities of Conjunctivitis

The pediatrician must consider conjunctivitis in terms of nonbacterial as well as bacterial causes. The latter usually responds to the available ocular medications containing antibiotics or sulfa. However, those cases which do not respond to this therapy may be caused by unrecognized nonbacterial causes. Patients who appear resistant to treatment may have been misdiagnosed because of peculiarities in clinical appearance, cursory examination, or insufficient laboratory studies. In infants, for example, foreign bodies under the lids may be found by everting the upper lid and examining the palpebral conjunctiva with adequate illumination and magnification. Omission of this maneuver might lead one to prescribe an antibiotic for a conjunctivitis which will not subside because it is the result of presence of a foreign body rather than an infection. The use of fluorescein dye will cause the areas of denuded epithelium to stain green when viewed under ultraviolet illumination in cases of conjunctivitis due to scratches or abrasions unrecognized under ordinary light. The persistence of watering and discharge requires a thorough inspection of the lacrimal punctum and canaliculus for evidence of obstruction. If none is apparent, attention should be directed toward ruling out other dis-

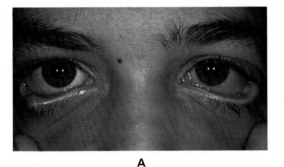

A
Conjunctivitis associated with chalazia.

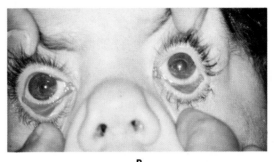

B
Stevens-Johnson's disease, 2 months old.

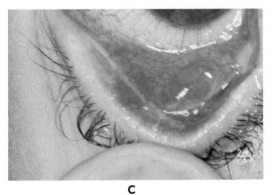

C
Stevens-Johnson's disease, close-up of case in *C.*

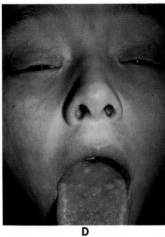

D
Stevens-Johnson's disease, with ulcerative tongue lesions and macular lesions on face.

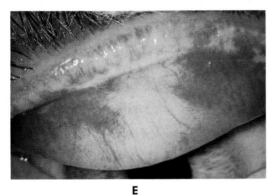

E
Stevens-Johnson's disease, scarred lid, 2 years old.

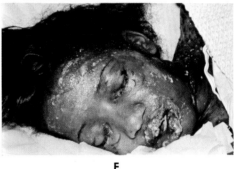

F
Stevens-Johnson's disease with fatal outcome.

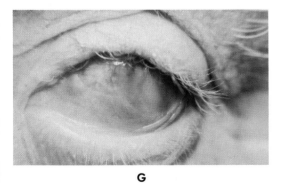

G
Ocular pemphigoid (note obliteration of formix and cul-de-sac).

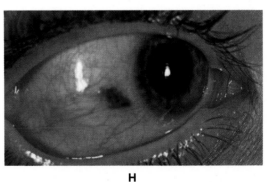

H
Pigmentation on the conjunctiva.

259

eases by noting the appearance of the size of the globe and luster of the cornea. Infants with congenital glaucoma have an enlarged eyeball with a cornea that has a bluish haze due to edema. The lids appear tightly apposed to the globe. Measuring the ocular tension with a Schiötz tonometer would be indicated. In young children, a thickened conjunctiva, with lid edema and heavy stringy discharge, is often associated with itching and the result of allergy. This is usually bilateral and responds to local antihistamines or steroids.

Unilateral conjunctivitis, associated with a thickened conjunctiva and upper lid edema, may produce the appearance of ptosis. Enlargement of the preauricular lymph node on the affected side is commonly present. The etiology is often difficult to ascertain because there are many viral, some fungal, and occasional rare types of bacteria that produce this clinical appearance. Viral disease of the cornea, epidemic keratoconjunctivitis, and certain adenoviruses cause a purulent discharge which is bacteriologically sterile. The disease resists treatment and lasts several weeks or months before finally resolving. Leptothrix infection, tularemia, and lymphopathia venereum are more remote causes of this so-called Parinaud's syndrome. In the latter condition the adenopathy may become suppurative. Obviously, serum samples should be obtained for adenovirus titers; cultures and smears should be made for bacteria, fungi, and cytology. Sometimes conjunctivitis may be persistent because of local drug toxicity. Ocular medications likely to be at fault are silver nitrate, neomycin, and the sulfonamides. Children under treatment for oculomotor disorders such as esotropia may exhibit conjunctival hyperemia or follicular conjunctivitis in response to miotics such as pilocarpine or Fluorpryl used to relax accommodation.

These brief remarks have concerned peculiarities of conjunctivitis in children; a more expansive discussion of the subject follows.

Symptoms

Conjunctivitis is an inflammation of the conjunctiva characterized by different degrees of hyperemia, discharge, and edema. The symptomatology varies from mild irritation and watering, to marked discomfort. There may be also present a profuse mucopurulent discharge associated with blurring of vision. In the absence of symptoms the inflammation is recognized by the objective signs of hyperemia and edema. In children, the disease is usually benign and of short duration, although it is often alarming to parents and teachers who are disturbed by the red watery appearance of the eyes and fear of contagion. In infants the disease is apt to be more serious and should be considered potentially dangerous. There are many causes for this disease both exogenous and endogenous, some depending on seasonal variation (such as allergic conjunctivitis and vernal catarrh) and others on geographic locale (such as trachoma and gonorrheal ophthalmia). What is dangerous about conjunctivitis is whether it is of type or severity to cause damage to other ocular structures (such as the cornea, for example) and result in visual impairment, or whether it is a premonitory sign or port of entry to systemic disease (as for example, meningitis). It is important, therefore, to make an etiologic diagnosis early in order that proper treatment be administered and complications avoided.

Classification

Conjunctivitis may be divided into two broad areas of classification:
1. Infectious
2. Noninfectious

Other classifications may be made on the basis of the duration of the disease (e.g., either acute, subacute, or chronic) or on the type of pathologic changes produced (e.g., follicular, papillary, cicatricial, and so on). Infectious types of conjunctivitis are those due to bacteria, viruses, fungi, and parasites. The noninfectious types of conjunctivitis include folliculosis, allergy, irritative-toxic, nutritional, and associative, i.e., as an added part of inflammation of the lids, cornea, or lacrimal apparatus. Also under this category are included those individuals whose eyes are anatomically predisposed to inflammation.

Diagnosis

The diagnosis of conjunctivitis requires obtaining an adequate history from the patient. This will often present clues that are helpful in narrowing down the differential diagnosis.

A history of trauma would suggest diligent search for a retained foreign body such as glass or wood. The presence of upper respiratory or sinus disease might indicate a secondary or an associated infectious type of etiology. Itching or rubbing the eyes with clenched fists suggests an allergic state. Crusting of the lid margins with difficulty opening the eyelids on awakening could mean that a chronic blepharitis with secondary infection was present. The examination requires patient cooperation and where this cannot be obtained the child should be sedated or even anesthetized. Adequate illumination with proper magnification is necessary. In infants and very young children, one may gain valuable information by immobilization and sedation in the operating room and use of the Zeiss operating microscope for examination.

In older children who are cooperative, the slit lamp biomicroscope is essential. This is an excellent means of determining the extent of an injury or searching for a retained foreign body. A magnifying loupe may be used if the other instruments are not available (Fig. 11–2).

Examination

In evaluating conjunctivitis one must make a thorough examination of the entire anterior segment including the lids, cornea, and adnexa.

Inspection — blink rate (infrequent, excessive).

Lids — margins, position-retracted, entropion, ectropion, gnarled, deformity.

Lashes — lack of, misdirected toward cornea, lice, scales, nits.

Skin — wrinkled, scaly, hyperemia, pallor, mascerated, excoriated, pigmentation, crusts.

Punctum — stenosed, pouting, slit, relation to lacrimal lake.

Conjunctiva — cul-de-sac — edema, hyperemia, follicles, papillae, concretions, foreign bodies, pigmentation, vascular congestion, forward extension of vessels in exposed area (interpalpebral), scars, symblepharon, discoloration, shrinkage of cul-de-sac.

Discharge — watery, purulent, mucoid, absence of, odor, discoloration.

Cornea — ulcers, dendritic or punctate stains, edema, infiltrates, pannus, photophobia, size, shape.

Palpation — tenderness, discharge on pressure over lids, canaliculi or sac, cysts, nodules.

Laboratory Procedures

It is common practice for many ophthalmologists when confronted with a case of conjunctivitis to resort to laboratory studies only when initial treatment has failed. Despite the fact that laboratory results are often negative, they are a valuable aid in establishing a diagnosis and selecting the proper therapeutic agents. Conjunctival smears and cultures should be made whenever possible. Cultures should be taken using a sterile cotton applicator, preferably moistened with sterile 5 per cent glucose or liquid medium, and rubbed gently against the bulbar and palpebral conjunctiva of the upper and lower fornices and of each eye separately. The swab should then be transferred directly to the appropriate bacteriologic media, i.e., blood agar or thioglycolate broth. If there is a delay in streaking or

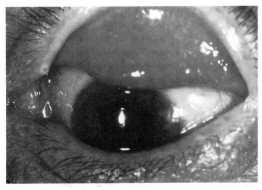

Figure 11–2   Acute conjunctivitis.

plating media, the swab should be suspended in a liquid medium until the bacteriologist can proceed further. Many negative cultures are the result of dry swabs and delay in transfer of material from the eye to the laboratory. Scrapings should be obtained by gently abrading the anesthetized conjunctiva (using Ophthaine or Ophthetic) with a sterile spatula and transferring to clean glass slides. The slides should be stained for bacteria and cytology, cultured on suitable media (B.B.L., blood agar, etc.), and sensitivity tested for antibiotic susceptibility. Scrapings may be transferred to HeLa cells, rabbit kidney cells or chick embryos, or other tissue culture media in suspected viral disease.

Neutralizing antibody titers should be made for specific adenovirus as well as group adenovirus titers from sera obtained from the patient during the acute phase of the disease and after it has subsided. Smears should be examined for predominant cell type, i.e., polymorphonuclear, lymphocytes, eosinophiles, mononuclears, giant cells, multinucleated giant cells, inclusion bodies, bacteria, hyphal elements, and yeasts.

It requires a great deal of time and patience to examine a slide, especially when searching for fungi or bacteria. Often, it is necessary to work in close cooperation with the hospital laboratory in order to increase the chance of positive findings. The etiologic agents which one suspects should be brought to the attention of the laboratory personnel so that appropriate stains and media are used.

Cellular reactions noted in conjunctival smears and scrapings include:

1. Polymorphonuclear reaction seen in:
   a. Bacterial infection, e.g., staphylococci, gonococci
   b. Viral infection — inclusion conjunctivitis, trachoma, lymphogranuloma
2. Mononuclear reaction
   Herpes simplex, epidemic keratoconjunctivitis
3. Eosinophilia — allergic states — vernal catarrh
4. Basophilia — allergic states — vernal catarrh trachoma
5. Plasma cells — trachoma

Environmental vs. Bacteriologic Causes of Conjunctivitis

The pollution of our atmosphere with sulfides, lead, and other industrial wastes has added additional noxious agents responsible for some cases of conjunctivitis in metropolitan areas. The use of aersol sprays for hair lacquers, body deodorants, room fresheners, and so forth have also become factors in the production of conjunctivitis. Eye make-up, mascara, eye shadow, contact lenses, false eyelashes, and the like are common offenders among teenagers as well as adults. The bacterial flora of the normal eye varies considerably. Most any organism might appear in culture in the absence of any clinical signs or symptoms of conjunctivitis. Repeat cultures may reveal a different bacteria or no growth in the absence of any treatment. In a bacteriologic study of over two thousand cases of conjunctivitis, Nicholas and Goolden of Los Angeles found the following:

47.8 per cent Coagulase-negative staph
14.7 per cent Coagulase-positive Staph aureus
13.4 per cent Corynebacterium
 8.6 per cent Alpha hemolytic strep
 1.4 per cent Pseudomonas

Less than 1 per cent included *Moraxella lacunata, Moraxella nonliquifaciens, Klebsiella pneumonia, Diplococcus pneumonia,* Mimea, Proteus, *Bacillus subtilis, Haemophilus influenzae, Neisseria catarrhalis.* Fourteen per cent of the cultures taken were negative.

Anatomic Predisposition to Conjunctivitis

In these cases there is a vulnerability for congestion which is related to the size of the globe, the amount of conjunctival exposure, the forward extension of bulbar conjunctival vessels toward the cornea, and the relationship of the lids and lid closure. The lower eyelids are usually recessed, exposing more conjunctiva below the limbus. There is also some disturbance in vasomotor tone so that the slightest irritant in the environment, be it dust, smoke, smog, or just fatigue, causes the eye to appear moderately inflamed.

These eyes may be protuberant, highly astigmatic, or myopic. No specific treatment is required. Decongestants have a limited transitory effect.

INFECTIOUS CONJUNCTIVITIS

Infectious conjunctivitis may be caused by numerous bacteria or viruses. Some of the important bacterial infections to be considered are as follows.

Bacterial Causes

Gonorrhea

The increase in gonorrhea in the United States has risen steadily over the past 5 to 6 years. Approximately one-half million cases were reported in one year. It is estimated that the true figure is perhaps three times that, since one survey of private physicians in the United States shows that probably no more than 17 per cent of treated cases of gonorrhea had been reported. Any case of hyperacute conjunctivitis with marked purulent discharge should be considered as gonorrheal in origin until proved otherwise.

A more common cause of ophthalmia neonatorum (gonococcal conjunctivitis), once considered solely the result of gonococcal infection and from which it must be differentiated, is inclusion blennorrhea or, as it is known today, inclusion conjunctivitis. *Chlamydia oculogenitalis* is the causal agent. Inclusion conjunctivitis is the most common type of ophthalmia neonatorum in the United States and the commonest cause of nongonococcal urethritis and cervicitis (Thygeson). Although a purulent papillary conjunctivitis similar to gonorrhea is found, its discharge and scrapings are bacteriologically sterile but exhibit cytoplasmic inclusion bodies.

This is a severe disease transmitted to the infant's eyes by contamination during passage through the infected birth canal at the time of delivery. It may occur at birth if there is premature rupture of the amniotic membranes. The incubation period is short (1 to 3 days) and the clinical signs are those of a profuse purulent discharge associated with marked edema and hyperemia of the eyelids and conjunctiva. The eyelids are often difficult to pry open due to the intense thickening and edema. The bacterial toxins are capable of destroying the cornea, with resulting perforation and blindness. The diagnosis can be made early by examining smears of conjunctival scrapings which show gram-negative intracellular diplococci. The organism may be identified in scrapings of the conjunctival cells before the organisms are released into the exudate. Cultures on chocolate agar and fermentation tests are necessary to differentiate the gonococcus from other members of the Neisseria group such as meningitidis. The Crede procedure of instilling 1 per cent silver nitrate into the infants eyes immediately after birth provides adequate prophylaxis. In children the disease occurs more commonly in girls, is less severe, and occurs from contamination and in association with a vulvovaginitis.

The finding that women may be asymptomatic carriers of the gonorrheal organism cultured from the cervix or rectum poses a further hazard to the spread of this disease.

Cervical and rectal swabs in the last trimester of pregnancy or immediately prepartum during labor may provide more useful information regarding those newborn infants likely to acquire the disease and requiring more diligent prophylaxis and observation.

Treatment with systemic and local penicillin and sulfonamides or tetracyclines is usually effective. Cases resistant to penicillin have been reported. Gonorrheal conjunctivitis must be differentiated clinically from other forms of purulent conjunctivitis which are produced by staphylococci, inclusion blennorrhea, silver nitrate, or other agents (Mimea, Candida, and Mycoplasma). The purulent conjunctivitis due to silver nitrate comes on 12 to 24 hours after instillation, lasts 24 to 48 hours, and is sterile. Inclusion conjunctivitis has a longer incubation period and smears of conjunctival scrapings show inclusion bodies in the cytoplasm.

Staphylococcus

This type of conjunctivitis may be either acute, producing a purulent discharge, or chronic conjunctivitis, with little or no discharge and associated with a chronic blepharitis. Scaling of the lid margins and yellowish crusts are present along with congestion of the conjunctival vessels. The fissuring and ulceration of the skin are not uncommon. The toxins also produce marginal corneal ulceration which responds to small doses of sulfa and steroid combinations. Neglected treatment of staph blepharitis in childhood may lead to adult chronic conjunctivitis which is disabling.

Pneumococcus

This is primarily a disease of school-age children and a prime cause of "pink eye." It is highly contagious. The severity of the conjunctivitis is dependent upon the virulence of the organism.

Hyperemia is usually marked along with petechial and subconjunctival hemorrhages. Pneumococcal conjunctivitis is usually catarrhal in type, is seldom purulent, and occasionally may form a pseudomembrane. Discharge is variable and may be either mucopurulent or sanious. The cornea is usually unaffected. An associated iridocyclitis may occur with severe forms of the disease. Chloromycetin, penicillin, and sulfa are effective.

Koch-Weeks Conjunctivitis

A similar conjunctivitis may be caused by the Koch-Weeks bacillus in warm tropical climates. Also known as *Haemophilus aegyptius*, its occurrence is notably in spring and fall. It may be associated with eye gnats. The conjunctivitis is severe with mucopurulent discharge, lid edema, photophobia, and blepharospasm.

Smears show a polymorphonuclear exudate. Gram-negative rods are found in epithelial cells taken from scrapings. The organism responds to 0.1 per cent polymyxin B sulfate.

Streptococcal Conjunctivitis

This condition often is catarrhal in type, but depending on the virulence of the organism, the toxin may produce a pseudomembrane or membranous conjunctivitis. Neomycin or chloramphenicol drops may be used, depending on sensitivity tests.

Meningococcal Conjunctivitis

This condition is rare. It may be a forerunner of meningitis and should be considered a serious infection. It occurs more often as an endogenous catarrhal conjunctivitis, complication meningitis, or septicemia but may occur as a primary infection which spreads to the meninges.

The organism may be found in smears of the conjunctival scrapings, emphasizing the importance of carrying out the laboratory procedure along with cultures early in the disease picture. Sulfonamides and tetracyclines should cure the infection.

Viral Causes

Inclusion Conjunctivitis

Inclusion conjunctivitis is a virus disease grouped among the PLT agents (psittacosis-lymphogranuloma-trachoma). Coupled with trachoma the agents are known as TRIC viruses. In infants the disease caused by the inclusion conjunctivitis agent *Chlamydia oculogenitalis* was previously known as inclusion blennorrhea. Clinically it has a somewhat longer incubation period than gonorrheal ophthalmia but in contrast to the latter runs a relatively benign and self-limited course. Recent evidence has been presented by Foster, Dawson, and Schacter that scarring and superficial pannus may occur following inclusion conjunctivitis of the newborn. Virus isolation may be made from scrapings taken from the anesthetized conjunctiva of the lower fornix with a platinum spatula and suspended in tissue culture maintenance media. There is a purulent discharge which is bacteriologically sterile. Stained smears of the conjunctival scrapings show numerous polymorphonuclear cells and cytoplasmic inclusions. Due to the lack of development of lymphoid tissue in the infant, follicles do not appear unless the disease persists for many weeks. (See Plate VII *G* and *H*, p. 329.)

In the adult the response to the virus is a follicular conjunctivitis. The preponderance of inflammatory follicular conjunctival change involves the lower lids, whereas in trachoma the upper eyelids and superior part of the cornea are affected. In adults inclusion conjunctivitis has been called "swimming pool conjunc - tivitis" because of its transmission in water. However, chlorination of swimming pools has eliminated the transfer of inclusion conjunctivitis by this route. Most "swimming pool conjunctivitis" is probably adenovirus infection (Thygeson).

The TRIC viruses have an affinity for the genital mucosa and conjunctiva. Oculogenital transmission may occur with or without water as a medium. The sulfonamides and tetracycline antibiotics are effective in controlling the disease.

Herpes Simplex

Herpes simplex produces a follicular conjunctivitis in association with follicles on the lids and margins. The cornea subsequently becomes involved with either punctate erosions or dendritic figures. The diagnosis is not difficult to make. Giant mononuclear cells are found in conjunctival scrapings and the virus can be isolated on tissue culture. The conjunctivitis is not serious; the corneal lesions are. Treatment consists of IDU every two hours and IDU ointment at night. This may be preceded by mechanical removal of the infected epithelial cells. Cycloplegics such as atropine or scopolamine are indicated to control the associated iridocyclitis. When severe iritis is present, small doses of steroids may be added to reduce the inflammation. Chemical cauterization with iodine is still advocated by some. There are enthusiastic reports of good results with the use of cryotherapy.

Measles

Measles virus produces a catarrhal conjunctivitis associated with a mucopurulent discharge. The diagnosis is made in association with the findings of Koplik's spots in the mucous membranes or conjunctiva near the caruncle. Skin rash, fever, and other constitutional symptoms are usually present. Photophobia is usually indicative of corneal involvement. No specific ocular therapy is necessary as a rule. An epidemic of measles in Haiti in 1966–1967 was associated with severe ocular involvement, with corneal ulceration in 25 patients, of whom 14 developed corneal perforation. Malnutrition was considered an important factor. The disease is seldom seen in the United States where vaccination is widely used. Measles conjunctivitis requires no specific treatment.

Varicella

Varicella or chickenpox seldom affects the conjunctiva, although vesicles may form on the lid margins. The vesicles may rupture and become pustular before undergoing resolution. The cornea is rarely involved. Prevention of secondary infection by instillation of sulfonamides is sometimes helpful.

Herpes Zoster

Herpes zoster seldom affects children and rarely produces lesions of the conjunctiva. Vesicular lesions erupt on the skin usually following the distribution of the frontal branch of the ophthalmic nerve. When the nasociliary branches are involved, ocular complications are usually produced. Treatment when ocular complications occur is aimed at reducing inflammation with steroids (local and systemic) and cycloplegics to alleviate iridocyclitis.

Chronic Conjunctivitis

Chronic conjunctivitis sometimes follows blepharitis, a very commonly encountered eye disease associated with seborrhea and diplobacillary bacteria (*Pityrosporon ovale*) (Fig. 11–3). Staphylococci are the most common contaminants of blepharitis, which not only leads to

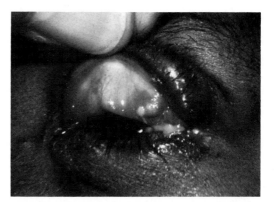

Figure 11–3   Chronic staphylococcic conjunctivitis.

chronic inflammation of the conjunctiva, but to styes, meibomitis, trichiasis, marginal corneal infiltrates and ulcers, epithelial keratitis, and a type of phlyctenulosis with pannus. Treatment of blepharitis early in childhood may avoid the development of the more serious complications mentioned here.

OCULAR COMPLICATIONS OF VACCINIA

Ocular complications occur approximately one in 40,000 vaccinations. The typical lesion is a white, umbilicated pustule on the eyelid surrounded by edema, redness, and preauricular adenopathy. The conjunctiva lesion is usually an excavated ulcer with a white necrotic center usually near the semilunar fold or caruncle. Treatment with hyperimmune vaccinia globulins is of value (Fig. 11–4).

Fungal Causes

Fungus infections of the conjunctiva are rare. Although fungi may commonly be found in the normal conjunctival cul-de-sac, they rarely act as pathogens. Their presence is usually the result of airborne contamination.

Aspergillus, Candida, Rhinosporidium, Blastomyces, Cephalosporium, and other species have been identified as causes of conjunctivitis. Diagnosis is made by examination of scrapings and smears of KOH preparation for yeast or hyphal elements. Amphotericin B, iodides, sul-

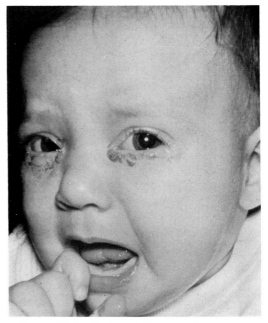

Figure 11–5 Conjunctivitis secondary to naso-lacrimal duct obstruction.

fonamides, pimaricin, and hamycin may be helpful. Conjunctivitis may occur secondary to canaliculitis caused by Actinomyces organisms. This is not a true fungus and responds to penicillin and sulfonamides. Treatment with these agents combined with irrigation of the canaliculi usually is sufficient.

Conjunctivitis Secondary to Nasolacrimal Duct Obstruction

Conjunctivitis may commonly be present in infants as a result of congenital membranous obstruction of the nasolacrimal duct, usually the canaliculus. This often causes persistent watering or mucopurulent discharge of the conjunctiva. Probing procedures may be deferred until after the infant is 6 months of age, since many of these cases clear spontaneously. Instillation of 0.1 per cent sulfacetamide several times a day will diminish chances of secondary infection, while irrigation with warm water or boric acid solution eliminates crusting of the purulent discharge (Fig. 11–5).

Retained intranasal foreign bodies may sometimes be causal in cases of unilateral conjunctivitis.

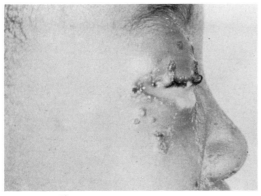

Figure 11–4 Vaccinia of lids.

MEMBRANOUS AND PSEUDOMEMBRANOUS CONJUNCTIVITIS

The pathologic reaction of the conjunctiva to certain bacteria and viruses is one of membrane or pseudomembrane formation. The pseudomembrane is a rich fibrin exudate which forms on the surface of the conjunctiva and is easily peeled off, leaving the surface smooth. Membrane formation is a result of deeper permeation of the exudate into the epithelium. It is removed with difficulty and leaves raw bleeding sites where the epithelium is dislodged. Some of the more common causes of membranous and pseudomembranous conjunctivitis are listed below:

Membranous Conjunctivitis	*Pseudomembranous Conjunctivitis*
Diphtheria Streptococcus	Corynebacterium diphtheria Streptococcus Pneumococcus Staphylococcus Herpes EKC Vernal catarrh, Stevens-Johnson disease Inclusion conjunctivitis

Membranous Conjunctivitis

Membranous conjunctivitis due to diphtheria is uncommon where immunization is widely practiced. The ocular reaction is one of swollen, red, tender lids with gray yellowish membrane formation of the conjunctiva. It is usually associated with inflammation of the upper respiratory passages. Cultures should be made on Löffler's medium or tellurite agar plates. Treatment requires the use of penicillin and diphtheria antitoxin (Fig. 11–6).

Stevens-Johnson Disease

This clinical entity is an eruption of erythema mutiforme involving the skin and mucous membranes of the mouth, conjunctiva, and urethrogenital areas. The lesions appear as red annular patches which form blisters and then ulcerate. The ocular involvement varies. It may be catarrhal, purulent, or a severe pseudomembranous type with marked swelling of the lids and profuse discharge. The cornea may also develop ulceration and even perforation. The acute ocular symptoms may last for several weeks. The etiology is not known. A virus has been suspected. The disease has also been linked with a sensitivity to certain drugs (aspirin, sulfa) and bacteria (strep, staph). Treatment is aimed at the prevention of secondary infection with antibiotics. Systemic steroids in large doses may be of value along with antibiotic administration to relieve the marked inflammatory changes in the tissues. Severe visual impairment and blindness commonly follow the pseudomembranous type.

When there is severe generalized involvement of the skin and mucous membranes, with bullous rupture, plasma loss, secondary infection and so on, the outcome is often fatal (Fig. 11–7).

FOLLICLES AND FOLLICULAR CONJUNCTIVITIS

Follicles are small, grayish, pinhead-sized aggregates of lymphocytes. They are avascular and smaller than the papillae, which contain a vascular tuft. In the newborn infant who lacks lymphoid tissue, there are no follicles present. Later follicles may occur normally at the lateral borders

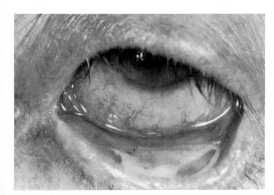

Figure 11–6 Pseudomembranous conjunctivitis.

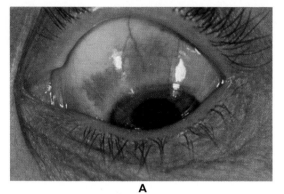

A

Pigmentation of the sclera.

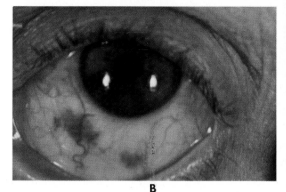

B

Melanosis oculi. (Deeper pigmentation involving iris 5 to 8 o'clock; pigmentation of sclera and conjunctiva.)

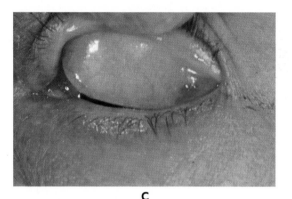

C

Conjunctival telangiectasia of medial aspect of upper lid.

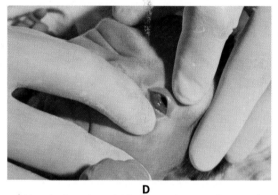

D

Chemical conjunctivitis in newborn 12 hours after silver nitrate.

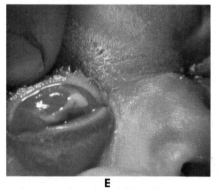

E

Gonococcal conjunctivitis. (Heavy purulent and intense hyperemia; conjunctival edema.)

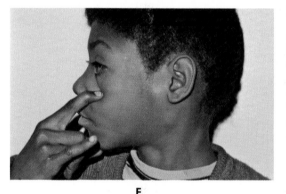

F

Cat-scratch fever. (Note preauricular and subauricular adenopathy.)

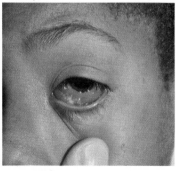

G

Cat-scratch disease. (Note granulomatous changes and chemosis of palpebral conjunctiva.)

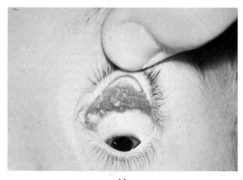

H

Parinaud's conjunctivitis.

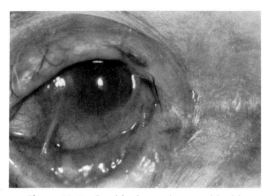

Figure 11–7 Symblepharon in pemphigoid.

of the upper tarsus and in the lower fornix. A noninflammatory follicular hypertrophy of the conjunctiva is common in children and is referred to as *folliculosis.* It is usually associated with hypertrophied lymphoid tissue of the tonsils and adenoids. No treatment is required, since the follicles tend to diminish over a period of time as other lymphoid tissue shrinks. Follicle formation of the conjunctiva in response to inflammation is known as follicular conjunctivitis and is a common manifestation of viral diseases such as inclusion conjunctivitis, adenoviruses, trachoma, and so forth. Chronic follicular conjunctivitis has been treated with cauterization by silver nitrate. This remains an effective form of therapy for the relief of symptoms in those cases in which the etiology is obscure and other medications have failed.

Follicular Conjunctivitis

Adenovirus infections of the conjunctiva generally produce a follicular conjunctivitis which then, depending on the type, affects the cornea. The latter becomes studded with epithelial lesions and subepithelial infiltrates which come and go over a period of weeks or many months. Type 8EKC is the most difficult to isolate. Types 3, 4, 5 and 9 produce cytopathic changes within 2 weeks on Maben cells, whereas type 8 requires more than 20 days. Neutralizing antibody titers in serum occur as early as 13 days, with the majority within 3 to 4 weeks after onset. In a child, adenovirus type 8EKC may manifest as a mild conjunctivitis in

association with an upper respiratory infection. There is little residual keratitis.

TRACHOMA

Trachoma is an ocular disease caused by a virus-like agent belonging to the psittacosis-lymphogranuloma group intermediate between rickettsiae and true viruses. The disease occurs widely in the Orient and Middle East countries. It is uncommon in the United States except in certain areas of the southwest, on Indian reservations of Arizona and New Mexico. Studies of Navajo Indians reveal that approximately 50 per cent of the adults indicated past or present infection with trachoma (Figs. 11–8 and 11–9).

Most trachoma currently seen in school population children is relatively mild. The high incidence of active disease is in the 14- to 19-year-old age group, with a rather marked predominance in girls. This finding suggests that transmission may occur via eye cosmetics.

Clinically the disease is characterized by progressive stages of acute catarrhal conjunctivitis, the development of follicles, papillary hypertrophy, and involvement of the cornea with vascular invasion, and ends with cicatricial changes and total vascularization of the cornea. The early stages are confined to the upper tarsal plate, with follicles predominant. The upper third of the limbus cornea is involved with epithelial keratitis and subepithelial infiltrates and extension of capillary loops. Laboratory studies include the examination of epithelial scrap-

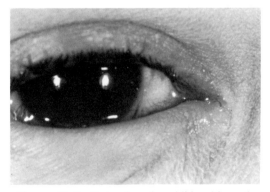

Figure 11–8 Entropion in child with active trachoma.

ings which are stained with Giemsa and demonstrate cytoplasmic inclusion bodies. Expressed follicle material reveals the presence of large macrophages (Leber cells) and lymphoblasts. This may serve to differentiate trachomatous from non-trachomatous follicles.

The agent can be grown on the developing chick embryo. Treatment includes systemic sulfonamides and antibiotics of the tetracycline group. Sulfonamides may be given systemically for 2 weeks, combined with topical administration of antibiotics four times daily for 6 weeks.

CRAB LOUSE INFESTATION

Conjunctivitis may be secondary to infestation of the eyelids with lice. The crab louse (*Phthirus pubis*) can be found in the base of the lashes along with nits (Figs. 11–10 and 11–11). The symptoms are usually intense itching and irritation. Treatment with 1 per cent gamma benzine hexachloride (Kwell cream) applied to the lid margins has been reported effective. Other treatment includes 3 per cent ammoniated mercury ointment or eserine (physostigmine) ointment.

PARINAUD'S CONJUNCTIVITIS

There are cases of unilateral conjunctivitis occurring in children that are associated with enlargement and tenderness of the preauricular nodes on the side affected. They are referred to as Parinaud's conjunctivitis. Apparently over the years

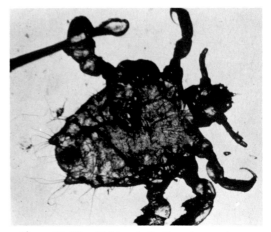

Figure 11–10   *Phthisus pubis* (louse) grasping eyelash.

this diagnosis has encompassed a number of etiologies. The conjunctivitis may be catarrhal or follicular and involves the palpebral conjunctiva sufficiently to give the appearance of ptosis of the upper lid. Some causes include adenovirus infection with associated keratitis, viral disease, *Pasteurella tuberculosis*, tuberculosis, Leptothrix transmission from contact with cats, lymphopathia venereum, cat-scratch fever, and others. The affection is therefore a nonspecific entity etiologically, but clinically it comprises the findings of conjunctivitis, preauricular adenopathy, and glandular enlargements (parotid). The adenopathy may become suppurative and the conjunctival lesions granulomatous.

CAT-SCRATCH DISEASE

In a series of 152 patients with cat-scratch disease, all had lymphadenopathy, but only 8.5 per cent of these cases progressed to suppuration. The infectious agent remains unknown. The most likely cause is thought to be a microorganism of the psittacosis-lymphogranuloma group.

A granulomatous lesion usually involving the conjunctiva of one eye was associated with preauricular adenopathy. Characteristically, there is minimal conjunctival erythema and no purulent exudate. In the above series, of 19 patients presenting with preauricular adenopathy, 6 had inoculation sites represented by granulomas in the eye. Association with

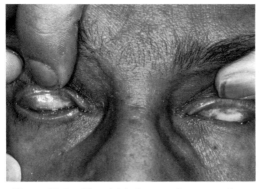

Figure 11–9   Cicatricial changes due to trachoma in boy 17 years old.

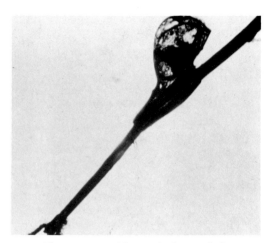

Figure 11–11 Nit attached to eyelash.

cats was reported in all but two cases in the series. Antibiotics and steroids did not prove to be of value (Carithers et al.).

TREATMENT

The treatment of conjunctivitis obviously depends on removal of the cause when known. Viral diseases are self-limited. TRIC viruses respond to sulfonamides and tetracyclines, and bacteria to the chemotherapeutic agent or antibiotic to which they are sensitive. The aim in treatment should be to give specific therapy in sufficient quantity. This means using multiple drops at frequent intervals (every hour or two) and ointment preparations at bedtime. Secretions or discharge should be gently irrigated with either saline or boric solution prior to instillation of medication. Care should be taken to avoid contamination of the dropper tip from contact with the lashes. The hands should be washed before and after handling the infected eyes to avoid spread of the infection. Compresses may be used cold or warm. Cold tends to reduce edema. Vasoconstrictors may be useful in nonspecific etiologies to reduce congestion and promote comfort. Steroids are of value in allergic cases but may be responsible for masking the toxic effect of certain antibiotics with which they are combined. In general treatment should be continued for 48 hours after the eyes revert to a normal appearance. One should avoid overtreatment and be constantly aware of drug toxicities. Patients who have been treated by a number of different antibiotic or chemotherapeutic combinations over a period of time often will improve by discontinuing all medications for several days and using plain lukewarm water compresses three or four times a day. When the skin of the lids is rough, excoriated, and irritated, a plain white vaseline may be applied sparingly two or three times a day. A fair number of recalcitrant cases will respond to this treatment. Chronicity should alert one to seek associated causes in the adnexal areas, lids, tear sac, and sinuses as well as environmental and systemic etiologies.

SUMMARY

It is obvious that conjunctivitis has many causes. In newborn infants with purulent discharge one should consider the more serious bacterial causes such as staphylococci, gonococci, meningococci, and Pseudomonas. Other etiologies should include inclusion conjunctivitis. In nonpurulent watery types of conjunctivitis a search for congenital abnormalities must be made. These are canalicular obstruction, absence or stenosis of the punctum, congenital glaucoma, and so on. Foreign bodies and abrasions along with chemical conjunctivitis due to silver nitrate are also to be considered. In older children bacterial and viral diseases are more common causes of conjunctivitis. Petechial or hemorrhagic types should make one suspect pneumonococcus, streptococcus or Koch-Weeks bacteria. Noninfectious hemorrhagic types may be caused by blood dyscrasias or other systemic disease. Purulent conjunctivitis may be staphylococcal, streptococcal, gonococcal, and so on. Sterile purulent discharge may be on the basis of viral, adenovirus, or epidemic keratoconjunctivitis infection. Follicular conjunctivitis is usually of viral etiology and one should consider the TRIC viruses in the differential diagnosis. Papillary conjunctivitis is more often allergic. Chronicity or history of trauma associated with poor response to medication is suggestive of fungus disease.

One cannot simplify the diagnosis when so broad a scope of causal agents may be responsible for this disease. Emphasis must be placed on thorough clinical examination and adequate laboratory tests (examination of smears, cytology, and cultures). The results are often rewarding when an adequate effort is made.

REFERENCES

Allen, J. H.: External Diseases of the Eye. *In* Liebman, S. D., and Gellis, S. S.: Pediatrician's Ophthalmology. St. Louis, The C. V. Mosby Co., 1966.

Carithers, H. A., Carithers, C. M., and Edwards, R. O. Jr.: Cat-scratch disease. J.A.M.A., *207*:312–316, January, 1969.

Dawson, C. R., Hanno, L., Wood, M.A.T.R., and Despain, R.: Conjunctivitis in the United States. III. Epidemiologic, Clinical and Microbiological Features. Amer. J. Ophthal., *69*:473–480, March, 1970.

Doggart, J. H.: Diseases of Children's Eyes. St. Louis, The C. V. Mosby Co., 1959.

Duke-Elder, S.: System of Ophthalmology. Vol. 3. Part I: Conjunctiva. St. Louis, The C. V. Mosby Co., 1965.

Ellis, P. P., and Smith, D. L.: Handbook of Ocular Therapeutics and Pharmacology. 3rd ed. St. Louis, The C. V. Mosby Co., 1969.

Foster, R. K., Dawson, C. R., and Schacter, J.: Late follow up of patients with neonatal inclusion conjunctivitis. Amer. J. Ophthal., *69*:467–472, March, 1970.

Frederique, G., Howard, R. O., and Boniuk, V.: Corneal ulcers in rubeola. Amer. J. Ophthal., *68*:996–1003, December, 1969.

Havener, W. H.: Ocular Pharmacology. 2nd ed. St. Louis, The C. V. Mosby Co., 1970.

Holt, L. B.: Pediatric Ophthalmology. Philadelphia, Lea & Febiger, 1964.

Leopold, I. H.: International Ophthalmology Clinics, Ocular Therapeutics. Boston, Little, Brown and Co., 1961.

Mitsue, Y., et al.: Association of adenovirus type 8 with epidemic keratoconjunctivitis. Special reference to the infantile form of the disease. Arch. Ophthal., *61*:891, 1959.

Mordhorst, C., and Dawson, C. R.: Sequelae of neonatal inclusion conjunctivitis and associated disease in parents. Amer. J. Ophthal., *71*:861–867, April, 1971.

New Orleans Academy of Ophthalmology: Infectious Diseases of the Conjunctiva and Cornea. St. Louis, The C. V. Mosby Co., 1963.

Nicholas, J. P., and Goolden, E. B.: Bacteriologic culture results in conjunctivitis. Arch. Ophthal., *75*:639, 1966.

Annual Review of Cornea. Arch Ophthal., 1971.

Thygeson, P.: Historical review of oculogenital disease. Amer. J. Ophthal., *71*:975–985, May, 1971.

Thygeson, P.: Ocular viral diseases. Med. Clin. N. Amer., *43*:(5):1419, 1959.

CHAPTER 12

DISEASES OF THE CORNEA

PETER R. LAIBSON, M.D.,
and GEORGE O. WARING, M.D.*

Diseases affecting the cornea and anterior segment in children differ little from disease in adults with the exception of the congenital and developmental abnormalities. There are, of course, specific diseases which first appear in infancy and childhood. Many corneal changes which are seen in the adult had their origins in childhood. If the patient had been examined during the original period of disease in childhood, the nature of the

*Authors' Comments: This discussion of congenital abnormalities of the anterior ocular segment consists of two portions: (1) a discussion of embryology in which developmental disorders are related to embryologic events, and (2) a discussion of specific congenital corneal abnormalities. Since concern is primarily with corneal disease, malformations of the iris, including aniridia, are excluded, except for incidental mention in the context of embryology.

The bibliography is limited to standard works on embryology and one or two articles on each abnormality discussed.

We gratefully acknowledge Miss Karen Albert, who did the drawings, and Dr. William Townsend and Dr. Arthur H. Keeney, who reviewed the manuscript. Illustrative photographs are acknowledged in the figure legends.

This work was suppported in part by Grant No. EY-00339-07 from the National Eye Institute (Dr. Laibson).

adult corneal disease would be better understood.

This chapter will delineate the common diseases of the earlier years of life which primarily affect the cornea, although they also may involve the surrounding structures such as conjunctiva, sclera, lids, and anterior chamber. The discussion will be divided into several areas:

   I. Embryology and developmental abnormalities
  II. Infections of the cornea
     A. Bacterial infections
     B. Viral infections
     C. TRIC agent infections
 III. Hypersensitivity manifestations of corneal disease
 IV. Corneal dystrophies and degeneration
  V. Corneal manifestations of systemic disease
 VI. Corneal injuries

EMBRYOLOGY AND DEVELOPMENTAL ABNORMALITIES

The anterior segment of the eye includes cornea, anterior chamber angle,

273

iris, and lens. Because several anatomic and physiologic systems are packed into a small space, its embryology and resultant malformations are difficult to understand. The use of multiple names for each malformation further complicates the picture. For example, mesodermal dysgenesis of the iris is also called Rieger's anomaly and includes both posterior embryotoxon and Axenfeld's anomaly. It sometimes co-exists with Peters' anomaly and may itself be a component of Rieger's syndrome. Confusion may be reduced by reviewing the development of the anterior segment and observing how each abnormality derives from arrested or aberrant growth. Once this anatomic basis is clear, descriptive and eponymic designations can be applied with better understanding (Table 12–1).

Most anterior segment congenital abnormalities are genetically determined defects of growth and differentiation. All developing tissues have a time during which they are maximally susceptible to injury and any agent interfering with proper differentiation at this sensitive period may produce an abnormality. Thus, similar malformations may result from the presence of abnormal genes, excess or inadequate metabolites, viral or other infectious agents, exogenous toxins, or mechanical insults. Likewise, the same agents insulting the developing fetus at different times will have different effects, depending on which tissues are most vulnerable.

The exact time during development at which malformations occur and the exact mechanism of aberrant development are unknown in many instances. However, the discussion that follows gives approximate times and speculative mechanisms to help the student of ocular embryology correlate developmental events with observed abnormalities. Against this approximate background he can refine chronology and etiology as more definite information becomes available.

Developmental periods are designated in weeks and months of gestation rather than the more exact crown-rump length, because the time periods have more meaning for the clinician.

General Development

In broad perspective, development of the globe consists of three major events (Fig. 12–1).

1. Invagination of neuroectoderm to form the optic vesicle and cup (complete by 6 weeks). This becomes the retina posteriorly and the epithelium of the ciliary body and iris anteriorly.

2. Invagination of surface ectoderm to form the lens vesicle (complete by 6 weeks).

3. Migration of the mesoderm which surrounds the mouth of the optic cup in four planes:

   a. Immediately beneath the surface ectoderm as two avascular waves to form the cornea (6th to 7th week).
   b. In front of the lens as a vascular wave to form the pupillary membrane, which later becomes the anterior iris stroma (7th week).
   c. Posteriorly around the outside of the optic cup to form the ciliary body, choroid, and sclera (2nd to 5th month).
   d. In the anterior chamber angle to form the trabecular meshwork and Schlemm's canal (6th to 8th month).

Cornea

The lens separates from the surface ectoderm at about 6 weeks. If this separation is incomplete, adhesion of cornea and lens may be present at birth. Delay of separation may block the ingrowth of mesoderm, producing a posterior corneal defect and corneal leukoma aligned with an anterior polar cataract (Figs. 12–18 and 12–19C).

Soon after the separation of the lens vesicle, a homogeneous acellular fibrillar membrane spreads beneath the epithelium. The origin of this primary stroma (or mesostroma) is not certain, but it may be secreted by the basal cells of the epithelium. It probably serves as a directional membrane along which corneogenic mesoderm migrates (Fig. 12–1A). This layer is prominent in lower animals, is difficult to see in primates, and may contribute to the formation of Bowman's membrane.

The first wave of mesoderm from around the optic cup sweeps between the primary stroma and lens at about 6 weeks to form the corneal endothelium, which will secrete its basement membrane (Desce-

TABLE 12–1 EPONYMS AND ANOMALIES

	Posterior Embryotoxon	Axenfeld's Anomaly	Axenfeld's Syndrome*	Rieger's Anomaly*	Posterior Keratoconus	Peters' Anomaly**	Mesodermal Dysgenesis of Iris and Cornea*
Developmental	Prominent Schwalbe's ring	Prominent Schwalbe's ring	Prominent Schwalbe's ring	Prominent Schwalbe's ring			Prominent Schwalbe's ring
		Iris strands to Schwalbe's ring	Iris strands to Schwalbe's ring	Iris strands to Schwalbe's ring			Iris strands to Schwalbe's ring
			Glaucoma	± Glaucoma (60%)		± Glaucoma	± Glaucoma
				Hypoplasia anterior iris stroma			Hypoplasia anterior iris stroma
Abnormality					Central posterior corneal depression	Central posterior corneal defect	Central posterior corneal defect
					Corneal leukoma	Corneal leukoma	Corneal leukoma
						Iris adhesions to leukoma	Iris adhesions to leukoma
						Lens adhesion to leukoma	

*May have systemic abnormalities.
**If inflammatory etiology, internal corneal ulcer of von Hippel.

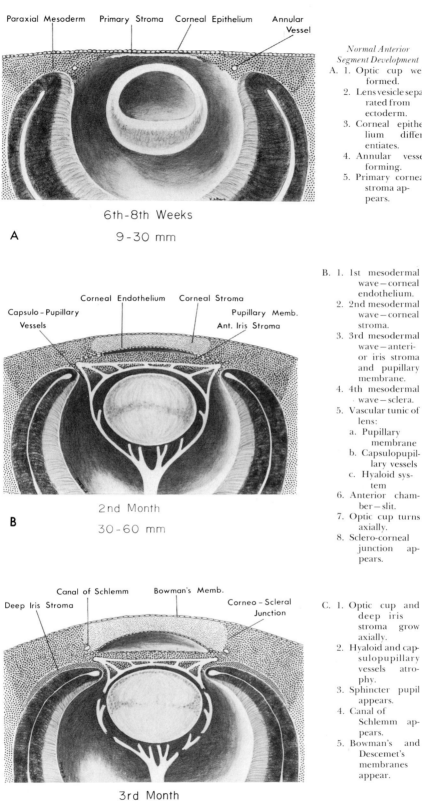

Paraxial Mesoderm   Primary Stroma   Corneal Epithelium   Annular Vessel

6th-8th Weeks

A   9-30 mm

Corneal Endothelium   Corneal Stroma

Capsulo-Pupillary Vessels

Pupillary Memb.

Ant. Iris Stroma

2nd Month

B   30-60 mm

Canal of Schlemm   Bowman's Memb.

Deep Iris Stroma

Corneo-Scleral Junction

3rd Month

C   60-70 mm

Normal Anterior Segment Development

A. 1. Optic cup well formed.
   2. Lens vesicle separated from ectoderm.
   3. Corneal epithelium differentiates.
   4. Annular vessel forming.
   5. Primary corneal stroma appears.

Possible Abnormalities (Chronology Speculative)

1. Absence of cornea.
2. Corneolenticular adhesion.

B. 1. 1st mesodermal wave—corneal endothelium.
   2. 2nd mesodermal wave—corneal stroma.
   3. 3rd mesodermal wave—anterior iris stroma and pupillary membrane.
   4. 4th mesodermal wave—sclera.
   5. Vascular tunic of lens:
      a. Pupillary membrane
      b. Capsulopupillary vessels
      c. Hyaloid system
   6. Anterior chamber—slit.
   7. Optic cup turns axially.
   8. Sclero-corneal junction appears.

1. Posterior corneal defect.
2. Mesodermal dysgenesis of iris (Rieger).
3. Corneal dermoids.
4. Anterior staphyloma.
5. Megalocornea.
6. Sclerocornea.

C. 1. Optic cup and deep iris stroma grow axially.
   2. Hyaloid and capsulopupillary vessels atrophy.
   3. Sphincter pupil appears.
   4. Canal of Schlemm appears.
   5. Bowman's and Descemet's membranes appear.

1. Aniridia.
2. Atypical iris coloboma, hole, corectopia, polycoria.
3. Microcoria.

Figure 12–1   Embryologic development of anterior ocular segment and malformations

(Illustration continued on opposite page.)

Figure 12–1 *Continued.*

Normal Anterior Segment Development	*Possible Abnormalities (chronology Speculative)*
D. 1. Corneal curvature increases. 2. Iris and ciliary body well developed. 3. Marginal sinus maximal. 4. Aqueous secretion begins. 5. Angle anterior chamber forming.	1. Cornea plana. 2. Corneal astigmatism. 3. Prominent Schwalbe's ring (posterior embryotoxon). 4. Microcornea. 5. Congenital iris cysts. 6. Iris-corneal adhesions.

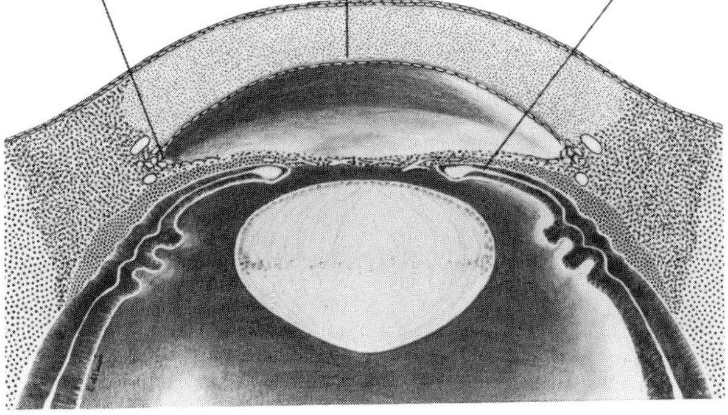

Angle Mesoderm   Descemet's Memb.   Iris Stroma

D   4th – 6th Months   70 – 200 mm

E. 1. Corneal epithelium 4 layers. 2. Mesodermal tissue in angle rarefying. 3. Trabecular meshwork forms. 4. Pupillary membrane atrophies.	1. Iris processes. 2. Prominent uveal trabecular meshwork. 3. Congenital glaucoma. 4. Persistent pupillary membrane.

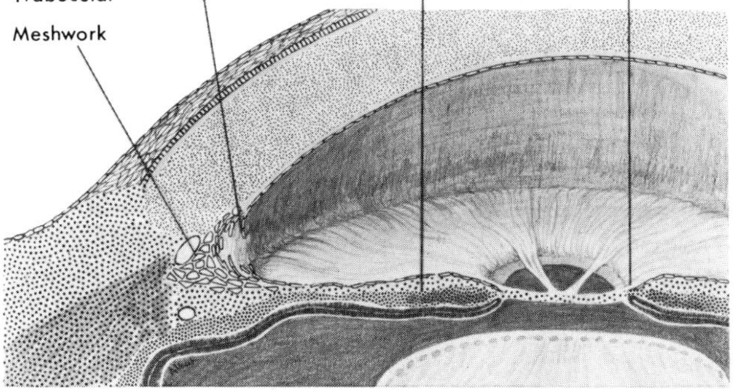

Angle Mesoderm – Endothelium   Superficial Iris Stroma

Trabecular Meshwork   Deep Iris Stroma

E   7th – 9th Months   200 – 300 mm

met's membrane) at about 3 months. The second wave of mesoderm follows quickly, migrating between the epithelium and endothelium to form corneal stroma (Fig. 12–1B).

The stroma early arranges itself in lamellar fashion. The fibroblasts of the posterior part of the cornea form their collagen fibers in a clearly organized fashion while those in the anterior portion produce a loose, less differentiated pattern. As the fibroblasts decrease in number, mucopolysaccharide content increases, first in the more organized posterior area, and later anteriorly. This two-layered pattern of development, which is evident in the adult cornea, may form the

basis for the limitation of some dystrophic processes to the anterior stroma (e.g., Reis-Bückler's dystrophy).

As the endothelium becomes more active, the cornea becomes dehydrated and more transparent while the sclera, with its irregular collagen fiber organization and lack of endothelium, becomes less transparent.

Incomplete migration of the first wave of mesoderm may leave a central defect in endothelium and Descemet's membrane which may couple with a stromal defect because of incomplete migration of the second wave. This central posterior corneal defect is called Peters' anomaly when inflammation is not present, and an internal ulcer of von Hippel when inflammation is evident (Figs. 12–9, 12–12, 12–15B, and 12–17A to C). An anterior staphyloma represents a more severe degree of failure of corneal mesoderm to form properly so that a thin, ectatic, leukoma lined by uveal tissue replaces the cornea (Fig. 12–19C).

Indistinct delimitation of cornea from sclera produces a scleralized cornea (Fig. 12–1B). Vascularized scleral tissue extends into the anatomic cornea, occasionally replacing it entirely (sclerocornea) (Fig. 12–27). The establishment of corneal margins is one factor determining corneal size.

Both ectodermal and mesodermal corneal tissues may become metaplastic during development. If the epithelium becomes keratinized and forms hair follicles, sebaceous glands, and sweat glands and if the mesoderm forms dense underlying fibrous tissue, the cornea is replaced by skin. This may be continuous with that of the face, sealing the globe beneath (cryptophthalmos). If this process is less extensive, a corneal dermoid results (Figs. 12–20 to 12–26).

By the 3rd month the structural cornea is present. Further development is largely related to corneal size and shape. At about 6 weeks the optic cup begins to grow forward and axially to form the pigmented epithelium of the ciliary body and iris (Fig. 12–1C). If the turning of the cup axially is delayed so that its mouth (ciliary ring) is large, the anterior segment will be enlarged (anterior megalophthalmos, megalocornea.) On the other hand, if the optic cup grows axially in a normal fashion to form a spherical globe, but growth of the anterior segment is then retarded (after the 5th month), microcornea may result.

Until 4 months, corneal and scleral curvature are the same. At that time the corneal growth rate accelerates, resulting in a greater corneal curve that produces the +43.00 diopters of corneal refraction. Arrest of this increased curvature results in cornea plana (Figs. 12–1C and D).

Iris

Paraxial mesoderm forms both the vascular and stromal portions of the iris.

Vascular elements first appear at 6 weeks. The annular vessel forms circumferentially around the mouth of the optic cup and is later replaced by the greater circle of the iris (Fig. 12–1A). From the annular vessel a series of vascular arcades accompanied by mesodermal stroma extend centrally between the lens and corneal endothelium to form the anterior portion of the vascular tunic of the lens (pupillary membrane), which later becomes the superficial layer of iris stroma (Fig. 12–1B). At the same time, the hyaloid artery has grown through the embryonic fissure of the optic stalk and across the vitreous cavity to the posterior aspect of the lens, where it ramifies as the posterior portion of the vascular tunic of the lens. The annular vessel sends branches posteriorly (between the rim of the optic cup and the equator of the lens) to anastomose with branches of the hyaloid vessel. These capsulopupillary vessels are the lateral portion of the vascular tunic of the lens. They are straight, do not anastomose with each other, and form a picket-fence-like enclosure for the lens (Fig. 12–1B).

Each of these three portions of the vascular tunic of the lens (anterior pupillary membrane, lateral capsulopupillary vessels and posterior hyaloid system) atrophies in later embryonic development, leaving the lens avascular in postnatal life (Figs. 12–1C and D). Failure of the anterior portion to atrophy produces a persistent pupillary membrane. If the posterior hyaloid vessels do not involute, persistent hyperplastic primary vitreous may result. Persistence of the capsulopupillary vessels extending from the iris to the lens may block the optic cup as it grows axially between the iris stroma and lens (Fig. 12–1C). This may influence the development of aniridia or atypical colobomas of the iris.

If the pupillary membrane fails to form primarily, the optic cup will lack a directional membrane, and only a rudimentary iris will develop (aniridia). Hypoplasia of this anterior leaf of iris stroma is part of the syndrome of mesodermal dysgenesis of the iris (Rieger's anomaly).

As the optic cup grows axially, it carries with it a layer of mesoderm which will become the deep stromal layer of the iris (Fig. 12–1D). This layer never extends past the margin of the pupil. A primary failure of the optic cup to grow in may result in a rudimentary iris (aniridia). The association of foveal hypoplasia with aniridia gives some evidence for this ectodermal theory.

As the optic cup grows between the lens and the pupillary membrane, it meets the barrier of tough, nondistensible fibrovascular capsulopupillary vessels (Fig. 12–1C). If these vessels atrophy, the cup can pass unimpeded. However, if they persist, aniridia may result. Some aniridic patients demonstrate these persistent vascular remnants. Others have a rudimentary iris doubled back on itself, as if it had hit a barrier and grown backward in the direction of least resistance.

Thus, three possible mechanisms may be implicated in the development of aniridia: (1) absence of the superficial stromal directional membrane, (2) primary failure of optic cup growth, and (3) persistence of capsulopupillary vessels.

Persistence of capsulopupillary vessels in a single area might block optic cup growth there, producing an atypical coloboma of the iris. (A typical iris coloboma results from failure of closure of the embryonic fissure inferonasally.) A wide variety of colobomatous defects may occur: a small notch in the pupil; a cleft in the iris extending partially to the periphery; a defect involving zonules, ciliary body, and choroid; a hole in the iris without a sphincter muscle (pseudopolycoria), as if the optic cup had grown around a capsulopupillary vessel; a separate pupil with a sphincter muscle (true polycoria), as if the optic cup had grown around a vessel at the time of iris sphincter formation; a defect over which a band of stroma extends (bridge coloboma); a distorted pupil (slit-shaped pupil, corectopia). All colobomatous and pupillary defects in iris development may result from primary dysgenesis of the mesoderm and neuroectoderm, and the mechanical role of capsulopupillary vessels is only inferential.

A number of other iris abnormalities may occur. Superficial epithelial cells at the margin of the optic cup differentiate to form the smooth muscle sphincter of the iris; its absence is rare (Fig. 12–1E).

Adjacent epithelial cells form the dilator muscle of the iris, absence of which produces congenital microcoria. As the space between the two layers of the optic cup obliterates, the marginal sinus of von Szily is produced at the mouth of the cup (Figs. 12–1C and D). If this persists, a marginal iris cyst results. Likewise, if the outer epithelial layer of the cup protrudes through the overlying stroma, an iris cyst may form. If the margin of the cup grows around the pupillary margin, sweeping up over the stroma, ectropion of the pigment border results.

At 6 months the anterior stromal layer (pupillary membrane) extends completely across the anterior chamber, and the posterior stromal layer overlying the optic cup extends to the pupillary margin (Fig. 12–12). Gradually, the vascular arcades of the superficial stroma atrophy, so that by birth the pupillary membrane has disappeared, resulting in the collarette of the iris, which lies approximately above the outer circumference of the sphincter (Fig. 12–1E). Remnants of the pupillary membrane may be seen in up to 90 per cent of newborns as strands originating from the collarette and extending across the pupil into the anterior chamber or to the cornea (with leukoma and/or internal ulcer) or to the lens with small anterior capsular opacities. Atrophy of the superficial stroma peripheral to the collarette forms the crypts of the iris, the tissue density depending on the degree of atrophy.

The chromatophores of iris stroma migrate from the neural crest, producing iris pigmentation in utero in black and yellow races and after birth in whites. The density of these melanin-containing cells dictates the color of the iris.

Anterior Chamber Angle

The anterior chamber is a thin slit completely lined by endothelium and containing albuminous fluid from 6 weeks until about 6 months, when the ciliary body begins to secrete aqueous humor (Figs. 12–1B and C). The embryonic cornea and iris lie in close apposition during this time. Failure of complete separation of the two produces absence of the anterior chamber (quite rare). Incomplete separation may leave iris processes bridging the anterior chamber to the cornea, either centrally associated with a posterior corneal defect and corneal leukoma (Peters' anomaly) or peripherally adherent to angle structures.

Mesoderm in the angle of the rudimentary anterior chamber forms Schwalbe's ring, the trabecular meshwork, and the scleral spur (Figs. 12–1*D* and *E*). At 4 months the angle is undifferentiated. The cornea is almost completely developed by this time. Six anatomic portions of the angle develop simultaneously up to the time of birth.

1. *Angle Recess.* The angle itself initially is filled with mesoderm up to the corneal margin. This gradually recedes until the recess of the angle extends out past the scleral spur at birth. This probably occurs because of increased rate of growth of the anterior segment with rarefaction of tissue spaces in the angle mesoderm. Atrophy (cell death) probably plays no role (Fig. 12–1*E*).

2. *Trabecular Meshwork.* The initially solid mesodermal tissue differentiates to form clefts between the collagen trabeculae. The exact nature of this process is unknown.

Two distinct groups of trabeculae form. The deep or outer layer between the cornea and sclera adjacent to Schlemm's canal (corneoscleral trabecular meshwork) is more compact and regular. The superficial or inner meshwork separating the anterior chamber from the corneoscleral meshwork (uveal trabecular meshwork) is looser and more irregular.

Some strands of mesodermal tissue will persist in the proximal portion of the angle extending from the iris base to Schwalbe's line, the trabecular meshwork, or the ciliary body. These are iris processes (Figs. 12–7, 12–11, and 12–17*E*) (sometimes incorrectly called peripheral anterior synechiae) and in lower mammals are uniformly present in a comblike configuration called pectinate ligaments.

The uveal trabecular meshwork extends from the ciliary muscle to end diffusely around Schwalbe's line. In most eyes these fibers are visible at slit lamp examination as a gray band on the endothelial surface (Fig. 12–5).

A system for aqueous drainage seems to be present by the 4th to 6th month, approximately the time the ciliary body begins to secrete aqueous. The facility of outflow increases gradually throughout gestation.

3. *Angle Endothelium.* The endothelial cell layer which overlies mesoderm gradually flattens. Fenestrations appear in the endothelial membrane at about the 8th month (Fig. 12–1*E*). Some endothelial cells bridge the spaces between trabecular fibers by long processes, and others migrate into the meshwork to cover the trabecular fibers. Persistence of the intact endothelial membrane at birth (possibly Barkan's membrane) may prevent the outflow of aqueous, resulting in congenital glaucoma.

4. *Schwalbe's Ring.* By 5 months, fibers can be identified at the peripheral end of Descemet's membrane which will become Schwalbe's anterior border ring. If these fibers are enlarged, Schwalbe's line will project into the anterior chamber as a prominent refractile ring. If it is positioned anteriorly, it may be visible through the cornea (posterior embryotoxon). Such anterior displacement usually carries uveal trabecular meshwork with it, producing a gray veil on the endothelial surface of the peripheral cornea, outlined centrally by the prominent white Schwalbe's line (Figs. 12–6, 12–9, 12–10, 12–14, and 12–17*E*).

5. *Canal of Schlemm.* A plexus of venous channels appears at the junction of the developing corneoscleral junction at about the 3rd month. It gradually takes on a more distinct structure as the canal of Schlemm.

6. *Scleral Spur.* After the canal of Schlemm forms, a triangle of scleral tissue forms behind it at the base of the developing meridional muscle of the ciliary body. This is the scleral spur. Until about the 7th to 8th month, the canal of Schlemm, scleral spur, and greater arterial circle of the iris are embedded in the mesoderm of developing sclera and ciliary body and are separated from the rudimentary anterior chamber by the mesoderm filling the angle recess. As rarefaction occurs and the angle recess forms, the canal of Schlemm gains access to the anterior chamber via the

trabecular meshwork, and the scleral spur is exposed in the recess. The greater arterial circle remains buried in the root of the iris, although in adults with deep angles some of its circumferential channels may appear as snakelike undulations in the recess.

Developmental Variations in Limbal Anatomy

The limbus is a junctional zone. Corneal epithelium and its basement membrane meet conjunctival epithelium and basement membrane. Corneal stroma juxtaposes sclera. Descemet's membrane meets Schwalbe's ring and the trabecular meshwork. Corneal endothelium becomes continuous with the endothelium covering the trabeculae.

These transitional zones form a number of circular structures which can be seen on slit lamp examination (Fig. 12–2), and variations in these structures are common in congenital malformations of the anterior segment.

EPITHELIUM. Corneal and conjunctival epithelia are continuous over the limbus.

Corneal epithelium has about five to eight regularly arranged layers of squamous cells lying on a smooth basement membrane which is supported by the acellular, regularly arranged stromal fibers of Bowman's membrane. The conjunctiva resembles skin with its multilayered epithelium lying on an undulating basement membrane, supported by irregular vascular subconjunctival connective tissue. At the limbus, the conjunctival epithelium forms a series of radially arranged digitations into the subepithelial connective tissue. Each of these is flanked by a vascular connective tissue peg which comes within a few cell layers of the surface. The pigmentation of the basal layers of the epithelial extensions into the connective tissue corresponds to the individual's skin pigmentation. When the basal cells are pigmented, a ring of radially arranged pigmented lines alternating with white spaces is formed at the limbus. The pigmented epithelial portion blends with the conjunctival margin while the white connective tissue projections blend with the corneal border. (These are called the limbal palisades of Vogt [Figs. 12–2 and

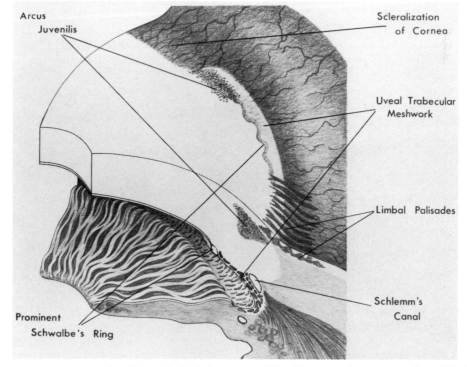

Figure 12–2 Developmental variations in limbal anatomy. This diagrammatic representation of limbal structures illustrates the appearance of each on the anterior surface and demonstrates the location of each in cross section.

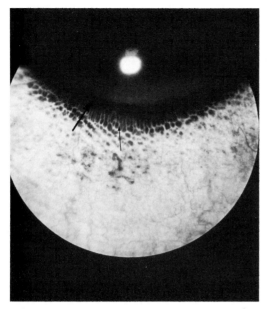

Figure 12–3 Limbal palisades of Vogt. This circle of white finger-like projections (small arrow) which breaks up the limbal pigment ring (large arrow) results from subepithelial connective tissue papillae pushing up near the surface, interrupting the pigmentation of the basal conjunctival epithelium.

12–3].) If the connective tissue projections are not prominent, the pigmented limbal epithelium will appear as a continuous dark brown circle at the corneal margin (Figs. 12–5 and 12–6). In whites, the structural limbal palisades can be seen on careful slit lamp examination, but they are devoid of pigment.

CORNEOSCLERAL JUNCTION. The essential components of both corneal stroma and sclera are collagen fibers, glycosaminoglycans, water, and some cells. Their differences are related to regularity of orientation of collagen fibers and degree of hydration (a dehydrated sclera is translucent). At the limbus, the cornea inserts into the sclera in either a wedge-shaped or oblique fashion. If the superficial rim of sclera extends centrally over the wedge of cornea, the limbus appears as a faint white translucent ring. This is usually the case superiorly and inferiorly, where the cornea is "scleralized" (Figs. 12–2 and 12–4). Thus, the vertical corneal diameter is about 1 mm. less than the horizontal when measured on the anterior surface. Also, deep limbal structures may be hidden from view superiorly and inferiorly while they are visible medially and laterally.

TRABECULAR MESHWORK. Careful slit lamp inspection of the deep corneal limbus nasally and temporally invariably reveals a thin semitransparent gray band which is denser near the limbus and fades gradually into the cornea. It may be hidden from view by scleral extension over the cornea. This is an anterior extension of the uveal trabecular meshwork up to and past Schwalbe's line. If a pig-

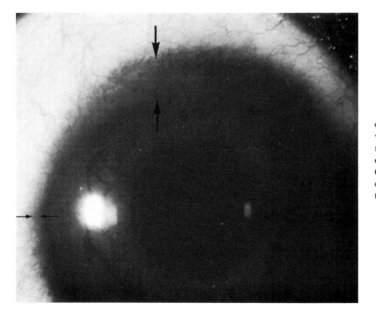

Figure 12–4 Scleralization of the cornea. At 12 o'clock the sclera and its vessels extend superficially into the cornea, hiding underlying iris and angle details (area between two large arrows). Compare the normal extent of sclera over the limbus at 9 o'clock (area between two small arrows).

mented ring is present in the limbal epithelium, the deeper uveal meshwork is set off by contrast and forms a striking gray arc immediately adjacent to the limbus (Figs. 12–2 and 12–5).

CORNEAL STROMA. Infiltration of the anterior and middle thirds of the corneal stroma superiorly and inferiorly with intracellular lipid granules results in a white bow-shaped opacity separated from the limbus by a clear area about 1 mm. wide. In children this anterior embryotoxon or arcus juvenilis corresponds histologically to the more common arcus senilis of adults. Occasionally it is associated with osteogenesis imperfecta, megalocornea, aniridia, or hyperlipemia (types 1 and 2) (Fig. 12–2).

SCHWALBE'S RING. At the deep limbus, corneal endothelium and Descemet's membrane meet the uveal trabecular meshwork at a junction designated as the anterior border ring of Schwalbe (also called Schwalbe's line). The ring is part of the uveal meshwork and has a structure similar to a trabeculum — a collagen-elastic core surrounded by thin leaves of the terminal portion of Descemet's membrane and covered on its inner surface by endothelium. Gonioscopically, it is appreciated as a change in texture from the refractile corneal endothelium to the reticulated translucence of the trabecular meshwork.

Schwalbe's ring may be thickened and positioned centrally, making it visible as an irregular refractile white line lying concentric to the limbus. This is most easily seen nasally or temporally. It may be broken or continuous and frequently has pigment spots on its inner surface representing prior attachment of iris processes. This centrally located prominent Schwalbe's ring is called a posterior embryotoxon (Gr., *embryon* = embryo; *toxon* = bow). If iris processes connect to it, it is known as Axenfeld's anomaly (Figs. 12–7 to 12–11, 12–17).

A prominent Schwalbe's ring is present in 8 to 15 per cent of normal eyes, but this high frequency is apparent only to those who look specifically for it. It may be associated with other ocular anomalies. Usually these involve malformations of mesodermal derivatives. Minor associated variants include hypoplasia of iris stroma, corectopia, polycoria, persistent pupillary membrane, iris colobomas, megalocornea, or high astigmatism. However, it may be part of more severe malformations such as Rieger's anomaly, aniridia, craniofacial dysplasia, and developmental glaucoma.

Mesodermal Dysgenesis of the Iris and Cornea

Since most anterior segment structures

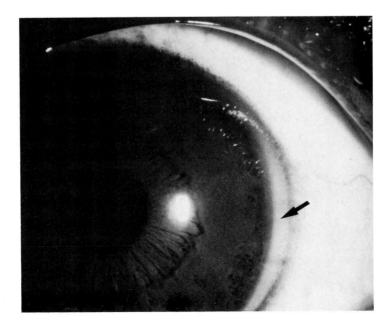

Figure 12–5 Prominent uveal trabecular meshwork. The limbus of this eye is demarcated by a pigment ring. Sclera extends up to but not beyond the ring. The light tissue lying central to the pigment ring (arrow) is uveal trabecular meshwork.

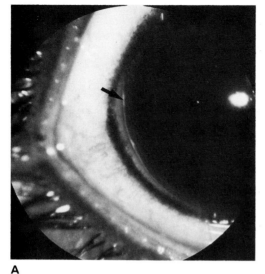

A

Figure 12–6 *A*, Prominent Schwalbe's ring (posterior embryotoxon). As in Figure 12–5, the limbal pigment ring and prominent uveal trabecular meshwork are present. The distinct white ring demarcating the uveal meshwork centrally is the enlarged, displaced Schwalbe's ring (arrow), which may be seen in about 10 per cent of normal eyes. *B*, Normal Schwalbe's ring (*S*). Cornea (*C*) and uveal trabecular meshwork (*T*) about at this juncture. *C*, Prominent Schwalbe's ring (posterior embryotoxon). Endothelium over the cornea (*C*) and the tubular Schwalbe's ring (*S*) has a cobblestone appearance. The trabeculae of the uveal meshwork (*T*) are also covered with endothelium. (Scanning electron micrographs courtesy of Dr. Morton Smith.)

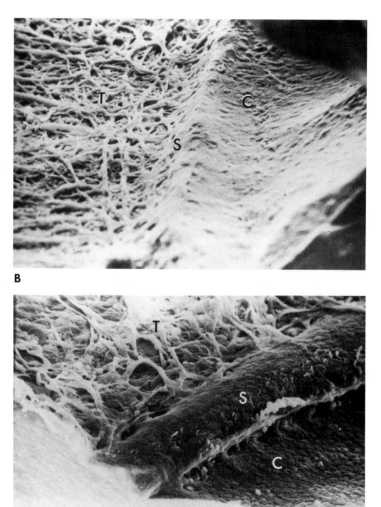
B

C

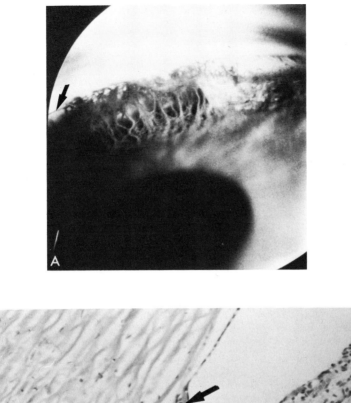

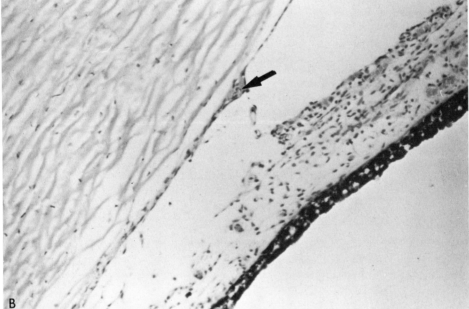

Figure 12–7 *A*, Axenfeld's anomaly. Gonioscopic view showing the angle recess filled with dense iris processes (persistent mesodermal tissue) which extend to a prominent Schwalbe's ring (arrow). This configuration may exist alone or as a part of a variety of iridocorneal dysgenesis. (Courtesy of Dr. Robison D. Harley.) *B*, Histologic section showing the prominent centrally displaced Schwalbe's ring (arrow) with iris processes extending to it (×64). (Courtesy of Dr. Merlyn Rodrigues.)

arise from the paraxial mesoderm, it is reasonable to expect that a defect in that germinal tissue would give rise to the co-existence of a number of abnormalities. This is the case in mesodermal dysgenesis

of the iris (Rieger's anomaly) and cornea (Peters' anomaly), sometimes referred to as the anterior chamber cleavage syndrome.

To clarify the relationship of the com-

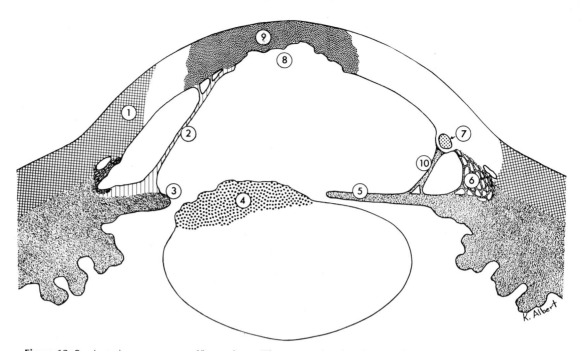

Figure 12–8 Anterior segment malformations. The composite drawing emphasizes that these anomalies are frequently found together. Some combinations have an eponymic designation, while others have no generally recognized name. Description of the individual components of a specific clinical case is of more value than applying blanket labels. (Modified after Reese, A. B., and Ellsworth, R. M.: Arch. Ophthal., 75:307, 1966.

1. Sclerocornea
2. Iris adhesion to corneal defect
3. Hypoiridia
4. Anterior polar cataract
5. Hypoplasia of anterior iris stroma
6. Persistent mesodermal tissue in angle
7. Prominent Schwalbe's ring
8. Central posterior corneal defect
9. Corneal opacity
10. Iris process to Schwalbe's ring

ponents of mesodermal dysgenesis of the iris and cornea, Table 12–1 correlates the developmental abnormality with the eponyms used clinically. Figure 12–8 is a composite drawing of these developmental abnormalities.

MESODERMAL DYSGENESIS OF THE IRIS (RIEGER'S ANOMALY). This anomaly includes nonprogressive hypoplasia of the anterior leaf of iris stroma accompanied by a prominent Schwalbe's ring to which iris strands are connected (Figs. 12–8 to 12–14).

Sex incidence is equal. Autosomal dominant inheritance can be demonstrated in 70 per cent of cases, with almost total penetrance of the gene but with a highly variable expressivity. Thus, surveys of families of persons with Rieger's anomaly will frequently reveal additional involved individuals, but a wide variation in the degree and type of iris and angle abnormality will exist (Figs. 12–9, 12–13,

12–14, and 12–17). About one third of cases are sporadic.

The clinical picture includes a high incidence of astigmatism and marked ametropia (about 50 per cent) and a similar incidence of strabismus (about 65 per cent). The sclera may appear blue and scleralization of the cornea is frequently present. This ill-defined corneal limbus might lead to the overdiagnosis of microcornea. Corneal size is normal in only about 65 per cent of patients, 25 per cent having megalocornea and 10 per cent having microcornea. Keratometry shows some shift toward corneal flattening.

The cornea may contain a posterior defect (Figs. 12–9 and 12–12). This defect of the endothelium, Descemet's membrane, and deep stroma may underlie clear cornea or it may be covered by a disciform leukoma which usually has iris processes extending to its borders. The presence of these corneal abnormalities in Rieger's

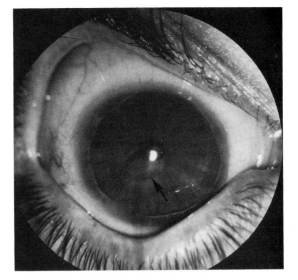

Figure 12–9 Rieger's anomaly with central posterior corneal defect. This right eye of a 23-year-old dwarf demonstrates a prominent Schwalbe's ring with iris process extending to it, an atrophic anterior iris stroma, and a central posterior corneal defect (arrow). Intraocular pressure was normal. Left eye appeared similar. (Courtesy of Dr. David Pao.)

mesodermal dysgenesis of the iris is what links it developmentally to Peters' mesodermal dysgenesis of the cornea. Otherwise, the entities are distinct.

Because the anterior iris stroma is absent, the usual appearance of Fuchs's crypts and vascular trabeculae is replaced by dull, slender, radial fibers of the deep stroma through which the iris sphincter and pigment epithelium are seen (Figs. 12–13 and 12–17*E*). Occasionally defects in the pigment epithelium are present.

Persistence of the pupillary membrane is rare.

Pupillary abnormalities are present in about 75 per cent of cases, including ectopic pupils (corectopia), abnormally shaped pupils (dyscoria), holes without a sphincter (pseudopolycoria), iridodiastasis, and ectropion of the pigment layer (Fig. 12–13).

A prominent Schwalbe's ring is always present with iris strands reaching to it (Axenfeld's anomaly) (Figs. 12–8, 12–10,

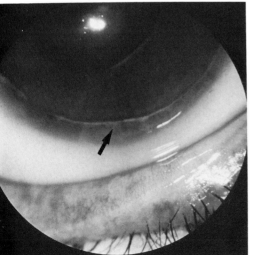

Figure 12–10 Rieger's anomaly. Close-up of 6 o'clock limbus of eye in Figure 12–8. Iris processes (arrow) extend to the irregular prominent Schwalbe's ring. (Courtesy of Dr. David Pao).

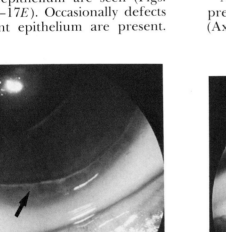

Figure 12-11 Angle in Rieger's anomaly. Gonioscopic appearance of eye in Figure 12–8 showing iris processes extending to Schwalbe's ring.

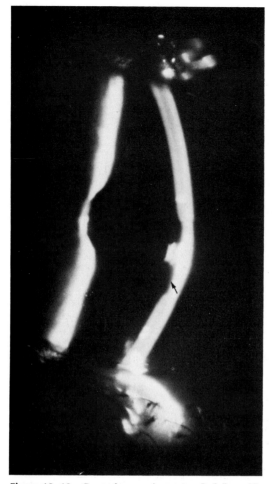

Figure 12–12 Central posterior corneal defect. Slit lamp view of eye in Figure 12–8 showing the depression in the posterior corneal surface (arrow). Cornea overlying it is clear and no iris processes extend to its margin. (Courtesy of Dr. David Pao.)

12–11, 12–13, 12–14, and 12–19D). The strands may extend from more central portions of the iris pulling the pupil out of shape. The root of the iris is hypoplastic with visible iridial vessels. A brownish-yellow tissue can sometimes be seen within the angle on gonioscopy, presumably persistence of endothelial and mesodermal tissue.

A variant of mesodermal dysgenesis of the iris is called iridogoniodysgenesis. It consists of hypoplasia of the anterior leaf of iris stroma, corectopia, and persistence of mesodermal tissue in the angle without a prominent Schwalbe's line or iris processes. Premature formation of cataracts is present. Inheritance may be autosomal recessive.

Apart from cosmetic appearance and occasional corneal opacities, Rieger's anomaly is of clinical significance because glaucoma is found in about 60 per cent of cases. The diagnosis of glaucoma should be made with caution, since one fourth of the patients have megalocornea which could be confused with buphthalmos. The glaucoma occurs presumably because of faulty angle development. However, congenital glaucoma with buphthalmos is rare in Rieger's anomaly. The onset of glaucoma is seldom before 5 years of age, and usually occurs from 5 to 20 years (juvenile glaucoma). After age 20 the frequency of onset is evenly distributed in each decade up to 50 years. The reason for delayed onset of developmental glaucoma is unknown. The clinical obligation to individuals with Rieger's anomaly is clear: they must be followed two or three times a year all their lives with measurement of ocular tension and plotting of visual fields to detect glaucoma at the earliest possible time. The clinical course of this non-buphthalmic glaucoma is similar to that of simple chronic open angle glaucoma.

Additional findings in Rieger's anomaly include pigment spots on the anterior lens capsule at the point of prior pupillary membrane attachments. Rarely, cataracts, subluxation of the lens, or colobomas of the lens margin are present. The choroid may be hypoplastic. The retina is usually normal. Facial malformations may be present (Rieger's syndrome). These include mandibular or maxillary hypoplasia, telecanthus, agenesis of dental elements to produce oligodontia vera, dysgenesis of dental elements to produce microdontia, conical teeth, or partial anodontia vera. Dental elements form at the same embryologic period as iris structures, and similar genetic factors may be at work to produce this association.

Differential diagnosis of mesodermal dysgenesis of the iris includes the following:

1. *Essential Progressive Iris Atrophy.* This acquired, unilateral, progressive disease is seen predominantly in young adult females and is manifested by iris atrophy, pupillary abnormalities, peripheral anterior synechiae, and glaucoma. No prominent Schwalbe's ring or peripheral iris strands are present.

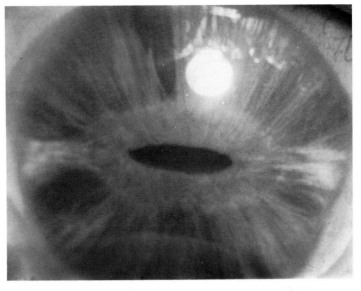

Figure 12–13 Rieger's syndrome. The right eye shows marked hypoplasia of the anterior iris stroma. The deep stroma is thin and fibrillary, revealing the underlying iris epithelium and pupillary sphincter. The pupil is slit-shaped and central. The prominent Schwalbe's ring is poorly illustrated. (Courtesy of Dr. George Spaeth.)

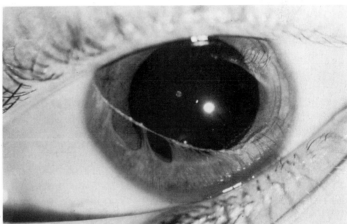

Figure 12–14 Rieger's anomaly. This 10-year-old white female presents a centrally displaced prominent Schwalbe's ring with iris processes extending to it from the angle recess and the collarette. Anterior iris stroma is absent at 11 o'clock. The configuration is accentuated by the dilated pupil. Intraocular pressure was normal. No other ocular anomalies existed. (Courtesy of Dr. Harold Koller.)

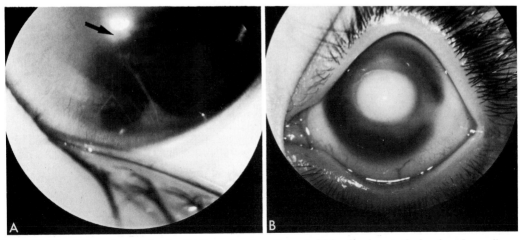

Figure 12–15 *A*, Peters' anomaly. A mild form showing attenuated iris adhesions to the border of a small corneal opacity (arrow). This was present bilaterally in this 9-month-old white female. *B*, Peters' anomaly. This 10-month-old white female had bilateral congenital central corneal opacities. During penetrating keratoplasty, iris adhesions were found extending from the pupillary margin to the borders of the opacity. An anterior polar cataract was present. (Courtesy of Dr. Harold Koller.)

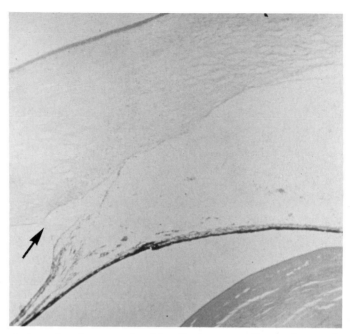

Figure 12–16   Histologic section demonstrating iris adhesions extending to the margin of a central posterior corneal defect. The overlying cornea is edematous (×6). (Courtesy of Dr. Robert D'Amico.)

2. *Primary Infantile Glaucoma.* This may be associated with iris atrophy, but is either autosomal recessive or sporadic, may be unilateral and is usually unaccompanied by a prominent Schwalbe's ring.

3. *Oculodentodigital Dysplasia.* In this defect, hypertelorism, small orbits, a narrow nose (Rieger's is broad), small teeth with enamel dysplasia, and malformation of the digits may be present. Microphthalmos may occur (seldom in Rieger's). Iris, pupillary, and angle abnormalities are absent.

MESODERMAL DYSGENESIS OF THE CORNEA. This ocular malformation, usually known as Peters' anomaly, is clinically and pathologically distinct from Rieger's mesodermal dysgenesis of the iris. It consists of a central posterior corneal defect (focal absence of endothelium, Descemet's membrane, and deep stroma), iris adhesions from the collarette to the border of this concavity, and an overlying opacity which presumably arises from aqueous penetrating the stroma (Figs. 12–15 to 12–17). Bowman's membrane is present peripher-

Figure 12–17   *A,* Mesodermal dysgenesis of iris and cornea. This 7-month-old male had bilateral megalocornea (13 mm. in diameter), a central posterior corneal defect with corneal leukoma in the right eye (*A* to *D*), and Rieger's anomaly of the left eye (*E* to *F*). (Courtesy of Dr. Turgut Hamdi.)

B, Keratoplasty for mesodermal dysgenesis of cornea. A penetrating keratoplasty was performed in the right eye at age 22 months and the graft remained clear for 5 months until graft rejection occurred. No iris processes extended to the corneal leukoma. An anterior polar cataract was discovered postoperatively.

C, Central posterior corneal defect with scarring. The corneal button shows that the central leukomatous portion (right side) is thickened from superficial fibrovascular invasion and deep stromal edema. In this area, Bowman's and Descemet's membranes are absent. The margin of the button (left side) shows more normal cornea with edematous stroma. Descemet's membrane is present in this area (arrow). (PAS stain, ×25.)

D, Central posterior corneal defect. The area of *C* in the box shows the transition (arrow) from intact Descemet's membrane peripherally to its replacement by fibrous tissue centrally. Only fragments of endothelium were seen. (PAS stain, ×250.)

E, Megalocornea and Rieger's anomaly. The left eye of this patient exhibited a 13-mm. cornea, a prominent Schwalbe's ring (arrow) with iris processes extending to it, and a hypoplastic iris stroma.

F, Iris processes in Rieger's anomaly. The angle is filled with delicate iris processes and mesodermal tissue extending up to the prominent Schwalbe's ring.

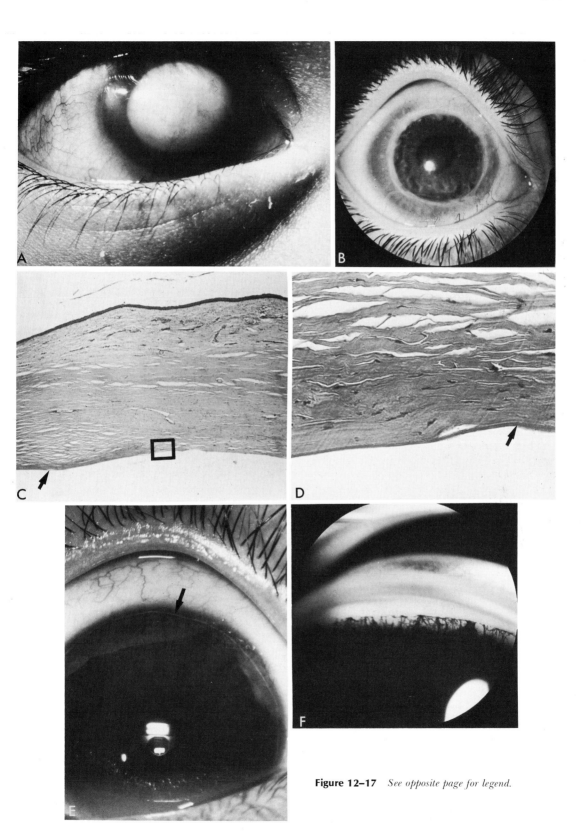

Figure 12–17 *See opposite page for legend.*

ally, but becomes thinned and is absent centrally. The stroma contains increased numbers of keratocytes and may or may not be vascularized. Descemet's membrane is present peripherally but absent centrally (Fig. 12–17). The endothelium is usually absent centrally also but may persist without Descemet's membrane. Connective tissue sometimes fills the central posterior corneal defect.

In contrast to Rieger's anomaly, mesodermal dysgenesis of the cornea is unilateral in about 20 per cent of cases, occurs sporadically or in an autosomal recessive pattern of inheritance, and seldom exhibits a prominent Schwalbe's ring, peripheral iris strands, iris hypoplasia, or pupillary abnormalities. It may be associated with microphthalmos or cornea plana. Like Rieger's, about 50 per cent of these patients have glaucoma, but in this case it is usually congenital, presenting a clinical picture of buphthalmos. Congenital cataract or microphakia may be present. The cataract may be anterior polar in line with the internal corneal defect, suggesting defective separation of lens from surface ectoderm. Rieger's and Peters' anomalies may coexist in the same eye.

The pathogenesis of this anomaly is unknown. This fact reemphasizes the point that multiple etiologies may produce similar pathologic results. This ignorance of pathogenic mechanisms has produced confusion in classifying types of mesodermal dysgenesis of the cornea. One approach to the classification of central posterior corneal defects is as follows (Fig. 12–8):

1. Posterior corneal depression with overlying clear cornea (localized posterior keratoconus) (Figs. 12–9 and 12–12).
2. Posterior corneal defect with leukoma (Fig. 12–17).
3. Corneal leukoma with iris adhesions to margin of posterior defect (Figs. 12–15 and 12–16).
   a. Probable developmental etiology (Peters' anomaly).
   b. Probable inflammatory etiology (internal ulcer of von Hippel).
4. Keratolenticular anomalies.
   a. Persistent corneal-lens adhesion (Fig. 12–18).
   b. Posterior corneal defect aligned with anterior polar cataract.

In most cases, the resulting clinical appearance is similar and its effect on the infant's visual development is devastating. Penetrating keratoplasty may preserve useful vision (Fig. 12–17).

A more severe form of corneal dysgenesis is congenital anterior staphyloma (Fig. 12–19). The cornea is opaque, irregular, and ectatic and protrudes between the lids. A bluish appearance may be present because of adherent iris. Histologically it is thin and vascularized, with Bowman's and Descemet's membranes present only peripherally. The lens may be present and cataractous or represented by remnants which are sometimes situated within the corneal tissue. Congenital glaucoma is frequently present,

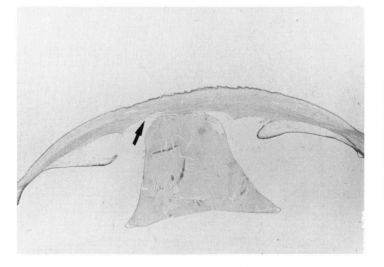

Figure 12–18 Congenital lens-corneal adhesion. The eye of this newborn demonstrates irregular and thickened corneal epithelium and stroma, central absence of Bowman's and Descemet's membranes, a central posterior corneal defect (arrow) with a lens-corneal adhesion, a conical cataractous lens, and malformation of the anterior chamber angles with adhesion of iris to cornea. (PAS stain, ×3.) (Courtesy of Dr. Charles G. Steinmetz.)

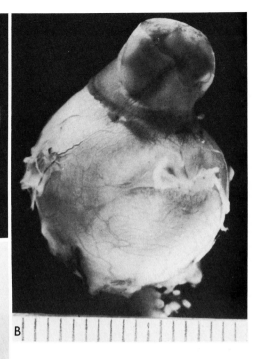

Figure 12–19   *A*, Congenital corneal staphyloma. This 5-day-old infant was born with a flat opaque right cornea. By 2 days of age, the cornea had become blue and ectatic as shown here. The left eye was normal except for persistent pupillary membrane. (Courtesy of Dr. Joseph H. Calhoun.) *B*, Gross appearance of globe. Ectatic area is limited to cornea. (Courtesy of Dr. Merlyn Rodrigues.) *C*, Histologic section of globe. Areas of the cornea are thin and ectatic. A superficial corneal abscess from exposure is present (arrow). Bowman's and Descemet's membranes are absent. A rudimentary lens is adherent to the central posterior cornea, blending with stroma tissue. Uveal tissue is firmly adherent to posterior cornea, sweeping down along the lens rudiment (Hematoxylin and eosin stain, ×3.) (Courtesy of Dr. Merlyn Rodrigues.)

presumably from malformation of and damage to angle structures. In most cases, treatment is futile, although surgical relief of the glaucoma and keratoplasty may preserve some visual function.

Mesodermal dysgenesis of the iris and cornea may coexist as shown in Figures 12–17 and 12–18.

These anomalies may be accompanied by a wide variety of other ocular and systemic abnormalities. Associated ocular defects include retinal dysplasia, persistent hyperplastic primary vitreous, retrolental fibroplasia, limbal dermoids, and cornea plana. They may be associated with isolated abnormalities of the central nervous, cardiovascular, urogenital, or digestive systems, or skull, face, and limbs. They may accompany more generalized syndromes: Marfan's, Weil-Marchesani, Klinefelter's, Lowe's, Norrie's, 13–15 trisomy, and rubella. In some of these the ocular abnormality provides the clue for thorough physical examination, laboratory investigation, and detailed genetic history in an attempt to uncover unsuspected or symptomatic disorders.

DERMOID TUMORS OF THE CORNEA. A corneal dermoid tumor is a solid congenital rounded mass consisting of keratinized epithelium overlying fibrofatty tissue which contains hair follicles, seba-

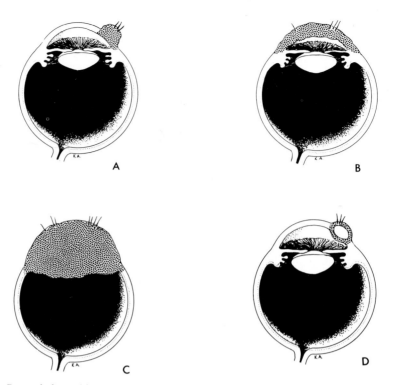

Figure 12–20   Corneal dermoids. *A*, Limbal dermoid tumor. *B*, Dermoid tumor replacing entire cornea. *C*, Dermoid tumor replacing entire anterior segment. *D*, Dermoid cyst of cornea. (After Ida Mann).

ceous glands, and sweat glands. It is usually a single unilateral pink-gray mass, 1 to 5 mm. in diameter, which straddles the limbus (Figs. 12–20 and 12–21). The clinical picture is highly variable, however. The masses may be multiple, bilateral, located on cornea alone or sclera alone, with or without visible hair, and either minutely small or large enough to obscure the entire cornea. The dermoid may extend into deeper layers of the corneal stroma and sclera but seldom grows into the angle structures. It is firmly fixed to the cornea.

Dermoids may enlarge slowly, especially at puberty or after trauma or irritation. Visual acuity is seldom affected, but if the tumor grows over the visual axis or produces significant corneal astigmatism, vision may fall. Dermoids contain considerable fatty tissue and a white arcuate haze of lipoid material extends into the corneal stroma in front of the tumor. This may encroach on the visual axis to blur vision.

Approximately one third of patients with limbal dermoids will have associated developmental anomalies. Among the most frequent is the constellation of epibulbar dermoids, auricular and vertebral anomalies (Goldenhar's syndrome) (Figs. 12–22 and 12–23).

In Goldenhar's syndrome the epibulbar dermoid straddles the limbus in the inferotemporal quadrant. It is bilateral in about 25 per cent of cases. A subconjunctival lipodermoid (lipoma covered by keratinized or nonkeratinized epithelium with hairs on the surface) is found in the superotemporal quadrant in about half the cases. This may blend with the epibulbar dermoid. Coloboma of the upper lid at the junction of the middle and inner third is present in about 25 per cent of cases. Other associated ocular anomalies include Duane's syndrome, lacrimal duct stenosis, and iris and choroidal colobomas.

The auricular anomalies are usually on the same side as the dermoid. These include preauricular appendages, posteriorly placed ears, microtia, and stenosis of the external auditory meatus. Vertebral anomalies occur in about two thirds of patients. The most frequent are fused cervical vertebrae, hemivertebrae, spina bifida, and occipitalization of the atlas.

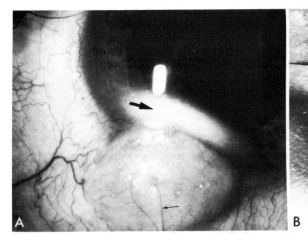

Figure 12–21 Limbal dermoid tumor. *A,* Vascularized limbal nodule with hair protruding from its surface (small arrow). A white lipid line in superficial corneal stroma extends centrally from the dermoid (large arrow). *B,* Tumor removed by superficial keratectomy. *C,* A significant corneal scar will remain.

Lumbosacral abnormalities occur as well. Facial malformations include micrognathia, macrostomia, dental abnormalities, and facial asymmetry. The diagnosis of Goldenhar's syndrome should lead to complete examination for associated systemic abnormalities, especially cardiovascular, renal, genitourinary, and gastrointestinal defects. Goldenhar's syndrome occurs sporadically, and there is generally no hereditary defect associated with it.

Limbal dermoids should be excised if they are producing visual disturbance, if they are irritated, or if they are cosmetically embarrassing. Small asymptomatic nodules may be observed. Surgical intervention should be tempered by two facts: (1) the cornea and sclera may be quite

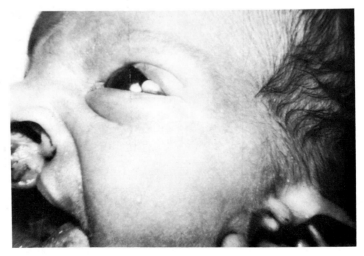

Figure 12–22 Goldenhar's syndrome. The limbal dermoid and preauricular skin tags are present in addition to a cleft lip. (Courtesy of Dr. Robison D. Harley.)

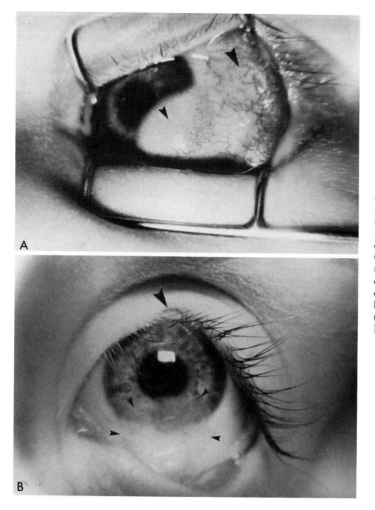

Figure 12–23 *A*, Goldenhar's syndrome. A lipodermoid of the conjunctiva (large arrow) and an epibulbar dermoid of the limbus (small arrow) are present concurrently in about half the cases. (Courtesy of Dr. Jules Baum.) *B*, Goldenhar's syndrome. A coloboma of the upper lid at the junction of the middle and inner thirds is present in about one fourth of cases (large arrow). The limbal dermoid tumor has been excised (small arrows). (Courtesy of Dr. Jules Baum.)

thin beneath the dermoid, increasing the possibility of corneal perforation at surgery; and (2) the scar remaining after excision will sometimes be as unsightly as the original tumor. Performing a lamellar corneal transplantation under the operating microscope may help minimize the dangers of ocular perforation and subsequent scar formation. It is worthwhile gonioscoping patients prior to or at surgery to discover possible angle involvement. A donor cornea should be available at the time of surgery in case the anterior chamber is entered. Dermoids do not recur.

Corneal dermoids take a wide variety of forms (Fig. 12–20). The simplest is the epithelial plaque, where a focal area of keratinized epithelium is present on the cornea. The limbal dermoid tumor is the next most complex form. It may occasion-

ally extend into angle structures and the anterior chamber.

Dermoid tissue may replace the entire cornea and limbus (Figs. 12–24 to 12–26). Clinically, the eye appears as a fibrofatty mass with hair which protrudes between the lids. In this case the underlying anterior chamber angle, iris, and lens are usually normal. A still more extensive dermoid replaces the entire cornea, iris, and lens, as if the primitive mesoderm became metaplastic and migrated between the ectoderm and the optic cup before the lens vesicle formed. This may be associated with retinal dysplasia. Rarely, a corneal dermoid cyst occurs. It is a sharply demarcated cystic mass in the corneal stroma which indents the anterior chamber. The cyst is lined by epithelium, is covered by connective tissue, and contains a milky fluid derived from sebaceous

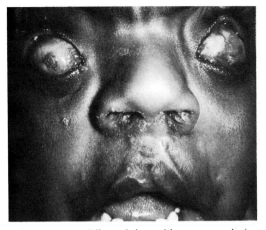

Figure 12–24 Bilateral dermoid tumors replacing entire cornea. This 3-year-old male was born with masses of vascularized tissue containing surface hair protruding grotesquely between his lids. He has had repair of cleft lip and palate.

glands and desquamating epithelium. The cyst may drain spontaneously either externally or into the anterior chamber where a toxic iridocyclitis results. Attempts to eliminate the cyst by surgical drainage are often frustrated by spontaneous reformation.

The etiology of dermoids is speculative. The metaplasia of the ectoderm to produce keratin and dermal appendages and of the mesoderm to produce fibrofatty tissue may be either a primary aberration of germinal tissue or a response to exogenous insult. The presence of eyelid colobomas just above limbal dermoids has

led to the speculation that amniotic bands notched the lid and caused a sequestration of dermal tissues at the limbus.

Dermoid tumors are not neoplasms. They are choristomas, that is, masses of histologically normal tissue in an abnormal location. Thus, they neither invade local structures nor metastasize to distant sites.

Because of the similarity of name, limbal dermoid tumors should not be confused with dermoid cysts of the orbit, brow, or lid, which are epithelial-lined cysts containing sebaceous fluid which may enlarge to produce exophthalmos; or with dermolipomas of the bulbar conjunctiva, which are nonprogressive fatty tumors covered with keratinized epithelium that extend back into the orbit and are usually only of cosmetic significance. Dermoids may also form on the caruncle and in the lacrimal gland.

The differential diagnosis of limbal dermoids may be difficult. In a child one should consider aberrant lacrimal gland, limbal teratoma, hemangioma, fibroma, congenital cyst, osteoma, or nevus. In an older individual, papilloma, pterygium, pinguecula, basal or squamous cell carcinoma, benign epithelioma, conjunctival xerosis or malignant melanoma become more likely, but the history of the presence of the nodule since childhood favors a diagnosis of dermoid.

It is important to differentiate large corneal dermoids from anterior staphylomas and extensive corneal leukomas (Table 12–3). All these may appear as a

Figure 12–25 Corneal dermoid, staphyloma, Axenfeld's anomaly. Right eye of patient shown in Figure 12–16. Cornea is replaced by a mass of vascularized connective tissue. Ectopic lacrimal gland is present at the limbus (large arrow). In this area the angle is deep and contains a prominent Schwalbe's ring with iris processes adherent to it (small arrow). A central corneal staphyloma is present. On one side, the iris stretches from the angle to the lip of the staphyloma; Descemet's membrane is present in this area. On the opposite side, iris lines the corneal defect and posterior cornea; Descemet's membrane is absent in these areas (Hematoxylin and eosin stain, ×3.)

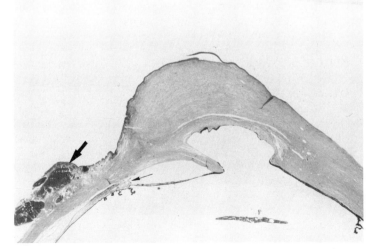

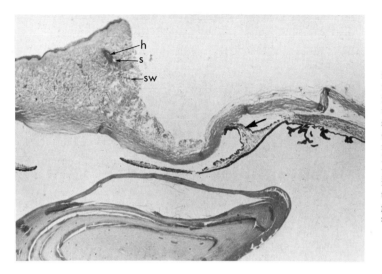

Figure 12–26 Corneal dermoid, iris-corneal adhesion. Left eye of patient in Figure 12–15. Anterior cornea is replaced by vascularized connective tissue containing hair follicle (*h*), sebaceous gland (*s*), and sweat gland (*sw*). A biopsy has been taken for diagnostic purposes, leaving a defect. Descemet's membrane is present peripherally but absent centrally. An iris adhesion (arrow) is present centrally. Angle structures are disorganized. (Hematoxylin and eosin stain, ×4.)

vascularized mass protruding between the eyelids. If the dermoid incompletely covers the cornea or has hair on its surface, little confusion occurs (Fig. 12–21). Staphylomas usually have a bluish color, because the underlying uveal tissue shows through the thin fibrotic cornea (Fig. 12–19). Corneal leukomas overlying posterior corneal defects may present as large masses (Fig. 12–15). Keloid scars may present at birth as white vascularized masses of the cornea. Presumably, they result from intrauterine corneal perforation with exuberant proliferation of connective tissue. Histologically they consist of a haphazard arrangement of fibroblasts, collagen bundles, and blood vessels covered by keratinized epithelium which does not contain dermal appendages. Iris and lens fragments may be found in the scar, suggesting perforation. The posterior cornea is often lined by iris, producing a thick staphyloma.

Ultrasound will indicate the thickness and density of the mass, the presence or absence of the lens, and the structural condition of the vitreous and retina. Biopsy of the mass will usually be diagnostic for corneal dermoid. If the anterior segment appears thin and ectatic, biopsy is unwarranted.

The distinction between these entities is important, since superficial dermoids leave the remainder of the globe intact and surgical excision with keratoplasty may preserve useful vision. This is especially important in bilateral involvement. Even extensive dermoids, staphylomas, and perforated corneal ulcers accompanied by angle and lens destruction may be approached surgically in selected cases, although enucleation is often advisable.

Congenital Abnormalities of Corneal Size and Shape

In general, uncomplicated variations in the size and shape of the cornea pose little threat to good visual acuity. Minor abnormalities act as warning signs which alert the ophthalmologist to search for unusual refractive errors, developmental glaucoma, or other ocular defects. Examination under anesthesia may be necessary to investigate a misshapen cornea.

In the newborn, the cornea is relatively large compared to the globe. It measures 9 to 10 mm. in horizontal diameter and usually grows to the adult size of 10.0 to 12.5 mm. between 6 and 12 months.

Corneal diameters are measured horizontally, where the corneoscleral junction is sharp. Vertically, the gradual extension of sclera over cornea makes precise identification of the limbus difficult. Measurement is performed with a millimeter rule braced on the bridge of the nose. A calibrated hand-held magnifier with a built-in metric scale may give more accurate and repeatable measurements than unaided visual inspection. Under anesthesia, calipers are used. Corneas smaller than 10 or larger than 13 mm. are abnormal.

ABSENCE OF CORNEA. This rare disorder occurs if the ectoderm fails to invaginate and mesoderm does not migrate across the mouth of the optic cup. A fibrous shell forms which is lined by retina and is devoid of cornea, iris, ciliary body, and lens. This should not be confused with corneal staphyloma (an ectatic cornea lined with uveal tissue protrudes between the lids), corneal dermoid (a skinlike mass replaces part of the cornea), sclerocornea (a scleralized cornea masks normal anterior segment structures), clinical anophthalmos or microphthalmos (the orbit may contain only shrunken rudiments of a globe), or cryptophthalmos (no eyelids are present and facial skin covers the orbit and fuses with the cornea).

MEGALOCORNEA (ANTERIOR MEGALOPHTHALMOS). Megalocornea is any cornea the horizontal diameter of which exceeds 13 mm. It may be as large as 18 mm. An enlarged cornea is present in four typical patterns:

1. Megalocornea unassociated with other ocular abnormalities. This may simply be a physiologically large cornea.

2. Megalocornea as part of general enlargement of the anterior segment (anterior megalophthalmos).

3. Megalocornea as part of general enlargement of the entire globe (megaloglobus).

4. Megalocornea as part of congenital glaucoma (buphthalmos).

Anterior megalophthalmos is usually inherited as an X-linked recessive and is thus limited to male members of a family (except for female homozygotes) without a pattern of male-to-male transmission. The cornea is clear, with distinct margins which frequently show a prominent Schwalbe's ring. High refractive errors are not usually present but a marked astigmatism is sometimes detected. If the anterior iris stroma is thin, the iris has a fibrillar appearance without crypts. A persistent pupillary membrane may be seen. Miosis is sometimes evident because of hypoplasia of the dilator of the pupil.

Enlargement of the anterior segment produces a deep anterior chamber. Since the lens is usually of normal size (as measured after intracapsular cataract extraction) it fits poorly in the enlarged ciliary ring. Thus, subluxation or frank dislocation and accompanying iridodonesis are common. Pigment dispersion from the iris epithelium produces a Krukenberg spindle. Cataracts occur more frequently and earlier (age 30 to 50) than in normal eyes. Cataract extraction, especially in the face of lens dislocation, is hazardous, but the use of cryoextraction and supportive devices like the Flieringa ring may reduce the incidence of complications. Congenital glaucoma is not present, but secondary glaucoma from anterior dislocation of the lens can occur. Persistent mesodermal tissue in the angle in the form of iris processes extending to the trabecular meshwork or Schwalbe's ring is sometimes seen on gonioscopy.

The corneal enlargement in buphthalmos is thought to result from the stretching caused by increased intraocular pressure. In this context, megalocornea with normal ocular pressure is considered a separate developmental abnormality. Table 12–2 lists the differentiating features of the two syndromes. Some individuals, however, consider the corneal enlargement in buphthalmos as a distinct developmental abnormality (keratodysgenesis) which occurs concomitantly with the angle abnormalities and glaucoma (goniodysgenesis). Evidence for this point of view includes (1) the occurrence of both isolated megalocornea in one eye and buphthalmos in the other eye of a single individual, and presence of both entities within a family; (2) common morphologic features in the angles of each (mesodermal remnants, deep angle); (3) a presumably normal rate of corneal growth in congenital glaucoma —the cornea started larger; (4) the presence of an enlarged cornea in some cases of buphthalmos before the intraocular pressure rises; (5) the contention that the breaks in Descemet's membrane in congenital glaucoma are developmental in origin, not from pressure stretching.

The management of congenital megalocornea includes the following:

1. Exclude congenital and developmental glaucoma utilizing the differential points in Table 12–2.

TABLE 12–2 DIFFERENTIAL DIAGNOSIS OF CONGENITAL GLAUCOMA AND ANTERIOR MEGALOPHTHALMOS (AFTER DUKE-ELDER)

Congenital Glaucoma (Buphthalmos)	Anterior Megalophthalmos (Megalocornea)
1. Elevated tension	1. Normal tension
2. Corneal size increases	2. Corneal size constant
3. Photophobia and epiphora	3. Asymptomatic
4. Corneal opacities (stromal edema, ruptures in Descemet's membrane)	4. Central cornea clear
5. Cornea flattened, astigmatism against the rule	5. Corneal curve normal or increased, astigmatism with the rule
6. Angle dysgenesis (mesodermal tissue obscures angle structures)	6. Angle normal, may contain iris processes
7. Cup/disc ratio may exceed 0.4	7. Cup/disc ratio less than 0.4
8. Bilateral in about two thirds of cases, but asymmetric	8. Bilateral and symmetric
9. May be autosomal recessive (60% males)	9. Sex-linked recessive (92% males)
10. Familial occurrence unusual	10. Familial occurrence common
11. Visual prognosis poor	11. Visual prognosis good

2. Follow-up annually because some individuals with megalocornea may develop glaucoma later.

3. Record associated ocular abnormalities, especially those of iridodonesis and lens position, since they are possible forerunners of lens dislocation. This may include ultrasound to exclude megaloglobus.

4. Examine other family members for similar abnormalities. Anterior megalophthalmos and congenital glaucoma may coexist in the same family.

5. Attend especially to the refraction with careful refinement of high cylinders.

6. Reassure the family of the nonprogressive nature of the findings if only isolated megalocornea is detected.

7. Be alert for the premature development of cataract and the need for extra caution during lens extraction.

MICROCORNEA. A cornea measuring less than 10 mm. in diameter with a normal-sized posterior segment represents pure microcornea. Corneal curvature is increased, and the resulting increased refractive power frequently produces a myopic refraction. However, if the eyeball is short (all components are proportional), the total refraction may be emmetropic, in which case the anomaly produces no functional impairment.

The chief concern about a patient with microcornea is the development of glaucoma, which is said to occur in 20 per cent of cases. Two mechanisms are possible:

(1) goniodysgenesis similar to other forms of developmental glaucoma; and (2) angle closure resulting from a relatively large lens pressing the iris forward against a relatively small anterior segment.

Associated ocular abnormalities include persistent pupillary membrane, corectopia, mesodermal remnants in the angle, congenital cataract, microphakia, typical colobomas, and small eyelids and orbits. If the entire globe is small, microphthalmos is present. The differential diagnosis of microcornea and microphthalmos may be established by axial ultrasound biometry.

Since microcornea is most often inherited as an autosomal dominent, family screening should be performed, especially to detect those who have microcornea with undiagnosed glaucoma.

CORNEA PLANA. Cornea plana gives the anterior segment a flat appearance, which is best appreciated on lateral viewing. The upper lid is poorly supported by the flat cornea and a pseudoptosis results. The limbus is poorly defined because vascularized scleral tissue extends onto the cornea, creating a gray peripheral circular zone. By transilluminating the globe, one can detect the true extent of the cornea beneath this gray band and can then measure the corneal diameter to find that it is well over 10 mm. Keratometric examination usually shows an anterior surface refractive power of less than 40 diopters. The anterior chamber is shallow. Bilaterally flat corneas are sometimes confused with microcornea because the limbus is scleralized, leaving a small transparent portion of the central cornea.

However, microcornea may be differentiated by its shorter radius of curvature, good support of the upper lid, sharp limbal margin, diameter under 10 mm., and refractive power greater than 40 diopters. Rarely, a true microcornea plana is found. In cornea plana, corneal growth continues, but the curvature is not formed; whereas in microcornea, the curve is formed, but growth is arrested (Figs. 12–1C and D).

With diminished corneal refractive power, one might expect high hyperopia, but since the globe itself may be elongated, refraction in cornea plana varies from hyperopia to myopia. Most patients are capable of having normal visual acuity.

Occasionally, aplasia of the retina and optic nerve accompany cornea plana. Clinical and electrodiagnostic acumen should identify this entity, since all refractive and surgical therapy is doomed to failure. Central corneal stromal opacities may be dense enough to produce amblyopia unless treated by keratoplasty. Congenital glaucoma is sometimes present. Other accompanying ocular abnormalities include: hypoplasia of the anterior iris stroma, iris and choroidal colobomas, aniridia, and congenital cataract.

Since the hereditary pattern is generally autosomal dominant, the probability of discovering other involved individuals during family screening is high.

SCLEROCORNEA. In this malformation scleral tissue accompanied by conjunctival and episcleral vessels extends across the limbus into cornea, obliterating the corneoscleral sulcus (Fig. 12–27). This disorder is usually bilateral, commonly asymmetric and nonprogressive. It may be unilateral. If the visual axis is clear, vision may remain unimpaired, but those eyes with a central opacity will develop amblyopia. A wide spectrum of clinical appearances occurs, from slight peripheral opacity to total replacement of the cornea.

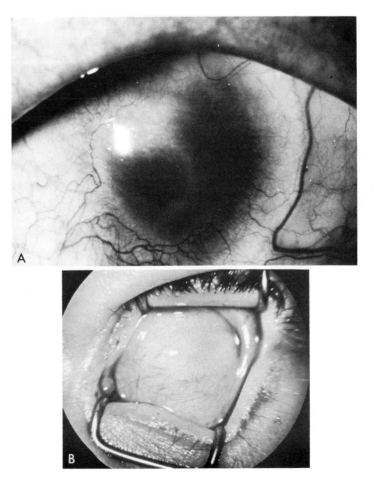

Figure 12–27 Sclerocornea. *A*, Scleral tissue extends in a geographic pattern toward central cornea. Some clear cornea remains centrally. *B*, Total replacement of the cornea by sclera. Penetrating keratoplasty was performed. Iris and lens were grossly malformed. (Courtesy of Dr. Joseph Calhoun.)

Corneal leukomas that overlie posterior corneal defects (Peters' anomaly) are often erroneously called sclerocornea. If the opacity is more dense centrally, it is probably not a true sclerocornea. In some cases a scleralized peripheral cornea meets the central leukoma of Peters' anomaly, and an exact clinical diagnosis is difficult.

The most common associated ocular anomalies are strabismus and nystagmus, which probably occur secondary to the amblyopia, and cornea plana with its associated blepharoptosis. Glaucoma may occur, but its evaluation is complicated by the altered rigidity of the sclerocornea and by the opacity obscuring the optic disc. Digital or Mackay-Marg tonometry may afford a better guide to intraocular pressure than applanation or indentation techniques. Other developmental anomalies of the anterior segment which sometimes accompany sclerocornea include a shallow anterior chamber with iris-corneal adhesions, atrophy of iris stroma, persistent pupillary membrane, corectopia, and posterior embryotoxon (see in the contralateral eye if the limbus is clear). High myopia and chorioretinal colombomas are occasionally present. Ultrasound can help clarify the refractive state and intraocular anatomy when the opacity prevents visualization.

Systemic abnormalities are rare. Craniofacial malformations and central nervous system anomalies may be present.

Sclerocornea is usually a sporadic finding and family studies can be expected to reveal few additional cases. Familial transmission has been described especially in the presence of cornea plana.

Histologically, the entire thickness of the cornea is replaced by vascularized sclera-like tissue. The collagen fibers are larger than those in normal cornea or sclera, and elastic fibers are present in the anterior stroma. The epithelium extends into the stroma. Bowman's membrane is absent. Descemet's membrane and endothelium are fragmented and replaced by fibrous tissue in some areas.

A penetrating keratoplasty is the only effective treatment, since the full thickness of cornea is involved. Even if this is carried out early enough to treat existing amblyopia, prognosis for useful vision is guarded because of associated glaucoma and possible high refractive error.

CORNEAL ASTIGMATISM. Astigmatism occurs when the refractive power of the cornea varies from one meridian to another, so that no point focus is formed on the retina. In approximately 90 per cent of children with astigmatism, the meridian of greatest curvature and greatest power is at 90 degrees (with-the-rule). The neutralizing minus cylinder will lie at axis 180 degrees to give minus power at 90 degrees. The explanation for this consistent orientation is classically that the lids compress the cornea enough to increase its vertical curvature, but equally likely is the speculation that the shape is a function of growth, the rate in one meridian differing slightly from that in another. Astigmatism is generated by the toric anterior surface of the cornea, average physiologic amounts ranging from 0.50 to 1.50 diopters. Mild refractive errors seldom exceed this amount, but in high degrees of ametropia, corneal astigmatism may be up to 8.00 diopters. Posterior corneal astigmatism is generally in the range of 0.50 diopters.

Corneal astigmatism may be inherited as an autosomal dominant with incomplete penetrance and variable expressivity.

DIFFERENTIAL DIAGNOSIS. The diagnosis of corneal opacities present at birth is challenging because of their rarity, their similarity of appearance, and the difficulties in examining infants. Table 12–3 presents some differentiating features of more common entities.

INFECTIONS OF THE CORNEA

Newborns and infants may develop conjunctivitis which may lead to corneal changes, either punctate keratitis or corneal ulceration. It is essential to perform scrapings of any corneal ulcer in order to establish, if possible, the organism responsible for the disease. Gram and Giemsa stains are preferred for the scrapings, and blood agar and broth tubes for cultures.

An antibiotic may be selected which will have greatest likelihood of controlling the corneal infection after the scrapings of the corneal ulcer are obtained. Severe bacterial infections caused by gram-negative organisms, particularly Pseudomonas,

TABLE 12-3 DIFFERENTIAL DIAGNOSIS OF COMMON CORNEAL OPACITIES PRESENT AT BIRTH

Type of Corneal Opacity	Laterality	Opacity	Ocular Pressure	Other Ocular Abnormalities	Course	Inflammation	Inheritance
Congenital glaucoma	Bilateral	Haze, focal	Elevated	Large cornea, photophobia, tearing, epithelial edema	Progressive	Uveitis	Autosomal recessive
Traumatic rupture of Descemet's membrane	Unilateral (or bilateral)	Haze, focal	Normal	Possible hyphema, epithelial edema	Spontaneous improvement in 3 weeks	None	Sporadic
Congenital hereditary endothelial dystrophy	Bilateral	Opaque, central and peripheral	Normal	None	Nonprogressive	None	Autosomal dominant or recessive
Sclerocornea	Unilateral (or bilateral)	Opaque, white, vascularized, peripheral	Normal (or elevated)	Cornea plana	Nonprogressive	None	Sporadic
Staphyloma	Unilateral	Opaque, bluish, ectatic	Elevated	Multiple	May ulcerate	Secondary	Sporadic
Epibulbar dermoid	Unilateral (or bilateral)	White, generalized or focal mass, hair, vascularized	Normal	None (or multiple)	Nonprogressive	Secondary	Sporadic
Peters' anomaly	Unilateral (or bilateral)	Haze, opaque, focal	Normal (or elevated)	None, Rieger's anomaly, lens adhesion	Nonprogressive	No	Sporadic (Autosomal recessive)
Corneal ulcer (bacterial, viral)	Unilateral (or bilateral)	Focal infiltrate, ulcer	Normal	None	May perforate	Yes	Sporadic
Congenital macular opacities	Bilateral	Central, diffuse maculae	Normal	None	Slowly progressive	No	Autosomal dominant or recessive

can rapidly destroy stromal tissue and lead to descemetocele and corneal perforation; therefore, it is essential to select an optimal antibiotic. If the scrapings of the corneal ulcer reveal gram-negative organisms, the antibiotic should be given by injection as well as topical therapy.

The examination of a young child is frequently difficult because of the child's pain, fright, and inability to cooperate. When it is not possible to examine the patient with a slit lamp, sedation is essential, so that the eye may be clearly seen. With medications such as ketamine, a child may be examined as an outpatient with enough anesthesia to allow corneal scrapings and subconjunctival or subtenons injections, if necessary, at the conclusion of the examination.

Conjunctival inflammation may extend to the cornea, resulting in either punctate keratitis or ulceration or both. A benign ocular disease then turns into a serious one. If adequate examination is performed early in the disease, severe corneal problems may be prevented and later disastrous corneal problems avoided. By not examining a child with appropriate thoroughness early in the disease, more harm is frequently done.

In discussing the appropriate diagnosis of conjunctival and corneal disease in children, examination of the cornea with a slit lamp is absolutely essential to rule out corneal disease. Frequently, small changes in the cornea that do not show up with a penlight are not seen until fluorescein dye is placed on the cornea. Once a diagnosis is made, medication should be started as quickly as possible. Corneal infections in children usually require the use of antibiotic medications in ointment form. Application of medicine is difficult for parents and the drop form of medication, properly applied, is wasted when the child squeezes or tears exces-sively, so that the drops are immediately diluted once they touch the eye. For this reason, ointments are preferred in infants and children for the treatment of corneal ulcerations. Despite theoretical slower re-epithelialization of corneal ulcers with ointment applications, the fact that ointments do remain in contact with the cornea longer makes this therapy better than drop medication. Parents must be instructed to use the drug properly, and if possible the ophthalmologist should show the parent how to use ointment during the initial office visit. Occasionally we have seen parents, when asked to demonstrate drug application, place the ointment onto their own fingers and then apply it to the lid margin or cheek. By demonstrating a technique of pulling the lid down putting the medication in the lower cul-de-sac and holding the lid open for 10 to 20 seconds, accurate drug application is achieved.

Bacteria which may cause corneal ulceration in children are similar to those that infect adults. Pneumococcus, Staphylococcus, Streptococcus, Pseudomonas, *Moraxella liquefaciens*, and *Klebsiella pneumoniae* are the more common bacteria which cause keratitis in children. The most common bacterial infection is due to *Staphylococcus aureus*, a gram-positive organism which usually causes a punctate keratitis in children. There is invariably a conjunctival element to this infection. The meibomian glands may be infected and serve as a reservoir for continued bacterial release and keratitis (Plate V-A).

Chronic staphylococcal blepharokerato-conjunctivitis in children is a problem and requires continued treatment until the source of infection is eradicated. Administration of sulfacetamide drops and ointment in conjunction with warm compresses and lid massage is the primary treatment for this disease in children. The newer

---

PLATE V

(*A*) Staphylococcal blepharitis with keratitis involving the lower and upper lids.

(*B*) Primary herpes simplex virus infection of the cornea and conjunctiva with numerous dendritic figures (Fluorescein stain.)

(*C*) Recurrent herpes simplex keratitis and geographic dendritic ulceration of the cornea. (Fluorescein stain.)

(*D*) Active chickenpox and limbal involvement with stromal inflammatory changes.

(*E*) Inclusion conjunctivitis of the newborn; no corneal changes were noted.

(*F*) Limbal vernal conjunctivitis with minimal vascularization but lymphoid hypertrophy at the limbus.

(*G*) Corneal ulcer due to marked papillary hypertrophy of the upper lid in vernal conjunctivitis.

(*H*) Phlyctenular conjunctivitis with phlyctenules at the limbus.

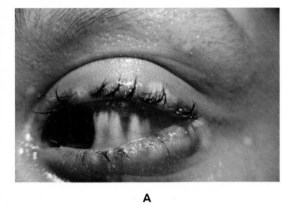

A

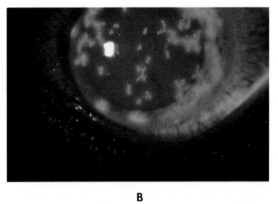

B

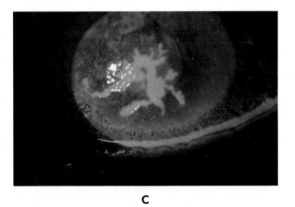

C

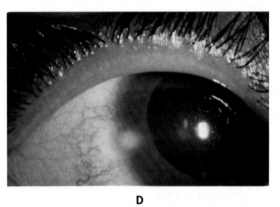

D

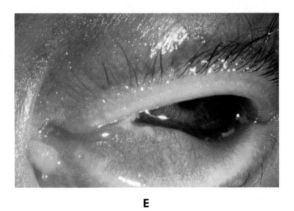

E

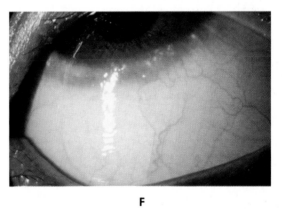

F

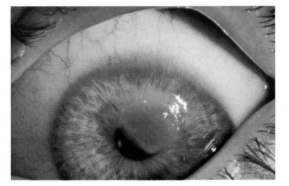

G

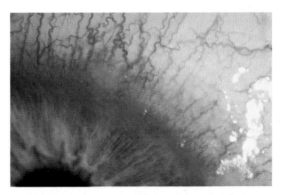

H

antibiotic gentamycin is effective for resistant strains of staph. With severe staphylococcal infection that does not respond to this treatment, the use of systemic antibiotics and local corticosteroids is frequently necessary. Staph desensitization may also be needed if it is found that the child has a marked hypersensitivity to the exotoxin produced by this organism. Other bacteria which may cause conjunctivitis and later keratitis are the *Haemophilus influenzae* and *Moraxella lacunata* organisms. Both are gram-negative, the first being a coccobacillus and the second a rod form of bacteria. Marginal ulcers are caused by each of these, and the Moraxella organism may cause an angular conjunctivitis.

Bacterial Corneal Infections

The most important anterior segment infection of the newborn is caused by *Neisseria gonorrhoeae*. This is a gram-negative diplococcus which appears in pairs and is intracellular. The infection, which is usually bilateral, may appear between 24 and 72 hours after birth. There is a severe purulent conjunctivitis while the cornea may ulcerate and perforate rapidly. The infection is acquired during the newborn's passage through the birth canal if the mother has been infected with the gonococcal organism. Many states require treatment of the newborn with 1 per cent silver nitrate (Credé method) in order to prevent this infection. Gonorrhea is increasing, and unfortunately, silver nitrate treatment is not universally performed prophylactically. The differential diagnosis includes chemical keratoconjunctivitis from faulty use of silver nitrate, inclusion conjunctivitis of the newborn, and other bacterial keratoconjunctivitides, particularly staphylococcal, which may also occur in epidemic proportions in a newborn nursery.

Viral Infections

Herpes simplex viral keratitis is the most severe form of corneal ulceration commonly seen in children in the United States, although trachoma (Chlamydia infection) is more prevalent around the world. The newborn may have maternal antibodies to HSV for the first 6 months of life, affording protection during this period from herpes simplex viral infection. After maternal antibodies are lost, the infant may acquire herpes simplex virus infection on the skin, in the eye, or systemically (Fig. 12–28). The infection is probably acquired by close contact with someone who has an active lesion either around the lids or fingers or elsewhere on the skin surface. Inapparent infection may also develop. The majority of children fall into this category.

Unfortunately, herpes simplex ocular infection is not readily diagnosed early in the course of the disease. The general practitioner or pediatrician usually sees the child first, and treatment is instituted for a red eye. This treatment may consist of an antibiotic-steroid combination to the detriment of the child. If there are

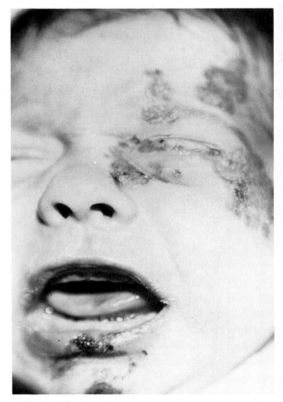

Figure 12–28 Primary herpes simplex keratitis involving the skin around the eye and lip in a 4-month-old child.

dendritic epithelial lesions forming on the cornea or conjunctiva (Plate V–B), the use of a local corticosteroid medication exacerbates the infection and causes wider spread as well as deeper involvement of the corneal tissue. After a week or more has passed and the infection is not controlled, the ophthalmologist may be consulted. At this time an uncooperative child is seen and slit lamp examination of the cornea is almost impossible. As previously mentioned, with a history such as this and poor response to medication, if the child is not able to be examined in the office, admission as an outpatient and examination under anesthesia is essential. Fluorescein dye must be placed on the cornea for evaluation of the disease, since small lesions are readily missed. Only with a combination of fluorescein and magnification such as is available with a slit lamp or operating microscope will lesions be visible. With examination under anesthesia or very heavy sedation, it is also possible to mechanically remove the dendritic or small geographic lesion at that time, if such is found. The antimetabolite 5-iodo-2′-deoxyuridine (IDU) in ointment form may be instilled at the end of examination. This ointment also should be prescribed for use every 4 hours at home. In addition, a cycloplegic should be used. Atropine sulfate, 1 per cent, is preferable in children.

Primary herpes simplex virus infection in the child is not the most serious form of this disease. Recurrent viral infection is common following the initial infection, and these recurrences are responsible for corneal scarring and visual loss (Plate V–C). Episodes of upper respiratory tract infections, high fever, and other debilitating diseases may initiate flare-ups of keratitis. Treatment for these recurrent herpetic infections is either repeated use of IDU ointment every 4 hours and/or mechanical debridement until the keratoconjunctivitis is under control. If the problem is not properly diagnosed, significant corneal scarring and vascularization occurs. Deeper corneal infection may ensue and contribute to the corneal disease. These deeper stromal diseases with corneal vascularization and disciform keratitis (Figs. 12–29 and 12–30) may require use of local corticosteroids even though this anti-inflammatory agent is contraindicated in superficial herpetic disease. Physicians should use great caution in treating a child's red eye with local corticosteroids, since herpes simplex virus infection may be the underlying cause. A minimal amount of steroid should be used when necessary, and frequent examinations are a necessity. The child should be seen at least twice a week during the first few weeks of this therapy, and medication must be tapered as soon as a response is achieved. In conjunction with steroid treatment, IDU ointment four times a day and an antibiotic ointment nightly should be

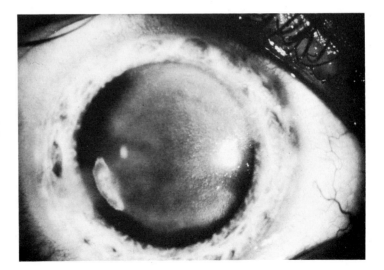

Figure 12–29 Disciform keratitis secondary to herpes simplex virus infection and recurrent disease.

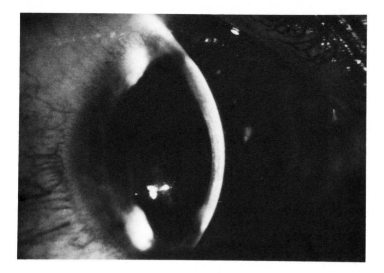

Figure 12–30   Slit lamp view of disciform keratitis in same patient as in Figure 12–29.

used. Allergy or toxicity to long-term use of IDU is a further problem, and in these cases hospitalization is often necessary.

Adenovirus Infections in Children

Corneal disease due to adenovirus infections in children are much less common than keratitis secondary to herpes simplex virus. Whereas in the adult form of adenovirus infection due to type 8 adenovirus (epidemic keratoconjunctivitis) there is typical superficial punctate keratitis followed by subepithelial corneal infiltrates (Fig. 12–31), in the child subepithelial corneal infiltrates are usually not seen. Marked follicular conjunctivitis, systemic symptoms, and preauricular adenopathy are seen in children but the cornea remains clear. Pseudomembranous conjunctivitis may be found accompanying adenovirus infections in children. Even with these marked conjunctival changes, the cornea may not develop infiltrates. Adenovirus types 2, 3, 5, 7, 8, and 11 have been isolated in children but the corneal changes are not commonly noted. In one large epidemic of adenovirus type 8, the youngest involved was 8 years of age and only 3 of 102 individuals were younger than 15 years of age. In a large study of the infantile form of adenovirus type 8, no instance of keratitis was noted, although follicular changes and pseudo-

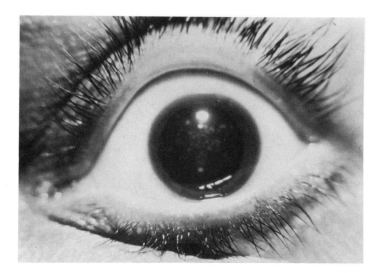

Figure 12–31   Subepithelial corneal infiltrates centrally in a case of adenovirus type 8 infection 3 months after the onset of disease.

membranes were prominent in the 12 cases. If corneal infiltrates do appear in children, they are transient and will disappear in time, leaving no corneal sequelae. The treatment of this disease requires local antibiotics alone in most cases to prevent secondary bacterial infection, which is not common. Local corticosteroids are only indicated in the more symptomatic cases.

Herpes Zoster Keratitis

The same viral agent which causes chickenpox also causes herpes zoster virus. Usually this virus is responsible for varicella in children and herpes zoster in the adult. There are many cases of herpes zoster keratoconjunctivitis in children, and this disease should not be overlooked. Unilateral facial and forehead blisters or similar lesions of the brow may be seen in children. When the nasociliary branch of the ophthalmic nerve is involved, there is a greater likelihood that there will be ocular involvement following herpes zoster infection. With inflammation of the nasociliary branch of this nerve, vesicles may appear on the tip or the side of the nose on the same side where skin vesicles appeared. Corneal involvement in herpes zoster may be seen as a punctate keratitis, stromal keratitis, and keratouveitis with conjunctivitis (Plate V-D).

Treatment of herpes zoster keratitis is the same for children and adults. Cycloplegia with atropine or scopolamine and local and systemic steroids may be necessary, depending upon the severity of ocular involvement. The use of systemic steroids should be approached with caution in children because of the possibility of systemic spread of this viral disease. Local corticosteroids are usually sufficient to quiet the corneal and anterior chamber inflammation.

Various forms of corneal involvement may occur in children with chickenpox. The mildest form is an epithelial keratitis which is self-limited and requires no treatment.

Severe corneal involvement may accompany varicella infection of the lid margins. Corneal ulcers, marginal corneal infiltrates, and interstitial keratitis have been noted following varicella infection in children. Observation may be all that is required in the benign cases. However, antibiotics, corticosteroids, and cycloplegics are frequently necessary with deeper corneal involvement.

Other viruses which may cause epithelial keratitis are rubeola and molluscum contagiosum. In molluscum, the skin nodules present on the lid margins can cause superficial keratitis. Epithelial keratitis is the most likely corneal manifestation in mumps, but cases of disciform keratitis have been reported and local therapy is usually all that is required. In most cases no residual scarring occurs.

Vaccinia

Vaccinial corneal ulcers can be severe in children. The disease is easily spread from the patient's own arm to his eyelid. Close contact with a recently vaccinated child or adult also may cause this problem. Corneal ulcers, disciform keratitis, and deep stromal scarring may be evident. Involvement of the eyelid with a typical vaccination mark with central ulceration and peripheral swelling and crusting should alert the physician to the possibility of vaccinial keratitis (Fig. 12–32). Treatment consists of local IDU ointment four times a day. In the severe cases, vaccine immune globulin may be obtained for intramuscular use. The local Red Cross supplies this drug in large cities.

TRIC Agent Keratitis

Trachoma is endemic in many parts of the world and in the southwest United States. In the Far and Middle East there are areas where 90 per cent of the population has trachoma. Although disease control may be possible in an isolated environment of children (boarding school), reinfection is common during visits to the family and local community. In childhood trachoma, there may be epithelial involvement in the upper half of the cornea in addition to superior limbal follicles. With further extension of corneal changes, subepithelial infiltrates and pannus may develop as the disease progresses (Fig. 12–33).

Control of this disease is essential, since it is by far the most common worldwide cause of corneal scarring and blindness.

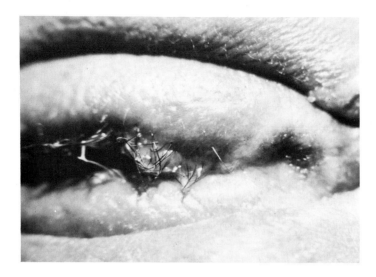

Figure 12–32 Vaccinial involvement of the outer canthus with lid swelling.

Estimates of disease prevalence in childhood and adult population range up to one quarter of a billion people.

Inclusion conjunctivitis (inclusion blennorrhea) of the newborn is seen throughout the United States (Plate V-E). The organism responsible is the TRIC agent. This disease should not be confused with gonorrheal ophthalmia, which appears within 2 days of birth. Usually inclusion conjunctivitis is noted between the 4th and 10th days of life. Inclusion conjunctivitis is acquired during passage through the birth canal. Corneal involvement, when keratitis does occur, is limited to the epithelium. There are few, if any, long-lasting corneal changes. The main form of disease is a purulent papillary and follicular conjunctivitis (Fig. 12–34). Sulfa drugs are the treatment of choice.

HYPERSENSITIVITY MANIFESTATIONS OF CORNEAL DISEASE

Vernal Keratoconjunctivitis

This is a disease of childhood, affecting males more frequently than females. Vernal conjunctivitis of the eye usually begins in the upper palpebral conjunctiva with papillary hypertrophy. Children with this problem have a history of allergy, although there is no definite etiologic basis for the papillary changes in the conjunctiva. The disease lasts for several years and may have remissions and exacerbations. The papil-

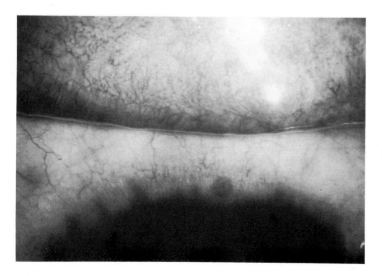

Figure 12–33 Superior limbal scarring and Herbert's pits in trachoma.

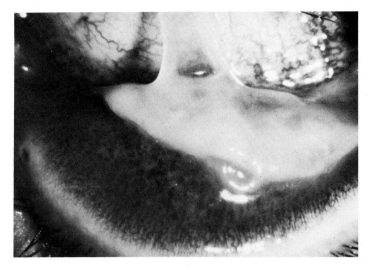

Figure 12–34 Purulent conjunctivitis and lid erythema in inclusion conjunctivitis.

lary excrescences in the upper lid, when large and cobblestone-like in appearance, may cause corneal ulceration and scarring (Figs. 12–35 and 12–36).

Usually local corticosteroid drops or ointment are sufficient for control of the vernal conjunctivitis, but occasionally very large papillary vegetations appearing in the upper lid must be removed by scraping. This must be done under heavy sedation or with general anesthesia. In some cases, the disease may be seen with pseudomembranous conjunctivitis. Eosinophils are seen on scrapings from the epithelial surface of the upper lid and are helpful in establishing the diagnosis.

Limbal vernal keratoconjunctivitis is another manifestation of vernal conjunc-

tivitis. Fine lymphoid follicles occur around the limbus (Plate V-F). These may appear yellow to light brown in color. The follicles do not stain with fluorescein nor do they become ulcerated. When these limbal changes are white or yellow-white hard dots, they are known as "Trantas' dots." Epithelial keratitis may accompany the limbal vernal conjunctivitis. Subepithelial stromal changes are not common. The typical corneal ulcer which is seen in vernal conjunctivitis secondary to palpebral changes is usually not seen with limbal vernal conjunctivitis (Plate V-G).

Phlyctenular Keratoconjunctivitis

This form of keratoconjunctivitis has in the past been thought to be due to hyper-

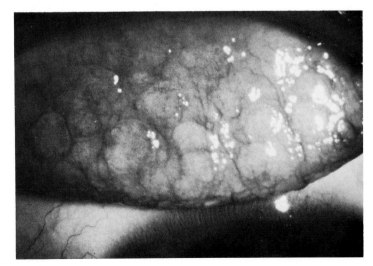

Figure 12–35 Large papillary, cobblestone excrescences in vernal conjunctivitis involving the upper lid.

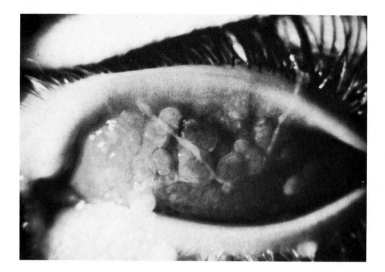

Figure 12–36   Individual giant follicles in vernal conjunctivitis with excessive mucus.

sensitivity to tuberculin protein, but a specific cause is not really known. Bacterial and viral cultures are negative and the disease is not specifically known to be due to a vitamin deficiency. Secondary staphylococcal infection may involve the phlyctenular changes but the disease is not primarily due to staphylococcal limbal invasion. The lesions are usually located at the limbus, are slightly elevated, and have a yellowish color (Plate V-H). At the head of the lesion a small corneal ulceration may occur and a fascicular ulcer encroaches on the cornea and extends centrally. Behind the head of the advancing lesion is a fascicle of blood vessels which appears as a leash pointing toward the head of the advancing ulcer. Other phlyctenules may appear around the cornea but usually only one advances across the cornea at a time. This disease usually responds to local corticosteroid therapy, leaving superficial stromal pannus and scarring.

Stevens-Johnson Disease and Drug Reaction

Stevens-Johnson syndrome is a severe systemic reaction which usually occurs following use of systemic sulfonamides or antibiotic drugs in children and young adults. Hypersensitivity to the drug administered may be responsible for the acute eruption. There are vesicular and bullous skin eruptions involving mucous membranes of the mouth and nose as well as conjunctival eruption. Mucopurulent and pseudomembranous conjunctivitis may be seen with ulcerations of the eyelid. The cornea is involved secondary to the lid reaction. Following healing of the lid margin, epidermalization occurs on the palpebral surface of the lid (Fig. 12–37). With continued irritation from the rough conjunctival surface, the cornea develops superficial punctate keratitis and pannus formation, usually inferiorly or superiorly. In severe cases cicatrization and symblepharon develop. Epidermalization may involve the corneal epithelium as well as conjunctival epithelium, so that the end result is a totally scarred conjunctiva and cornea, with firm adhesions of the lid margin to the cornea itself (Fig. 12–38). Corneal transplantation in these cases is the only hope for vision, but even with this procedure the prognosis is poor. Treatment of the acute disease is difficult. Only systemic and local corticosteroids offer any hope of aborting the more severe, later consequences. When symblepharon and epidermalization occur, scleral or soft contact lenses can be applied to protect the cornea. Reformation of the inferior cul-de-sac may be necessary when symblepharon forms.

Epidermolysis Bullosa

The cornea is involved in the severest form of this disease. Corneal clouding in the region of Bowman's membrane and epithelium occurs. Bullae similar to those

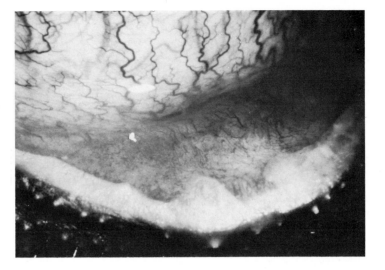

Figure 12–37 Epidermalization of the palpebral conjunctiva of the lower lid in Stevens-Johnson disease. This is a keratinization of the normal smooth, glistening palpebral conjunctiva.

found in the skin result in corneal ulceration, and perforation of the cornea can occur.

CORNEAL DYSTROPHIES AND DEGENERATION

Corneal dystrophies are unusual and quite dramatic when seen against a background of clear corneal tissue. Some degree of corneal opacification or clouding is present in these diseases. Dystrophies are bilateral, are hereditary in nature, occur more centrally than peripherally, are nonvascularized, and usually do not manifest inflammatory signs and symptoms. On the other hand, corneal degen-

erations are unilateral more often than bilateral, involve the peripheral as well as the central cornea, and often follow inflammation of the cornea. They are not hereditary and occur following other ocular or systemic disease.

The corneal dystrophies are not limited to childhood and, although occasionally beginning in childhood, most are first seen in the teenage or later years. They become progressively worse during mid adult life. Those corneal dystrophies first seen in childhood will be emphasized in this section.

Anterior Corneal Dystrophies

The anterior corneal dystrophies include those which involve the epithelium,

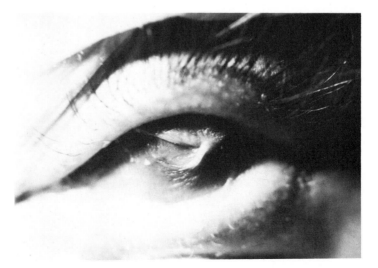

Figure 12–38 Lid changes in Stevens-Johnson disease with total scarring and symblepharon involving the lid and cornea.

basement membrane, and Bowman's membrane with very superficial stromal changes, but they are not primarily in the stroma.

Hereditary Juvenile Epithelial Dystrophy of Meesmann

Meesmann's dystrophy is a dominant epithelial dystrophy seen in early childhood, usually by 3 or 4 years of age. Visual acuity is not seriously affected, although vision may be reduced to 20/50 or less. The corneal lesions appear as small cystic changes in the deep epithelium and are noted best at the slit lamp on retroillumination. The disease is not progressive, and if vision is reduced to less than 20/60, a lamellar corneal transplant may be performed to replace the pathologic superficial cornea. Corneal sensitivity is reduced in Meesmann's dystrophy. Grossly, the cornea may appear slightly hazy, but only at the slit lamp is the disease readily evident.

Hereditary Epithelial Dystrophy of Stocker and Holt

Stocker and Holt described 20 individuals in one family in four generations manifesting these changes. The earliest involvement was noted at several months of age and the inheritance was a dominant pattern. Vision varied from slight clouding to almost total corneal opacification. The cornea had punctate gray opacities causing the epithelial surface to appear irregular at the slit lamp in mild involvement, while in more advanced cases the epithelium had marked changes, with thickening and thinning resulting in irregular astigmatism and visual loss. Corneal sensitivity was reduced. With severe corneal changes, a lamellar corneal transplant was the treatment of choice.

Reis-Bückler Dystrophy

This is a dominant hereditary dystrophy which is first seen early in life, usually by 3 to 4 years of age. The corneal changes in the beginning appear as gray, geographic clouded areas in the deep epithelium, Bowman's membrane, and the basement membrane. The epithelium gradully becomes irregular as the opacification and geographic changes on the corneal surface increase (Plate VI-A). This leads to decreased vision, 20/200 or less in later years. Later in the pathologic course, the midstroma may be involved. Corneal sensitivity is reduced when the corneal changes occur. Recurrent corneal erosion resulting in severe inflammatory changes and vascularization of the cornea occurs later in the disease. Treatment during the recurrent erosion stage is similar to that for recurrent erosion. Topical atropine, antibiotics, steroids, and pressure patching is indicated. When the cornea heals, a soft contact lens may be used to reduce the irregular astigmatism and improve vision. With severe changes in the anterior stroma, a lamellar corneal transplant is the treatment of choice.

Hereditary Anterior Membrane Dystrophy of Grayson and Wilbrandt

This dystrophy, which usually is seen by 10 years of age, causes gradual loss of vision. There may be occasional pain and inflammation but these are not major problems. Corneal sensitivity is normal. Regular opacities are noted at slit lamp examination between Bowman's membrane and the epithelium. The corneal nerves are usually prominent. Other anterior corneal dystrophies such as microcystic dystrophy are usually not seen in infancy and childhood.

PLATE VI

(*A*) Reis-Bückler corneal dystrophy involving the superficial cornea, epithelium, Bowman's membrane, and sub-Bowman's stroma. Note irregular astigmatism, as shown by the reduplicated light reflex.
(*B*) Granular corneal dystrophy in the early part of the third decade. This was first seen during the late teen years.
(*C*) Hereditary corneal dystrophy with a clear penetrating corneal transplant.
(*D*) Marked hydrops in a patient with Down's syndrome who had keratoconus.
(*E*) Corneal clouding and thickening in Hurler's disease.
(*F*) Bitot spot of the conjunctiva adjacent to the cornea. Note the glistening area here which represents degenerated epithelial cells.
(*G*) Kayser-Fleischer ring in Wilson's disease. This orange brown ring is noted for 360 degrees around the periphery.
(*H*) Slit lamp view of Kayser-Fleischer ring in Wilson's disease to show the deposition in the region of Descemet's membrane in the cornea.

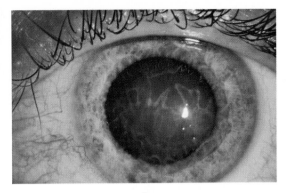

A

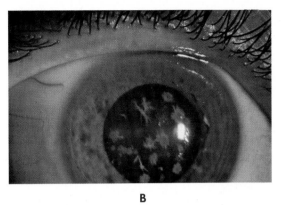

B

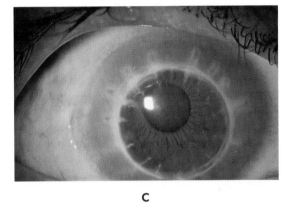

C

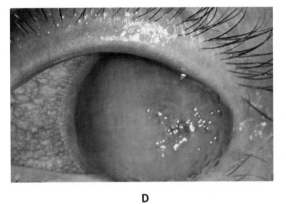

D

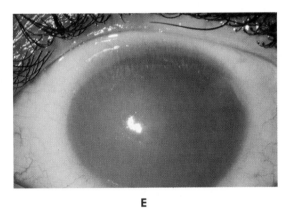

E

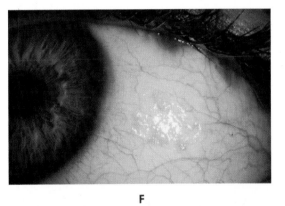

F

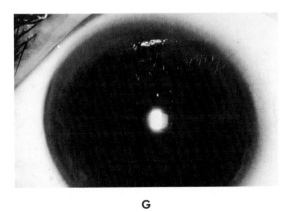

G

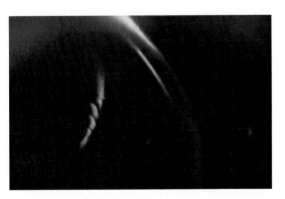

H

Stromal Corneal Dystrophies

The three common corneal dystrophies — granular, lattice, and macular — are not usually seen in infancy.

Granular Dystrophy

Granular dystrophy may be seen late in the first decade, but visual acuity is not decreased. There is relatively good vision in the first four or five decades because the lesions are discrete and sharply outlined, leaving clear cornea around them (Plate VI-B). This dystrophy, which does not cause epithelial irregularity and has normal corneal sensitivity, is dominant in its mode of inheritance. It does not lead to corneal vascularization or corneal erosion. Histopathologic findings have revealed that the abnormal tissue represents a hyalin degeneration in the stroma.

Lattice Dystrophy

Lattice dystrophy also is dominant in its pattern of inheritance and appears earliest toward the end of the first decade. The corneal epithelium is spared and therefore vision is good until the third or fourth decade. There is progressive opacification in a linear pattern in the superficial stroma, usually in the central region of the cornea (Fig. 12–39). Corneal sensitivity is decreased when more pathologic changes occur, but this does not occur in adolescence. The lesions appear as irregular thick opacified linear changes which can not be followed to the limbus and therefore are not blood vessels or corneal nerves. They may be mistaken for hypertrophic corneal nerves or vessels if careful slit lamp examination is not done. The stroma around these pathologic changes remains clear until later in life when recurrent erosion and opacification reduces vision to less than 20/200. A penetrating corneal transplant is indicated if vision deteriorates and the disease involves most of the corneal stroma. The histopathologic changes in the cornea indicate that the abnormal material is an amorphous hyalin material in the stroma. In addition to the hyalin there may be amyloid present in the cornea. Amyloid is not seen in granular and macular corneal dystrophies.

Macular Corneal Dystrophy

Because of the recessive mode of inheritance, macular dystrophy is seen early in life, during the first decade, and leads to more severe corneal scarring than the other two dystrophies. The lesions are not clearly circumscribed as they are in the granular and lattice dystrophies. They appear dirty gray in color, with poorly defined edges varying in size and shape in the stroma. When subjected to histopathologic examination, the corneal opacification reveals deposits of acid mucopolysaccharide located throughout the stroma, even involving the endothelium. This dystrophy is rarely seen because of its recessive nature. Penetrating corneal transplantation is necessary early in life if good vision is to be expected.

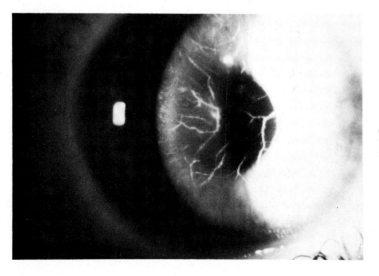

Figure 12–39 Lattice dystrophic changes in the corneal stroma. These were found in a 19-year-old with a family history of lattice dystrophy.

Crystalline Dystrophy of Schnyder

This dystrophy, an autosomal dominant one, may be seen early in infancy or at birth. The lesions are bilateral in nature and consist of many fine, small crystals located in the region beneath Bowman's membrane. Corneal sensitivity is normal. There is slow progression of the dystrophy with no vascularization. Vision remains good throughout life despite the crystalline changes in the cornea.

Dsytrophies involving the endothelium are not common in early life. Alterations in Descemet's membrane may be seen at birth, but these are either changes from congenital glaucoma or birth injuries or are developmental changes rather than corneal dystrophies or degenerations.

Congenital Hereditary Corneal Dystrophy

Full-thickness clouded corneas seen at birth in both eyes may represent congenital hereditary corneal dystrophy. The opacities can occur in early infancy and not be present at birth. This is a dominant hereditary dystrophy with incomplete penetrance, since it is much less common than the usual dominant corneal dystrophies. The corneal appearance at birth may be mistaken for congenital glaucoma, but the intraocular pressure obtained under anesthesia is normal. There is full-thickness corneal edema and epithelial edema although the anterior chamber, iris, and angle are normal. An interesting finding in this disease is the thickening of collagen fibrils. This is not present in any other

corneal dystrophy. The endothelium was abnormal in several cases examined after keratoplasty, and in others it was missing when the button was subjected to histopathologic examination.

Unfortunately, penetrating corneal transplantation in this disease is not uniformly successful (Plate VI-C). There is generally less than a 50/50 chance of success when a keratoplasty is done for hereditary corneal dystrophy. Repeat transplantation also has a small chance of remaining clear. Corneal sensitivity is normal. Electron microscopic findings have been reported, but the cause of this dystrophy is unknown.

Corneal Degeneration

The most common corneal degeneration in early adolescent years is keratoconus. This is a bilateral noninflammatory disease which affects both sexes but is more common in women. It may occur at puberty in women. It is difficult to see in the adolescent years, and progression occurs toward the late teens and in the early twenties. Unilateral keratoconus also may be seen but bilateral cases are far more frequent.

In childhood the earliest changes are characterized by distorted images at the keratometer and with the Placido disc. When the patient undergoes retinoscopy for refraction there is an uneven motion or slit with the retinoscope. This has been described as a scissors motion (Fig. 12–40).

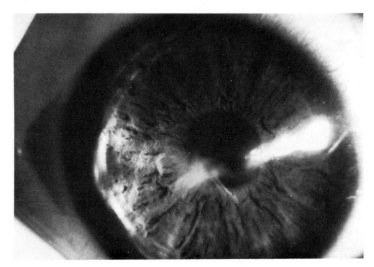

Figure 12–40 Keratoconus with abnormal light reflex off the surface of the cornea owing to the central cone.

With the ophthalmoscope there is also a more dense irregular dark reflex in the center of the fundus reflex which causes distortion of the fundus picture. Slit lamp examination reveals very early central or paracentral thinning but this is hard to detect in the earlier stages. There may be deep corneal stroma striae, and with careful slit lamp examination a Fleischer ring can be found at the upper or lower border of the early cone. Acute hydrops or edema of the cornea following breaks in Descemet's membrane are not usually seen in the first decade but may occur in the mid or late teens (Fig. 12–41). It is usually not necessary to perform a penetrating corneal transplant during adolescence for keratoconus. If the cone progressively thins, treatment with corneal, soft, or scleral lenses is not adequate to restore good vision, and a corneal transplant is necessary. Keratoconus may be seen with other conditions such as retinitis pigmentosa or Down's, Marfan's, and Alport's syndromes (Plate VI-D). Keratoconus can be associated with atopic dermatitis, and many children with keratoconus have some history of allergy. Frequently these children rub their eyes excessively. There is no successful treatment to prevent progression of keratoconus and only corneal transplantation offers the opportunity to restore vision in the severest cases. Corneal transplantation in appropriate cases is 90 per cent successful but is rarely necessary in childhood.

Calcific Degeneration of the Cornea

Calcific degeneration of the cornea in children usually is secondary to other corneal disease. In the young child, injuries with alkaline materials such as cement, lye, and ammonia are not uncommon and this severe chemical trauma may quickly lead to secondary calcific changes in the cornea, sometimes within two or three weeks of the original injury. Treatment with chelating agents such as EDTA will enhance removal of the calcium when it is in the region of Bowman's membrane and the superficial epithelium.

Systemic diseases with hypercalcemia may result in calcium deposits in the cornea. Hyperparathyroidism, vitamin D toxicity, milk-alkali syndrome, renal rickets, and hypophosphatasia, which result in elevations of blood calcium, may also induce calcific degeneration in the cornea.

Calcium in the cornea appears as either paralimbal, slight gray opacification in the region of the basement or Bowman's membrane, nasally and temporally, or in a band-shaped distribution across the central cornea. There may be small holes in the degenerative area which are characteristic of calcific degeneration. This corneal degeneration may also result from inflammatory diseases of the anterior segment such as uveitis and trauma. It is unusual for children to have long-standing anterior segment disease and therefore secondary calcific degeneration is not

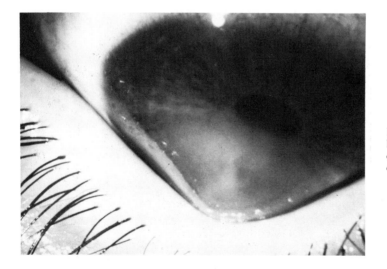

Figure 12–41 Acute hydrops in keratoconus, Munson's sign; the lower lid is pushed away from the cornea owing to the cone formed by the edematous stroma.

common in this age group. There is, however, an idiopathic hypercalcemia in children and band keratopathy secondary to chronic polyarthritis or Still's disease.

CORNEAL MANIFESTATIONS OF SYSTEMIC DISEASE

The corneal changes seen in systemic diseases of infancy and childhood may or may not affect vision in the young patient. Many of these diseases are rare in children and may have been described only in one or two cases, in either English or foreign literature. The more common systemic conditions will be mentioned as seen in infancy and childhood rather than the adult forms.

Diseases of the Cornea Due to Abnormalities in Carbohydrate Metabolism

The mucopolysaccharidoses are a group of diseases with definite systemic physical characteristics. They are described elsewhere. Hurler's disease, MPS I, is important in that the disease may be confused with congenital glaucoma and general hereditary corneal dystrophy and possibly interstitial keratitis. The cornea is hazy, with edema and thickening (Plate VI-E). The disease has many systemic characteristics, and demonstration of mucopolysaccharides in the urine aids in making the diagnosis. The cornea may be clear at first but becomes diffusely clouded in time, without signs of inflammation or vascularization. In Hunter's disease, MPS II, clouding of the cornea is present as well as multiple systemic abnormalities. In addition to the corneal changes, pigmentary degeneration of the retina may be responsible for visual loss. Sanfilippo's syndrome, MPS III, does not show corneal changes, whereas Morquio's syndrome, MPS IV, does show corneal clouding.

Scheie's syndrome, MPS V, is present in affected cases by 7 or 8 years of age. The cornea undergoes progressive clouding and becomes thicker. In Maroteaux-Lamy syndrome, MPS VI, corneal opacities are seen early.

It is evident that with clouded corneas early in life, urine analysis as well as testing the intraocular pressure is essential before a specific diagnosis can be made.

Diseases of Abnormal Protein Metabolism in Children

Cystinosis (Fanconi's syndrome) is a disease of altered amino acid metabolism. There is normal growth and development, usually until the 6th month of life when growth fails to continue and muscular weakness develops. Deposits of soluble cystine crystals in the conjunctiva, cornea, sclera, and choroid are found. The cornea is clouded and has very tiny glistening punctate dots which are the crystals reflecting light from the cornea. They are noticed throughout the full thickness of cornea; however, there is a concentration of crystal toward the corneal periphery. The disease is transmitted either as a dominant or autosomal recessive. Other diseases of the cornea with crystals are not seen in childhood; these are gout and dysproteinemia.

Inborn errors of metabolism with corneal changes are rarely seen. In phenylpyruvic oligophrenia, corneal opacities are present as well as cataracts. In porphyria, another inborn error of metabolism, the cornea may show ulceration and vascularization as well as keratomalacia. The full-blown picture appears later in life.

Diseases of Lipid Metabolism in Children

Corneal changes accompanying abnormal lipid metabolism are not usually seen in infancy and childhood. Arcus juvenilis has previously been described in the section on developmental abnormalities.

In Fabry's disease, a sex-linked, recessively transmitted disease, are abnormal lipid storage and corneal changes. In the epithelium of the cornea, fine pinpoint opacities involving the central and peripheral cornea may be found. The changes radiate from the central cornea to the periphery in a fanlike fashion. The first manifestations of this disease may be the corneal opacities. Although they appear in early childhood and are asymptomatic they are significant in that later systemic changes will occur which may herald the full-blown disease and early death. There are other ocular signs including focal vascular dilatations of the conjunctiva and retinal vessels.

In Hand-Schüller-Christian disease, corneal disease is rare. Corneal infiltration at the limbus and stromal lipid deposits have been described. Corneal changes in juvenile xanthogranuloma are also rare but may occur.

Corneal Changes in Avitaminosis

In severe malnutrition corneal changes from vitamin A deficiency may be seen. Keratomalacia with thickening of the corneal epithelium, epidermalization, and keratinization can occur. In the late stages, Bowman's membrane is replaced by pannus, and the cornea may appear hazy and thickened. The Bitot spot, a surface foamy conjunctival change temporal to the limbus, is also seen in vitamin A deficiency (Plate VI-F).

In riboflavin deficiency a superficial punctate keratitis may be evident which causes photophobia. Vascularization of the cornea is seen in the later stages.

Interstitial Keratitis of the Cornea Secondary to Systemic Cause

The most common cause of interstitial keratitis in children is congenital syphilis. The corneal manifestations of this disease acquired in utero occur in the first decade of life. Corneal changes are uncommon at birth or in the early infancy years. Congenital syphilis is first seen in the cornea as a rapid progression of corneal edema involving the cornea diffusely. Following this, vascularization of the deep cornea occurs, which is characteristic of the residual changes in the cornea noted later in life. The corneal vascularization may take on a salmon pink color because of the marked vascularization which lasts for several weeks. Later, gradual clearing of these corneal vessels occurs over a period of weeks to months. Ghost vessels remain in the deep cornea. The lines of clearing in the deep cornea are called Fuchs's lines and are characteristic of congenital syphilis. Treatment in this early stage of corneal involvement consists of topical corticosteroids and systemic therapy for the congenital syphilis. Dilatation of the pupil and antibiotics to prevent secondary infection are also used. During later years of life, if vision is significantly involved because of the corneal scarring, a penetrating corneal transplant may be done. It is important to examine the lens for opacities and the retina for changes which may cause visual loss.

Since the incidence of syphilis is increasing at the present time, the ophthalmologist should be aware of the corneal changes in this disease as well as Hutchinson's triad, which consists of corneal changes, abnormal dentition, and a flat bridge of the nose, all due to congenital syphilis.

Tuberculosis

Interstitial keratitis due to tuberculosis was more prevalent in the past when tuberculosis was a common disease. The disease in children, although not rare, is uncommon. Corneal changes include nodular corneal lesions with dense residual scarring and opacities following clearing. In children with undiagnosed corneal lesions and midstromal vessels, a tuberculin test and chest x-ray should be obtained.

Viral Interstitial Keratitis

Interstitial keratitis due to herpes simplex virus is probably more common than either of the two preceding diseases. In addition to herpes simplex virus, other viral infections, particularly mumps, measles, and vaccinia, may cause these stromal changes. Herpes zoster and varicella keratitis also can cause interstitial keratitis.

Wilson's Disease

Hepatolenticular degeneration is a disease of abnormal protein metabolism. There are liver and extrapyramidal changes which, if not corrected early in life, lead to permanent brain damage. Decrease in the ceruloplasmin is associated with an increase in the serum copper which is not bound to protein. In addition, there is an increase of copper secretion in the urine as well as copper deposition in various tissues such as liver and cornea.

The corneal changes are diagnostic of this disease. An orange-brown ring in the periphery of the cornea, called the Kayser-Fleischer ring, is the characteristic feature (Plate VI-G). The ring is deposited in the deep stroma in and around Descemet's membrane (Plate VI-H). There is a clear zone separating Descemet's membrane from the limbus. It is essential that all children manifesting mental or other systemic disease be examined with the slit lamp for early signs of this Kayser-Fleischer ring.

Refsum's Syndrome

Retinitis pigmentosa is part of this autosomal recessive disease in addition to other findings such as chronic polyneuritis. The corneal changes may consist of epithelial thickening and degeneration, with pannus formation in the region of Bowman's membrane. Hypertrophy of corneal nerves is present in this disease but the corneal changes are not the cause of the marked visual loss.

Keratoconjunctivitis Sicca

This is an unusual finding in children, although dry eyes should not be overlooked in a differential diagnosis of irritative phenomena in older children. Punctate keratitis, and very rarely filamentary keratitis, may be seen in older children with decreased production of tears. In addition, there is an excess of mucus in the precorneal tear film and an increase in viscosity of the tear film itself. Keratoconjunctivitis sicca may be found accompanying Still's disease or rheumatoid arthritis in children, and in lupus erythematosus, among other collagen diseases.

Familial Dysautonomia (Riley-Day Syndrome)

In early infancy this disease may first be seen in a child with failure to thrive. The ocular changes include an absence of tearing and corneal anesthesia due to the absence of corneal nerves. Corneal changes may be varied and include ulceration, resembling neuroparalytic keratitis and keratomalacia. Symptoms may be mild, such as punctate keratitis seen in exposure keratitis, or there may be more severe involvement. The prognosis is poor later in life and the ocular problem becomes less important as systemic changes occur.

CORNEAL INJURIES IN CHILDREN

Unfortunately corneal injuries in children may lead to significant or total visual loss as well as psychological problems due to severe corneal scarring and disfigurement. Ocular injuries in adults resulting from accidents may be prevented by the use of safety lenses. In children, these accidents are tragic, since they may be prevented by keeping harmful chemicals, sharp pointed toys, and instruments out of reach.

Corneal lacerations with sharp instruments, such as pencils, darts, and scissors, usually strike the lens also, and the additional problem arises of how to handle the secondary cataract and iris in the corneal wound. Fortunately, in children the lens material frequently resorbs, leaving a thin secondary membrane. If the laceration is paracentral, the midcornea, which is used for visual purposes, may be clear after injury, allowing a satisfactory image to form on the retina. If the scar is centrally located (Fig. 12–42) and the corneal

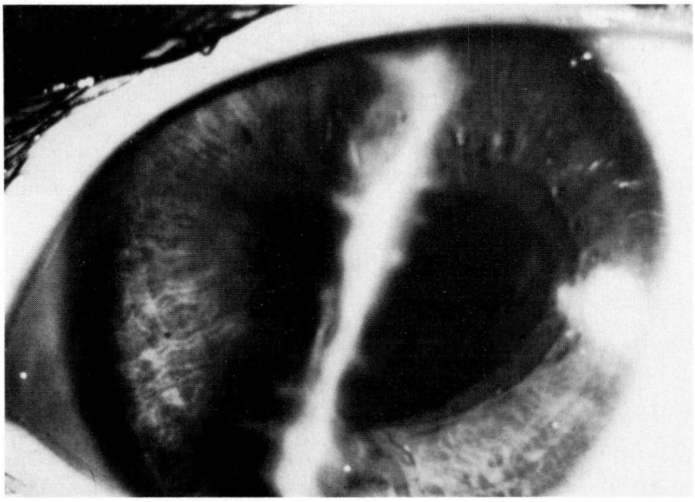

Figure 12–42 Central linear healed laceration which involved the cornea and did not strike the lens, therefore leaving a clear pupillary opening.

periphery is clear, a rotating autokeratoplasty after the initial trauma may be helpful in rotating the central scar out of the pupillary axis. This should be done before the secondary cataract is incised, since the secondary membrane is a useful barrier to prevent vitreous from coming forward. Others advocate incision of the secondary membrane at the time of keratoplasty in order to clear the pupillary area and enhance vision following surgery. During initial laceration repair it is best to attempt removal of anterior synechia to the back of the cornea. This may be done through the wound itself by passage of a synechiolysis spatula through the wound to sweep iris or lens remnant from the back of the cornea. It is important to do this to prevent vascularization or retrocorneal membrane formation (Fig. 12–43).

Chemical injuries may be serious in children, particularly alkali burns of the cornea and sclera. The common household cleaner ammonia is exceedingly dangerous and is easily accessible to children, since it is usually stored in a cabinet beneath the sink or on a low shelf. Within seconds of splashing ammonia on the eye the pH in the anterior chamber may climb to 12.0, causing denaturation of stromal protein as well as inflicting permanent damage on the iris and lens. The iris may balloon forward and touch the back of the cornea. Lens opacities develop rapidly in these accidents, and the healing stage is exceedingly long, frequently years after injury. Calcific degeneration may occur following alkali burns in small children. This complication must be looked for by slit lamp examination, so that proper therapy is instituted. Alkali burns in children are treated similarly to those in adults but therapy is difficult with children, since they are invariably uncooperative. Collagenase inhibitors in addition to conventional treatment is indicated. EDTA is used to remove secondary calcific degeneration. Soft contact lenses are now used to promote re-epithelialization. In addition to ammonia, lye, cement, grout, and lime may be found around the house. Acids cause corneal burns but are not nearly as severe as alkali chemical injuries of the cornea. All chemicals should be kept out of the reach of children, including turpentine, shellac, paints, and other fluids which may be ingested or splashed into the eye.

Blast injuries of the cornea, secondary to air guns such as B-B guns or pellet guns fired at close range, do great injury to a child's eye. Pellets have considerable range and may cause perforation of the cornea even at 50 yards. At present, tear gas pen guns are readily available to children and have caused injury to the

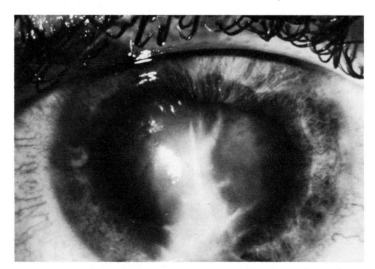

Figure 12–43   Central corneal laceration with lens opacification and anterior synechia.

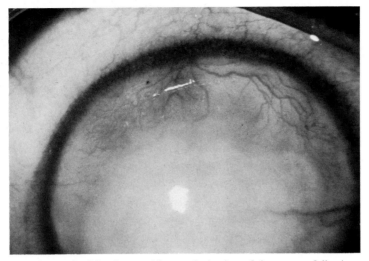

Figure 12–44 Total organized hyphema with vascularization of the cornea following corneal injury.

eyes. Most states have no law prohibiting sale or use of such guns. Injuries are caused by the blast when the gun is shot within 1 to 2 feet of the face. The blast comes from the gun powder which is used to propel the gas. Particles of gas which are over two years of age may act as missiles and cause corneal perforation. In addition, the plastic housing may be split and the plastic itself can also act as a missile at very close range. It is important to recognize that, in addition to corneal lacerations, contusions of the cornea with deep folds in Descemet's membrane and anterior chamber hemorrhage may occur from these injuries (Figs. 12–44 and 12–45). Recession of the angle, macular edema, and retinal hemorrhages have also been found.

Injury to children's eyes are handled as are injuries to adults. It is important to thoroughly examine the child's eye. If this is impossible by coaxing, general anesthesia should be used for careful operating microscope examination at the earliest time.

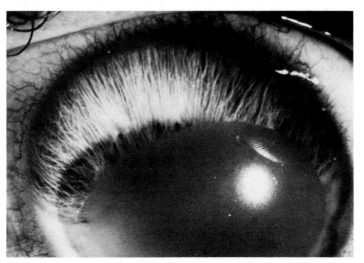

Figure 12–45 Blood staining of the cornea following total hyphema with resolution of the peripheral blood staining of the cornea.

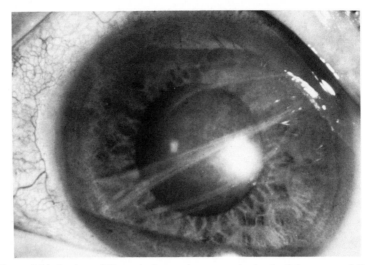

Figure 12–46 Linear folded tubes of Descemet's membrane on the back of the cornea following birth trauma. This patient's vision was 20/30 despite these corneal changes.

Birth Trauma

Trauma at birth is usually caused by forceps application in which one of the blades may be placed across the cornea. This results in excessive pressure to the cornea and breaks in Descemet's membrane. These breaks lead to corneal edema at birth which will clear in the first months of life. The breaks in the cornea, which are usually vertical or slightly off the vertical, will persist and appear as ridges of folded Descemet's membrane attached at both ends to the cornea in later life (Figs. 12–46 and 12–47). Good visual acuity may be obtained but usually there is some visual loss and in some cases it is severe. Corneal edema from endothelial decompensation may occur in the third or fourth decade. Penetrating keratoplasty has been successful in restoring some vision to these eyes.

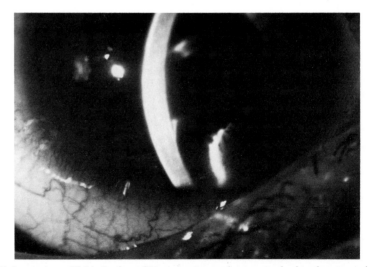

Figure 12–47 Slit lamp view of folded tubes of Descemet's membrane attached to the cornea inferiorly and in the anterior chamber centrally.

REFERENCES

Alkemade, P. P. H.: Dysgenesis Mesodermalis of the Iris and the Cornea. A Study of Rieger's Syndrome and Peters' Anomaly. Assen, Netherlands, Royal Vangorcum, 1969.

Allen, L., Burian, H. M., and Braley, A. E.: A new concept of the development of the anterior chamber angle. Arch. Ophthal., 53:783, 1955.

Barber, A. N.: Embryology of the Human Eye. St. Louis, The C. V. Mosby Co., 1955.

Barkan, O.: Pathogenesis of congenital glaucoma. Amer. J. Ophthal., 40:1, 1955.

Baum, J. L., and Feingold, M.: Ocular aspects of Goldenhar's syndrome (91 references). Amer. J. Ophthal., 75:250, 1973.

Burian, H. M., Braley, A. E., and Allen, L.: External and gonioscopic visibility of the ring of Schwalbe and the trabecular zone. Trans. Amer. Ophthal. Soc., 52:389, 1955.

Dailey, E. G., and Lubowitz, R. M.: Dermoids of the limbus and cornea. Amer. J. Ophthal., 53:661, 1962.

Donaldson, D. D.: Atlas of External Diseases of the Eye. Vol. I. Congenital Anomalies and Systemic Diseases, 1966; Vol. III. Cornea and Sclera, 1971. St. Louis, The C. V. Mosby Co.

Duke-Elder, S.: System of Ophthalmology. Vol. III. Embryology. St. Louis, The C. V. Mosby Co., 1963.

Falls, H. F.: A gene producing various defects of the anterior segment of the eye. Amer. J. Ophthal., 32:41, 1949.

Feigin, R. D., and Caplan, D. B.: Corneal opacities in infancy and childhood. Pediatrics, 69:383, 1966.

Goldstein, J. E., and Cogan, D. G.: Sclerocornea and associated congenital anomalies. Arch. Ophthal., 67:762, 1962.

Hamburg, A.: Incomplete separation of the lens and related malformations. Amer. J. Ophthal., 64:729, 1967.

Hansson, H., and Jerndal, T.: Scanning electron microscopic studies on the development of the iridocorneal angle in human eyes. Invest. Ophthal., 10:252, 1971.

Hay, E. D., and Revel, J.: Fine Structure of the Developing Avian Cornea. New York, S. Karger, 1969.

Henkind, P., and Friedman, A. H.: Iridogoniodysgenesis. Amer. J. Ophthal., 72:949, 1971.

Howard, R. O., and Abrahams, I. W.: Sclerocornea. Amer. J. Ophthal., 71:1254, 1971.

Jacobs, H. B.: Posterior conical cornea. Brit. J. Ophthal., 41:31, 1957.

Jerndal, T.: Goniodysgenesis and hereditary juvenile glaucoma. Acta. Ophthal. (Suppl.) 107:1, 1970.

Karlsberg, R. C., Emery, J. M., Green, W. R., Valdes-Dapena, M., and Coulombre, A. J.: Anomalies of iris and anterior chamber angles. Arch. Ophthal., 86:287, 1971.

Kenyon, K. R., and Antine, B.: The pathogenesis of congenital hereditary endothelial dystrophy of the cornea. Amer. J. Ophthal., 72:787, 1971.

Larsen, V., and Eriksen, A.: Cornea plana. Acta Ophthal., 27:275, 1949.

Mann, I.: The Development of the Human Eye. 2nd ed. London, British Medical Association, 1949.

Mann, I.: Developmental Abnormalities of the Eye. 2nd ed. London, British Medical Association, 1957.

O'Grady, R. B., and Kirk, H. Q.: Corneal keloids. Amer. J. Ophthal., 73:206, 1972.

Reese, A. B., and Ellsworth, R. M.: The anterior chamber cleavage syndrome. Arch. Ophthal., 75:307, 1966.

Smelser, G. K., and Ozanics, V.: Morphological and functional development of the cornea. In Duke-Elder, S., and Perkins, E. S. (eds.): The Transparency of the Cornea. Oxford, Blackwell Scientific Publications, 1960.

Smelser, G. K., and Ozanics, V.: The development of the trabecular meshwork in primate eyes. Amer. J. Ophthal., 71:366, 1971.

Smelser, G. K., and Ozanics, V.: Development of the cornea. Symposium on the cornea. Transactions of the New Orleans Academy of Ophthalmology. St. Louis, The C. V. Mosby Co., 1972, pp. 20–29.

Sugar, H. S.: The oculoauriculovertebral dysplasia of Goldenhar. Amer. J. Ophthal., 62:678, 1966.

Townsend, W. M.: Congenital corneal leukomas. I. Central defect in Descemet's membrane. Amer. J. Ophthal., 77:80–86, 1974.

Townsend, W. M., Font, R. L., and Zimmerman, L. E.: Congenital corneal leukomas. II. Histopathologic findings in 19 eyes with central defect in Descemet's membrane. Amer. J. Ophthal., 77:192–206, 1974.

Vail, D. T.: Adult hereditary anterior megalophthalmus sine glaucoma: a definite disease entity, with reference to the extraction of the cataract. Arch. Ophthal., 6:39, 1931.

Waardenburg, P. J.: Gross remnants of the pupillary membrane, anterior polar cataract and microcornea in a mother and her children. Ophthalmologica, 118:828, 1949.

CHAPTER 13

DISORDERS OF THE UVEAL TRACT

JOSEPH W. HALLETT, A.B., M.D.

INFLAMMATIONS — UVEITIS

Inflammation of the uveal tract may be purulent or nonpurulent. Purulent inflammations in the form of endophthalmitis or panophthalmitis are associated with similar involvement of the retina, vitreous, and outer coat of the eye. Occasionally metastatic, they are mostly the result of exogenous infection following wounds or intraocular surgery and will be considered elsewhere in this volume.

Incidence

Nonpurulent or endogenous uveitis is far and away the most common affection of the uveal tract, yet it is comparatively rare in children. At the Hospital for Sick Children in Toronto 43 per 100,000 admissions are for the treatment of clinically manifest uveitis. At the Wills Eye Hospital about 150 admissions per year are for the diagnosis and treatment of uveitis; of these cases 10 per cent are in the pediatric age group. It must be realized, however, that adults with uveitis are often treated as outpatients, but children are almost always hospitalized. Among our admissions, boys outnumbered girls in a ratio of 63 to 37 per cent, which is almost exactly the same sex ratio as in our adult admissions. Seven per cent of all enucleations in children are a consequence of uveal inflammation.

In our pediatric group 47 per cent had binocular involvement as compared to 32 per cent of our adult patients. This significantly higher percentage of bilateral involvement in children probably reflects their increased ocular hypersensitivity and capacity to react. It is generally accepted that young tissues respond to noxious stimuli more vigorously and extensively than older ones.

Classification

It is common to classify uveitis as acute or chronic iritis, cyclitis, or choroiditis, depending upon the portion of the uveal tract affected. Panuveitis refers to a diffuse involvement of the entire tract. Peripheral uveitis is a special, but important, type that occurs in the extreme fundus periphery and may eventually involve the contiguous structures. In children the ratio of predominantly anterior uveitis to predominantly posterior uveitis to panuveitis has been reported to be approximately 2:1:1. Of 32 children studied by Coles, 17 had anterior uveitis, 13 posterior uveitis, and 2 panuveitis. In general, the younger the child the more diffuse the inflammation.

The division of uveitis into granulomatous and nongranulomatous varieties seems to be dependable only in anterior involvement of the eye. We consider choroiditis to be granulomatous in the vast majority of instances. Accordingly, in our group we found 40 children with granulomatous, 31 with nongranulomatous, and 8 with unclassified uveitis. In addition, 15 cases were diagnosed as peripheral uveitis. Adding to this the 8 cases of unclassified uveitis, which are mostly instances of peripheral uveitis, gives approximately a 25 per cent incidence of peripheral uveitis in the pediatric group. This order of magnitude is quite in accord with the report from the Wilmer Institute, where out of 22 cases of peripheral uveitis one third occurred in children under 10 years of age. Hogan (1959) states that peripheral uveitis comprises 16 per cent of all uveitis in children and 80 per cent of them are bilateral.

General Pathology

Inflammation of the iris dilates the iris vessels through which a protein-rich exudate and inflammatory cells pass into the aqueous. This produces a flare in the anterior chamber and keratic precipitates (K.P.). Polymorphonuclear cells and lymphocytes form into fine K.P., and epithelioid cells form large mutton-fat K.P. (Fig. 13–1). Adhesions may form at the angle (peripheral anterior synechiae) or centrally at the pupillary margin (posterior synechiae). Posterior synechiae around the entire circumference of the pupil produce seclusio pupillae (Fig. 13–2), secondary glaucoma, and a forward bowing of the iris (iris bombé) (Fig. 13–3). Occasionally a pupillary membrane forms which obscures the pupil (occlusio pupillae). Lymphocytes

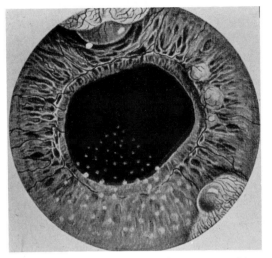

Figure 13–1   Anterior granulomatous uveitis—mutton-fat keratic precipitates and iris nodules.

and plasma cells may infiltrate anywhere in the iris stroma and produce nodules. Rarely are such nodules typically granulomatous lesions such as tubercle or sarcoid nodules. Local necrosis of the iris leads to iris atrophy and fibrosis. The iris thins, flattens out, and loses its pigment. Later a neovascular membrane may grow over the anterior iris surface (rubeosis iridis) and evert the pigment epithelium (ectropion pupillae).

Inflammation of the ciliary body makes it edematous and provokes exudation of protein-rich fluid into the posterior

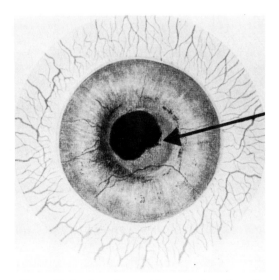

Figure 13–2   Anterior uveitis—seclusion of pupil.

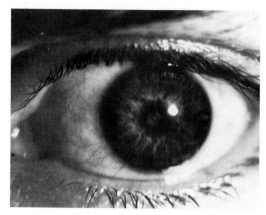

Figure 13–3 Iris bombé.

aqueous and anterior vitreous. A fibrous cyclitic membrane may develop behind the lens, in which complicated cataract may appear. As the cyclitic membrane contracts the pars plana and anterior choroid can detach. Finally, the ciliary body becomes atrophic, fibrotic, and hyalinized.

In the choroid the blood vessels dilate and pour out inflammatory fluid and cells. Inflammatory retinal detachment may develop. If necrosis of tissue ensues, the retina is destroyed and patches of chorioretinitis and vitreous opacities appear. With healing, prechoroidal fibrosis and chorioretinal adhesions appear along with pigment proliferation. Severe inflammation destroys both retina and choroid, resulting in a white patch surrounded by pigment clumps.

Symptoms and Signs

In adults the symptoms of uveitis are pain, photophobia, lacrimation, and visual disturbance. The same signs pertain to the disease in children, with two points worthy of emphasis: First, children frequently do not complain of visual difficulties, which may not even be suspected until strabismus develops; second, photophobia, which is usually most prominent in anterior uveitis, is often very severe in children, resulting in marked blepharospasm. The latter makes it extremely difficult to pry the lids open for examination of the eyes.

Of the manifold signs of uveitis, among which K.P., synechiae, vitreous opacities, and chorioretinal lesions are of major significance, none are particularly characteristic of childhood involvement except for band keratopathy. This is a progressive superficial deposition of calcium in a band-like zone across the central cornea in the exposed area of the palpebral orifice. Although it may occur in any long-standing uveitis at any age, it commonly appears early in juvenile iridocyclitis and has been described principally in association with juvenile rheumatoid arthritis (Still's disease).

Some other secondary complications occur with greater regularity and much earlier in the course of the disease than in adults. Posterior synechiae are frequently well formed by the time the child is first seen. Complicated cataract tends to develop early and to mature rapidly. Children seem to have a predilection for vitreous opacities and cyclitic membrane. Massive exudation in the fundus, as seen in Coats's disease, is more a juvenile than an adult trait. Hypopyon, which is an uncommon sign but does occur typically in Behçet's disease and in lens-induced uveitis, may also be associated with retinoblastoma. Mention of the latter brings to mind two cases of retinoblastoma seen at Wills Eye Hospital which presented initially as diffuse granulomatous uveitis.

Glaucoma occurs so commonly in adults with uveitis that it becomes mandatory to check the intraocular tension routinely and often. Though not easy to do in children, the few instances in which we have investigated it the tensions have almost always been low. The consequences of uncontrolled glaucoma are, however, so severe that at least a finger tension, despite its inaccuracy and inadequacy, should be included in the routine management of uveitis in children.

PLATE VII
- (*A*) Flocculi of iris, congenital excrescences of pigmented iris epithelium completely occluding the pupil.
- (*B*) Brushfield's spots in Down's syndrome.
- (*C*) Congenital posterior staphyloma.
- (*D*) Aniridia with anterior polar cataract associated with Wilms' tumor.
- (*E*) Heterochromia, congenital.
- (*F*) Waardenburg's syndrome with heterochromia.
- (*G*) Inclusion bodies from inclusion blenorrhea (see section on Inclusion Conjunctivitis, p. 264, for discussion). (Courtesy of Dr. Phillips Thygeson.)
- (*H*) Clinical appearance of inclusion blenorrhea (p. 264). (Courtesy of Dr. Phillips Thygeson.)

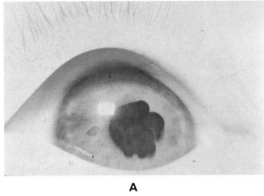

A

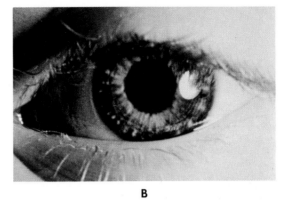

B

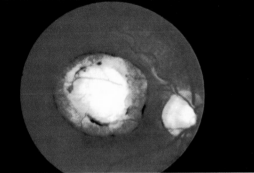

C

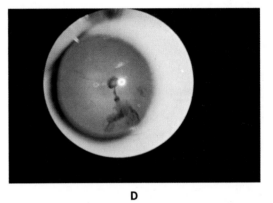

D

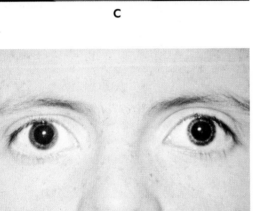

E

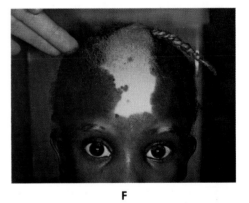

F

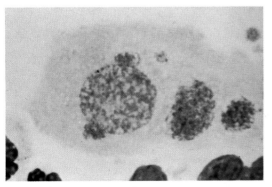

G

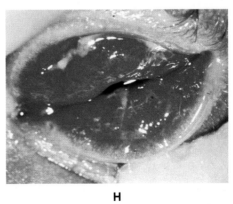

H

TABLE 13–1 DIAGNOSTIC PROCEDURES IN CHILDHOOD UVEITIS

Complete blood count, including platelets
Urinalysis
Erythrocyte sedimentation rate
Total serum protein and A/G ratio
Serologic test for syphilis
Toxoplasmosis hemagglutination test
Histoplasmosis complement fixation test
Latex agglutination test
X-ray of skull, chest, and small bones
Skin tests—tuberculin, histoplasmin, streptococci, allergens
Stool examination for ova and parasites
Lymph node and conjunctival biopsies

Diagnostic Studies

Routine uveitis surveys are designed to disclose the various etiologic agents that have been incriminated in that disease. An entire survey in a child may be too formidable a task and perhaps sufficient information can be obtained from a careful history and specifically directed laboratory tests. In Table 13–1 are listed the procedures routinely ordered at Wills Eye Hospital. This is supplemented, of course, by other specific examinations whenever indicated.

Etiology

The presumed etiologic diagnoses change with advancing knowledge. Some of the more recent reports, along with our findings, are listed in Table 13–2. Toxoplasmosis is the major cause of posterior uveitis. Still's disease, herpes simplex, and sarcoid command most attention in anterior involvement. Undetermined etiologies run from 20 to 50 per cent in various series. Peripheral uveitis, which is diagnosed with increasing frequency, is completely enigmatic, although *Toxocara canis* larva was recently identified in the eye of a 6-year-old girl, presenting as a peripheral uveitis. The role of trauma is hard to evaluate because these cases are not listed under the often associated uveitis.

Special Forms of Uveitis

Toxoplasmosis

Toxoplasma gondii is an obligate intracellular protozoan parasite. Its mode of spread is unknown despite its frequent and widespread occurrence in man and in wild and domestic animals. Infection may be congenital or acquired. The mother gives no evidence of illness when the congenital variety is passed to the fetus through the placental circulation. It is very rare for subsequent offspring to be infected.

Retinochoroiditis is present in 80 per cent of children with toxoplasmosis and is bilateral in 85 per cent of these cases. It occurs typically in the macular area as a large, poorly defined, elevated focus associated with copious exudation into the vitreous. Small satellite foci are common. In about 2 to 4 months, healing may set in and the lesions become atrophic, pale, punched-out, and bordered with dense pigment. Additionally, cerebral calcifica-

TABLE 13–2 ETIOLOGY OF UVEITIS IN CHILDREN

	Kimura (1964)	Sachsenweger (1964)	Coles (1963)	Wills (1961–64)
Toxoplasmosis	60	2	10	45
Still's disease	11	—	1	—
Sarcoid	3	—	2	1
Tuberculosis	1	1	2	5
Herpes simplex	5	—	1	—
Sympathetic ophthalmia	2	2	—	—
Behçet's syndrome	1	—	—	—
Vogt-Koyanagi-Harada	1	—	—	—
Trauma	1	—	—	—
Peripheral uveitis	41	—	—	15
Fuchs's heterochromia	7	—	—	—
Ankylosing spondylitis	1	—	—	—
Congenital syphilis	—	2	—	1
Metastatic suppurative	—	9	—	—
Histoplasmosis	—	—	—	2
After BCG inoculation	—	1	—	—
Ulcerative colitis	—	—	1	—
Undetermined	48	20	15	10
Total	182	37	32	79

tion, convulsions, jaundice, fever, anemia, and hepatosplenomegaly all point to the diagnosis of toxoplasmosis. Strabismus, nystagmus, and poor vision from macular scarring are common (Fig. 13–4).

Acquired acute toxoplasmic focal retinochoroiditis appears between 11 and 40 years of age. There is no predilection for the macula as in the congenital variety. Systemic manifestations are just about nil, yet local reactivation is frequent, suggesting that a hypersensitivity mechanism is in force.

In addition to the clinical picture the diagnosis is based primarily on the Sabin-Feldman methylene blue dye test and on the toxoplasmin skin test, both of which at this writing are not commercially available. The skin test becomes positive 4 to 12 months after acute infection. If positive, no further studies need be done to make the diagnosis. A dye test titer as low as 1:8 must be considered significant in a child who presents the typical fundus findings. The indirect hemagglutination test and the indirect fluorescent antibody test are easier and safer to do than the dye test and are probably just as accurate (Fig. 13–5).

Specific therapy with pyrimethamine (Daraprim), sulfonamide, and corticosteroid should start to show some improvement in 1 to 2 weeks and may be continued up to about 8 weeks. The absorption of Daraprim from the gastrointestinal tract tends to be poorer in children so they should receive somewhat more than the

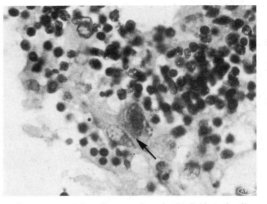

Figure 13–5 Small cytoplasmic inclusion bodies (arrow) in cytomegalic inclusion disease could be mistaken for Toxoplasma organisms (1000x). (From Smith, Zimmerman, and Harley.)

usual reduced pediatric dosage. Depression of the leukocytes and platelets should be checked for once or twice weekly and should be treated promptly with calcium Leucovorin, 5 to 15 mg. daily. Lesions resistant to treatment may quiet down under cryotherapy. Photocoagulation around inactive lesions is claimed to prevent recurrences.

Peripheral Uveitis

Next to toxoplasmosis, peripheral uveitis or pars planitis is the most common type of juvenile uveitis. It usually starts between the ages of 6 and 10 years as a mild chronic cyclitis characterized by a myriad of punctate opacities in the retrolental space and anterior vitreous. It may begin in the peripheral choroid and pars plana in the region of attachment of the vitreous base. Some cases present as a peripheral vasculitis and retinitis.

Most cases smoulder on in a chronic form for many years, some subside, a few develop choroidal and retinal detachment or proceed to occlusion of the retinal vessels. Children often develop a massive yellow-gray exudate over the inferior ora serrata. This gradually becomes vascularized via the ciliary body and proliferates onto the posterior capsule of the lens, producing a cyclitic membrane.

The etiology is profoundly mysterious, and treatment, even with corticosteroids, lacks value. Wong and Hersh were able to control some cases with methotrexate, which can hardly qualify as a drug for routine administration.

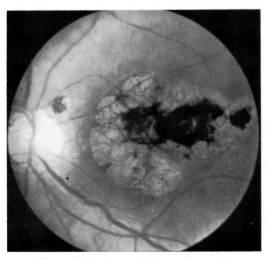

Figure 13–4 Congenital toxoplasmosis.

Rheumatoid Arthritis in Children (Still's Disease)

Up to 20 per cent of children with Still's disease develop chronic anterior uveitis. The ocular inflammation may antedate the joint manifestations by several years. Almost invariably both eyes are ultimately involved. The triad of band-shaped keratitis, severe iridocyclitis, and complicated cataract was formerly considered pathognomonic for Still's disease, but it is now evident that many forms of anterior uveitis in children eventually develop the same clinical picture. Posterior segment inflammation is rare. There is no specific treatment for the ocular component of rheumatoid arthritis.

The role of *autoimmunity* in uveitis may appropriately be considered here, since the *collagen diseases*, which include rheumatoid arthritis and *systemic lupus erythematosus*, are suspected to be autoimmune diseases. In this regard we found the latex agglutination test, which is positive in 90 per cent of rheumatoid arthritis patients and in only 1 per cent of a normal control group, to be positive in 20.5 per cent of endogenous uveitis cases. We further found that a complement fixation test using antigens from normal human liver and kidney was positive in 52 per cent of a group with uveitis and in only 5 per cent of a healthy control group.

Tuberculosis

The incidence of tuberculous uveitis is not proportional to the incidence of the systemic disease. The eyes seem to become involved during the course of systemic tuberculosis only in the case of miliary dissemination. The modern belief is that most tuberculous uveitis occurs on the basis of an allergic hypersensitivity reaction from some extraocular form of tuberculosis rather than being the result of direct organismal invasion.

In 1917 about 70 per cent of school children had a positive tuberculin skin test, whereas recently only 5 per cent are positive. Consequently, a negative tuberculin test is now of considerable help in ruling out tuberculosis as a possible etiologic factor in uveitis. We have found the Middlebrook-Dubos hemagglutination test to be valueless in the diagnosis of tuberculous uveitis.

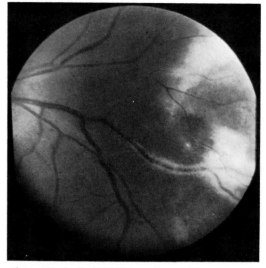

Figure 13–6   Periphlebitis, tuberculosis suspected.

Other than the soft yellow-white miliary tubercles of the choroid there is no typical clinical picture of tuberculous uveitis. Iridocyclitis may be acute nongranulomatous or chronic granulomatous. Choroiditis may be exudative, severe, spreading, juxtapapillary, and associated with retinal periphlebitis (Figs. 13–6, 13–7, and 13–8.)

Treatment by tuberculin desensitization should be considered when there is a high degree of sensitivity. A focal reaction in the eye concomitant with the skin test may be indicative of such hypersensitivity. Isoniazid is well tolerated by children in

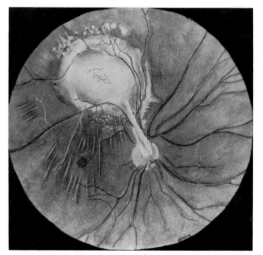

Figure 13–7   Giant conglomerate tubercle in 9-year-old boy from Panama.

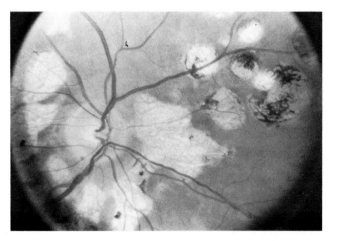

Figure 13–8 Disseminate chorioretinitis, tuberculosis suspected.

the adult dosage of 100 mg. t.i.d. and need not be reduced unless the child's weight is under 60 pounds. A dramatic improvement in the eye after 1 or 2 weeks of treatment may be considered corroboration of the etiology. In association with para-aminosalicylic acid, 150 mg. per kg. of body weight, divided into three parts and taken with meals, treatment should be extended for 2 years to prevent relapse of active tuberculosis and for at least 1 year as a preventive measure. Streptomycin has been too toxic in our experience to continue its use.

Sarcoid

Sarcoid is a chronic granulomatous disease that may involve almost any structure in the body. Of unknown etiology, it has a striking predilection for Negroes in the United States. The most frequent ocular manifestation is granulomatous anterior uveitis characterized by huge mutton-fat keratic precipitates and nodules of various sizes on and in the iris. Large inferior vitreous opacities may be found, often occurring in chains. Occasionally the fundus presents retinal periphlebitis and the characteristic "candle wax drippings" around the retinal veins (Fig. 13–9.)

The diagnosis is based on an elevated erythrocyte sedimentation rate, reversal of the serum A/G ratio, hypercalcemia, relative anergy to tuberculin, a positive Kveim test, and typical x-ray findings in the lungs and punched-out lesions in the phalanges. Positive lymph node biopsy is most incontrovertible.

Treatment is entirely nonspecific and consists of vigorous mydriasis and intensive local and systemic corticosteroid therapy.

Viral Uveitis

This diagnosis rests almost entirely upon association of the uveitis with a recognizable viral disease; for example, *herpes simplex* of the cornea is often associated with anterior uveitis. The herpetic virus has, however, been recovered from the aqueous in acute iritis without associated keratitis. Cogan diagnosed a case of herpes simplex chorioretinopathy and meningitis in an infant on the basis of a significant rise in specific antibodies

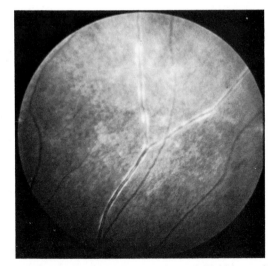

Figure 13–9 Sarcoid—retinal periphlebitis and "candle wax drippings."

against the virus during the course of the disease.

HERPES ZOSTER. Herpes zoster characteristically involves the eye along with the cutaneous eruption in the distribution of the ophthalmic division of the trigeminal nerve. Usually only a keratitis is present; however, especially if the ala nasi is involved, recurrent granulomatous iridocyclitis and secondary glaucoma are common. This relationship is explained by the fact that the nasociliary nerve is the sensory nerve to the ala nasi and to the uveal tract. Systemic corticosteroid, immune serum, and gamma globulin alleviate the condition along with appropriate local treatment.

CYTOMEGALIC INCLUSION DISEASE. Cytomegalic inclusion disease is caused by a virus which primarily affects stillborn babies, infants, and children under 12 years of age. It involves many organs, including the uveal tract and retina, as well as exhibiting cerebral calcifications. This is a source of confusion with toxoplasmosis. Inclusion bodies have been found in the urine and aqueous humor.

Cytomegalic inclusion disease is characterized by the formation of large cells with intranuclear and cytoplasmic inclusions. The causal cytomegalovirus (CMV) passes transplacentally from an asymptomatic mother to the fetus. A recent study in Nova Scotia showed that 60 per cent of the women of childbearing age had no antibodies to CMV. This would establish a degree of susceptibility greater than that to rubella and, since CMV is constantly present, it may prove to be more important than rubella as a cause of congenital disease. In the same study, 34 per cent of newborns had antibodies to CMV. Stillbirths are frequent. Microcephaly, mental retardation, and spastic diplegia are common, and many organs may be involved.

Although anterior uveitis, cataract, and optic atrophy have been reported, the most consistent eye findings are multiple, small, diffuse areas of retinochoroiditis. These may coalesce as activity continues to form one large necrotic area similar to that of toxoplasmosis, differentiation from which is even more difficult because of the intracranial calcification found in both diseases. There may even be histopathologic confusion, inasmuch as the cytoplasmic inclusions can be mistaken for Toxoplasma.

Diagnosis is aided by culturing CMV from the urine, tears, conjunctival scrapings, cerebrospinal fluid, or liver biopsy. Inclusions may be found in urine sediment, conjunctiva, and liver. No treatment is dependable, although steroids have been moderately successful.

BEHÇET'S SYNDROME. Behçet's syndrome of recurrent uveitis, often with hypopyon associated with ulcers of the mucous membranes, inflammatory polyarthritis, phlebitis, and skin and neurologic complications, is claimed to be caused by a virus.

CONGENITAL RUBELLA SYNDROME. In the congenital rubella syndrome an active iridocyclitis is found in most eyes. Lens surgery in these eyes releases a large dose of virus into the surrounding intraocular tissues and an often intractable endophthalmitis results.

INFLUENZA. Influenza apparently varies in its different epidemics: in some epidemics, uveal manifestations prevail; in others, an unusual frequency of ocular paralysis or optic neuritis has been registered. Acute nongranulomatous anterior uveitis is the usual picture. Secondary glaucoma is frequent. Fibrinous exudate in the anterior chamber and even hypopyon may occur.

MUMPS. Mumps may cause iritis at the climax of the general disease or with the beginning of convalescence. The development is rapid and the outcome benign. Since it occurs during the course of epidemic parotitis, it should not be confused with *uveoparotitis of Heerfordt*. This is a chronic inflammation of the uvea and parotid glands often accompanied by dacryoadenitis and paralysis of the facial nerve.

CHICKENPOX. Uveitis during the course of *chickenpox* is extremely rare. It is usually anterior, mild, and favorable in prognosis. I reported such a case which appeared two days after the exanthem in a 7-year-old boy.

SUBACUTE SCLEROSING PANENCEPHALITIS (SSPE). SSPE is a slowly progressive fatal neurologic disease caused by the measles virus. It usually occurs between the ages of 4 and 16 years and affects males predominantly, in a ratio of 4 to 1. It may

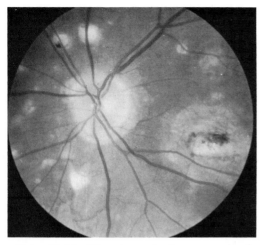

Figure 13–10 Histoplasmosis—large macular lesion and smaller, discrete, sparsely pigmented choroidal lesions.

present as a focal low-grade chorioretinitis. There is no vitreous involvement. Nystagmus, cortical blindness, papilledema, and optic atrophy may also occur. Progressive neurologic and mental deterioration terminate in death within 6 months to 3 years. The complement fixation test for measles in the cerebrospinal fluid is almost always positive.

Fungus Infections

With the possible exception of *Histoplasma capsulatum*, fungi are rare causes of uveitis in children. Histoplasmosis characteristically presents a clear vitreous; disciform detachment of the macula or perimacular area, with or without subretinal hemorrhage; and small, discrete, sparsely pigmented choroidal lesions or scars in the central, mid- or peripheral fundus. (See Figure 13–10.) A positive histoplasmin skin test corroborates the clinical impression, though it should be noted that skin testing of 1924 elementary school children in Maryland revealed 34.8 per cent positive. This increased with age, amounting to 42.4 per cent in the sixth-graders compared to 26.5 per cent in the second-graders. The histoplasmin complement fixation test may be of value when the skin test is falsely negative, and the blood for the test should be drawn before the skin test is administered.

Though effective, amphotericin B is too nephrotoxic for control of this disease. Prompt use of corticosteroids may abort an attack. Active lesions away from the fovea can be successfully engulfed by photocoagulation. Prophylactic histoplasmin desensitization may protect the second macula when the other is scarred.

Fungus infections may occur in the eye following injuries, operations or during the course of other fungal infections such as actinomycosis of the lung, mucormycosis of the sinuses, sporotrichosis and aspergillosis. Similar mycotic infections occur without knowledge of the portal of entry or without other evidence of systemic mycotic disease. The uveitis following such an infection begins insidiously with visual clouding from a profusion of vitreous opacities, pain, redness, and chemosis.

There may be an attempt of the tissue to "wall off" an involved area during the early stages. The uveitis develops into an endophthalmitis in most instances with loss of the eye. However, the tissue damage even after repair leads to extensive alteration in the function of the eye and may result in glaucoma, cyclitic membrane, occlusion of the pupil, and retinal separation.

Numerous recent reports reflect the aggressiveness with which these conditions are being managed. Though extremely irritating locally, amphotericin B has been injected sub-Tenon and even intravitreally. Valuable vision has been reportedly salvaged, thereby justifying the treatment.

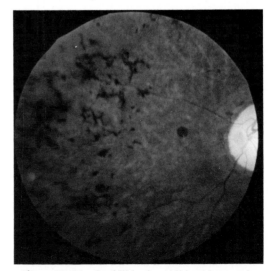

Figure 13–11 Syphilitic choroiditis with secondary pigmentary degeneration of the retina, resembling retinitis pigmentosa.

Congenital Syphilis

Chorioretinitis is the most common ocular picture seen in congenital syphilis. The salt-and-pepper variety is often confined to the periphery, produces little visual impairment and is not progressive. In secondary pigmentary degeneration of the retina the process tends to be diffuse and exhibits pigmentary cuffing of the blood vessels, often in a bone corpuscle configuration reminiscent of retinitis pigmentosa (Fig. 13–11). Patchy and diffuse loss of vision and visual field results. After the age of 4 years, interstitial keratitis makes its appearance and is always associated with uveitis.

A positive serologic test for syphilis in both child and mother will clinch the diagnosis. The serum fluorescent treponemal antibody absorption (FTA-ABS) test is often positive in congenital syphilis when the routine serologic tests are usually negative. Specific treatment has prospects of success only in very young children; in later years antiluetic therapy has no influence on the progress of the disease. Prompt treatment of the infected mother during pregnancy prevents or attenuates eye disease in the offspring.

Leprosy

Leprosy is a chronic infection caused by the *Mycobacterium leprae*, which chiefly affects superficial neural and epithelial tissues. Children are more susceptible to infection than adults. The disease is not congenital and infants removed from their leprous mother have not contracted the disease, according to a series from Panama.

Superficial punctate keratitis and chronic recurrent iritis are early signs of the disease. Choroiditis is not common in leprosy. Diagnosis is made by the identification of the acid-fast bacilli found in the serum of lepromatous skin lesions. Diaminodiphenylsulphone (DDS) has been an effective therapeutic agent in conjunction with atropine and cortisone topically.

Jensen's Juxtapapillary Choroiditis

Jensen's juxtapapillary choroiditis consists of circumscribed inflammatory changes of the choroid adjacent to the disc. A large sector-shaped field defect stretches out from the blind spot. The etiology is unknown.

Vogt-Koyanagi-Harada Disease

Vogt-Koyanagi-Harada disease is a relatively rare condition of unknown etiology characterized by uveitis, alopecia, poliosis, vitiligo, tinnitus, deafness, and signs of meningoencephalitis (Fig. 13–12). The uveitis may become severe and bilateral symmetrical, inferior, retinal detachments can be observed. The optic disc may appear hyperemic and the veins engorged. The uveitis clears in about 50 per cent of the patients and the detachment subsides. Complications of glaucoma, cataract, and phthisis bulbi may develop. The poliosis and deafness seem to be permanent. There are some similarities to sympathetic ophthalmia, suggesting a uveal pigment sensitivity.

Fuchs's Heterochromia

Fuchs's syndrome presents as a mild persistent cyclitis associated with atrophic alterations of the iris in the affected eye. The radial markings of the pupillary zone become less prominent and the pigment layer often has a moth-eaten appearance. No posterior synechiae are found, complicated cataract usually develops, and secondary glaucoma is common. It is not fully established whether the heterochromia is congenital or not. Both cause and effect treatment elude us.

Lens-Induced Uveitis

Rupture of the lens capsule liberates lens material into the eye cavities. This results in one or the other of two different types of uveitis that subsides when the lens or lens substance is removed. The uveitis is often associated with glaucoma.

The *phacotoxic reaction* usually occurs in the presence of a hypermature cataract. The lens material acts as a chemical irritant probably directly on the iris and ciliary body. Macrophages come in to engulf the liberated material. No polymorphonuclear cells are seen.

Endophthalmitis phacoanaphylactica results from an underlying sensitivity to lens protein probably amplified by bacteria or their toxins. The typical picture consists of a break in the lens capsule of one eye by operation or injury. After the inflammation has quieted down in this first eye, the second eye, which always shows a mature or hypermature cataract, develops

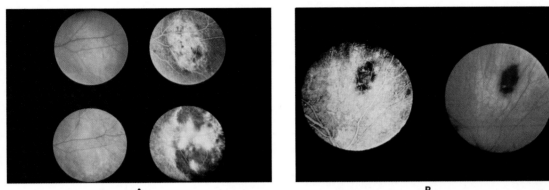

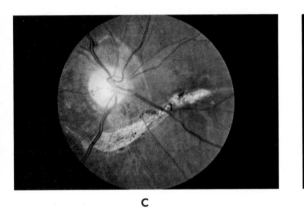

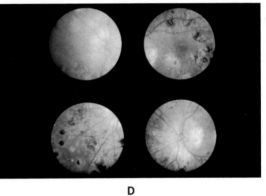

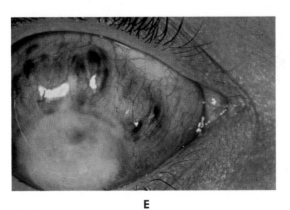

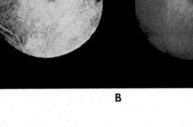

PLATE VIII

(A) Hemangioma of the choroid before and after treatment with photocoagulation.

(B) Choroidal nevus and the appearance with fluorescein angiography.

(C) Choroidal rupture resulting from blunt trauma (white male, age 12).

(D) Uveitis, syphilitic.

(E) Intercalary staphyloma following severe sclerokeratitis (white male, age 14).

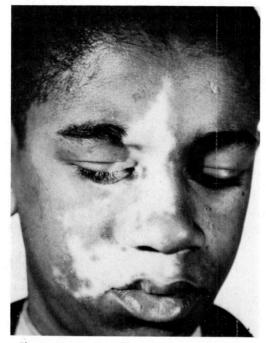

Figure 13–12 Vogt-Koyanagi-Harada disease, illustrating poliosis and vitiligo with bilateral uveitis.

a spontaneous rupture of the lens capsule and a severe anterior granulomatous uveitis. Polymorphonuclear cells and macrophages are found in the aqueous, iris, and lens.

Visceral Larva Migrans

This is a syndrome of early childhood resulting from ingestion of dirt. It is caused by the larvae of *Toxocara canis* and *cati*, the common intestinal roundworm of dogs and kittens. In the eye it may produce chronic endophthalmitis, solitary retinal granuloma, or peripheral retinitis. The diagnosis is established only by histopathologic examination. Most cases occur in the 4- to 6-year age group. There is no specific treatment.

Sympathetic Ophthalmia

Fortunately rare, this disease tends to occur most commonly in children. The dreaded clinical picture is that of a bilateral generalized ocular inflammation following a perforating wound of one eye. A positive diagnosis can only be made histologically: granulomatous aggregates of epithelioid and giant cells thicken the choroid; the choriocapillaris is free of infiltration; small foci of epithelioid cells (Dalen-Fuchs nodules) lie under a mound

of retinal pigment epithelium; inflammation extends via the emissary vessels and nerves through the sclera; necrosis is rare; and the retina is often not affected. Prophylactic enucleation of severely traumatized eyes is the best treatment. Corticosteroids may help some cases, others require immunosuppressive drugs.

Glaucomatocyclitic Crises

These are unilateral recurrent attacks of acute noncongestive glaucoma associated with signs of mild cyclitis. Tensions of 40 to 60 mm. may persist from a few hours up to two weeks or more. Small, flat, round K.P. and a trace of flare and cells appear transiently. Posterior synechiae do not form and the angles remain open. Treatment is with mild miotics, topical corticosteroids, 10 per cent phenylephrine and systemic carbonic anhydrase inhibitors. Surgery is not indicated.

Acute Posterior Multifocal Placoid Pigment Epitheliopathy

This newly described entity occurs primarily in young adults who are otherwise healthy. Rapid loss of central vision results from multifocal, yellow-white placoid lesions at the level of the pigment epithelium and choroid, and all posterior to the equator. The lesions tend to clear, and vision returns to essentially normal after a period of several months, despite residual marked pigmentary alterations in the pigment epithelium. The etiology is obscure and treatment is symptomatic.

Treatment of Uveitis

In the discussion of special forms of uveitis specific treatment, if any, was listed. In most cases adjuvant nonspecific measures are also advisable. In the many instances in which no etiology can be established, nonspecific treatment is all that can be offered. This comes in local or systemic varieties.

Local Treatment

MYDRIATICS. *Mydriatics* constitute a time-honored remedy for uveitis. Two obvious advantages accrue from their use: first, it makes observation of the fundus easier; second, posterior synechiae may be released or be prevented from developing. Ocular discomfort is often ameliorated when the uvea is relaxed by mydriatics. Anterior uveitis demands more strenuous and prolonged mydriasis than posterior uveitis. I prefer 10 per cent phenylephrine and 1 per cent cyclopentolate for rapid and vigorous pupillary dilation. To maintain prolonged mydriasis 0.5 to 1 per cent atropine solution or ointment once or twice daily is effective. Some children flush up readily with atropine and may even develop fever and delirium. One can then substitute 0.12 to 0.25 per cent scopolamine, 2 to 5 per cent homatropine, or 0.5 per cent cyclopentolate. Dark glasses, of course, are a comfort in the presence of dilated pupils. Unyielding posterior synechiae may be lysed by subconjunctival injection of 2 minims each of 1 per cent atropine, 2 per cent cocaine and 1:1000 epinephrine.

HEAT. In the form of moist packs, electric pad, infra-red, or diathermy, heat can be very comforting and is claimed to aid absorption of inflammatory products.

CORTICOSTEROIDS. Corticosteroids as drops or ointments are effective, particularly in anterior uveitis. Very frequent applications are advised initially and treatment should continue 1 to 3 weeks after all activity of the disease has disappeared. Cortisone and hydrocortisone have been almost entirely replaced by the newer synthetics such as prednisone, dexamethasone, and fluprednisolone. Subconjunctival injection, usually in the form of 0.5 cc. of depot 6 methyl prednisolone, is often resorted to when systemic steroid therapy has to be supplemented or replaced. It is particularly helpful in the lysis of recent dense posterior synechiae. Additional injections, if needed, may be given in 1 or 2 weeks.

PARACENTESIS. Anterior chamber puncture or paracentesis with release of aqueous is occasionally utilized in uveitis. Study of the fluid may help to establish the etiology. The increased antibody content of the secondary aqueous is theoretically beneficial. Secondary glaucoma can be transiently controlled. I have seen dramatic improvement result from aspiration of the milky aqueous in phacotoxic uveitis.

IRIDECTOMY. Iridectomy is mandatory for control of secondary glaucoma associated with iris bombé. Occasionally a chronic or recurrent iridocyclitis will respond favorably only to an iridectomy performed at the site of a persistent posterior synechia. The laser beam or photocoagulator may be superior modalities for this procedure.

GLYCERINE. Glycerine or hypertonic saline or glucose drops are often useful in clearing corneal edema due to secondary glaucoma or following extensive endothelial damage from K.P.

CHELATING AGENTS. Chelating agents such as Versenate can clear superficial calcific corneal deposits in band-shaped keratopathy. Prior light curettage of the affected area is helpful.

ANTIGLAUCOMA DROPS. *Pilocarpine* and other antiglaucoma drops are at times required to control secondary glaucoma. To minimize posterior synechia formation, alternate daily use of these drops along with mydriatics is effective. To the same end more emphasis may be placed on epinephrine drops rather than the miotics. Iridectomy, as mentioned above, and even filtering operations are occasionally in order.

OTHERS. *Photocoagulation* and *transscleral cryotherapy* have each been successfully employed to terminate or to prevent the spread of active lesions of chorioretinitis due to such agents as toxoplasmosis and histoplasmosis. Similarly, *trapdoor diathermy* beneath the exudative mounds of peripheral uveitis reduces the inflammation.

Systemic Treatment

CORTICOSTEROIDS. Corticosteroids are the most popular drugs in the modern management of uveitis. ACTH or the synthetic steroids may be chosen. The oral preparations are frequently given in the morning, daily or every other day. A high dosage level at the start should continue until there is obvious improvement and then be tapered off gradually. If no benefit derives from one compound, others should be tried. A child may properly take an oral dosage of 2 mg. prednisone or its equivalent per kilogram per day.

ANALGESICS. Analgesics, such as salicylates, are commonly prescribed. At times, narcotics are indicated for relief of discomfort. Phenylbutazone is claimed to have a weak cortisone-like effect in uveitis.

FOREIGN PROTEIN THERAPY. Foreign protein therapy, which includes intra-

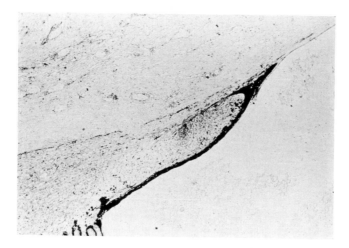

Figure 13–13 Anterior synechia in aniridia.

muscular whole milk or intravenous typhoid vaccine, has been largely supplanted by the steroids.

IMMUNOSUPPRESSION. Immunosuppressant agents such as methotrexate and cyclophosphamide have recently been promulgated for the containment of severe or recalcitrant uveitis as exemplified by sympathetic ophthalmia or peripheral uveitis. Though effective where nothing else works, the serious side-effects of these drugs severely limit their widespread use. Accordingly, the chelating agent, *penicillamine*, which can dissociate abnormal globulins in rheumatoid arthritis and, therefore, has theoretically possible advantages in uveitis, was investigated as a substitute for the immunosuppressants. It improved 6 out of 8 stubborn cases, but the side-effects, particularly on the blood picture, were also too severe to recommend it.

OTHERS. *Carbonic anhydrase inhibitors* and osmotherapeutic agents may be most effective in the management of secondary glaucoma, especially when mydriasis must be maintained to counteract posterior synechiae.

CONGENITAL AND DEVELOPMENTAL ANOMALIES

Iris

Aniridia

Aniridia is the apparent absence of the iris on clinical examination. Actually, a

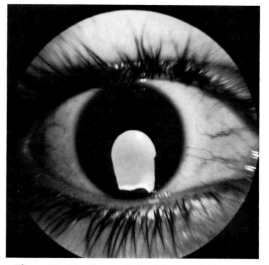

Figure 13–14 Congenital coloboma of iris, typical position.

rudimentary iris hidden behind the corneoscleral margin is always present (Fig. 13–13). The pupil occupies the entire area of the cornea. There is usually photophobia and poor vision and frequently nystagmus. Other ocular deformities such as aplasia of the macula, lens opacities, and retinal dystrophy are commonly present. Secondary glaucoma develops in many cases. The inheritance of this defect is on the basis of a dominant characteristic. There appears to be a causal relationship between aniridia and Wilms' tumor.

Coloboma

Coloboma is a common anomaly of the iris that may be transmitted as a dom-

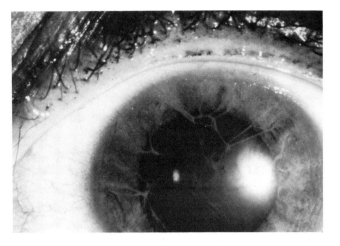

Figure 13–15 Persistent pupillary membrane.

inant characteristic. The typical position is inferior, indicating its relationship to anomalous closure of the fetal cleft. Coloboma of the lens and choroid is often associated. Atypical coloboma may occur anywhere else in the iris. A great variety of shapes and sizes occurs; even colobomatous holes exist, which produce a pseudopolycoria (Fig. 13–14).

Persistent Pupillary Membrane

Persistent pupillary membrane is very common. It may be confused with hyperplasia of the mesoderm, in which the anterior layer of the iris, instead of terminating at a distance from the pupillary margin, encroaches upon the pigment border or even the pupil. Similarly the pigment layer of the iris may be con-

genitally hypoplastic, as in albinism, or hyperplastic, as in flocculus or exuberant pigment fringe at the margin of the pupil. Heterochromia may be associated with uveitis (Figs. 13–15 and 13–16).

Pupillary Anomalies

Pupillary anomalies may appear in several different guises. Polycoria, or multiple pupils, each surrounded by a sphincter, is rare. More commonly, partial aniridia produces holes in the iris and a pseudopolycoria. Corectopia, eccentric displacement of the pupil, is transmitted as a dominant factor and may be associated with other anomalies, most often subluxation of the lens. Microcoria is congenital miosis, has been found in association with ophthalmoplegia and is usually transmitted as a recessive characteristic. Anisocoria, pupils of unequal size, is a frequent

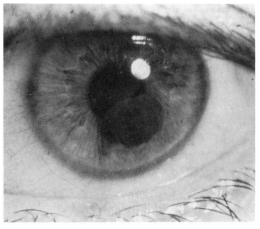

Figure 13–16 Flocculus of iris, congenital excrescences of pigmented iris epithelium.

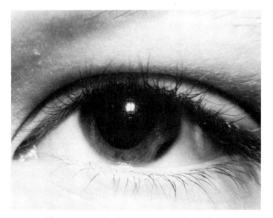

Figure 13–17 Traumatic iridodialysis.

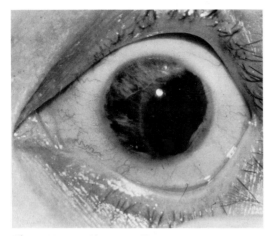

Figure 13–18 Circumpupillary aplasia of the iris.

sign of craniocerebral trauma. Iridodialysis, iridodonesis, radial tears of the iris, and iritis may all result from blunt injuries to the eye (Fig. 13–17).

In circumpupillary aplasia of the iris, the defect involves the mesodermal layers, the pigment epithelium, and the sphincter muscle. It probably represents an incomplete form of aniridia and is genetically determined (Fig. 13–18).

Choroid Coloboma

Choroid coloboma is typically situated inferiorly and often involves the lower portion of the disc. The margins are usually sharp and pigmented. The floor tends to be on a lower level than the rest of the fundus. Coloboma is atypical and rare when it occurs elsewhere in the fundus. Macular coloboma, if unilateral, usually provokes strabismus soon after infancy.

The venae vorticosae normally drain the posterior choroid but very occasionally a *choroidovaginal vein* takes over that function. It appears as a broad, flat, dark vessel lying deep to the retina and it disappears over the edge of the disc.

Gyrate Atrophy

Gyrate atrophy of the choroid is a slowly progressive patchy atrophy of choroid, pigment epithelium, and retina. It starts in the periphery and eventually all the fundus disappears. The macular area becomes involved late in the disease process.

The prominent symptoms are night blindness and gradually increasing visual failure. Constricted retinal vessels, pale discs, cataracts, and progressive myopia are frequent concomitants. The disease is hereditary.

Choroideremia

Choroideremia is a congenital absence of the choroid and retinal pigment epithelium. A central patch of choroid persists with intact macula and disc. The obvious symptoms are tubular vision and night blindness. It is bilateral and occurs only in males (Figs. 13–19 and 13–20).

Choroidal Sclerosis

Choroidal sclerosis may begin in either juvenile or adult life. In the juvenile variety, extensive macular changes occur with yellow spots, which eventually produce atrophy of the choroid and destruction of the pigment epithelium. Generalized choroid sclerosis is usually transmitted as an autosomal dominant but other pedigrees have suggested transmission by a recessive gene or even a sex-linked gene.

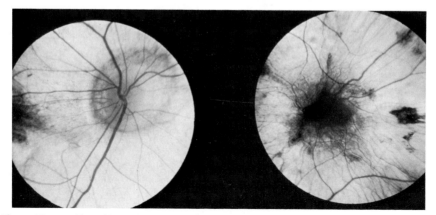

Figure 13–19 Choroideremia—only a central patch of choroid persists with intact macula.

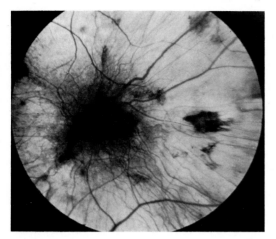

Figure 13–20　Choroideremia—Same case as in Fig. 13–19, close up.

CYSTS AND TUMORS

Iris

Cysts

Clear cysts of the iris are believed to result from trauma such as perforation of the cornea, which permits the corneal epithelium to invaginate into the anterior chamber. Slow growth over a period of years eventually distorts the iris. The treatment is iridectomy.

Congenital cysts of the iris appear as semitransparent vesicles lying in the mesodermal layers of the iris or as pigmented cysts on the posterior surface of the iris.

Spontaneous cysts of the iris stroma are uncommon. Half of them occur before the tenth year of life, which indicates their probable developmental etiology. They appear as gray or dark spots in the iris stroma, which grow slowly to form transparent vesicles.

Tumors

Hemangioma of the iris is rare, but dilated iris vessels are often seen in children with angioma of the eyelids. The abnormal vessels may not be recognized until they block the angle and produce secondary glaucoma.

Neurofibroma of the iris is seen only in association with generalized neurofibromatosis. Multiple, small, yellow-brown, asymptomatic plaques are noted. No treatment is usually required.

Nevi are the most common tumors of the iris. They usually appear just before puberty as pigment freckles, which may lie within the stroma or appear as raised spots on the surface. They never attain great size and treatment is not indicated. A change in size or degree of pigmentation need not indicate a malignant change, but this should be suspected, even though it is rare, whenever there is a change in pupillary function (Fig. 13–21).

The *nevus of ota* is a benign unilateral melanosis of the skin in the areas innervated by the ophthalmic and maxillary divisions of the fifth nerve; it is associated with irregular pigmentation of the episclera and uveal tract on the same side and may extend to the optic disc. It is also known as oculodermal melanocytosis. The onset is usually prior to age 1, but may occur up to puberty.

Uveal malignant melanoma is by far the most common intraocular tumor of adults,

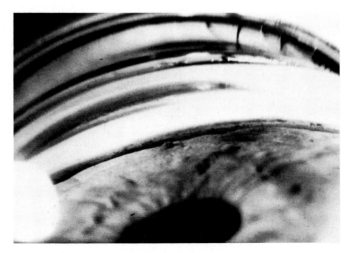

Figure 13–21　Iris nevi, gonioscopic view.

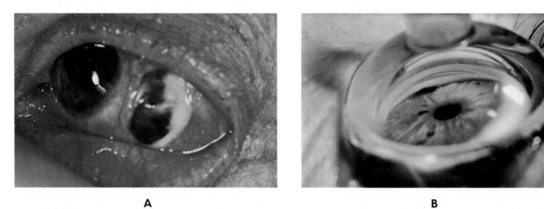

A

B

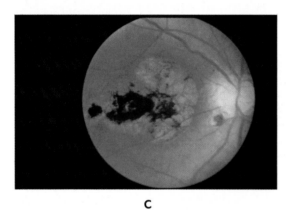

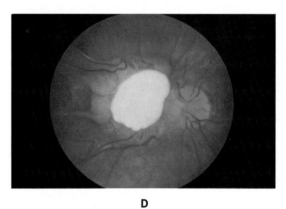

C

D

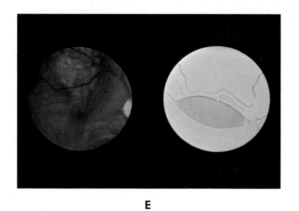

E

PLATE IX

(*A*)   Scleromalacia perforans in rheumatic arthritis.
(*B*)   Malignant melanoma of iris, gonioscopic view.
(*C*)   Toxoplasmic chorioretinopathy (white female, age 3).
(*D*)   Intraocular parasite, *Toxocara canis* suspect (white male, age 6).
(*E*)   Malignant melanoma of choroid; rapid growth in teenage girl.

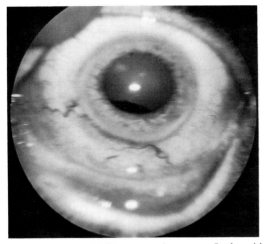

Figure 13–22 Malignant melanoma of choroid grossly visible through pupil.

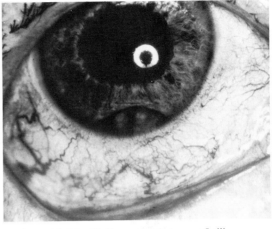

Figure 13–23 Malignant melanoma of ciliary body.

but less than 1 per cent of the cases are found during the first two decades. A considerably greater proportion, 41 per cent, arise in the iris as compared to 7 per cent in adults. This reflects the well-known fact that patients with iris tumors are usually younger than patients with melanomas of the choroid and ciliary body. The tumor invades the iris muscles and deforms the pupil. Wide excision can result in complete cure, unless the angle has been invaded, which demands enucleation.

Xanthogranuloma of the iris (nevoxantho-endothelioma) occurs in infants. It appears as a yellowish plaque or fleshy iris mass, which produces recurrent unilateral hyphema and eventually secondary glaucoma. It is often mistaken for an iris melanoma. The skin of the chest, axillas, or face often presents associated xantho-

granulomas, which usually clear spontaneously. The iris lesions respond well to about 400 R. of radiation, and if treated promptly obviate the need for enucleation.

Ciliary Body

Diktyoma is a rare epithelial tumor probably derived from the medullary layer of the embryonic retina. It usually makes its appearance around the age of 5 years. Locally invasive and slow-growing, it may block the aqueous drainage channels and produce secondary glaucoma. Ophthalmoscopic and slit lamp examinations reveal a mass in the ciliary body, pushing the iris forward and narrowing the anterior chamber. Enucleation is indicated.

Choroid

Hemangioma is rare and, unless associated with generalized angiomatosis, is

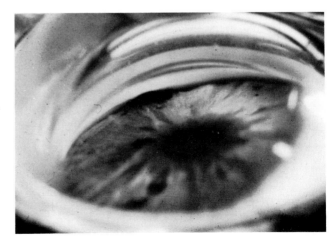

Figure 13–24 Malignant melanoma of iris invading iridocorneal angle, goniophotograph.

difficult to differentiate clinically from a malignant melanoma. Intravenous fluorescein is retained in the dilated vessels of a hemangioma, but malignant melanoma is unchanged. Pressure on the globe may blanch an angioma but not a malignant melanoma. P^{32} is taken up by a malignant melanoma, not by angioma.

Nevi or benign melanomas of the choroid are congenital, flat, blue-gray, well-circumscribed areas in the posterior fundus. They are asymptomatic and no diagnostic problem during childhood, but in adults they must be differentiated from malignant melanoma.

Malignant melanoma of the choroid is extremely rare in childhood. The clinical features are similar to those presented by adults and Callender's classification of cell types has the same prognostic significance as in melanoma of adults (Figs. 13–22, 13–23, and 13–24).

REFERENCES

Cleasby, G. A.: Nevoxanthoendothelioma (juvenile xanthogranuloma) of the iris. Diagnosis by biopsy and treatment with x-rays. Trans. Amer. Acad. Ophthal. Otolaryng., 65:609–613, 1961.

Cogan, D. D., Kuwabara, T., Young, G. F., and Knox, D. L.: Herpes simplex retinopathy in an infant. Arch. Ophthal., 72:641–645, 1964.

DiGeorge, A., and Harley, R.: Aniridia and Wilm's tumor. Arch. Ophthal., 75:796, 1966.

Embil, J., Haldane, E., MacKenzie, R., and Van Roogen, C.: Prevalence of cytomegalovirus infection in a normal urban population in Nova Scotia. Canada Med. Assoc. J., 101:78, 1969.

Gills, J. P.: Combined medical and surgical therapy for complicated cases of peripheral uveitis. Arch. Ophthal., 79:723–728, 1968.

Hallett, J. W., Wolkowicz, M. I., Leopold, I. H., and Wijewski, E.: Latex agglutination test in uveitis. Arch. Ophthal., 64:133–134, 1960.

Hallett, J. W., Wolkowicz, M. I., Leopold, I. H., and Wijewski, E.: The Middlebrook-Dubos test in uveitis. Arch. Ophthal., 63:1016–1017, 1960.

Hallett, J. W., Wolkowicz, M. I., Leopold, I. H., Canamucio, C., and Wijewski, E.: Autoimmune complement fixation test in endogenous uveitis. Arch. Ophthal., 68:168–171, 1962.

Harley, R. D.: Ocular leprosy in Panama. Amer. J. Ophthal., 29:295, 1946.

Harley, R. D., and Wedding, E. S.: Syndrome of uveitis meningoencephalitis, alopecia, poliosis and dysacousia. Amer. J. Ophthal., 29:524, 1946.

Hogan, M. J., Kimura, S. J., and Thygeson, P.: Signs and symptoms of uveitis. Amer. J. Ophthal., 47:155–170, 1959.

Kimura, S. J., and Hogan, M. J.: Uveitis in children: Analysis of 274 cases. Trans. Amer. Ophthal. Soc., 62:171–192, 1964.

Smith, M., Zimmerman, L., and Harley, R. D.: Ocular involvement in congenital cytomegalic inclusion disease. Arch. Ophthal., 76:696, 1966.

Soll, D. B., and Turtz, A. I.: Retinoblastoma diagnosed as granulomatous uveitis. Arch. Ophthal., 63:687–691, 1960.

Welch, R. B., Maumenee, E., and Wahlen, H. E.: Peripheral posterior segment inflammation, vitreous opacities, and edema of the posterior pole. Arch. Ophthal., 64:540–549, 1960.

Wong, V. G., and Hersh, E. M.: Methotrexate in the therapy of cyclitis. Trans. Amer. Acad. Ophthal. Otolaryng., 69:279–293, 1965.

Yanoff, M., Schaffer, D. B., and Scheie, H. G.: Rubella ocular syndrome. Correlation of clinical, viral and pathologic studies. Jr. Amer. Acad. Ophthal., 72:896, 1968.

CHAPTER 14

DISEASES OF THE RETINA AND VITREOUS

WILLIAM TASMAN, M.D.

CONGENITAL RETINOSCHISIS

Congenital retinoschisis is an inherited ocular disorder transmitted as a sex-linked recessive trait, occurring in males. It is characterized by splitting of the retina into an inner and outer layer at the level of the nerve fiber layer (Yanoff et al., 1968). The most characteristic ophthalmoscopic finding is an elevation of the inner layer of the retinoschisis, usually in the inferotemporal quadrant. The anterior limit of the retinoschisis seldom extends to the ora serrata while the posterior limit may extend to the optic disc. Inner layer breaks are common and appear as large round or oval-shaped holes (Plate X-A). In some eyes the inner layer breaks are so large that only remnants of the inner layer remain. In eyes with breaks in the outer layer as well as the inner layer an associated retinal detachment may develop.

Macular lesions are a consistent finding with congenital retinoschisis and have a typical appearance. Usually there is a cystoid macular change which has a spoke-wheel configuration. When seen in the young male, this sign should alert the observer to the possibility of the peripheral changes seen in congenital retinoschisis. In addition, the ERG will frequently show a subnormal B wave in the presence of a normal A wave (Krill et al., 1972). Vitreous membranes are associated with retinoschisis in about 50 per cent of cases. Some of these may occur secondary to vitreous hemorrhage but similar membranes have been seen in babies before any vitreous hemorrhage has occurred.

The natural history of retinoschisis is that of a stationary or slowly progressive disease. When retinoschisis is limited to the peripheral retina, reasonably good central vision can be maintained for several decades. The most important manifestation of progressive disease is an increase in the extent or the height of the retinoschisis bulla. It is important to realize that progression of congenital retinoschisis may be followed by spontaneous partial regression.

Differential diagnoses include retinal detachment, posterior hyperplastic vitreous, Wagner's disease, and Favre's disease. Retinal detachment in a child may be differentiated from congenital retinoschisis in that the latter is always bilateral.

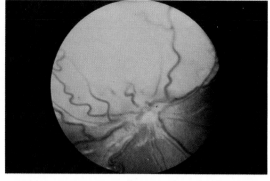

A

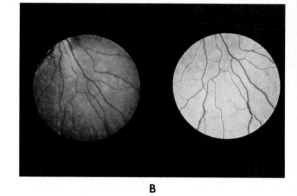

B

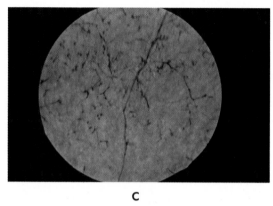

C

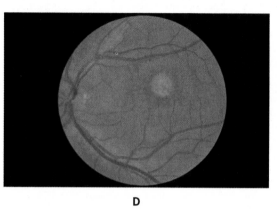

D

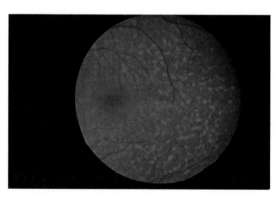

E

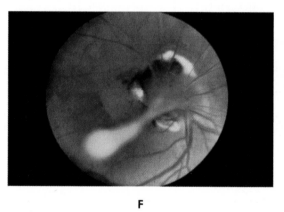

F

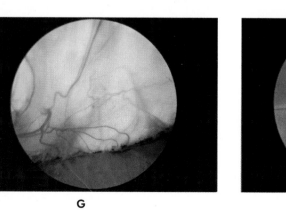

G

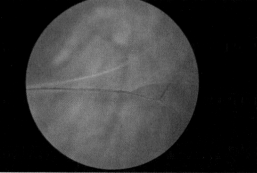

H

Secondly, retinal detachment, unlike congenital retinoschisis, usually extends to the ora serrata. In some cases of hyperplastic vitreous, extensive hyaloid remnants which are adherent to the disc and inferior retina may contract and cause an inferior retinal detachment with or without visible retinal breaks. This condition is generally unilateral and is neither familial nor hereditary. Wagner's vitreoretinal degeneration affects the entire fundus without a predilection for the lower half. It is transmitted as an autosomal dominant and is characterized by avascular preretinal membranes, usually without holes, which cause kinking of retinal vessels and may lead to retinal detachment. The vitreous is liquefied and detached. Retinal pigmentation similar to retinitis pigmentosa, sheathed vessels, and cataracts are also seen, but the macula is usually normal. Favre-Goldmann vitreoretinal degeneration is transmitted as an autosomal recessive. The disease is characterized by night blindness and fundus changes typical of retinitis pigmentosa. Cataract, peripheral retinoschisis, and chorioretinal degeneration are also present. The vision may remain stationary for the first two or three decades before further progression of visual loss occurs (Krill et al., 1972).

As long as congenital retinoschisis is not accompanied by frank retinal detachment, no operation of any kind is indicated. Recurrent vitreous hemorrhages are best treated conservatively, but when retinal detachment develops, operation is indicated.

CHOROIDAL COLOBOMA

During normal development, the fetal fissure closes by fusion of the two layers of the optic cup. The inner layer and the outer pigment epithelium layer fuse with their counterparts on each side of the fissure in a regular fashion. This process begins at the equator and proceeds anteriorly and posteriorly as if a zipper were being closed in each direction. The location of this fissure is characteristically inferior and slightly nasal so that typical fissural defects are below the disc. When the regular process of fusion of layers at the fissure does not occur properly, colobomatous defects result.

The mature colobomatous defect shows absence of the pigmented and vascular tunics (Plate X-B). At the margin of the defect there is usually an abrupt return of choroid and pigment epithelium, the retina being closely applied over the scleral edge of the coloboma. The retina is not bound or attached to the margins of the defect throughout, although there is frequently an incomplete line of hyperpigmentation suggesting an attachment. The defect may be limited in extent to the lower fundus or may include the disc or even part of the fundus above it. The macula may be eliminated by inclusion in the defect.

Jesberg and Schepens (1960) observed two types of retinal detachment associated with choroidal coloboma. The first type includes eyes with retinal detachment in which the coloboma is no more than an incidental finding. Obvious retinal breaks were found, apparently unrelated to the coloboma, and their closure resulted in reattachment of the retina. The second type of retinal detachment appeared to be definitely related to the choroidal coloboma. In this group the retinal detachment was either inferotemporal with demarcation lines or it was total, and it was thought that the detachment was due to a break or breaks located in the colobo-

---

PLATE X

(A) Inner layer dehiscences in congenital retinoschisis.

(B) Congenital coloboma of the pigment epithelium and choroid. The superior border of the coloboma is demarcated by pigment.

(C) Persistent hyperplastic vitreous emanating from the disc.

(D) Flecked retina appearance of fundus flavimaculatus.

(E) Vitelliform macular degeneration with egg yolk appearance. This picture is commensurate with good visual acuity.

(F) Retinitis pigmentosa with typical bone corpuscular pigment.

(G) Oguchi's disease light adapted on left. Dark adapted retina is seen on right demonstrating Mizuo's phenomenon.

(H) Large retinoblastoma with tortuous nutrient vessels.

matous area. Such breaks easily escape visual detection because of lack of contrast between the white scleral background and diaphanous retinal membrane.

POSTERIOR HYPERPLASTIC VITREOUS

The most constant feature in persistent hyperplastic vitreous is a dense white vitreous band which usually extends from the disc to the fundus periphery or to the lens (Plate X-C). It may occur in any meridian but is most common nasally. Limited retinal detachments or other evidence of vitreoretinal traction, such as traction folds, macular pigmentary degeneration, or pigmented demarcation lines, are often associated findings. Prominent uveal processes and relative microphthalmos are also characteristic of hyperplastic vitreous.

As with other anomalous vascular systems posterior hyperplastic vitreous can vary in degree. The spectrum includes Bergmeister's papilla, vitreoretinal veils around the disc and macula, vitreous stalks and hyaloid remnants, and retinal folds. Each is related to the other and to congenital abnormalities of the anterior primary vitreous.

FAMILIAL EXUDATIVE VITREORETINOPATHY

Criswick and Schepens (1969) recently described a disease of the vitreous and retina which they term familial exudative vitreoretinopathy. It is familial in nature and features certain aspects of retrolental fibroplasia, Coats's disease, and peripheral uveitis. The history and findings, however, remain distinct from these diseases and for this reason they consider it a separate entity. The disease is inherited with an apparently autosomal dominant irregular mode of inheritance.

The vitreous cavity features organized membranes in all quadrants both peripherally and centrally which appear to be intimately bound to the retina and often contain large new blood vessels. The striking ophthalmoscopic feature is peripheral retinal exudation. It is subretinal and

intraretinal and, unlike peripheral uveitis, occurs posterior to the ora serrata, most commonly on the temporal side. Localized retinal detachment, often forming a broad fold, usually extends temporally from the disc. New retinal vessels in the periphery are subject to recurrent vitreous hemorrhage. The ocular changes are slowly progressive and tend to run a downhill course, with increasing proliferation of blood vessels, increasing exudation, membrane formation, and retinal detachment.

MEDULLATED NERVE FIBERS

Not all lesions in the fundus cause visual disturbance. For example, medullated nerve fibers, which are a developmental disorder, appear during the first year of life and rarely affect vision. They occur predominately among males and, although bilateral cases occur, unilaterality is the rule. The medullated fibers have a feather-like appearance and are usually adjacent to the disc. Sometimes they are located away from the optic nerve, but unless the macula is affected, vision is preserved. If inherited, the mode of transmission is usually autosomal dominant.

APLASIA AND HYPOPLASIA OF THE MACULA

Aplasia of the macula is often associated with gross ocular deformities such as microphthalmos, aniridia, coloboma of the optic nerve, monocular myopia, and medullated nerve fibers. Hypoplasia of the macula, another rare entity, has been suggested as a possible cause for certain forms of amblyopia. In this condition the central retina does not differentiate completely and is usually arrested at 6 to 8 months of intrauterine development.

HETEROTOPIA OF THE MACULA

Displacement of the macula from its anatomically normal location can be unilateral or bilateral, and it may be in any direction, although it is most common inferotemporally (Grondahl, 1963). A pseudostrabismus and abnormal angle kappa are often attendant findings.

Heterotopic maculas may result from irregular growth of the posterior segment of the eye, or disturbances in maturation of retinal structures, particularly when other congenital malformations such as persistent hyaloid artery, coloboma, or microcornea are present. The most common cause, however, is traction. Traction may result from prenatal inflammatory processes, bleeding, or developmental anomalies. The most important pathologic findings are the vitreoretinal adhesions which are common to persistent hyperplastic vitreous, retrolental fibroplasia, trauma, congenital retinoschisis, and retinal detachments.

CONGENITAL OPTIC PITS

Congenital optic pits are usually located on the temporal side of the disc. Many have associated macular lesions which have been described as having the characteristic appearance of central serous retinopathy (Sugar, 1964). A well-visualized channel between the optic pit and the elevated macula is usually observed and can be demonstrated with fluorescein dye, suggesting that the macular lesion may be the result of a leak from the optic pit into the subretinal space.

FUNDUS FLAVIMACULATUS

Fundus flavimaculatus affects males and females equally. Usually the disease is stationary or only slightly progressive. Characteristically, the retinas of these patients show yellow, irregularly shaped spots, sometimes in the central area of the retina where they can seriously affect central vision (Plate X-D).

The lesions are thought to be acid mucopolysaccharide in the pigment epithelium (Krill et al., 1972) and do not transmit fluorescein. Later, however, the lesions may disappear as the acid mucopolysaccharide leaves the pigment epithelial cell.

BEST'S VITELLIFORM DEGENERATION

In 1905, Best reported eight members of one family with an interesting macular dystrophy, now called vitelliform degeneration. The transmission in this disease is usually autosomal dominant, but there may be a decreased penetrance and variable expressivity in the transmission. Vitelliform macular degeneration has a very distinct appearance. It is characterized by a sharply defined discoid formation in or immediately adjacent to the macula (Plate X-E). It is usually yellow, orange, or pinkish-yellow and varies in size from 0.5 to 4.0 disc diameters. There are no blood vessels over the lesion. The abnormality is subretinal and resembles the yolk of a poached egg. It is usually diagnosed between the ages of 5 and 15 years and is bilateral, although unilateral cases have been reported. The condition is very slowly progressive. Gradually the homogeneous content of the vitelliform disc may form a sediment that becomes fragmented, leaving fairly marked pigmentation and, in some cases, even a focus of chorioretinal atrophy. The macular picture at that point is often indistinguishable from other types of macular degeneration and it is in this stage that serious loss of vision occurs. Braley (1966) has suggested that the yolklike lesion eventually scrambles, leading to the pigmentation which ensues.

The electroretinogram response is normal, as are the peripheral visual fields. Central scotomas cannot be elicited in eyes with normal visual acuity but are present late in the disease. Dark adaptation is normal. However, the electro-oculogram is always abnormal in patients with vitelliform macular degeneration as well as in carriers of the condition who do not demonstrate fundus abnormalities (Krill et al., 1972). Thus, this test has become extremely helpful in making the diagnosis of carrier states and, as a result, is helpful in genetic counseling, since a carrier can be told he definitely harbors the trait and has a reasonable chance of passing it on to one of his offspring.

The pathogenesis of vitelliform degeneration is still rather confused, although it seems probable, as stated by Francois

(1968), that an unknown abnormal substance is responsible. Francois localizes the lesion to the pigment epithelium, Bruch's membrane, or the potential space between the pigment epithelium and Bruch's membrane.

Braley (1966) concluded that the vitelline dystrophy of the macula is present at birth and that if no change is visible postnatally the disease will not develop later. Falls also agrees that the absence of ophthalmoscopic findings is a definite prognostic sign and that Best's disease is present at birth (Braley and Spivey, 1963). He postulated a cystic pooling of semi-liquid exudate between the lamina vitrea and the pigment cell layer of the retina and suggested that the visual acuity remained excellent so long as the pigment cell layer remained intact. Blodi (1966) found that the early appearing cyst has the characteristics of a circumscribed detachment of the pigment epithelium. Visual loss usually appears upon rupture of the cyst when destruction of the retinal elements occurs.

Vitelliform macular degeneration must be differentiated from *cone dysfunction syndromes* which, in general, are heralded by photophobia and severe color vision loss in the face of good central vision. Often these patients will develop an acquired nystagmus which is not seen in vitelliform macular degeneration. Furthermore, affected individuals have characteristic ERG findings, in which there is usually a severe abnormality of the cone portion of the test in relation to the rod or scotopic portion of the test, even in very early cases (Krill et al., 1972). Examination of the fundi usually reveals a bull's eye appearance, in which the foveal area is reddish with a depigmented area surrounding it. Fluorescein angiography in such patients will reveal transmission of the fluorescein through the depigmented area, giving a halo type of configuration around the fovea. This condition is an autosomal dominant condition when it occurs in a hereditary fashion, but may occur sporadically.

STARGARDT'S DISEASE

Stargardt's disease was first described by Stargardt in 1909. The original article actually described what we know now as fundus flavimaculatus and atrophic macular degeneration. Today, however, Stargardt's disease is more often thought of as an autosomal recessive condition which usually appears between the ages of 8 and 14, is bilateral, is slowly progressive, and is sometimes associated with macular degeneration. Characteristically the foveal reflex is absent or grayish in color. Pigmentary spots sometimes develop in the macula area and may accumulate irregularly. Eventually a circular area of depigmentation and chorioretinal atrophy of the macula area follows in some cases. The evolution is slow and progressive unless hemorrhage occurs to accelerate visual loss. Usually by the age of 30 the disease is well established and, even though the vision may be decreased to 20/200, total blindness does not occur.

Paufique and Hervouet (1963), in a pathologic study, found a complete absence of all visual cells in the macular area. The pigment epithelium had completely disappeared and, slightly to the side of the macula, newly formed connective tissue had replaced the sensory elements of the retina. The nuclear and ganglion cell layers were normal. Blodi (1966) noted a similar disappearance of the visual elements in the macular area, as well as loss of the pigment epithelium.

DOYNE'S CHOROIDITIS

Doyne's honeycombed choroiditis manifests itself between the ages of 12 and 19. The disease is bilateral and more frequent in women. It is characterized by large, circular, colloid-like deposits in the perimacular area. It is accompanied by an eventual loss of central vision and is a primary familial tapetoretinal degeneration. The basic lesions of the disease are large drusen-like bodies. They appear as round and yellowish foci with sharp lines of demarcation. There is little pigment proliferation but hemorrhages may occur in older cases. The visual acuity remains normal or nearly normal for many years until crystalline material begins to accumulate. At that point, visual function becomes affected.

PRIMARY AND SECONDARY RETINAL PIGMENTARY DISORDERS

Given the name "retinitis pigmentosa" by Donders in 1855, this condition is probably more accurately called pigmentary retinal dystrophy. It is often hereditary and is characterized by progressive deterioration of the visual cells, pigment epithelium, and choroid. Clinically, a thinning of the retinal vessels, waxy pallor of the optic disc, and the appearance, initially at the equator, of "bone-corpuscle" pigment have been described as the typical findings. Choroidal sclerosis is commonly seen late in the disease. The condition is always bilateral in familial cases, but sporadic unilateral cases have been noted. The pigmentary changes typically become visible during the first decade of life and may begin as fine dots which gradually assume the spidery bone-corpuscle appearance (Plate X–F). As the disease progresses, the equatorial girdle widens and a ring scotoma in the visual field is produced.

Of greater importance in the diagnosis is the electroretinogram. In primary pigmentary degeneration of the retina, the ERG response is subnormal or absent, a change which appears before the subjective visual deterioration or ophthalmoscopically visible changes. The electroretinogram is also helpful in the differential diagnosis of primary and secondary retinitis pigmentosa unless the secondary form is very far advanced.

Histology reveals a general disappearance of the neuroepithelial elements, proliferation of glial cells, changes in the pigment epithelium, and an obliterative sclerosis of the retinal vessels. First to be affected are the rods, as opposed to the ganglion cells and nerve fiber layer, which may remain unaffected, even when the eye is blind. The migration of pigment into the retina, aided by macrophages, follows the degeneration.

Three basic modes of inheritance are recognized: autosomal recessive, autosomal dominant, and sex-linked. The first is the most common and the sex-linked form is often the most disabling.

Significant ocular associations include posterior cataract, glaucoma, myopia, and keratoconus. Well-established extraocular accompaniments include deafness, diencephalic and endocrine anomalies, oligophrenia, ophthalmoplegia, and the lipidoses (Table 14–1). Friedreich's ataxia, amyotrophic lateral sclerosis, and progressive muscular atrophy have also been associated with retinitis pigmentosa.

Perhaps the best known condition in the differential diagnosis of retinitis pigmentosa is the syndrome of Laurence-Moon-Biedl, which embraces the picture of mental retardation, hypogenitalism, polydactyly, shoulder and hip girdle obesity, retinal changes, and a recessive inheritance pattern. It occurs predominately among males and the retinal changes may simulate typical retinitis pigmentosa or may be characterized by macular degeneration. A third form appears as a disseminated choroidal sclerosis.

Leber's congenital amaurosis is characterized by near congenital blindness or reduced vision. Ophthalmoscopically, the fundus at first may appear normal or salt and pepper changes may be found. Pigmentary changes become more obvious as time passes, the disc becomes atrophic, and macular degeneration develops. Keratoconus and cataracts are often associated with Leber's disease, and the condition is transmitted as an autosomal recessive. A particular characteristic of Leber's congenital amaurosis is the oculodigital reflex, which consists of excessive rubbing of the eyes, with production of phosphenes.

Finally, retinal pigmentation occurs in lues, and in the peripheral retina of patients with juvenile cystinosis.

ALBINISM

Albinism occurs as a sex-linked trait in which the eye presents a pigmentary deficiency. In males visual acuity is generally quite poor but in the heterozygous female the retinal physiology is normal. Nystagmus is common and the inheritance pattern is sex-linked. The heterozygous female may disclose ophthalmoscopic changes characterized by milder manifestations of the presence of the disease. These changes usually take the form of a cocoa brown pigmentation of the retina that is sparsely distributed and that is

TABLE 14–1 RETINITIS PIGMENTOSA AND ASSOCIATED SYSTEMIC DISORDERS

1. Lipidoses
   a. Gaucher's disease
   b. Amaurotic family idiocy
      A constant finding in the juvenile form (Batten-Mayou disease, Spielmeyer-Vogt disease), but a variable finding in the late infantile form (Jansky-Bielschowsky disease), in which ocular signs may vary between the infantile and juvenile forms.
2. Late form of Pelizaeus-Merzbacher disease (a form of sudanophilic cerebral sclerosis)
3. Progressive familial myoclonic epilepsy
4. Spinopontocerebellar degenerations
   a. Marie's ataxia
   b. Friedreich's ataxia
   c. Unclassified spastic paraplegias
   d. Charcot-Marie-Tooth disease
   e. Progressive pallidal degeneration with retinitis pigmentosa
   f. Hereditary muscular atrophy, ataxia, and diabetes mellitus
5. Specific syndromes with progressive external ophthalmoplegia and retinitis pigmentosa
   a. Progressive external ophthalmoplegia (progressive nuclear ophthalmoplegia ocular myopathy)
   b. Retinitis pigmentosa, external ophthalmoplegia, and heart block
   c. Retinitis pigmentosa, ophthalmoplegia, and spastic quadriplegia
   d. Abetalipoproteinemia (Bassen-Kornzweig syndrome, acanthocytosis).
   e. Refsum's syndrome
6. Generalized muscular dystrophy
7. Myotonic dystrophy (Steinert's disease)
8. Syndromes in which a hearing loss is a prominant finding
   a. Hallgren's syndrome
   b. Refsum's syndrome
   c. Usher's syndrome
   d. Retinitis pigmentosa with deafness of varying severity
   e. Cockayne's disease (Cockayne-Neill disease, Neill-Dingwall syndrome)
   f. Alstrom syndrome (retinitis pigmentosa, deafness, obesity, and diabetes)
9. Syndromes with renal disease as a prominent feature
   a. Familial juvenile nephrophthisis (Fanconi's nephrophthisis)
   b. Hereditary nephritis, retinitis pigmentosa, and chromosomal abnormalities
   c. Cystinuria
   d. Cystinosis (Fanconi syndrome I)
   e. Oxalosis
10. Syndromes in which bone disease is a prominent feature
    a. Paget's disease
    b. Osteogenesis imperfecta (Lobstein's syndrome)
    c. Marfan's syndrome
    d. Osteopetrosis "familiaris" (marble bone, osteosclerosis fragilis generalisata, Albers-Schönberg disease)
11. Syndromes with skin disease
    a. Werner's disease
    b. Psoriasis
12. Laurence-Moon-Biedl syndrome
13. Dresbach's syndrome (elliptocytosis, ovalocytosis)
14. Klinefelter's syndrome
15. Mucopolysaccharidoses—Retinal degenerations have now been reported in types I, II, III, and V
16. Hooft's disease (hypolipidemia syndrome)

*From Krill, A. E.: Sight Saving Review, *42*:26, Spring, 1972.

arranged in clusters, especially in the macular area.

CONGENITAL MELANOSIS

Melanosis of the retina or grouped pigmentation of the retina is characterized by clusters of black pigment arranged in bear track distribution throughout the fundus. Sometimes a considerable portion of the retina will be affected. The condition may be bilateral. The visual acuity and visual fields are normal and there is no known hereditary transmission.

OGUCHI'S DISEASE

Oguchi's disease is a stationary form of congenital night blindness which is usually distinguishable from other types of nyctalopia by a combination of two readily observable phenomena. First is the unusual color of the fundus, which has been described as ranging from various shades of gray white to yellow. The area involved by the abnormal color may be limited to a small section of the midperiphery or may extend throughout the entire fundus in a discontinuous or homogeneous pattern. The second unique characteristic of Oguchi's disease is Mizuo's phenomenon which is a change in the color of the fundus in the dark-adapted state. When light is prevented from entering the eye, the fundus color is transformed from the light shade seen initially to a reddish, more normal appearance (Plate X-G). The time necessary to elicit this color change varies among patients.

RETINOBLASTOMA

Retinoblastoma is a highly malignant, congenital tumor which characteristically arises multicentrically in one or both retinas. The tumor usually remains confined to the eye for relatively long periods of time, i.e., months or several years, but then metastasizes rapidly, via direct extension into the optic nerve, hematogenously from the retina or choroid, and occasionally by way of the lymphatics, if the orbit is involved.

Retinoblastoma occurs once in every 20,000 to 25,000 births, and the frequency appears to be relatively constant in various parts of the world. Approximately 30 per cent of the cases involve both eyes. It is inherited as an autosomal dominant characteristic, and the average penetrance is about 60 per cent. Only 8 to 10 per cent of all new cases have a family history. The remainder represent spontaneous mutations, giving rise to the first affected individual in the family line. The cause of this mutation is unknown.

The penetrance of this gene seems to vary. The offspring of any survivor of bilateral retinoblastoma will have approximately a 50 per cent chance of developing the tumor, whereas only about 10 per cent of the progeny of survivors of unilateral retinoblastoma will have the disease. In genetic counseling, an average penetrance of 80 per cent has been assumed to stress the hereditary implication of this disease. Survivors of retinoblastoma are told that there is an overall possibility of 40 per cent that any children born to them will have retinoblastoma. When a child with retinoblastoma is born to normal parents with no family history of the disease, there is a 4 per cent chance that a subsequent child will have retinoblastoma. Furthermore, there is a 6 to 7 per cent chance that there will be a subsequent affected child somewhere in the ensuing family line.

Macroscopically, retinoblastomas have been divided into two groups. The first appears to originate in the internal nuclear layers of the retina, and then extends into the vitreous cavity, where it can be readily seen with the ophthalmoscope (Plate X-H). This is the most common pattern and is called the endophytum type. When the tumor arises in the external nuclear layers, it may grow in the subretinal space, detaching the retina ahead of it, and producing an exophytum type of retinoblastoma. The exophytum type gives rise to more errors in diagnosis, since the tumor is obscured by overlying detachment.

The most common presenting sign of retinoblastoma is a white or "cat's eye" reflex in the pupil. When a tumor is present in the macula, a white reflex may be apparent when the tumor is small, but when the tumor arises in the retinal periphery, it may grow to considerable size before it can be viewed through the pupil and then is seen only when the child looks in a particular direction. The reflex is much more obvious when the pupil is dilated and, for this reason, mydriatic drops are a mandatory part of ocular examination. The second most frequent presenting sign is strabismus due to involvement of the macula. It is well to consider that any child with strabismus and a poorly fixing eye has retinoblastoma until it is proved otherwise. A third and not generally appreciated sign of retinoblastoma is a red, painful eye due to inflammatory reaction. This results from spontaneous necrosis or hemorrhage from the tumor and may be accompanied by secondary glaucoma.

Retinoblastomas are usually creamy pink in color and frequently there is neovascularization on the surface. Microaneurysmal and telangiectatic vessels may be seen and the nutrient vessels may be extremely large, simulating a retinal angioma (Plate X-H). Retinoblastoma has no predilection for any particular area of the retina but commonly occurs in the region of the ora serrata. It is essential, therefore, to examine children under anesthesia with careful scleral indentation. More than three-fourths of all patients with retinoblastoma will have more than one tumor in any involved eye. When the child is first seen, the entire retina must be carefully surveyed and all the tumors noted as to size and precise location. Retinoblastoma occurs in eyes of normal size and microphthalmos is rarely, if ever, present. Cataracts are never seen with retinoblastoma except as a late complication of hemorrhage or inflammatory disease.

Two features of retinoblastoma are almost pathognomonic. The first of these is calcification and the second is seeding of tumor cells into the vitreous. Calcification may occur as the result of any type of advanced hemorrhagic or inflammatory disease, but the particular pattern of calcification in retinoblastoma is typical. This can be appreciated either with the ophthalmoscope or by x-ray. When the calcium is on the surface of the tumor, it is sharply demarcated and glistening white, and resembles cottage cheese. When the calcium occurs deeper within the tumor, it is seen as a gray-white translucent area with vague outlines.

Since the most common presenting sign of retinoblastoma is a white pupil, the differential diagnosis includes larval granulomatosis, uveitis, Coats's disease, angiomatosis retinae, metastatic retinitis, persistent hyperplastic primary vitreous, retrolental fibroplasia, retinal dysplasia, vitreous hemorrhage, massive retinal fibrosis, medullated nerve fibers, coloboma, and high myopia.

The most significant factor in the treatment of retinoblastoma is the stage of the disease at the time treatment is undertaken. The following classification by Ellsworth and Reese has been generally adopted to evaluate the results of treatment (Reese, 1963):

Group I — Very Favorable
    a. Solitary tumor, less than 4 disc diameters (D.D.) in size, at or behind the equator
    b. Multiple tumors, none over 4 D.D. in size, all at or behind the equator

Group II — Favorable
    a. Solitary tumor, 4 to 10 D.D. in size, at or behind the equator
    b. Multiple tumors, 4 to 10 D.D. in size, behind the equator

Group III — Doubtful
    a. Any lesion anterior to the equator
    b. Solitary tumors larger than 10 D.D. behind the equator

Group IV — Unfavorable
    a. Multiple tumors, some larger than 10 D.D.
    b. Any lesion extending anterior to the ora serrata

Group V — Very Unfavorable
    a. Massive tumors involving over half the retina
    b. Vitreous seeding

Unilateral Cases

Unilateral retinoblastoma is probably best treated by prompt enucleation after the fellow eye has been thoroughly studied and a search for metastasis is negative. In unilateral cases, the tumor has usually grown to considerable size before the diagnosis is made and the risks involved with treatment can hardly be justified in the presence of a normal fellow eye.

Bilateral Cases

In bilateral retinoblastoma, the eye which led to the detection of the disease is generally far advanced and usually comes to enucleation, whereas the remaining eye has a more favorable prognosis and is amenable to treatment. This type of asymmetrical bilateral involvement is the rule in retinoblastoma.

The following modalities are available for the treatment of retinoblastoma:
  1. *General Agents* — treating the entire retina
    a. Radiation
    b. Chemotherapy
  2. *Local Measures* — treating only the tumor-bearing area of the retina
    a. Diathermy

b. Radon seeds, cobalt-60 applicators
c. Light coagulation
d. Cryotherapy

Ellsworth and Reese treated all cases in Groups I, II and III with radiation alone, and radiation is combined with intracarotid triethylene melamine in Groups IV and V. Light coagulation, cryotherapy, and radioactive cobalt applicators are extremely valuable adjunctive measures in the management of tumor recurrence.

RETINAL DYSPLASIA

Retinal dysplasia is a nonspecific pathological term that has been applied to a syndrome producing retinal folds in association with other systemic anomalies. Some, if not all, of these cases have 13–15 trisomy, and common associated anomalies include cerebral agenesis, internal hydrocephalus, anomalies of the heart and vascular system, polydactylism, harelip, cleft palate, and malrotation of the gut.

METASTATIC RETINITIS

Metastatic retinitis refers to spread of infectious emboli to the eye during the course of one of the exanthematous diseases of childhood, producing widespread, virulent chorioretinitis with severe vitreous reaction and yellow-white opaque tissue behind the lens. Although this entity unquestionably exists, it is rare, and the history linking the eye disease to a foregoing viral disease is helpful in making the diagnosis.

COATS'S DISEASE

Coats, in his original description of the condition, described three stages of the disease. The first stage emphasized primarily exudative change in the fundus, with little or no telangiectasis (1908). His last stage was angiomatosis of the retina, a fact which Coats himself realized in his second report, published in 1912 (see References). Since that time, the term "Coats's disease" has been variously used, but most authorities now agree that Coats's original description of exudation between the retina and choroid and of telangiectasis are essential clinical features of the disease.

Apparently two forms of the disease exist. One occurs primarily in children, the other in adults. The adult form, though similar in appearance to the juvenile disease, probably occurs secondary to an intraocular inflammation. In addition, the serum cholesterol has frequently been reported as elevated in affected adults, a finding not noted in children.

Incidence is greater among males and the condition is most often unilateral. However, bilateral cases are sometimes seen and the disease certainly occurs in females too.

Frequently the disease is first recognized in older children because they complain of visual impairment. This is often due to exudation in the posterior pole. Associated with the exudation are the typical "light bulb" or grape clusters of telangiectasis (Plate XI-A). Sometimes the vascular malformations are quite small and hard to find, a fact which may help to explain why Coats emphasized the presence of a first stage of the disease with little or no vascular involvement.

Fluorescein dye is a helpful adjunct in studying patients with Coats's disease, since it demonstrates leakage from the telangiectatic vessels and obscure, fine arteriovenous networks. Early macular involvement can also sometimes be noted with fluorescein before exudation in the posterior pole occurs. As Coats's disease progresses, it may lead to secondary retinal detachment. Generally no retinal break is present, but this is not always the rule.

Hogan and Zimmerman (1969) describe the characteristic retinal lesion of telangiectasis as numerous small well-defined red globules resembling capillary aneurysms. On microscopic examination, the capillary channels in the inner retinal layers are dilated and thin-walled. Eosinophilic PAS-positive exudate is common in the retina, particularly in the outer half.

The differential diagnosis of Coats's disease includes angiomatosis retinae, retinoblastoma, persistent hyperplastic

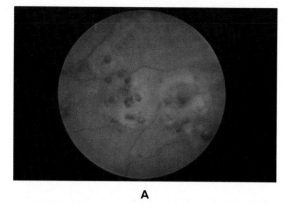

A

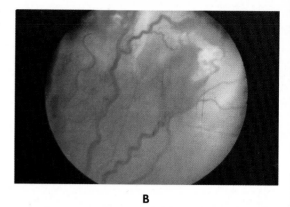

B

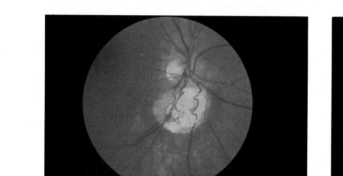

C

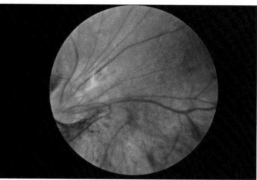

D

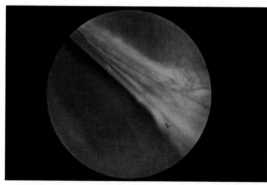

E

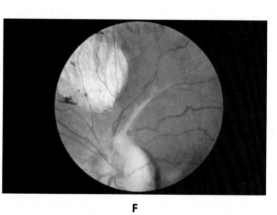

F

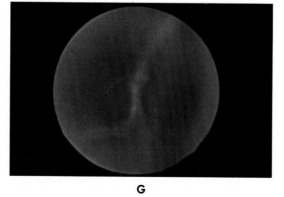

G

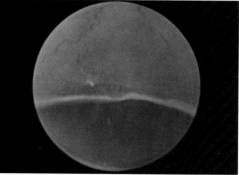

H

vitreous, retrolental fibroplasia, larval granulomatosis, metastatic retinitis, familial exudative vitreoretinopathy, massive retinal fibrosis, Eales's disease, sickle cell retinopathy, leukemia, and anemia.

The treatment of Coats's disease has pros and cons, since all cases may not be progressive. Morales (1965) followed 22 of 51 cases of Coats's disease for an average of 5 years. During this interval about half the cases developed progressively more severe ocular signs, while in the other half the retinopathy stayed the same. A second major consideration is the calculated risk that treatment may aggravate the condition rather than improve it. To obviate these possibilities, documented progression of the Coats's disease by color and fluorescein photography is extremely helpful.

Coats's disease is most commonly treated by photocoagulation. Burns are applied to the telangiectatic areas in an effort to eliminate them and thereby halt progression of the disease, so that the ultimate end results—subretinal fibrosis and retinal detachment—do not occur. If the retina is too elevated to obtain a photocoagulation burn, a scleral buckling procedure consisting of diathermy over the telangiectatic areas, drainage of subretinal fluid, and encirclement of the globe may be indicated. Cryotherapy is also effective in the treatment of Coats's disease, and in the future argon and krypton lasers, which operate between 4880 Å and 5145 Å, may provide additional modalities for eliminating the vascular malformations.

The effectiveness of therapy can be evaluated by how successfully the telangiectases have been eliminated. Frequently a treated area appears to demonstrate an adequate chorioretinal scar, but after injection of fluorescein, leakage at the edges of the scar is seen. Further photocoagulation of such leaking sites is then indicated. Two other good barometers of effective treatment are resorption of the exudate and reattachment of the retina if it has been detached. Once the telangiectatic areas are destroyed, exudate begins to disappear within 8 weeks after treatment. Resorption may then continue over the next 7 to 12 months before it completely disappears. Conversely, the reappearance of exudate usually indicates further activity of the disease and a new area of telangiectasis which must be searched out and treated. For this reason, patients with Coats's disease should be rechecked at least every 6 months.

EALES'S DISEASE

Eales's disease is a retinal vascular disease which affects young males. The characteristic changes are bilateral involvement in the absence of any systemic disease and perivasculitis along the retinal vessels. Frequently arcades of neovascularization are present which may lead to vitreous hemorrhaging. This condition should not present a differential diagnostic problem with Coats's disease, since it rarely occurs before the age of 19 years.

PHAKOMATOSES (HAMARTOMATOSES)

The term "phakomatosis" has been used to embrace primarily four conditions with intracranial, cutaneous, and ocular manifestations. They include Sturge-Weber disease, retinal angiomatosis and cerebellar angioma (von Hippel-Lindau disease), tuberous sclerosis (Bourneville's disease), and neurofibromatosis (von Recklinghausen's disease).

PLATE XI

(*A*) Typical light bulb telangiectatic vascular changes of Coats's disease.

(*B*) Retinal angioma with dilated and tortuous afferent and efferent vessels.

(*C*) Mulberry type tumor occurring in tuberous sclerosis.

(*D*) Dragged retina in retrolental fibroplasia. In 80 per cent of cases dragging is to the temporal side.

(*E*) Temporal retinal fold in retrolental fibroplasia.

(*F*) Chorioretinal scarring typical of retrolental fibroplasia. These scars are frequently confused with those due to toxoplasmosis or cytomegalic inclusion disease.

(*G*) Large peripheral vitreous membrane in young adult with retrolental fibroplasia.

(*H*) Typical retinal dialysis following blunt trauma.

In 1879 Sturge presented a hemiparetic and epileptic patient with a facial nevus flammeus and buphthalmos to the Clinical Society of London. He suggested that the neurological component of the syndrome in this case was due to a nevus condition of the brain similar to that on the patient's face. Later, Weber's name became linked with the disease because of his description of the radiological appearance in a case similar to that of Sturge.

Clinically, Sturge-Weber disease is characterized by cutaneous angiomatosis (nevus flammeus, capillary nevus) affecting the face, particularly in its upper part. Epilepsy is present in almost every case and begins early in life. Gyriform calcifications become radiologically visible after infancy and in a significant number of cases buphthalmos or glaucoma may also be present. Mental retardation, often to a marked degree, is almost always the rule and hemiparesis contralateral to the facial nevus is frequently present. Homonymous hemianopia can also sometimes be found when confrontation field testing is done.

The essential pathologic features of the disease are the facial nevus flammeus and the leptomeningeal angiomatosis, but not glaucoma or buphthalmos. The leptomeningeal angiomatoses are made up of a network of small thin-walled vessels different from those of racemose angioma and arterialized angioma. The intracerebral calcifications are probably secondary to this superficial angiomatosis, since they appear in cerebral tissue underlying the vascular anomaly. The affected hemisphere often shows an overall stunted growth, although the calcification and angiomatosis are usually confined to the posterior half of the brain.

Epilepsy has been a finding in nearly all cases of Sturge-Weber disease in which the essential lesions of the condition are present. The onset of seizures may be the symptom which brings the patient to the doctor's office, and a bout of convulsions may be followed by an abrupt slowing of intellectual development. Convulsions generally begin during the first year of life in those patients with the more extensive facial nevi and by the age of 2 years when the facial nevus is less marked. The convulsions are frequently focal on the side of the body contralateral to the nevus, but may become generalized.

When the facial nevus encompasses one or both lids, the conjunctiva and sclera may show some degree of angiomatosis. Buphthalmos or glaucoma occurs in some, but by no means all, cases of Sturge-Weber disease. The etiology of the buphthalmos or glaucoma is still unknown. The most striking fundus changes are in the choroid. Frequently the fundi have a dark appearance. This is thought to be the result of a uveal angioma which fluoresces markedly. Dunphy (1934), in a summary of ocular histological examinations in Sturge-Weber disease, noted that choroidal angioma was the most frequent pathologic finding.

In von Hippel-Lindau disease (angiomatosis retinae) 20 per cent of patients will develop central nervous system involvement, characteristically the cerebellar hemangioblastoma, although hemangioblastomas of the medulla, pons, spinal cord, and more rarely of the cerebrum also occur (Lindau, 1927). Of all intracranial tumors, these are the most favorable for surgery, for more than 80 per cent of patients may be saved by operation. Microscopically the hemangioblastoma is a mass of capillary vessels lined with endothelium running in collagenous fibrous tissue. These tumors do not metastasize, but produce symptoms secondary to the cyst size. Paroxysmal headaches secondary to coughing, sneezing, and position change, as well as nausea, vomiting, giddiness, unsteady gait, and clumsiness of the fingers are all common symptoms. Successful surgical treatment requires drainage of the cyst, removal of the tumor nodules, and, if possible, removal of the entire wall of the cyst (Craig et al., 1941).

The average age of onset is 25 years, but one-fourth of all cases have been described in the pediatric age group. It is generally inherited as an autosomal dominant trait with incomplete penetrance and delayed expression (Jesberg et al., 1968; Nicol, 1957). Pheochromocytoma may be associated with von Hippel-Lindau disease or neurofibromatosis.

The classic fundus lesion is an angiomatous round or oval globular reddish nodule which may be so small that it is not noted clinically. On the other hand, it may be several disc diameters in size and project 8 to 10 disc diameters into the vitreous.

Some lesions may have a yellow or gray cast secondary to exudation and gliosis. Others may have many small vessels and hemorrhages on their surfaces. Passing to the angioma are a pair of retinal vessels, an artery, and its accompanying vein. They are enormously dilated and tortuous, showing focal swellings, kinkings, and sausage-like constrictions (Plate XI-B). The artery in the earlier stages may be smaller and less tortuous than its fellow vein, although frequently the two vessels appear indistinguishable. The lesions of angiomatosis retinae are multiple in one-third or more cases and bilateral in about one-half.

Although not malignant, the tumors of angiomatosis retinae undergo changes which can destroy the eye. Shining white or yellow spots of exudate and retinal edema appear around the lesions, between or along the dilated feeder vessels, around the disc and, for unknown reasons, in the macula well away from the angioma. Hemorrhages into the subretinal space, retina or vitreous, secondary gliosis, and retinal detachments may develop secondary to the retinal tumors. As late sequelae, iridocyclitis with extensive posterior synechiae, rubeosis and secondary glaucoma, cataract, staphylomas, or phthisis bulbi may occur.

Fluorescein angiography of the fundus in angiomatosis retinae has proved a valuable tool for the clinician concerned with the pathogenesis, clinical manifestations, and treatment of the disease. The characteristic mural lamellar flow in the early venous filling period clearly denotes which vessel is the vein and which is the artery. Absence of fluorescence of the lesions and feeder vessels after treatment denotes that therapy has been complete. Perhaps most significantly fluorescein studies demonstrate that a profuse and continuous leakage occurs from the angiomatous tumor. Such leakage explains how exudative material may overlie the tumor and lead to gliosis and retinal detachment.

Of all the phakomatoses, von Hippel-Lindau disease has been most amenable to treatment, in both its central nervous system and ocular involvement. The presence of discrete peripheral retinal lesions composed of thin-walled new-formed vessels has encouraged the use of various modalities to destroy them. The advent of photocoagulation provided a new means for successfully treating angiomatosis retinae and offered significant advantages over diathermy (Guerry et al., 1958; Meyer-Schwickerath, 1956). In the first place, by requiring no conjunctival incision and causing no necrosis of sclera, photocoagulation therapy of a large angioma or multiple angiomas could be spread out over a period of months. Because photocoagulation allows for multiple treatments with gradual shrinkage of the tumor, there is less risk of complicating hemorrhage. It can be accurately applied to the surface of the angioma or between feeder vessels, thus avoiding severe hemorrhage, and may be used to treat lesions in the vicinity of the disc or macula. Since new tumors may develop over years of follow-up, a definite cure is rarely obtained by treatment at one sitting. Photocoagulation is, of course, not completely free of complications. Retinal and vitreous hemorrhages, transient exudative retinal detachments, and traction on the retina may follow treatment.

A recent review of the results of photocoagulation has shown that 80 per cent of the treated eyes were saved (Wessing, 1967). In early cases, success by photocoagulation alone was found to be achieved nearly all the time, while those cases with secondary changes responded about 50 per cent of the time.

Cryotherapy has also been used to treat angiomas and shows promise of being an effective way of eliminating the tumors. Frequently even large tumors can be eradicated with only one treatment when the individual lesion is frozen on three separate occasions for a full minute each time.

Neurofibromatosis of von Recklinghausen's disease is characterized by developmental anomalies and tumors of the nervous system, skeleton, and viscera and by pigmentary lesions of the skin. Malformations and tumors of the eye and orbit are frequent and important manifestations of the syndrome. The disease is congenital and is essentially a disturbance in the development of ectodermal and mesodermal tissues. Manifestations of the disorder may be apparent at birth, but often the signs develop later in life and progress with age, especially during puberty and pregnancy. Heredity is an important factor in the development of the disease and transmission is usually as a simple dominant, though familial evidences of the disease are often subtle and show great variability (Chao, 1959; Marshall, 1953).

The characteristic tumor of von Recklinghausen's disease is the neurofibroma which may affect any of the cranial nerves, the spinal cord, the spinal roots and peripheral nerves, and the sympathetic system. The tumors consist of whorl-like proliferations of Schwann cells which produce diffuse or focal thickening and tortuosity of the affected nerve. They are not encapsulated and tend to extend and invade through tissue spaces.

Cutaneous manifestations, principally café au lait spots, may indicate the presence of the disease immediately at birth or, like the other signs, may appear later. They occur on any part of the body but are more frequently found on the unexposed areas. These melanotic spots are not specific for von Recklinghausen's disease, since they also occur in normal individuals and in tuberous sclerosis.

The eyelids are a common site of extensive plexiform neuromas which produce ptosis and disfiguring enlargement of the lids and adjacent areas of the face. Exophthalmos in von Recklinghausen's disease results from neurofibromas within the soft tissues of the orbit, from tumors of the optic nerve, and from abnormalities of the bony structure of the orbit (Brewer and Kierland, 1955; Dabezies and Walsh, 1961). Congenital absence or erosion of the bones by tumor allows protrusion of the brain through the defect.

Neurofibromatous involvement of the choroid and ciliary body produces diffuse or localized thickening of these tissues. Although frequently difficult to appreciate clinically, they have characteristic histological features (Wolter, 1965; Wolter et al., 1962). The tumor tissue is very cellular and contains hyperplastic Schwann cells, abundant melanocytes, meshworks of nerve fibers, and ovoid bodies. The ovoid bodies are lamellar structures composed of concentric layers of Schwann cells, with hyalinization of the core cells and with nerve fiber branches extending into the interspaces. Uveal tract neurofibromatosis is frequently associated with glaucoma.

Retinal lesions in von Recklinghausen's disease are rare, although tumor masses resembling the hamartomas of Bourneville's disease do occur (Block, 1948; Frenkel, 1967; Hales, 1963; Van der Hoeve, 1923 and 1932). Ophthalmoscopically they generally appear as small, discrete, moderately elevated lesions. They may be single or multiple and are usually grayish-white or yellow. Microscopically the masses are primarily proliferations of glial cells of the nerve fiber layer, with branching astrocytes and ganglion cells.

Tumors of the optic nervehead occur in von Recklinghausen's disease, and both the ophthalmoscopic and histological features of the lesions have been reported (Copeland et al., 1934; Goldsmith, 1949; Stallard, 1938; Trueman and Rubin, 1953; Van der Hoeve, 1921). The tumors may be gliomas or meningiomas. Gliomas usually develop in the first 10 years of life, are slowly progressive, and may eventually show sarcomatous changes. Meningiomas appear at a later age and are more likely to invade non-neural tissue. The tumors of the optic nerve and chiasm produce loss of vision and field, papilledema, or optic atrophy, and may produce enlargement of the optic foramen by extension. Proptosis and limitation of motility favor intraorbital involvement.

Bourneville's tuberous sclerosis is a complex disorder characterized principally by multiple tumors of the nervous system, mental deficiency and epilepsy, and specific cutaneous lesions. Manifestations of the disorder usually become apparent in infancy or early childhood. There is then progressive mental and physical deterioration and death usually occurs before the age of 25 years in the fully developed syndrome.

The characteristic lesions of the central nervous system are the cortical "tubers" and the subependymal "candle drippings." The "tubers" are pale firm areas within the gyri, often extending over several adjacent convolutions. In these areas there is proliferation of glial elements and disturbance of the normal structure of the gray matter. The "candle drippings" are nodules of neuroglial overgrowth which project into the ventricles, most often near the foramen of Monro, producing a diagnostic picture with air encephalography. The lesions frequently undergo cystic degeneration and secondary calcification, which may be seen on x-ray.

Mental deficiency is usually obvious by the third year, when patients begin to exhibit dullness and disordered behavior. At the same time epilepsy may develop, and status epilepticus may ultimately cause death.

Cutaneous manifestations of tuberous sclerosis consist of adenoma sebaceum of the face, fibromas of the trunk, shagreen patches, and sometimes café au lait or depigmented spots and nevi. Adenoma sebaceum is the pathognomonic skin lesion of tuberous sclerosis and appears as a reddish-brown or yellowish papular rash, the nodules being somewhat firm and sometimes confluent. The rash occurs in a butterfly distribution over the face, and the papules consist of hyperplastic connective tissue.

The major ocular abnormalities are tumors of the disc and retina which are best classified as hamartomas. These lesions may occasionally cause secondary glaucoma, intraocular inflammation, or hemorrhage, while the intracranial lesions may produce papilledema or optic atrophy. Giant drusen are also associated with tuberous sclerosis. Van der Hoeve (1921, 1923 a and b, 1932) has provided the classic ophthalmoscopic and microscopic descriptions of the fundus lesions and, moreover, has emphasized the significance of these ocular lesions in making a diagnosis of tuberous sclerosis, especially in the early or incomplete forms of the disease. The distinctive ocular lesion of tuberous sclerosis is the refractile multinodular tumor of disc or retina, appropriately likened to an unripe mulberry or to clumps of tapioca or frogs' eggs (Plate XI-C). Unfortunately, not all the ocular tumors of tuberous sclerosis present in this easily recognized form. Sometimes the retinal tumors have a smooth contour and appear as flat white or yellow spots in the fundus.

The mulberry type lesions most often arise from the disc or from the retina near the disc. They may be one-half to two or more times the diameter of the disc, and they may protrude as much as 4 or 5 diopters into the vitreous.

Microscopically all types of disc and retinal tumors have certain basic similarities. The masses are composed of proliferations of pleomorphic cells and their processes are thought to be elements of the glial series (Garron and Spencer, 1964; McLean, 1956; Messinger and Clarke, 1937). The proliferations are usually confined to the nerve fiber layer but may extend into other layers of the retina or into the substance of the optic nerve. The cells are usually elongated and often have indistinct walls, giving the appearance of a syncytium. Intracytoplasmic fibers can often be seen. The cell type is frequently difficult to classify, but in some cases the cells have been identified as astrocytes (Garron and Spencer, 1964; McLean, 1956). The tumor masses frequently contain cystic spaces and areas of calcification or ossification.

The effects of the ocular and intracranial lesions on visual function are variable and essentially unpredictable. The hamartomas of disc and retina do not necessarily produce significant loss of vision. Their size and location are critical factors in determining their effect on function and, fortunately, they do not usually occur in the macula. More commonly, loss of vision results from the intracranial lesions which cause papilledema and later optic atrophy. Very rarely, vision may be impaired by secondary glaucoma, inflammation, or intraocular hemorrhage.

RETROLENTAL FIBROPLASIA

Once it was established that oxygen administered in high amounts was the cause of retrolental fibroplasia, the importance of monitoring oxygen concentration became more apparent. At first, ambient oxygen levels were limited wherever possible to 40 per cent and measurements of oxygen concentration were made by oxygen analyzers and flowmeters. In spite of these precautions, retrolental fibroplasia continued to occur, and often 40 per cent oxygen was not sufficient to relieve the respiratory distress syndrome. More recently, the important relationship between blood oxygen tension (Po_2), the respiratory distress syndrome, and retrolental fibroplasia has been shown (Patz,

1967 a and b; Robertson et al., 1968; Silverman, 1968 and 1969 a and b, Smith, 1964). It is estimated that 10 per cent of all infants under 2500 gm. birth weight are afflicted with the respiratory distress syndrome (Patz, 1967a). In the United States alone this accounts for about 40,000 infants yearly who develop the condition. The exact cause is unknown, but a combination of cardiopulmonary abnormalities deprives the infant in respiratory distress of an adequate tissue oxygen supply, so that high concentrations of oxygen are required. For example, an infant with respiratory distress may require 100 per cent oxygen to achieve the same arterial Po_2 level as the normal infant breathing room air. Since the cardiopulmonary deficiencies in distress infants may disappear at any time, high ambient oxygen concentrations in the incubator can result in sharply elevated arterial Po_2. Thus, the importance of monitoring the arterial Po_2 to avoid potentially retinotoxic oxygen levels becomes obvious.

The techniques for measuring Po_2 are time-consuming and require a highly skilled pediatric team, as well as specially trained technicians and expensive instrumentation. In addition, even with frequent sampling, it is extremely difficult to keep the Po_2 within normal limits. Because of this and because the majority of hospitals do not monitor arterial oxygen, the ophthalmologist may make an important contribution to safer oxygen therapy. Examination of the retina for retinal vasoconstriction can provide a general guideline as to the arterial oxygen levels that have been maintained.

Careful ophthalmoscopy should be repeated at the time of discharge from the nursery and again at 5 months of age. The latter date is selected because previous studies failed to demonstrate active retrolental fibroplasia developing after this age (Patz, 1967a). As will be shown, however, periodic examinations are indicated during the growth years because of the progressive nature of the cicatricial stage.

As currently described by the National Society for the Prevention of Blindness, the earliest sign of the active phase of retrolental fibroplasia is transient attenuation of the retinal vessels. This is followed by Stage 1 of the disease, in which the vessels become dilated and tortuous. Hemorrhages may or may not be present, and early neovascularization, especially in the fundus periphery, is sometimes visible. As Stage 2 ensues, neovascularization becomes more obvious and the peripheral retina appears clouded. Although vitreous haze may be a feature of this stage, spontaneous regression is still possible. Peripheral retinal detachment develops in Stage 3 and, as it extends, leads to Stage 4. When the entire retina becomes detached, the disease has reached its fifth and most active stage.

The active stages of retrolental fibroplasia are followed later by varying degrees of scarring which are divided into five categories of severity. The mildest cicatricial phase (Grade 1) is characterized by pale fundi, attenuated vessels, small areas of opaque tissue in the peripheral fundus, and irregular retinal pigmentation. In Grade 2 the opaque tissue occupies more of the peripheral fundus and is associated with some localized retinal detachment. The disc is distorted by traction, usually toward the temporal side. Grade 3 patients usually have a retinal fold which extends to the peripheral opaque tissue from the disc. Whereas patients with the first two grades of retrolental fibroplasia have useful vision, patients with Grade 3 retrolental fibroplasia may have visual acuity varying from 5/200 to 20/50. In Grade 4, retrolental tissue covers part of the pupil and only a small area of attached retina or red reflex is visible. Finally, in Grade 5 the retrolental tissue covers the entire pupillary area and no fundus reflex is present. These five categories of cicatricial retrolental fibroplasia as outlined by the National Society for the Prevention of Blindness can now be described more adequately because of better examination techniques.

The most common finding in cicatricial retrolental fibroplasia is myopia. Although this does not represent a specific change in retrolental fibroplasia alone, there appears to be a significant relationship between the degree of myopia and the severity of the retrolental fibroplasia. Myopia associated with retrolental fibroplasia is seen early and falls into the congenital group. Generally it is discovered before age 6 years and most commonly between 4 and 6 years of age. The relationship of the degree of myopia to the severity of retrolental fibroplasia is also important, since retinal detachment, a serious consequence of cicatricial retrolental fibroplasia, occurs most often in highly myopic eyes.

The vitreoretinal changes in cicatricial retrolental fibroplasia may be divided into those which occur between the posterior pole and the vortex ampullae, i.e., the posterior fundus, and those found peripheral to the vortex ampullae. Through the years, "dragged discs" have been considered almost a characteristic change in Grades 1 and 2 cicatricial retrolental fibroplasia. Usually, but not always, the displacement is to the temporal side (Plate XI-D). On histological examination of eyes with dragged retina, several interesting observations can be made. Most important is the fact that the retina is folded over the optic nerve, while the nerve itself may show little or no displacement. Because the histological appearance correlates with the clinical picture of retinal displacement rather than optic nerve displacement, the term dragged retina is suggested as a replacement for dragged disc.

In more severe cases of cicatricial retrolental fibroplasia, dragging of the retina assumes the shape of a retinal fold, again most commonly to the temporal side (Plate XI-E). Usually the fold runs radially through the macula toward the fundus periphery, where it fans out to become confluent with gliotic tissue near the posterior border of the vitreous base. The cortical vitreous is thickened over the fold and is adherent to it, causing traction toward the temporal side. Retinal vessels which are incorporated into the retinal fold give the surrounding fundus a relatively avascular appearance. Because the retinal folds frequently run through the macular area, ocular nystagmus and vision less than 20/800 may be associated findings.

Alterations in the pigmentation of the fundus are common in cicatricial retrolental fibroplasia and may occur in the periphery as well as in the posterior fundus. Essentially the pigmentation takes two forms. The first consists of discrete patches characterized by apparent loss of the pigment epithelium and outer sensory retinal layers. These lesions may be confused with the chorioretinal scars seen in toxoplasmosis or cytomegalic inclusion disease (Plate XI-F). Less commonly the alteration in fundus pigmentation is in the form of clumping.

In addition to the striking changes in the posterior fundus, lesions anterior to the vortex ampullae are equally as characteristic of retrolental fibroplasia and perhaps even more common than those in the posterior fundus. Pigmentary changes similar to those already described occur with equal frequency in the peripheral retina. Equatorial folds also occur between the equator and the ora serrata, and may be the only retinal finding consistent with cicatricial retrolental fibroplasia. Recognized as one or more ridges in the retina, equatorial folds are often associated with small discrete areas of chorioretinal scarring. Again, the cortical vitreous is thickened and adherent to the folds and on histological examination may appear as a membrane attaching to the crest of the fold. Just as with temporal retinal folds, it seems reasonable to assume that attachment of the cortical vitreous to the underlying retina is a contributing etiologic factor to equatorial folds.

Retinoschisis may present a differential diagnostic problem from rhegmatogenous retinal detachment and equatorial retinal folds in cicatricial retrolental fibroplasia. Usually it is associated with the presence of areas of white without pressure due to vitreous traction on the retina. Clinically the retinoschisis seen in cicatricial retrolental fibroplasia is similar to senile retinoschisis with retinal splitting apparently between the inner and outer nuclear layers. The retinal vessels usually travel in the inner retinal layers but may on occasion cross from the inner layer through the schisis cavity to the outer layer. Intraretinal exudates in the inner retinal layers are common. Appearing as small, discrete, whitish spots in the inner retinal layer, intraretinal exudates sometimes are also seen in areas of white without pressure. Occasionally these are arranged in circular fashion and may be mistaken for the borders of a retinal break. Similarly, outer layer retinal breaks may be confused with a retinal hole through full thickness retina.

Lattice degeneration in cicatricial retrolental fibroplasia is similar to that seen in the eyes of patients who have no history of prematurity. Generally there is thinning of the inner retinal layers coupled with vitreous condensation over the area of lattice degeneration.

A less common peripheral retinal finding is neovascularization. When it occurs, neovascularization is often in close proximity to areas of the retina in which there are occluded peripheral retinal vessels.

Elevated retinal vessels are another change found in cicatricial retrolental fibroplasia. Vitreous hemorrhage frequently precedes recognition of the elevated vessel which cannot then be identified until later, when the media has cleared. Usually the vessel leaves the retina and runs along the posterior surface of the vitreous gel, which in the area of the elevated vessel has contracted and moved away from the retina. The vessel may be a terminal branch or may be pulled from the retina for part of its course before returning to the inner retinal layers once again.

The presence of peripheral avascular vitreous membranes in cicatricial retrolental fibroplasia is one of the most consistent findings. The membranes are most commonly temporal and are located just anterior to the equator. Some are thin and gossamer in appearance, while others are thicker and quite dense (Plate XI-G). Often one end of a vitreous membrane can be traced to a retinal insertion or to a gliotic vitreoretinal condensation confluent with the vitreous base.

Another important vitreous change is syneresis of the vitreous gel. This is most common in the central vitreous and appears as optically empty cavities on slit lamp biomicroscopy. The syneresis cavities are sometimes bridged by vitreous fibrils which have condensed to form thin bands. These bands may exert traction on the retina when the syneresis cavity is located peripherally or posteriorly.

One of the most serious complications of cicatricial retrolental fibroplasia is rhegmatogenous retinal detachment. The characteristics of this type of detachment are discussed in the section on juvenile retinal detachment.

The predilection for temporal retinal involvement in retrolental fibroplasia may be related to retinal development. The retina is unique in that it is completely devoid of its own blood vessels until the fourth month of gestation, at which time vessels from the embryonic hyaloid vascular stalk in the optic nerve extend into the adjacent retina and start growing forward to the anterior part of the retina. The observation that the full-term infant's anterior retina is still avascular (Cogan, 1963), especially on the temporal side, may account for more cicatrization on that side than on the nasal side.

The presence of peripheral vitreous membranes as a significant finding in cicatricial retrolental fibroplasia is understandable on the basis of delayed vascularization of the peripheral retina in premature babies. The fact that it may be a more common finding than dragged retina in the posterior pole emphasizes the need for careful examination of the peripheral fundus before ruling out the diagnosis of cicatricial retrolental fibroplasia.

RETINAL DETACHMENT

Retinal detachment due to retinal breaks is fortunately rare in children. Although there is universal agreement that trauma is the most common cause of retinal detachment in children, the incidence of the other causes of juvenile detachment is controversial. Some authors feel that prematurity is the second most common cause (Tasman, 1967) while others favor myopia (Hilton and Norton, 1969). However, most investigators agree that, not including trauma, prematurity, myopia, aphakia, inferior temporal dialysis, lattice degeneration, and uveitis are the conditions most frequently associated with rhegmatogenous detachment in children, regardless of the incidence.

The fact that trauma is the most common cause of juvenile detachment helps to explain the greater incidence of this condition in males as compared to females. Blunt trauma and penetrating injuries can both cause detachment. However, in the case of blunt trauma there may be a latent period of several months or even years between the injury and diagnosis of the detachment (Cox et al., 1966). This is understandable for two reasons: often children are reluctant to report an injury or symptom, and, secondly, many traumatic detachments start inferiorly and do not cause a subjective awareness until the macula is threatened.

Because traumatic retinal detachments may be initially asymptomatic, one or more demarcation lines are often present and, when found, confirm a duration of at least several months. A multiplicity of demarcation lines indicates successive increases in the size of the detachment and is evidence that chorioretinal adhesions cannot be counted on to wall off a detachment. The detachments are seldom bullous but tend instead to be smooth and flat. Fixed star folds are rare, although they may occur, and intraretinal cysts may be present if the detachment is old. These disappear spontaneously in a few days if the retina reattaches after surgery.

Typically, the retinal break seen after blunt trauma begins as a tear along the posterior border of the vitreous base. Gradually the break takes on the classic configuration of a dialysis (Plate XI-H). These tend to occur primarily in the inferotemporal and superonasal quadrants. Of course, any of the other quadrants, and sometimes more than one, may be the site of a dialysis, so careful searching of the ora serrata, 360 degrees, is imperative. When the retina tears along both the anterior and posterior borders of the vitreous base, the vitreous base itself is avulsed and may hang like a pigmented loop in the vitreous cavity with its underlying strip of attached retina. When avulsion of the vitreous base is present superonasally, it is pathognomonic of traumatic retinal detachment.

Another form of traumatic peripheral retinal damage is extensive detachment of the ora serrata, with retinal breaks in the nonpigmented epithelium of the pars plana ciliaris along the anterior border of the vitreous base. Pars plana breaks appear as small or large dialyses and cannot usually be seen without scleral depression. Although the epithelium of the pars plana ciliaris is thin and may appear more translucent than the posterior retina, this difference in thickness may not be striking enough to identify the ora serrata. The position of the ora, however, may be made more obvious by a variable amount of pigment which has been dragged from the underlying pigment epithelium. Another clue to the position of the ora is the presence of cystoid degeneration, which differentiates the extreme periphery of the retina from the epithelium of the pars plana. The contrast between retina and thin pars plana is more marked in the folds of the often tented ora serrata, so that light reflected from the uveal blood vessels is transmitted as a reddish color through these tented areas which can easily be mistaken for triangular breaks.

Traumatic retinal detachments with dialysis have a favorable surgical prognosis. Usually they do not settle during bed rest, but when the subretinal fluid is drained the retina flattens nicely.

The age at which retinal detachment occurs in the cicatricial retrolental fibroplasia group ranges from 10 to 19 years, with an average of 13.5 years, a fact which emphasizes that cicatricial retrolental fibroplasia may be a progressive disease characterized by vitreous shrinkage and vitreoretinal adhesion (Tasman, 1970). The actions of vitreous membranes which attach to the retina undoubtedly also contribute to traction on the peripheral retina. Ultimately this may lead to retinal breaks and equatorial folds near the retinal breaks when the retina detaches.

Multiple rather than single breaks appear to be the rule in retinal detachment which occurs with retrolental fibroplasia. Usually the retinal breaks are round or oval in appearance and equatorial in location. They are most common on the temporal side and occasionally may occur in an area of lattice or pigment. Free-floating opercula are generally not present, and just posterior to the retinal breaks, marked equatorial folds indicative of severe vitreous traction are common.

The remaining causes of rhegmatogenous retinal detachment in children include congenital inferotemporal dialysis, myopia, aphakia, lattice degeneration, uveitis, and congenital retinoschisis. Congenital dialyses usually occur bilaterally and are located inferotemporally along the posterior border of the vitreous base. Like traumatic dialyses, they have an excellent surgical prognosis.

REFERENCES

Block, F. J.: Retinal tumor associated with neurofibromatosis (von Recklinghausen's disease). Report of a case. Arch. Ophthal., *40*:433, 1948.

Blodi, F. C.: The pathology of central tapeto-retinal dystrophy (hereditary macular degenerations). Trans. Amer. Acad. Ophthal. Otolaryng., *70*:1058, 1966.

Braley, A. E.: Dystrophy of the macula. Amer. J. Ophthal., *61*:1–24, 1966.

Braley, A. E., and Spivey, B. E.: Hereditary vitelline macular degeneration (possibly of vitelliform origin): A clinical and functional evaluation of a new pedigree with variable expressivity and dominant inheritance. Trans. Amer. Ophthal. Soc., *61*:339, 1963.

Bruwer, A. J., and Kierland, R. F.: Neurofibromatosis and congenital unilateral pulsating and nonpulsating exophthalmos. Arch. Ophthal., *53*:2, 1955.

Chao, D.: Congenital neurocutaneous syndromes in childhood. I. Neurofibromatosis. J. Pediat., *55*:189, 1959.

Coats, G.: Forms of retinal diseases with massive exudation. Roy. London Ophthal. Hosp. Rep., *17*:440, 1908.

Coats, G.: Weber retinitis exudativa. Arch. Ophthal., *81*:275, 1912.

Cogan, D. G.: Development and senescence of the human retinal vasculature. Trans. Ophthal. Soc. U.K., *83*:465, 1963.

Copeland, M. M., Craver, L. F., and Reese, A. B.: Neurofibromatosis with ocular changes and involvement of the thoracic spine. Arch. Surg., *29*:108, 1934.

Cox, M. S., Schepens, C. L., and Freeman, H. M.: Retinal detachment due to ocular contusion. Arch. Ophthal., *76*:678, 1966.

Craig, W. M., Wagener, H. P., and Kernohan, J. W.: Lindau-von Hippel disease. A report of four cases. Arch. Neurol. Psychiat., *46*:36, 1941.

Criswick, V. G., and Schepens, C. L.: Familial exudative vitreoretinopathy. Amer. J. Ophthal., *68*:578, 1969.

Dabezies, O. H., Jr., and Walsh, F. B.: Pulsating exophthalmos in association with neurofibromatosis of the eyelid. Trans. Amer. Acad. Ophthal. Otolaryng., *885*, 1961.

Dunphy, E. B.: Glaucoma accompanying nevus flammeus. Trans. Amer. Ophthal. Soc., *32*:143, 1934.

Francois, J.: Vitelliform degeneration of the macula. Bull. N.Y. Acad. Med., *44*:18, 1968.

Frenkel, M.: Retinal angiomatosis in a patient with neurofibromatosis. Amer. J. Ophthal., *63*:804, 1967.

Garron, L. K., and Spencer, W. H.: Retinal glioneuroma associated with tuberous sclerosis. Trans. Amer. Acad. Ophthal. Otolaryngol. *68*:1018, 1964.

Goldsmith, J.: Neurofibromatosis associated with tumors of optic papilla. Report of a case. Arch. Ophthal., *42*:718, 1949.

Grondahl, J.: Heterotopia of the macula. Probably caused by ablatio falciformis congenita. Acta Ophthal. (Kovenhavn), *41*:259, 1963.

Guerry, D., III. Wiesinger, H., and Ham, W. T.: Photocoagulation of the retina. Report of a successfully treated case of angiomatosis retinae. Amer. J. Ophthal., *46*:463, 1958.

Hales, R. H.: Glioma of the optic disc. Arch. Ophthal., *70*:648, 1963.

Hilton, G. F., and Norton, E. W. D.: Retinal detachment in juveniles. *In* Dufour, R., Fison, L., and Meyer-Schwickerath, G. (Eds.): Med. Problems in Ophthalmology, *8*:325, 1969.

Hogan, M., and Zimmerman, L. E.: Ophthalmic Pathology 2nd ed. Philadelphia, W. B. Saunders Co., Figures 143 and 568, 1969.

Jesberg, D. O., and Schepens, C. L.: Retinal detachment associated with coloboma of the choroid. Arch. Ophthal., *65*:163, 1960.

Jesberg, D. O., Spencer, W. H., and Hoyt, W. F.: Incipient lesions of von Hippel-Lindau disease. Arch. Ophthal., *80*:632, 1968.

Krill, A. E., and Deutman, H. F.: Variations of juvenile macular degeneration. Trans. Amer. Ophthal. Soc., (in print).

Lindau, A.: Zur Frage der Angiomatosis Retinae und ihrer Hirnkomplikationen. Acta Ophthal., *4*:193, 1927.

Marshall, D.: Glioma of the optic nerve as a manifestation of von Recklinghausen's disease. Trans. Amer. Ophthal. Soc., *51*:117, 1953.

McLean, J. M.: Glial tumors of the retina in relation to tuberous sclerosis. Amer. J. Ophthal., *41*:428, 1956.

Messinger, H. C., and Clarke, B. E.: Retinal tumors in tuberous sclerosis. Review of the literature and report of a case, with special attention to microscopic structure. Arch. Ophthal. (Chicago), *18*:1, 1937.

Meyer-Schwickerath, G.: Prophylactic treatment of retinal detachment by light coagulation. Trans. Ophthal. Soc. U.K., *76*:739, 1956.

Morales, A. G.: Coats' disease. Amer. J. Ophthal., *60*:855, 1965.

Nicol, A. A.: Lindau's disease in five generations. Ann. Hum. Genet., *22*:7, 1957.

Patz, A.: New role of the ophthalmologist in prevention of retrolental fibroplasia, Arch. Ophthal., *78*:565, 1967(a).

Patz, A.: Oxygen administration in the premature infant: a two-edged sword, Amer. J. Ophthal., *63*:351, 1967(b).

Paufique, L. et Hervouet, F.: Anatomie pathologique d'un cas de maladie de Stargardt. Bull. Soc. Ophtal. Franc., *76*:108, 1963.

Reese, A. B.: Tumors of the Eye. 2nd ed. New York, Harper & Row (Hoeber), 1963.

Robertson, N. R., Gupta, J. M., Dahlenburg, G. W., and Tizard, J. P. M.: Oxygen therapy in the newborn, Lancet, *1*:1323, 1968.

Silverman, W. A.: Oxygen therapy and retrolental fibroplasia, Amer. J. Pub. Health, *58*:2009, 1968.

Silverman, W. A.: Diagnosis and treatment. Oxygen therapy and retrolental fibroplasia. Pediatrics, *43*:88, 1969(a).

Silverman, W. A.: Oxygen and retrolental fibroplasia in neonates. Pub. Health Rep., *84*:16, 1969(b).

Smith, C. A.: Diagnosis and treatment: use and misuse of oxygen in the treatment of prematures. Pediatrics, *33*:111, 1964.

Stallard, H. B.: A case of intra-ocular neuroma (von Recklinghausen's disease) of the left optic nerve head. Brit. J. Ophthal., *22*:11, 1938.

Sugar, H. S.: An explanation for the acquired macular pathology associated with congenital pits of the optic disc. Amer. J. Ophthal., *57*:833, 1964.

Tasman, W. S.: Vitreoretinal changes in cicatricial retrolental fibroplasia. Trans. Amer. Ophthal. Soc., *68*:548, 1970.

Tasman, W.: Retinal detachment in children. Trans. Amer. Acad. Ophthal. and Otolaryngol., *71*:455, 1967.

Trueman, R. H., and Rubin, I. E.: Tumor of the optic disc associated with neurofibromatosis: Presentation of a case. Arch. Ophthal., *50*:468, 1953.

Van der Hoeve, J.: Augengeschwulste bei der tuberosen Hirnsklerose (Bourneville). Arch. Ophthal. (von Graefe's), *105*:880, 1921.

Van der Hoeve, J.: Augengeschwulste bei der tuberosen Hirnsklerose (Bourneville), und verwandten Krankheiten. Arch. Ophthal. (von Graefe's), *III*:1, 1923(a).

Van der Hoeve, J.: Eye diseases in tuberous sclerosis of the brain and in Recklinghausen's disease. Trans. Ophthal. Soc. U.K., *43*:534, 1923(b).

Van der Hoeve, J.: The Doyne Memorial Lecture: Eye symptoms in phakomatoses. Trans. Ophthal. Soc. U.K., *52*:380, 1932.

Wessing, A.: 10 Jahre Lichtkoagulation bei Angiomatosis Retinae. Klin. Mbl. Augenheilk, *50*:57, 1967.

Wolter, J. R.: Nerve fibrils in ovoid bodies with neurofibromatosis of choroid. Arch. Ophthal., *73*:696, 1965.

Wolter, J. R., Gonzales-Sirit R., and Mankin, W. J.: Neurofibromatosis of the choroid. Amer. J. Ophthal., *54*:217, 1962.

Yanoff, M., Rahn, E. K., and Zimmerman, L. E.: Histopathology of juvenile retinoschisis. Arch. Ophthal., *79*:49, January, 1968.

CHAPTER 15

DISORDERS
OF THE LENS

P. ROBB McDONALD, M.D.

INTRODUCTION

Cataracts in children may be developmental, acquired (inflammatory or metabolic), or traumatic. This presentation is concerned principally with their management rather than a detailed description of the various types of developmental cataracts and the causes of uveitis and other pathological conditions. Cordes (1957) and Francois (1959) have more than adequately covered the subject of congenital or developmental cataracts, though for the sake of completeness one must mention the variations in size, shape, and opacification of the lens. The normal structure of the lens is schematically depicted in Figure 15–1.

Congenital aphakia is extremely rare and when it occurs is usually associated with a grossly underdeveloped or rudimentary eye. The shape of the lens may vary—in spherophakia it is more spherical than normal. It is usually bilateral and may be an incidental defect. It is seen in Marchesani's syndrome. Iridodonesis is present and the lens may spontaneously dislocate into the anterior chamber.

Colobomas of the lens can also occur. Zonular fibers are usually absent in the

region of the coloboma which may be outlined with some fine dustlike opacities. When the coloboma is inferior, it is usually in conjunction with other colobomatous defects of the eye.

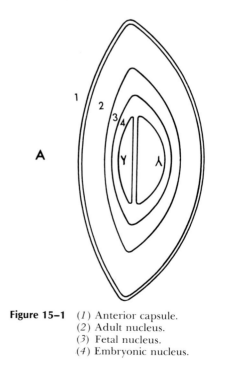

Figure 15–1 (*1*) Anterior capsule.
(*2*) Adult nucleus.
(*3*) Fetal nucleus.
(*4*) Embryonic nucleus.

370

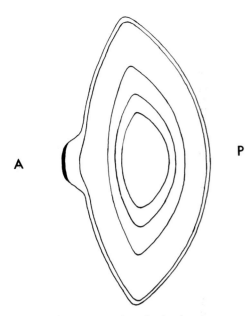

Figure 15–2 Anterior lenticonus.

Additional congenital defects in the shape of the lens are anterior (Fig. 15–2) and posterior lenticonus (Fig. 15–3); the latter is much more common. They resemble small central ectasias of the anterior or posterior portion of the lens. They give rise to a marked visual disturbance because of the refractive error as well as the frequent association of lens opacities.

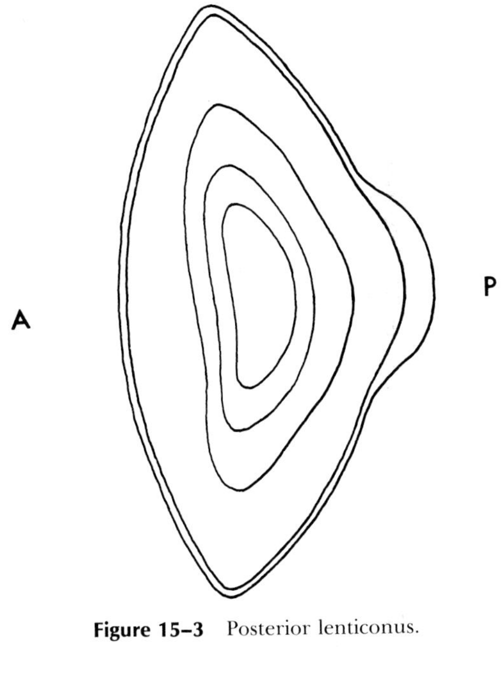

Figure 15–3 Posterior lenticonus.

Anomalies in the position of the lens, subluxation, are seen most frequently in Marfan's or Marchesani's syndrome. Marfan's syndrome (arachnodactyly), caused by a defect of connective tissue, is characterized by increase in skeletal length, spider fingers, scoliosis, and disturbances in the larger blood vessels. Marchesani's syndrome is a hyperplastic form of congenital mesodermal dystrophy. Those affected are short in stature and have short stubby fingers.

CATARACTS

There are several different types of congenital cataract and many variations of each type. Only the more common forms will be considered at this time (Table 15–1).

The term developmental would appear to be more acceptable than congenital. Congenital to most readers implies inheritance or phenotype, whereas developmental includes the phenotype or phenocopy, the latter resembling the first but is not genetically transmitted.

Embryological Development of the Lens and Hyaloid System

With even a superficial knowledge of embryology, one cannot help but marvel at the development of the human embryo. By the seventh week, the embryo has the full complement of organs. The critical period for gross congenital abnormalities is over by the fourth to fifth week, although after this time there may be changes in the organs already formed as a result of noxious effects of disease. The most noticeable examples are the serious sequelae of rubella. It would be interesting to note why the virus of rubella affects primarily the organs of sight and hearing.

The development of the *lens* can be divided into two phases: the formation of the lens vesicle and the development of the lens fibers with formation of the nuclei. The lens arises from ectoderm that is in contact with the neural ectoderm of the optic bulb and stalk. The lens plate invaginates into the lens pit to form the lens vesicle. It is closed in by the 8 mm.

TABLE 15–1   MORPHOLOGICAL CLASSIFICATION OF CONGENITAL CATARACTS

Anterior Axial Embryonic Cataract: Anterior axial embryonic cataracts were described by Vogt (1919). The opacities are usually but not invariably bilateral and consist of a number of small white dots situated in the neighborhood of the anterior Y suture, sometimes anterior and at times posterior to this suture. They have been reported as a frequent occurrence in children. The condition is nonprogressive and rarely causes any disturbance of vision.

Sutural (Stellate) Cataract: This cataract usually affects either one or both of the Y-shaped sutures of the fetal nucleus. It is stationary and almost always bilateral. Usually the opacity is made up of fine white or bluish dots which may assume a feathery configuration but sometimes they are dense and consist of calcareous-like deposits taking on many different shapes. The cataracts are transmitted with autosomal dominance.

Congenital Morgagnian Cataract: This cataract shows the same characteristics as observed in the long-standing cataract of the adult. The condition is rare in the child. The cortex is liquefied into a milky white fluid containing the free-floating nucleus. The toxic effects from the cortical material may excite the development of a uveitis. At times a spontaneous absorption may occur so that only the anterior and posterior capsules remain. When this occurs it may be referred to as a membranous cataract.

Lamellar (Zonular) Cataract: This form of cataract is characterized by a circumscribed zone of opacity consisting of fine opaque-white spots arranged in concentric layers. When the pupil is dilated there is a clear rim of cortex present about the periphery. From the surface of the cataract a number of projections arise resembling the spokes of a wheel. They are known as "riders" and vary considerably in size and shape. Zonular cataracts display a large variety of forms recognizable by slit lamp. Most cases appear to be inherited as an autosomal dominant.

Congenital Floriform Cataract: These opacities are most common in the axial portions of the lens and are seen most typically in the anterior and posterior fetal sutures. The cataract appears to consist of a number of oval elements grouped together, resembling the petals of a flower. Transmission has been reported as an autosomal dominant.

Central Pulverulent Cataract: (Also Nuclear or "Coppock" Cataract): This type of cataract is limited to the embryonic nucleus. It is nonprogressive and always bilateral in occurrence. The opacity consists of minute discrete white dots giving an appearance of a granular disc. Vision is rarely affected unless the pupil is extremely small. Sometimes a larger area than usual is affected and the opacity becomes more dense, resembling a nuclear cataract. This latter form may reduce visual acuity considerably. Most cases of this type are inherited as autosomal dominant and exceptionally as a recessive character.

Congenital Anterior Pyramidal (Polar) Cataract: This cataract may occur as a congenital defect or it may be formed postnatally. In the former case it is thought to be the result of an aberration at the time of formation of the lens vesicle from the surface epithelium and involves primarily the anterior capsule but may penetrate into the lens substance. The postnatal anterior polar cataract may occur as a sequela of an ulceration of the cornea. The opacities involve the anterior lens capsule and are sharply circumscribed. They are small, round, white opacities which vary in size from a pinpoint to an area readily visible to the naked eye. However, the involved area is seldom, if ever, as large as the pupil. In some instances there may be a conical projection rising above the level of the normal lens capsule. The lesion usually remains stationary, although it may occasionally progress to complete opacification of the lens (Fig. 15–4).

Congenital Posterior Polar Cataract: This opacity can be recognized as a dense, saucer-shaped opacity covering the posterior pole and may be considered to be a very mild form of a persistent hyperplastic vitreous. A disturbance of the lens fiber directly beneath the lesion may result in a marked interference with vision and necessitate extraction if the cataracts are bilateral.

Mittendorf's Dot With Hyaloid Artery Remnants: The remnant of the attachment of the hyaloid artery is seen as a fairly large dot (about 1 mm. in size) on the posterior pole. A free-floating thread or a number of corkscrew-shaped threads may be seen suspended in the vitreous attached to the hyaloid face. Seen with the ophthalmoscope, vascular remnants on the posterior surface of the lens are found in nearly 2 per cent of all individuals. With the slit lamp, remnants are noted in many individuals.

Congenital Posterior Lenticonus (Lentiglobus): This lesion is seen as a large congenital globular protuberance on the posterior surface of the lens, extending back into the vitreous. It is usually associated with a posterior lens opacity and is often associated with a remnant of the hyaloid artery. It has been suggested that the cause of the malformation is an undue pull on the zonular fibers during the development of the lens.

Congenital Coralliform Cataract: This is an unusual form of cataract, inherited as an autosomal dominant, consisting of rounded and oblong opacities grouped toward the center of the lens, resembling a piece of coral. Failure of the anterior surface to close may be the cause of this condition. The opacities may extend from the anterior to the posterior capsule.

TABLE 15-1 *Continued*

Congenital Punctate Cerulean Cataract: This condition is seen frequently as small, scattered, bluish opacities throughout the lens. In Mongolian idiocy a similar type of cataract is seen, occurring at puberty. These opacities may represent late-formed fibers which have broken down into granular debris and are subsequently surrounded by healthy fibers. The opacities lie in the superficial layers of the fetal nucleus and in the adolescent cortex. The cataracts are bilateral, nonprogressive, and in general cause minimal loss in vision.

Congenital Disciform (Annular) Cataract: In this form of cataract, the nucleus is lacking and the lens is represented by a flattened disclike structure, surrounded by a ring of clear cortex. The central disc structure may become ectopic and frequently is displaced to the upper, nasal quadrant. It has been found that this type of cataract may be associated with macular hypoplasia, so that the prognosis following surgery may be poor.

stage and becomes round. The cells of the posterior wall of the hollow sphere elongate and fill the vesicle. By the third month, the embryonic nucleus has formed and secondary fibers develop that form the fetal nucleus. The lens capsule is now formed and the sutures are apparent beneath the capsule (Fig. 15–8).

The following zones of discontinuity may be recognized in the adult lens, according to Duke-Elder:

Nuclei: 1. The embryonic nucleus, an optically clear central area formed during one to three months of embryonic life and constituting the primary lens fibers.

2. The fetal nucleus, formed from secondary fibers during

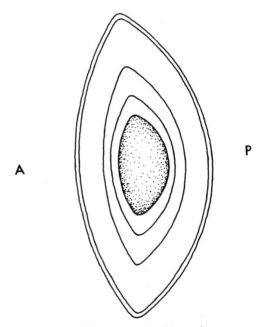

Figure 15-5 Coppock or dustlike nuclear cataract.

the third to eighth month of fetal life.

3. The infantile nucleus, formed during the last weeks of fetal life and continuing to puberty.

4. The adult nucleus, formed during adult life.

Cortex: The cortex represents the the soft superficial fibers formed after puberty and deposited between the nuclei and the subcapsular epithelium.

The *hyaloid system* develops in the primary vitreous and forms a vascular network which envelops the lens (tunica vasculosa lentis). These vessels begin to disappear by the fifth month and the

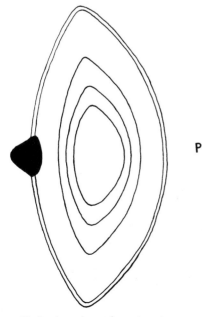

Figure 15-4 Anterior polar cataract.

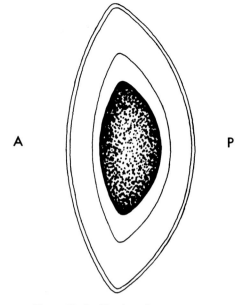

A   P

Figure 15–6   Total nuclear cataract.

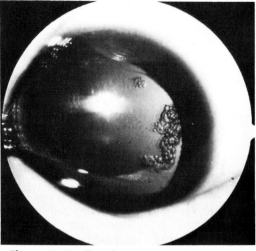

Figure 15–8 Transient cataract in premature. This baby boy was born after 34 weeks of gestation. On routine eye examination, 19 days after birth, both lenses had multiple small bubbles or blister-like opacity clustered in the mid periphery, deep in the posterior subcapsular space. (Courtesy of Dr. Guy H. Chan. From McCormick, A.: Canad. J. Ophthal., 3:202, 1968.)

entire hyaloid system should disappear normally by the seventh or eighth month. In a similar fashion, the primary vitreous should shrink and disappear by the eleventh week, since its persistence will interfere with normal vision (Fig. 15–9).

Transient cataracts of prematurity have been observed on several occasions (Figs. 15–8 and 15–9). The lens opacities appear as discrete, grapelike clusters in the posterior subcapsular space and disappear gradually over a period of 6 to 12 months.

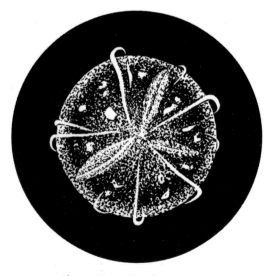

Figure 15–7   Zonular cataract.

Leukokoria (White Pupil) – Differential Diagnosis

In leukokoria, babies are born with a white pupillary reflex or acquire it at a later date. When a child is born with bilateral white pupillary reflexes, one should first consider the possibility of *rubella infection in the mother*. These babies are usually small, ill-nourished, and difficult to feed. Some of them have other congenital abnormalities related to the heart or auditory apparatus. Recovery of the virus or a positive serological test from the child confirms the diagnosis. The other consideration is the child with disc-shaped cataracts whose normal development was disturbed in embryo during the fifth week of life.

Retrolental Fibroplasia

Children with *retrolental fibroplasia* do not have a white pupillary reflex at birth. Subsequently an amaurotic pupillary reflex may be observed while the lens usually remains relatively clear. Examination of the fundus together with the history of prematurity, low birth weight, and exposure to additional oxygen usually helps confirm the diagnosis. Frequently some peripheral elevation of the retina may be observed which may progress to complete

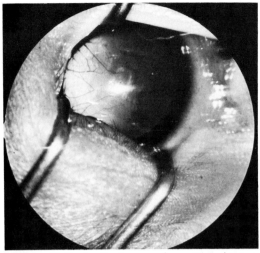

Figure 15–9 Lenticular vascular pattern in premature. This baby girl, 30 weeks after gestation, was examined four days after birth. A network of fine vessels was noted to extend from the periphery of the lens centrally. All vessels were deep and adjacent to the posterior lens capsule. (Courtesy of Dr. Guy H. Chan.)

retinal detachment. The preretinal membrane formation may resemble that seen in hyperplastic primary vitreous or retinal dysplasia. The eyes of these children are frequently microphthalmic, the anterior chamber may be shallow, and they frequently have nystagmus and photophobia. Should the fundus be visible there is usually dragging of the disc and a disturbance of the peripheral retina.

Retinal Dysplasia

Retinal dysplasia is rare. There are developmental abnormalities at birth that consist of ocular abnormalities which may resemble severe retrolental fibroplasia, as well as diffuse systemic malformations. The condition is usually bilateral: the children are usually full term. The eyes may be slightly microphthalmic, the anterior chamber is usually shallow, and the iris may be immobile because of anterior synechiae. The lens is clear at birth and one can see a white mass of vascularized tissue in the retrolental space. The lens eventually becomes opaque. The association of other systemic malformations helps distinguish it from persistent hyperplastic primary vitreous.

Persistent Hyperplastic Primary Vitreous

The best description of *persistent hyperplastic primary vitreous* (PHPV) is offered by Reese (1955). The condition occurs in full term infants and is usually unilateral. The defect occurs in fetal life, sometime between the fourth and sixth month, and is noticed immediately after birth or several months later. It may vary greatly from a mere persistence of a Mittendorf dot or persistence of the hyaloid artery or both. This condition should be suspected in children with unilateral cataract or in those children in whom a mature cataract developed rather rapidly in the postnatal period. The vascular attachment may cause a lenticular hemorrhage or rupture of the posterior capsule, with rather rapid maturation of the cataract, which may go on to spontaneous absorption.

Retinoblastoma and Pseudoglioma

Two other causes of an amaurotic pupillary reflex are *retinoblastoma* and so-called *pseudoglioma*. These are not usually present at birth. The differential diagnosis may be difficult, but since the lens is usually clear at the onset, further discussion is not germane to this presentation. It has been stated that a retinoblastoma has never been observed in a clinically observable microphthalmic eye. With the advent of ultrasound diagnostic measurements of the anterior-posterior diameter of the globe, this may no longer hold true, though the clinical appearance of microphthalmos will still hold true.

The term *pseudoglioma* is used to denote any condition in the posterior segment that might simulate a retinoblastoma. It is purely a descriptive clinical term to signify an inflammatory process in the posterior pole such as may occur with *Coats's disease*. On occasion, pseudoglioma may present as a dense cyclitic membrane in the posterior segment. Careful examination will usually reveal the true nature of the condition.

Congenital Cataracts

Children with *congenital cataracts* are usually full term. The opacities may vary from a few dustlike spots to a completely dense white opacity. They may be caused by an inherited defect in the germ plasm or some environmental influence affecting the normal germ plasm. They are frequently associated with other obvious congenital ocular defects such as nystagmus and microphthalmos as well as anomalies affecting other parts of the body. It has been estimated that at least 50 per

TABLE 15–2 ETIOLOGICAL CLASSIFICATION OF CATARACTS IN CHILDREN

1. *Hereditary:* Frequently autosomal dominant in conjunction with associated ocular abnormalities or included in a syndrome with systemic disorders.
2. *Embryopathic:* Nongenetic conditions affecting human embryo during intrauterine life.
   a. Viruses—rubella, rubeola, chickenpox, smallpox, herpes zoster, poliomyelitis, influenza, hepatitis, and infectious mononucleosis
   b. Bacteria—syphilis
   c. Protozoa—toxoplasmosis and cytomegalic inclusion disease
   d. Helminthiases—Gescheidt (1883) found 4 Distoma worms in congenital cataracts of a 5-month-old child
3. *Drug-induced Lens Changes and Toxic Agents*
   a. Systemic corticosteroids
   b. 2–4 Dinitrophenol
   c. Triparanol (MER-29)
   d. Trichlorobutyl alcohol
   e. Maternal drug therapy has been suspect for wide range of drugs (Hertzberg, Australia)
   f. Chlorpromazine hydrochloride (Thorazine)
   g. Naphthol and naphthalene
   h. Vitamin D excess
4. *Prematurity:* Cataractous changes have been observed in the absence of retrolental fibroplasia. Persistence of pupillary membrane may be confusing.
5. *Deficiency Factors:* Produces cataracts.
   a. Diet deficient in tryptophan in white rats (Pike, 1950)
   b. Hypoxia in utero may result in cataracts in rats
   c. Vitamin A deficiency in mice
   d. Deficiency of vitamins B_{12}, C, D, and pantothenic and folic acids according to animal experiments
6. *Metabolic Disturbances*
   a. Galactosemia (galactose-1-phosphate uridyl transferase deficiency)
   b. Diabetes mellitus
   c. Hypoparathyroidism and pseudohypoparathyroidism
   d. Homocystinuria (cystothionine synthetase deficiency)
   e. Wilson's disease (chalcosis lentis)
   f. Fabry's disease (ceramide trihexosidase deficiency)
   g. Refsum's disease (excess phytanic acid)
   h. Primary amyloidosis
7. *Chromosomal Disturbances*
   a. Down's syndrome (mongolism), 21 Trisomy
   b. 13–15 Trisomy
   c. 16–18 Trisomy
   d. Turner's syndrome
8. *Cataracts Secondary to Ocular Disease*
   a. Trauma
   b. Retrolental fibroplasia
   c. Persistent hyperplastic primary vitreous
   d. Congenital glaucoma
   e. Retinoblastoma
   f. Uveitis
   g. Retinal detachment
   h. Retinitis pigmentosa
9. *Ionizing Effect of Radiation (Excessive Dosage):* Direct effect and secondary to chromosomal aberrations and fetal changes.
10. *Congenital Cataracts Secondary to Ocular Anomalies*
    a. Microphthalmos/microcornea
    b. Keratoconus
    c. Sclerocornea
    d. Anterior cleavage syndrome
    e. Coloboma
    f. Aniridia
    g. Heterochromia
    h. Persistent pupillary membrane
    i. Ectopia lentis
    j. Retinal dysplasia
    k. Associated motility disturbances
    l. Megalocornea
11. *Cataracts in Association with Systemic Syndromes*
    a. ALPORT'S SYNDROME: Anterior lenticonus, cataracts, chronic nephritis, and deafness. Inherited as autosomal dominant.
    b. MATERNAL RUBELLA SYNDROME: Ocular and cardiac defects, deafness, and mental retardation. From St.

TABLE 15–2 ETIOLOGICAL CLASSIFICATION OF CATARACTS IN CHILDREN — *Continued*

Christopher's Hospital for Children, 118 patients exhibited the syndrome:
(1) Serological confirmation 70%
(2) Ocular manifestations 68%
(3) Retinopathy...52%
(4) Microphthalmos..41%
(5) Abnormal irides (poor dilatation response)..38%
(6) Cataracts (bilateral or unilateral)..32%
(7) Nystagmus 30%
(8) Strabismus 9%
(9) Glaucoma.. 8%

c. Down's Syndrome (Mongolism): Strabismus, cataract, Brushfield's spots, mental retardation, dwarfism, hyperextensibility of joints, drooling, open mouth, and large tongue.

d. Bonnevie-Ullrich's Syndrome (Turner's Syndrome): Webbed neck, lymphangioedema of hands and feet, coarctation of aorta, cataracts, strabismus, epicanthus, and lacrimal system abnormalities. XO chromosomal pattern diagnostic.

e. Hallermann-Streiff Syndrome: Dyscephaly, dwarfism, cutaneous atrophy, dental abnormalities, microphthalmos, and cataracts. Differentiate from progeria, Franceschetti's syndrome, and cleidocranial dysostosis.

f. Sjögren's Syndrome: Bilateral congenital cataracts and oligophrenia.

g. Marinesco-Sjögren's Syndrome: Similar to Sjögren's. Bilateral congenital cataracts, oligophrenia, spinocerebellar ataxia, and mental retardation.

h. Dermatological Disorders (Syndermatotic Congenital Cataracts):
   (1) *Rothmund's Syndrome:* Bilateral cataracts either congenital or developing in third to fifth year of life, telangiectases, brownish skin pigmentation, hypogenitalism, and poikiloderma atrophicans vasculare.
   (2) *Schäfer's Syndrome:* Congenital cataracts, palmoplantar keratosis with hyperhidrosis, small foci of alopecia, pachyonychia (thick nails), oligophrenia, and hypogenitalism.
   (3) *Congenital Ichthyosis:* Hyperkeratosis involving articular folds, palms, and soles; hyperhidrosis and sebaceous secretion. Congenital cataracts may occur.
   (4) *Siemen's Syndrome:* Congenital cataracts, atrophy or hypoplasia of skin.
   (5) *Incontinentia Pigmenti of Bloch-Sulzberger:* Slate-gray cutaneous pigmentation in patches and streaks, hypohidrosis or anhidrosis, dental anomalies, alopecia in females, congenital cataract, nystagmus, strabismus, and persistent hyperplastic primary vitreous.
   (6) *Atopic Dermatitis:* Eczematoid lesions of skin, especially on exposed parts. Skin becomes thickened, reddened, and dry. Cataracts may develop, bilateral, keratoconus.

i. Congenital Cataracts and Oxycephaly: Usually zonular cataracts accompanied by other ocular manifestations due to oxycephaly such as optic atrophy and exophthalmos.

j. Congenital Cataracts and Acrocephalosyndactylism: (Apert's Syndrome): Cataracts associated with tower skull, wide-placed eyes, strabismus, ptosis, and syndactyly.

k. Congenital Stippled Epiphyses (Conradi's Syndrome): Congenital calcifying chondrodystrophy, kyphoscoliosis, digital anomalies, articular dysfunction, craniofacial anomalies, congenital cardiopathies, and cataracts.

l. Laurence-Moon-Bardet-Biedl Syndrome: Cataracts, retinitis pigmentosa, nystagmus, strabismus, obesity, hypogenitalism, mental retardation, polydactyly.

m. Congenital Hemolytic Icterus: Bilateral congenital cataracts, microphthalmia, and icterus with splenomegalic anemia. Abnormal fragility of red cells.

n. Lowe's Syndrome (Oculocerebrorenal): Congenital cataracts, glaucoma, mental deficiency, retarded psychomotor development, aminoaciduria, renal rickets, and muscular hypotonia.

o. Weil-Marchesani Syndrome: Lenticular myopia, ectopia lentis, spherophakia, microphakia, brachydactyly, subnormal growth, and decrease in joint flexibility.

p. Marfan's Syndrome: Myopia, strabismus, blue sclera, spherophakia, high refractive error, cataract, arachnodactyly, relaxed ligaments, congenital heart disease, dissecting aneurysm, and subnormal muscular development.

q. Van der Hoeve's Syndrome (Osteogenesis Imperfecta): Blue sclera, cataract (rare), bones easily fractured, deafness (60 per cent), dental defects, hyperflexibility of ligaments, and fineness of hair.

r. Ectodermal Dysplasia: Cataracts, microphthalmos, anhidrosis, hypotrichosis with absence or underdevelopment of the teeth.

s. Myotonic Dystrophy (Steinert's Disease): Cataracts, ptosis, pigmentary retinopathy, myotonia, muscular wasting, gonadal, and other endocrine abnormalities.

t. Albers-Schönberg Disease: Osteopetrosis (hard and brittle bones), cataracts, optic atrophy, hepatosplenomegaly, and deafness.

u. Trisomy D (13–15): Microphthalmia, corneal opacities, cataracts, retinal dysplasia, flexion contracture of fingers, cleft palate, and congenital heart disease.

v. Oculodentodigital Dysplasia (Meyer-Schwickerath Syndrome): Typical facies presenting thin nose, hypoplastic alae and narrow nostrils, microcornea, iris anomalies, syndactyly, and camptodactyly of fourth and fifth fingers, enamel hypoplasia, and congenital cataract.

w. Craniofacial Dysostosis (Crouzon's Disease): Acrocephaly, break-nose, hypoplastic maxilla, exophthalmos, strabismus, and occasionally cataracts.

TABLE 15–2 ETIOLOGICAL CLASSIFICATION OF CATARACTS IN CHILDREN—*Continued*

x. OTHER ASSOCIATIONS:
   (1) Epilepsy
   (2) Cortical agenesis
   (3) Meningoencephalocele
   (4) Hydrocephalus (congenital)
   (5) Tuberous sclerosis
   (6) Hurler's disease
   (7) Mandibulofacial dysostosis
   (8) Polydactyly/syndactyly
   (9) Plagiocephaly

cent of these children have associated ocular defects. They are also associated with many other syndromes, including mongolism (Down's syndrome) (Table 15–2).

The parents will usually consult an ophthalmologist because they were sent by their physician, who probably observed a white pupillary reflex and suspected some visual impairment. The child should be thoroughly examined, under general anesthesia if necessary. Should a minimal opacity be found which will not prove to be a visual handicap, it may be well to refer to this as a spot on the lens rather than as a cataract. The latter term may connote blindness to the already distraught parents. Should the opacification obviously affect the visual acuity, the problem should be thoroughly discussed with the parents. Certainly any child with cataractous changes deserves the benefit of a careful survey by a pediatrician with access to a good laboratory. Some effort must be made to make an etiological classification of the disorder. A careful history with background information concerning the various family relatives can be most rewarding.

One of the most common causes of cataracts that we have seen in the Philadelphia area has been the *maternal rubella syndrome*, involving the heart, eyes, and ears and frequently associated with mental retardation. The serological test acts as an accurate guide for diagnosis. Metabolic disorders must be searched for routinely even though *galactosemia, diabetes mellitus, hypoparathyroidism,* and *homocystinuria* are uncommon in the ordinary practice. The unusual feature of the galactosemia cataract is that it can be reversed if detected sufficiently early to remedy the diet. Diabetic cataracts occur in the young as scattered, snowflake opacities, but they have a tendency to mature and become a total opacity very rapidly. I have observed

this phenomenon accompanied by considerable imbibition of fluid, to take place within a few months.

Zonular cataracts associated with tetany characterize *hypoparathyroidism*, which can be easily confirmed. *Pseudohypoparathyroidism* may cause cataracts in older children. Many skin lesions including severe *atopic dermatitis* may be a cataractogenic factor. *Corticosteroids* administered over a long period have been a cause in our experience. Chronic inflammatory diseases such as *toxoplasmosis, cytomegalic inclusion disease,* and *histoplasmosis* must be considered in cases in which the etiology is uncertain.

If the child seems to be progressing satisfactorily and can see the normal objects for his age, there is no immediate urgency to operate on the cataracts. Two or three decades ago, it was felt that the best results were obtained if one waited until the child was at least 2 years of age. This has all changed with the newer operative techniques which have been developed. *One must never lose sight of the fact that one cannot estimate the visual acuity in incomplete cataracts.* Opinion as to surgery should depend on the visual response expected from a child of the same age group. In the case of complete cataracts, there is no question as to what should be done.

Prognosis for Vision

Frequently, one finds references indicating that children with corrected vision of 20/50 or 20/70 do not require surgery, since this degree of visual acuity is preferable to having the aphakic eye with reduced visual fields, heavy corrective lenses, and potential postoperative complications. This statement presumes a measurement of visual acuity which is rarely possible in the younger patients. Good judgment on the part of the surgeon and comparison of the visual responses of the child to those of a child of similar development are the best indications for intervention.

When nystagmus accompanies cataract, distance visual acuity can rarely be improved more than 20/70, yet the near visual acuity is often better.

In several large series, visual results in patients under age 2 have been poorer than visual results in the 3- to 5-year age group. This comparison is probably not valid, since the younger group undoubtedly presented with bilateral complete cataracts so frequently associated with other anomalies, including mental retardation. Certainly, microphthalmos and nystagmus were common in the rubella series, which made up our larger group.

From a survey of 100 congenital cataracts, 10 per cent obtained visual acuity of 20/40 or better and only one child was 2 years of age; the remainder were in the 3- to 6-year age period.

Using our present statistics, it is unlikely that one can achieve better visual results than 20/200 in 50 per cent of our patients with congenital cataracts.

Whether or not amblyopia can be fully prevented by removal of the congenital cataract early, followed by the fitting of a contact lens, is not known, but work in this area is being pursued at present.

I have frequently been perplexed by the activity of the 2-year-old aphakic child who removes his thick glasses and seems to function visually as though he had a full correction. By the time such a child has another birthday, he will usually be wearing his aphakic correction.

Preoperative Considerations

There is a difference of opinion regarding surgery in the case of *rubella cataracts.* Scheie (1967), who has the largest published series of case reports, feels that an iridectomy should be the first surgical procedure, followed at the age of 18 months by aspiration. Parks and Von Noorden et al. (1969), however, do not agree with this and feel that these children should undergo surgery as soon as the diagnosis is made. Scheie et al. (1967) and Yanoff et al. (1968) recovered the virus from lens material in a large number of their patients and feel that this accounted for a 40 per cent incidence of complica-

tions. The author has seen such patients who, when operated on at the age of 6 months, go on to develop phthisis bulbi within a matter of weeks, despite an uneventful surgical procedure. It may be that a more virulent virus was present in some areas or that the more cortical material removed the less chance for the severe toxic reaction to occur.

Complicated Cataracts

The occurrence of uveitis in children fortunately is not too frequent. It is estimated that about 5 per cent of patients with uveitis are under 16 years of age (Makley et al., 1969; Mazon, 1969; Schlaegel, 1969). The workup of these patients is usually unrewarding and for the most part they are treated empirically with local medication and deposit or systemic steroid therapy.

Cataracts do develop in such patients and their removal is indicated when vision is seriously impaired. They should be operated on during a period of quiescence and should be adequately treated with steroids pre- and postoperatively. The surgical technique should be the same as that for congenital cataracts, with freeing of all posterior synechiae, combined with sphincterotomies if necessary. The sub-Tenon's capsule injection of steroids at the conclusion of the procedure is most efficacious in reducing the inflammatory response.

The surgical procedures now to be recommended are an optical iridectomy or discission and aspiration. Simple discission, which may have to be repeated, and linear extraction are now seldom employed. Little has been written lately about optical iridectomies. Patients with congenital miosis and a dense central anterior polar cataract will certainly not be harmed by having an iridectomy as an initial procedure. It is possible that the midportion of the lens and equator are clear and the child may be able to see and still maintain his power of accommodation.

The aspiration technique has been described by Scheie (1960), Parks (1967), and others (McDonald, 1965). The author is of the opinion that this is not an operation for the occasional surgeon and that it

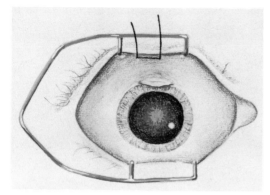

Figure 15–10 Thin wire speculum and small limbal incision at 12 o'clock.

should be done under the operating microscope.

Operative Technique

The eye to be operated on should be fully dilated with atropine, Cyclogyl, and Neo-Synephrine drops prior to surgery. The strength of the atropine solution should vary depending on the age of the patient. General anesthesia with intubation of the patient should be employed in all cases.

The speculum should be lightweight; the thin wire speculum is excellent, in that there is no pressure on the eyeball. A superior rectus suture is essential and an inferior rectus suture may help steady the eyeball.

A small 3-mm. conjunctival flap is prepared at 12 o'clock and dissected to expose the limbus (Fig. 15–10). A beveled

knife needle tract is then made at 4:30 or 7:30 o'clock and directed toward 6 o'clock. This is for the introduction of a 25-gauge scalp vein needle into the anterior chamber. The wing tips are cut off and the connecting tubing is connected to a container of Ringer's solution. The flow is easily controlled by the gauges on the connecting polyethylene tubing (Fig. 15–11). Wong (1967) suggested a similar contrivance utilizing a 30-gauge needle connected with tubing to a 20-cc. syringe. This requires another assistant as well as considerable force to keep the anterior chamber filled.

Once the scalp vein needle or the fine polyethylene tubing has been introduced into the anterior chamber, one is ready to incise the anterior capsule. The proper selection of a knife needle is important. The blade should be no more than 3 mm. and there should not be any heel to the blade. Swan (1959) has described such a blade and another one is available.*

The knife needle should enter the eye at the limbus at 3 or 9 o'clock. The needle should be held in the plane of the iris as a Graefe knife. The initial incision should be from 6 to 12 o'clock, then 5 to 10 o'clock, and 7 to 2 o'clock so as to open up the anterior capsule like petals in a flower (Fig. 15–12). This can be accomplished with a short blade without danger of inadvertently cutting the cornea and enlarging the incision. The knife needle is withdrawn and a small amount of saline is injected through the tract in case cap-

---

*Greishaber & Company, Chicago, Illinois.

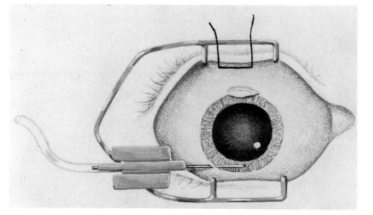

Figure 15–11 Introduction of needle into anterior chamber to maintain steady flow of saline.

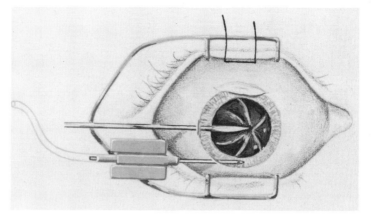

Figure 15–12 Discission of the anterior capsule in several meridians.

sule was drawn into the wound. This can usually all be accomplished without refilling the chamber from the suspended Ringer's solution. Another alternative is to introduce a Sato needle at 12 o'clock where the flap has been prepared and incise the capsule from 6 to 10 o'clock and 6 to 2 o'clock. The lens may be stirred up with the same needle, and then the anterior capsule may be completely aspirated.

At this time a limbal incision with a 2-mm. keratome (Fig. 15–13) or knife needle should be made at 12 o'clock where the limbus was exposed, and an 18-gauge needle on a glass syringe should be introduced into the anterior chamber. The tip of the needle should be honed down so that it is not sharp, or a side opening needle, as described by Gass (1969), should be employed. Glass syringes are much better than plastic ones, since they do not stick.

Once the needle is introduced, gentle suction should be started and the flow of Ringer's solution regulated to provide constant maintenance of the anterior chamber (Fig. 15–14). When using the operating room microscope almost all the cortical material can be removed (Fig. 15–15). One can get under the iris and dislocate cortical material with ease.

In the author's opinion, a complete iridectomy should always be performed. In the case of congenital miosis, a sphincterotomy should also be performed at 5 and 7 o'clock with Barraquer scissors.

At the conclusion of the operation the wound at 12 o'clock should be closed with a 6-0 or 7-0 gut suture. This is also used to close the conjunctiva. Following or preceding this the anterior chamber should be filled with air.

At the conclusion of the procedure 1 cc. of a soluble steroid combined with one drop of atropine is injected beneath Tenon's capsule, above or below.

Figure 15–13 Anterior chamber at 12 o'clock may be entered with small keratome or an enlarged knife needle incision.

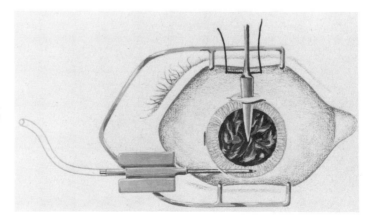

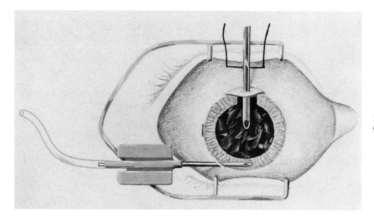

Figure 15–14 Introduction of 18-gauge needle through preplaced incision.

Following this, drops are instilled 2 or 3 times a day and the patient may be discharged in 4 or 5 days.

According to Parks and Hiles (1967) and Van Noorden et al. (1969), these patients may be fitted for contact lenses within a few weeks. In the case of monocular cataracts an occluder lens may be fitted on the phakic eye.

Recently, several additional modalities for cataract extraction have been introduced. Phacoemulsification employs the use of high frequency sound waves to fragment and emulsify lens cortical material. By means of a large needle introduced through a 2-mm. limbus opening, a fine jet stream of saline is introduced and then aspirated with the finely emulsified lens material. Advantages are inherent in the small opening required, which permits early ambulation. Disadvantages and complications can be minimized with frequent use of the instrument and special care.

The Douvas Roto-Extractor functions on a different principle. A special needle can be introduced into the eye at the limbus or at the pars plana. The needle contains a fine cutting mechanism in the tip. Fluid enters and is aspirated from the eye. Gentle suction applied draws the desired tissue (cataract, capsular remnant, or PHPV) into a hole with access to the rotating cutting mechanism, and the tissue is immediately excised in fine particles and aspirated. Advantages of the Roto-Extractor are similar to those of the phacoemulsifier.

Both instruments illustrate innovative advances in anterior segment surgery.

TRAUMATIC CATARACTS

Traumatic cataracts in children pose somewhat similar problems as to the timing of the operative procedure. As a general rule there is no urgency. Should

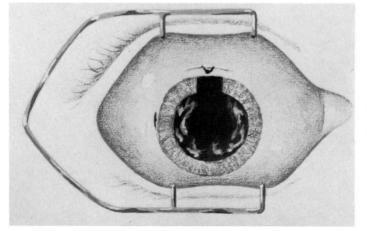

Figure 15–15 Completion of procedure; suture through cornea sclera at 12 o'clock, suture at 9 o'clock incision if necessary. Minimal amount of cortical material remains.

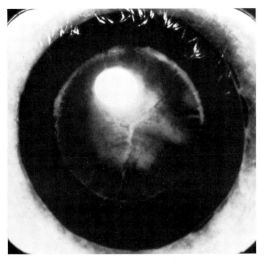

Figure 15–16 Lamellar (zonular) cataract.

there be a corneal perforation with a laceration of the capsule, repair of corneal laceration and freeing of the anterior synechia should come first. Should there be a lot of free cortical material in the anterior chamber, as much as is conveniently possible should be removed at this time. In some cases, however, the laceration has transfixed the lens and vigorous irrigation or aspiration will result in filling the anterior with formed vitreous. Delay of a few weeks may permit the formation of a posterior capsule-vitreous membrane. Then an aspiration as described for congenital cataracts may be carried out with less risk.

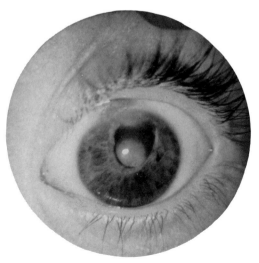

Figure 15–17 Typical rubella cataract in microphthalmic eye following iridectomy.

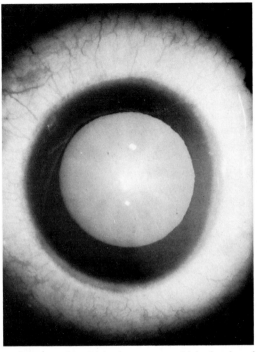

Figure 15–18 Diabetic cataract which developed to maturity in 8-year-old girl.

Children are also subject to contusion cataracts. These may not be obvious until any hyphema has cleared. When the trauma has subsided, consideration should be given to aspiration of the cataract. Should the child be under 6 years of age, treatment should not be delayed beyond 6 months after the injury if feasible, since amblyopia may develop. After this age time is not a critical factor and aspiration of the cataract may be performed when convenient.

One must not forget that these are traumatized eyes. They may have suffered perforating injuries, hyphema, or hemorrhage into the posterior segment. Gonioscopy and ophthalmoscopy should be performed under general anesthesia if necessary. There may be recession of the angle and/or damage to the posterior segment. In the past it has been the policy of many ophthalmologists to adopt a "hands off" policy. However, with the new surgical techniques and the ability to fit these children with contact lenses, one's thinking about these cases should change.

The surgical technique should be essentially that employed for congenital cataracts. It can be used successfully even if the lens is partially dislocated.

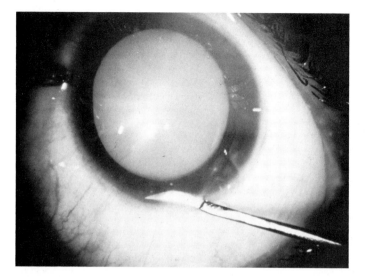

Figure 15–19 Intracorneal incision in cornea at 6 o'clock prior to insertion of #20 polyethylene tubing to keep chamber formed.

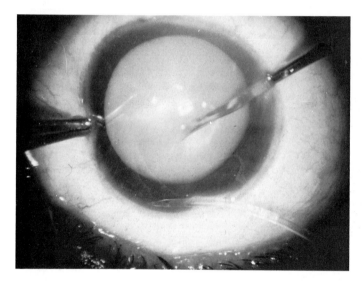

Figure 15–20 Cruciate on **V**-shaped incision through anterior capsule.

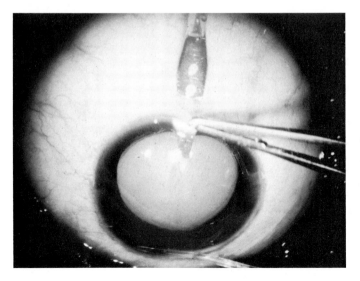

Figure 15–21 Narrow-bladed keratome incision into anterior chamber beneath conjunctival flap.

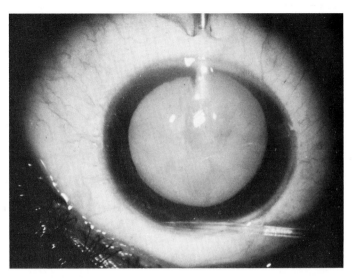

Figure 15–22 Introduction of small beveled 19-gauge needle into anterior chamber.

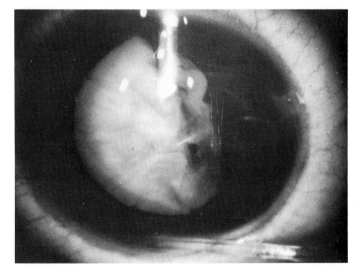

Figure 15–23 Gentle push-pull movement of plunger aspirates cataract readily.

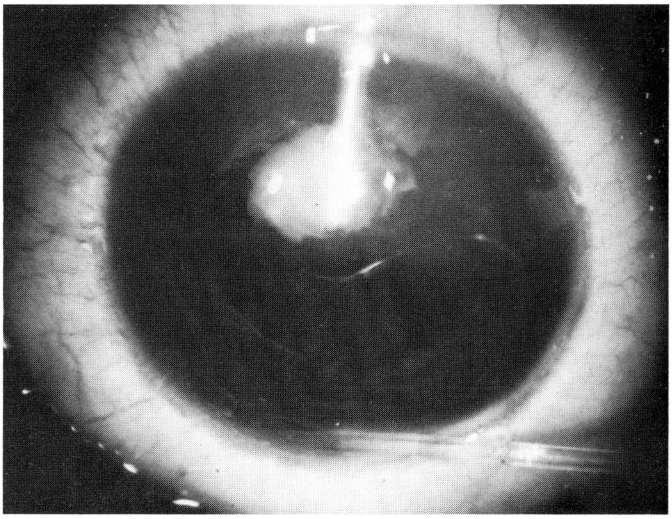

Figure 15–24 Cataract almost completely aspirated.

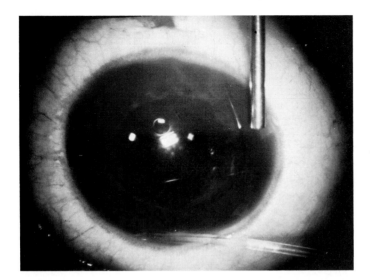

Figure 15–25 Cataract aspirated, few capsular remnants peripherally.

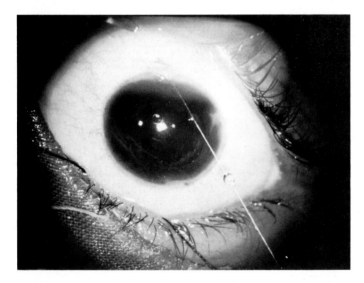

Figure 15–26 Conjunctival flap closed with 8–0 virgin silk.

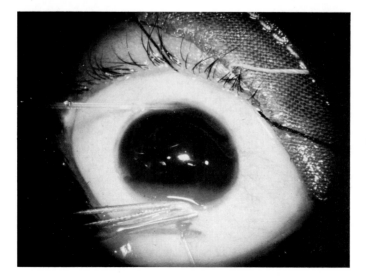

Figure 15–27 Sector iridectomy at conclusion of aspiration.

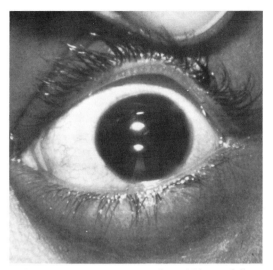

Figure 15–28 Appearance of eye 24 hours following aspiration.

THE DISLOCATED LENS

A subluxated lens in children is usually associated with trauma or with *Marfan's* or *Marchesani's* syndromes. Some may also occur in association with *homocystinuria*. In many instances the visual impairment can be at least partially corrected with the appropriate corrective lenses. Should the phakic refraction be unsatisfactory, photocoagulation of the iris to simulate an iridectomy may permit the wearing of a phakic correction in spectacles or contact lenses. Patients with Marfan's syndrome may frequently have an associated congenital miosis (Table 15–3).

Surgical Treatment

Should the vision be reduced to a handicapping level despite these measures, surgery of the lens should be considered. The 2-needle discission technique (Kirby, 1950) is not too satisfactory, though in certain instances the lens may shrivel up, permitting the wearing of an aphakic correction. The double-pronged needle of Calhoun may be employed when it is passed through the pars plana from one side of the eye to the other to trap and support the dislocated lens. It is applicable to luxations in the anterior chamber and serves to fixate the lens until it can be removed by the cryoprobe with a minimal loss of vitreous.

Maumenee and Ryan (1969) have recently suggested the aspiration of such clear lenses. This method is certainly superior to the previous techniques that have been reported. One must not let one's enthusiasm for trying this procedure outweigh the more conservative approach of attempting to improve the vision by less dramatic methods.

Postoperative Complications

The most common complications following cataract surgery in children are glaucoma and retinal detachment. Glaucoma is most frequently caused by pupillary block. This may be unrecognized if the iris is bound down to a posterior capsule which retards or inhibits the

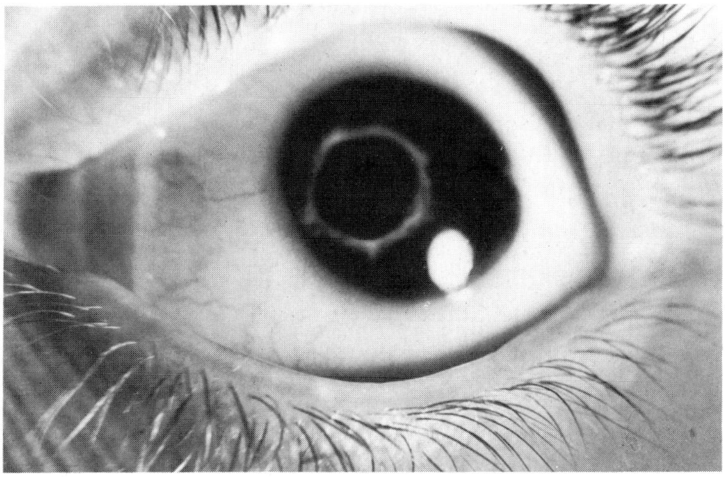

Figure 15–29 Unusual demonstration of Wieger's capsulohyaloid ligament following cataract aspiration in an eye with congenital aniridia. Dense circular ring is at the level of the posterior capsule. (Courtesy of Dr. A. H. Keeney.)

TABLE 15–3 DISLOCATED LENSES ASSOCIATED WITH SYSTEMIC CHANGES

Conditions and Changes	Frequency
1. Marfan's Syndrome (skeletal and cardiovascular)	75%
2. Homocystinuria (thromboses, retardation, skeletal)	90%
3. Weil-Marchesani Syndrome (brachymorphia)	50%
4. Sulfite Oxidase Deficiency (neurological, decerebrate behavior)	100%
5. Osteogenesis Imperfecta (multiple fractures, blue sclera, deafness)	Rare
6. Ehlers-Danlos Syndrome (fibrodysplasia elastica)	Rare
7. Scleroderma (induration and firmness of skin)	Rare
8. Hyperlysinemia (ocular, mental, and physical retardation)	Rare

formation of a shallow anterior chamber (Maumenee and Ryan, 1969). This is seen less frequently with the aspiration technique and the prolonged use of a cycloplegic and local steroid medication. The only way to detect it, however, is to take postoperative tensions at intervals of a few months following the surgical procedure.

Retinal detachments may or may not be related to the surgical procedure or procedures. The loss of vitreous most certainly predisposes to this complication. Patients with congenital cataracts, however, are known to have other congenital abnormalities.

The finding of extensive lattice degeneration is not uncommon. The children are also subject to more direct trauma to the head and bodies in their formative years which may be a precipitating factor.

Another, though less serious complication, is condensation of the posterior capsule or the formation of Elschnig pearls. The latter can be irrigated free of the pupillary space with ease (McDonald, 1965). The secondary cataract can usually be satisfactorily dealt with by a discission of the capsule with a sharp knife needle. Upon withdrawing the needle, a small bubble of air should be injected through the tract into the anterior chamber to free any strand of capsule or vitreous that might be withdrawn with the knife needle.

SUMMARY

The outlook for children with congenital cataracts has improved considerably during the past decade. The incidence of their occurrence and the associated congenital defects have not decreased. Progress has been made in improved surgical techniques and the ability to fit contact lenses on the infants. This hopefully overcomes the amblyopia that frequently develops as the result of delayed surgery or the ineffectiveness of occlusion when wearing the regular cataract glasses.

The surgery is delicate, is best performed under high magnification, and had best be done by surgeons familiar with the technique and who have facilities for fitting infants with contact lenses.

REFERENCES

Chandler, P. A.: Surgery of the lens in infancy and childhood. Arch. Ophthal., 45:125, 1951.

Chandler, P. A.: Choice of treatment in dislocation of the lens. Arch. Ophthal., 71:765, 1964.

Chandler, P. A.: Surgery of congenital cataract. Trans. Amer. Acad. Ophthal. Otolaryng., 72:341, 1968.

Cordes, F. C.: Symposium on Diseases and Surgery of the Lens. St. Louis, The C. V. Mosby Co., 1957.

Duke-Elder, S., and Cook, C.: Normal and Abnormal Development. Part I: Embryology. St. Louis, The C. V. Mosby Co., 1963.

Francois, J.: Les Cataractes Congénitales. Paris, Masson & Cie, 1959.

Francois, J.: Heredity in Ophthalmology. St. Louis, The C. V. Mosby Co., 1961.

Francois, J.: Syndromes with Congenital Cataract. 16th Jackson Memorial Lecture. Amer. J. Ophthal., 52:207, 1961.

Gass, J. D. M.: Lens aspiration using a side opening needle. Arch. Ophthal., 82:87, 1969.

Harley, J. D., and Farrar, J. F.: Maternal drug therapy and congenital cataracts. Med. Aust., 51:212, 1964.

Kirby, D. B.: Surgery of Cataract. Philadelphia, J. B. Lippincott Co., 1950.

Knapp, A.: Operative treatment of congenital subluxation of the lens. Arch. Ophthal., 27:158, 1942.

Leibman, S. D., and Gellis, S. S.: The Pediatrician's Ophthalmology. St. Louis, The C. V. Mosby Co., 1961.

Makley, T. A., Jr., Long, J., and Suie, T.: Uveitis in children. J. Pediat. Ophthal., 6:136, 1969.

Maumenee, A. E., and Ryan, S. J.: Aspiration technique for dislocated lens. Amer. J. Ophthal., 68:808, 1969.

Mazow, M. L.: Chronic cyclitis. J. Pediat. Ophthal., 6:73, 1969.

McDonald, P. R.: Symposium on Cataracts. St. Louis, The C. V. Mosby Co., 1965.

Nelson, W. E., Vaughan, C. C., and McKay, R. J.: Textbook of Pediatrics. Philadelphia, W. B. Saunders Co., 1969.

Parks, M. M.: Personal communication.

Parks, M. M., and Hiles, D. A.: Management of infantile cataracts. Amer. J. Ophthal., 63:10, 1967.

Reese, A. B.: Persistent hyperplastic primary vitreous. Trans. Amer. Acad. Ophthal. Otolaryng., 59:271, 1955.

Reese, A. B., and Blodi, F. C.: Retinal dysplasia. Amer. J. Ophthal., 33:23, 1950.

Reese, A. B., and Straatsma, B. R.: Retinal dysplasia. Amer. J. Ophthal., 45:199, 1958.

Scheie, H. G.: Aspiration of congenital or soft cataracts: A new technique. Amer. J. Ophthal., 50:1048, 1960.

Scheie, H. G., and Albert, D. M.: Adler's Textbook of Ophthalmology. Philadelphia, W. B. Saunders Co., 1969.

Scheie, H. G., Rubenstein, R. A., and Kent, R. B.: Aspiration of congenital or soft cataracts: Further experience. Amer. J. Ophthal., 63:3, 1967.

Scheie, H. G., Schaffer, D. B., Plotkin, S. A., and Kertesz, E. D.: Congenital rubella cataracts: Surgical results and virus recovery from intraocular tissue. Arch. Ophthal., 77:440, 1967.

Schlaegel, T. F., Jr.: Uveitis in childhood. J. Pediat. Ophthal., 6:66, 1969.

Swan, K. C.: Modified knife and techniques for discission. Amer. J. Ophthal., 47:56, 1959.

Von Noorden, G. K., Ryan, S. J., and Maumenee, A. E.: Management of congenital cataracts in children. Trans. Amer. Acad. Ophthal. Otolaryng., 1969 (in press).

Wong, V. G., and Collier, R. H.: Maintenance of the anterior chamber depth during anterior segment surgery. Arch. Ophthal., 77:384, 1967.

Yanoff, M., Schaffer, D. B., and Scheie, H. G.: Rubella ocular syndrome: Clinical significance of viral and pathological studies. Trans. Amer. Acad. Ophthal. Otolaryng., 72:896, 1968.

CHAPTER 16

GLAUCOMA IN INFANTS AND CHILDREN

ROBISON D. HARLEY, M.D., F.A.C.S.,
and DONELSON R. MANLEY, M.D.

Definition

Glaucoma can be defined as an abnormally high intraocular pressure. It may be primary, it may be associated with other congenital ocular abnormalities, or it may be associated with a systemic disease or syndrome. Secondary glaucoma develops from conditions other than developmental abnormalities such as inflammation, trauma, and tumors.

Buphthalmos (oeil de boeuf) is frequently used to describe primary infantile glaucoma. Hydrophthalmos (hydrophthalmia) is an older term which was used because of the supposed similarity to hydrocephalus. Buphthalmos and hydrophthalmos describe the anatomically enlarged eye which results from distention and remains the most conspicuous feature. Since the underlying cause of all the symptoms and signs is the increased intraocular pressure, the term primary developmental glaucoma is preferable.

PRIMARY DEVELOPMENTAL GLAUCOMA

Primary developmental glaucoma is caused by a developmental abnormality in the iridocorneal angle of the eye which impairs aqueous outflow from the eye. The remainder of the eye is normal. Included within this classification are the congenital, infantile, and juvenile forms of glaucoma.

Congenital glaucoma may be inherited as an autosomal recessive with variable penetrance, but more commonly the disease occurs without known antecedent inheritance. Typical signs of congenital glaucoma may be present at birth in 35 per cent of cases, at 6 months of age in over 70 per cent, and by 12 months of age in approximately 80 per cent. An additional 10 per cent of glaucoma cases occur between 1 and 3 years of age. After age 3, the cornea and sclera are more resistant to stretching. About 75 per cent have the disease bilaterally, and the majority of the cases occur in males. It has been stated that approximately 10 per cent of the children in schools for the blind were admitted with uncontrolled glaucoma. Glaucoma occurs in about 0.05 per cent of all newborns.

Infantile glaucoma, which develops during the first three years after birth, may present some difficulty in diagnosis. Photophobia, tearing, and blepharospasm are the commonest initial signs and should alert the mother or pediatrician to the disease.

Juvenile glaucoma appears after 3 years of age and is often used to describe any glaucoma (Axenfeld, pigmentary, or Sturge-Weber syndrome) occurring from about 3 years up to young adulthood. Since the common denominator is the age of onset rather than etiology, the term juvenile glaucoma, although frequently used, is generally not preferred.

The Clinical Picture

Early Signs

Photophobia and blepharospasm often occur together (Fig. 16–1). Photophobia is usually the initial sign but is not enough by itself to arouse suspicion in most cases. It is thought to be caused by irritation of the corneal epithelium which occurs as a result

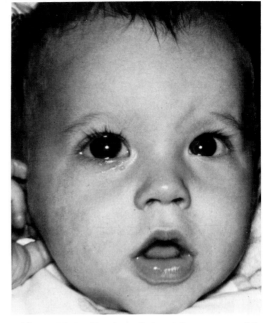

Figure 16–2 Tearing of the right eye caused by glaucoma. Note the increased corneal diameter of the right eye.

of the elevated intraocular pressure. Mild photophobia may be evident only when the infant is outdoors in bright sunlight. The parents may notice the baby keeping its eyes closed, and their usual reaction is to provide some shade, in the belief that the baby is merely showing normal sensitivity to sunlight. Moderate photophobia will be noticed indoors as well; the baby will often keep its eyes closed, even while eating. Severe photophobia will cause the baby to keep its eyes closed constantly, and it may keep its head buried in a pillow. During periods of discomfort the baby will be seen to rub its eyes.

Tearing usually accompanies photophobia and blepharospasm, and is also caused by irritation of the corneal epithelium (Fig. 16–2). Tearing may vary during the day and increase during periods of photophobia.

The infant with photophobia, blepharospasm, and tearing should be evaluated carefully, for there are other conditions that may cause similar clinical signs. Corneal irritation may be caused by abrasions, foreign bodies, and inflammations. A thorough examination can be performed in the office and should include eversion of the

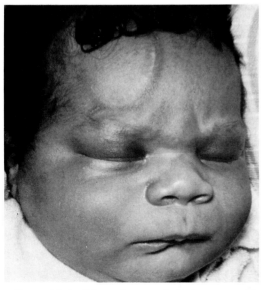

Figure 16–1 Bilateral congenital glaucoma with intense photophobia and blepharospasm.

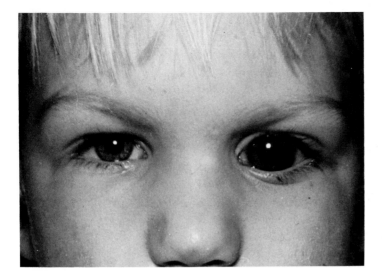

Figure 16–3 Corneal enlargement of left eye that developed slowly over a period of 2 years. Child was first evaluated because of failing vision test. Generalized corneal haziness was present.

lids to examine the palpebral conjunctiva. One should look for abrasions or foreign bodies of the cornea. The eyelashes may be turned inward against the cornea as a result of epiblepharon or misdirection of their growth. It is not uncommon for an infant with early glaucoma to be treated for what is thought to be an allergy, and one should look carefully for typical limbal vegetations and conjunctival changes that are associated with allergy. Blockage and infection of the nasolacrimal duct may be thought to be present, and this should be carefully evaluated. Pressure should be applied over the tear sac to determine if purulent material can be expressed from the puncta. More than one infant has been probed and irrigated when early glaucoma was actually the cause of the tearing. The tearing that accompanies glaucoma is clear, and it is helpful to keep in mind the general rule that a "wet" eye with a "wet" nose may indicate glaucoma whereas a "wet" eye with a "dry" nose may indicate blockage of the nasolacrimal duct. Any child undergoing a probing and irrigation of the nasolacrimal duct should have routine measurements taken of the ocular tension and corneal diameters.

Corneal edema is the sign which usually arouses suspicion. It is present in 25 per cent of cases at birth and in over 60 per cent by the sixth month. At first it is epithelial, but later there is stromal involvement, and permanent opacities may occur.

Corneal enlargement (Figs. 16–3 and 16–

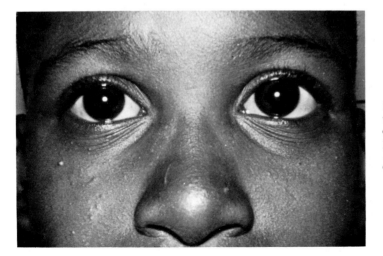

Figure 16–4 Megalocornea in an 11-year-old boy. Corneal diameters were 14 mm., and no breaks in Descemet's membrane were present. Applanation tension in the right eye was 14 mm., and in the left, 16 mm. No cupping of the optic discs was present.

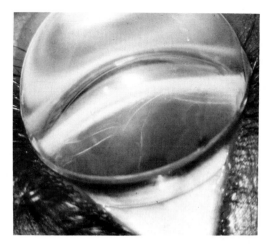

Figure 16–5 Breaks in Descemet's membrane seen through a Koeppe lens. The sharp linear edges of the breaks are evident.

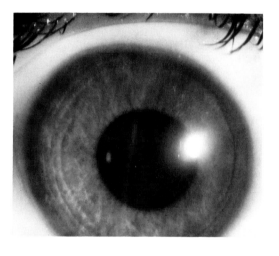

Figure 16–6 Forceps injury to the right cornea at birth resulted in a single linear break in Descemet's membrane running vertically across the pupil.

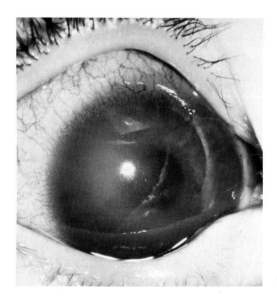

Figure 16–7 Temporal corneal clouding of the right eye which occurred following a break in Descemet's membrane.

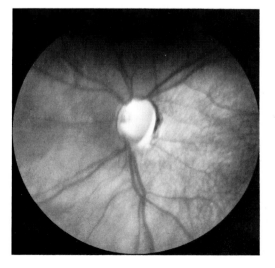

Figure 16–8 Same child as in Figure 16–4. Visual acuity in left eye was light perception. Advanced cupping and atrophy of the left disc were present. The right eye was normal.

4) occurs along with enlargement of the globe, especially when the onset is before age 3. After that the distensibility of the globe is more limited and the increased intraocular pressure is manifested by cupping of the optic disc. Normal infant corneas measure 10.5 to 11 mm. in the horizontal meridian. Corneal diameters measuring 12.5 to 13 mm. are easily recognized, especially if they are unilateral.

Tears or breaks in Descemet's membrane (Figs. 16–5 to 16–7) occur because it is less elastic than the corneal stroma. The tears are usually peripheral and concentric with the limbus. Others may be horizontal. The endothelium lays down a new membrane over the defects, but the edges of the tears usually remain visible. The stroma over these tears may be permanently opacified.

The *anterior chamber increases* in depth.

Cupping and atrophy of the optic nerve (Fig. 16–8) may occur, especially after the third year. It is not normal for an infant to have cupping. When the tension can be normalized early, the cupping may be reduced or disappear completely.

Late Signs

1. The cornea becomes hazier and larger. Corneal diameters measuring 17 or 18 mm. have a poor visual prognosis. As the ciliary ring enlarges, iridodonesis and subluxation of the lens may occur. Since these eyes are easily traumatized, corneal ulceration, hyphema, rupture, and phthisis may result.

2. Even if the intraocular pressure is controlled, there may be anisometropia and corneal scarring, which can result in amblyopia.

Ocular Examination

A complete examination of the eyes must be performed on each child suspected of having glaucoma. (See Figures 16–9 to 16–14.) The examination must include the following:

1. A careful inspection of the external eye, lids, and face for hemangioma, antiridia, café au lait spots, nevi, or skin neurofibromas.

2. Corneal diameter (Fig. 16–11).

3. Microscopic exam for inspection of corneal haze and breaks in Descemet's membrane.

4. Tonometry (Fig. 16–10).

5. Gonioscopy (Fig. 16–13).

6. Ophthalmoscopy (Fig. 16–14).

Pathogenesis

The defect is thought to be in the microanatomical pathways of the outflow mechanism. The explanation should be consistent with clinical, anatomic, and surgical facts, but the pathogenesis of primary developmental glaucoma is not yet fully understood.

There is general agreement that congenital glaucoma arises from an abnormality or an arrest in development of mesoderm of the corneoscleral junction. This results in a structural defect in the region of the filtration angle, causing an obstruction to the drainage of aqueous humor.

Barkan believed that infantile glaucoma was due to the obstruction of aqueous outflow caused by a transparent membrane representing a forward extension of the uveal meshwork with an abnormal insertion on the angle wall.

Maumenee has observed the following abnormalities, which suggest a different view of the pathogenesis:

1. In congenital glaucoma there is a failure of the iris and ciliary body to separate from the trabecular fibers.

2. The ciliary processes and ciliary body are pulled centrally, possible as the result of microphakia, so that the ciliary processes are central to an imaginary line that passes vertically through the posterior end of Schlemm's canal.

3. The longitudinal and circular muscle fibers insert further forward and to a greater extent than normally into the corneoscleral portion of the trabeculae.

4. The scleral spur is displaced forward and is therefore more difficult to visualize.

Such features represent a failure of cleavage of the iris from the cornea. It is suggested that the abnormal pull of the meridional fibers of the ciliary body closes the trabecular sheets. A goniotomy cuts the trabecular ends of these fibers, thus opening the spaces.

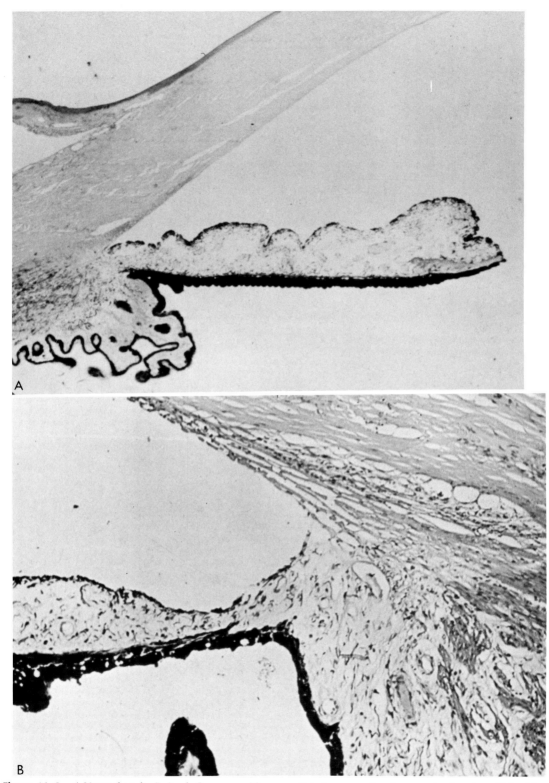

Figure 16–9 *A*, Normal angle. *B*, Angle from eye with congenital glaucoma, showing anterior location of iris with abnormal tissue inserting on trabecular meshwork and absence of angle recess.

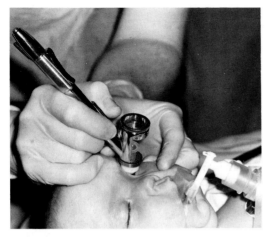

Figure 16–10 Ocular tension being measured with the Halberg applanation tonometer. (Rynco Scientific Co., New York.)

Gonioscopic Anatomy

The deep anterior chamber and flat iris plane are similar to that in an aphakic eye. The anterior iris mesoderm tends to be hypoplastic and the radial iris vessels prominent, especially if the pressure is elevated. The angle is usually wider than 45 degrees. The flat insertion of the iris into the trabecular meshwork is the most characteristic of the findings (Fig. 16–9). The angle recess which is beginning to form in most normal newborn eyes is not seen in the eye with infantile glaucoma. In the less pronounced cases, there may be only 0.1 mm. difference in normal and abnormal iris insertions. The peripheral iris and its radial vessels lift slightly at their juncture with the trabecular meshwork. The blood vessels then arch backward toward the ciliary body.

The trabecular surface glistens, reminiscent of stippled cellophane. The trabecular sheets are much more transparent than the adult tissues with which the examiner is so familiar. In the normal infant eye there is little angle recess, but the anterior ciliary body and its insertion on the scleral spur are clearly visible. In the eye with infantile glaucoma the trabecular sheets seem to be thicker. Schwalbe's line is in its normal location. Pigmentary arcades are frequently observed at the periphery of the iris.

Tonometry

Every child suspected of glaucoma must have a careful tonometric evaluation under deep general anesthesia supplemented by a topical anesthetic to the cornea.

Halothane has been credited with a re-

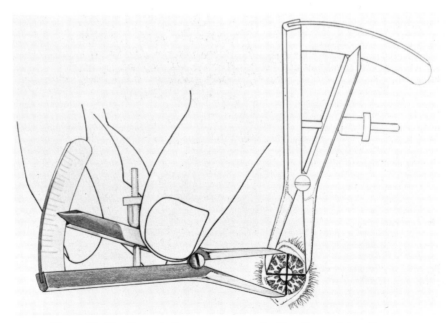

Figure 16–11 Corneal diameters measured with a Castroviejo caliper.

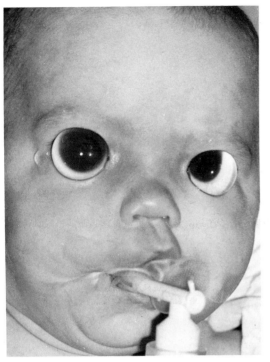

Figure 16–12 Placing Koeppe lenses over both eyes allows rapid evaluation of the angles.

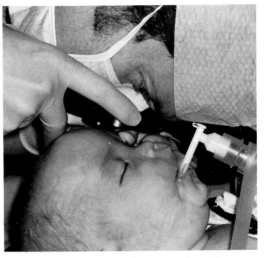

Figure 16–14 Ophthalmoscopy may be performed, and the appearance of the disc should be studied. Drawings of the cupping are helpful, as are photographs which allow future comparisons to be made.

duction of intraocular pressure after an initial increase in the early stage of anesthesia.

Ketamine has been shown to average higher tension readings, especially during light anesthesia. Whenever there is uncertainty concerning borderline readings, repeated tensions should be taken.

A tension reading should take place first, before any ocular manipulations and certainly prior to gonioscopy. Because scleral rigidity affects the Schiotz tonometer, hand-held applanation instru-

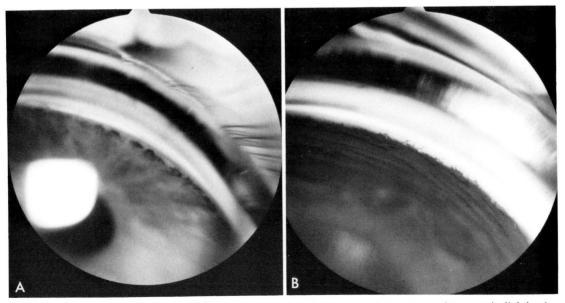

Figure 16–13 Goniophotographs of eyes with congenital glaucoma. *A,* Appearance often seen in lightly pigmented races, showing black segments separated by thin bands of light connective tissue which run outward from the surface stroma of the iris. Vessels crossing the angle are frequently present (Lister lens). *B,* Anterior insertion of the iris with numerous iris processes inserted onto the tissue in the angle recess. This type is more commonly seen in heavily pigmented eyes.

ments, such as the Draeger or Halberg tonometer, are superior. The MacKay-Marg has also been shown to compare favorably with other tonometers.

Dehydration for infants can be a factor in reduction of intraocular pressure and can produce false tonometric readings. Ocular changes observed in infantile glaucoma are often more severe than the pressure would indicate, and the surgeon's judgment must be influenced by other characteristic signs and symptoms.

Differential Diagnosis

A wide variety of disorders may simulate congenital glaucoma. Some of these are discussed here to demonstrate the differentiating features (see Table 16–1).

Megalocornea and High Myopia

In the differential diagnosis of an enlarged cornea, one must consider megalocornea and high myopia (Fig. 16–4). *Megalocornea* is a congenital, nonprogressive, bilateral and symmetrical developmental anomaly of the eyes in which there is a primary overgrowth of the anterior segment and the posterior portion is of normal size. The corneal diameters are between 13 and 17 mm. The corneas are clear, the anterior chamber is deep, the intraocular pressure is normal, and there is no glaucomatous cupping of the optic disc. Iris findings have included miosis due to poor development of the dilator muscle, stromal atrophy, and iridodonesis. Gonioscopic findings have been reported and include widening of the angle, a deep anterior chamber, a prominent scleral spur, and increased pigmentation of the trabeculum and the posterior surface of the cornea (Krukenberg's spindle). As a result of enlargment of the anterior scleral ring, the zonules may be stretched, and subluxation or dislocation of the lens may occur. Secondary glaucoma may occur if the lens then causes a pupillary block or angle closure. Changes in the corneal curvature may cause astigmatism, which may decrease visual acuity. Cataracts have been reported in early adult life. Megalocornea occurs predominately in males (92 per cent) and is usually transmitted as a recessive X-linked type. Some reports of autoso-

TABLE 16–1 DIFFERENTIAL DIAGNOSIS IN INFANTILE GLAUCOMA*

Inflammation
  Intrauterine corneal inflammation
    Congenital syphilis, interstitial keratitis, nonluetic interstitial keratitis, rubella keratitis
  Infantile corneal inflammation
    Chemical keratitis
  Herpes simplex
  Varicella herpes zoster
  Variola and vaccinia
  Trachoma
  Mumps keratitis
  Staphylococcal
  Inclusion conjunctivitis
  Measles keratoconjunctivitis

Systemic Diseases
  Corneal lipidosis
  Hyperlipemia
  Hereditary dystopic lipidosis (Fabry's disease)
  Lignac-Fanconi syndrome (cystinosis)
  Disorders of calcium metabolism
  Mucopolysaccharidoses (MPS)
  Congenital porphyria
  von Gierke's glycogen storage disease
  Hand-Schüller-Christian disease
  Morquio Ullrich's syndrome
  Osteogenesis imperfecta (blue sclerotic syndrome)
  Riley-Day syndrome (familial dysautonomia)
  Cogan' syndrome
  Bloch-Sulzberger syndrome·
  Wilson's disease

  Other Systemic Disorders
    Benign mucosal pemphigoid
    Erythema multiforme
    Rosacea
    Sjögren's keratoconjunctivitis sicca
    Leprosy

Trauma
  Rupture of Descemet's membrane
  Postnatal trauma

Skin Disease
  Congenital ichthyosis
  Congenital dyskeratosis

Corneal Dystrophy
  Congenital hereditary corneal dystrophy
  Congenital idiopathic corneal edema

Genetic Disorders
  Down's syndrome (mongolism)
  13–15 Trisomy syndrome

Birth Anomalies
  Congenital corneal leukoma
  Persistent hyperplastic primary vitreous
  Large cornea of high myopia
  Megalocornea

*Modified after Kwitko, M. L.: Glaucoma in Infants and Children. New York, Appleton-Century-Crofts, 1973.

mal dominant transmission have been made. Families have been reported in which one child had megalocornea while another of the sibship had typical congenital glaucoma. This has led some ophthalmologists to believe that these two entities represent different stages of the same condition.

High myopia may result in enlargement of an eye, although this does not always occur. Refraction will reveal any enlargement, and examination should show a clear cornea, normal intraocular pressure, and no glaucomatous cupping of the optic disc. Although both myopia and congenital glaucoma may appear clinically as an enlarged eye, the difference is that in myopia the post-equatorial region is affected first, while in congenital glaucoma many of the early changes take place in the anterior portion of the globe.

Inflammation

The interstitial keratitis of congenital syphilis generally manifests itself between 5 and 15 years of age. There is intense photophobia and lacrimation. The cornea becomes vascularized and hazy, and folds in Descemet's membrane are often present. Blepharitis, keratoconjunctivitis, and keratitis may be seen in the newborn child on a chemical, allergic, bacterial, or viral basis.

Metabolic Disorders

Familial lipoidosis may give a cloudy appearance to the cornea. Cystinosis, or cystine storage disease, is a generalized disturbance of the amino acids, appearing as an aminoaciduria with the accumulation of cystine in the liver, spleen, lymph nodes, kidneys, bone marrow, and ocular tissues, including the cornea, conjunctiva, and sclera. The corneal crystals are not present at birth, but begin to develop between the third and sixth months of life. They increase progressively and may give rise to a "glare" type of photophobia.

Hurler's syndrome, MPS IH, must be differentiated from congenital glaucoma. Hurler's syndrome consists of mucopolysaccharide infiltration of many body tissues, including the cornea, giving it a ground glass appearance. Chondrodystrophic skeletal changes, dwarfism, kyphosis, large head, grotesque face, and short claw fingers make up the syndrome. Pigmentary retinopathy has been described. Related conditions are Scheie's syndrome (MPS I S), Morquio's syndrome (MPS IV), and Maroteaux-Lamy syndrome (MPS VI), which have corneal involvement and must be differentiated from glaucoma.

Congenital Hereditary Corneal Dystrophy

In this disorder the corneal opacities are frequently present at birth. The condition is bilateral and exhibits a ground glass appearance which varies from a slight haze to dense white and involves the entire thickness of the stroma. There is no photophobia, and corneal sensitivity is normal. Intraocular pressure measurements are within normal limits. The clinical appearance of this condition bears some resemblance to congenital glaucoma.

Congenital Idiopathic Corneal Edema

Corneal edema in an infant may represent early changes in a metabolic disorder or may be a dystrophy which commenced during fetal life. Some forms of corneal edema may be self-limiting or respond to local steroids. Corneal sensitivity and intraocular pressure are normal.

Hereditary epithelial corneal dystrophy may develop during the early months of life.

Blue Sclerotic Syndrome

Reduction of collagenous fibers with thinning of the sclera allows the uveal pigment to be seen more readily. Buphthalmia also leads to thinning of the scleral coat, but as a secondary phenomenon. Therefore, there is a need for noting the differentiating points. Other features of the blue sclerotic syndrome include fragilitas ossium, dislocation and subluxation of the joints, and deafness.

Riley-Day Syndrome

The Riley-Day syndrome consists of deficient lacrimation, excess sweating and salivation, abnormal reaction to minimal emotional stress, skin blotches, motor incoordination, and thickened speech. There are two constant ocular findings: defective lacrimation and corneal hypesthesia. The corneal lesions may be divided into three types: severe central lesions, mild lesions resembling exposure keratitis, and faint scarred areas of the lower cornea.

Anterior Corneal Staphyloma

Corneal perforation from injury or ulceration causes a protrusion of the corneal stroma with adherence of the iris. The presence of iris tissue gives the cornea a blue color. Anterior synechiae may result in secondary hypertension. Whereas the buphthalmic eye develops a uniform enlargement of the cornea, the staphyloma may be irregular and conical. Even when the staphyloma is extensive, a peripheral zone of normal cornea is usually present.

Keratectasia

When the cornea is weakened by inflammation, e.g., interstitial keratitis or ulceration, the normal intraocular pressure may be too high for the cornea to withstand, and protrusion may take place. There is no perforation, and the iris is free of the cornea, as opposed to corneal staphyloma where the iris forms much of the protuberant scar. If protrusion is extensive, Descemet's membrane may rupture, giving a picture not unlike that seen in congenital glaucoma.

Keratoconus

While the cornea and neighboring sclera are greatly enlarged and the cornea flattened with ocular hypertension, keratoconus represents a form of keratectasia in which only the central cornea bulges forward, becoming thin and prominent, and often surrounded by a pigment ring. The characteristic appearance distinguishes the condition from congenital glaucoma even though tears in Descemet's membrane appear frequently. A marked astigmatism is present. Keratoconus may occur at birth and may be associated with congenital cataract, aniridia, and ectopia lentis.

Other types of corneal deformities include *keratotorus*, in which there is a toric or vaultlike ectasia, and *keratoglobus*, in which the cornea is enlarged, globular, and protruding, with a thinning of the peripheral stroma.

Cornea Plana

Flattening of the cornea may occur in varying degrees, including involvement of the anterior sclera. Other features include opacification of the corneal stroma, shallow anterior chamber, and astigmatism. Cornea plana is due to defective development during fetal life and may be associated with other anomalies, including coloboma of the iris, congenital cataract, and ectopia lentis. Glaucoma may occur if the filtration angle is involved.

Bloch-Sulzberger Syndrome

The Bloch-Sulzberger syndrome, or incontinentia pigmenti, was described in 1926. There are two types: patchy pigmentary dermatosis, which occurs at birth, and a reticular form, which begins after the age of 2. Most of the cases occur in young females. Anomalies of the eye occur in one quarter of the cases. The eye conditions may include corneal opacities, congenital cataract, iris malformation, persistent hyperplastic primary vitreous, pseudoglioma, pre- and postnatal uveitis, and retinal detachment. The skin lesion consists of wavy striae of slate gray color. More recently corneal lesions have been observed. The disease may be inherited as an autosomal or sex-linked dominant. Glaucoma can occur if outflow is impaired.

Birth Injury

Breaks in Descemet's membrane due to trauma, such as from a difficult forceps delivery (Fig. 16–6), may simulate the breaks in Descemet's membrane seen in congenital glaucoma. If damage to the endothelium is extensive, the cornea may become cloudy. There may be photophobia and tearing, and the clinical picture may present a problem in differentiation from congenital glaucoma. The breaks in Descemet's membrane resulting from trauma tend to be linear and oblique in their course in the cornea. Astigmatism and amblyopia are commonly observed.

SECONDARY GLAUCOMA IN INFANTS AND CHILDREN

Elevation of intraocular pressure in infants may occur secondary to a wide variety of ophthalmic conditions (see Table 16–2).

Inflammatory diseases such as fetal or neonatal keratitis or uveitis may also exhibit a rise in intraocular pressure. Ger-

TABLE 16–2 SECONDARY GLAUCOMA IN INFANCY AND CHILDHOOD*

Inflammation
1. Chemical
2. Infection (bacterial and parasitic)
3. Rubella and other viral diseases
4. Nonspecific inflammatory diseases

Trauma
1. Nonpenetrating wounds
2. Penetrating wounds
3. Phakoanaphylactic endophthalmitis
4. Foreign bodies
5. Sympathetic ophthalmia

Carotid-Cavernous Sinus Fistula

Tumors
1. Retinoblastoma
2. Diktyoma

Other Disorders
1. Retrolental fibroplasia
2. Juvenile xanthogranuloma (nevoxanthoendothelioma)
3. Metabolic disorders
4. Lens-induced glaucoma
5. Norrie's disease
6. Spontaneous rupture of the eyeball
7. Administration of steroids

*Modified after Kwitko, M. L.: Glaucoma in Infants and Children. New York, Appleton-Century-Crofts, 1973.

man measles contracted during the first trimester has long been noted to give rise to glaucoma as part of the rubella syndrome. It has been suggested that this form of infantile hypertension differs from primary congenital glaucoma.

Congenital tumors such as retinoblastoma and diktyoma may be associated with a rise in ocular tension. Trauma may also have a similar effect. Retrolental fibroplasia and infantile xanthogranuloma (nevoxanthoendothelioma) are also known to be associated with glaucoma.

Steroid-induced glaucoma has been observed in children from the prolonged topical application of medication containing cortisone. The condition usually subsides with discontinuation of the medicine.

LOCAL OCULAR ABNORMALITIES

A wide variety of ophthalmic conditions occurring in children have an elevated intraocular pressure as part of the clinical picture. Associated glaucoma is related to obstruction of aqueous drainage caused by a developmental anomaly in the eye (see Table 16–3).

TABLE 16–3 DEVELOPMENTAL ANOMALIES ASSOCIATED WITH INFANTILE GLAUCOMA*

Corneal Anomalies
1. Sclerocornea
2. Microphthalmos
3. Cornea plana
4. Anterior chamber cleavage syndrome
5. Peter's anomaly (mesodermal dysgenesis of the cornea)
6. Rieger's disease
7. Axenfeld's syndrome

Iris Anomalies
1. Aniridia
2. Coloboma of the iris
3. Persistent pupillary membrane
4. Corectopia
5. Polycoria
6. Essential iris atrophy

Lens Anomalies
1. Congenital aphakia
2. Congenital cataract
3. Subluxation of the lens
4. Anterior lenticonus, lentiglobus
5. Persistent hyperplastic primary vitreous (PHPV)

Hamartomatoses
1. Von Recklinghausen's disease
2. Von Hippel-Lindau disease
3. Blue nevus of Ota
4. Sturge-Weber syndrome

Mesodermal Anomalies
1. Marfan's syndrome
2. Weill-Marchesani syndrome

Metabolic Disease
1. Oculocerebrorenal syndrome (Lowe's syndrome)
2. Homocystinuria
3. Sulfite oxidase deficiency

Other Genetically Determined Diseases
1. Turner's syndrome
2. Hereditary oculodentodigital dysplasia
3. Pierre Robin syndrome

Other Conditions
1. Hemangioma of the choroid
2. Pigmentary glaucoma
3. Rubinstein's syndrome (broad thumb syndrome)
4. Mongolism (Down's syndrome)
5. Conradi's syndrome
6. Hallermann-Streiff syndrome
7. Werner's syndrome

*Modified after Kwitko, M. L.: Glaucoma in Infants and Children. New York, Appleton-Century-Crofts, 1973.

Aniridia (Irideremia)

In aniridia there is a complete or partial absence of iris tissue. There is usually a rudimentary band of iris present which may be pulled up toward the line of Schwalbe, thus sealing the angle. This condition is said to have an incidence of 0.04 per cent; it may be associated with congenital cataract, microphakia, ectopia lentis, retinal aplasia, nystagmus, corneal opacities, and aplasia of the macula, as well as congenital glaucoma. The surgical treatment of glaucoma associated with congenital aniridia is generally not considered satisfactory, although Barkan described the use of the goniotomy procedure to release the adhesions of the iris stump. Cyclodiathermy has been advocated as the operation of choice. Aniridia probably represents an arrest in the differentiation of the optic cup at the 70 to 80 mm. stage. DiGeorge and Harley reported on the association of aniridia with Wilms' tumor.

Coloboma of the Iris

Coloboma of the iris is found when there is faulty development of the eye during the stage of closure of the fetal fissure, so that the location of the coloboma is downward and nasal. Although a large segment may be absent, the remainder of the iris is normal. A typical coloboma of the iris may result when there is an abnormal persistence of fetal blood vessels at the edge of the optic cup.

Polycoria

Polycoria is another defect associated with congenital glaucoma. There is actual reduplication of the pupil and the sphincter muscle. Frequently, an anterior polar cataract is present, with congenital corneal opacities. True polycoria must be differentiated from dehiscence and diastasis of the iris. False polycoria may be seen after a severe anterior segment injury and is also associated with elevated intraocular pressure.

Pigmentary Glaucoma

Pigmentary glaucoma may be seen as early as 12 years of age. Loose pigment particles find their way by aqueous fluid currents into the filtration angle and may cause a secondary glaucoma. Krukenberg's pigment spindle is present on the posterior corneal surface; the characteristic appearance is due to anterior chamber aqueous flow dynamics.

Adhesions Between Iris and Cornea

Adhesions between the iris and the cornea may obstruct the filtration angle and give rise to an elevated intraocular pressure. The cause of this anomaly may be a perforation of the cornea during fetal life, with anterior synechia formation.

Microcornea (Microphthalmos)

This condition is based upon a defect in embryological development occurring around the fourth month of fetal life, when the cornea and the sclera have the same curvature. If development of the sclera continues while the corneal curvature is retarded, cornea plana results. If scleral growth is retarded and the corneal curvature develops normally, microphthalmos occurs. Glaucoma is not uncommon. Associated findings consist of shallow anterior chamber, cataract, and retinal dysplasia.

The Anterior Chamber Cleavage Syndrome (Reese and Ellsworth)

Congenital central anterior synechia. Adhesions between the iris collarette and the paracentral cornea are associated with dense corneal opacities, which together may produce decreased visual acuity and glaucoma.

Posterior embryotoxon (Axenfeld's Syndrome). Axenfeld's syndrome or mesodermal dysgenesis may be properly classified under the anterior chamber cleavage syndrome. It is recognized as an anterior displacement of Schwalbe's line, which is thickened and easily recognized with the slit lamp microscope.

The trabeculum is long and there are varying degrees of iris adhesions to Schwalbe's line. Obstructions to the filtration angle contribute to elevated intraocular tension. The condition is inherited as an autosomal dominant. There are a wide range of anterior segment disturbances which characterize the anterior chamber cleavage syndrome: dyscoria, pseudopolycoria and polycoria, corectopia, iridotasis, iris dehiscences, prominence of the iris sphincter, aplasia of the mesodermal leaf of the iris ectropion uveae, congenital corneal opacification, anterior polar cataract, and ectopia lentis.

Rieger's anomaly. This condition, known as mesodermal dysgenesis of Rieger, represents another variation of the chamber cleavage disorder. It is inherited through autosomal dominant genes. The iris may show hypoplasia of the anterior stromal leaf, iridotrabecular adhesions, and posterior embryotoxon. Other gross deformities may occur in the iris, such as corectopia, coloboma, and those listed under Axenfeld's syndrome. Glaucoma is a common sequela as a result of defective angle filtration

Dental anomalies in the form of oligodontia and anodontia together with dysplasias of the skull and skeleton have been recorded.

Von Hippel's internal corneal ulcer (keratoconus posticus). This condition represents an involvement of the posterior cornea associated with posterior keratoconus. Reese and Ellsworth classify it as yet another member of the anterior chamber cleavage dysgenesis group.

Sclerocornea. Sclerocornea and cornea plana were noted in one third of anterior chamber cleavage syndrome groups by Reese and Ellsworth. Glaucoma was present in 3 of 7 cases reported by Goldstein and Cogan. Embryotoxon represents the mildest form of the cleavage disorders and appeared in the fellow eye of a patient with sclerocornea.

Associated ocular defects include cornea plana, embryotoxon, glaucoma, microphthalmos, microcornea, and nystagmus. Systemic abnormalities involve the skin (dermatitis), skull (brachycephaly), and cerebellum (ataxia). Sclerocornea must be differentiated from other forms of vascular pannus, including vascular keratitis.

Peter's anomaly. Peter's anomaly is a congenital disorder in which there is a central opacity with abnormalities of the posterior stroma and a local absence of Descemet's membrane. Glaucoma is common. Various defects of the anterior segment, including microphthalmos and sclerocornea, have been recorded.

Spherophakia

Malformation of the lens may cause glaucoma as a result of blockage of the outflow channel in the pupillary area (pupillary block).

Anterior Lenticonus

Anterior lenticonus is a congenital anomaly characterized by an anterior lens surface which protrudes to assume a conical (lenticonus) or spherical form (lentiglobus). It is easily recognized by a slit lamp. It is usually seen in males as a bilateral defect but may also occur unilaterally as part of Alport's syndrome.

Persistent Hyperplastic Primary Vitreous (PHPV)

The persistence of hyperplastic primary vitreous is seen as a fibrous tissue mass located behind the lens to which retinal elements and ciliary processes extend. Hemorrhage may be present at the periphery of the tissue. The lens may become cataractous, or spontaneous absorption may take place. A sustained rise in intraocular pressure may lead to buphthalmos in the infant.

Congenital Cataract

A lens opacity combined with a defective iridocorneal angle may occur as an isolated anomaly, although it is usually seen as part of some other syndrome.

Retinitis Pigmentosa

An association of microphthalmia, retinitis pigmentosa and glaucoma are genetically determined. Glaucoma is nearly four times more frequent in retinitis pigmentosa than in the general population.

ASSOCIATED SYSTEMIC ANOMALIES

A wide variety of ophthalmic conditions occurring in children have an elevated intraocular pressure as part of the clinical picture; some typical disease entities will be discussed here.

Marfan's Syndrome

The outstanding features of Marfan's syndrome are arachnodactyly, loose-jointedness, long thin bones, pectus excavatum, hypoplasia of skeletal muscle and subcutaneous fat tissue, dilation or dissecting aneurysm of the aorta, striae distensae, subluxation of the lens, and glaucoma. Burian and Wachtel have both shown that the filtration angle in Marfan's syndrome is often deformed, with the majority of fibers arising from the meridional portion of the ciliary muscle inserting into the trabecular meshwork anterior to the scleral spur and Schlemm's canal.

Homocystinuria

Homocystinuria is a genetically transmitted enzymatic fault, in which the metabolic pathway from methionine to cystine is disturbed by a deficiency in cystathionine synthase.

Schimke and McKusick identified 38 sufferers in 20 families by urine assay for homocystine. Formerly confused with Marfan's syndrome, homocystinuria is distinguished by nontraumatic dislocation of the lens, mental retardation, and a typical malar flush. Other signs and symptoms include glaucoma, a tall body (notably larger below the waist), long limbs, flat turned-out feet, osteoporosis and scoliosis with a tendency to vertebral fracture, and a variety of cardiovascular abnormalities. Venous thrombosis and pulmonary embolism are frequently noted. The oldest patient in this series was 45 years of age; 10 patients had died by the age of 28. Glaucoma may occur secondary to the lens subluxation or cataract formation.

Weill-Marchesani Syndrome

The condition is characterized by brachycephaly, short pyknic build, short fingers and toes, good musculature, tight joints, ectopia lentis after age 25, microphakia, and spherophakia. It has been reported as both autosomal recessive and dominant. Death occurs by cardiovascular disease, usually in the fifties. Glaucoma may develop secondary to a subluxated lens.

Sturge-Weber Syndrome (Encephalotrigeminal Angiomatosis)

The Sturge-Weber syndrome is characterized by a port-wine facial hemangioma involving the lid, orbit, and scalp, ipsilateral choroidal hemangioma, ipsilateral meningeal hemangioma, epilepsy, intracranial calcification, and congenital glaucoma. Glaucoma is thought to result from choroidal angiomata or angle abnormalities. However, chorodial hemangiomas cannot be identified regularly with flourescein, and the angle is usually open but with excessive vascularity.

Neurofibromatosis

Neurofibromatosis of the eyelid and orbit is a well recognized but uncommon manifestation of von Recklinghausen's disease. Other changes include café au lait spots and multiple tumors of peripheral nerves. The disease, which often commences in early childhood, may be accompanied by tumor-like masses in the temple, side of the face, and orbit. Glaucoma probably develops as a result of several factors, including infiltration of the angle by neurofibromatous material and fibrovascular tissue together with a thickening of the ciliary body with forward displacement and narrowing of the angle.

Lowe's Syndrome

Lowe and co-workers described a syndrome in 1952 which they called the "oculocerebrorenal syndrome." The ophthalmic findings included cataracts, nystagmus, steamy corneas, blue sclerae, microphthalmia, and glaucoma. The syndrome was characterized by a decreased ability of the kidney to fabricate ammonia, organic aciduria, systemic acidosis, mental retardation, and osteomalacia. Glaucoma develops in over half of the cases as a probable result of a poorly developed filtration angle. Glaucoma may be seen in the microphthalmic eye. Males are primarily affected; the female carriers show scattered punctate lens opacities.

Pierre Robin Syndrome

The Pierre Robin syndrome is characterized by three defects: micrognathia, cleft palate, and glossoptosis. Other abnormalities include flattening of the root of the nose, finger, and toe anomalies, cardiac murmurs, hearing loss, and hydrocephalus. Ocular pathology includes high myopia, retinal detachment, congenital glaucoma, congenital cataract, and microphthalmia. Gonioscopy revealed a thin, grayish, nearly translucent membrane over the trabeculum in one child with congenital glaucoma and in another who exhibited only high myopia (Smith).

Turner's Syndrome

Turner's syndrome involves a diverse clinical picture including infantilism, webbing of the skin of the neck, and cubitus valgus occurring in undersized postadolescent girls with amenorrhea and an absence of secondary sexual characteristics. Congenital glaucoma has been reported as an associated anomaly. Other eye findings include ptosis, cataract, strabismus, epicanthus, blue sclera, color blindness, and corneal nebulae.

Trisomy 13 Syndrome

Trisomy 13 syndrome results from the presence of an extra autosomal chromosome of the 13–15 or D group. The following abnormalities have been noted: mental retardation, deafness, heart defects, hemangiomata, cleft lip, cleft palate, motor seizures, low-set ears, polydactyly, and horizontal palmer creases. The ocular findings include microphthalmia, iris coloboma, persistent pupillary membrane, congenital cataract, retinal dysplasia, corneal opacities, and hyperplastic primary vitreous. Cogan and Kuwabara have noted the apparent characteristic of a cartilage mass extending from the retrolental region to the sclera in the region of the coloboma. Glaucoma may develop as a result of a poorly developed filtration angle.

Trisomy 18 Syndrome

Trisomy 18 is characterized by failure to thrive, mental retardation, low-set ears, cardiac defects, flexion deformity of fingers, and partial syndactyly of toes. Ocular defects include congenital glaucoma, optic atrophy, lens opacities, and ptosis.

Down's Syndrome
(Trisomy 21; Mongolism)

This disorder is characterized by mental retardation, elasticity of joints, large tongue, small little finger, Brushfield's spots on the iris, and simian crease. Congenital cataract is common and congenital glaucoma has been described.

Hallermann-Streiff Syndrome

This syndrome is characterized by dyscephaly, birdlike facies, localized hypotrichosis and atrophy of the skin, and bilateral microphthalmos. Congenital glaucoma may develop. The cataracts have been known to undergo spontaneous absorption.

Juvenile Xanthogranuloma
(Nevoxanthoendothelioma)

This is a self-limited condition affecting predominantly the skin about the scalp and face, but occasionally appearing on the trunk and extremities. Lesions on the iris appear salmon pink, elevated, and distinct from normal iris. The lesion is prone to bleed and may present as a spontaneous anterior chamber hemorrhage. Glaucoma may develop.

Congenital Rubella Syndrome

Characteristic findings include cardiac complications, deafness, and ocular complications. Ocular abnormalities include cataract, retinopathy, microphthalmos, hypoplastic iris, strabismus, and glaucoma. The anterior chamber angle may be altered as a result of the infiltrating viral inflammatory process.

Idiopathic Infantile Hypoglycemia

Hypoglycemia occurring prior to 2 years of age responds favorably to ACTH, with a tendency toward spontaneous recovery. Scheie reported ocular complications including congenital cataracts, nasolacrimal duct obstruction, optic atrophy, and congenital glaucoma.

Oculodermalmelanocytosis
(Nevus of Ota)

This condition consists of a unilateral pigmentation involving the sclera, uveal tract, and skin of the periorbita. Bilateral cases may occur. Glaucoma has been reported. Examination of the filtration angle reveals sporadic hyperpigmentation which is believed to be related to elevated intra-ocular pressure. Normal angle structures may be completely obscured by pigment.

Hereditary Oculodentadigital Dysplasia

Meyer-Schwickerath, Gruterich, and Weyers (1957) described two patients with microphthalmos, dental anomalies, and a deformity of the fifth fingers bilaterally, consisting of a camptodactylia. The alae nasi were small with anteverted nostrils. One of the patients, a 13-year-old girl, had bilateral glaucoma. The glaucoma is prob- ably related to a defective angle formation in a microphthalmic eye.

TREATMENT OF GLAUCOMA IN INFANTS AND CHILDREN

General Principles

The diagnosis of infantile glaucoma is an indication for immediate surgical inter-vention. Final visual results depend on early diagnosis and the successful control

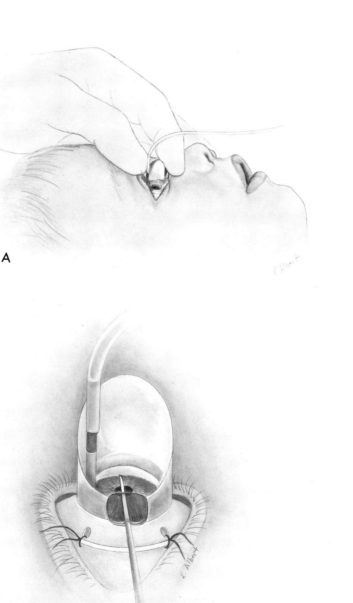

A

B

Figure 16–15 Goniotomy: Worst lens. *A*, The lens is placed over the eye and sutured in place. The lens is held by the surgeon, and saline may be in-troduced through a tube to maintain optical clarity at the interface between the lens and the cornea. *B*, Close-up view of the lens. The goniotomy knife enters the anterior chamber just an-terior to the limbus, and a goniotomy may be performed under direct visual-ization.

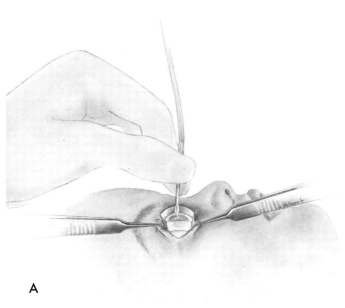

A

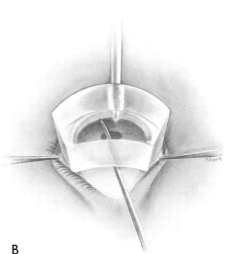

B

Figure 16–16   Goniotomy: Lister lens. *A*, Fixation of the eye is obtained by the assistant grasping the vertical rectus muscles at their insertions. This holds the lids away from the lens and steadies the eye. The surgeon places the lens on the cornea and observes the angle opposite to him by focusing the operating microscope. A second assistant introduces saline through the tube to maintain optical clarity. This lens has the advantage of not requiring suturing to the eye. *B*, Close-up view showing the knife in the anterior chamber. Care must be taken to avoid the iris and lens. *C*, Post goniotomy, showing cleft to the left.

of the tension before the disease becomes advanced.

Medical management is of limited value. Miotics have no useful long term effect. Carbonic anhydrase inhibitors such as acetazolamide effect a significant lowering of intraocular pressure when used every 6 hours. This drug can be helpful in the diagnosis if the corneal clouding clears and may also have some usefulness in resistant cases that have not been completely controlled surgically.

The prognosis for a good visual result is poor for infants who are born with enlarged globes or who have developed enlarged eyes prior to surgical management.

Surgical Management
(Figs. 16–15 to 16–20)

The primary objective in the surgical management of infantile glaucoma is the normalization of intraocular pressure as quickly and as permanently as possible.

Since the principal fault in infantile glaucoma is the problem of outflow resulting from inadequate filtration via the trabeculum into Schlemm's canal, our primary concern must focus on improving filtration through the trabecular meshwork.

It is not well understood at present

(Text continued on page 411)

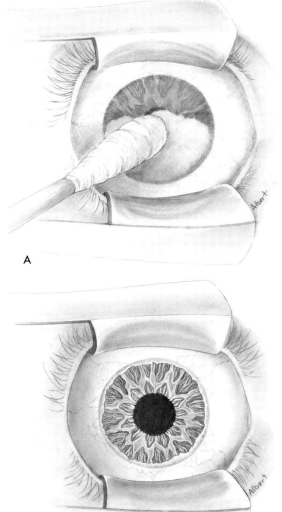

A

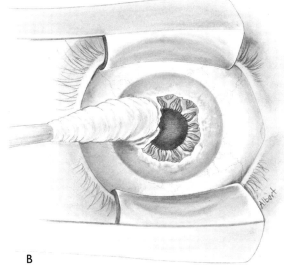

B

C

Figure 16–17 Removal of the corneal epithelium may be necessary if the clouding prevents adequate visualization of the angle. *A*, 95 per cent alcohol is placed on a cotton swab and dabbed on the cornea. The epithelium becomes more cloudy. *B*, After 1 to 2 minutes the epithelium can be easily peeled off of Bowman's membrane by lightly rubbing the swab on the corneal surface. *C*, The epithelium has been removed.

Figure 16–18 Trabeculotomy. *A*, A limbus-based conjunctival flap is made, 4 to 5 mm. from the cornea. A 2 × 2 mm. wide limbus-based scleral flap is made extending one-half to two-thirds the thickness of the sclera. *B*, Cut-away view of the scleral flap showing the posterior extension of the cornea into the sclera. The location of the canal of Schlemm is indicated. *C*, Using high magnification, a scratch-down incision is made just over the junction of the blue cornea and white sclera. Aqueous may be seen to escape when the canal has been cut. The location of the canal is shown in dotted lines. *D*, Vannas scissors are introduced into both cut ends of the canal, which is then enlarged 2 mm. to either side. *E*, A trabeculotomy probe is placed into one side and rotated into the anterior chamber, thus rupturing through the inside wall of the canal, the trabecular meshwork, and the pretrabecular tissue. The probe is then passed in a similar manner in the other cut end of the canal. *F*, The scleral flap is then closed with interrupted 10–0 Ethilon sutures and the conjunctiva is closed with 8–0 white silk suture.

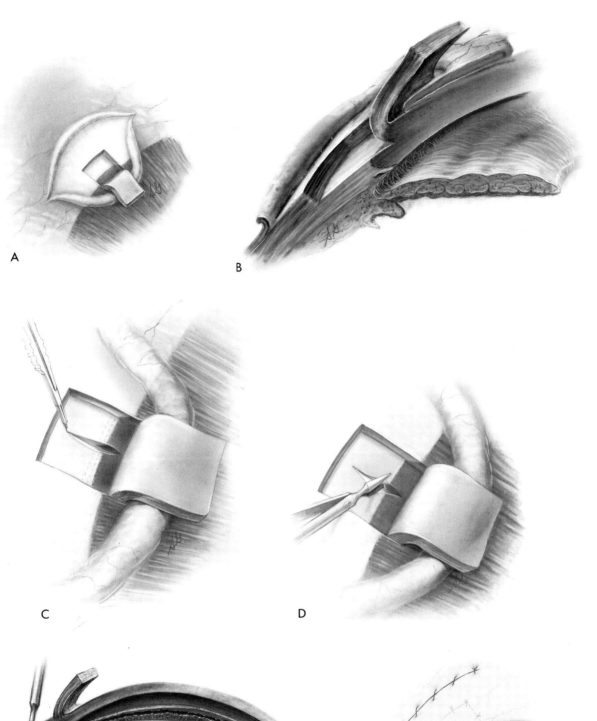

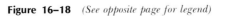

Figure 16–18   *(See opposite page for legend)*

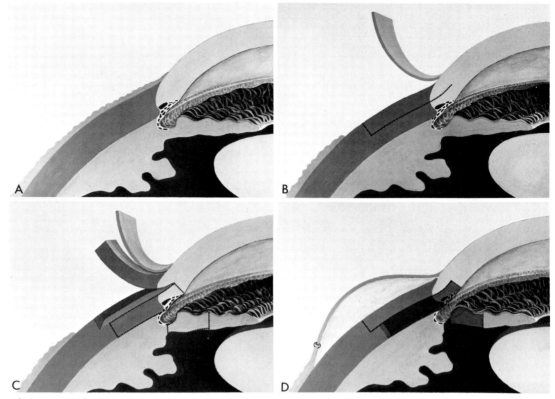

Figure 16–19   Trabeculectomy. *A*, Schlemm's canal and trabecular network. *B*, Initial lamellar incision illustrating superficial corneoscleral lamellae. *C*, Excised corneal and scleral tissue containing Schlemm's canal and trabecular meshwork. Peripheral iridectomy performed. *D*, Scleral lamella replaced and sutured at corners. Overlying conjunctiva sutured.

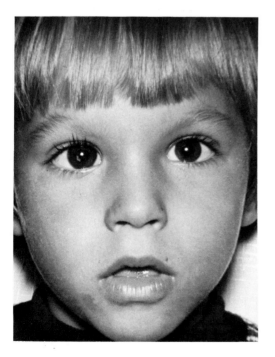

Figure 16–20   Same patient as in Figure 16–2 (now 6 years of age). The intraocular pressure was normalized after one goniotomy. The cornea remained enlarged, and refractive error was OD −4.00 sph. and OS +1.50 sph. Glasses and occlusion was started, and corrected visual acuity in the right eye is now 20/80.

whether success results from incising an impermeable structure (membrane or the trabeculum itself) or incising a forward displacement of the anterior limiting membrane of the iris on the trabeculum. In either instance, the surgical attack on the trabeculum to improve the facility of outflow is direct and logical.

The most significant advance in the surgery for infantile glaucoma has been the development of the goniotomy or trabeculotomy procedure by Barkan, which should have a success rate of at least 80 per cent with experienced surgeons. It has been shown to have relatively small risk to the infant eye and may be repeated at least four times before proceeding to a different method.

Various other surgical methods have been devised for the control of intraocular pressure in congenital glaucoma. These procedures may be generally classed as follows:

1. *Trabeculotomy*—the slitting open of the trabecular meshwork obstruction.
2. *Trabeculectomy*—the removal of a section of the trabeculum and the adjacent Schlemm's canal.
3. *Filtration procedures*—an externalized by-pass fistula.
4. *Combination of trabecular and filtration procedures.*

Trabecular surgery includes the following:

1. *Internal trabeculotomy or goniotomy* (Barkan).
2. *Internal direct trabeculotomy or goniotripsy* (Urrets; Zavalia, Kwitko, and Galin).
3. *Abexterno trabeculotomy* (Allen and Burian).
4. *Trabeculectomy* (Dellaporta and Fahrenbruch).

Filtration procedures included the following:

1. *Scleral cautery with iridectomy* (Scheie).
2. *Limboscleral trephine* (Sugar).

A combination procedure involving trabecular and filtration methods is the *gonio puncture* (Scheie).

Trabecular surgery must receive first consideration. Goniotomy or internal trabeculotomy offers good results, but other surgeons claim equally good results with abexterno trabeculotomy and trebeculectomy.

Filtering procedures should be reserved for those cases which have not responded to trabecular surgery or the gonio puncture.

REFERENCES

Allen, L., and Burian, H. M.: Trabeculotomy abexterno. Amer. J. Ophthal., 53:19, 1962.

Barkan, O.: Pathogenesis of congenital glaucoma, gonioscopic and anatomic observations of the angle of the normal eye and congenital glaucoma. Amer. J. Ophthal., 40:1, 1955.

Barkan, O.: A new operation for chronic glaucoma, restoration of physiological function by opening Schlemm's canal under direct magnified vision. Amer. J. Ophthal., 19:951, 1936.

Burian, H. M.: A case of Marfan's syndrome with bilateral glaucoma. Amer. J. Ophthal., 50:1187, 1960.

Cogan, D. G., and Kuwabara, T.: Ocular pathology of the 13–18 trisomy syndrome. Arch. Ophthal., 72:246, 1964.

Dellaporte, A., and Fahrenbruch, R. C.: Trapanotrabeculectomy. Trans. Amer. Acad. Ophthal. Otolaryng., 75:283, 1971.

DiGeorge, A. M., and Harley, R. D.: The association of aniridia, Wilms' tumor and genital abnormalities. Trans. Amer. Ophthal. Soc., 63:64, 1965.

Goldstein, J. E., and Cogan, D. G.: Sclerocornea and associated congenital anomalies. Arch. Ophthal., 67:761, 1962.

Kwitko, M. L.: Glaucoma in Infants and Children. New York, Appleton-Century-Crofts, 1973, pp. 186–189, 390–391, 483–489.

Kwitko, M. L., and Galin, M. A.: Direct goniotomy for congenital glaucoma. Excerpta Medica. In press.

Lowe, C. V., Terrey, M., and MacLachlan, E. A.: Organic aciduria, decreased renal ammonia production, hydrocephalus and mental retardation, a clinical entity. Amer. J. Dis. Child., 83:164, 1952.

Maumenee, A. E.: The pathogenesis of congenital glaucoma, a new theory. Trans. Amer. Ophthal. Soc., 56:507, 1958.

Meyer-Schwickerath, G., Gruterich, E., and Weyers, H.: Mikrophthalmos syndrome. Klin. Monatsbl. Augenheilkd., 131:18, 1957.

Reese, A. B., and Ellsworth, R. M.: The anterior chamber cleavage syndrome. Arch. Ophthal., 75:307, 1966.

Scheie, H. G.: Congenital glaucoma—congenital anomalies of the eye. Trans. New Orleans Acad. Ophthal. St. Louis, The C. V. Mosby Co., 1968, pp. 342–372.

Scheie, H. G., and Albert, D. M.: Adler's Textbook of Ophthalmology. 8th ed. Philadelphia, W. B. Saunders Co., 1969, pp. 354–360.

Scheie, H. G.: Goniopuncture, an evaluation after eleven years. Arch. Ophthal., 65:38, 1961.

Scheie, H. G.: Filtering operation for glaucoma. A comparative study. Amer. J. Ophthal., *53*:571, 1962.

Scheie, H. G., Rubinstein, R. A., and Albert, D. M.: Congenital glaucoma and other abnormalities with idiopathic infantile hypoglycemia. J. Pediat. Ophthal., *1*:45, 1964.

Schimke, R. N., McKusick, V. A., Huang, T., and Pollack, H. D.: Homocystinuria, a study of 38 cases in 20 families. J.A.M.A., *193*:711, 1965.

Shaffer, R. N.: Microsurgery of the outflow channels, conclusions. Trans. Amer. Acad. Ophthal. Otolaryng., *76*:411, 1972.

Smith, J. L., Cavanaugh, J. J. A., and Stone, F. C.: Ocular manifestations of the Pierre Robin syndrome. Arch. Ophthal., *63*:984, 1960.

Sugar, H. S.: Juvenile glaucoma with Axenfeld's syndrome: a histologic report. Amer. J. Ophthal., *59*:1012, 1965.

Sugar, H. S.: Further experience with limboscleral trephination. Eye, Ear, Nose and Throat Monthly, *417*:31, 1968.

Urrets-Zavalia, A.: Goniotripsy: an operation for congenital glaucoma. Ophthalmologica, *140*:14, 1960.

Wachtel, J. G.: The ocular pathology in Marfan's syndrome. Arch. Ophthal., *76*:512, 1966.

CHAPTER 17

TRAUMA OF THE GLOBE, ADNEXA, AND ORBITAL WALLS: PROPHYLAXIS AND IMMEDIATE THERAPY

ARTHUR H. KEENEY, M.D.

INTRODUCTION AND EXTENT OF THE PROBLEM

Frequently the ophthalmic practitioner —like many general surgeons—feels that *trauma* is a problem for someone else. This may embrace incorrect rationalizations such as that it is "infrequent," "basically simple," or "should be handled by a junior man." Such thinking may also espouse a few very correct points as "it could have been prevented" or, less nobly, "it interrupts my schedule." The National Society for the Prevention of Blindness under-scores current data indicating that "half of all blindness is preventable." With specificity in relation to age, more individually lost eyes (monocular blindness) occur during the first decade of life than during any subsequent decade (Slusher-Keeney, 1965). Nearly one third of the lost eyes in this first decade follow trauma. Blind school populations reflect a lower incidence of traumatic cause, because these children present bilateral impairments which, in early life, rarely stem from injuries.

Ocular injuries are strongly correlated with sex and appear in a male:female distribution from 3 to 1 for falls and up to 8 to 1 for blinding wounds. Thus, control programs and efforts surrounding the activities of boys will give a higher yield than will efforts equally invested for boys and girls.

This chapter will cover recent developments in prevention of trauma. It will also cover the frequently encountered mechanisms and types of injuries. It defers encyclopedic tabulation of each possibly injurious element and compound to such bibles of ocular toxicology as that by Morton Grant (1962) or the Toxicity Bibliography of the National Library of Medicine (1968). It avoids exciting but rare esoterica such as cosmic ray damage to the eyes in space travel, blowout fractures confined to the orbital roof (Smith, in press), or drug-related sun staring with self-induced solar burns of the retina (Anaclerio and Wicker, 1970).

Both skillful salvage and progressive prophylaxis are incumbent obligations of the ophthalmologist.

PREVENTION OF INITIAL AND SECONDARY INJURIES

Protective Lens Materials

Major industry has dramatically demonstrated that impact-resistant lenses for spectacles and goggles have enormous value in reduction of injuries. Early advances in such preventive ophthalmology were achieved with heat-tempered glass of approximately 3 mm. thickness. This continues to be a valuable lens material for industrial and general purposes, even in rough and tumble boys. It is adequately described and standardized by the American National Standards Institute (ANSI) Z87.1–1968 code for "Occupational and Educational Eye and Face Protection." Unfortunately, such crown glass safety lenses are heavy by virtue of their minimal 3 mm. thickness and this is compounded by refractive prescriptions of high diopter powers. Lens weight can be reduced about 50 per cent with use of so-called hard resin plastic lenses made from allyl diglycol carbonate or CR-39 (Columbia Southern Resin 39). These resin lenses have even greater impact resistance than do corresponding tempered glass lenses, par-

ticularly in high minus cylinders. Surface scratching of allyl resin lenses, however, is more of a problem than with glass and necessitates rinsing the lenses in water and wiping them with a clean soft tissue rather than rough cloth. Use of allyl resin lenses (Armorlite, Durikon, Aolite, Saf-T-Vis, Ortholite, Cristyl, Enduron) has steadily increased since their introduction in the early 1940s, but the advent of less expensive polycarbonate lenses in the late 1960s has challenged their leadership.

No lens is truly *shatterproof* and therefore this term must be avoided. All spectacle, sunglass, and goggle lenses, however, should be made of some protective material exceeding the strength of conventional crown glass. Currently, hard resin (ASTM Class I plastics) lenses afford the widest range of resistance to both small and large missiles at high and low velocity and are therefore particularly suitable for active boys, though surface scratching may occur more rapidly than with glass. Mars and scratches, though affecting the optical excellence of the lens surface, do not significantly reduce the impact resistance of plastic lenses. Heat-tempered glass, however, may be grossly weakened by pits or scratches which interrupt or ventilate the compressed skin surface of these lenses; such defects are germinal centers for fracture systems, and therefore heat-tempered glass lenses should be discarded when flawed.

As a compromise from the weight and thickness of heat-tempered industrial or occupational glass lenses, all manufacturers now provide semi-ophthalmic thickness or "dress safety" glass lenses having a minimum thickness of 2 mm. (Benson, Hardrx; American Optical, Tempross; Bausch and Lomb, Safe-Rex). This gives an intermediate level of protection, particularly in plus spherical lenses but less so in high minus lenses and least in high minus cylinders. Specifications for these lenses are established by the American National Standards Institute Z80.1–1972 code for First Quality Ophthalmic Lenses.

Lens strength increases with:
1. Thickness
2. Temperature
3. Increasing sphericity

4. Decreasing cylindricity
5. Inherent resilience or energy-absorbing capacity of the lens material
6. Freedom from flaws, pits, or scratches, especially in glass lenses
7. Roundness or symmetry of the lens configuration (eyepiece shape)
8. Uniformity of support or tension in the lens mounting

Thus, in prescribing spectacle lenses one must consider not only the optical components but also the lens material (heat-tempered glass or hard resin plastic) and the range of thickness (industrial or semi-ophthalmic).

Spectacle Mountings or Frames

RETAINING LIP DESIGN. A major advance in protective design has occurred in the last few years by improved frame construction with a posterior lip on the eyepiece requiring that lenses always be inserted from the front. This lip on the face side of the spectacles extends 0.1 mm. further toward the center of the eyepiece than does the anterior or front lip. Thus, a retaining edge or lip of 0.1-mm. height gives even, circumferential back support to the lens, reducing the likelihood of injurious posterior displacement.

MOUNTING TENSION EXERTED ON THE LENS. Metal or wire rims usually have a set screw for tightening the frame or eyewire about the lens. Such frames have a long history of use in industry and contributed to the early success of reducing eye injuries in conjunction with heavy occupational lenses. Tightening such metal eyepieces, however, can set up weakening torques or strains in the lens, particularly in odd-shaped, thinner, or cylindrical heat-treated glass. By changing to the evenly resilient or elastic mounting of a plastic eyepiece, uniform retention force is distributed over the entire circumference of the lens. Such uniform edge compression does not impair the stress-strain system established in heat-treated glass lenses, and in spherical powers it may actually increase the impact resistance.

FRAME MATERIALS. The advance from wire frames to even-tension plastic mountings brought with it the question of dangerous flammability. Frames made of cellulose nitrate are highly flammable and burn with vicious splattering of flaming particles over a distance of a few feet. Just as the motion picture industry abandoned the risk of a guncotton-derived plastic for film, so the Optical Manufacturers Association of this nation has required the elimination of cellulose nitrate from the frame industry. Unfortunately, some foreign manufacturers still import these attractive and easily polished frames which can be ignited by a match or cigarette. The Food and Drug Administration, through its Hazardous Substance Branch, has acted against these imports, and the American National Standards Institute (ANSI) has excluded them from "first quality" codes. All frames should be of slowly combustible or fire-retardant plastic; this commonly is cellulose acetate or cellulose butyrate.

Secondary Missiles and Secondary Ocular Injuries

The previously discussed principles of (1) impact-resistant lens materials, (2) using plastic rather than wire rims to avoid undesirable torque in the lenses, and (3) added support of lenses by posterior lips on the eyepieces of frames are all spectacle factors in *protecting* the eyes from foreign bodies and blast or splash trauma. Hazards due to the spectacles themselves are (1) flammability of frame materials and (2) the injurious potential of displaced or broken lenses. Apparently owing to poor reporting and failure of ophthalmic surgeons to identify mechanisms and materials of injury, previous textbooks (Duke-Elder, 1954) have disclaimed a major or consecutive role of spectacles in producing eye trauma. Both personal and institutional experience here are distinctly to the contrary (Keeney and Estlow, 1971) (Fig. 17–1).

Nonheat-tempered crown glass, as also used in both the front and back glass layers of laminated lenses, tends to spall into multiple, sharp, slender, and vicious fragments when it is broken (Keeney, 1965). These may easily penetrate the cornea and anterior ocular components or perforate the globe with deep and serious lacerations. Heat-tempered glass lenses, however, like similarly tempered glass in side windows of automobiles, tend to

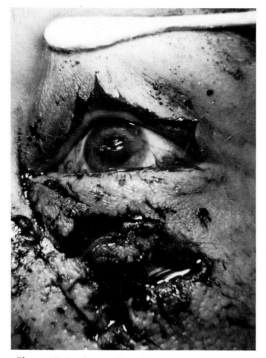

Figure 17–1 Lacerations from spectacle glass fragments deep into the cornea, sclera, and both lids, penetrating to the periosteum.

crumble into thicker and more obtuse fragments when their limit of elasticity is exceeded. These are less likely to penetrate or perforate the globe and may actually be rolled in one's hand with general impunity.

The nonsafety lens, like flammable frames, not only fails to provide protection but of itself becomes a dangerous device which can send secondary missiles of glass fragments deep into the eye (Keeney, 1965) or lead to facial or fatal burns (Van Portfliet and Fralick, 1951). Fragmentation of the softer or less brittle allyl resin lenses, when it does occur, generally yields a small number of relatively large fragments which are not saber-like in configuration. These plastic lenses, when impacted at energy levels above their modulus of rupture, may show only a linear crack or two with the fragments sometimes clinging together in the frame after having prevented perforation. When small fragmentation occurs, as in the contact area from a relatively small and high-energy missile, again rather obtuse and crumblike fragments are produced. These do not easily penetrate the eye.

Not only prescription lens fragments from nonheat-treated glass but also segments of thin and inexpensive acrylic plastic lenses have been extracted from their lacerations deep into the globe or orbit on numerous occasions. Even the inexpensive sunglasses found on a display card in gas stations or drug stores can be a valuable protection to the human eyes or can be a hazardous source of secondary missiles. All lenses worn on the face should be impact-resistant shields, particularly in the case of children, workers in hazardous occupations, individuals who have lost effective sight in one eye, or those who drive or ride in automobiles. The American National Standards Institute Z80.3–1972 code for sunglasses and fashion eyewear, for the first time, sets minimal safety performance standards for such lenses.

Automotive Injuries to the Eyes

The most common cause of childhood injury is agreed by nearly all investigators to be the automobile. Automobile crashes are reported to be the leading cause of death from ages 1 to 24 (Snyder, 1969). Factors in automotive crash causation are legion, generally multiple in any crash, and enormously difficult to prove or tabulate in verified rank of importance (Keeney, 1964). In childhood it is thus particularly necessary to establish measures for injury reduction and attenuation of the "second impact" within the vehicle or, with five times greater tragedy, on ejection from the vehicle. Though the child is removed from the special risks of the driver (steering column impalement, greater exposure), he presents both inferior skull resistance to impact and a disproportionate head-to-body mass which increases the frequency and severity of head injuries (Snyder, 1969).

Statistical tabulations from the Automotive Crash Injury Research Program at Cornell confirm that about 75 per cent of all body damage in auto crashes involves head injury. About 10 per cent of all body injuries involve the eye or adnexa (Garrett, 1963). This is nearly five times more frequent than ocular injuries among battlefield casualty survivors in Vietnam. The "battered child syndrome" has been widely described in medical, sociologic, and lay presses as a result of adult abuse, and yet the "neglected child syndrome" of an unrestrained child in an automobile crash accounts for 250,000 to 1,000,000 injured children each year. The Trauma Research Group at UCLA has shown that usually *two* children are damaged in each injury producing crash and that each child averages two significant types or sites of injury. Most injuries are at impact speeds under 40 miles per hour, and the speed of 30 m.p.h. generally divides fatal from non-fatal injuries (Siegel et al., 1968). Though windshields continue to be a major source of face and head trauma, introduction in 1966 of the new high penetration resistance (HPR) glass with the plastic interlayer (polyvinylbutyral) increased from 0.015 to 0.030 inch (0.38 to 0.76 mm.) thickness has produced a major reduction in ocular and facial lacerations. Further reductions in eye and head injuries by improved glazing are available at the engineering level (Van Laethan, 1968).

In spite of safety improvements in vehicle design during the last four years, it is still essential to utilize restraint systems for children and to recognize the greater susceptibility to head damage as a result of the center of gravity being several inches higher than in adolescence. Thus, the lap-belted child tends to go into forward head rotation more rapidly than does the adult who has a lower center of gravity.

In general, some type of harness, safety vest, or multiple element system with wider load distribution than conventional 2-inch wide lap belts is needed for children under 4 to 6 years of age. For infants to the age of about 6 months, a car bed-bassinet offers some security if placed on the rear seat in line with the length of the car. The rear supports, generally left folded, can be secured with the center rear lap belt, and the usually extended front supports can be secured by threading the center front lap belt through them. The infant should be placed feet forward and a sturdy netting secured over the bassinet. In 1969, General Motors introduced its lightweight (6 lb.) and inexpensive "Infant Safety Carrier," which is basically a double shell, molded, deep plastic pan secured to the car seat with a standard lap belt (Sierent,

1969). The infant faces rearward, and the belt does not touch his body. It is designed for infants up to about 9 months of age or 20 lb. weight. On to the age of 1 or 2 years, a vest* or upper and lower torso harness** should be worn by the child and when in the car this is coupled to a vertical harness looped around the seat back and anchored through the floor.

After the age of 1½ or 2 years, a molded plastic seat and restraint device anchored by the conventional lap belt offers good protection.† The Ford Motor Company "Tot-Guard" (1967) affords particularly good head and eye protection. The General Motors Child Safety Seat (Model II, 1968) is slightly more complicated with upper torso webbing and less potential protection to the face. The Union Carbide Corporation Astro-Guard Seat II (1966) available in many department stores needs a seat back loop as well as the standard lap belt and provides double shoulder restraint but is the most expensive of this group (Fredericks, 1969). The Firestone-Hamill "Protecta-Tot" metal tubing and cushioned seat introduced in 1971 for use with the standard adult lap belt also serves as a child's seat for table use. Other encouraging designs are "The Guardian," "Auto-Safe," and "Bobby Mac Chairs."

After the age of 3 or 4, the adult lap belt should be used and may offer more acceptable visibility if combined with a firm, backless cushion 6 to 9 inches high. A bandolier or single oblique shoulder harness should *not* be used with the lap belt for either short adults or children under a height of about 4½ feet because of increased potential for neck and laryngeal injury.

Although the search for completely passive restraint systems—requiring no action on the part of vehicle occupants—is being strongly pushed and even date-

---

*Irvin Child Safety Harness, Irving Air Chute Company, Lexington, Kentucky; Sears, Roebuck and Company.

**Castiglione "Tot-Trava-Safe," Tulareloft, Inc., Tulare, California.

†National Highway Traffic Safety Administration, FMVSS, Standard No. 213, which became effective April 1, 1971, prescribes minimal performance standards for such seating systems for children between the ages of 6 months and 3 years.

lined by the U.S. National Highway Safety Administration, the most widely useful and statistically validated safeguard against crash injury is the occupant-coupled, appropriate, multiple webbing restraint. In the adult, this is the double shoulder, inverted Y harness and seat belt. In children, further research is still needed in both design and production, but at all times in all automobiles children must be safeguarded against the needless horrors of second impacts within the car and the even worse ejections beyond the car.

EXAMINATION OF THE INJURED EYE

As in all medical and ocular problems, both urgency and efficiency require a division of approach into *preliminary* and *definitive* or *detailed* phases. This applies to the history, physical examination, and even answering of phone inquiries. In an office well attuned to patient needs, the receptionist knows that the essential response to a mother's phone call for aid in the case of chemical splash into a child's eye is not to ask the name and address but rather to interrupt the distraught mother with calm yet firm instructions to flush the eye immediately under a water tap, after which the mother should call back promptly and arrange for emergency medical treatment.

Similarly, the ophthalmologist begins significant portions of his examination simply upon first seeing the patient and *simultaneously* acquires preliminary items of the history (Paton and Goldberg, 1968). In minor injuries, such as those from wind-blown foreign bodies, the steps of history taking and examination are undertaken as the usual procedures in elective office consultation. In contrast, with massive middle-third facial injuries, as from an unrestrained child being crushed into an automobile dashboard, immediate concern is with the airway and vital signs.

The following is the usual progression of steps in reception of a child with ocular injury. Preliminary history is taken in accord with the exigency of the child's condition. Usually, details of the offending instruments and mechanism are re-

vealed better as examination and understanding of the injuries unfold. Thus, whether an intraorbital pellet, clearly expected by history or demonstrated by x-ray, is copper-coated, lead, or steel is best established by a relative bringing in samples of the ammunition used. Whether glass fragments found in the globe come from nonsafety spectacles or a wind-shield—of importance in prophylactic programing, though not in individual ocular repair—can be established later by "search and rescue" of the spectacles or a photograph of the windshield.

1. *General Condition.* Airway, vital signs, and head injuries.

2. *Preliminary History.* Circumstances and position during injury; previous general health (diabetes, seizures, nephritis, or the like); ocular health (strabismus, amblyopia, congenital defects, glasses); and current medications or drug sensitivities.

3. *Preliminary Inspection of Ocular Adnexa.* Lids, glabella, orbital rims, and so on, and their obscuration by edema, ecchymosis, or emphysema.

4. *Topical Anesthetic.* In the responsive—and always apprehensive—child, these are called "feel better drops," and the first ones are instilled over the *closed* lid borders before attempting to open them. Avoid pontocaine which burns and compounds patient fears. Avoid cocaine, which softens the epithelium and may give confusing pupillary dilatation.

5. *The Globes.* Damage, position, rotation. When major lacerations, large foreign bodies, or prolapse of ocular contents are detected, further details of examination should be deferred until full arrangements and instrumentation are available for repair.

6. *Laboratory Work.* Hemoglobin, type and cross-match, and so forth as may be needed for general condition or for surgery.

7. *Visual Acuity.* Without and with glasses, as appropriate. Even in extensive injuries, try to establish pupillary reactions, differentiate light perception and projection, or determine better degrees of vision, such as counting fingers at a specified number of feet from the patient.

8. *Fluorescein Staining.* Use individually packaged, dry, sterile fluorescein paper strips rather than aqueous solutions, which

are notorious for growing *Pseudomonas aeruginosa*. Remember it is the intact and exposed Bowman's membrane which stains intensively with fluorescein, and if this layer has been destroyed in a chemical burn, the corneal stroma stains diffusely but less intensively. Damage or loss of epithelium in the bulbar conjunctiva yields a yellowish coloration to fluorescein.

9. *Detailed Bulbar Examination.* This should begin with oblique focal illumination and never a glaring source directed frontally and painfully into the eye. The examiner should be wearing a loupe both to minimize subsequent steps and, in some minor cases, to detect an offending small foreign body under the upper lid, with possible completion of care by removing it on the tip of his thumb in continuation of the eversion maneuver. In suspect and frank perforations, caution must be exercised to avoid any pressure on the globe by the examiner's fingers or by the patient involuntarily squeezing his lids. This can cause irreparable loss of vitreous or lens, with needless complication of the original laceration.

At times, a facial nerve block of the Atkinson type is both a safeguard and an aid to inspection. Two per cent lidocaine with epinephrine can be injected painlessly if a perfectly sharp, small (26 or 27 gauge) needle is used with flooding both before the skin is entered and continuously during advancement.

Instrumental procedures should not be more extensive than indicated by the child's condition. Some elegant steps are contraindicated in early phases of trauma management. Thus, scleral depression for indirect ophthalmoscopy of the periphery is deferred following anterior segment lacerations; gonioscopy in search of angle recession is similarly deferred during the days after a small initial hyphema has cleared. On the other hand, several valuable but simple procedures are frequently overlooked. Transillumination (with a Finoff tip) of the lid may reveal an embedded radiolucent foreign body; transscleral transillumination (Finoff or Mira tip) may similarly localize a foreign body in an opaque lens or differentiate a pigmented but translucent inclusion cyst from a similarly dark-colored but completely opaque hematoma or malignant melanoma. Inspection with the ultraviolet Wood's or Hague light may precisely identify a luxated lens or lens fragment by its fluorescence. On the rare occasion when eye surgeons make use of this light, however, they fail to obtain its value because they don't pause to achieve their own dark adaptation. When working under the high luminance of surgical lights, an ophthalmologist is incapable of detecting low-intensity fluorescence, unless he both closes his eyes and pauses for a few minutes with the operating lights off.

Don't hesitate, even with a 1 or 2 year old child, to attempt indicated slit lamp study with the child in the parent's arms. Gonioscopy and tonometry can be done after the age of $3\frac{1}{2}$ or 4 with repeated instillations of topical anesthetic, so that you truthfully stick by your promise not to hurt. Even incisional removal of corneal foreign bodies can be done at the slit lamp with the stable 5 or 6 year old and a mature, comforting ophthalmologist. Many embedded foreign bodies can be removed this way safely and more quickly for the patient, and in a more easily familiar approach for the physician.

10. *X-ray Examination.* In the presence of airway impairments, facial fractures, or corneal lacerations (constituting about two thirds of penetrating bulbar wounds), it is often unwise to position a patient face down for usual PA and Water's views. A compromise may be achieved if the x-ray equipment affords these views in the sitting position for the cooperative youngster in neither shock nor syncope. Frequently, the hydrostatic needs for closing corneal wounds transcend any technical urgency or medicolegal routinism in obtaining scout films for unlikely foreign bodies. However, in a properly planned search for minute, anterior bulbar foreign bodies, even of such low radiopacity as glass, a bone free study (Vogt) using a small dental film pressed into the inner canthal area must be included. Adequate low density definition is assured if the film shows individual cilia.

Skull films in various PA and ipsilateral projections may not reveal small orbital cracks and bone defects or soft tissue density foreign bodies such as wood and glass. In these cases, PA and lateral laminagrams, or preferably the newer hypocycloidal tomograms, may be needed, particularly to demonstrate blowout fractures of the orbital floor. A submento-vertex projection should be ordered to identify suspect fractures of the zygomatic arch or medial orbital wall.

MINOR DISTURBANCES OF INJURY THAT MAY CONCEAL MORE EXTENSIVE INJURIES

1. *"Black Eye" (Lid Ecchymosis).* All such patients should be examined for evidence of blowout fractures of the orbit, as well as contusion damage to the globe (hyphema, iridodialysis, dislocation of the lens, retinal edema, choroidal rupture).

2. *Small Conjunctival Laceration.* Critical fundus search for edema or perforation should be made beneath such a wound. During cleansing under topical anesthetic, the surgeon must be certain there is no underlying scleral laceration, and this may require extending the conjunctival wound for direct visual exploration.

3. *Conjunctival Hemorrhage.* This is rarely spontaneous in the child without hematologic disease. It may obscure a foreign body which is suggested by a telltale spot of yellowish stain after fluorescein at a site of perforation.

4. *Subconjunctival Hemorrhage.* This is generally darker than the conjunctival hemorrhage, but either may result from contusion. A hemorrhage appearing or progressing deep in a canthal recess many hours after initial head trauma suggests anterior cranial fossa fracture. Usually, it is impossible to see beyond or proximal to these deep hemorrhages, and the conjunctiva may be moved over them by traction on the lid.

5. *Small Perforating Wound.* If corneal, this may be produced by a small glass or metallic fragment which becomes hidden behind the limbus, usually inferiorly. This may be evidenced months later by localized recurrent bullous keratopathy or by color changes in the iris or lens capsule due to chalcosis or hemosiderosis from copper or iron. Such wounds in the sclera demand careful search for particles in the posterior globe. Iron is the most common domestic offender, particularly destroying the ganglion cells and pigment epithelium leading to irreversible retinal impairment which a child may not acknowledge so long as he has good vision in the other eye.

6. *Conjunctivitis Secondary to Embedded Foreign Body.* This may mask a small or large foreign body in the upper cul-de-sac not apparent on single eversion of the lid. Woody or weedy fragments commonly lodge here as a running child falls in brush. Other items such as BB's or "lost" contact lenses may hide or embed in the far recess of the upper cul-de-sac. Double eversion with a Walker or Desmarres everter is always needed to inspect this recess, and at times an incision into an apparent granuloma is necessary.

7. *Retinal Edema.* Contusion, either direct or by blast (shock) effect, which is sufficient to cause edema anywhere in the fundus may produce traumatic retinal detachment, particularly in the inferior temporal periphery in children. After initial edema has subsided during 5 to 10 days of curtailed activity, careful inspection of the peripheral retina, ora, and pars plana should be done with appropriate scleral indentation. Early retinopexy of a small hole or dialysis may avoid a more extensive procedure or even macular detachment later.

Diffuse retinal edema or associated hemorrhage into the vitreous may initially obscure more significant contusion rupture of the choroid. Usually this appears as irregular white arcs beneath the retina and concentric to the disc (Fig. 17–2). Pigment

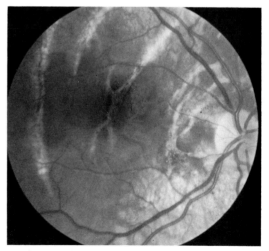

Figure 17–2 Multiple choroidal ruptures and associated retinal edema from recent contusion injury.

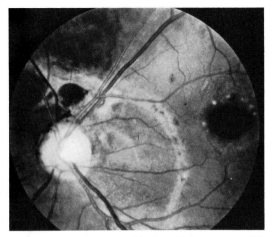

Figure 17–3 Large, old choroidal rupture with secondary pigmentary scarring and permanent reduction of central visual acuity.

may accumulate in these "cracks" with the passage of weeks (Fig. 17–3).

8. *Perforating Injuries of Posterior Orbit into the Brain.* An external wound in the lid or the conjunctiva may appear insignificant unless a history of "perforation in depth" has been obtained. Small children playing with long, sharp objects frequently provide no history. The sudden onset of acute meningitis may be the first sign that the injury was indeed serious.

9. *Traumatic or Contusion Hyphema.* Seriousness of bleeding within the closed space of the anterior chamber has long been recognized and the statistically worsened prognosis with recurrent bleeding is well documented. Recently, however, there has been good evidence correlating the extent of traumatic angle recession (by number of quadrants involved) with the magnitude of hyphema and associated damages, such as lens dislocation and iris tears.

TRAUMATIC OR CONTUSION HYPHEMA

Traumatic hyphema or contusion hyphema is always a serious intraocular disturbance signaled by the presence of blood in the anterior chamber. This characteristically results from blunt injury to the eye as distinguished from lacerating or perforating injuries, whether accidentally or surgically sustained. One unique property of this injury is sometimes characterized as "closed space injury" or "closed space bleeding." The offending agent may be no more than the flipped end of a washcloth, necktie, or similar item. It may be a toy, a small ball, a clod of dirt, or a thrown rock. The injury is distinctly more frequent in males than in females, and when resulting from simple accidents, such as falls, occurs in a male-to-female distribution of approximately 3 to 1; its relationship to more aggressive behavior, such as fists, BB's, and ice balls, appears in a male-to-female distribution of approximately 8 to 1. The mechanics of injury may be likened to the deformation of a ping-pong ball under localized pressure followed by prompt reformation of the ball on release of the pressure.

Accumulated evidence from post-injury gonioscopy and histologic specimens indicates that the overwhelming anatomical cause of such anterior segment bleeding is a tear in the ciliary body. This usually disrupts an anterior ciliary artery branch such as an arterial twig to the ciliary muscles or one of the 10 to 12 recurrent choroidal arteries; one of the large efferent veins from the ciliary body to the episcleral plexis may instead be torn. Far less frequently than tears into the anterior ciliary body, there may rarely be cyclodialysis, with avulsion of the anterior ciliary muscle insertion from the scleral spur. The presence of associated ocular injuries is directly proportional to the number of quadrants involved in the ciliary body tear. These associated anterior segment injuries include ruptures of the iris sphincter, iridodialysis, traumatic cataract, subluxation of the lens, luxation of the lens, and subconjunctival scleral rupture. Generally, as most anterior segment surgeons well realize, bleeding is not evoked by dialysis of the thin iris root from its usual insertion into the ciliary body, or from division of the iris sphincter. Except in the presence of iris or vascular disease such as rubeosis, severed blood vessels in the iris promptly retract and are sealed by the elastic architecture of the iris. Surgeons concerned with contusion injury hyphema are therefore concerned with both location and extent of ciliary body tears and their disruption of vessels proximal to the anterior chamber angle.

Prognosis is related to the extensiveness

of the ciliary body tear and roughly to the amount of blood in the anterior chamber. Thus, minute amounts of bright blood in the anterior chamber, though always of potentially serious consequence, offer less immediate concern than do large hemorrhages. Similarly, large hemorrhages not quite filling the anterior chamber present less threat of overwhelming glaucoma than do black hyphemas (eight-ball hemorrhages) completely occupying the chamber.

Although prognosis for a small initial hyphema is encouraging with no more than supportive care, this prognosis abruptly changes in the presence of secondary bleeding, which usually occurs between the second and sixth days following injury and may at times recur over several episodes.

Blood in the anterior chamber may preclude visualization of associated injuries and does contraindicate the manipulations of gonioscopy which are ultimately necessary to assess the total injury. Generally, gonioscopy is not done for a period of two or three weeks following complete absorption of blood and quieting of the eye.

The secondary glaucoma accompanying traumatic hyphema may be due to initial contusion damage to the trabecular meshwork, which in turn is further decompensated by red blood cells and their breakdown products occluding the trabecular interstices. As a third factor, the volume of blood liberated into the closed space of the globe may directly increase hydraulic pressure within the eye, compounding this glaucoma. If unrelieved, ultimate organization and fibrosis of a large blood clot filling the chamber spells loss of sight and eye.

Although hyphema may prevent visualization of anterior segment details, the physician first examining such an injured eye must also make complete and gentle examination to rule out associated foreign body injuries, hidden cul-de-sac wounds, or other orbital disorders such as anterior cranial fossa fracture with deep subconjunctival or orbital bleeding progressing from the nasal aspect of the orbit as much as 36 hours after injury.

Nausea and vomiting often compound the ocular disturbance. Transient increases in intrathoracic pressure associated with vomiting increase venous pressure and

distention in the neck and head, thus favoring further intraocular bleeding. Nausea and vomiting produced by the glaucoma of traumatic hyphema may mislead the general physician into search for abdominal distress.

Treatment

The isolated, *traumatic hyphema* with or without nausea and vomiting, is best treated by bed rest, sedation, and removal of the patient from a congested environment. If added support and comfort can be brought to a youngster, either at home or under hospital care, binocular patches may be used to achieve quietude of the eyes as well as of the body. In a highly apprehensive youngster, it is better to leave the uninjured eye open. Television and the distraction of other individuals should be reduced, but a bedside radio may offer considerable comfort.

When there is no glaucoma, as is commonly true with small, initial, or primary hemorrhages, antiglaucomatous medications should not be used prophylactically because their potential for reducing intraocular pressure may foster further bleeding. Likewise, surgical evacuation is contraindicated as long as intraocular tension is normal or can be normalized.

The greatest concern in treatment is to avoid secondary hemorrhage and complications of secondary glaucoma. The eye of the child or young adult will generally not stand abrupt elevations of intraocular pressure for a period exceeding 24 to 48 hours without serious damage. When such eyes ultimately clear, if not going on to phthisis, they show the stigmata of the postcongestive triad: (1) iris atrophy, (2) synechia, and (3) glaucoma flecken. Tragically, this triad is often worsened by concurrent optic nerve damage from ischemia.

When secondary glaucoma supervenes, efforts should be made to control it by oral Diamox or glycerin. This may be augmented by topical Levo-epinephrine 2 per cent two or three times a day, but its effectiveness is limited and slow in onset. Keratocentesis as a temporizing measure may, in a child, require general anesthetic, which distinctly compounds the risk and problems of care in a procedure which is of transient value only. When the chamber is so completely filled with blood that no iris details are visible and secondary glaucoma is not controllable by oral medication, the surgeon then has only a day or two to temporize before evacuating the clot surgically. Sears (1970) has well pointed out that if pressure can be normalized, clot retraction is optimal at four days after bleeding, and this timing mechanically facilitates freeing of the clot from the iris and occasionally delivering an intact "collar button clot." Here the anterior and posterior chamber blood clots are united by a narrow band through the pupillary aperture. Delay to the fourth day, however, may increase the possibility of intraocular ischemic damage if ocular tension is not normalized.

Surgical removal of a large anterior chamber clot or "eight ball" should be done through an adequate limbal incision, affording the introduction of an irrigating tip or rarely a cupped capsule forceps to assist in withdrawing the clot. The use of a cryoextractor (Hill, 1968) cannot be easily controlled and may cause fractionation of the clot or engagement of the iris. Kelman experimentally used a vibrating tip at 25,-000 cycles per second through a small incision in an effort to break down organized clots (Kelman and Brooks, 1971). The potential hazards and quantitation of energy delivered to the anterior chamber structures by such an instrument are not yet critically determined.

At irrigation of a large clot, it is not unusual for ischemic iris to prolapse. When the iris does appear white and devoid of its blood supply, it is preferable to excise the iris minimally rather than to reposition it repetitively. If the prolapsed iris is of healthy coloration and apparently with good arterial supply, the surgeon may evaluate the added trauma of reposition versus ease in completion of the clot delivery. After clearing the chamber, there is a potential for further hemorrhage attendant upon both reduction of intraocular pressure and the reopening of injured sites. At this point, the surgeon, however, gains visible control of the anterior chamber, even though semicontinuous lavage may be necessary to maintain visibility. It may be possible to identify a limbal location beneath which blood is issuing. If this can be done, partial-penetrating diathermy may be applied to the sclera 2 to 4 mm.

from the limbus through a small conjunctival incision. With luck, this may control further bleeding. On closure of the incision, the surgeon should instill a large bubble of air into the anterior chamber approaching the stage of air block glaucoma again in an effort to avoid further bleeding.

The complication of *blood staining to the cornea* relates to damaged endothelium, such as that caused by traumatic indentation, or to protracted and severe elevation of intraocular pressure. Usually a combination of the two elements facilitates diffusion of breakdown blood products into the corneal stroma. If intraocular pressure is normalized, this reddish-brown discoloration of the cornea slowly absorbs from the periphery and assumes a round or disclike configuration which may require two or three years to clear. Lesser degrees, of course, clear in a matter of months. Blood staining of the cornea is not of itself an indication for surgical intervention or for corneal transplantation.

Late evaluation necessitates careful gonioscopy through 360 degrees to assess the amount of ciliary body tear and consequent angle recession. This appears as a deepened ciliary body band in the anterior chamber angle, or rarely as a light gray or whitish area extending proximal to the scleral spur when the ciliary body has been dialyzed from its normal insertion. The ciliary body tear is not responsible for glaucoma but is an index of associated damage, particularly to the trabecular area. Such eyes may have secondary glaucoma not only in the acute throes of the trauma but by insidious onset as late as 10 or 12 years following damage.

Long-term management also requires careful indirect ophthalmoscopy of the peripheral fundus to search for associated retinal dialysis and traumatic holes. When found, these must be treated according to their own indications.

ORBITAL FRACTURES

The classic division of the face into lower, middle, and upper thirds commits the ophthalmologist, literally, to deep involvement in both middle third and upper third fractures, because the floor of the orbit is the dividing line between these two major areas. The traditional French classification of fractures by La Forte at the turn of the century defines the La Forte II as a middle-third fracture extending through the inferior orbital rims, orbital floors, glabella, and zygomaticomaxillary suture lines. The La Forte III generally involves the orbits more posteriorly through the ethmoids and sphenoids as well as the zygomaticofrontal and maxillofrontal sutures. This latter fracture gives a craniofacial dysjunction or detachment of the midfacial bones from the cranium, with major neurological concerns of brain injury and cerebrospinal rhinorrhea.

The British classification of middle-third facial fractures, evolved during World War II, gives more completely detailed classification by division into *central* and *lateral* with first, second, and third degrees of severity. Though these have progressive ophthalmic significance (first-degree central is limited almost exclusively to nasolacrimal damage), primary management is usually in the province of the maxillofacial surgeon. The ophthalmologist, however, should be cognizant of ramifications and difficulties of orbital and zygomatic fractures, so that in a time of need he may be able to handle them alone. When teeth are present and alveolar arch fractures coexist, it is wise to have these secured first to establish a baseline for further alignments (Georgiade, 1969).

Somewhat more than a half century after La Forte's studies, it became clearly apparent that midthird fractures of the face could consist of orbital floor, less commonly medial wall, or rarely roof fractures, without breaks in the orbital rim. These are the *blowout* fractures caused by force transmitted through an intact globe. The striking object, commonly a fist or ball, generally has a radius of curvature of about 1 but less than 2 inches. The radius of the orbital entrance varies between 15 and 20 mm. If the radius of curvature of the striking object is about 2 inches or greater, it is essentially impossible to intrude on the orbital contents, and the impact from such an object is taken by the heavy orbital rim. Orbital wall fractures, of course, can be produced by objects of this or greater radius, but they are associated with rim fractures.

The clinical findings in orbital blowout fracture are

Periorbital swelling and ecchymosis	100 per cent
Vertical diplopia	75 per cent
Fracture seen on tomography	60 per cent
Enophthalmos	50 per cent
Positive forced duction test	50 per cent
Infraorbital nerve hypoesthesia	40 per cent
Fracture seen on plain x-ray	35 per cent
Serious ocular injury	10 per cent

Orbital or periorbital emphysema may be present when the fractures involve the ethmoid air cells or the medial orbital wall.

Treatment

When there is vertical diplopia, significant enophthalmos, limitation of forced ductions, or distinct x-ray evidence of orbital tissue incarcerated into the orbital floor (as by the "bomb-bay" or downward convexity of the antral roof mucosa into the antrum), orbital floor exploration is indicated. In the absence of enophthalmos, and with adequate forced rotations, it is doubtful that either diplopia or x-ray demonstration of fractures warrants intervention. Although children begin bone repair as early as five days post-injury, it is technically feasible to postpone orbital floor repair for four to six days if post-injury swelling or timing of patient transfer so dictates. Delay of a few weeks, however, complicates the outlook for easy freeing of incarcerations, functional elimination of vertical imbalances, or control of enophthalmos. After a few months, it becomes even more difficult but not impossible.

Current surgical practice is to insert the thinnest possible sheet of Teflon or Silastic as a subperiosteal implant to bridge the floor defect. This should be sufficiently posterior to avoid any tensions in closing of the periosteum and more superficial tissues. When definite enophthalmos is a complicating factor, implants up to 3 mm. in thickness or plastic enucleation conformers can be introduced to cover the defect and to lift the globe upward as well as forward.

Among the serious orbital injuries, upper-third facial fractures represent the area of greatest risk of associated brain injury. Schultz (1969) reported 36 of these within his series of 1042 consecutive facial injuries. Seventy-two per cent of the 36 resulted from automobile injuries, usually from the dashboard or lower windshield (an additional 14 per cent came lately from motorcycle injuries). Hospitalization tended to be about three times as long as for the average facial injury. All the patients presented periorbital ecchymosis, and 90 per cent had lacerations of the brow or upper lid. Restrictions of bulbar movement and diplopia were almost always associated with supraorbital fractures, but bulbar lacerations were infrequent. Satisfactory x-rays are often difficult to obtain at the time of injury because of airway problems and difficulty in positioning the face against x-ray film for PA exposure. Open exploration and reduction must be done (1) through an incisional extension of the laceration, (2) through a brow incision and exploration, or (3) by development of a thick forehead (scalp) flap. Bone fragments may commonly be found driven deep into the orbit, and such circumstances necessitate search for levator and superior rectus lacerations which require initial suturing. Bone fragments should be preserved and replaced under direct vision whenever possible. Secondary plastic repairs, split rib grafts, or medium hard block dimethyl polysiloxane (Silastic) implants may be anticipated in about one fourth of cases.

OCULAR BURNS AND NEWER CONCEPTS IN THEIR TREATMENT

Burns may be considered on the basis of their origin as *chemical, thermal, electrical,* and *radiational,* though principles of care are similar (Roper-Hall, 1965). In childhood, burns are nearly always the result of household chemicals* and frequently the consequence of unguarded action by busy mothers. The prime consideration of *immediate* copious irrigation with water has been stressed. This is repeated under topical anesthesia by the receiving or emergency room staff and the ophthalmologist, who presses the search for hidden particu-

*Ammonia, lime, alkalis, liquid soaps, Drano, Liquid-plumr.

late chemical or associated foreign matter. The extent of damage is assessed by (1) area and intensity of fluorescein stain, (2) area and intensity of ischemia in the pericorneal bulbar conjunctiva, and (3) degree of corneal opacification. When there is only epithelial involvement of the cornea and when hyperemia has not given way to ischemia of the bulbar conjunctiva, almost any noninjurious management will be followed by satisfactory healing.

Major challenges present themselves when ischemia affects half or more of the perilimbal conjunctiva and there is diffuse, though light, fluorescein staining of most of the cornea associated with opalescence and impaired ability to visualize iris details. In these major burns several new techniques now give promise of improved salvage.

1. *Constant Irrigation.* A perforated silicone T tube may be inserted through a stab wound of the lower cul-de-sac and then attached to a suspended intravenous bottle of sterile Ringer solution containing an antibiotic and sometimes steroids (Stokes and Houser, 1969). This provides constant irrigation without frequent nursing attendance and without digital opening of lids which may also present burned and sensitive surfaces. Alternatively, a channeled silicone ring (like the solid acrylic Walser ring conformer) or a tubed contact lens conformer may be inserted to maintain the cul-de-sacs and concurrently provide constant conjunctival irrigation from an intravenous drip.

2. *Subconjunctival Injection of the Patient's Own Blood (Novosibirsk Procedure).* This is used immediately to (1) nourish ischemic tissues, (2) provide a compatible buffer solution, (3) dilute the invading chemical, and (4) act as a barrier to deeper penetration. This is not in the vague concept of "autohemotherapy" and the Russian theory of biotherapy. Final results of these and other measures are difficult to assess in relation to precise degrees of burn.

3. *Removal of Necrotic and Chemical Impregnated Tissues.* This may be easily decided upon and carried out in the lower conjunctiva in some cases, but often it is uncertain. Emergency keratoplasty (keratoplasty au chaud) (Alberth, 1968) has similar value when Bowman's membrane and stromal tissue are lost and the corneal surface is irregularly pocked. Such heroic

measures also necessitate full lavage of the anterior chamber, which many surgeons are reluctant to do by puncture through devitalized limbal tissues. A living homograft offers relatively enhanced resistance to neovascularization, whereas the results of late grafting through densely vascularized tissue are known to be poor.

4. *Chelation of Calcific Deposits.* For unknown reasons, healing of chemical burns in children may be accompanied by early and superficial calcific scarring. This seems to exert a vasotrophic influence, but the deposits may be removed by disodium versinate (Versene or EDTA) drip for 5 to 15 minutes over the area after de-epithelialization. Such procedures may have to be repeated a few times over the months of healing.

5. *Flush-fitting Scleral Shells or Scleral Flange Contact Lenses (Ridley).* These acrylic lenses can be made from molds by a skilled technician within a couple of hours, and when elected for major corneal or cul-de-sac burns, they should be prepared immediately or within a few days after the initial edema subsides. Deep sedation or even general anesthesia may be required in the restive child. They aid in maintenance of the cul-de-sacs and prevention of adhesion between burned surfaces. Good exchange of tears and liquid medications is afforded both beneath the shells and well into the fornices. Inspection is facilitated. Patient comfort is surprising and gratifying.

6. *Maintenance of Lacrimal Puncta.* Too frequently, punctal preservation is neglected in the face of major corneal and conjunctival burns. Stenosis is less likely if some firm material is inserted immediately through the punctal site when the lid border in this area is burned or stains with fluorescein. Gelatin rods of 1-mm. diameter (Foulds, 1961) or nonchromicized catgut suture material of 1- or 2-gauge diameter is suitable for this purpose and has the advantage of spontaneous absorption in 10 to 15 days. There is no concern with possible loss or displacement of such materials as there is with silicone or polyethylene.

OCULAR LACERATIONS

A disproportionate incidence of ocular lacerations occurs in children, particularly in the first decade of life and decreasing by almost half in the second decade. Most of these are associated with play and not with the retained small metallic foreign bodies seen in adult male workers. The male preponderance increases with the potentially predatory nature of activities. Thus, bow-and-arrow, BB, and even occasional 0.22-calibre gun wounds are represented far more frequently in males than are the injuries from falls and auto crashes.

Several factors in management of ocular lacerations have been well established in the decades following World War II.

Gains Established in the Postwar Decade

1. Direct suturing should almost completely supersede the use of conjunctival flaps.

2. Infection should be essentially eliminated by prophylactic administration of penicillin and other antibiotics systemically and subconjunctivally.

3. Principles of debridement have been established for each type of ocular tissue. Bulbar conjunctiva may be debrided, excised, and mobilized liberally. Lid, tarsal, and scleral tissue should be minimally debrided, and corneal tissue should almost never be excised, except in preparation for full-thickness donor grafting. Irregular or complex skin and lid wounds may be reduced by excision to eliminate jagged tear lines and obtain simple linear closures.

4. Self-sealing linear corneal wounds, usually under 3 mm. in length, or small tongue wounds with good reformation of the anterior chamber and no uveal incarceration should be left unsutured.

5. Complete reformation of the anterior chamber with air rather than fluid after direct suturing greatly reduces the incidence of adherent leukoma, anterior synechia, and closed angle glaucoma. Iris bombé in a child's eye will almost certainly lead to loss of the eye, regardless of further surgical interventions (Reinecke and Beyer, 1966). Both Roper-Hall (1959) and Reinecke have recorded the statistically improved salvage with this technique. Air may be injected through the original wound using a small right-angle cannula as designed by Rycroft (1957) or through a knife needle or Wheeler knife track made in a contralateral limbal site over the intact iris. This latter technique reduces the undesirable potential of air behind the iris.

Newer Concepts of the 1960s

1. *Anterior Vitrectomy.* Until recent years, vitreous loss and the adverse effects of incarceration were expected concomitants of (1) removal of dislocated lenses, (2) removal of traumatic cataracts with through-and-through perforations, and (3) repair of major anterior segment lacerations with uveal prolapse and lens disorganization. Such eyes are now treated by appropriate direct surgery plus planned removal of anterior vitreous through the wound or limbal incision until the anterior vitreous surface falls posterior to the iris plane and preferably appears concave. Small triangular cellulose sponges (Edward Weck & Co., Inc.), individually mounted on short plastic handles, are tipped into the anterior vitreous, where they swell and engage the gel sufficiently to draw forward a segment which can be excised proximally. In young and healthy vitreous, a dozen or more such sponges may be used successively until adequate vitreous has been removed. This precludes vitreo-endothelial adhesions, with their later vitreous tug and adverse effect on the macula and other portions of the retina. This may well supersede attempts to avoid such vitreous adhesions by wiping the wound with a sponge moistened in hyaluronidase.

2. *Microsurgical Techniques.* The recent development of practical binocular magnification of about 10X at a working distance of 30 cm. has made possible increased accuracy of about 8-fold in corneal suturing. It also makes possible the identification of defects in the vitreous face and localization of sites of origin in vitreous presentation. Microsurgery, on the other hand, exacts its cost in reduced field; altered subjective projection; increased light requirements, with greater drying effects; and increasingly complex mechanical apparatus, foot controls, and optical systems. The novitiate entering eye surgery quickly masters this system, and the mature surgeon adapts in a short time if he uses it regularly. The uniform use of general anesthesia in children makes adoption of microsurgery easier than with adult patients, for whom traditional local anesthesia perpetuates occasional problems of head stability and maintenance of field. Microsurgery has yielded an incidental byproduct of increased stability and precision by forcing ocular surgeons to the seated position and to reliance on finger rather than hand or wrist movements.

3. *Finer Sutures and Needles.* The suture and needle industry has moved slightly ahead of the surgical microscope developers in affording consistent and dependable sutures of 7-0 to 10-0 size. Six-0 materials should now be the largest used in closing lid and facial skin. Seven-0 should be the largest used in corneal repairs, and even with intermediate levels of magnification (head-mounted Beckerscope; portable, table-mounted Codman operating microscope), the advantages of more closely spaced and less traumatic 8-0 and 9-0 sutures can be gained with relative facility.

4. *Reduced Incidence of Sympathetic Ophthalmia.* This former plague of the limbal or ciliary body wound was particularly fostered by inaccurate closures, uveal incarcerations, and delayed healing. It has always been less common in pigmented races, such as Negroes and Asians, but in recent years it has become more rare even in Caucasians. It is essentially unknown in lower animals. Though long-term treatment or control has been improved by steroid therapy, greater gains have apparently been made in prophylaxis. More accurate and more prompt closures seemingly contribute to this decrease. Because uveal pigment is of low antigenicity, the pathogenic concept of hypersensitivity alone seems marginally plausible in explaining the devastating effects in this most unique of paired organ disturbances. Additional factors include a hypothetical chromatotropic virus which may be inhibited, as the trachoma virus, by widespread use of antibiotics. Whatever the mechanism in reduction of sympathetic ophthalmia, it does embolden the surgeon to repair increasingly severe lacerations and to refrain from early enucleation.

5. *Tetanus Immunization.* In the past 30 years, tetanus toxoid has been available, and active immunizations with appropriate courses of injection have produced effective levels of antibody titer (above 0.01 antibody units [AU] per ml. of serum) for many years. Booster injections have been widely used, especially in the United States, not only by physicians treating injuries but by camp and school directors as routine admission requirements. During the 1960s, however, an increasing number of tetanus toxoid reactions were reported. Frequently

repeated boosters, even with the dose reduced from 0.5 to 0.1 cc., seem to be associated with decreasing or ultimately no gain in antibody unit (AU) levels and increasing incidence of reactions. Sampling of serum titers in 143 children in a suburban pediatric practice revealed levels from 0.0025 AU or less up to 50 AU per ml. (Peebles et al., 1969). This is a range greater than 20,000-fold. Therefore, if a validated history of full immunization is available (three injections, not less than a month apart in infancy and reinforced with a fourth about 1 year later, and a booster injection on first entering school), no further injection should be given for 10 or 12 years. Subsequent booster injections should be no more frequent than every 10 years.

When there has been no active immunization, and the child is seen on the day of injury with a dirty wound, 250 units of tetanus immune globulin (human) should be injected. If there has been delay of a day or more, this dose should be doubled. In either case, active immunization should be started concurrently with 0.5 cc. (4 or 5 Lf units) of aluminum phosphate precipitated toxoid. Passive protection from tetanus immune globulin (human) lasts about 3 weeks, or more than twice as long as that from the older bovine or equine tetanus antitoxin (5000 units). The latter should be avoided because of sensitization and serum reactions (Beneson, 1970).

REFERENCES

Alberth, B.: Surgical Treatment of Caustic Injuries to the Eye. Budapest, Akademiai Kiado, 1968.

Anaclerio, A. M., and Wicker, H. S.: Self induced solar retinopathy by patients in a psychiatric hospital. Amer. J. Ophthal. 69:731, May, 1970.

Beneson, A. S. (Ed.): Control of Communicable Diseases in Man. 11th ed. New York, American Public Health Association, 1970.

Duke-Elder, W.: Textbook of Ophthalmology. Vol. VI. St. Louis, The C. V. Mosby Co., 1954, p. 5729.

Foulds, W. S.: Intra-canalicular gelatin implants in the treatment of kerato-conjunctivitis sicca. Brit. J. Ophthal., 45:625, 1961.

Fredericks, R. H.: Research in Child Restraint Development. American Association for Automotive Medicine, 13th Proceedings (n.p.), 1969, pp. 207–212.

Garrett, J. W.: Oculo-orbital injuries in automobile accidents. Bulletin Auto. Crash Injury Research, No. 4, March, 1963.

Georgiade, N. G.: Plastic and Maxillofacial Trauma Symposium. Vol. 1. St. Louis, The C. V. Mosby Co., 1969.

Grant, W. M.: Toxicology of the Eye. Springfield, Ill., Charles C Thomas, 1962.

Hill, K.: Cryoextraction of total hyphema. Arch. Ophthal., 80:368, September, 1968.

Keeney, A. H.: Automotive Trauma—The Second Impact. In New Orleans Acad. of Ophthal.: Industrial and Traumatic Ophthalmology, St. Louis, The C. V. Mosby Co., 1964, pp. 57–64.

Keeney, A. H.: Lens materials and the prevention of eye injuries. Trans. Amer. Ophthal. Soc., 54:521, 1965.

Keeney, A. H., and Estlow, B. R.: Spectacle glass injuries to the eye. Amer. J. Ophthal., 72:152, July, 1971.

Kelman, C. D., and Brooks, D. L.: Ultrasonic Emulsification and Aspiration of Traumatic Hyphema. Amer. J. Ophthal., 71:1289, June, 1971.

Paton, D., and Goldberg, M. F.: Injuries of the Eye, the Lids, and the Orbit. Philadelphia, W. B. Saunders Co., 1968.

Peebles, T. C., Levine, L., Eldred, M. C., and Edsall, G.: Tetanus-Toxoid Emergency Boosters. New Eng. J. Med., 280:575, March, 1969.

Reinecke, R. D., and Beyer, C. K.: Lacerated Corneas and Prevention of Synechia. Amer. J. Ophthal., 61:131, January, 1966.

Roper-Hall, M. J.: The treatment of ocular injuries. Trans. Ophthal. Soc. (U.K.), 79:57, 1959.

Roper-Hall, M. J.: Thermal and chemical burns. Trans. Ophthal. Soc. (U.K.), 85:631, 1965.

Schultz, R. C.: Upper Third Face Fractures from Vehicle Accidents. American Association for Automotive Medicine, 13th Proceedings (n.p.), 1969, pp. 109–130.

Sears, M. L.: Surgical management of black ball hyphema. Trans. Amer. Acad. Ophthal. Otolaryng., 74:820, July-August, 1970.

Siegel, A. W., Nahum, A. M., and Appleby, M. R.: Injuries to Children in Automobile Collisions. Proceedings of the 12th Stapp Car Crash Conference, New York, Soc. Auto. Engineers, 1968, pp. 1–48.

Sierent, G. W.: Infant Safety Carrier (G. M.). American Association for Automotive Medicine, 13th Proceedings (n.p.), 1969, pp. 213–220.

Slusher, M. D., and Keeney, A. H.: Monocular blindness—Analysis of etiology and preventive needs in 424 cases. Sight-Saving Rev., 35:207, Fall, 1965.

Smith, R. R. and Blount, R. L.: Ptosis, superior gaze paresis, pulsating exophthalmos, and blow-out fracture of the orbital roof. Amer. J. Ophthal., 71:1052, May, 1971.

Snyder, R. G.: Impact Injury Tolerances of Infants and Children. American Association for Automotive Medicine, 13th Proceedings (n.p.), 1969, pp. 131–164.

Toxicity Bibliography, National Library of Medicine. Washington, D.C., U.S. Government Printing Office, Vol. 1, No. 1, January, 1968; and following.

Van Laethen, R.: A New High Safety Glazing for Automobiles and Other Vehicles. Proceedings of the 12th Stapp Car Crash Conference, Soc. Auto. Engineers, New York, 1968, p. 360.

Van Portfliet, P., and Fralick, F. B.: Inflammability of Plastic Eyeglass Frames. Amer. J. Ophthal., 34:1727, December, 1951.

CHAPTER 18

PEDIATRIC NEURO-OPHTHALMOLOGY

LOIS J. MARTYN, M.D.

Section I

Ophthalmic Manfestations of Central Nervous System Disorders in Children

The Evaluation of Signs and Symptoms

VISION ABNORMALITIES

For physicians interested and engaged in the evaluation and treatment of disease of the central nervous system, the diagnosis of lesions involving the visual pathways is a primary concern. For the patient—child or adult—few disorders are more distressing or have greater significance than those which adversely affect visual function. For the ophthalmologist, no endeavor is more commanding than the preservation of vision, unless it be the ophthalmic detection of potentially incapacitating or life threatening neurologic or systemic disease.

Affections of the visual pathways may manifest as deficiency or loss of visual acuity, as impairment of special visual functions such as color perception or dark adaptation, as localizing field defects, or as abnormal visual sensations. The evaluation of these abnormalities is infinitely more challenging in the child than in the adult. Whereas both subjective and objective information is crucial to complete assessment of these various alterations in all age groups, in the very young, ill, or mentally deficient patient, accurate diagnosis may be totally or almost totally dependent on objective observations. In addition, the presenting signs and symptoms of vision

429

alterations in childhood vary significantly with the age and abilities of the child, with the acuteness of the affection, and with the severity and laterality or symmetry of the defect. In the infant, the presenting manifestation of a vision deficit may be nystagmus or strabismus, the underlying vision impairment passing unrecognized for weeks or months. In the pre-verbal toddler, the presenting clue may be behavior change, irritability, timidity, or clumsiness. In the older child, the initial manifestation may be disinterest or deterioration in school work unless the child promptly recognizes and verbalizes his visual problem. In the event of a slowly progressive loss of vision or field, the defect may be inapparent to both child and parents until it has become severe; similarly, asymmetric or strictly unilateral involvement may exist undetected for years.

In the differential diagnosis of lesions affecting the visual pathways in childhood, greater emphasis is placed on congenital defects, on genetically determined hereditary metabolic and degenerative processes, and on tumors that tend to be occult and insidious. As the principal step in the assessment of these disorders is topographical diagnosis, information pertaining to visual field abnormalities is presented first; visual acuity deficiencies, special visual function disturbances, and abnormal visual sensations are described subsequently.

Visual Field Defects

The significance of visual field defects in ophthalmoneurologic diagnosis lies in the organization and distribution of both the percipient and conductive elements of the visual pathway. As a frame of reference for discussion of pathological field changes, it is appropriate here to review the salient anatomic features of the visual pathway and the essential characteristics of the normal visual field.

The visual pathway consists of sensory receptor cells that lie completely within the retina and a three-neuron arc that conveys the visual impulse from the retinal photoreceptors to the occipital visual cortex. The sensory cells are the rods and cones; it is their outer segments that contain the photopigments which initiate the excitatory visual responses to light. The rod and cone cell bodies comprise the outer nuclear layer of the retina, and their axon processes extend into the outer plexiform layer where they synapse with the dendrites of the first order neurons of the conducting system. The *first order neurons* are the bipolar cells; their cell bodies lie in the inner nuclear layer and their axons extend into the inner plexiform layer where they synapse with dendrites of the second order neurons. The *second order neurons* are the ganglion cells that lie in the inner retina. The ganglion cell axons form the nerve fiber layer of the retina, continue as the nerve fibers of the optic nerve, extend through the chiasm and optic tract, and terminate in the lateral geniculate body where they synapse with the third order neurons. The *third order neurons*, whose axons form the optic radiations of the cerebral hemispheres, extend to the occipital lobe where they terminate in the visual cortex, the area striata.

Regional organization and segregation of importance in topographical diagnosis begin in the retina. Consideration must be given (1) to division of the retina into two major regions—central and peripheral, and (2) to division of the retina into four major quadrants—upper and lower temporal and upper and lower nasal.

The central retina, also referred to as the area centralis or macular area, is a region approximately 5.5 mm. in diameter, with its center located 4 mm. temporal to the center of the optic disc and 0.8 mm. below the horizontal meridian. The area is further subdivided into the fovea, parafovea, and perifovea, the central fovea being 1.5 mm. in diameter and the concentric parafoveal and perifoveal bands being, respectively, 0.5 mm. and 1.5 mm. in width. The extent of the macula and its subdivisions is determined by histologic features; the structure of the central retina is specially differentiated to subserve the highest visual acuity. A principal feature is dense concentration of cones throughout the macular region. The photoreceptor population of the most central 0.5 to 0.6 mm. of the fovea is pure cone; beyond the rod-free area, cones are interspersed with rods, and within a short distance beyond the macula, rods become more numerous than cones. In the visual field, the most central rod-free area corresponds to 1°40′ to 2°, or approximately 1° to either side of fixation, while the macular area in its entirety corresponds to 18°20'.

The peripheral retina is the whole rest of the retina beyond the macula. In contrast to that of the central retina, the photoreceptor population of the peripheral retina is predominantly rod. The peripheral retina is particularly adapted for scotopic vision whereas the central retina is particularly adapted for photopic vision.

The four quadrants of the retina are determined by vertical and horizontal meridians that pass through the center of the macula. As will be clarified in the description of the retinal nerve fiber pattern and its projection through the visual pathway, impulses initiated in the upper retinal quadrants are relayed to the upper visual cortex and impulses initiated in the lower quadrants are relayed to the lower visual cortex; those initiated in the temporal quadrants are relayed to the homolateral cortex, while those initiated in the nasal quadrants are relayed to the contralateral cortex.

Nerve fibers arising from the macula and from the retina between the disc and macula pass directly into the temporal aspect of the optic disc as the papillomacular bundle. Fibers arising in the temporal retina peripheral to the macula take an arched course, passing above and below the macula to attain the disc, entering the disc in its upper and lower poles. The nasal fibers maintain a radial course into the disc.

In the distal portion of the optic nerve, the arrangement of nerve fibers corresponds generally to the nerve fiber pattern of the retina. The papillomacular bundle, carrying approximately 65 per cent of the retinal nerve fibers, occupies a temporal sector-shaped area measuring one quarter to one third the disc area. The upper quadrant fibers occupy the dorsal portion of the nerve and the lower quadrant fibers occupy the ventral portion of the nerve, with the fibers from the peripheral nasal quadrants lying medial to those from the peripheral temporal quadrants.

In the more proximal portion of the optic nerve (proximal to the level of entrance of the central retinal vessels) the papillomacular bundle attains a more central position, with the fibers from the nasal portion of the macula lying medial to the fibers from the temporal portion of the macula. Fibers from the peripheral retina maintain their relative positions, upper remaining dorsal, lower remaining ventral, and nasal and temporal maintaining their respective sides.

Approaching the junction of the optic nerve and chiasm, nasal and temporal fibers begin to separate, fibers from the nasal hemiretina coursing in the medial and medioventral part of the nerve, and fibers from the temporal hemiretina coursing in the lateral and dorsolateral part of the nerve.

In the optic chiasm, fibers from the nasal hemiretina decussate to pass into the contralateral optic tract, while fibers from the temporal hemiretina remain uncrossed and pass into the ipsilateral optic tract. The decussating ventral fibers (representing the lower nasal retinal quadrants) cross anteriorly in the chiasm, looping anteriorly into the terminal portion (junction zone) of the opposite nerve before coursing posteriorly into the tract. The decussating dorsal fibers (representing the upper nasal retinal quadrants) cross more posteriorly in the chiasm to enter the dorsomedial aspect of the tract. The hemidecussation involves both peripheral and central (macular) fibers. Macular fibers that cross do so in the central and posterior portions of the chiasm, mostly posteriorly.

Each optic tract carries fibers from the temporal half of the homolateral retina and fibers from the nasal half of the contralateral retina. Fibers from the upper retinal quadrants course dorsomedially and fibers from the lower retinal quadrants course ventromedially to terminate in the lateral geniculate body. The slight rotation of the visual fibers evident in the tract is also seen in the geniculate body, where upper retinal fibers become situated medially and lower retinal fibers become situated laterally. This rotation becomes "straightened out" in the geniculocalcarine pathway.

From the lateral geniculate body, located on the posterolateral part of the pulvinar of the thalamus, visual fibers of the optic radiation traverse the external sagittal stratum in the white matter of the cerebral hemispheres to reach the striate area of the occipital lobe. The upper fibers of the optic radiation (geniculocalcarine pathway), representing the upper retinal quadrants, pass in a relatively direct course posteriorly through the temporoparietal area to the occipital lobe. The lower fibers, particularly those lowermost, loop forward toward the anterior pole of the temporal lobe before turning back to course into the occipital lobe; the temporal loop bears the name of Meyer.

The visual cortex, area striata or area 17, is situated along the superior and inferior lips of the calcarine fissure. Fibers representing the upper retinal quadrants terminate in the superior portion of the visual cortex; fibers representing the lower retinal quadrants terminate in the inferior portion of the visual cortex. The left visual cortex represents the left half of each retina, and the right cortex represents the right half of each retina. The macular quadrants are represented posteriorly in the poles.

The outward projection of all retinal points from which vision can be initiated is the visual field. The normal monocular field is a slightly irregular oval which from the point of fixation extends approximately 60° upward, 60° inward (nasally), 70 to 75° downward, and 90 to 95° or more outward (temporally). Within each field, the projection of the disc forms a vertically oval blind spot, 5.5° wide and 7.5° high, with its center located 15.5° temporal to fixation and 1.5° below the horizontal meridian.

The combination of the right and left monocular fields—the binocular field—is roughly an oval with a horizontal span of approximately 190° and a vertical span of approximately 130°. The area of overlap of the two monocular fields is roughly circular, with a diameter of approximately 120°. Unpaired temporal crescents, representing the far peripheral nasal retina, extend approximately 30° beyond the paired or overlapped binocular portion.

Each field can usefully be divided into the central field, that area lying within 25° of fixation, and the peripheral field, that area lying beyond 25°. Alternatively, each field can be divided into four zones. The central zone reaches to the inner side of the blind spot; it encompasses the area of macular vision. Surrounding the central zone is the cecal zone, which starts at the inner side of the blind spot and extends to the 25° circle. Concentric to the cecal zone is the intermediate zone, the region between 25 and 50°; beyond 50° is the peripheral zone.

Evaluation of the visual field involves determining its peripheral extent and exploring the sensitivity throughout its extent, processes referred to as *perimetry* and *scotometry*. In the classical method, the field is delineated on an arc or portion of a sphere. As the patient fixates a central point on the arc, the visual stimulus (test object) is moved toward fixation from the periphery, and the patient reports the points of appearance and disappearance of the stimulus. By using several stimuli of different size, intensity, color, or contrast, the points of the retina just sensitive to a given threshold are delineated and recorded. The lines joining points of equal sensitivity are referred to as isopters. For detailed evaluation of the central field, a process called *campimetry*, a flat screen—usually the tangent screen—is employed; by increasing the test distance, central field defects can be magnified and more accurately elucidated.

In pediatric practice, precise measurement of the fields by instrumentation is often impossible. In such situations, confrontation and attraction techniques are useful and can be effective in even the very young, ill, inattentive, or retarded patient. In standard confrontation, the examiner compares the patient's field with his own; the examiner faces the patient, each fixates the other's eye, the examiner moves a stimulus in from the periphery equidistant between himself and the patient, and the patient reports when he sees the stimulus. In an often-used variation of the confrontation test, an object is brought from behind the patient's head and he reports when the target comes into view. With this technique, an optically elicited movement can be used in lieu of a verbal response; the child may show his attraction to the stimulus by turning his eyes or head toward the target or by reaching for the stimulus. Toys, lollipops, lights, and faces are particularly effective stimuli for eliciting attraction responses in children.

Visual field defects take many forms, and each must be analyzed according to its position, shape, size, intensity, uniformity, margins, onset, and course. Position and configuration of the field defect are of utmost importance in topographical diagnosis. Size is less crucial in diagnosis, but changes in size of the defect can be important in assessing the course of progression or recovery of a lesion. The intensity, the uniformity, and the margins of a defect provide information concerning the extent to which a lesion has affected a given portion of the visual pathway, and can provide information as to the course and nature of the disease process. For example, the margins of a field defect caused by intracranial tumor are generally sloping, attesting to varying degrees of compression or destruction in and around the site of the lesion, whereas the margins of a defect caused by vascular occlusion or incision tend to be steep or sharp. With regard to onset and course, defects generally develop slowly when due to tumor, and rapidly or precipitously when due to vascular processes (e.g., hemorrhage, thrombosis) or trauma.

As the configuration and position of field defects are of greatest significance in topographical diagnosis, these characteristics are used here in classifying the most common field abnormalities and their implications.

HEMIANOPIAS AND QUADRANTANOPIAS

The term hemianopia describes a defect of the half-field. The boundary may be the vertical meridian, delimiting a right or left temporal or nasal hemianopia, or the horizontal meridian, delimiting a superior or inferior altitudinal hemianopia. When the defect is confined by both the vertical and horizontal meridians, the term quadrantanopia is applied. Such sector defects, whether they involve all or less than the half-field, or all or less than a quadrant, may be either central, peripheral, or combined.

A unilateral hemianoptic defect is indicative of pathologic change affecting the visual fibers anterior to the chiasm, in either the optic nerve or retina. Bilateral hemianopia is the hallmark of a lesion affecting the visual fibers more posteriorly, i.e., in the chiasm, in the tract, or in the geniculocalcarine pathway. This is not to infer, however, that all bilateral hemianoptic defects are of posterior origin; it is not impossible for the disease affecting one retina or optic nerve to affect the other simultaneously, or even symmetrically.

When corresponding half-fields — that is, the right halves of both fields or the left halves of both fields — are affected, the hemianopia is said to be homonymous. If the field defect of one eye is identical to that of the other eye in all characteristics, excepting the difference in size produced by the unpaired temporal crescent, the homonymous hemianopia is said to be congruous.

When noncorresponding half fields — that is, both inner halves or both outer halves — are affected, the hemianopia is said to be heteronymous, and is designated as either binasal or bitemporal.

The various types of hemianopias require further comment with regard to their diagnostic significance.

Homonymous Hemianopias

Homonymous hemianopias are characteristic of pathologic change affecting the visual fibers posterior to the chiasmal hemidecussation. Distinguishing features of the hemianopia and associated neurologic signs vary, depending on the site of the lesion; i.e., according to whether it is in the optic tract or in the various portions of the geniculocalcarine pathway.

With optic tract involvement, the hemianopia tends to be irregular and incongruous, unless, of course, the lesion is total in its effect, producing a complete and absolute homonymous hemianopia. An associated sign of value in topographical diagnosis of tract involvement is Wernicke's hemianoptic pupil, an afferent pupil dysfunction corresponding to the hemianoptic field defect; the pupil sign, however, may be difficult to demonstrate.

Hemianopias of temporal lobe involvement also tend to be incongruous, provided they are incomplete. As the lower geniculocalcarine fibers course forward into the temporal lobe (Meyer's loop), the typical hemianoptic defect of this region is an upper quadrantanopia; frequently it is a small upper sector defect, the so-called "pie in the sky," having a triangular shape with its apex directed toward fixation. Paroxysmal visual hallucinations, frequently highly differentiated, taking the form of objects or scenes, are also common with temporal lobe involvement. In addition there may be uncinate fits (paroxysmal olfactory or gustatory hallucinations), fugue or dream-like states, the déjà vu phenomenon, and psychomotor epileptic seizures. With a pathologic process on the dominant side there may also be sensory aphasia in the form of impaired comprehension of speech or difficulty in finding appropriate words.

Hemianopias that occur with parietal lobe involvement tend to be more congruous than those of more anterior origin, and the defect frequently is a lower quadrantanopia. In some cases, particularly with lesions of the parieto-occipital area, the defect takes the form of "visual inattention" or "visual extinction" in the homonymous half-fields; this impairment is detected by simultaneous stimulation of both half-fields. Depending on which particular area of the parietal lobe is affected, there may be a variety of associated signs. Anterior lesions involving the posterior central gyrus produce sensory jacksonian fits. Lesions affecting the angular gyrus and the neighboring regions on the dominant side result in various combinations of alexia, agraphia, acalculia, right-left disorientation, finger agnosia, and right homonymous hemianopia, whereas angular involvement on the nondominant side produces topographical agnosia and left homonymous hemianopia. With involvement of the white matter of the parieto-occipital region, there frequently is impairment of optokinetic nystagmus on rotation of the targets toward the side of the lesion.

Hemianopias of occipital origin characteristically are congruous; they may "split" or "spare" fixation. Except for the field changes, occipital lesions tend to be neurologically "silent," though often with extension forward there may be involvement of the peristriate and the neighboring parieto-occipital regions, resulting in alexia without agraphia (in the case of dominant hemisphere involvement), topographic agnosia (nondominant hemisphere involvement), visual object agnosia, achromatopsia, and visual irreminiscence. Bilateral occipital lobe involvement, producing double homonymous hemianopia, may result in bilateral blindness, occasionally accompanied by the patient's denial or unawareness of the blindness, a phenomenon referred to as Anton's syndrome. There may be visual hallucinations; these generally are unformed, primitive light sensations.

Double Homonymous Hemianopia

This defect signifies bilateral involvement of the visual pathways posterior to the chiasmal hemidecussation. If the causative pathologic process is total in its effect, bilateral blindness results. More selective involvement may result in double homonymous hemianoptic central or paracentral scotomas; alternatively, the hemianoptic defects may be peripheral.

In most instances, double homonymous hemianopia is the result of pathologic change affecting both occipital lobes simultaneously. Many pathologic processes, including inflammation, degeneration, tumor, and trauma, may be responsible for bilateral occipital involvement, but a primary etiologic factor is hypoxia or anoxia, and cerebral circulation can be compromised in many ways.

In children it is not uncommon to find a double homonymous hemianopia amounting to cerebral or cortical blindness secondary to hydrocephalus, meningoencephalitis, toxic or hypertensive encephalopathy, trauma, or diffuse demyelinating degenerative disease.

Crossed Quadrantanopia

This is a rare field defect in which diagonally opposite quadrants are affected. Such a defect can result from disease affecting the upper calcarine cortex on one side and the lower calcarine cortex on the opposite side. The crossed quadrantanopia may be a stage in the development or resolution of a double homonymous hemianopia.

Crossed quadrantanopias are also ascribed to the chiasmal compressive syndrome wherein a lesion displaces the chiasm from the lateral side or below, compressing it against the opposite internal carotid artery.

Crossed quadrant defects may also result when simultaneous bilateral lesions produce sector defects in opposite quadrants of the two fields, as may occur with glaucoma or juxtapapillary inflammation.

Altitudinal Hemianopia

Altitudinal hemianopia, a defect of the superior or inferior half-field bounded by the horizontal meridian, indicates selective involvement of those visual fibers that represent, respectively, only the lower or only the upper half of the retina.

Unilateral altitudinal hemianopia necessarily is a prechiasmal defect. Excluding a retinal disorder such as detachment, it indicates involvement of the optic nerve somewhere in its orbital, canalicular, or intracranial course. A prime cause of altitudinal defects is optic nerve ischemia from vascular disease; however, this is a major concern in the older age group rather than in the pediatric age group. A major cause of altitudinal defects in all age groups is optic nerve trauma, particularly at the level of the canal or its foramen. Tumor or other mass lesion involving the optic nerve may also give rise to altitudinal defects. Another consideration is bony deformities, and a loss of upper field is described in oxycephaly.

Bilateral altitudinal defects, in the absence of bilateral retinal or optic nerve abnormalities as just described, are generally caused by damage to the chiasm, particularly trauma, or by disease affecting the occipital area. The bilateral altitudinal hemianopia of occipital origin is in effect a double homonymous quadrantanopia produced by a lesion affecting either both upper or both lower lips of the calcarine cortex; such defects may occur particularly with ischemia, trauma, or tumor. Inflammatory and demyelinating lesions are not principal considerations, as they tend to produce rather irregular defects.

Binasal Hemianopia

This defect requires simultaneous involvement of the temporal fibers bilaterally.

Presumably a mass lesion in the region of the chiasm or a dilated third ventricle can displace the temporal chiasmal or prechiasmal fibers laterally, compressing them against the carotid arteries. In clinical practice, however, the importance of this mechanism as an explanation for selective binasal field loss is disputed. An alternative explanation for production of binasal defect by a single lesion is displacement of the chiasm laterally against one carotid artery by a tumor or aneurysm arising on the contralateral side of the chiasm, thus affecting the temporal fibers of both sides simultaneously.

As with other bilateral field defects, the cause may be bilateral retinal, optic nerve, or tract disease. Retinal detachment, bilateral developmental anomalies of the disc, and demyelinating disease affecting temporal fibers in both optic nerves or in the tract must be considered. Of particular importance is the fact that binasal field defects may develop consequent to papilledema that has damaged the temporal fibers by compression and ischemia at the disc.

Bitemporal Hemianopia

Bitemporal hemianopias are typical of lesions affecting the median aspect of the optic chiasm, wherein nasal fibers from both eyes decussate. This is not to infer that all chiasmal field defects are clear-cut bitemporal hemianopias, nor that all bitemporal hemianoptic defects necessarily are of chiasmal origin, but it should be noted that the chiasm is the only region where a single lesion can affect the nasal fibers from both eyes simultaneously.

In the event of median chiasmal pressure from below—particularly when the lesion is situated relatively anteriorly—the field loss tends to commence in the upper temporal quadrants, progressing clockwise in the field of the right eye and counterclockwise in the field of the left eye; the loss may be scotomatous or nonscotomatous, symmetric or asymmetric. In the event of median chiasmal pressure from above, the field loss begins in the lower and outer quadrants, and progresses counterclockwise in the field of the right eye and clockwise in the field of the left; that is, in the reverse direction to that of pressure from below. With relatively posterior median chiasmal interference, involvement of the central field is usual, as the macular fibers that cross do so in the more posterior portions of the chiasm.

In childhood, the usual cause of a chiasmal bitemporal hemianopia is craniopharyngioma or optic glioma; pituitary adenoma, so frequent a cause of bitemporal hemianopia in the adult years, is rare in childhood. An occasional cause of bitemporal hemianoptic defects is compression of the chiasm by a dilated third ventricle; the child with posterior fossa tumor or an intraventricular lesion may develop bitemporal depression consequent to hydrocephalus. Trauma, inflammatory processes, and demyelinating lesions of the chiasm are less commonly encountered causes of bitemporal hemianopia in childhood.

Not to be confused with classical bitemporal hemianopia of chiasmal origin are bitemporal defects associated with simultaneous bilateral involvement of the nasal fibers elsewhere. Demyelinating disease can affect the nasal fibers of the optic tracts or optic nerves bilaterally. Developmental optic nerve abnormalities such as hypoplasia, dysversion, or drusen, may produce bitemporal defects when present bilaterally, as may bilateral retinal disease. Accurate perimetry and critical ophthalmoscopy are essential to proper differentiation.

Junction Scotoma

This is a special type of hemianopia caused by a lesion at the anterior angle of the chiasm, where optic nerve fibers continue into the chiasm. At this level homolateral nasal and temporal fibers are well separated and can be affected selectively; also, looping into this region ventrally are crossed nasal fibers from the contralateral side.

As originally described, the junction scotoma of Traquair is a temporal hemianoptic scotoma ipsilateral to a lesion involving the nasal fibers at the point where the optic nerve joins the chiasm. A lesion situated at the inner anterior angle of the chiasm frequently also involves the crossed nasal fibers, producing a peripheral upper temporal defect in the opposite field. As it progresses, the angle lesion may ultimately produce blindness of the homolateral eye combined with the peripheral temporal defect in the contralateral field.

Primary causes of junction and angle involvement in childhood are optic glioma and craniopharyngioma.

CENTRAL SCOTOMAS

Certain defects of the central portion of the field are classified as *central, paracentral,* or *pericentral scotomas* on the basis of their relationship to the point of fixation, while those involving the normal blind spot are designated *cecal.* A defect encompassing both the fixation area and the blind spot is referred to as *centrocecal.*

Central Scotoma

A central scotoma is a defect that involves the point of fixation and the immediately surrounding area. The defect may be minute or large, absolute or relative. The configuration generally is round or irregularly oval.

A unilateral central scotoma is characteristic of disease involving the macula itself or the central fibers (papillomacular fibers) as they traverse the retina or optic nerve. As it is not uncommon for disease that affects one macula or optic nerve to affect the other simultaneously, bilateral central scotomas also are frequently of peripheral origin. Alternatively, bilateral scotomas can develop as the result of disease affecting the optic chiasm or more posterior portions of the visual pathway. Critical examination of bilateral central scotomas may show the defects to be double homonymous hemianoptic scotomas, as may occur with occipital pole disease.

Paracentral Scotomas

Paracentral scotomas lie immediately adjacent to fixation, the greater part being to one side. Paracentral defects are further described as supracentral, infracentral, nasocentral, or temporocentral, depending on their position relative to fixation.

Like true central scotomas, paracentral defects commonly are of retinal or optic nerve origin, but careful evaluation for hemianoptic characteristics suggestive of disease of the chiasm or posterior visual pathways is essential.

Pericentral Scotomas

Pericentral scotomas involve the area immediately and equally around fixation, leaving the point of fixation relatively unaffected.

The significance of pericentral scotomas parallels that of central and paracentral scotomas.

Centrocecal Scotomas

Centrocecal scotomas are characteristic of papillomacular fiber bundle damage. The defect encompasses the area from fixation to the normal blind spot.

Optic neuritis or toxic amblyopia is the usual cause of centrocecal scotoma.

CECAL SCOTOMAS

Cecal scotomas are field defects involving the area of the normal blind spot. A common form of cecal scotoma is the enlargement of the normal blind spot that occurs with papilledema. Another is the glaucomatous nerve fiber bundle defect that extends from the blind spot.

A special form of cecal scotoma is the cecocentral scotoma, a papillomacular defect that extends from the blind spot to fixation. This defect is commonly seen with retrobulbar optic neuritis or toxic amblyopia.

ARCUATE SCOTOMAS: NERVE FIBER BUNDLE DEFECTS

Field defects that accurately conform to the anatomic configuration of the retinal nerve fiber pattern are referred to variously as arcuate, scimitar, comet, Seidel, or Bjerrum scotomas.

The classic nerve fiber bundle scotoma, usually called a Bjerrum scotoma, arches around fixation from the blind spot to the horizontal raphe in the nasal field, where it ends in a sharply demarcated horizontal or nasal step. Rarely does a nerve fiber bundle scotoma extend temporally from the blind spot, or temporally above or below the blind spot in a radial, straight, or wedge form. The variations in the shape and position of these scotomas are determined by the site and extent of the nerve fiber damage.

Nerve fiber bundle defects are the typical field defects of glaucoma, but any pathologic process that interferes with nerve fiber bundles either in the retina or in the optic nerve can produce arcuate scotomas. They are sometimes found with developmental defects of the disc, particularly pits and drusen.

RING SCOTOMAS

A field defect that completely or partially encircles the fixation point at some distance from it is called an annular or ring scotoma. A ring type defect can be produced by a double arcuate scotoma involving symmetrical nerve bundles above and below the disc, but such symmetry is rare. The term ring scotoma generally describes a defect which does not conform to the retinal nerve fiber pattern and does not include the blind spot in its course. Conforming to this latter definition is the typical field defect of retinitis pigmentosa and its variants.

The ring scotoma of retinitis pigmentosa develops in the mid-periphery, corresponding to the areas of retinal degeneration. The field loss may be patchy initially, but as the disease progresses the defect tends to become more complete and to expand outward, inward, or in both directions. Expanding outward, the ring scotoma may "break through" the periphery, leaving a severely contracted field centrally.

GENERALIZED FIELD DEPRESSION, PERIPHERAL DEPRESSION, AND CONCENTRIC CONTRACTION

Generalized field depression refers to a reduction in sensitivity throughout the field. When the sensitivity of only the peripheral isopters is reduced, the term generalized peripheral depression is appropriate. When the sensitivity of certain peripheral isopters is reduced to absolute blindness, leaving the whole field equally restricted, generalized peripheral contraction or concentric contraction exists.

Generalized field depression can be demonstrated in normal persons by reducing the intensity of the stimuli. Pathologic field depression can be seen in patients with unclear media and in patients with diffuse optic atrophy.

Peripheral depression and concentric contraction may develop with prolonged papilledema, and when contraction does occur consequent to papilledema, the prognosis is poor. Another condition productive of concentric contraction is retinitis pigmentosa; as a ring scotoma "breaks through" the periphery, it may leave a markedly constricted field. Toxic drugs, also, can be responsible for peripheral depression or contraction; quinine, for example, can produce field loss ranging from slight generalized peripheral depression to contraction of the field to within a few degrees from fixation.

To be differentiated from peripheral depression and contraction of organic origin are concentric field defects of psychogenic origin. The so-called "tubular" field found in hysterical or malingering patients typically is a small circular field that does not change appropriately when the stimulus size or test distance is changed. Commonly the size of the tubular field determined by formal perimetry is inconsistent with the facility with which the patient travels and the ease with which he detects unexpected peripheral distractions. Psychogenic tubular fields and spurious defects of various types are not uncommon among school-age children. Also common is the so-called spiral field of fatigue; in nervous, tired, or bored children, a progressive contraction is often recorded as the examination progresses.

Common Vision Disorders: Definitions and Clinical Considerations

Whereas most vision disorders of neurogenic origin can be described in terms of specific visual field defects, many vision abnormalities, particularly visual acuity defects, special visual function impairments and abnormal visual sensations, are best described in terms of their general symptomatology, their mode of onset, and their course.

Amblyopia

In its broadest sense, the term amblyopia is properly used to describe many types of vision deficiency of both organic and functional origin. However, the term is preferably used to denote subnormal visual acuity in the absence of an ophthalmoscopically detectable retinal abnormality or afferent visual pathway disease that would adequately explain the vision deficit. It generally implies a vision defect due to sensory stimulus deprivation (disuse) or inhibition (misuse) occurring early in life.

As the many developmental and neurologically benign forms of amblyopia are discussed fully in Chapter 7, only comments pertaining to neurologic differential diagnosis will be made here. Indeed, only a few words of caution are in order.

Because certain nervous system diseases of childhood, particularly tumors and degenerative processes affecting the visual pathway, can be insidious and can progress for long periods without producing associated ophthalmoscopic, pupillary, ocular motor, or general neurologic evidence of

their presence, a high level of suspicion must be maintained in evaluating all children with subnormal visual acuity. Further, it is not uncommon to find functional amblyopia due to stimulation deprivation or inhibition coexistent with or secondary to organic disease. What appears to be a benign strabismic amblyopia may in fact be due to an insidious optic glioma that has not yet produced optic atrophy. Alternatively, what appears to be an acquired loss of vision may in fact be a longstanding, previously undetected benign amblyopia. Only precise documentation of the mode of onset and course of vision defects combined with critical examination for both ocular and neurologic abnormalities will differentiate the neurologically benign amblyopia from the vision deficit due to progressive disease.

Amaurosis

The term amaurosis, derived from the Greek word meaning dim, is generally defined as total or partial loss of vision; by common usage, the term has come to imply profound deficiency of vision—that is, blindness or near blindness.

With the exception of those cases in which the etiology of the vision deficit is readily explained by objective examination of the eye itself, the differential diagnosis of amaurosis in childhood requires consideration of the innumerable neurologic disorders that affect the visual pathways (Table 18–1).

When the amaurosis exists from birth, primary consideration must be given to (1) developmental malformations of the brain and optic nerves; (2) cerebral and optic nerve damage consequent to gestational and perinatal infection and inflammatory processes, metabolic disturbances, anoxia, or hypoxia; (3) perinatal trauma involving the visual pathways; and (4) certain genetically determined optic atrophies and retinal degenerations that manifest early. Among the neurologic causes of congenital amaurosis, cerebral impairment resulting from anoxia, the congenital infection syndromes (principally rubella, cytomegalovirus, toxoplasmosis, and syphilis), hydrocephalus, porencephaly, and microcephaly are relatively frequent, as are Leber's congenital retinal amaurosis and severe optic nerve hypoplasia.

TABLE 18–1 CHILDHOOD AMAUROSIS: PRINCIPAL NEUROLOGIC CONSIDERATIONS

Congenital Malformations
Optic nerve hypoplasia
Congenital hydrocephalus
Hydranencephaly
Porencephaly
Micrencephaly
Encephalocele, particularly occipital type

Phakomatoses
Bourneville's tuberous sclerosis
von Recklinghausen's neurofibromatosis
 (special association with optic glioma)
Sturge-Weber syndrome
von Hippel-Lindau disease

Tumors
Retinoblastoma
Optic glioma
Perioptic meningioma
Craniopharyngioma
Cerebral glioma
Posterior and intraventricular tumors when
 complicated by hydrocephalus

Neurodegenerative Diseases: Abiotrophies
Cerebral storage disease
 Gangliosidoses, particularly Tay-Sachs disease
 (infantile amaurotic familial idiocy),
 Sandhoff's variant, generalized
 gangliosidosis
 Other lipidoses, particularly the late onset
 amaurotic familial idiocies such as those of
 Jansky-Bielschowsky and of Batten-Mayou-
 Spielmeyer-Vogt
 Mucopolysaccharidoses, particularly Hurler
 syndrome and Hunter syndrome
Leukodystrophies (dysmyelination disorders),
 particularly metachromatic leukodystrophy and
 Canavan's disease
Demyelinating scleroses (myelinoclastic diseases),

Neurodegenerative Diseases: Abiotrophies (Continued)
 especially Schilder's disease and Devic's
 neuromyelitis optica
 Special types: Dawson's disease, Leigh's disease,
 the Bassen-Kornzweig syndrome, Refsum's
 disease
 Retinal degenerations of obscure pathogenesis:
 "retinitis pigmentosa" and its variants, and
 Leber's congenital type
 Optic atrophies of obscure pathogenesis: congenital autosomal recessive type, infantile and
 congenital autosomal dominant types, Leber's
 disease, and atrophies associated with
 hereditary ataxias—the types of Behr, of
 Marie, and of Sanger-Brown

Infectious Processes
 Encephalitis, especially in the prenatal infection
 syndromes due to *Toxoplasma gondii*, cyto-
 megalovirus, rubella virus, *T. pallidum*
 Meningitis; arachnoiditis
 Optic neuritis
 Chorioretinitis

Hematologic Disorders
 Leukemia with CNS involvement

Vascular and Circulatory Disorders
 Collagen vascular diseases
 Arteriovenous malformations—intracerebral
 hemorrhage, subarachnoid hemorrhage

Trauma
 Contusion or avulsion of optic nerves or chiasm
 Cerebral contusion or laceration
 Intracerebral, subarachnoid, or subdural
 hemorrhage

Drugs and Toxins

Amaurosis that develops in an infant or child who once had useful vision has somewhat different implications. When the amaurosis develops rather rapidly, it may be indicative of an encephalopathy as might occur with hypertension, infectious or para-infectious conditions, vasculitis, leukemia, toxins, or trauma. It may be due to acute demyelinating disease affecting the optic nerves, chiasm, or cerebrum. In some cases, precipitous loss of vision is explained by rapidly progressive hydrocephalus (or shunt dysfunction) and other types of increased intracranial pressure that may produce an ischemia of the visual areas. More slowly progressive loss, by contrast, is suggestive of tumor or neurodegenerative disease.

Optic nerve and chiasmal gliomas and craniopharyngiomas are primary considerations in children who show progressive loss of vision, with or without other neurologic signs, while cerebral tumors are less frequently responsible for amaurosis in childhood. Whereas some tumors produce amaurosis by rather direct involvement of the visual pathways, others, such as intraventricular and posterior fossa tumors, may indirectly affect the visual pathways by causing hydrocephalus and increased intracranial pressure. Finally, the neurodegenerative diseases to be considered are many of the sphingolipidoses and amaurotic familial idiocies, and certain of the mucopolysaccharidoses.

In each case, the primary step in differential diagnosis is topographical classification of the amaurosis, with proper interpretation of the ophthalmoscopic findings and associated neurologic signs. It is useful to first classify the amaurosis as pregeniculate or postgeniculate on the basis of the pupillary findings. Because the afferent pupil fibers from the retina travel the visual pathway only to the level of the lateral geniculate body, afferent conduction, as reflected in the pupillary response to light, is impaired by pregeniculate lesions that are of sufficient magnitude to cause amaurosis, but is not affected by postgeniculate (geniculocalcarine) lesions. There may, of course, be combined pre- and postgeniculate involvement and concurrent efferent pupillomotor dysfunction that would complicate the picture, but in "pure" lesions of either the pregeniculate or postgeniculate pathways, the distinction made on the basis of the pupillary response to light is valuable.

Once the integrity of the afferent pupillary system has been determined, the significance of the ophthalmoscopic findings can be appropriately assessed. In the absence of hysteria or malingering, normal ophthalmoscopic findings in a patient with amaurosis and normal pupillary responses to light indicate the presence of cerebral disease; such could be the case with anoxia, encephalitis, or trauma. When there are ophthalmoscopic signs of fundus abnormality in an amaurotic patient with normal pupillary responses to light, the fundus changes, though not directly responsible for the vision deficit, may provide evidence as to the nature of the postgeniculate pathology; such could be the case with congenital infection syndromes, hypertensive encephalopathy, or the hamartomatoses. Normal ophthalmoscopic findings in a patient with amaurosis and afferent pupillary dysfunction suggest pathologic change in the retrobulbar area, such as optic neuritis or a chiasmal or parachiasmal lesion that has not yet produced disc changes; this combination of signs may even be found with intrinsic retinal disorders (such as Leber's congenital retinal degeneration) before the pigmentary changes develop. When there are ophthalmoscopic signs of fundus disease in combination with afferent pupillary dysfunction, the pertinent question is whether the disorder is confined to the anterior visual pathway or whether the fundus changes are the visible expression of widespread disease.

More often than not, the complete delineation of childhood amaurosis and its etiology requires extensive investigation involving electrophysiologic tests, neuroradiologic procedures, chemical and enzyme assays, and genetic studies.

Obscurations

Transient episodes of vision loss or blurring that last only seconds or minutes have rather special diagnostic implications. Of primary importance are the visual obscurations and "amblyopic attacks" of papilledema consequent to increased intracranial pressure; these must be differentiated from the visual symptoms of migraine and cerebrovascular insufficiency.

Obscurations associated with papilledema characteristically are fleeting, usually lasting less than 30 seconds and rarely more than a minute. They begin abruptly and end abruptly. Though usually sporadic, they may be precipitated by sudden changes in posture or by excitement. The sensation is one of a hazy clouding, darkening, or total blackout of vision in one or both eyes; there may be associated flashes of light or color (photopsias). As a rule, there is complete restoration of vision after each attack. The precise mechanism of these attacks is not known; they are generally attributed to transient ischemia, possibly related to changes in orbital blood flow evoked by the effects of intracranial pressure on cerebrovascular regulatory mechanisms. When the increased intracranial pressure is relieved, the attacks cease. Obscurations in themselves are not predictive of the ultimate visual outcome in patients with papilledema, even when the attacks are frequent and repetitive.

Obscurations that occur as a migraine phenomenon generally persist many minutes, frequently 15 to 20 minutes or more. While scintillating scotomas and fortification figures confined to the half-fields are the typical symptoms of migraine, some patients do experience less distinctive episodes of blurring, even temporary total amaurosis. The visual symptoms may occur with or without headache, and with or without other migraine symptomatology such as nausea, vomiting, photophobia, paresthesias, or hemiparesis. The periodicity of migraine is an important distinguishing feature.

Other causes of transient visual obscurations in childhood are unusual. Carotid insufficiency, so common in adults, is characterized by unilateral blackouts of vision lasting only 2 to 3 minutes or 5 to 10 minutes, and the visual symptoms of the transient cerebrovascular insufficiency are often accompanied by transient motor or sensory loss on the contralateral side of the body.

Photopsias

Photopsias are abnormal visual phenomena that take the form of sparks, lightning flashes, luminous rings, fiery globes, and other primitive light sensations. Typical of photopsias are the positive visual phenomena that occur with mechanical stimulation of the retina—traction on the retina by detachment or scarring, or pressure on the eye through closed lids.

Photopsias have no specific localizing value, as they may arise from involvement of the visual pathways anywhere from the retina to the occipital cortex. Some occur in association with obscurations or amblyopic attacks, as with papilledema (increased intracranial pressure) or migraine. Some show transition to formed hallucinations and may signify cerebral disease.

Visual Hallucinations

A visual hallucination is the apparent perception of an external object when no such object is present. The visual phenomenon may be simple—an unformed hallucination or photopsia consisting of primitive light sensations, or complex—a formed or cinematographic hallucination consisting of differentiated figures, animals, persons, or entire scenes having extension in time or space.

Hallucinations may arise from disturbances in the visual pathways anywhere from the retina to the occipital lobe. They have no precise localizing value. Formed hallucinations, however, are usually indicative of temporal lobe involvement, in which case they may be associated with dreamy states and with olfactory and gustatory hallucinations. By contrast, the hallucinations of occipital lesions generally are unformed and simple, as are the hallucinations of anterior visual pathway lesions.

Hallucinations may arise from functional as well as organic disturbances. Psychosis must be considered in the differential diagnosis. Hallucinogenic drugs, notably mescaline, cannabis, and lysergic acid, must also be considered. Several drugs regularly used in ophthalmic practice, notably atropine, scopolamine, and cyclogyl, also have hallucinogenic properties, and children receiving these drugs topically may experience hallucinations, confusion, and excitement; the effect is transitory.

Micropsia, Macropsia, and Metamorphopsia

Micropsia is a disturbance of vision wherein objects appear smaller than their actual size. *Macropsia* is a disturbance of vision wherein objects appear larger than their actual size. *Metamorphopsia* is a disturbance of vision wherein objects and lines appear distorted and irregular.

These vision disturbances may be of central or peripheral origin, and have no localizing value. They may occur with deep-seated cerebral lesions, with migraine, or with epilepsy, and even with tumor near the chiasm. They may also occur as the result of retinal disease, particularly macular degeneration or central retinitis wherein retinal elements are displaced by edema or scarring. Alternatively, the cause may be an optical abnormality.

Night Blindness: Nyctalopia

Nyctalopia or "night blindness" refers to vision deficiency in reduced illumination. It generally implies an impairment in rod function, particularly dark adaptation time or threshold, but a variety of factors may contribute to night vision difficulties. Delineation of the problem may require a number of special tests, including dark adaptometry, electroretinography, electrooculography, and even an assessment of the effects of glare, in addition to a basic evaluation of visual function under mesopic and scotopic conditions.

For clinical purposes, it is useful to categorize night vision problems according to whether they present as stationary or progressive conditions of congenital or acquired type, with or without ophthalmoscopically evident abnormalities.

STATIONARY CONGENITAL NIGHT BLINDNESS WITH NO ASSOCIATED FUNDUS ABNORMALITIES occurs as a hereditary disorder transmitted as either a dominant, autosomal recessive, or X-linked recessive condition. In all three inherited types, there is inability to see in the dark because of the absence of rod adaptation. The dark adaptation curve characteristically is monophasic, lacking the scotopic or rod component. There may also be mild to moderate photopic abnormalities, with the monophasic cone adaptation curve frequently being slow and elevated. The visual field and color vision are normal, but visual acuity varies with the genetic pattern; it is normal in the dominant form, normal or occasionally abnormal in the autosomal recessive form, and subnormal (20/40 to 20/200) in the X-linked form. Myopia is regularly associated with the X-linked form, and is frequently present in the autosomal recessive form with poor vision.

The exact pathogenesis of these hereditary forms of congenital stationary night blindness is not clear, but it appears to be postreceptoral; rods and visual pigments are not lacking.

STATIONARY CONGENITAL NIGHT BLINDNESS OCCURRING IN ASSOCIATION WITH FUNDUS ABNORMALITIES suggests principally two conditions: fundus albipunctatus and Oguchi's disease.

Fundus albipunctatus is distinguished by the presence of discrete white dots in the retina, a finding present from infancy. Most patients show delayed dark adaptation, although some show no secondary or rod adaptation. Visual acuity, fields, and color vision are normal. The etiology is obscure. The inheritance is generally autosomal recessive.

Oguchi's disease is distinguished by the presence of a yellowish or gray-white metallic retinal sheen that may disappear after a prolonged period in the dark—a phenomenon referred to as Mizuo's phenomenon—only to reappear soon after exposure to light. Two major forms of the disorder occur. In type 1 Oguchi's disease, rod adaptation is severely retarded, often requiring 2 to 4 hours or even as long as 24 hours, with the final threshold normal or elevated; the fundus discoloration and Mizuo's phenomenon typically are present in type 1. In type 2, there is no rod dark adaptation, the fundus discoloration tends to be less prominent, and Mizuo's phenomenon may be slight (type 2a) or absent (type

2b). In both forms, daylight visual acuity, fields, and color vision are normal. The pathogenesis is not known. The condition is inherited as an autosomal recessive and it is most frequently seen in the Japanese.

PROGRESSIVE NIGHT BLINDNESS, as a rule, is indicative of a primary or secondary pigmentary retinal degeneration, a choroidal atrophy, or a vitreoretinal degeneration. Although the night blindness of these conditions is often referred to as acquired, because the symptoms appear at varying times after birth, the underlying disorder often is genetically predetermined and congenital in nature.

In the pigmentary retinal degenerations there is progressive deterioration of retinal neuroepithelium, the rods generally being affected first. Impairment of night vision, often the initial clinical manifestation, usually becomes evident during childhood. Peripheral field depression, typical ring scotomas, and eventually marked constriction of the field develop. Central visual acuity may be affected early or late in the disease, generally later. With time, significant retinal signs develop. Retinal pigment migration and aggregation, clump and spicular formation, especially in the midperiphery and along veins, are typical, though in some cases pigment changes are minimal or absent. Retinal arteriolar attenuation and some degree of optic pallor are evident in most cases. The ERG characteristically is abnormal.

Pigmentary retinal degenerations productive of night blindness (including classical retinitis pigmentosa and its variants, such as inverse retinitis pigmentosa, degeneration sine pigmento, retinitis puncta albescens, and even Leber's congenital retinal degeneration) are inherited most commonly as autosomal dominant or X-linked recessive conditions, and may occur as primary retinal diseases without associated abnormalities. Alternatively, night-blinding progressive retinal degeneration may occur in association with a variety of neurologic and somatic abnormalities, often secondary to a genetically determined metabolic disorder. Representative of the many neurologic and systemic disorders associated with night-blinding retinal degeneration are the Hurler, Hunter, Scheie, and Sanfilippo syndromes (mucopolysaccharidoses), juvenile amaurotic familial idiocy of Batten-Mayou-Spielmeyer-Vogt (lipidosis), the Bassen-Kornzweig syndrome (abetalipoproteinemia and acanthocytosis), Tangier disease (α-lipoprotein deficiency), Refsum disease (phytanic acid storage), Hallervorden-Spatz (extrapyramidal system degeneration), the Laurence-Moon-Biedl syndrome (obesity, hypogonadism, and mental retardation), and Usher's syndrome (deafness). With regard to ophthalmoneurologic diagnosis, it is the recognition of these associations that is of great importance.

Conditions other than the genetically determined retinal and choroidal degenerations included in the differential diagnosis of progressive impairment of night vision are vitamin A deficiency and retinal damage related to toxins and drugs.

Vitamin A deficiency of sufficient degree to cause night vision complaints may occur in patients suffering from prolonged or chronic gastrointestinal, pancreatic, or liver disease that interferes with fat absorption and transport. It can be added here that the progressive night-blindness of the Bassen-Kornzweig syndrome is related to vitamin A deficiency secondary to the abetalipoproteinemia, and it may be improved with vitamin A therapy.

A drug of particular concern as a potential cause of progressive night blindness is quinine. In toxic doses it produces progressive retinal degeneration with pigmentary and arteriolar changes. Unfortunately quinine has been used as an abortifacient, producing retinal damage not only in the adult but also in the infant, should it survive the abortion attempt.

Also to be included in the differential diagnosis of progressive night blindness is optic nerve disease. There may be some impairment of night vision consequent to optic neuritis and optic atrophy.

Not to be confused with the foregoing types of night blindness are the common night vision disturbances of myopia and cataract.

Day Blindness: Hemeralopia

Day blindness—deficient vision in good illumination with comparatively better vision in dim illumination—is unusual. Most commonly it is a congenital disorder, inherited as an autosomal recessive condition. Its etiology and pathogenesis are unknown. Generally there is associated amblyopia and color vision deficiency.

In some cases, day blindness is acquired. It may develop as the result of disorders that damage foveal cones; it occurs in association with macular degeneration. It can develop in toxic amblyopia.

A relative day blindness may result from central opacities of the cornea or lens.

Color Vision Disorders

As color vision disorders, particularly the congenital dyschromatopsias, are described thoroughly in Chapter 19, they will be discussed here only as they pertain to ophthalmoneurologic diagnosis.

In lesions of the visual pathways, vision for colors may be impaired before vision for white and form are affected. This fact is of particular importance in detection of visual field defects; a loss not evident when white test objects are presented to the subject may become obvious when colored test objects are used, and the diagnostic implications of *hemiachromatopsia* (inability to discern color in the visual half-field) correspond to those of hemianopia. Furthermore, it is frequently stated that lesions of the conducting system tend to impair red-green discrimination, whereas affections of the percipient elements impair blue-yellow discrimination.

Loss of ability to recognize colors, a condition called *color agnosia*, and inability to recall or name colors, referred to as *amnestic color aphasia*, may result from cerebral affections that do not involve the visual radiations directly.

One congenital color vision disorder merits comment here; this is *achromatopsia*, a recessively inherited condition wherein color vision is absent and vision is monochromatic. It is associated with subnormal vision, nystagmus, and photophobia. This diagnosis must be considered in children with unexplained pendular nystagmus and defective vision; it is not uncommon for the color vision defect to pass unrecognized for years while the family searches for an explanation for the photophobia, abnormal eye movements, and vision deficit. The family should be informed that the condition is nonprogressive and neurologically benign, but that it is hereditary.

Diplopia

Diplopia or double vision is the abnormal subjective sensation of seeing one object as two. Diplopia is usually a binocular phenomenon, but may be uniocular; when both occur in the same patient there may be triplopia or even quadrilopia, and many of the causes of uniocular diplopia may produce multiple images or polyopia.

Pathological binocular diplopia occurs as the result of misalignment of the visual axes due to displacement or deviation of the eye (heterophoria, heterotropia, strabismus, squint). The object of regard stimulates the fovea of one eye (true image) and an eccentric retinal point of the fellow eye (false image). The diplopia is described as horizontal when the images are side by side, vertical when one image is above the other, and torsional when an image is tilted. The false image is projected in a direction opposite to the displacement or deviation of the eye. If the eye is deviated upward, its image is projected downward. If the eye is deviated inward (nasally), its image is projected outward (temporally). In convergent strabismus the diplopia is uncrossed or homonymous, whereas in divergent strabismus the diplopia is crossed or heteronymous. In nonparalytic or comitant strabismus the diplopia is constant in all fields of gaze, whereas in paralytic or noncomitant strabismus, the diplopia worsens (i.e., the separation of images increases) in the fields of action of the faulty muscle. These features are determined by measurement of the diplopia in the cardinal positions of gaze, utilizing red-green goggles, a single red lens, or the Maddox prism to distinguish the images of the two eyes.

In ophthalmoneurologic diagnosis, pathologic binocular diplopia is of greatest significance as a symptom of extraocular muscle paralysis (particularly when it is of recent onset), and other ocular motor disturbances such as convergence spasm or paralysis of convergence or divergence. It is not uncommon for diplopia to be the presenting symptom of increasing intracranial pressure, anterior or posterior fossa tumor, meningitis, neurodegenerative disease, myasthenia gravis, or other equally serious neurologic disease.

An important distinguishing feature of pathological binocular diplopia of organic origin is the fact that the diplopia disappears when one eye is covered. Though a child may not be able to verbally express diplopia, he quickly learns to alleviate the bothersome double vision by squinting one eye closed, by covering one eye with a hand, or by assuming compensatory head positions. The development of these mannerisms in a child should be heeded as a clue to the presence of binocular diplopia and the possibility of neurologic disease.

Uniocular diplopia (or polyopia) may be due to optical abnormalities such as irregularities in the cornea, dislocation or subluxation of the lens, cataractous changes in the lens, or bubbles, crystals, or foreign bodies in the aqueous or vitreous. It may also result from retinal detachment. In rare instances, uniocular diplopia is of central origin; it may be due to cerebral disease, but often it is of hysterical or psychogenic origin.

Oscillopsia

Oscillopsia is the illusory sensation of movement of a stationary object. It is important as a subjective symptom of acquired nystagmus and certain other abnormal eye movements. This disturbance may herald the presence of brain stem or vestibular disease.

Alexia and Dyslexia

Not to be confused with vision defects arising directly from visual pathway affections are sensory visual aphasia and agnosias caused by disturbances in higher centers.

Alexia, commonly referred to as word blindness, is the inability to appreciate the meaning of written words or of musical or mathematical symbols. Dyslexia implies partial impairment; the patient may appreciate letters but not words, words but not numbers, and so forth. The defect may be cortical or subcortical. In cortical alexia, writing also is affected; that is, there is alexia with agraphia. This occurs with lesions in the region of the angular gyrus of the dominant hemisphere. There may be, in addition, object agnosia, spatial agnosia, and other defects. When the lesion is entirely subcortical, deep to the angular gyrus, writing may be preserved. Alexia without agraphia occurs most commonly with cerebrovascular accidents involving the left occipital lobe and splenium of the corpus callosum. Often there is also interruption of the visual pathway, resulting in an associated contralateral homonymous quadrantanopia.

Psychogenic Vision Disturbances

Vision abnormalities due to either malingering or hysteria are not uncommon in school-age children. These disturbances generally follow one of several patterns that can be readily recognized.

Willful feigning of partial vision loss in one or both eyes is one of the more frequently encountered problems. In the event of monocular or asymmetric vision impairment, the spurious nature of the deficiency can best be demonstrated by having the child read a polarized vision chart with both eyes simultaneously. Alternatively, the vision of the better eye can be gradually (and secretively) blurred with high plus lenses as the child reads the Snellen chart with both eyes open. When bilateral vision impairment is claimed, it is often possible to demonstrate telltale inconsistency between distance and near visual acuity. The central visual field findings generally fail to correlate with the declared visual acuity, as the patient usually does not report an appropriate central scotoma. Also, the patient's history of activities often belies the declared vision disability; the child who claims difficulty with school reading may show no disability in reading comics, sports news, movie magazines, or T.V. listings.

Rarely, the problem is one of total blindness in one or both eyes as a manifestation of either hysteria or malingering. In addition to using the aforementioned methods, the examiner can often prove the presence of vision by eliciting normal optokinetic nystagmus or by eliciting following movements by tilting a mirror back and forth before the eye in question.

Field constrictions are relatively frequent problems in this category, and may reflect hysteria, anxiety, fatigue, or simply willful fabrication. Again, the history and observations of the patient's activities and capabilities often belie the declared disability. Also, in formal testing, the linear dimensions of the field may remain remarkably constant when the stimulus size and test distance are significantly changed, and this type of field contraction is referred to as a tubular field. Spiral contraction of the field is also commonly found, especially with fatigue; as the examination proceeds, the field becomes progressively more constricted. Suggestibility is frequently evident.

Whatever the pattern of the manifestation, the examiner must undertake to demonstrate and deal with the problem without exposing the child to ridicule or punishment. As a rule, the children do well with reassurance and positive suggestion; less often does the problem require formal psychiatric care.

PUPIL ABNORMALITIES

The significance of pupillary signs in neurologic disease lies in the protracted course and anatomic distribution of the afferent and efferent pupillary pathways.

The afferent pathway—the retinomesencephalic arc—arises in the receptors of the retina and traverses the optic nerve, chiasm, and optic tract. Leaving the anterior visual pathway before the lateral geniculate body, the afferent pupil fibers traverse the brachium of the superior colliculus and synapse in the pretectal nucleus adjacent to the posterior commissure.

Efferent innervation is mediated by two pathways, one sympathetic, the other parasympathetic. The final common efferent pathway for the dilator pupillae is a three-neuron sympathetic arc. Arising in the hypothalamus, the first sympathetic neuron travels through the brain stem to synapse in the ciliospinal center. From the ciliospinal center the second neuron traverses the sympathetic chain to attain the superior cervical ganglion, where it synapses. The postganglionic sympathetic pupillomotor fibers then accompany the internal carotid artery into the skull, follow the ophthalmic division of the trigeminal nerve (cranial nerve V) into the orbit, and reach the iris dilator via the nasociliary and long ciliary nerves.

For the sphincter pupillae, the final common efferent pathway is a two-neuron parasympathetic arc. The parasympathetic fibers arise in the Edinger-Westphal nucleus just dorsal and rostral to the main oculomotor nuclear mass in the rostral midbrain, and traverse the oculomotor nerve (cranial nerve III) to the ciliary ganglion in the orbit; after synapsing in the ciliary ganglion, the postganglionic parasympathetic fibers reach the iris sphincter via the short ciliary nerves.

Evaluation of pupil abnormalities requires a systematic assessment of pupil shape, position, size, the direct and consensual reaction to changing illumination, and the response to near vision effort, with careful attention to the symmetry and equality of the pupils under all conditions.

Irregularity or distortion of the pupil shape is referred to as *dyscoria*, and displacement or eccentricity of the pupil is termed *corectopia*. Both corectopia and dyscoria may occur as congenital anomalies, but they may also result from local iris abnormality such as posterior synechiae, traumatic iris tears, or iris atrophy. Of neurologic significance is the fact that lesions of the mesencephalon can cause migration of the pupil, leading to corectopia. Detection and clarification of dyscoria and corectopia often depend on careful slit lamp examination. Old photographs may be of help in determining the age of onset.

Abnormalities in the size of the pupils are described by the terms miosis and mydriasis. *Miosis* is a state of excessive constriction of the pupils, generally to less than 2 mm. It may result from irritative lesions of the efferent parasympathetic pathways, as in encephalitis and meningitis, and in inflammation within the cavernous sinus, superior orbital fissure, or orbit. Miosis also can occur as the result of local irritation of the sphincter, as in iritis. It may also result from paralytic lesions of the sympathetic pathways and dilator pupillae. In addition, there is a condition called congenital miosis that is attributed to congenital absence of the iris dilator.

The opposite pupillary state, *mydriasis*, is excessive dilatation of the pupil. It may result from irritative lesions of the efferent sympathetic pathways, but it more commonly results from paralytic lesions of the parasympathetic fibers as they course through the oculomotor nerve from the midbrain to the eye, and a very common cause of paralytic mydriasis is increasing intracranial pressure. The oculomotor pupillary fibers are also vulnerable to disease in the cavernous sinus, in the superior orbital fissure, and in the orbit. Should there be simultaneous paralysis of both oculo-motor parasympathetic pupillary fibers and sympathetic fibers in the cavernous sinus and sphenoidal areas, the mydriasis will be of only moderate degree. Mydriasis may also result from trauma to the eye and from eye disease that affects the iris, the sphincter, or its innervation.

Inequality of pupil size is referred to as *anisocoria*. A principal question to be answered in each case is whether the larger or the smaller pupil is abnormal. As a rule, if the anisocoria is more pronounced in bright light, the larger pupil is abnormal, and if the anisocoria is maximum in dim light, the smaller pupil is abnormal. Although many individuals have a mild degree of "physiologic" pupillary inequality, all anisocoria requires investigation or at least explanation. Anisocoria signifies efferent or effector dysfunction; anisocoria is not a feature of pure afferent lesions.

Defects in specific functions of the pupil, as determined by responses to changes in illumination and near vision effort, are designated by a variety of terms. The term *iridoplegia* describes paralytic rigidity of the pupil to light and near; it denotes a defect in the sphincter or in the parasympathetic efferent pathway, but it does not indicate the specific site of the lesion. Iridoplegia combined with *cycloplegia* (paralysis of accommodation) is referred to as *internal ophthalmoplegia*. In situations where the reaction to near is better than the reaction to light, the term *light-near dissociation* is used; this can occur with afferent conduction defects and with some efferent parasympathetic defects, particularly ciliary ganglion defects, but the light-near dissociation phenomenon is a special feature of pretectal rostral mesencephalic lesions. Numerous eponyms, too, are used to denote certain types of pupillary dysfunction. Preferred terms are those which designate the pathogenesis or site of origin of the defect.

Afferent Pupillary Defects

The pupillary signs of an afferent conduction defect are decreased amplitude of the contraction to light, prolonged latency in the reaction to light, and pupillary escape on prolonged stimulation with light. Both the direct and consensual responses are affected. In pure afferent lesions there is, of course, no defect in the pupil response to near. It hardly seems necessary to add that the pupillary response to light can be perfectly normal in complete blindness. Because the afferent pupillary light fibers depart from the visual pathways anterior to the lateral geniculate body, damage to the postgeniculate visual pathways does not produce defects in the pupillary response to light; only lesions of the pregeniculate pathways or of the pretectal region produce afferent defects in the pupillary light reflex.

In testing for afferent conduction defects, it is essential to avoid misinterpreting a near response as a true light response; in patients able to cooperate, this is accomplished by controlling fixation, whereas in infants the differentiation depends on careful timing of the stimulus and the response.

The amaurotic pupil of an eye that is blind as the result of retinal or optic nerve involvement is characterized by the following: on direct stimulation of the blind eye with light, neither the pupil of the blind eye nor the pupil of the fellow eye responds; on stimulation of the intact eye, however, both pupils respond and they respond equally. It is often stated that the pupil of an amaurotic eye is larger than the pupil of the fellow intact eye; however, in pure afferent defects, the pupils should be of equal size under all conditions. In bilateral blindness of the pregeniculate type, the pupils do tend to be large, but symmetrically so.

Marcus Gunn's pupil sign indicates a unilateral or asymmetric conduction defect in the afferent pathways anterior to the chiasm. It is a valuable objective sign of optic nerve disease in children, and it is particularly useful in the diagnosis of retrobulbar neuritis and optic nerve tumor when the disc appears normal. The conduction defect is demonstrated by the so-called swinging flashlight test, a simple technique for comparing the pupillary constriction elicited by light stimulation of one eye relative to that produced by equal light stimulation of the fellow eye. With the patient looking straight ahead under conditions of constant moderate diffuse illumination, a flashlight (pen light) is swung back and forth from one eye to the other, alternately illuminating each eye several times for 5 to 10 seconds. When light is directed into the normal or better eye, both pupils respond briskly, constricting fully and symmetrically. When light is directed into the affected eye, the pupillary constriction is faulty, reflecting the degree of afferent impairment, and both pupils will show incomplete constriction because of the consensual effect. Thus, on moving the light from the intact eye to the affected eye, both pupils will dilate, and on moving the light from the affected eye to the normal eye, both pupils will constrict to a greater degree. If the afferent prechiasmal conduction defect is pure (i.e., uncomplicated by an efferent innervational or effector defect), there will be isocoria regardless of which eye is illuminated, and the pupil response to near vision will be intact. A modification of the swinging flashlight test may also be effective in demonstrating the asymmetric conduction defect. On monocular occlusion of the normal eye, the pupil of the exposed affected eye will be large, but on occlusion of the abnormal eye, the pupil of the exposed normal eye will be relatively smaller.

Wernicke's hemianoptic pupil sign is indicative of a lesion in the afferent fibers of the optic tract, between the chiasm and the lateral geniculate body. If the sign can be demonstrated or detected, it is useful in distinguishing the homonymous hemianopia of a tract lesion from the homonymous hemianopia of an optic radiation lesion. The sign consists of impaired reaction of both pupils when light is directed onto the blind half of either retina, and intact reaction of both pupils when light is directed onto the seeing half of either retina. This hemianoptic pupil reflex is difficult to elicit because of diffusion of light throughout the eye; more controlled stimulation of the hemiretinas may be accomplished by using the slit lamp beam. In determining the validity of the sign, it is also important to remember that stimulation of the nasal half of the retina normally evokes a better pupillary response than does stimulation of the temporal retina.

Pretectal Pupillary Defects

As already mentioned, the axons of the retinal ganglion cells that mediate the pupillary light reflex synapse in the pretectal nucleus in the rostral midbrain. Intercalated neurons for the light reflex then extend ventrocaudally around the periaqueductal gray from the pretectal nucleus to the Edinger-Westphal nucleus, with a hemidecussation in the posterior commissure. These pretecto-oculomotor light reflex fibers attain the Edinger-Westphal nucleus on the dorsal side, while the near vision fibers approach the nucleus slightly more ventrally. Thus, pathologic changes in the rostral midbrain, particularly lesions infiltrating from a dorsal aspect, can produce defects in the light reflex with sparing, or relative sparing, of the pupillary component of the near reflex. Light-near dissociation of mesencephalic origin is seen in Parinaud's syndrome and in the sylvian aqueduct syndrome or Koerber-Salus-Elschnig syndrome. Also, the classic Argyll Robertson pupil of syphilis is attributed, at least in part, to pretectal involvement. It must be noted, however, that there are forms of light-near dissociation, the so-called pseudo-Argyll Robertson or Argyll Robertson-like pupils, that are not due to mesencephalic disease, but to more peripheral dysfunction; pretectal disease is just one consideration in the differential diagnosis of light-near dissociation.*

Light-near dissociation in aqueductal syndromes in children occurs as the result of pinealomas or other tumors of the pineal region and as the result of chronic hydrocephalus of aqueductal stenosis. By definition, the reaction of the pupils is better to near than to light,† and the pupils are usually large. The range of signs that can be produced by lesions in the area of the rostral midbrain and aqueduct include, in addition to light-near dissociation, corectopia, accommodative defects (particularly spasm of accommodation with impairment of accommodative amplitude), lid retraction, ptosis, nuclear oculomotor paresis, convergence palsy or convergence spasm, vertical gaze palsy, and vertical nystagmus or convergence retraction nystagmus. In various combinations, these signs comprise Parinaud's syndrome and the sylvian aqueduct syndrome. Some clinicians restrict the use of the term Parinaud's syndrome to the combination of vertical gaze palsy, mesencephalic pupillary defects, and nuclear oculomotor paresis, and use the Koerber-Salus-Elschnig eponym to designate the more extensive aqueductal syndrome.

Argyll Robertson pupils are a classic sign of neurosyphilis. Although this condition is not a pediatric disease, description of the characteristics of Argyll Robertson pupils is necessary for purposes of differential diagnosis, as so many disorders produce light-near dissociation. In their fully developed classic form, Argyll Robertson pupils do not react to light directly or consensually, although the retina is sensitive to light. They do react to near, except in the terminal stages when the pupils may become fixed to all stimuli. Typically, the pupils are miotic and dilate poorly in response to reduced light, mydriatics, and psychosensory stimuli. It is useful to remember that the light-near dissociation pupils of neurosyphilis are small, whereas those of pineal area tumors and of Adie's syndrome are large. As a rule, Argyll Robertson pupils are bilateral, but the involvement may be asymmetric. The signs develop gradually rather than abruptly, and therefore incomplete and incipient signs must not be overlooked. In many cases there is dyscoria and iris atrophy.

Efferent Pupillomotor Defects: Parasympathetic Types

Although the motor functions of the pupil are controlled by both parasympathetic and sympathetic innervation, the activity of the sphincter and its parasympathetic innervation predominate. Lesions affecting the parasympathetic pupillomotor outflow in the midbrain or anywhere in the peripheral course to the sphincter pupillae can produce complete or partial pa-

---

*Conditions to be considered in the differential diagnosis of light-near dissociation in adults are syphilis (Argyll Robertson pupil), diabetes (tabes diabetica), pituitary tumor (tabes pituitaria), pinealomas and other lesions in the region of the posterior commissure, Adie's syndrome (tonic pupil) and aberrant regeneration of the third nerve, primary amyloidosis, and myotonic dystrophy. Few of these conditions occur in childhood.

†In pretectal lesions, the dissociation of the light and near responses may be reversed, resulting in decrease of the near reaction and preservation of the light reaction. Accommodative disturbances usually accompany this type of pupillary dissociation.

ralysis of pupillary constriction; there is not only impairment of the pupil response to all stimuli but also dilation of the pupil. In many cases the parasympathetic fibers for accommodation are simultaneously involved, producing internal ophthalmoplegia, the combination of iridoplegia and cycloplegia. Topical diagnosis of the parasympathetic lesion then depends on associated localizing signs, but it is to be emphasized that isolated involvement of the parasympathetic pupillomotor fibers can occur anywhere from the midbrain to eye. Of course, a local ocular pathologic process, particularly old iris trauma, and the deliberate or accidental use of mydriatic or cycloplegic drugs must be considered in every case of pupillary paralysis before embarking on an investigation for neurologic disease. While biomicroscopy is the essential procedure for detection of iris damage, the test useful in differentiating neurogenic pupillary paralysis from that due to cycloplegics is the instillation of pilocarpine (4%). Pilocarpine will effect pupillary constriction in the presence of neurogenic paralysis, but not in the presence of pharmacologic blockade.

Hutchinson's pupil is the dilated pupil of third nerve compression that occurs with expanding supratentorial lesions. This pupillary disturbance is always associated with decreasing level of consciousness and other evidence of increasing intracranial pressure. As intracranial pressure rises, the uncus of the temporal lobe wedges through the tentorium, compressing the oculomotor nerve against the dorsum sella or petroclinoid ligament; the ipsilateral pupil dilates and eventually becomes completely unreactive to light and near. This progressive pupillary paralysis is a valuable sign of the need for surgical decompression, and a unilateral Hutchinson's pupil is frequently a reliable indication of the side of an expanding supratentorial mass, such as a hematoma or tumor. Bilateral pupillary paralysis with increased pressure is a graver sign, usually indicating coning and mesencephalic compression. There may be recovery of pupillomotor function if the pressure is relieved and the patient survives.

Adie's pupil or the Holmes-Adie Pupil is the familiar designation for pupillotonia,

a special type of efferent pupillomotor dysfunction due to postsynaptic parasympathetic denervation. The preferred term for this condition is simply "tonic pupil." The affected pupil shows an absent or markedly defective response to light or only a segmental response to light, delayed slow constriction on near gaze, and sluggish redilation after relaxation of the near vision effort. Under conditions of ordinary diffuse room illumination, the affected pupil may be the smaller one because of its slow redilation to reduced illumination. The tonic pupil does dilate normally to mydriatic drops and to psychosensory stimulation. Also, the consensual responses of the fellow pupil are intact.

As a rule there is an associated defect in accommodation; there may be impaired amplitude or sluggish relaxation of accommodation with resultant complaints of blurred vision.

A distinctive feature of the tonic pupil is its sensitivity to methacholine (Mecholyl), a cholinergic substance. The tonic pupil constricts to topical methacholine (2.5%), whereas the normal pupil does not constrict to methacholine of even higher concentrations. This hypersensitivity reaction may also be seen after instillation of 0.25% pilocarpine. The cholinergic supersensitivity persists for years, providing a valuable diagnostic test for this condition.

The tonic pupil is caused by a lesion of the ciliary ganglion, and the disorder is most often unilateral. The condition may be viral in origin, and it may be associated with involvement of dorsal root ganglion elsewhere. The combination of hypoactive deep tendon reflexes (particularly hypoactive knee and ankle jerks) and tonic pupil is generally referred to as Adie's syndrome or pupillotonic pseudotabes. This condition occurs most commonly in females 20 to 30 years of age, but it may occur in children. In children, a tonic pupil with hypersensitivity to methacholine occurs in familial dysautonomia, the Riley-Day syndrome.

Efferent Pupillomotor Defects: Sympathetic Types

Lesions of the sympathetic pupillomotor pathways produce less profound effects on pupillary function than do lesions of the parasympathetic pathways. Irritative lesions are uncommon, but they are characterized by pupillary dilatation and often an associated elevation of the lid and increased sweating on the same side. More common are paralytic lesions, and the effects of oculosympathetic paralysis are referred to as Horner's syndrome.

Horner's syndrome consists of miosis, ptosis, and facial anhidrosis due to homolateral oculosympathetic paralysis. There may also be ipsilateral ocular hypotony, increased amplitude of accommodation, and hypopigmentation of the iris. The syndrome is more frequently incomplete than complete, and the signs are often subtle. The affected miotic pupil constricts to light and to near vision effort, but it fails to dilate fully in reduced illumination. Hence the miosis and anisocoria are maximum in dim light or darkness and become less obvious in bright light or on near gaze. The ptosis is slight, usually less than 2 mm., and may escape detection. It is best seen on forward gaze, as it is caused by impairment of sympathetic flow to Müller's muscle, a smooth muscle of the lid that affects lid position; there is no defect in levator palpebrarum action. Owing to lack of sympathetic tone in its smooth muscle, the lower lid also may be higher than normal, further contributing to narrowing of the palpebral fissure. The fissure narrowing gives an illusion of enophthalmos; true enophthalmic recession of the globe into the orbit is disputed. In the typical Horner's syndrome, there is also a defect in sweating and in vasoconstriction of the face and neck, making these areas warm, dry, and flushed initially. In some cases sweating is preserved, and in others the

hypohydrosis is limited to the forehead.* If the oculosympathetic paralysis is congenital or develops in the first year or two of life, there is likely to be hypopigmentation of the homolateral iris. It is unusual for depigmentation to occur as the result of Horner's syndrome acquired later in life.

Pharmacologic tests are important in the diagnosis and localization of an oculosympathetic paralysis. If there is a lesion of the first or second sympathetic neuron, the miotic pupil will not dilate to 1% epinephrine drops. If there is a lesion of the second or third sympathetic neuron, the miotic pupil will not dilate to 4% cocaine drops (Table 18–2).

In children, Horner's syndromes are most often seen as the result of birth injury to the brachial plexus; less often are they due to pulmonary disease or thoracic or cervical surgery. Since a subtle congenital Horner's syndrome may go unnoticed for long periods, it is important to try to document the age of onset of the palsy by examining old photographs and all available records before launching an extensive investigation for acquired disease or tumor.

EYE MOVEMENT DISORDERS

Abnormalities of eye movement are cardinal manifestations of neurologic disease.

---

*The sympathetic fibers reach the head as a plexus around the carotid artery. Fibers that control sweating and vasomotor tone to the face leave the oculosympathetic fibers to distribute via the external carotid artery. Therefore Horner's syndrome without sweating may result from a lesion in the sympathetic pathway in its internal carotid course.

TABLE 18–2   OCULOSYMPATHETIC PARALYSIS: PHARMACOLOGIC RESPONSES*

Testing Agent	First Neuron Lesion (from hypothalamus to ciliospinal center)	Second Neuron Lesion (from ciliospinal center to superior cervical ganglion)	Third Neuron Lesion (from superior cervical ganglion to eye)
Atropine 1%	+	+	+
Cocaine 4%	++	−	−
Epinephrine 1%	−	−	+++
Neo-Synephrine 10%	+	+	+++

*plus (+) = dilation
minus (−) = failure to dilate

The extensive anatomic ramifications of the ocular motor system and the complexity of the afferent and efferent mechanisms that govern eye movement provide unlimited opportunity for disturbance of ocular motor functions by all manner of pathologic processes. In children, ocular motor disorders are particularly important clues to brain tumor, inflammatory disease, neurodegenerative disease, and developmental defects. Depending on the site of involvement, ocular motor system dysfunctions present as extraocular muscle palsies, conjugate gaze disorders, nystagmus, and a number of other abnormal movements, some of which have special diagnostic implications. Determining the source and significance of these movement disorders requires careful analysis of their objective characteristics, precise documentation of their mode and age of onset, and assessment of associated signs and symptoms.

Extraocular Muscle Palsies

Extraocular muscle palsies are defects in the action of individual extrinsic ocular muscles due to processes in the final common pathway for eye movement; the dysfunction is in the nuclear or infranuclear portion of the innervating cranial nerve, in the neuromuscular junction, or in the muscle itself. Whereas the primary effect of an ocular muscle palsy is limitation of movement of the eye in the field of action of the affected muscle, the equally important secondary effect is disturbance of the parallelism of the eyes on forward gaze. Because of the action of the antagonists of the paretic muscle, ocular muscle palsies give rise to strabismus (heterotropia or heterophoria), and paralytic strabismus characteristically is incomitant; the dissociation or deviation increases on gaze in the field of action of the paretic muscle, and the secondary deviation (the angle of squint measured with the paretic eye fixing) is greater than the primary deviation (the angle of squint measured with the sound eye fixing). These signs may be overt or subtle, depending on the severity of the muscle weakness. As a rule, in the event of complete or relatively complete paralysis, there is marked strabismus with obvious limitation of movement of the eye in the field of action of the involved muscle. In less severe cases there may be minimal limitation of movement or only muscle paretic nystagmus (a jerking of the eye on movement in the field of action of the affected muscle) with or without strabismus on forward gaze.

The subjective manifestation of ocular muscle paresis is diplopia. This disturbing sensation is a most valuable clue to ocular motor disorders, and it is often the first symptom to convey the need for medical attention. Children often cannot verbalize diplopia, but they will squint, cover one eye with a hand, or assume compensatory head and eye positions to avoid double vision; the development of any such peculiar mannerisms in children should be promptly heeded as a warning of ocular motor disturbance. In patients capable of cooperating, the diplopia can be utilized in identifying the faulty muscle, as separation of the images increases in the field of action of the paretic muscle. Measuring the amount of diplopia in the six cardinal positions of gaze (to the right, to the left, up to the right, up to the left, down to the right, down to the left) is referred to as plotting diplopia fields; the test is performed with the patient wearing a red glass or Maddox prism over one eye (or red-green goggles over both eyes) to differentiate the images of the two eyes.

Identification of the paretic muscle or muscles generally presents no problem; it depends only on results of the motility tests combined with knowledge of the basic anatomy and functions of the extraocular muscles (Table 18–3). More difficult, however, is the delineation of the pathogenesis of the palsy and its significance to the patient.

The causes of extraocular palsies are protean (Table 18–4). Muscle disorders must, of course, be considered in the differential diagnosis of ocular muscle palsies; congenital dysplasia of the muscles for eye movement is uncommon, and the muscular dystrophies of childhood only infrequently involve the muscles for eye movement, though they commonly do affect the muscles for lid movement. A special group of conditions, seemingly heredodegenerative, and all related by chronic progressive external ophthalmoplegia (PEO), may be the exception to this statement. In some instances, the progressive external ophthalmoplegia is of myogenic

TABLE 18–3 THE EXTRAOCULAR MUSCLES

Ocular Muscle	Innervation	Functions
Lateral rectus	Abducens (cranial nerve VI)	Abduction — moves eye outward.
Medial rectus	Oculomotor (cranial nerve III)	Adduction — moves eye inward.
Superior rectus	Oculomotor (cranial nerve III)	Elevation: action increases as eye is abducted; becomes nil when eye is adducted. Intorsion: action increases as eye is adducted. Adduction.
Inferior rectus	Oculomotor (cranial nerve III)	Depression: action increases as eye is abducted; becomes nil when eye is adducted. Extorsion: action increases as eye is adducted. Adduction.
Inferior oblique	Oculomotor (cranial nerve III)	Extorsion: action increases as eye is abducted. Abduction. Elevation: action increases as eye is adducted; becomes nil when eye is abducted.
Superior oblique	Trochlear (cranial nerve IV)	Intorsion: action increases as eye is abducted. Abduction. Depression: action increases as eye is adducted; becomes nil when eye is abducted.

origin, but in others the condition is of neurogenic origin. Progressive external ophthalmoplegia is associated with a variety of other defects (Tables 18–5 and 18–6), and many of these conditions are manifested in childhood.

A more common cause of ocular muscle palsies in children is neuromuscular transmission disease, namely myasthenia gravis, and the ophthalmic signs are often the presenting manifestations of the condition. Characteristically the muscle weaknesses of myasthenia fluctuate, worsening with fatigue and improving with rest, and as a rule, the diagnosis can be promptly established by demonstration of improved muscle strength on administration of edrophonium (Tensilon) intravenously, or preferably Prostigmin intramuscularly.

The greater number of extraocular muscle palsies are resolvable in terms of cranial nerve dysfunction and neurologic disease. Tumor, inflammatory disease, infectious and para-infectious conditions, degenerative and demyelinating processes, vascular disorders, and trauma can affect the cranial nerves anywhere in their course from the brain stem to the eye. With few exceptions, acquired cranial nerve palsies in children are ominous signs of a serious pathologic process, whereas congenital cranial nerve palsies generally are indicative of birth trauma, congenital infection syndromes, or developmental anomalies (aplasia or hypoplasia) of the cranial nerve nuclei or fibers, in which case there may be associated aberrant innervations and paradoxical movements.

Oculomotor (Cranial Nerve III) Palsies

Paralysis of the third cranial nerve has a profound effect on ocular motility, as this nerve supplies four of the muscles that move each eye: the medial rectus, the superior rectus, the inferior rectus, and the inferior oblique. With complete paralysis of the third nerve, the ocular motor signs are inability to rotate the eye medially and inability to elevate or depress the eye, with diplopia in both the horizontal and vertical directions. Also, the eye will be deviated laterally because of action of the intact lateral rectus, and deviated downward and intorted as the result of action of the intact superior oblique. In addition to the ocular motor disturbances, with complete paralysis there will be ptosis, iridoplegia (paralysis and dilatation of pupil), and cycloplegia (paralysis of accommodation). Varying degrees and varying combinations of these

Congenital Ocular Motor Paralyses
Developmental abnormalities of ocular motor nerves and extraocular muscles:

Absence or hypoplasia of cranial nerve nuclei or nerve fibers.
Aberrant innervation.
Dysgenesis (absence or hypoplasia) of extraocular muscle.
Abnormal muscle insertion.
Fibrous substitution of extraocular muscle.
Fascial defects (sheath and check ligament abnormalities).

Special examples:
Möbius syndrome.
Duane's retraction syndrome.
Brown's tendon sheath syndrome.
Strabismus fixus.

Developmental abnormalities of brain affecting ocular motor pathways:
Syringobulbia.
Congenital hydrocephalus.
Hydranencephaly.
Porencephaly.
Hindbrain deformity: Arnold-Chiari Syndrome.

Other congenital and developmental disorders:
"Congenital static familial ophthalmoplegia."
Progressive external ophthalmoplegia.
Myasthenia congenita.
Cyclic oculomotor paralysis.

Acquired Ocular Motor Palsies
Neurogenic
Infections and para-infectious processes:
Encephalitis: brain stem involvement.
Acute viral or bacterial encephalitis or meningoencephalitis.
Postfebrile or post exanthem encephalitis or encephalopathy, as with measles, German measles, chicken pox, or mumps.
Postvaccinial encephalitis, as may occur after immunization with rabies, smallpox, influenza, poliomyelitis, or pertussis vaccines.
Encephalitis related to infection with infectious hepatitis viruses, mononucleosis, or adenovirus infections.

Neuritis: cranial nerve trunk involvement.
Acute neuritis secondary to basal meningitis, intracranial sinusitis, petrositis (Gradenigo's), accessory nasal sinusitis, orbital periostitis, or orbital abscess.
Special types related to infection:
Polyradiculoneuritis (Guillain-Barré).
Acute infective ("rheumatic") polyneuritis.
Benign sixth nerve palsy.

Toxic phenomena related to infection.
Ophthalmoplegia due to toxins of certain bacterial infections such as diphtheria, tetanus, botulism.

Acute inflammatory conditions of uncertain etiology.
Sarcoidosis.
Collagen vascular diseases.

Acquired Ocular Motor Palsies *(Continued)*
Recurrent multiple cranial nerve palsies, "allergic."

Tumors.
Tumors causing direct involvement of ocular motor nerves or nuclei: brain stem gliomas, chordomas, basal meningiomas, neurinomas (von Recklinghausen's).
Tumors causing indirect involvement through hydrocephalus and increased intracranial pressure: chiasmal and parachiasmal, cerebral, intraventricular, and cerebellar tumors.

Vascular disorders.
Arteriovenous malformations, arteriovenous aneurysms, venous and arteriovenous angiomas, intracranial or intraorbital.
Intracerebral, subarachnoid, subdural bleeds.
Thrombosis, embolism.
Vasculitis, arteritis.
Migraine, ophthalmoplegic.

Degenerations.
Demyelinating diseases.
Schilder's disease.
Multiple sclerosis.
Devic's disease.
Leigh's disease.
Dawson's disease.

Systemic metabolic disorders.
Dysthyroidism.
Diabetes.
Deficiency diseases, such as beriberi (thiamine), pellagra (nicotinic acid), and scurvy (ascorbic acid).

Hematologic disorders.
Anemias.
Leukemias.

Trauma.
Craniocerebral.
Orbital.

Intoxications from exogenous poisons.
Metallic — lead.
Organic substances.
Venoms — snake, wasp.
Drugs and spinal anesthetics.

Neuromuscular
Myasthenia gravis.

Myogenic
Primary muscle dystrophies.
Myotonic dystrophy.
Certain forms of progressive external ophthalmoplegia.
Myositis
Collagen vascular diseases.
Myopathy
Dysthyroidism (exophthalmic ophthalmoplegia).
Muscular degeneration.
Fatty degeneration.
Hyaloid degeneration.
Amyloidosis.
Muscular infiltrations.
Reticuloses, particularly the leukemias.

TABLE 18–5 SYNDROMES EXHIBITING PROGRESSIVE
EXTERNAL OPHTHALMOPLEGIA (PEO)*

1. **Progressive External Ophthalmoplegia (Alternatively, Progressive Nuclear Ophthalmoplegia or Ocular Myopathy)**
   - PEO in pure form, or combined with facial or proximal limb weakness, or with pharyngeal weakness, generalized myopathy, pigmentary retinal degeneration, heart block or other cardiac abnormalities, or mental retardation.
   - In this form, PEO probably is myopathic rather than neuropathic.

2. **Oculopharyngeal Dystrophy (of Victor et al.)**
   - Ptosis or PEO combined with dysphagia and dysphonia (pharyngeal weakness).
   - Occurring primarily as a restricted familial condition, suggesting a transmitted single gene defect.
   - In sporadic cases, sometimes combined with facial and limb-girdle weakness.

3. **Chronic Progressive External Ophthalmoplegia and Muscular Dystrophy (of Lind and Prame)**
   - PEO combined with a range of abnormalities including pharyngeal, facial, and proximal limb weakness, retinal degeneration, cardiac conduction defects, mental deficiency, small stature, spinal fluid protein elevation, and EEG abnormalities.

4. **Muscular Dystrophy Including Features of Ocular Myopathy, Distal Myopathy, and Myotonic Dystrophy (of Schotland and Rowland)**
   - PEO combined with dysphagia, facial weakness, cervical muscle weakness, and sometimes distal limb weakness.
   - Occurring in an autosomal dominant pattern.

5. **Ocular Myopathy Associated With Retinitis Pigmentosa**
   - PEO combined with pigmentary retinal degeneration and occasionally also with pharyngeal weakness, hearing loss, vestibular dysfunction, cerebellar ataxia, small stature, delayed sexual development, spasticity.

6. **Retinitis Pigmentosa, External Ophthalmoplegia, and Heart Block (of Kearns and Sayre)**
   - PEO combined with pigmentary retinal degeneration and cardiac conduction defects.
   - Sometimes additional features such as unsteadiness of gait, hearing loss, short stature, delayed sexual development.

7. **Retinitis Pigmentosa, Ophthalmoplegia, and Spastic Quadriplegia (Alfano and Berger and Walsh)**
   - PEO combined with pigmentary retinal degeneration, spastic weakness of limbs, and dysphagia.

8. **Abiotrophic Ophthalmoplegia Externa (Cogan)**
   - PEO combined with other degenerative abnormalities, particularly retinal degeneration.
   - Sometimes with spinal fluid protein elevation, cardiac conduction defects, facial weakness, cervical muscle weakness, EEG abnormalities.

9. **Retinitis Pigmentosa, Acanthocytosis, and Heredodegenerative Neuromuscular Disease (Bassen-Kornzweig Syndrome)**
   - Intestinal malabsorption, abetalipopro-

After Drachman, *in* Smith (ed.): Neuro-Ophthalmology. Vol IV. St. Louis, The C. V. Mosby Co., 1968.

*Progressive external ophthalmoplegia has been recognized as a feature in numerous syndromes exhibiting a variety of manifestations of degenerative disease patterns. Many of the syndromes do not appear to be clear-cut entities since it has not been firmly established that the disease classifications are etiologically separate conditions. However, it is valid to recognize and enumerate associated defects which accompany progressive external ophthalmoplegia in the hope of enlightened identification. Ultimately, the discovery of specific metabolic defects may help settle the issue.

signs occur in partial oculomotor paralysis.

Third nerve palsies occur with a variety of inflammatory, infectious, and para-infectious processes, vascular lesions, tumors, and degenerative and demyelinating diseases that may involve the nerve anywhere from the mesencephalon to the eye. With expanding supratentorial lesions such as hematomas, tumors, cerebral edema, or hydrocephalus, the third nerve is particularly vulnerable to compression by herniation of the temporal lobe, and it would seem that most third nerve palsies in children are the result of increasing intracranial pressure or trauma. In contrast to the situation in adults, oculomotor palsies due to diabetes are not a problem in children, and aneurysms, so frequently a cause of oculomotor palsy in adults, are rare in children. Episodic oculomotor palsy may be seen in children with ophthalmoplegic migraine, but this condition is unusual. In all of these conditions, the oculomotor involvement may be complete or incomplete. Paralysis of only those fibers supplying the extraocular muscles is referred to as external ophthalmoplegia; paralysis of fibers mediating pupillary constriction is referred to as iridoplegia; paralysis of fibers mediating accommodation is

TABLE 18–5 SYNDROMES EXHIBITING PROGRESSIVE
EXTERNAL OPHTHALMOPLEGIA (PEO)* *(Continued)*

9. **Retinitis Pigmentosa, Acanthocytosis, and Heredo-degenerative Neuromuscular Disease (Bassen-Kornzweig Syndrome)** *(Continued)*
   teinemia, acanthocytosis, and progressive ataxic neuropathic disease leading to areflexia, proprioceptive defects, cerebellar dysfunction, Babinski's sign and cutaneous sensory defects.
   — Pigmentary retinal degeneration.
   — Ptosis and PEO in some cases.

10. **Spongiform Encephalopathy With Chronic Progressive External Ophthalmoplegia (Daroff et al.)**
    — PEO with proximal limb weakness, hyporeflexia, heart block, pigmentary retinal degeneration, small stature, delayed sexual development, seizures, spinal fluid protein elevation, EEG abnormalities.
    — Extensive vacuolar changes in many areas of brain and spinal cord, including nuclear and supranuclear ocular motor areas.

11. **Generalized Disorder of Nervous System, Skeletal Muscle, and Heart Block Resembling Refsum's Disease and Hurler's Disease (Shy et al.; Gonatas)**
    — PEO and ptosis, proximal limb weakness, areflexia, pigmentary retinal degeneration, myopathy, neuropathy, cerebellar ataxia, abnormalities of heart rhythm, hearing loss, mild dementia, spinal fluid protein elevation, EEG abnormalities.
    — Lipid accumulation and mitochondrial abnormalities in muscle.
    — Endoneural fibrosis and so-called zebra bodies in peripheral nerves.

12. **Refsum's Syndrome**
    — Peripheral polyneuropathy, cerebellar ataxia, retinitis pigmentosa, spinal fluid protein elevation.
    — In some cases, ichthyosis.
    — In certain instances, PEO.
    — Autosomal recessive disorder of lipid metabolism.
    — Elevated serum phytanic acid levels.
    — Lipid granules in neurons, astrocytes, perivascular macrophages, meninges, and in hepatic and renal cells.
    — "Onion bulb" changes of peripheral nerves.

13. **Hereditary Ataxia of Sanger-Brown**
    — Spinocerebellar degeneration.
    — PEO and ptosis.
    — Sometimes also dysarthria, dysphagia, weakness, hyperreflexia, choreiform movements, optic atrophy, dementia.

14. **Familial Ataxia, Neural Amyotrophy, and External Ophthalmoplegia**
    — PEO.
    — Cerebellar ataxia.
    — Peripheral neuropathy.
    — Sometimes hyporeflexia, pes cavus.
    — Pathologic changes including myopathy of ocular muscles, demyelination of peripheral nerves, loss of anterior horn cells and of cells of Clark's column, and demyelination of dorsal columns.

referred to as cycloplegia; the combination of iridoplegia and cycloplegia constitutes internal ophthalmoplegia, and the combination of internal and external ophthalmoplegia is total or complete ophthalmoplegia. Whether complete or incomplete, internal or external, isolated oculomotor palsies are of limited localizing value. Associated signs are essential to topographical diagnosis. Syndromes of special diagnostic importance with regard to oculomotor involvement are the Benedikt, Weber, and Nothnagel syndromes. Syndromes of multiple cranial nerve palsy involving the oculomotor nerve are the cavernous sinus syndrome, the superior orbital fissure syndrome, and the orbital apex syndrome.

Benedikt's syndrome is indicative of a lesion in the dorsal area of the cerebral peduncle involving the third nerve fibers and the red nucleus or its connections in the brain stem. The syndrome consists of ipsilateral oculomotor signs and contralateral tremor of the face and limbs. If in addition there is lemniscus involvement, there may be contralateral hemianesthesia.

Weber's syndrome results from a destructive pathologic process in the posterior end of the crus cerebri involving the ventral fascicular portion of the third nerve and the pyramidal tract; it may also be produced by a space-taking lesion close to the peduncle, involving the third nerve after it has left the brain stem. The syndrome is characterized by ipsilateral oculomotor signs and contralateral hemiplegia.

Nothnagel's syndrome is caused by a lesion involving the emerging third nerve

TABLE 18–6 CLINICAL FEATURES ASSOCIATED WITH PROGRESSIVE EXTERNAL OPHTHALMOPLEGIA

Pigmentary retinal degeneration
Optic atrophy
Cardiac conduction defects and other cardiac abnormalities
Hearing loss and vestibular dysfunction
Facial weakness
Pharyngeal weakness
Limb-girdle weakness
Hyporeflexia
Spasticity
Ataxia, dysmetria
Mental deficiency
Seizures
EEG abnormalities
Small stature
Delayed sexual development
Spinal anomalies
Hereditary tendencies
Spinal fluid protein elevation
Phytanic acid elevation
Acanthocytosis and abetalipoproteinemia
Reduced steroid excretion

fibers, the superior cerebellar peduncle, and the red nucleus. The syndrome consists of ipsilateral oculomotor signs and ataxia of the limbs contralateral to the lesion.

The cavernous sinus syndrome is characterized by involvement of cranial nerves III, IV, V, and VI, singly or in various combinations, with signs of congestion of the cavernous sinus and its associated venous channels. There may be complete immobility of the eye, ptosis, pupillary rigidity, loss of accommodation, marked edema and venous engorgement of the lids and conjunctiva, and congestion of the orbital tissues with proptosis. There may or may not be evidence of venous engorgement in the fundus. Most complete forms of the syndrome occur with cavernous sinus thrombosis resulting from inflammation or from invasion of the sinus by tumor. As a rule, cavernous sinus syndromes in childhood are of the septic variety, arising from infection in the adjacent sinuses or ear, with accompanying pain and systemic signs of sepsis. Cavernous sinus signs may also develop with carotid aneurysm within the sinus or with carotid-cavernous fistula; important distinguishing signs of the latter are the presence of bruit and signs of arterialization of the lids and conjunctival vessels due to shunting of arterial blood into the venous channels. Whether the etiology is inflammation, tumor, or vascular conditions, the cavernous sinus signs will vary depending on the degree of sinus involvement and the predominant site of the disease. In the anterior form of the syndrome, only the first branch of the trigeminal nerve is affected, whereas in the posterior form, the first and second branches, and sometimes even the third, are affected. In lesions of the sinus and sphenoidal region, the oculomotor fibers for the extrinsic ocular muscles are apt to be involved before those for the intrinsic ocular muscles. Also, there is likely to be only moderate dilatation of the pupil if there is simultaneous involvement of the oculomotor fibers and the sympathetic fibers.

The superior orbital fissure syndrome consists of unilateral oculomotor, trochlear, and abducent paresis combined with involvement of the first branch of the trigeminal nerve without signs of venous congestion. In the superior orbital fissure region, there may be preferential involvement of the oculomotor fibers for the internal ocular muscles. A mass lesion in the region of the superior orbital fissure is a principal cause of this syndrome, though it may also occur with inflammation or trauma. Clinically, one often cannot differentiate the superior orbital fissure syndrome from an anterior cavernous sinus syndrome.

The orbital apex syndrome consists of paresis of the third, fourth, fifth (first branch), and sixth cranial nerves, and proptosis combined with signs of optic nerve involvement. There may be disc edema, retrobulbar neuritis, or optic atrophy, and there may be either central or peripheral visual field defects. As with the cavernous sinus syndrome, the principal etiologies are inflammation or tumor.

Trochlear (Cranial Nerve IV) Palsies

Paralysis of the fourth nerve affects the function of only the superior oblique muscle. As the principal functions of the superior oblique are depression of the eye in adduction and intorsion in abduction, fourth nerve paralysis produces hypertropia (upward deviation) of the affected eye, limitation of depression that worsens on inward rotation, and extorsion that worsens on outward rotation of the involved eye. There is commonly a compensatory head tilt toward the opposite shoulder, with some depression of the chin. Diagnosis of the palsy is easily confirmed by the Bielschowsky head tilt test; when the head is tilted toward the affected side, the involved eye makes an upward movement. The presence or absence of torsion of the eye can be detected by observing selected iris markings or conjunctival blood vessels, or by placing moistened filter paper markers on the cornea or limbus.

Fourth nerve palsies are not common in children, and isolated fourth nerve palsies are of no particular localizing value. Like the third and sixth nerves, the fourth nerve can be involved in cavernous sinus, superior orbital fissure, and orbital apex syndromes. However, the fourth nerves are particularly vulnerable to damage as they emerge from the mesencephalon dorsally and decussate in the anterior medullary vellum. They can be injured in head trauma that produces contusion of the medullary vellum or by blunt forces that displace the brain stem against the tentorium or the cerebellum against the floor of the posterior fossa. They can also be affected by tumor in the region of the roof of the midbrain; thus fourth nerve palsy in children may be indicative of pinealoma. To be differentiated from true fourth nerve palsy are the mechanical disorders of superior oblique function that result from damage to the trochlea or tendon of the superior oblique, as may occur with frontal sinus surgery, superior orbital rim trauma, or inflammation; Brown's tendon sheath syndrome is one such disorder.

Abducens (Cranial Nerve VI) Palsies

Paralysis of the sixth nerve affects the function of only the lateral rectus muscle. As the sole function of the lateral rectus is abduction, sixth nerve paralysis produces limitation of lateral movement of the affected eye, convergent strabismus, homonymous horizontal diplopia that worsens on gaze toward the involved side, and often also a compensatory face turn toward the side of the paretic muscle.

Abducent palsies occur with relative frequency in children, and with few exceptions, they are indicative of serious neurologic disease. Because the course of the sixth nerve from the pons to the eye is quite long, the nerve is apt to be affected by increasing intracranial pressure; thus, abducent paralysis is often a nonspecific, nonlocalizing sign of hydrocephalus, intracranial tumor, intracranial hemorrhage, or cerebral edema of any origin. The nerve may also be involved more directly by tumor in the brain stem, by tumor along the base of the skull, by nasopharyngeal tumors, or by parasellar lesions. The abducent nerve is also particularly vulnerable to trauma, especially because its course over the temporal bone is sharply angulated. Like the oculomotor and trochlear nerve, the abducent nerve is also subject to the effects of meningitis and other intracranial inflammatory diseases, degenerative and demyelinating diseases, vascular processes, and neurotoxins. Within the cavernous sinus it is vulnerable to inflammatory, thrombotic, and neoplastic processes, and it is also frequently damaged by the pressure of carotid-cavernous fistula. It can similarly be involved in superior orbital fissure and orbital apex syndromes. Developmental and congenital abnormalities of the abducent nerve and its effector muscle are also relatively common. Syndromes of particular importance in the differential diagnosis of abducent paralysis in children are the Möbius syndrome, Duane's syndrome, Gradenigo's syndrome, and the benign sixth nerve palsy syndrome. Syndromes of topographical significance are the Foville, Millard-Gubler, and Raymond-Cestan syndromes.

Foville's syndrome is indicative of a pathologic process in the lower part of the pons at or just above the level of the abducent nucleus, involving also the fibers of the facial nerve and pyramidal tract. It is characterized by ipsilateral lateral rectus palsy and loss of conjugate gaze to the same side, and hemiplegia of the contralateral limbs. There may also be a Horner's syndrome.

The Millard-Gubler syndrome is caused by a lesion in the pons below the abducent nucleus, involving the abducent nerve, the facial nerve, and the pyramidal fibers. The syndrome consists of lateral rectus palsy and peripheral facial palsy ipsilateral to the lesion, and paresis of the limbs contralateral to the lesion. In contrast to Foville's syndrome, there is no gaze paresis, since the association fibers of the abducent nucleus are not involved.

The Raymond-Cestan syndrome is characterized by ipsilateral lateral rectus palsy and contralateral hemiplegia; it is indicative of a lesion involving the abducent nucleus and pyramidal fibers in the pons.

Möbius syndrome is the familiar eponym for congenital facial palsy with inability to abduct the eyes beyond the midpoint. The facial palsy is usually bilateral, frequently asymmetric, and often incomplete, tending to spare the lower face and platysma. Typically there is a masklike expression, but sagging of the face is not a prominent feature of this congenital facial palsy, in contrast to acquired facial palsy in adults. Corneal complications and epiphora are variable. As a rule, the abduction defect (whether unilateral or bilateral) is complete, but convergent deviation on gaze forward is not regularly present. Characteristically there is no diplopia, and usually there is no amblyopia. There may be a compensatory face turn. In most cases vertical movements, convergence, and adduction for lateral gaze are intact, but there may be variable defects in each of these. In addition to the abnormalities of eye and facial movements, there may be other associated developmental defects, including ptosis, palatal and lingual palsy, deafness, absence of vestibular responses, deficiencies of pectoral and lingual muscles, micrognathia, syndactyly, supernumerary digits, and even absence of hands, feet, fingers, and toes.

The pathogenesis of the Möbius syndrome and its associated anomalies is unsettled. There is some evidence that the oculofacial motor abnormalities are due to a disorder of supranuclear mechanisms, but muscle defects and hypoplasia of cranial nerve nuclei have also been implicated.

Duane's syndrome (Stilling-Türk-Duane syndrome) is a congenital deficiency of abduction with an associated retraction of the globe on adduction. Typically the retraction is accompanied by narrowing of the palpebral fissure. There may also be deficient adduction of the affected globe, with vertical or oblique movement of the eye on attempted adduction.

The deficiency of abduction can be partial or complete, unilateral or bilateral. There is often a compensatory face turn toward the side of the affected lateral rectus, with the eyes preferentially turned toward the unaffected side. On gaze forward the eyes may be orthotropic or esotropic. Diplopia and amblyopia are not regular features of the syndrome. The associated retraction and fissure narrowing vary in amount; they may be pronounced or barely detectable.

There has been controversy as to whether Duane's syndrome is caused by primarily mechanical, muscular, or neural defects. Paradoxical innervation of the extraocular muscles has been demonstrated in Duane's syndrome, and aplasia of the abducens has been reported in a necropsy study; an anomaly of innervation may explain the paradoxical innervation.

This ocular motor disorder may occur as an isolated congenital defect in otherwise normal individuals, but it has been seen in association with the Klippel-Feil syndrome and other congenital disorders. In some instances it is familial.

Gradenigo's syndrome consists of an acquired abducens palsy with pain in the distribution of the homolateral trigeminal nerve. It indicates disease involving the petrous portion of the sixth nerve and the adjacent gasserian ganglion. The principal signs and symptoms are lateral rectus weakness and diplopia, eye and facial pain, photophobia, lacrimation, and sometimes corneal hypesthesia. There may also be involvement of the seventh nerve, producing an associated facial palsy. The usual source of the syndrome is otitis media and mastoiditis with inflammation extending into the petrous bone, its meninges, and the inferior petrosal sinus. There may be clinical signs or cerebrospinal fluid evidence of meningitis. Extradural abscess, even subdural abscess, and brain abscess should be considered. In some cases the syndrome is indicative of tumor.

Benign sixth nerve palsy has been described as a distinct clinical entity in children. It is a painless acquired abducent palsy that clears without residua. The palsy typically develops 1 to 3 weeks after a nonspecific febrile or upper respiratory illness. Improvement in the palsy usually begins within 3 to 6 weeks after its onset, and resolution is usually complete within 10 weeks. This transient benign palsy is thought to represent the neurotropic effect of a viral infection. It may, however, represent a process similar to that of Gradenigo's syndrome, a thrombophlebitis of the inferior petrosal sinus. Cerebrospinal fluid changes are not usually present, but relative lymphocystosis of the peripheral blood has been found in a number of children with benign sixth nerve palsy.

This benign cranial nerve syndrome is an exception to the rule that the development of a cranial nerve palsy in a child is an ominous event, usually indicating intracranial tumor, hydrocephalus, meningitis, or demyelinating disease.

Conjugate Gaze Disorders

In contrast to extraocular muscle palsies that signify defects in the final common pathway for the action of individual extrinsic ocular muscles, disturbances of the conjugate and disjunctive movements of the eyes—that is, the paired movements of the two eyes in gaze upward, downward, laterally, and in convergence and divergence—are signs of disorder in the supranuclear centers and pathways that govern physiological directional movements of both eyes in unison. Depending on the site and nature of the lesion, there may be paralysis of gaze in a given direction, conjugate deviation of the eyes (paralytic or spastic), or dissociated movements, such as skew deviation or internuclear ophthalmoplegia. In each instance, only the function or activity represented in the particular region involved is impaired; other movements, though they require the same extrinsic ocular muscles, remain intact. Thus in supranuclear paralysis of right lateral gaze, the left medial rectus fails to adduct on attempted right gaze, but it can adduct normally for convergence.

Although the complex central mechanisms and pathways for the supranuclear control of conjugate and disjunctive eye movements will not be reviewed in detail here, an attempt is made to incorporate this information in the descriptions of specific conjugate gaze disorders that follow.

Horizontal gaze palsies are manifested by inability to look laterally toward the right or left with both eyes; characteristically there is no diplopia, as the two eyes are affected symmetrically. There may be impairment of voluntary and command movements, of pursuit movements, of optically induced movements, or of reflex vestibular movements selectively or in combination, and an analysis of the elements involved is of importance in topographical diagnosis. Voluntary and command movements are tested by asking the patient to look in a given direction. Pursuit movements are tested by having the patient fixate and follow a slowly moving target. Optically induced movements and the reflex of regard are tested by attempting to attract the patient's attention to a target brought in from the periphery of his field. Vestibular and proprioceptive reflex movements are tested by quickly flexing, extending, or rotating the patient's head.

A palsy of voluntary and command movements with preservation of the other components of lateral gaze and reflexive horizontal movements suggests a lesion in the cortical gaze center of the frontal lobe (Brodmann's area 8) or in the corresponding internal capsule. Paralytic lesions in these areas produce a defect in gaze toward the contralateral side. Initially there may be a conjugate deviation of the eyes toward the side of the lesion because of the unopposed effect of the intact contralateral oculogyric center, and there may be an accentuation of the fixation and proprioceptive reflexes. As a rule, the gaze palsy of hemisphere lesions is of relatively short duration. In association with the gaze palsy of a frontal lesion there will often be facial palsy and hemiplegia on the side contralateral to the lesion.

Defects in movements induced by visual stimuli (that is, pursuit movements, the optically elicited reflex of regard, and the fixation movements of optokinetic nystagmus) occur with more posterior lesions of the hemispheres, principally with lesions of the occipital centers (Brodmann's areas 18 and 19).

Impairment of all components of lateral gaze, including the movements in response to proprioceptive stimuli, points to a lesion in the supranuclear horizontal gaze centers of the pons and in the adjacent posterior longitudinal bundle. In contrast to gaze palsies of cortical and subcortical origin, the gaze defect of a pontine lesion is toward the side of the lesion; the associated conjugate deviation is toward the side opposite the lesion. Also, pontine gaze palsies tend to be more enduring than cortical and subcortical gaze palsies, and bilateral gaze palsies are more apt to be of pontine origin. Pontine horizontal gaze palsies are often accompanied by homolateral peripheral facial palsy, homolateral abducens palsy, and contralateral hemiplegia (the Foville-Millard-Gubler syndrome). The primary consideration in children with these signs is pontine glioma; tumors of adjacent regions also may produce these signs by pontine compression. A special type of horizontal gaze disorder seen in children is congenital ocular motor apraxia.

Congenital ocular motor apraxia is a disorder of voluntary horizontal gaze movements that is distinguished by the presence of compensatory head thrusts. The classic clinical picture is unmistakable, but the condition may be subtle in some cases. Typically the child with congenital ocular motor apraxia is unable to look quickly toward either side voluntarily, either in response to command or in response to attraction by an eccentrically situated visual stimulus; he may, however, be able to follow a slowly moving visual target to either side, and he characteristically shows retention of random and involuntary (reflexive) lateral movements. To compensate for the defect in purposive lateral gaze, the child thrusts his head laterally to divert the eyes to the desired point of fixation. In so doing, he induces a contraversive deviation of the eyes, necessitating an overshoot with the head thrust to attain fixation; when the desired position of the eyes is achieved, the child corrects his head position. The head thrust or head jerking in many cases is the most conspicuous manifestation of the disorder, and it is often the feature which draws attention to the gaze defect. Obligate contraversive deviation of the eyes (Roth-Bielschowsky deviation) in response to body rotation, and absence of the fast phase of nystagmus on rotation and on optokinetic nystagmus testing are regular features of congenital ocular motor apraxia. There may also be blinking of the eyes as the child attempts eccentric gaze to either side. Often the condition becomes less conspicuous with age.

The pathogenesis of this disorder is obscure; it may possibly be due to delayed myelination of the ocular motor pathways for conjugate lateral gaze. It occurs more frequently in males than in females, and familial instances of ocular motor apraxia have been reported, speaking for genetic determination. The gaze defect is not regularly associated with other neurologic defects, but affected children do tend to be clumsy, and they quite naturally have difficulties in reading efficiently.

Gaze disorders like congenital ocular motor apraxia have been described in association with agenesis of the corpus callosum, macrocephaly, tumor of the medulla and cerebellum, and kernicterus. Also, an acquired ocular apraxia due to bilateral lesions of the frontal eye fields may be seen in adults, but this type is usually not associated with the typical head thrust, though there may be apraxia of the head and limbs.

Vertical gaze palsies are characterized by inability to look up or down fully with both eyes. In most cases there is inability to look up; less often there is inability to look up and down; rarely is there selective impairment of gaze down. As with horizontal gaze palsies, various components of vertical gaze may be affected. For example, there may be loss of voluntary vertical gaze movements with retention of pursuit and reflex movements, or there may be loss of both voluntary and pursuit movements with retention of only reflex movements in response to proprioceptive and vestibular stimulation. The supranuclear nature of a vertical gaze palsy can be demonstrated by eliciting a Bell's phenomenon (upward rotation of the eyes during lid closure) or by eliciting vertical eye movements in response to flexion and extension of the head as proof of the integrity of the ocular motor nuclei and infranuclear pathways.

As a rule, vertical gaze palsies are indicative of a lesion in the mesencephalic tegmentum or adjacent structures; clinically significant vertical gaze palsies are rarely of cortical or subcortical origin. A principal cause of vertical gaze palsies in children is tumor in the third ventricle or midbrain, particularly tumor of the pineal gland. Aqueductal stenosis and hydrocephalus also produce vertical gaze palsies in children. Other causes include trauma with contusion of the midbrain, degenerative and demyelinating disease, encephalitis, and vascular disorders.

Signs commonly associated with vertical gaze palsies due to disease in the area of the midbrain include pupillary abnormalities such as light-near dissociation, general pupillomotor rigidity, corectopia and dyscoria, and accommodation disturbances, particularly spasm of accommodation with impairment of accommodative amplitude. There may be pathological lid retraction, ptosis, extraocular muscle paresis, and convergence palsy. In some cases there are spasms of convergence, convergent retraction nystagmus, and vertical nystagmus, particularly on attempted vertical gaze. Combinations of these signs in association with vertical gaze palsies are variously described as the Koerber-Salus-Elschnig syndrome or the sylvian aqueduct syndrome. The customary eponymic designation for an isolated vertical gaze palsy or a vertical gaze palsy associated with only pupillary abnormalities and nuclear oculomotor paresis is Parinaud's syndrome.

Convergence palsy, in pure form, is inability to adduct the two eyes to fix on a near object in the absence of medial rectus palsy or paralysis. There is horizontal diplopia on attempted near gaze, and small degrees of base-out prisms produce diplopia, as adduction for convergence is all but impossible. True convergence palsy must be differentiated from convergence insufficiency. In convergence insufficiency, some degree of convergence is usually present, and some adduction for near can be effected with base-out prisms. Also, convergence insufficiency tends to be less constant than true convergence palsy.

Convergence palsy occurs with tumors of the midbrain and third ventricle, particularly pinealomas, and it is often combined with vertical gaze palsy. It is also seen with encephalitis, demyelinating diseases, vascular lesions, and head trauma.

Divergence palsy is inability to abduct the eyes into a parallel position in the absence of lateral rectus palsy or paralysis. There is homonymous diplopia for distant gaze. This condition may be seen in encephalitis, in multiple sclerosis, and with head trauma.

Internuclear ophthalmoplegia is usually described as failure of adduction on conjugate gaze in association with dissociated jerk nystagmus of the abducting eye as the result of a lesion in the medial longitudinal fasciculus. There are, however, two descriptions and classifications of internuclear ophthalmoplegia in current usage; both are presented here.

According to the Cogan classification, internuclear ophthalmoplegia denotes a lesion of the medial longitudinal fasciculus (MLF) characterized by subnormal adduction of the medial rectus ipsilateral to the lesion, on horizontal gaze toward the side opposite the lesion, with jerk nystagmus of the abducting fellow eye. If there is concomitant impairment of adduction on convergence, the internuclear ophthalmoplegia (INO) is referred to as an anterior INO, signifying a lesion in the midbrain. If adduction on convergence is preserved, the INO is referred to as a posterior type, indicating a more posterior lesion, and there may be superimposed involvement of abducent and lateral gaze function with a lesion at the level of the fourth ventricle. The internuclear ophthalmoplegia is further named according to the side of the affected medial rectus, and this terminology in effect designates the side of the lesion. Thus, in a right posterior internuclear ophthalmoplegia, Cogan classification, there is normal convergence, but on left conjugate gaze there is incomplete adduction of the right eye and jerk nystagmus of the left eye, and the lesion is in the right portion of the MLF.

In the Lutz classification, anterior INO denotes supranuclear paresis of adduction on lateral gaze with nystagmus in the abducting eye, and posterior INO denotes supranuclear paresis of abduction on lateral gaze. Thus many clinicians use the term anterior internuclear ophthalmoplegia for adduction failure on lateral gaze with or without convergence impairment, and reserve the term posterior internuclear ophthalmoplegia for supranuclear failure of abduction on lateral gaze with preservation of abduction in response to vestibular stimulation.

Diagnosis of the classic forms of internuclear ophthalmoplegia is not difficult. Detection of less obvious cases may be enhanced by testing horizontal optokinetic responses. When the targets are moved in the direction of the involved medial rectus (toward the lesion), the amplitude of response is greater in the contralateral eye. In a bilateral INO, on rotation of targets from left to right, the nystagmus is greater in the left eye, and on rotation of targets from right to left, the nystagmus is greater in the right eye. There may also be dysmetria, an ataxic overshoot of the eye opposite to that showing the medial rectus involvement on lateral gaze. Vertical nystagmus, usually evoked by upward gaze, and skew deviation are also seen with internuclear ophthalmoplegia.

In general, bilateral internuclear ophthalmoplegia is most often associated with demyelinating disease, whereas unilateral INO is most often due to vascular disease. In children, INO may be a presenting or prominent sign of tumor involving the brain stem. Infrequently, myasthenia gravis may produce ocular motor disturbances mimicking INO.

Skew deviation is the term applied to divergence of the eyes in the vertical plane; it is due not to an isolated extraocular muscle palsy or orbital defect, but to a supranuclear lesion in the central nervous system. Often there is intorsion of the lower eye and extorsion of the higher eye, or it may just appear that one eye is deviated down and in, and the other, up and out. The deviation may remain constant or it may vary in different directions of gaze, and in some cases it may resemble an alternating hypertropia, with right hypertropia on gaze to one side and left hypertropia on gaze to the other side. As a rule, there is vertical diplopia.

Skew deviation occurs with lesions at many sites in the brain stem, particularly with lateral lesions of the pontine tegmentum. It also occurs with disease of the cerebellum or vestibular apparatus. Often the etiology is tumor, as with pontine skew deviation in particular, but skew may also result from vascular disease and less grave problems. It has been seen as the result of acute cerebellar lesions, particularly after trauma or posterior fossa surgery, and it

may be transient. Skew is also associated with the Arnold-Chiari malformation. Depending on the site of the lesion, there may be other signs, such as internuclear ophthalmoplegia. It is often said that the side of the hypotropic eye is the side of the lesion.

Spastic deviations — tonic or clinic deviation of the eyes — occur in several situations. First, in any case of conjugate gaze paralysis there may be spastic deviation of the eyes in the opposite direction as the result of unopposed activity of intact mechanisms. Pure types of spastic deviation, however, may result from irritative conditions of the central nervous system; they occur with such processes as meningitis, encephalitis, hemorrhage, trauma, and epilepsy. A common type of spastic deviation is that which occurs as part of an adversive seizure, a focal motor seizure that involves the frontal oculogyric center, producing tonic and clonic contractions of the extraocular muscles with deviation of the eyes toward the side contralateral to the irritative focus. It is usually accompanied by facial twitching, by turning of the head, and by jacksonian involvement of the extremities on the side contralateral to the epileptic focus. Another important type of spastic deviation is the so-called oculogyric crisis, in which there is sporadic tonic deviation of the eyes, most commonly upward. The exact mechanism of oculogyric crisis is unclear, but it is generally attributed to disturbances in the extrapyramidal system and it is seen most commonly in postencephalitic parkinsonism. Spastic deviations of this type may result from certain phenothiazines, and it is important to consider the effects of drugs in evaluating spastic deviations in children.

A spastic deviation of considerable interest in children is spasm of convergence. Like other spastic deviations, convergence spasms may result from inflammatory, traumatic, and other irritative lesions, but rhythmic tonic or clonic convergent movements are a particularly important feature of the aqueductal syndromes. Very commonly, however, convergence spasms are on a voluntary or psychogenic basis as part of spasm of the near reflex, in which cases the diagnosis can be made by the use of +3.00 lenses or cycloplegic drops.

Nystagmus

Nystagmus is defined as involuntary rhythmic oscillations of one or both eyes in any or all fields of gaze. The term usually connotes a pathologic state of the complex afferent and efferent systems controlling ocular tonus and the position of the eyes, but it must be remembered that there also are physiologic and induced forms of nystagmus that may be elicited by appropriate stimuli.

Before discussing the significance and classification of specific types of nystagmus, it is appropriate to review the terminology applied to the analysis of the objective characteristics of the oscillations.

There are just two principal morphologic types of nystagmus—pendular and jerk. *Pendular nystagmus* is characterized by oscillations of approximately equal speed in both the to-and-fro direction, like the even swing of a clock pendulum. *Jerk nystagmus* is characterized by a biphasic rhythm, with a slow component in one direction and a rapid component in the opposite direction. Jerk nystagmus is customarily named according to the direction of the rapid phase. Thus, right jerk nystagmus describes an oscillatory cycle composed of a slow swing toward the left and a rapid movement toward the right.

The oscillations of pendular and jerk nystagmus are further described according to their plane, their amplitude, and their rate. The plane of the oscillations may be horizontal, vertical, or rotary (torsional), or of a mixed type such as horizontal-rotary or oblique. The amplitude may be fine (excursions of less than 3 degrees), medium (excursions of 5 to 15 degrees), or coarse (excursions of more than 15 degrees), and the rate or frequency of the oscillations may be rapid or slow. In general, the rate varies with the amplitude; the faster the rate, the finer the amplitude, and vice versa.

Nystagmus may also be graded on the basis of its severity or prevalence in various directions of gaze; this terminology applies primarily to jerk nystagmus of constant direction, but it may be useful in following the course of disease. If the nystagmus occurs only on gaze in the direction of the quick component, it is referred to as *first degree nystagmus.* If the nystagmus occurs on gaze in the direction of the quick component and on gaze forward, it is *second degree nystagmus.* If the nystagmus is present on gaze to both sides and on forward gaze, it is *third degree nystagmus.*

The essential techniques of nystagmus evaluation are observation, characterization, and recording of its basic features, noting how the nystagmus behaves in all directions of gaze, how it responds to vestibular stimulation and postural changes, and how it is influenced by visual fixation. Clinical observation of the oscillations can be augmented by the use of lenses to magnify the ocular movements; a loupe, Bartels' spectacles, Frenzel goggles, or even the slit lamp or ophthalmoscope can be used for this purpose. More exact analysis and permanent objective recording of the ocular movements can be accomplished by electronystagmography; this technique allows not only accurate recording of the spontaneous oscillations with the eyes open and closed but also the responses to optokinetic tests and to caloric, rotational, galvanic, and compression tests. The results of these observations convey information as to the source or mechanism of the eye movements, and the ultimate purpose of the analysis of the nystagmus is to determine its significance to the health of the patient.

Physiologic Nystagmus

The clinically important types of physiologic and induced nystagmus are optokinetic nystagmus, evoked vestibular nystagmus, end-position nystagmus, and voluntary nystagmus.

Optokinetic nystagmus is a biphasic jerky nystagmus induced by watching a series of objects moving across the field of vision. The slow phase is produced as the eyes involuntarily pursue one of the objects to the limit of view or to the limit of comfortable conjugate gaze. The jerk phase is produced as the eyes make a rapid corrective movement in the opposite direction to fixate another target in the sequence. A common example of optokinetic nystagmus (OKN) is train or railroad nystagmus, produced when an individual in a moving vehicle watches the passing scenery. For clinical purposes, OKN is elicited by a sequence of stripes or figures on a rotating drum or strip of cloth; even a newspaper headline can be used. The response depends on many factors, including the patient's vision and attention, the adequacy of the stimuli, and the integrity of the ocular motor pathways. Although OKN is dependent on vision, it is not dependent specifically on intact central vision or intact visual fields; it can be elicited in the presence of variable degrees of central vision and field defects. It is important, however, that the size and separation of the targets be suitable to the degree of vision; the response will not be elicited if the visual angle subtended by the target is too small or if the rotation is too fast. Since the presence of the OKN response indicates that some vision is present, the OKN test can be useful in demonstrating and calibrating vision in infants, in handicapped or retarded children, and in malingerers. The principal clinical use of OKN testing, however, is the detection and localization of lesions involving the ocular motor pathways, since lesions in various portions of the brain may alter either phase of the OKN response. Lesions involving the white matter of the parietotemporal or parieto-occipital region, in or about the supramarginal gyri, are particularly apt to alter the OKN response. With lesions in this area, the response is defective on rotating the drum toward the side of the lesion, and hemianopia per se is not the determining factor. As a rule, a defective or asymmetric horizontal OKN response ("positive" OKN sign) in the presence of a hemianopia indicates a lesion in the white matter of the parietotemporal or parieto-occipital region involving the middle or posterior part of the optic radiations, whereas a normal or symmetric horizontal OKN response ("negative" OKN sign) in the presence of a hemianopia suggests that the lesion is in more anterior regions of the optic radiations, in the lateral geniculate body or optic tract, or possibly in the cortex itself, near the calcarine fissure. An asymmetric disturbance of vertical responses as compared to horizontal responses suggests the possibility of a brain stem lesion. Also, a dissociated horizontal OKN response may be seen with medial longitudinal fasciculus lesions and internuclear ophthalmoplegia; on rotation of targets toward the side of the lesion, the nystagmus will be greater in the unaffected eye than in the eye with the impaired adduction.

Evoked vestibular nystagmus is a jerk nystagmus induced in normal individuals by displacement of endolymph in the semicircular canals. It can be produced by acceleration and deceleration of the head on rotation of the body, and by irrigation of the ear with cold or warm water. It can also be produced by compression and suction techniques and by galvanic stimulation. The slow phase is the vestibulogenic phase; it is dependent on the impulses from the semicircular canals and its direction is always in the direction of flow of the endolymph. The rapid phase is the corrective movement, and the jerk is in the direction opposite to the flow of the endolymph. Thus, irrigation of an ear with cold water will produce nystagmus toward the opposite side, and irrigation of an ear with warm water will produce nystagmus toward the side of the irrigated ear ("COWS" = cold, opposite; warm, same). Pure horizontal vestibular nystagmus can be produced by rotation in the upright position with the head flexed 30° on the chest, and vertical nystagmus can be produced by rotation with the head tilted toward either shoulder. The anatomic and physiologic facts governing vestibular responses are readily available in basic texts.

End-position nystagmus describes the unsustained jerky oscillations that commonly occur on extreme lateral gaze. True end-position nystagmus appears only when the object of regard is beyond the binocular field of vision on horizontal gaze; it does not normally occur on vertical gaze. Typically there are only 10 to 15 oscillations, and the jerk is always in the direction of gaze. The nystagmus generally is symmetrical, though it tends to be greater in the abducting eye. End-position nystagmus is of no pathological significance. It occurs in healthy individuals, and it is often seen in tired and nervous individuals.

Voluntary nystagmus is a rapid pendular ocular tremor that certain individuals can induce by will or physical effort. This feat usually requires voluntary fixation and convergence effort, but it can be produced by other means. The oscillations can rarely be sustained for more than brief periods of time, and they can rarely be maintained in all positions of gaze. An intent expression, tensing of muscles, squinting and tearing, and exhaustion of the phenomenon are clues to the volitional nature of this nystagmus. Children may learn this trick early in life; they use it to amuse their friends, to distress their parents, and to confuse their doctors.

Pathological Nystagmus

Although our knowledge of the complex mechanisms underlying various types of nystagmus is incomplete, all spontaneous and pathological nystagmus can be related to a disturbance in one of three basic mechanisms that regulate the position and movement of the eyes. Nystagmus may arise from defects in the fixation mechanisms, from defects in the conjugate gaze mechanisms, or from defects in the vestibular system.

Nystagmus from defects in the fixation mechanisms typically is present on forward gaze. It tends to be variable and it diminishes when fixation is abolished. The nystagmus of imperfect fixation may arise from a disorder of the visual sensory portion or the motor portion of the system for fixation. If the defect is within the eye itself or in the afferent visual pathways anywhere from the retina to the visual cortex and its association areas, the nystagmus is commonly referred to as "ocular" nystagmus, and it tends to be basically pendular more often than jerky. If the imperfect fixation is due to a lesion in the posterior fossa or motor pathways, the nystagmus is often referred to as a "neurologic" type of fixation nystagmus; it may be either pendular or jerky, and it may develop at any age.

The "ocular" types of fixation nystagmus include:

1. Pendular nystagmus of subnormal vision and ocular defects. As a rule, pendular nystagmus will develop secondary to poor central vision if the vision deficit has been congenitally determined or if the vision has been lost in the first year or two of life, and pendular nystagmus may in fact be the presenting sign of a vision defect or ocular abnormality in an infant. The nystagmus is usually a horizontal pendular type, and it remains horizontal pendular on upward and downward gaze. On lateral gaze it con-

verts to jerk nystagmus, with the jerk in the direction of gaze. It characteristically is seen in association with congenital optic atrophy and with morphologic and functional abnormalities of the macula, as in chorioretinitis and coloboma involving the macula, and in albinism, in aniridia, and in achromatopsia; it is also seen with high refractive errors and with opacities of the media that interfere with normal fixation.

2. Hereditary pendular nystagmus. Congenital pendular nystagmus may be seen in families without overt evidence of an ocular abnormality, in which case it is simply called hereditary pendular nystagmus. It may be inherited as a dominant or sex-linked trait, and it appears within the first few months of life. Like the nystagmus of ocular disease, it is a horizontal pendular nystagmus that remains horizontal pendular on vertical gaze and converts to directional jerk nystagmus on lateral gaze. It may be accompanied by some rhythmic contraversive head movements. The nystagmus persists throughout life, though it may lessen with age. There is no oscillopsia.

3. Latent nystagmus. A conjugate nystagmus evoked by occlusion of one eye is a latent nystagmus. This is a congenital condition and it is usually bilateral. It is often associated with strabismus, particularly esotropia and double hypertropia with monocular amblyopia. The nystagmus elicited is a jerky nystagmus with the jerk toward the fixing eye, and the nystagmus is greatest when gaze is directed toward the open eye. This jerk nystagmus may be superimposed on a pendular nystagmus. The visual acuity is better with both eyes open than with either eye occluded.

4. Spasmus nutans. In its complete form, spasmus nutans is characterized by the triad of pendular nystagmus, head nodding, and torticollis. The etiology of this acquired condition is obscure, but the clinical features are distinctive, and the diagnosis can often be made even when only one or two elements of the triad are present. The condition develops within the first year or two of life, lasts only a matter of months, and does not signify disease. The nystagmus of spasmus nutans characteristically is a very fine and extremely rapid horizontal pendular nystagmus that is variable in different directions of gaze. It tends to be asymmetric, and it may be unilateral. Poor illumination and deprivation have been implicated in the etiology of the nystagmus, but its true cause is unknown and vision is usually quite normal upon recovery. The head nodding is variable. It is usually oblique or horizontal, and of moderate rate and amplitude. Head nodding is not compensatory for the nystagmus and it may occur independently of it. The head tilt or turn is also variable and often subtle. Although classical spasmus nutans does not signify disease, in rare instances a developing intracranial lesion may produce signs that mimic spasmus nutans.

5. *Miner's nystagmus.* Miners working in inadequate illumination have been known to develop a horizontal or oblique pendular nystagmus that disappears with adequate illumination. It is usually restricted to the upper fields of gaze. Miner's nystagmus is mentioned here only because it attests to the fact that a fixational nystagmus can be induced by adverse circumstances, which may be of significance in considering the possible etiology of spasmus nutans.

6. *Acquired unilateral pendular nystagmus of poor vision.* A unilateral pendular nystagmus may develop with loss of vision in that eye, especially if it is the patient's remaining eye. This nystagmus is usually a vertical pendular nystagmus of slow rate and medium amplitude.

7. *Congenital jerk nystagmus.* Congenital jerk nystagmus is characterized by horizontal jerky oscillations with a directional preponderance. The nystagmus is coarser in one direction of gaze than in the other, and the jerk is toward the direction of gaze; there is a point of reversal in which the nystagmus lessens. The vision is best in the position of least nystagmus, and a head turn to bring the eyes into the position of least nystagmus is a characteristic feature of this type of nystagmus. The nystagmus remains horizontal in vertical gaze and there is no oscillopsia. Congenital jerky nystagmus develops early, and persists throughout life. Its etiology is unknown; in some cases it is hereditary. Whether it should be classified as a sensory or motor type of fixational nystagmus is debatable,

but it properly belongs with the "ocular" types, as it does not signify threatening disease.

The "neurologic" types of fixation nystagmus include:

1. *Acquired fixational nystagmus of neurologic disease.* A fixational nystagmus of the pendular or jerky type in the horizontal or vertical plane may develop at any age as the result of posterior fossa disease; it is an ominous sign and often indicates demyelinating disease of the brain stem. There usually is oscillopsia, and, unlike the congenital types of fixational nystagmus, this nystagmus will usually convert to a directional jerk nystagmus on upward and downward gaze.

2. *See-saw nystagmus.* An unusual nystagmus generally classified as a fixational type is the see-saw nystagmus of Maddox, which is a disjunctive pendular nystagmus. As one eye elevates, the other depresses, and the vertical eye movement is often accompanied by a torsional movement of each eye. The etiology of this nystagmus is obscure, but it is often associated with bitemporal field defects and chiasmal lesions.

Nystagmus from defects in the gaze mechanisms is probably the most common form of nystagmus. It is characterized by jerky oscillations that are evoked by gaze (or attempted gaze) in one or more directions, with the rapid component varying according to the direction of gaze. There characteristically is a rest point at which the nystagmus ceases. Gaze-evoked nystagmus may signify an abnormality in either the central or peripheral elements of the conjugate gaze mechanisms. Clinically important types of gaze-evoked nystagmus are:

1. *Gaze paretic nystagmus.* Gaze-evoked nystagmus of varying severity is often the expression of an incomplete paralysis of conjugate gaze arising from a variety of lesions affecting the central pathways. Owing to weakness of conjugate gaze, the eyes drift back toward the primary position and there is then a quick corrective movement in the opposite direction. Such nystagmus is most often due to brain stem disease, in which case the rapid

component is directed toward the side of the lesion. It may also occur with cerebellar disease. Less often it is due to cerebral disease, but in cases of gaze paretic nystagmus of cortical origin, the jerk phase is directed to the side opposite the lesion.

2. Toxic gaze-evoked nystagmus. Certain drugs, particularly barbiturates and dilantin, can produce gaze nystagmus in the horizontal or vertical plane. This effect is important to remember in children with seizures, and a history of drug ingestion is required in every case of gaze nystagmus. This nystagmus disappears within a few days after cessation of the drug.

3. Dissociated nystagmus of internuclear ophthalmoplegia. Jerking nystagmus of the abducting eye on lateral gaze is a classic feature of internuclear ophthalmoplegia, the ocular motor sign of medial longitudinal fasciculus disease.

4. Muscle paretic nystagmus. On gaze in the field of action of a paretic muscle there may be dissociated jerky nystagmus of the affected eye; the direction of the nystagmus corresponds to the direction of action of the paretic muscle. The muscle paresis may be of neural, synaptic, or end organ origin.

Nystagmus from defects in the vestibular system characteristically is a jerky nystagmus of constant direction. It is independent of visual stimuli, and it is greatest when the stabilizing effect of fixation is eliminated. The slow component is the vestibulogenic phase, whereas the rapid phase is the corrective movement. The two types of spontaneous vestibular nystagmus to be differentiated are:

1. The nystagmus of peripheral vestibular dysfunction. Disease of the labyrinth or its neural connections to the brain stem is characterized by a horizontal-rotary jerky nystagmus of constant direction. It is usually associated with tinnitus and deafness, and vertigo is a prominent symptom. The nystagmus and vertigo of peripheral disease are maximal at the outset and tend to disappear within weeks of the onset, even if the underlying cause continues.

2. The nystagmus of central vestibular dys-

function. Disease of the vestibular nucleus in the brain stem or of the central connections of the vestibular nuclei is characterized by a horizontal-rotary jerk nystagmus that may change direction on right and left gaze and may become vertical on upward and downward gaze. Tinnitus and deafness are not regular features of central vestibular disease, and vertigo is not a prominent symptom. The nystagmus of central vestibular disease tends to persist as long as the underlying cause continues. Central vestibular nystagmus commonly occurs with demyelinating disease, with encephalitis, and with tumor. It may also be seen with the Arnold-Chiari malformation and platybasia.

Special Types of Abnormal Ocular Movements

Several types of abnormal eye movements that are often included in discussions of nystagmus are best described separately, as they are morphologically distinctive and often have special diagnostic significance. These conditions are opsoclonus, ocular motor dysmetria, flutter, ocular bobbing, downbeat nystagmus, nystagmus retractorius, and periodic alternating nystagmus.

Opsoclonus and "ataxic conjugate movements of the eye" are terms used to describe spontaneous nonrhythmic, multidirectional chaotic movements of the eyes. The oscillations may be nearly constant, or periodic and recurrent; they characteristically persist in sleep and they may persist unchanged during caloric testing. The eyes appear to be in a state of agitation, with irregular bursts of almost violent horizontal, vertical, and even rotary or oblique movements of varying amplitude. These eye movements are always conjugate with no diplopia; there may be subjective blurring or oscillopsia. There are often concurrent myoclonic jerks of the face, trunk, and extremities, but the muscular twitches are not necessarily synchronous with the eye movements.

Opsoclonus is most often associated with encephalitis marked by restlessness, malaise, fatigability, low grade fever, and tremulousness or widespread myoclonus. The sensorium may be clear. There may be minimal spinal fluid changes. Usually there is recovery in a matter of weeks or months.

In some cases, opsoclonus is the presenting sign of an occult neuroblastoma, one of the most frequent malignancies of childhood. Appropriate diagnostic studies for neoplasm are essential in patients with opsoclonus.

The exact pathogenesis of opsoclonus is unclear, but these abnormal conjugate eye movements generally indicate brain stem disease.

Ocular motor dysmetria indicates a lack of precision in performing movements of refixation. It is analogous to dysmetria of the limbs. On change of fixation from one point to another there is an overshoot (or undershoot) of the eyes. The overshoot is corrected by several to-and-fro oscillations or dampening movements that progressively diminish in amplitude until desired fixation is attained. The phenomenon may occur equally on looking to either side, it may be greater to one side than to the other, or it may occur on looking to one side only. The dysmetria is often more obvious on change of fixation from an eccentric position back to the primary position than on movement from the primary position toward an eccentric point. This ocular motor abnormality is a sign of cerebellar and cerebellar pathway disease, and it is most commonly seen with acute conditions.

Flutter-like oscillations of the eyes are rapid horizontal pendular oscillations that occur in bursts lasting only a few seconds. These intermittent to-and-fro movements come on spontaneously, interrupting maintained fixation, or occurring on change of fixation. Vision is usually momentarily blurred during the bouts of flutter. Like ocular motor dysmetria, flutter-like oscillations are characteristic of cerebellar disease. They may be seen with degenerative and demyelinating disease. They commonly occur with acute cerebellar disease and after surgery upon the cerebellum.

Ocular bobbing is an unusual type of spontaneous vertical oscillation of the eyes, seen in patients with extensive disease of the pons. The eyes intermittently dip downward and then return again to the midposition. The initial downward movement is brisker and more jerk-like than the slow return movement upward, and the bobbing may occur at regular or irregular intervals. This phenomenon is seen in stuporous or comatose patients who show total paralysis of spontaneous and reflexive eye movements in the horizontal plane; it has been reported in association with pontine infarction and hemorrhage, and even in a child with extensive pontine tumor.

Downbeat nystagmus consists of downward jerking of the eyes. Characteristically the jerking movements occur on gaze downward, but they may occur on gaze forward or in other directions; always, however, the fast component is downward. Often the downbeat phenomenon varies with head position, being worse with the head erect, hyperextended or retroflexed, and less with the head supine. The oscillations may produce oscillopsia, a subjective sensation of movement of the environment, or "jumpy" vision that can interfere with reading. As a rule, downbeat nystagmus is indicative of lesions in the lower end of the brain stem or cerebellum. It occurs most commonly in platybasia, in the Arnold-Chiari syndrome, or in association with the Klippel-Feil anomaly and superior cervical deformities. It has also been described with ependymoma of the posterior fourth ventricle, with tumor extending into the pontine cistern, and with arachnoidal adhesions in the posterior fossa.

Nystagmus retractorius is characterized by repetitive jerking of the eyes into the orbits with slower return movements to the original position. As a rule, this phenomenon is associated with gaze palsies, particularly vertical gaze palsies; the jerking movements usually appear on attempted gaze in the involved direction, but they may appear spontaneously. Nystagmus retractorius is indicative of lesions in the region of the sylvian aqueduct between the third and fourth ventricle or in the region of the corpora quadrigemina, and the phenomenon is an important feature of the Koerber-Salus-Elschnig syndrome. Although the causal condition may be neoplastic, vascular, or inflammatory, nystagmus retractorius in children suggests particularly the presence of pinealoma and hydrocephalus.

Periodic alternating nystagmus is a rhythmic jerk-type nystagmus that undergoes phasic or cyclic changes in amplitude and direction. After jerking in one direction for a minute or two, the eyes may remain still for a few seconds and then begin jerking toward the opposite side. This phenomenon has been described in patients with vascular and degenerative disease of the brain stem or its cerebellar connections.

ABNORMALITIES OF LID FUNCTION

Disorders of lid posture and movement rank in importance with abnormalities of ocular motility in the diagnosis of nervous system disease, yet evaluation of lid function is an often neglected part of the ophthalmic examination. Assessment of the resting position of both the upper and lower lids, evaluation of lid opening and closing—not only in voluntary movements but also in spontaneous and reflexive movements—and evaluation of the coordination of eye and lid movement in all directions of gaze are essential to proper neuro-ophthalmic examination.

Serving lid functions are three final common pathways: the orbicularis oculi muscle innervated by the facial nerve (cranial nerve VII) for closure of both lids; the levator palpebrae superioris innervated by branches of the superior division of the oculomotor nerve (cranial nerve III) for elevation of the upper lid; and the accessory muscle of Müller supplied by the cervical sympathetic system to augment opening of the lids. Also participating in the control of lid movements are cortical and supranuclear mechanisms. Thus abnormalities of lid posture and movement can arise from defects affecting any portion of the several cerebral, brain stem, and peripheral neural mechanisms governing lid functions; the most common of these abnormalities are ptosis, lid retraction, paradoxical lid movements, lagophthalmos, blepharoclonus, and blepharospasm.

Ptosis

Ptosis—more correctly, blepharoptosis—is drooping of the upper eyelid below its normal position. Many varieties of ptosis occur and the etiologies of this condition are diverse. In pediatrics, the differential diagnosis of congenital ptosis is of paramount interest and warrants special comment, but acquired ptosis of childhood demands even greater attention, as it usually signifies potentially serious nervous system disease. Of primary importance in neurologic diagnosis are the paralytic, neuromuscular, and sympathetic types of ptosis. To be differentiated from these types are mechanical ptosis and pseudoptosis. Inflammation, swelling, scar tissue, vascular lesions, tumor, and structural defects can all produce varying degrees of lid droop, and careful inspection and palpation of the lids for these conditions are essential. Also, true ptosis must be distinguished from voluntary or involuntary pseudoptosis effected by orbicularis oculi contraction or spasm; in these cases, wrinkling of the lids is usually evident, the orbicularis contraction generally worsens on attempted lid opening, the spasm often can be relieved by pressure on the supraorbital notch, and there may be associated vision and field defects of psychogenic origin.

Paralytic Ptosis

Paralytic ptosis is the lid droop that results from innervational defects in the pathways governing the function of the levator palpebrae superioris—namely, the oculomotor nerve, its nucleus, and its supranuclear and cerebral connections. In general, those principles which apply to topographical diagnosis of extraocular muscle palsies of oculomotor (third cranial nerve) origin also apply to the topographical diagnosis of paralytic ptosis. In peripheral oculomotor lesions, the involvement is commonly unilateral or asymmetric, the ptosis often is just one feature of an ophthalmoplegia, and rarely does the lid droop appear before other oculomotor signs such as extraocular muscle paralysis, paralytic mydriasis or cycloplegia. In the orbit, the branch of the third nerve destined for the levator can be affected selectively or in combination with involvement of the oculomotor supply for the superior rectus, but multiple involvement is more common. In syndromes of the sphenoidal region, particularly in the cavernous sinus syndrome, ptosis is usually accompanied by other signs of oculomotor palsy and by paresis of the fourth, fifth, and sixth cranial nerves. In basal lesions giving rise to paralytic ptosis, there is commonly combined involvement of the third, fifth, sixth, seventh, and eighth nerves. In contrast to paralytic ptosis of peripheral type, the ptosis of nuclear origin characteristically is bilateral and relatively symmetrical; the ptosis may well precede other signs of oculomotor dysfunction and may even occur as an isolated condition, though other nuclear third nerve signs are usual. Because the levator portion of the oculomotor nucleus is the caudal portion, there is also often associated involvement of the fourth nerve nucleus. In addition to nuclear and peripheral types of paralytic ptosis, there are supranuclear types of ptosis. Lesions in the mesencephalon in the region of the posterior commissure can produce ptosis (generally a mild one) that is often associated with impairment of upward gaze and small unreactive pupils. As there is also cortical representation for lid opening near the frontal oculogyric center, there may be slight droop of the lid contralateral to a cerebral lesion. So-called cortical ptosis is a rare condition, but it does occur with epileptic seizures, and mild bilateral ptosis may be observed with frontal lobe disease.

As with extraocular muscle palsies of oculomotor origin, the causes of paralytic ptosis include the general effects of increasing intracranial pressure, direct involvement by trauma, demyelinating and degenerative diseases, vascular lesions and hemorrhage, inflammatory and infectious processes, and the effects of drugs and toxins. Especially pertinent to the diagnosis of congenital paralytic ptosis is the fact that there may be dysgenesis (aplasia or hypoplasia) of the oculomotor nuclei; also, the third nerve may be damaged by intrauterine infections and by birth trauma. Old photographs are particularly helpful in differentiating congenital ptosis from acquired ptosis.

Neuromuscular Ptosis

There are two principal types of neuromuscular ptosis: the ptosis of myasthenia gravis, a myoneural transmission defect, and the ptosis of the myopathies or muscular dystrophies. Both types can present in childhood.

Characteristically, myasthenic ptosis is variable and asymmetrical; it worsens with fatigue and improves with rest or after administration of Prostigmin or Tensilon. Sustained upward gaze is often effective in demonstrating the lid weakness of myasthenia; although the lids may elevate fully initially on upgaze, the lids tend to droop on prolonged upward gaze. Another useful diagnostic sign is Cogan's lid twitch sign; on return of gaze from infraversion to the primary position, a momentary upward twitch or overshoot occurs in myasthenic patients.

In contrast to the ptosis of myasthenia, the ptosis of myopathy is usually bilateral, symmetrical, and chronically progressive. Ptosis of this type is often associated with external ophthalmoplegia in the conditions described as the PEO syndromes (p. 455). Myotonic dystrophy (Steinert type) may lead to ptosis; this condition is rarely congenital but it does manifest in childhood. Congenital myotonia (Thompson's disease) also is associated with ptosis, and this condition is congenital.

Sympathetic Ptosis

Sympathetic ptosis is drooping of the upper lid due to the loss of tone in Müller's muscle that results from oculosympathetic paralysis. Since Müller's muscle is an accessory rather than a primary muscle for elevation of the upper lid and since it also provides tone for retraction of the lower lid, several features serve to distinguish sympathetic ptosis from paralytic ptosis and levator paralysis. Sympathetic ptosis characteristically is mild, rarely more than one or two millimeters, whereas the ptosis of neurogenic or myogenic levator paralysis can be severe or complete. In sympathetic ptosis the lid fold is retained and there is no lid lag on upward gaze; in paralytic or neuromuscular ptosis there is diminution or absence of the lid fold, and on upward gaze lid lag and accentuation of the ptosis with dissociation of eye and lid movement often are evident. With sympathetic ptosis there is usually accompanying elevation of the lower lid margin contributing to narrowing of the palpebral fissure and an appearance of enophthalmos, a pseudo-enophthalmos; pure oculomotor or levator paralysis has no effect on the position of the lower lid. Most helpful to the diagnosis of sympathetic ptosis, however, are accompanying signs of oculosympathetic paresis comprising the Horner's syndrome; these are relative miosis, defective sweating, transitory dilatation of the ocular and facial vessels, increased temperature, and occasionally lowered ocular pressure or even depigmentation of the iris, all homolateral to the ptosis and ipsilateral to the lesion.

Sympathetic ptosis may result from lesions involving the sympathetic pathways anywhere in their course from the hypothalamus through the brain stem and upper spinal cord, in the cervical nerve roots or ascending sympathetic chain, or in the intracranial or orbital ramifications. In children, tumors affecting the hypothalamic region, medulla, or spinal cord, in addition to inflammatory and degenerative diseases of the brain stem and cord, must be considered. Pulmonary and mediastinal disease, particularly inflammatory and neoplastic conditions, retropharyngeal tumor, and swelling of the cervical lymph nodes of various etiologies, are important causes of sympathetic ptosis. Cavernous sinus and orbital disease, principally inflammatory and infectious processes in children, is also to be considered. Before embarking on extensive investigation for a pathologic process, however, it is essential to differentiate acquired from congenital sympathetic paresis. It is not uncommon for the minimal ocular signs of congenital sympathetic paralysis to be overlooked for months or years and then suddenly noted. Old photographs are often helpful in establishing the presence or absence of ptosis in infancy. Also helpful in the differentiation is the fact that hypopigmentation of the iris is more often a sign of congenital than of acquired sympathetic denervation. Many cases of sympathetic ptosis are congenital, the result of birth injury to the brachial plexus, and there may be associated signs of Klumpke's paralysis.

Congenital Ptosis

This is a relatively common condition of diverse etiologies. The most common type, often referred to as simple ptosis, is due to dysplasia or faulty differentiation of the levator palpebrae superioris muscle. This defect frequently occurs as an autosomal dominant condition. The ptosis typically is unilateral more often than bilateral, the lid lacks a normal tarsal fold, and the skin of the lid appears smooth and unwrinkled. There may be associated deficiency of the superior rectus muscle. Some cases are complicated by other developmental deformities of the lids such as epicanthus or blepharophimosis.

Clinically similar to cases of simple congenital ptosis due to faulty muscle differentiation are cases due to dysplasia (aplasia or hypoplasia) of the oculomotor nucleus or its peripheral third nerve fibers. There is a hereditary tendency for these innervational defects also; they may be recessive or dominant traits. In these cases the ptosis commonly is bilateral and there may be other signs of oculomotor dysfunction or associated signs referable to defective development of other cranial nerves.

Occasionally congenital ptosis is due to birth trauma. There may be direct trauma to the levator during delivery, and in the history it is important to seek evidence of damage to the lid from forceps. In some cases there may be damage to the intracranial portions of the oculomotor nerve; in particular, there may be damage to the third nerve before its entrance into the cavernous sinus consequent to traction or tearing of the tentorium near its attachment to the posterior clinoid process. With birth injury to the third nerve, there may be signs of reinnervation in 4 to 6 weeks and the ptosis may improve with time, but sometimes there is aberrant regeneration resulting in paradoxical movements of the ptotic lid.

To be differentiated from the foregoing types of ptosis are the congenital types of neuromuscular ptosis. In some cases myasthenia, the muscular dystrophies, or the PEO syndromes present with ptosis at birth (p. 540). Also to be differentiated is the mild ptosis of congenital sympathetic palsy, commonly the result of birth injury to the brachial plexus.

More unusual types of congenital ptosis are the periodic and synkinetic types, some of which are explained by aberrant innervation. These are described on p. 473.

Common to many types of congenital ptosis of moderate to severe degree are compensatory habits. With time, children learn to assume a compensatory posture with the head tilted backward, and they learn to utilize the frontalis muscle to help lift the ptotic lid. In evaluating levator function it is important to keep the patient's head erect and to eliminate the frontalis effect by firm pressure on the brow.

Lid Retraction

Lid retraction is inappropriate or excessive elevation of the upper lid sufficient to bare the sclera above the upper limbus on forward gaze. The phenomenon produces an expression of fear or surprise and often also an illusion of exophthalmos. On upward gaze, the retraction usually is exaggerated; in some cases, lagging of the lid behind the eye on downward gaze also accentuates the effect. To be differentiated from pathologic lid retraction are certain physiologic phenomena. During the act of staring or as an exaggerated act of attention or surprise, there may be temporary lid retraction; thus visual effort should be eliminated during evaluation of the resting lid position. In persons suffering progressive vision loss, there may be chronic lid retraction as an accompaniment of the effort to see. Also, the normal lid posture in infants must not be confused with pathologic lid retraction; in newborns the upper lid commonly rises above the upper limbus and the lower lid skirts the lower limbus, whereas later the lids cover both the superior and inferior limbal arcs on forward gaze.

Pathologic lid retraction may arise from disease affecting the lid musculature or from disorders of lid innervation.

Spastic Lid Retraction

This is the retraction produced by levator contraction as the result of inappropriate excitation of levator innervation. Rarely is this phenomenon the result of a third nerve lesion, though clonic spastic retraction may occur in incomplete paresis. More commonly, spastic lid retraction is indicative of a lesion affecting the corticonuclear pathways of the mesencephalon. Whereas lesions in the upper part of the mesencephalon in the region of the posterior commissure commonly produce ptosis associated with small unreactive pupils and loss of conjugate upward gaze, lesions situated anterior to the posterior limit of the posterior commissure may produce lid retraction associated with enlarged reactive pupils, with or without deficiency of upward gaze. Meningitis, degenerative processes in the upper brain stem, dilatation of the third ventricle or aqueduct, pinealomas, or pressure from other tumors in the posterior region of the third ventricle or rostral midbrain are the usual causes of spastic lid retraction. In these cases, the retraction is often extreme, with the lid margin tucked under the infra-orbital skin fold. Characteristically the retraction is sustained on forward or upward gaze, and the disparity between the limbus and lid margin usually increases on upward gaze. On downward gaze, however, the levator tone decreases and the lids follow the eyes downward in the normal manner. This supranuclear type of lid retraction is also referred to as posterior fossa stare, tucked lid, or Collier's sign. The lid retraction of the setting sun sign in infants with hydrocephalus is probably of this type.

Sympathetic Lid Retraction

This type is the result of contraction of Müller's muscle due to stimulation of the sympathetic innervation. With excitatory lesions of the oculosympathetic pathways there is not only widening of the palpebral fissure resulting from retraction of both lids but also dilatation of the homolateral pupil, vasoconstriction, sweating, and lowering of the temperature of the side of the face ipsilateral to the lesion. The principles which apply to the topical diagnosis of oculosympathetic paresis or Horner's syndrome (p. 450) apply to the differential diagnosis of sympathetic excitation.

Neuromuscular Lid Retraction

Neuromuscular lid retraction occurs in disease states that produce hyperexcitability of the levator fibers or the neuromuscular function. Often the effect is asymmetric or unilateral, and in addition to retraction on forward and on upward gaze, there is usually lid lag, a failure of the lid to descend normally on downward gaze. Representative of the neuromuscular type of lid retraction is the retraction that occurs with administration of certain drugs. Prostigmin and Tensilon can produce lid retraction in patients with myasthenic levator involvement. Succinylcholine in subparalytic doses may produce lid retraction, as can topical sympathetic drugs such as phenylephrine that may affect the levator fibers as well as the smooth muscle fibers. Thyroid extract in excessive amounts also may produce retraction and lid lag, and in infants the same effect can be seen as the result of maternal hyperthyroidism, though the effect on the neonate is transient, disappearing in 2 to 3 weeks.

Unlike the lid signs of neuromuscular excitation, the retraction and lid lag of myopathic disease usually are due to mechanical changes. In myopathy of dysthyroidism there is pathologic shortening and fibrosis of the levator fibers; true thyroid myopathy is not apt to occur in childhood, but retraction due to sympathetic stimulation in acute thyrotoxicosis does occur in children.

Paradoxical Lid Movements and Phasic Lid Phenomena

The term paradoxical lid movement refers to lid retraction or ptosis that occurs inappropriately in association with certain eye movements or with other activity such as jaw movement. These unusual and abnormal lid-oculomotor and lid-jaw synergies may occur as both congenital and acquired phenomena. The most common of these disorders are the Marcus Gunn jaw-winking phenomenon, the inverse Marcus Gunn phenomenon, and the lid signs of third nerve misdirection. To be differentiated from these synergies are the phasic movements of cyclic oculomotor paralysis or "spasm."

The Marcus Gunn Jaw-Winking Phenomenon

This phenomenon is characterized by involuntary spasmodic retraction of the up-per lid that occurs synergically with certain movements of the jaw. In most cases the upward jerk of the lid occurs in association with movements that involve external pterygoid contraction; in such cases, moving the mandible to the contralateral side, projecting the mandible forward, or opening the jaw widely may produce the retraction. Less often the phenomenon occurs during contraction of the internal pterygoid; the lid may elevate on closing the mouth, specifically on clenching the teeth. The involved lid is often ptotic, but may appear normal or even somewhat retracted when the jaw muscles are inactive. There may be associated congenital limitation of eye movement on the same side.

The pathogenesis of the trigeminooculomotor synkinesis is unknown, but in most cases the condition is congenital. In rare instances the condition is familial. The phenomenon is usually detected in infancy as it so often manifests during the act of sucking. There is a general tendency for the condition to become less conspicuous with age, and sometimes it disappears.

"Inverse Marcus Gunn Phenomenon"

"Inverse Marcus Gunn phenomenon" is the term applied to ptosis that occurs synergically with opening of the mouth; there is paradoxical inhibition of the levator palpebrarum during mouth opening. The condition is congenital and it is to be distinguished from other congenital types of paradoxical ptosis, as paradoxical levator inhibition may also occur in association with ocular adduction or supraduction.

Aberrant Regeneration of the Third Nerve

Aberrant regeneration of the third nerve — misdirection of regenerating fibers following oculomotor paralysis — is a phenomenon characterized by a variety of paradoxical oculomotor effects, a principal one being paradoxical lid retraction. During healing of an oculomotor paralysis, the levator palpebrarum may receive regenerating fibers originally destined for other of the extrinsic ocular muscles normally innervated by the third nerve; similarly, fibers intended for the medial rectus might be misdirected to the superior rectus or inferior oblique, the sphincter pupillae could receive fibers intended for the inferior rectus, and so forth. Thus there may result inappropriate elevation of the lid on attempted gaze medially, or constriction of the light-paretic pupil on gaze downward. The paradoxical lid retraction occurring in association with ocular movement (or attempted ocular movement) subsequent to oculomotor paralysis is known as Fuch's phenomenon. If the lid retraction occurs specifically on attempted infraduction, the phenomenon is referred to as the pseudo-Graefe sign.* Although aberrant regeneration may follow oculomotor paralysis of diverse etiologies, the condition is most apt to develop consequent to traumatic paralysis. The congenital levator-oculomotor synergies of this type are usually attributed to trauma, generally birth trauma. As a rule, the manifestations of misdirection persist.

Cyclic Oculomotor Spasm

This is a rare and curious phenomenon characterized by phasic activity of intra- and extraocular muscles alternating with signs of oculomotor paresis. Phasic retraction of the lid alternating with ptosis is a prominent manifestation of the condition. During the "spastic" phase there may be constriction of the pupil, convergent deviation of the eye, and spasm of accommodation as well as retraction of the lid; the "spastic" or miotic phase may be accentuated by attempted adduction. During the alternate paralytic phase there is ptosis, mydriasis, and paralysis of eye movement. The rhythmic cyclic changes continue through both sleeping and waking hours. As a rule the condition is congenital, and persists throughout life. The etiology of the disorder is unknown, but it has been speculated that part of the oculomotor nucleus has suffered aplasia or degeneration, with the remaining nuclear cells showing a certain irritability. The condition usually is unilateral, and it is more common in females than in males.

---

*The lid lag of myopathic disease—in particular that of dysthyroidism—is designated Graefe's sign. In myopathic lid lag, the upper lid pauses and then follows the eye downward; there is normal levator inhibition during downward gaze; the restriction of lid relaxation is mechanical.

Lagophthalmos

Lagophthalmos is inability to close the lids. Although defective lid closure can result from structural lid abnormalities or mechanical restrictions, lagophthalmos usually signifies orbicularis oculi paralysis of myogenic or neurogenic origin. The muscular dystrophies, the progressive external ophthalmoplegias (p. 540), and myasthenia gravis (p. 541) can give rise to orbicularis weakness, and these conditions may present in childhood. More frequently, however, orbicularis paralysis results from a lesion of the seventh nerve or its central connections. As a rule, neurogenic paralysis of the orbicularis oculi is just one feature of a facial palsy, and the clinical picture of the palsy will vary, depending on the site of involvement. As there is bilateral central representation for the muscles of the upper face, central lesions have little effect on the orbicularis oculi, whereas peripheral lesions involve the upper and lower facial musculature equally. In supranuclear pyramidal lesions, only voluntary movements of the orbicularis and other upper facial muscles are affected, and they are impaired to only a small degree owing to the bilateral cortical representation for voluntary movements; emotional movements are unimpaired, as they are subserved by a separate supranuclear pathway. Hemiplegia frequently accompanies the facial paralysis of supranuclear pyramidal origin. In lesions of the pons affecting the facial nerve or its roots, there is usually involvement of neighboring structures, particularly the abducent nerve, its nucleus or its association fibers, and the pyramidal fibers. Thus with the facial palsy of a pontine lesion there may be an associated homolateral lateral rectus palsy, loss of conjugate gaze toward the same side, and hemiplegia of the contralateral limbs (Foville's syndrome, p. 457), or these same signs without paralysis of conjugate gaze (Millard-Gubler syndrome, p. 457). In children, these pontine signs suggest the possibility of pontine glioma or degenerative disease, though vascular lesions and inflammatory processes are also to be considered; there are also congenital forms of facial palsy in association with abducent palsy (Möbius syndrome, p. 458). Basal lesions affecting the seventh nerve root also commonly involve neighboring cranial nerves, particularly the eighth nerve and the intermediary nerve of Wrisberg, resulting in accompanying loss of hearing, loss of taste in the anterior two thirds of the tongue, and sometimes a diminution of tear secretion. Such involvement is apt to occur with basal meningitis, neuromas, or basal fractures.

Paralysis of the facial nerve due to lesions in the petrous temporal bone is distinguished by alterations in functions subserved by fibers that become associated with the seventh nerve in this part of its course. Parasympathetic fibers for lacrimation join the facial nerve probably just distal to the facial nucleus and leave the facial nerve at the geniculate ganglion as the greater superficial petrosal nerve in the petrous canal. Thus a lesion of the seventh nerve between its nucleus and the geniculate ganglion can impair lacrimation, whereas a lesion in the nucleus or its supranuclear pathways or in the nerve peripheral to the geniculate ganglion does not impair tear secretion. Secretory fibers for the sublingual and submaxillary glands are also associated; they arrive in the intermediate nerve of Wrisberg which runs between the seventh and eighth nerves, reach a cell station in the geniculate ganglion, and leave the nerve within the facial canal above the stylomastoid foramen in the chorda tympani. Fibers for the sense of taste in the anterior two thirds of the tongue traverse a similar route. Fractures of the petrous temporal bone, occasionally herpes zoster infection spreading to the geniculate ganglion, and otitis media can involve the facial nerve and its associated fibers in the petrous temporal bone and its facial canal. A special type of facial palsy localized to the petrous temporal portion of the nerve is Bell's palsy.

Bell's Palsy

Bell's palsy denotes a peripheral facial palsy of relatively sudden onset arising from inflammation of the seventh nerve within the facial canal in the petrous temporal bone. The paralysis most probably is due to compression of the nerve fibers by the edema of an interstitial neuritis confined by the rigid bony canal. In most cases the etiology of the inflammation is ob-scure, but the condition is usually attributed to a viral infection or a vascular-ischemic process. The sudden onset is a characteristic feature; there is usually no warning and no accompanying neurologic deficits, though in some cases there is mastoid pain. The involvement is usually unilateral. As a rule there is recovery with return of function varying from weeks to months, but in some cases there is permanent weakness. As with any type of peripheral facial palsy, in Bell's palsy there may be epiphora and paralytic ectropion, though these problems are not as severe in childhood as they are in later life. More worrisome are possible complications of lagophthalmos. With defective lid closure, the cornea may be exposed to desiccation, ulceration, and secondary infection. Depending on the severity and duration of the lagophthalmos, the cornea can be protected by one or more of the following: methylcellulose drops or bland ointments, an airtight shield (Buller shield) to retain moisture, or tarsorrhaphy. In unconscious patients, the lids can often be kept closed by tape, which is preferable to improper patching with a gauze pad that could abrade the cornea.

Classical Bell's palsy does occur in childhood, but the onset of a facial palsy in a youngster should always suggest the possibility of other processes, particularly myasthenia gravis, tumor (especially pontine glioma or posterior fossa neuroma), or extension of infection from an otitis media. Extracranial involvement of the seventh nerve may occur with parotid disease or with suppuration of nodes at the angle of the jaw.

Blepharospasm, Blepharoclonus, and Lid Tics

Abnormal tonic and clonic contractions of the orbicularis oculi occur in a variety of organic and psychogenic disorders. Blepharospasm is an involuntary tonic contraction of the orbicularis producing forcible closure of the lids; the spasm may be repetitive or persistent, lasting minutes, days, months, or even years. Blepharoclonus, on the other hand, is an increased rate of blinking. Both blepharospasm and blepharoclonus may occur reflexly as the result of sensory irritation mediated by the trigeminal nerve, or directly as the result of pathologic stimulation of the seventh nerve or its central connections. Irritation of painful ocular disease and those ocular conditions characterized by photophobia (albinism, achromatopsia, aniridia, and so forth) are common causes of organic blepharospasm and blepharoclonus. Neurologic causes are less common, though pontine tumor may produce myotonia of the lids progressing to spasm, zoster of the geniculate ganglion may produce clonic contractions, and irritative frontal lobe lesions may produce spasmodic contralateral lid closure as part of an adversive seizure. Abnormal orbicularis oculi contraction can also result from the neuromuscular hyperexcitability of hypoparathyroidism, hyperventilation, or tetanus, and there may be myotonia of the lids in myotonic dystrophy. In children particularly, tremulousness of the lids may be seen with opsoclonus and encephalopathy.

To be differentiated from organic types of blepharospasm and blepharoclonus are the lid contractions of psychogenic origin. Blepharospasm of psychogenic origin is not uncommon in adults, but in children the more usual lid phenomenon of psychogenic origin is a spasmodic tic characterized by repetitive blinking—a psychogenic blepharoclonus. Tics may date from an irritation, with the spasm being perpetuated long after the initiating stimulus has disappeared. To some extent, tics are controlled by will; they can usually be voluntarily initiated or imitated and they cease in sleep or with diversion. As a rule, the psychogenic tics of childhood are easily recognized and they usually abate in time if they are not compounded by too much attention on the part of parents, teachers, and doctors.

FUNDUS ABNORMALITIES: OPTIC NERVE AND RETINAL MANIFESTATIONS OF NEUROLOGIC DISEASE

Readily accessible to objective examination, and capable of exhibiting a wide variety of pathologic processes of both focal and systemic nature, the fundus oculi commands special attention in neurologic diagnosis.

Of primary importance are affections of the optic nerve that are evident at the disc. Included here are papilledema and other forms of disc edema, papillitis (optic neuritis), optic atrophy, and several conditions that may be confused with the aforementioned abnormalities. Prenatal malformations of the optic disc that occur as isolated ocular defects or as manifestations of extensive nervous system malformation are described in Section II of this chapter (pp. 493–495).

Equally important are the retinal manifestations of systemic and neurologic disease, such as retinal pigmentary degeneration including the special macular degenerations of childhood, retinitis and chorioretinitis, vascular retinopathy, and phakomata.

Papilledema

Whereas "disc edema" is the unrestricted general term for optic nervehead swelling of diverse etiologies (Table 18–7), papilledema is the preferred designation for the forms of disc swelling that result from increased intracranial pressure.

In its fully developed form, papilledema or "choked disc" is characterized by edematous blurring of the disc margins, edematous elevation of the nervehead, partial or complete obliteration of the disc cup, capillary congestion and hyperemia of the disc, generalized engorgement of the veins, loss of the venous pulsation, nerve fiber layer hemorrhages around the disc, and peripapillary exudates. In many cases, retinal exudates extending into the macula take the form of fan- or star-shaped figures. In addition, concentric peripapillary retinal wrinkling frequently is evident. Typically there is generalized enlargement of the normal blind spot, and there may be transient obscurations of vision lasting only seconds, but the visual acuity generally is normal. Lesser degrees and various combinations of these signs and symptoms occur in early, less completely developed papilledema, and the diagnosis of early or incipient papilledema frequently is difficult. The use of fluorescein angiography can be helpful; in the presence of capillary

TABLE 18–7   DISC EDEMA: DIFFERENTIAL DIAGNOSIS

Ocular Conditions
  Sudden decrease of intraocular pressure (ocular hypotony)
    Perforation of globe; fistula (accidental or surgical)
  Acute increase of intraocular pressure
    Generalized edema of ocular tissues
  Retinal vasculitis
  Neuroretinitis
  Uveitis

Orbital Conditions
  Orbital tumor
  Abscess
  Aneurysm
  Nerve sheath hemorrhage
  Venous congestion (as with cavernous sinus thrombosis)
  Endocrine exophthalmos

Intracranial Conditions
  Increased intracranial pressure: true papilledema
    Intracranial tumor
    Hydrocephalus
    Brain abscess
    Encephalitis, meningitis
    Encephalopathy, as with infectious or para-infectious processes, degenerative diseases (e.g., Schilder's disease), toxins (e.g., lead), trauma, vascular and ischemic disorders
    Intracranial hemorrhage—intracerebral, subarachnoid, subdural, epidural
    Dural sinus thrombosis
    Pseudotumor cerebri
  Decreased intracranial space
    Cranial dysostosis (oxycephaly)
  Cerebrospinal fluid abnormalities: protein elevation, increased viscosity
    Guillain-Barré syndrome (with or without increased intracranial pressure)

Systemic Conditions
  Vascular hypertension
    Renal disease
  Blood dyscrasias
    Anemias, leukemias, thrombocytopenia, polycythemia, macroglobulinemia
  Cardiopulmonary disorders and ventilatory insufficiency states (hypercapnia and chronic respiratory acidosis)
    Congestive failure, congenital heart disease
    Cystic fibrosis
    Pickwickian syndrome
  Endocrine disorders
    Hyperthyroidism, hypoparathyroidism, Addison's disease
  Collagen vascular diseases

stasis in papilledema, fluorescein will fill the dilated capillaries and leak into the extravascular tissues, "staining" the tissues for periods as long as 10 minutes.

As a rule, when the increased intracran-ial pressure is alleviated, the papilledema resolves, and the disc may return to a normal or nearly normal appearance within 6 to 8 weeks. Sustained chronic papilledema of unrelieved longstanding increased intracranial pressure, however, leads to involutional and atrophic changes of the disc, permanent nerve fiber damage, and impairment of vision that may progress to blindness.

In childhood, papilledema develops most frequently and most rapidly as the result of posterior fossa tumor or intraventricular tumor with obstructive hydrocephalus. In cases of supratentorial lesions, particularly intracerebral tumors, the development of papilledema tends to be a later sign. Pronounced papilledema commonly is seen in children with pseudotumor or with encephalopathy of various types. Whatever the etiology, however, the disc signs of increased intracranial pressure in childhood may be modified by the distensibility of the young skull. In the early years, before firm closure of the cranial sutures, papilledema may be minimal, delayed, or absent in the presence of markedly elevated intracranial pressure; this is not to imply, however, that spreading of the sutures precludes the development of papilledema.

At the present time, knowledge concerning the pathogenesis of papilledema is incomplete, but certain factors are evident. With increased intracranial pressure there is elevation of pressure within the intravaginal space surrounding the optic nerve, and it has been demonstrated that increased pressure within the intravaginal space is an essential factor in the production of papilledema. With increased intravaginal pressure, there occurs congestion of capillary circulation in the region of the scleral canal and optic nervehead; the capillaries affected are those derived from the arterial circle of Zinn and Haller. Ultimately, congestion in the capillary circulation of the disc results in intracellular glial swelling. Intracellular swelling in the glia-lined interstices of the lamina cribrosa compounds the regional microcirculatory disturbance. Although dilatation of the veins and capillaries is a principal feature of papilledema, there is no evidence that the orbital venous pressure is elevated in patients with increased intracranial pressure. It is proposed that variations in the occurrence, symmetry, and severity of papilledema are explained by variations in the patency of the intravaginal space, or in the patency of the intracanalicular channels through which cerebrospinal fluid must pass to flow into the intravaginal space.

Optic Neuritis

Optic neuritis is the general term for involvement of the optic nerve by inflammation, degeneration, or demyelinization, with attendant impairment of function. The process may begin near the surface of the nerve or within the core of the nerve; it may begin anteriorly, within or near the globe, or as far posteriorly as the chiasm. When the involvement is far enough behind the lamina cribrosa so that its early effects are not ophthalmoscopically evident at the nervehead, it is referred to as *retrobulbar neuritis*. When the ophthalmoscopically visible part of the nervehead is affected, the process is referred to as *papillitis* or *intraocular optic neuritis*, which is characterized by various degrees of disc swelling, often with hemorrhages and exudates. When both the retina and neural tissue of the disc are involved, the term *optic neuroretinitis* is applied. Selective involvement of the papillomacular bundle is called *axial neuritis*, while involvement of the extramacular portions of the nerve is *periaxial neuritis*. When there is inflammatory involvement of the optic nerve sheaths, the term *optic perineuritis* or *perioptic neuritis* is used.

In most instances, optic neuritis is an acute process. It is more commonly unilateral than bilateral. The principal clinical manifestation is loss of vision that commences rather abruptly and progresses rapidly. The involved eye may become blind or almost blind in a matter of hours or days, but commonly the vision loss is less profound (20/200 or better). As a rule, the vision loss is painless, though in some cases there is pain on movement of the globe or on palpation of the globe for 1 or 2 days before the vision loss commences. In most cases of acute optic neuritis there is some improvement in visual acuity beginning 1 to 4 weeks after the onset, and the vision

may improve to normal or near normal level within weeks or months. Rarely there is delayed improvement. In a certain percentage of cases there is permanent impairment of vision.

Field defects of various types occur in optic neuritis, but the usual defect is a central scotoma that characteristically is more pronounced for color than for white, and more pronounced for red than for blue test objects. The defect usually is large and roughly circular. In some instances the field defect is paracentral, altitudinal, or arcuate, or, in the event of chiasmal involvement, hemianoptic or junctional.

In childhood, optic neuritis rarely occurs as an isolated entity; rather, it usually is an expression of more widespread neurologic or systemic disease. It may develop as part of an acute meningitis. It may develop consequent to a viral infection, often as a complication of encephalomyelitis following an exanthem. Alternatively, it may signify one of the many demyelinating diseases of childhood, particularly Devic's neuromyelitis optica or Schilder's disease. In other instances the cause is an exogenous toxin or toxic drug; to mention just a few possibilities, neuritis may develop with lead poisoning, or as a complication of long term, high dose chloramphenicol treatment (as for pulmonary disease in cystic fibrosis), or as the result of the use of illicit drugs.

Pseudopapilledema and Pseudoneuritis

A common pitfall in ophthalmoneurologic diagnosis is misinterpretation of certain disc anomalies that bear superficial resemblance to papilledema. These conditions preferably are referred to simply as elevated disc anomalies, though it has been customary to apply the nonspecific term "pseudopapilledema" to anomalous disc elevations unaccompanied by vision changes, hemorrhages, venous congestion, or exudates, and to apply the term "pseudoneuritis" to anomalous disc elevations accompanied by vision or field defects, retinal vessel abnormalities, and hyperplastic glial tissue.

Anomalous elevation of the disc that can be confused with papilledema is seen in certain cases of hyperopia of moderate to severe degree. Such elevation lacks true venous dilatation, edema, hemorrhages, and exudates; the general good health of the patient, the normal size of the blind spot, and the unchanging appearance of the abnormality on serial examination should be sufficient to suggest that the elevation is an anomaly.

Hyperplastic glial tissue located on the disc surface in one or both eyes also may be confused with papilledema. This abnormality commonly occurs in association with persistent hyaloid remnants, including the so-called Bergmeister's papilla. The disc surface may appear white or gray; the cup may be obliterated, the emerging retinal vessels may be obscured by the hyperplastic glial tissue, and anomalous branching of the vessels is common. Capillary congestion, exudates, and hemorrhages are not present. Frequently there is a mild degree of amblyopia.

Frequently confused with papilledema is anomalous elevation of the disc associated with intrapapillary drusen. Drusen are round or globular bodies composed of concentric lamellae of hyalin material. Their pathogenesis is unknown, but they tend to occur as a familial disorder transmitted as an irregular dominant. The condition generally is bilateral. When they are buried within the optic nervehead, drusen commonly produce a smooth or irregular elevation of the disc; this frequently is the situation early in life. With advancing age, intrapapillary drusen tend to become visible at the surface of the disc. Completely or partially exposed drusen appear as glistening yellowish bodies that resemble tapioca pearls, varying in size from minute granules to globules 2 or 3 times the diameter of a vein. The presence of hyalin bodies can often be well demonstrated by transillumination with oblique light, as the more superficial drusen glow in the light. Especially helpful in the diagnosis of buried drusen in a child with a confusing picture of disc elevation is detection of ophthalmoscopically visible drusen in other family members. In some instances drusen are associated with nerve fiber bundle or sector field defects, enlargement of the blind spot, decreased visual acuity, and even with small nerve fiber layer hemorrhages adjacent to the disc. The condition can be perplexing. Though intrapapillary drusen may well explain elevation of the disc, in certain cases the possibility of the coexistence of intrapapillary drusen and intracranial disease must be considered, especially in the presence of decreased vision. In addition, drusen may be associated with tuberous sclerosis.

Optic Atrophy

When insult to the optic nerve, whether of traumatic, inflammatory, degenerative, neoplastic, or vascular origin, results in irreparable damage to optic nerve fibers leading to degeneration of axons and attendant loss of function, optic atrophy exists.

It is customary to classify optic atrophy as ascending or descending, and as primary ("simple") or secondary, though there are certain problems inherent in the application of these terms.

"Simple" or "primary" optic atrophy connotes a degeneration of optic nerve fibers accompanied by minimal glial proliferation and essentially no mesenchymal reaction. There is disappearance of axis cylinders and myelin sheaths, and resultant shrinkage of the optic nerve. At the nervehead there is loss of nerve substance and lack of glial or mesenchymal compensation; the process leads to a deepening and widening of the optic cup and a baring of the lamina cribrosa. The prototype of primary optic atrophy is syphilitic optic atrophy.

The term secondary optic atrophy denotes an atrophy characterized by a significant degree of reactive alteration in the glial and mesenchymal tissues of the nervehead; the essential degenerative features may be obscured by the proliferation of astrocytes, fibrous connective tissue, and blood vessels. Such reaction is apt to occur when the primary process is an acute inflammatory or vascular lesion located close to the globe. Alternative terms for this type of optic atrophy are postneuritic and postinflammatory.

In addition to the primary and secondary types of optic atrophy, there is a third pathologic type, referred to as cavernous optic atrophy. The cavernous type is characterized by mucoid degeneration of the glia in association with the disappearance of optic nerve fibers without proliferative reaction by the glial or connective tissue elements. The mucoid degeneration leads to the formation of mucoid-filled lacunae within the compartments previously occupied by nerve fibers. Cavernous type atrophy most commonly is the result of glaucoma.

Ascending optic atrophy or consecutive atrophy results from disease affecting the retinal ganglion cells, the retinal nerve fiber layer, or the intraocular portion of the optic nerve, leading to an ascending degeneration of axons within the optic nerve. The process may be focal or generalized.

Descending optic atrophy occurs with lesions affecting the intraorbital, intracanalicular, or intracranial portions of the nerve, resulting in progressive degeneration of the nerve fibers distally, and generally also proximally.

As viewed with the ophthalmoscope, optic atrophy is characterized by various degrees of diminished vascularity of the disc, pallor and loss of substance and cupping of the nervehead, with or without glial proliferation.

As indicated in the introduction, optic atrophy is not a disease in and of itself; rather, it is the common expression of a wide variety of pathologic processes that may be either congenital or acquired. Although an exhaustive review of the pathologic causes of optic atrophy in childhood is not attempted here, certain types of optic atrophy, particularly the heredodegenerative types, require special comment.

Leber's hereditary optic atrophy is a degenerative or abiotrophic disorder of the optic nerve having distinctive clinical features. The condition occurs predominantly in males during early life. It is characterized by profound bilateral loss of vision and large central scotomas that persist.

The classical manifestations most frequently develop between 18 and 23 years of age, though the disease may make its appearance considerably earlier, or later. The initial symptom is blurring of vision in one eye, followed within a few days or a few weeks by similar involvement of the fellow eye. The vision loss is rapidly progressive, becoming profound within the period of a week or two. During the initial stage of the disease, the disc may appear normal or there may be a picture of optic neuritis with low grade or pronounced swelling of the discs, sometimes with hemorrhages and exudates. Pallor of the disc generally develops within a few weeks of the onset of the vision disturbance. Commonly the entire disc is involved; in some cases only the papillomacular region is severely affected. Ultimately the disc appearance is that of a "primary" optic atrophy. Following the initial downhill course of weeks or even months, there is in a certain percentage of cases some degree of improvement. The final vision, however, rarely is better than 20/200, and in the majority of cases the process ends in complete or almost complete blindness.

Histopathologic studies of this condition have shown reduction in the size of the optic nerve, destruction of axis cylinders, and breakdown of myelin sheaths. Atrophy of the papillomacular bundle may be pronounced. Thinning of the nerve fiber layer of the retina, as well as destruction of the ganglion cells with atrophy of these cells most pronounced about the fovea, has been observed. In some cases of Leber's disease there has been arachnoid thickening with cyst formation about the sella region.

The etiology of the disorder is not known, and even its genetic transmission is not fully understood. Although the disease is often described as a sex-linked recessive condition, there is evidence that it is not a simple or true sex-linked recessive disorder.

Neurologic abnormalities reported to occur in association with Leber's optic atrophy include spasticity, paraplegia, dementia, deafness, migraine, vertigo, and episodic loss of consciousness.

Behr's optic atrophy is a hereditary type of optic atrophy that is associated with hypertonia of the extremities and increased deep tendon reflexes, mild cerebellar ataxia, bladder disturbances, some degree of mental deficiency, and possibly external ophthalmoplegia. The disorder affects principally males in the 3- to 11-year age group. There is similarity between this condition and some cases of hereditary cerebellar ataxia of the Marie and Friedreich types.

Autosomal recessively inherited congenital optic atrophy is a rare condition that is evident at birth or develops at a very early age. It is characterized by pronounced loss of vision; there may be complete or almost complete blindness. In cases of incomplete vision loss, severe color vision defects (achromatopsia) and restriction of the visual field are common. As viewed with the ophthalmoscope, the atrophy appears to be complete, and there may be pronounced arteriolar narrowing. The condition tends to be static. Nystagmus generally is present.

Dominantly inherited infantile optic atrophy is a relatively mild type of heredodegenerative optic atrophy that tends to be progressive through childhood and adolescence. As a rule the eyes appear normal at birth; frequently the defect is not detected until the child reaches school age. The visual acuity remains between 20/20 and 20/60 in a high percentage of cases; only rarely is there a severe deficiency of vision, approaching 20/200 or worse. Commonly only the temporal or papillomacular region of the disc is pale and atrophic. The usual field defect is a paracentral or central scotoma. In many instances there is inability to perceive the color blue. Night vision complaints are not unusual.

Gray Pseudo-Optic Atrophy (Myelogenous Dysgenesis)

Gray pseudo-optic atrophy, or myelogenous dysgenesis, is a condition described as occurring primarily in premature infants. The child is born blind, but partially or completely recovers vision within a period of months. At birth the disc is gray, the fundi are hypopigmented, the eye movements are uncoordinated, and the pupils are unreactive to light.

This condition has been attributed to delayed myelination of the optic nerve fibers. Reportedly the ERG and VER improve with time, as does the vision. The prognosis generally is favorable.

Pigmentary Retinal Degeneration: "Retinitis Pigmentosa" and Its Variants

Whereas pigmentary retinal degeneration commonly occurs as a primary ocular disorder having no systemic or neurologic implications, it frequently occurs in association with other abnormalities as an expression of systemic metabolic or neurologic disease or as one feature of a multifaceted syndrome.

Whether occurring as a primary or secondary process, pigmentary retinal degeneration in its typical form is characterized by progressive disorganization of the normal retinal pigmentary pattern, arteriolar attenuation, usually some degree of optic atrophy, and impairment of visual function. Dispersion, migration, and aggregation of pigment produce a variety of ophthalmoscopically visible changes, ranging from fine granularity or coarse irregularity of the pigmentary pattern to distinctive focal pigment aggregates having the configuration of bone corpuscles and perivascular spicules. Pigment changes usually appear first in the mid- or far periphery, though in some instances the central retina is affected first ("inverse" type); there usually is progression to generalized retinal involvement. Depending on the areas and cell layers of retina predominantly affected, the attendant visual impairment may be primarily night blindness, peripheral field loss (ring scotoma or concentric contraction), reduction of visual acuity, or impairment of color perception, singly or in various combinations. Retinal function as measured by the ERG may be reduced early or late in the disease.

The list of conditions with which pigmentary retinal degeneration is associated is seemingly endless (see Chapters 14 and 19). The following selected examples of neurologic and systemic disorders associated with pigmentary retinal degeneration appearing in childhood merely attest to the diversity of the spectrum. Pigmentary retinal degeneration occurs in association with mental retardation, obesity, hypogonadism, and polydactyly in the Laurence-Moon-Biedl syndrome; with ataxic neuropathic disease, abetalipoproteinemia, and acanthocytosis in the Bassen-Kornzweig syndrome; with progressive cerebellar ataxia and peripheral polyneuropathy in the Refsum syndrome; with rigidity, hyperkinesia, and mental retardation in Hallervorden-Spatz disease; with cerebellar ataxia and spasticity in the syndromes of Sanger-Brown and of Marie, and with cerebellar ataxia and hypotonia in Friedreich's disease; with deafness in Usher's syndrome and in Cockayne's syndrome; with ophthalmoplegia and heart block in the Kearns-Sayre syndrome; with generalized mucopolysaccharidosis, as in the syndromes of Hurler, Hunter, Scheie, and Sanfilippo; with neuronal lipidosis and psychomotor deterioration, as in the juvenile amaurotic familial idiocy of Batten-Mayou-Spielmeyer-Vogt and in the late infantile form of Jansky-Bielschowsky. Thus, in each case of pigmentary retinal degeneration, consideration must be given to the possible systemic, neurologic, and genetic implications of the ocular manifestation.

To be differentiated from the diffuse pigmentary retinal degenerations are pigmentary retinopathies due to inflammatory and infectious processes, such as rubella and syphilis.

Macular Degenerations

In many instances, retinal degeneration signifying systemic or neurologic disease presents as a focal macular degeneration; the macular lesion may occur alone or as the dominant feature of a diffuse retinal degeneration.

Excluding the many lipidoses that are associated with retinal degeneration presenting as a macular cherry-red spot (described separately), diseases that commonly exhibit or present with macular degeneration in childhood are the late onset amaurotic familial idiocies, namely the late infantile cerebromacular degeneration of Jansky-Bielschowsky and the juvenile cerebromacular degeneration of Batten-Mayou. In both of these conditions, obtunding of the foveal light reflex, grayness of the macular region, and progressive pigmentary alteration of the macula may be the early signs of diffuse neurodegeneration that eventually will lead to blindness, dementia, paralysis, and ultimately death. Although the macular

change may precede or for a time dominate the ophthalmic picture in these neuronal storage diseases, there commonly is progression to diffuse pigmentary retinal degeneration with arteriolar attenuation and optic atrophy.

Pigmented macular degeneration may also be seen in the Sjögren-Larsson syndrome and in subacute sclerosing panencephalitis of Dawson (van Bogaert's disease, p. 529).

To be differentiated from the macular degenerations having systemic and neurologic implications are the hereditary macular dystrophies of childhood that are not regularly associated with other abnormalities, such as those of Stargardt and of Best (see Chapter 14).

Cherry-Red Spot

Because of the special histologic features of the macular region,* certain pathologic processes affecting the retina produce a distinctive sign referred to as the cherry-red spot. Ophthalmoscopically, the cherry-red spot is a bright to dull red area at the center of the macula surrounded by a concentric grayish white or yellowish halo. The halo is the result of swelling and loss of transparency of the multilayered ganglion cell ring of the macula caused by either edema, abnormal lipid accumulation, or a combined effect of the two. The central red area is the normal choroidal vascular blush of the less cellular macular center, its redness markedly accentuated by the dull or creamy pallor of the surrounding halo.

A typical cherry-red spot occurs in several of the neuronal lipid storage diseases, specifically in certain of the sphingolipidoses. Cherry-red spots characteristically develop in virtually all cases of Tay-Sachs disease (G_{M2} type I) and in the Sandhoff variant (G_{M2} type II); as a rule, the fundus

---

*Throughout most of the retina the ganglion cells form a single cell layer. In the macular region, however, the ganglion cells increase to 8 to 10 layers, diminishing again in number toward the fovea where they disappear entirely. In addition, the inner plexiform layer and the inner nuclear layer diminish toward the center of the macula and are absent within the fovea.

sign is present by the time other signs of psychomotor retardation and neurologic deterioration become apparent in infancy, and the spot usually is dramatic in its appearance, though in later stages of the disease it may become less distinct as neurodegenerative changes progress. Cherry-red spots also develop in many cases of generalized gangliosidosis (G_{M1} type I) and in some cases of metachromatic leukodystrophy (sulfatide lipidosis). Macular changes similar to those of a cherry-red spot may develop in certain cases of neuronopathic Niemann-Pick disease (principally type A, possibly type C), and in certain mucolipidoses, namely Farber's disease and Spranger's disease; in these disorders, the morphologic changes at the macula as seen with the ophthalmoscope generally are not as distinctive as those of the Tay-Sachs prototype.

To be differentiated from the cherry-red spot occurring as a cardinal sign of metabolic neurodegenerative disease is the cherry-red spot that develops as the result of retinal ischemia secondary to central retinal artery occlusion, vasospasm, or ocular contusion.

As a general rule, the macular cherry-red spot—whether it is due to ganglion cell storage, cellular edema, and destruction occurring as part of generalized neuronal lipidosis, or as the result of cloudy swelling due to local circulatory disturbances—is merely the focal ophthalmoscopically visible evidence of pathology that generally involves the extramacular and peripheral regions of the retina as well. In addition, in the lipidoses, the disease may not be limited to the ganglion cell layer but may also involve the inner nuclear and inner plexiform layers.

Phakomata

Herald lesions of the eye, commonly referred to as phakomata, occur in a number of hamartomatous disorders, including Bourneville's disease, von Recklinghausen's disease, von Hippel-Lindau's disease, the Sturge-Weber syndrome, and the Wyburn-Mason syndrome. These conditions are described in detail in Section II of this chapter (pp. 511 and 543); only the fundus lesions are reviewed here for purposes of ophthalmoneurologic differential diagnosis.

The distinctive ocular lesion of Bourneville's disease (tuberous sclerosis) is usually described as a refractile yellowish, multinodular cystic mass resembling an unripe mulberry or clump of tapioca arising from the disc or retina. Equally characteristic and infinitely more common are flatter and duller yellow or whitish lesions of the retina. They occur in various sizes ranging from minute dots to lesions approaching the size of the disc. They may be single or multiple, unilateral or bilateral. The lesions appear to be glial hamartomas composed of astrocytic or pleomorphic cells.

Retinal and optic disc lesions similar to the smooth, less elevated lesions of tuberous sclerosis occur in von Recklinghausen's disease (neurofibromatosis), but with less frequency than in tuberous sclerosis.

In von Hippel-Lindau's disease (angiomatosis of the retina and cerebellum) the distinctive fundus lesion is a hemangioblastoma of the retina. This vascular lesion usually is a reddish globular mass accompanied by large paired arteries and veins that pass to and from the lesion; in some cases the lesion is less distinct because of exudation and gliosis. The hemangioblastomas may be found in any region of the fundus, but they most commonly lie temporally, anterior to the equator. They occur in various sizes, and may be single or multiple, unilateral or bilateral.

The fundus lesion in the Sturge-Weber syndrome (encephalofacial angiomatosis) is a choroidal hemangioma; it may impart a dark color to the fundus, but it is best seen with fluorescein angiography.

In the Wyburn-Mason syndrome, the characteristic fundus sign is a racemose angioma of the retinal vessels. This vascular anomaly can be rather extensive and dramatic, the fundus showing a tangle of dilated and tortuous vessels.

APPENDIX TO SECTION I   NEURO-OPHTHALMIC SIGNS

Sign	Description	Significance
Adie's Tonic Pupil	A large pupil with delayed, deficient reaction to light, a slow reaction to near, and delayed redilation. Most often unilateral. Hypersensitivity to 2.5% methacholine; otherwise normal reactions to miotics and mydriatics.	Attributed to denervation secondary to ciliary ganglion lesion, possibly viral. Commonly associated with decreased deep tendon reflexes in young females.
Anton's Syndrome	Cortical blindness with denial of the blindness; amnestic aphasia, loss of recent memory and retention, and confabulation.	The result of occipital cortex disease (bilateral homonymous hemianopia); commonly of vascular origin.
Argyll Robertson's Pupil	Diminished or absent pupil reactions to light with intact reactions to near; miosis and anisocoria; failure to dilate to atropine; also iris atrophy. Usually bilateral.	Characteristic of neurosyphilis. Atypical forms, i.e., Argyll Robertson-like pupils associated with lesions affecting the midbrain.
Balint's Syndrome	Psychic paralysis of visual fixation with optic ataxia and disturbances of visual attention.	Occurs with bilateral occipitoparietal lesions.
Bell's Phenomenon	Upward (or, less commonly, in other directions) deviation of eyes on efforts to close lids against resistance.	An associative facio-ocular movement. A valuable sign of integrity of the brain stem and infranuclear pathways for elevation of the eyes.
Benedikt's Syndrome	Oculomotor palsy with contralateral dyskinesia (hyperkinesia, ataxia) and intention tremor of the arm, sometimes with hemianesthesia.	Indicative of lesion in the area of the red nucleus affecting fascicular fibers of the third nerve as they pass ventrally in the midbrain.
Brun's Syndrome	Paroxysmal episodes of vertigo, headache, vomiting and blurring of vision or transient blindness on change of head position. Freedom from symptoms between attacks. Protective splinting of head between attacks.	Due to obstruction of CSF pathways with sudden increased intracranial pressure. Occurs most commonly with tumors in fourth ventricle, in third or in lateral ventricles.
Cavernous Sinus Syndrome (Spheno-Cavernous Syndrome)	Complete or partial paralysis of third, fourth, and sixth cranial nerves, often with involvement of fifth, and venous congestion.	Associated with tumors, infection, thrombosis in cavernous sinus; also with carotid-cavernous fistula.
Cogwheel Eye Movements	Saccadic, jerky, inaccurate ocular pursuit movements.	Related to acute cerebellar dysfunction, or with disruption of smooth conjugate gaze functions at any level.
Collier's Sign ("Posterior Fossa Stare"; "Tucked Lid")	Symmetrical upper eyelid retraction on gaze upward and on gaze forward, but not on gaze downward. Sometimes in association with vertical gaze paresis.	A supranuclear lid retraction associated with lesions of the posterior portion of the third ventricle, the cerebral aqueduct, and the rostral midbrain. Commonly a feature of the Koerber-Salus-Elschnig syndrome.
Dalrymple's Sign	Abnormal wideness of the palpebral fissure.	Thyroid myopathy.
Doll's Eye Movements	Contraversive movements of the eyes on passive movement of the head.	Reflexive vestibular and cervical eye movements. Pathologic in the conscious, seeing patient. Useful in assessing brain stem and infranuclear pathway integrity in the unconscious patient. Occur in decerebrate state. Associated with pseudobulbar syndromes.

APPENDIX TO SECTION I   NEURO-OPHTHALMIC SIGNS (Continued)

Sign	Description	Significance
Duane's Syndrome (Stilling-Türk-Duane Syndrome)	Deficiency of abduction with retraction of eye on adduction.	A congenital condition generally attributed to a co-contraction phenomenon or anomalous innervation, possibly nuclear hypoplasia (VI).
Foster-Kennedy Syndrome	"Primary" optic atrophy with loss of vision on one side and concomitant papilledema on the other side. Often with impairment of sense of smell ipsilateral to the optic atrophy. Sometimes with exophthalmos.	A sign of baso-frontal lesions, especially meningiomas of sphenoid ridge and olfactory groove, and frontal lobe tumors. Also with suprasellar tumors; even with dilatation of third ventricle affecting chiasm.
Foville Syndrome	Abducent and horizontal gaze palsy with homolateral facial palsy; also ipsilateral Horner's syndrome (oculosympathetic paralysis), ipsilateral analgesia of face and loss of taste from anterior two thirds of tongue, and ipsilateral peripheral deafness.	Indicative of a lesion in the dorsal lateral pontine tegmentum: the "anterior inferior cerebellar syndrome."
Gerstmann's Syndrome	Right-left confusion, dysgraphia, dyscalculia, and finger agnosia, often with homonymous hemianopia and positive OKN sign.	Indicative of lesion involving posterior central gyrus of dominant hemisphere.
Gifford's Sign	Difficulty in eversion of upper eyelid.	The result of shortening of the levator occurring in dysthyroidism.
Gradenigo's Syndrome	Complete or partial paralysis of abducens with pain or hypesthesia in the face and eye; also photophobia, lacrimation, and facial paralysis.	Occurs with ipsilateral inflammation of the apex of the petrous bone and its meninges—thrombophlebitis of inferior petrosal sinus—usually originating with otitis media, mastoiditis; rarely tumor.
Graefe's Sign	Lid lag on gaze downward.	A neuromuscular phenomenon occurring in dysthyroidism, occasionally in myotonia dystrophica.
Hertwig-Magendie Syndrome (Skew Deviation)	Vertical divergence of eyes, comitant or incomitant. Lower eye often intorted; higher eye often extorted. May be unilateral supranuclear vertical palsy.	Occurs with lesions in medulla, pons, or rostral midbrain, and with cerebellar lesions. Lower eye often homolateral to lesion.
Horner's Syndrome	Miosis with ipsilateral ptosis and dyshidrosis; also ocular hypotony, increased amplitude of accommodation, and iris hypopigmentation.	Oculosympathetic paralysis. Localization dependent on pharmacologic test (Table 18–2) and associated signs.
Hutchinson's Pupil	Fixed dilated pupil in association with signs of increasing intracranial pressure.	Occurs with compression of third nerve pupillomotor fibers consequent to increased intracranial pressure. Paralyzed pupil often homolateral to expanding supratentorial lesion.
Koerber-Salus-Elschnig Syndrome (Sylvian Aqueduct Syndrome)	In complete form, characterized by: (1) Supranuclear vertical gaze palsy, often with vertical nystagmus; (2) Tonic or clonic convergent movements; (3) Nystagmus retractorius; (4) Pupillomotor abnormalities; (5) Nuclear oculomotor palsies; (6) Supranuclear upper lid retraction.	Indicative of sylvian aqueduct lesion or periaqueductal lesion.

(Appendix continues on following page)

APPENDIX TO SECTION I NEURO-OPHTHALMIC SIGNS *(Continued)*

Sign	Description	Significance
Marcus Gunn Jaw-winking	Ptosis with inappropriate elevation of ptotic lid on opening of mouth or on side to side movement of jaw.	Aberrant innervation phenomenon; trigemino-oculomotor synkinesis.
Marcus Gunn Pupil Sign	Deficient direct and consensual pupil responses to stimulation of one eye with light, with intact direct and consensual pupil responses to stimulation of fellow eye with light of equal intensity. Best demonstrated by so-called swinging flashlight test, repeatedly stimulating the two eyes alternately for a few seconds with light of constant intensity, watching for constriction of both pupils equally on stimulation of normal eye and relative dilatation of both pupils on stimulation of affected eye. Isocoria.	Characteristic of an asymmetric or wholly unilateral afferent conduction defect, prechiasmal.
Millard-Gubler Syndrome	Abducent palsy and ipsilateral facial palsy with contralateral hemiplegia.	Indicative of ventral paramedian pontine lesion involving the sixth nerve nucleus, the seventh nerve fibers and the pyramidal tract fibers.
Möbius Syndrome	Facial diplegia, often asymmetrical, with abducent paralysis. Range of associated findings includes lingual palsy, external ophthalmoplegia, malformations of extremities and digits, branchial malformations, pectoral muscle defects, mental deficiency.	A congenital condition generally attributed to aplasia of brain stem nuclei (VI and VII).
Nothnagel's Syndrome	Ipsilateral oculomotor palsy with cerebellar ataxia.	Indicative of lesion in the area of the brachium conjunctivum, involving the fascicular portion of one oculomotor nerve (III).
Nystagmus Retractorius	Retraction or convergent-retraction nystagmus on attempted or prolonged upward gaze or near gaze.	Indicative of sylvian aqueduct and periaqueductal lesions. A feature of the Koerber-Salus-Elschnig syndrome; also the Parinaud syndrome.
Ocular Bobbing	Spontaneous vertical oscillations of eyes in a setting of paralysis of horizontal eye movement; downward excursion more brisk than upward excursion.	Occurs with extensive pontine disease; usually hemorrhage or infarction, rarely tumor.
Ocular Dysmetria	Overshoot or undershoot of eyes on conjugate lateral gaze, with several corrective or dampening pendular oscillations terminating in fixation. Often best demonstrated on gaze from eccentric point back toward primary position.	A sign of acute cerebellar dysfunction. Overshoot commonly toward the side of the lesion. Analogous to dysmetria of the limbs.
Ocular Flutter	Intermittent bouts of to and fro pendular oscillations, lasting only seconds, occurring on change of fixation or spontaneously. Productive of momentary blurring of vision.	Indicative of cerebellar disease.
Ocular Motor Apraxia of Cogan —Congenital	Defect of voluntary horizontal gaze with retention of reflexive eye movements. Characteristic head thrust. Absence of fast phase of nystagmus on OKN testing and on rotational testing.	Congenital; often familial. May be a clue to agenesis of corpus callosum and to lesions in region of pons or rostral midbrain.

APPENDIX TO SECTION I   NEURO-OPHTHALMIC SIGNS *(Continued)*

Sign	Description	Significance
Oculogyric Crisis	Spasmodic conjugate deviation of eyes, usually upward, for seconds, minutes, or hours.	A manifestation of disease of the basal ganglia and upper midbrain. Seen in Parkinson's disease, encephalitis. Can be drug-induced.
Orbital Apex Syndrome	Complete or partial paralysis of third, fourth, and sixth cranial nerves, with involvement of fifth (neuralgia in region of ophthalmic branch, corneal and lid hypesthesia) in association with exophthalmos and optic nerve involvement (disc edema, optic neuritis, optic atrophy) and loss of vision or field.	Indicative of tumor or infection in apex of orbit.
Parinaud's Syndrome	Supranuclear vertical gaze paresis with nuclear oculomotor pareses and pupillomotor abnormalities.	Associated with midbrain tegmentum, periaqueductal and posterior commissure lesions. In children, seen especially with pinealoma and aqueductal stenosis.
Pseudo-Graefe's Sign	Inappropriate elevation of upper eyelid on attempted gaze downward following oculomotor paralysis.	A third nerve misdirection phenomenon.
Raeder's Paratrigeminal Syndrome	Pain in the eye (first division V) with Horner's syndrome (oculosympathetic paralysis).	A sign of disease in the cavernous sinus or superior orbital fissure; commonly infection. Rarely a migraine in childhood.
Raymond Syndrome	Abducent palsy with contralateral hemiplegia, sometimes with hemianesthesia.	Indicative of ventral paramedian pontine lesion involving sixth nerve nucleus and pyramidal tract fibers.
Setting Sun Sign	Staring expression with upper eyelid retraction and deficient upward gaze.	Seen in hydrocephalus.
Stellwag's Sign	Retraction of the upper eyelid associated with infrequent or incomplete blinking.	A myopathic sign in dysthyroidism.
Superior Orbital Fissure Syndrome	Complete or partial paralysis of third, fourth, and sixth cranial nerves, and involvement of first division of fifth with hypesthesia and decreased corneal sensation; also exophthalmos.	A sign of superior orbital fissure disease, commonly granuloma or tumor, especially meningioma.
Uncinate Fit	Paroxysmal, usually unpleasant olfactory, gustatory, auditory, or visual hallucinations; often with fugue state or déjà vu.	A sign of irritative temporal lobe pathology—sometimes neoplasms, sometimes birth injury. Look for "pie in sky" homonymous superior quadrantanoptic field defect.
Weber's Syndrome	Oculomotor paralysis, often complete, with contralateral hemiplegia.	Indicative of lesion below the red nucleus affecting the fascicular fibers of the third nerve as they exit from the midbrain.
Wernicke's Hemianoptic Pupil Sign	Homonymous hemianoptic pupillary defect—deficient pupillary response to light falling on affected corresponding hemiretinas in presence of homonymous hemianopia, with normal pupillary response to light falling on nonaffected hemiretinas.	Signifies optic tract affection. Useful in differentiating tract from radiation hemianopias.

Section II

Disorders of the Nervous System in Childhood

HYDROCEPHALUS

The term hydrocephalus denotes dilatation of the cerebrospinal fluid pathways produced by abnormal accumulation of cerebrospinal fluid under increased pressure. This pathologic condition is not a disease in itself, but rather the common expression of a wide variety of disorders that may be either congenital or acquired (Table 18–8).

TABLE 18–8   PRINCIPAL CAUSES OF HYDROCEPHALUS*

Tumors
  Gliomas of cerebellar or pontomedullary origin, dermoids or choroid plexus adenomas obstructing the fourth ventricle or caudal end of the aqueduct of Sylvius
  Gliomas of the midbrain and basal ganglia or pineal tumors obstructing the posterior third ventricle and aqueduct
  Craniopharyngiomas and gliomas obstructing the foramen of Monro or anterior portion of the third ventricle
  Gliomas of the diencephalon and optic pathways or congenital lesions obstructing the interpeduncular cistern

Congenital Malformations
  Spina bifida and cranium bifidum
      Arnold-Chiari malformation
  Aqueductal atresia, stenosis or forking; gliosis of the aqueduct; congenital septa of the aqueduct
  Congenital cysts
      Porencephalic cysts within the brain
      Arachnoid cysts above or below the tentorium
      Posterior fossa cysts due to prenatal occlusion of the foramina of Magendi and Luschka: Dandy-Walker syndrome
  Vascular malformation
      Arteriovenous malformation (involving posterior cerebral artery and vein of Galen or straight sinus) occluding aqueduct

Inflammation
  Hemorrhage, leading to fibrosis and thickening of leptomeninges and obliteration of subarachnoid pathways
  Infection, with meningitis, leading to obliteration of subarachnoid pathways or blockage of aqueduct or basal cistern

*Adapted from Matson.

The mechanism of the hydrocephalus is usually (a) an obstruction to cerebrospinal fluid flow somewhere between the principal site of fluid formation within the ventricular system and the principal site of fluid absorption in the subarachnoid space over the cerebral surface, or (b) an impairment of cerebrospinal fluid absorption; rarely is the mechanism an excessive formation of cerebrospinal fluid.

GENERAL MANIFESTATIONS.   The effects of hydrocephalus are essentially those of increased pressure modified by the distensibility of the young skull. The clinical findings and appearance are characteristic.

The head enlarges at an abnormal rate, disproportionate to the growth of the body. There is expansion of the cranium with progressive thinning of the calvarium and spreading of the cranial sutures. The forehead tends to become prominent, the orbits laterally displaced, and, in contrast to the expanded cranium, the face appears small. The scalp becomes stretched and thinned, and the veins become prominent. There is often a staring expression, with retraction of the lids and downward deviation of the eyes. Characteristically the fontanelles are distended and tense. A peculiar hollow or cracked pot sound (Macewen's sign) can often be elicited by percussion of the head. The head may transilluminate.

The children tend to be feeble, feed poorly, and fail to thrive. Irritability is typical, and crying often is high pitched. With increasing degrees of uncompensated pressure, vomiting, disorganized motor activity, convulsions, spasticity, and paralyses may develop. There often is progression to a state of somnolence. With decompensation, disturbances of respiration and circulation occur.

Depending on the severity of the process, the nature of the causative condition, and the effectiveness of treatment, varying degrees of physical and mental disability may result. Spastic paraparesis and psychomotor retardation are common. Often the deficits are profound, though some patients may show minimal or no disability.

OPHTHALMIC MANIFESTATIONS. A variety of neuro-ophthalmic abnormalities occur, particularly in advanced cases and during periods of decompensation.

Loss of visual acuity and field due to pressure, ischemia, and even stretching of the optic nerves, chiasm, or tracts is common, and the pregeniculate vision defects can be symmetrical or asymmetrical. Pressure and ischemia can also damage the posterior visual pathways; homonymous hemianoptic defects and cortical blindness may result.

The vision loss of hydrocephalus can develop acutely with decompensation and be reversible with control, but prolonged or repeated episodes of pressure and ischemia often produce permanent damage to the visual pathways. Multiple surgical procedures, infections, seizures, and hypoxia contribute significantly to deterioration of vision and field in hydrocephalus, and control of these complications is vital in the management of children with hydrocephalus.

The usual ophthalmoscopic sign of hydrocephalus is optic atrophy of varying severity resulting from slowly progressive or repeated insults to the pregeniculate fibers. Less commonly there is papilledema of increased intracranial pressure; this may resolve with control, but postpapilledema optic atrophy may develop. Sometimes the discs are normal.

Ophthalmoscopic clues to causes of hydrocephalus, such as hamartomas and congenital infections, may be evident in some cases.

Pupillary abnormalities are variable and unpredictable. Often there are afferent conduction defects due to the anterior pathway damage, while normal pupillary light responses are retained in the cases of pure cortical blindness. Signs of efferent pupillomotor dysfunction frequently are present, occurring with decompensation and compression of the third nerve. Commonly there is a combination of these pupillary effects.

Disturbances of ocular motor function are especially frequent and important signs of hydrocephalus. Abducens palsies are common, and intermittent or progressive esotropia with or without frank paralysis of abduction can be a presenting sign of the increasing pressure. Exotropia, convergence deficiency, spasms of convergence, nystagmus, and gaze palsies also are common. A typical finding is the "setting sun" sign, characterized by a staring expression with retraction of the upper lids baring the upper sclera, and downward deviation of the eyes with deficiency of upgaze. In the event of amaurosis, there may be oculovestibular or random purposeless eye movements.

PRENATAL MALFORMATIONS

Anomalies of the nervous system and eye resulting from aberrations of development occurring during intrauterine life are among the most frequent abnormalities encountered in pediatric practice. They range in severity from minor stigmata (such as small retinal or optic nerve colobomata) having little or no deleterious effect on function, to gross malformations, such as anencephaly or cyclopia, that are incompatible with life.

Despite repeated observations and intensive investigations on the mechanisms of abnormal development, the pathogenesis of prenatal malformations in man remains largely undetermined. While genetic factors and endogenous defects of the germ plasm would seem to be of primary importance in the determination of many defects, it is known that the same defects may be effected by exogenous factors. Understanding of the mechanisms of prenatal malformations is further complicated by the fact that the ultimate form of the anomaly does not necessarily give precise indications as to the stage of development at which the aberration commenced; a malformation may be the end stage of a gradual retardation of development or the consequence of an abrupt insult to development. Because of such problems in the etiologic and pathogenetic classification of prenatal malformations, at the present state of our knowledge anomalies of the nervous system are best classified on the basis of morphologic features alone.

Since the common anomalies of the globe and adnexa are presented in other

(Text continued on page 493.)

TABLE 18-9 CONGENITAL STRUCTURAL MALFORMATIONS OF THE BRAIN AND ITS COVERINGS

Designation	Description	Ophthalmic Signs	Associated Abnormalities and Clinical Effects
Septo-Optic Dysplasia (de Morsier)	Agenesis of the septum pellucidum with malformation of the optic chiasm and agenesis of the corpus callosum.	Optic atrophy, optic nerve hypoplasia, colobomata (disc or choroidal), microphthalmos or anophthalmos. Defective vision, possibly bitemporal deficit. Hypertelorism.	Associated midline facial anomalies; cleft lip and palate, hypoplasia or absence of nose. Hypopituitarism and growth failure.
Arrhinencephaly	Aplasia of olfactory bulbs and tracts. Connotes a spectrum of teratisms characterized by olfactory aplasia combined with median dysplasia of face.	Spectrum of graded severity from extreme hypotelorism (a single median orbit and fused eye—cyclopia) to hypertelorism. Possibly anophthalmos, microphthalmos, colobomata, or optic atrophy.	Range of facial abnormalities that includes arrhinia with proboscis, bilateral or median cleft lip and palate, micrognathia. Retardation of various degrees.
Holoprosencephaly	Tendency for prosencephalon to remain incompletely cleft and undifferentiated into complex cerebral hemispheres. Connotes a spectrum of median faciocerebral deformities of graded severity.		
Macrencephaly	Enlarged brain with thickened cortex and elaborate convolutions.	Defective vision. Optic atrophy.	Mental deficiency and motor retardation. Convulsions. Enlarging head not to be confused with hydrocephalus: ventricles not enlarged.
Micrencephaly (microcephaly vera)	Smallness of brain with resultant smallness of calvarium. Inherent poor development of cortical cells. Head at least two standard deviations below mean for age and sex.	No constant defect, but reported range includes epicanthus, microphthalmos, microcornea, colobomata, persistent vascular remnants, cataract, aplasia of macula, gliosis, and pigmentary degeneration of retina.	Hereditary tendency common: autosomal recessive. All grades of mental deficiency, motor disturbances, and epilepsy. Sometimes blind, deaf, and dumb.
Lissencephaly (agyric micrencephaly)	Absence of fissures and sulci of cerebral cortex—"smooth brain". In less severe form, microgyria.	Possibly microphthalmos, maldevelopment of retina (aplasia or glial changes with rosettes), but no constant malformation. Little response to visual stimuli owing to cerebral deficiency.	True agyria incompatible with prolonged life. Lesser maldevelopment (microgyria) associated with various grades of psychomotor retardation and failure to thrive. Seizures. Sometimes micrognathia, low-set ears, wide-set eyes, and upward slanting palpebral fissures.

Hydranencephaly	Maldevelopment of brain in which cerebral hemispheres are reduced to membranous sacs filled with cerebrospinal fluid. In contrast to anencephaly, meninges and cranium are intact, and in contrast to hydrocephalus, head size is normal or only slightly enlarged.	Cortical blindness is usual. Sometimes retinal or optic "atrophy" – ? truly hypoplasia ?	Limited life span; death usually occurring in infancy or early childhood. Psychomotor retardation and growth retardation. Seizures. Head transilluminates
Porencephaly	Cystlike cavity of cerebral hemisphere connecting with ventricular system; often bilateral and symmetrical.	Congenital hemianopias and other vision defects. Sometimes optic pallor. Strabismus.	Hemiplegias and sensory deficits, seizures, mental deficiency. Sometimes asymmetry of head.
Syringomyelia, syringobulbia	Congenital affection characterized by glial proliferation and cavity formation in central portions of spinal cord; when medulla involved, syringobulbia exists.	Sometimes optic atrophy, possibly related to an accompanying arachnoiditis or hydrocephalus. Oculosympathetic paralysis (Horner's syndrome) if cervical area affected and enlarged. Commonly nystagmus. Occasionally impaired corneal sensitivity or ocular motor paralysis.	Congenital sensory defects, progressive muscle atrophy, trophic changes and scoliosis.
Craniorachischisis (cranium bifidum)	Maldevelopment of cerebral portion of neural tube in which neural tube fails to close and to separate from surface ectoderm, and mesoderm that forms bony covering of CNS fails to meet over the defect. Dysplasia ranging from anencephaly to cranium bifidum occulta. Most frequently occipital, and commonly associated with Klippel-Feil anomaly.	May be those of anencephaly or of encephalomeningoceles. With occipital type in particular, possibly cortical blindness.	May be those of anencephaly or of encephalomeningoceles.
Anencephaly	Absence or gross deficiency of cranial vault and overlying skin, with absence or gross maldevelopment of cerebral hemispheres, with or without maldevelopment of cerebellum, basal ganglia, brain stem, cord, and spine.	Aplasia or hypoplasia of retinal ganglion cells and nerve fibers (optic nerve aplasia or hypoplasia); less commonly colobomata, microphthalmos, or anophthalmos. Deformity of orbits.	Incompatible with life.
Encephalo-meningocele	Protrusion of brain substance and its meninges through defect in skull.	Possibly microphthalmos or apparent anophthalmos, optic atrophy, or nerve fiber aplasia or coloboma; rarely papilledema. With trans-sphenoidal encephalocele in particular, colobomatous defects of optic disc, and hypertelorism. With orbital type, proptosis (usually pulsating) and limitation of eye movement.	Frequently associated abnormalities include hydrocephalus, spina bifida, club feet, cleft lip and palate. Possibly hypopituitarism.

(Table continues on following page)

TABLE 18–9 CONGENITAL STRUCTURAL MALFORMATIONS OF THE BRAIN AND ITS COVERINGS (*Continued*)

Designation	Description	Ophthalmic Signs	Associated Abnormalities and Clinical Effects
Arnold-Chiari Deformity	Malformation of hindbrain characterized by (1) downward displacement of cerebellar tonsils through foramen magnum (tongue of cerebellar tissue adherent to dorsal surface of upper cervical cord); (2) elongation and downward displacement of medulla oblongata and fourth ventricle through foramen magnum, with downward displacement of upper cervical cord; (3) partial or total obstruction to communication between fourth ventricle and basal cistern; and (4) hydrocephalus.	Nystagmus; usually vertical, often down-beat. Ocular motor palsies with diplopia; sometimes skew deviation.	Cerebellar ataxia and pyramidal tract signs. Signs of hydrocephalus.
Dandy-Walker Syndrome	Cerebellar dysraphia and pseudocyst of cisterna cerebellomedullaris in association with atresia of foramina of Luschka and Magendi. Cystlike enlargement of fourth ventricle displaces and in part replaces midline structures of cerebellum. Pons, medulla and upper cervical cord broader than normal and displaced anteriorly. Dilatation of aqueduct of Sylvius and of third and fourth ventricles.	Ophthalmic effects of increased intracranial pressure (hydrocephalus): optic atrophy (or papilledema), pupillary dysfunction, abducent paralysis, nystagmus.	Regularly associated with obstructive hydrocephalus and enlargement of head with prominence of occiput. Psychomotor retardation. Sometimes seizures.

chapters, emphasis is here placed on pre-natal malformations of the optic nerve and on structural defects of the brain and its coverings (Table 18–9).

Optic Nerve Hypoplasia

Optic nerve hypoplasia is a congenital deficiency of optic nerve fibers; although other explanations are proposed, this anomaly is generally attributed to a primary failure of development of the retinal ganglion cells and their axons.

Differentiation of the retinal ganglion cells normally occurs at about 6 weeks of life or at the 17 mm. stage of development; growing into the primitive papilla to form the neural elements of the optic nerve, the ganglion cell axons normally reach the optic chiasm by the 18 mm. stage, and the lateral geniculate body by the 25 mm. stage. Complete or partial failure of this process results in varying degrees of optic nerve hypoplasia, with distinctive morphologic and clinical manifestations.

In optic nerve hypoplasia, the nerve-head characteristically is small, occupying only a fraction of the usual disc area, leaving a pale or pigmented halo of sclera between the margin of the nerve and the border of the pigmented retinal epithelium and choroid. Commonly the halo is bordered on either side by a rim of pigment, forming the so-called double-ring sign. The nervehead is often pale, but sometimes pink. A true paucity of nerve substance is a more reliable diagnostic criterion of optic nerve hypoplasia than is disc color. There is usually a corresponding deficiency of the macular ganglion cell ring, with the macular contour appearing flat and poorly differentiated on ophthalmoscopic examination. The major retinal vessels are generally normal, however, since they develop independently of the retinal ganglion cells; growth of mesoderm is not affected in optic nerve hypoplasia.

The primary clinical significance of this developmental anomaly is the attendant abnormality of vision. Depending on the degree of hypoplasia, the vision defects range from blindness to peripheral field defects with preservation of central vision. The manner of clinical presentation varies with the severity, laterality, and symmetry of the condition. Unilateral and asymmetric hypoplasia commonly presents as heterotropia; the ocular deviation usually develops early in life, but commonly the underlying vision defect is not suspected by the parents. Bilateral hypoplasia of relatively severe degree typically manifests in infancy; ocular nystagmus is often the presenting sign, and the vision defect is usually apparent to the family early. Less severe hypoplasia often exists unrecognized for years.

Pupillary evidence of the afferent conduction defect, normal ERG responses, and subnormal VER are expected findings with significant degrees of hypoplasia. The optic canals may be small or normal in size.

Optic nerve hypoplasia may occur unilaterally or bilaterally as an isolated anomaly in otherwise normal individuals. It may also occur in association with other developmental abnormalities, including microphthalmia, cyclopia, anencephaly, hydrocephalus, and orbital encephalomeningocele. It is an important feature of septo-optic dysplasia, a developmental disorder characterized by anomalies of the midline structure of the brain in association with abnormalities of the optic nerves, optic chiasm, and optic tracts. Typically there is agenesis of the septum pellucidum and malformation of the fornix, which does not become attached to the corpus callosum. There commonly is enlargement or dilatation of the chiasmatic cistern. There may also be anormalities of endocrine functions, presumably as the result of extension of the midline defect into the hypothalamus. Growth failure may result. Thus the presence of optic nerve hypoplasia in a youngster should alert one to the possibility of growth hormone deficiency and midline brain defects.

Optic Nerve Aplasia

True aplasia of the optic nerve is a very rare anomaly in which there is complete absence of the optic nerve and the retinal vessels. The condition presumably results from failure of the paraxial mesoderm to grow into the optic stalk before closure of the fetal fissure.

Normally, following formation of the

embryonic fissure along the ventrolateral surface of the optic cup and stalk, mesodermal tissue invades the optic cup through the fissure, filling the cup with embryonic blood vessels and the hyaloid system, and forming the primitive papilla. If for some reason the growth of mesoderm into the embryonic fissure is delayed, the fissure may fuse completely, preventing the hyaloid and retinal vessels from entering the eye, resulting in complete aplasia of the optic nerve with absence of the papilla, the retinal vessels, and the retinal ganglion cell layer. The affected eye is blind.

This developmental defect almost never occurs in otherwise normal individuals. It is usually associated with gross malformation of the globe, or with malformation of the brain.

Optic Nerve Colobomata

The typical coloboma is a developmental malformation of the eye related to incomplete or anomalous closure of the embryonic fissure. The defect may involve the iris, ciliary body, choroid and retina, optic nerve, or any combination thereof, depending on the site and extent of the aberration.

Closure of the embryonic cleft begins at the 10 to 11 mm. stage of development (during the fifth week of life); fusion commences in the midportion of the fissure and proceeds both distally and proximally, reaching the anterior rim of the optic cup by the 15 mm. stage and the proximal end of the fissure by the 20 mm. stage. At some point during the process, excessive eversion and hyperplasia of the neural layer and nonclosure may occur. When the proximal portion of the fissure fails to close properly, the retina and choroid around the nerve may be affected—the nerve itself being normal and sharing passively in the deformity—or the nerve itself or its sheath may be involved. Rarely is the coloboma entirely contained within the nerve sheath; in such a case the primitive epithelial papilla of Bergmeister suffers aplasia, and the extreme end of the fissure remains widely open. The anatomic condition often cannot be predicted by the ophthalmoscopic findings, but patholog-

ically the distinction is the relation of the vaginal sheath to the ectasia. An ectasia which comes into relation with the vaginal sheath from its outer side is a coloboma of the fundus, whereas one which comes into relation with the sheath from its inner side is a coloboma of the nerve. In some instances there is combined involvement.

The clinical appearance of colobomatous defects in and about the optic nerve varies considerably. There may be deep colobomatous cupping of the disc or merely an irregularity or pit of the disc margin. There may be ectasia of the colobomatous area in or adjacent to the disc, forming a large retrobulbar cystlike cavity with marked distortion and maldirection of the disc entrance. There may be chorioretinal defect extending down from or surrounding the disc (peripapillary coloboma), the nerve itself being normal.

A scotoma corresponding to the area of the colobomatous defect is usually present.

Coloboma of the optic nerve may occur in an otherwise normal eye, or in association with other anomalies such as microphthalmia, cyclopia, or anencephaly. The association of optic nerve colobomata and trans-sphenoidal encephalocele has been reported.

Optic Nerve Pit

Congenital pit or "hole" of the disc is a developmental defect of the optic nerve that is considered to be a minimal coloboma.

The ophthalmoscopic appearance is distinctive. The disc defect is usually oval or slitlike, resembling a fish mouth with its long axis concentric with the disc margin, but it may be round, irregular, or even triangular in shape. Often the cavity is filled or covered by a veil of tissue that is gray, pigmented, or transparent. Sometimes there is a vessel dipping into or emerging from the defect. Occurring more often unilaterally than bilaterally, this anomaly most frequently is situated in the lower temporal quadrant of the disc, close to or touching the rim, but never extending beyond the margin of the disc. Rarely is a pit centrally located. Varying in size from a minute hole to a large fossa or crater, a pit may range from a shallow depression to a cavity several diopters deep. In some instances the pit may look like a protrusion rather than a cavity; binocular ophthalmoscopy and biomicroscopy are invaluable in the diagnosis.

The pathologic appearance of this defect conforms with the herniation of neural ectoderm and the proliferation of retinal tissue associated with typical colobomata. The pit is formed of rudimentary retinal tissue, irregular glial elements, and remnants of nerve fibers and pigment epithelium; dipping down through a defect in the lamina cribrosa, these anomalous tissues extend into the optic nerve toward the vaginal sheath and come into relation with its inner aspect. The defect is limited within the dural sheath; the nerve fibers from the retina skirt the defect on their way into the optic nerve, and the choroid is uninvolved.

Vision and field defects are sometimes associated with optic nerve pit. The defect in the nerve can give rise to central or peripheral scotomas, arcuate or sector field defects, and enlargement of the blind spot.

An important complication of this anomaly is serous detachment of the macula, occurring most commonly in the second or third decade of life. The pathogenesis of central serous retinopathy in association with optic pit is not clear, but it may produce visual symptoms; fortunately the prognosis for recovery of vision is good.

An association of hole in the optic disc, nasopharyngeal trans-sphenoidal encephalocele, and agenesis of the corpus callosum has been reported.

Dysversion of the Optic Nervehead

Dysversion is a maldirection of the optic nervehead commonly described as tilting of the disc; the condition is generally attributed to anomalous insertion of the optic stalk into the optic vesicle. Commonly there is a nasal tilt, with the central retinal vessels emerging toward the nasal side rather than toward the temporal side. More rarely, there is downward or oblique tilting. The condition usually is bilateral.

The significance of the dysversion in ophthalmoneurologic diagnosis is that it may result in vision and field defects, not infrequently bitemporal or altitudinal defects, that must be differentiated from those of acquired or progressive disease. In addition, the distortion can be confused with papilledema.

PRENATAL INFECTION SYNDROMES

A significant proportion of infant morbidity and mortality is the result of prenatal infection with one of several agents that are capable of traversing the placental barrier and establishing active disease in the developing embryo or fetus. The agents most frequently responsible for prenatal infection are the rubella virus, cytomegalovirus, *Toxoplasma gondii*, and *Treponema pallidum*. With the exception of syphilis (*T. pallidum*), infection with these agents is commonly innocuous or inapparent in the pregnant woman, whereas it is potentially disastrous in the developing embryo or fetus.

Manifestations in the infant are influenced by several factors, including the time at which the infection exerts its greatest effect, the virulence of the agent, and the immunity response of the mother and infant. The result may be fulminant, possibly lethal infection, subacute or chronic disseminated or multifocal infection that may persist long after birth, or a variety of permanent inflammatory sequelae ranging in severity from minor stigmata to disabling abnormalities; in certain instances, especially in the case of rubella, there are teratogenic as well as inflammatory consequences.

Highly vulnerable to the damaging effects of prenatal infection are the nervous system and eye. The resulting neurologic and ophthalmic abnormalities quite frequently are the predominant manifestations. In certain instances the ocular findings are distinctive, having great significance in the differential diagnosis of the various congenital infection syndromes.

The Congenital Rubella Syndrome

In its most severe and complete form, the congenital rubella syndrome is characterized by signs of disseminated virus infection, disturbances of somatic growth, and anomalies of development. Cataracts, pigmentary retinopathy, deafness, psychomotor retardation, congenital heart defects, and growth failure are major stigmata of the disease, and systemic manifestations of continuing virus infection are often present in the neonatal period, with persistence of the virus in the infant long after birth.

GENERAL MANIFESTATIONS. Consequences of this transplacental infection are determined primarily by the timing of the viral insult; infection at any time during the first 4 or 5 months of gestation may result in widespread or multifocal inflammatory disease of varying severity, but infection in the first 6 or 8 weeks presents the greatest hazard to organogenesis and life, as a result of cell damage and necrosis. The heart, for example, is especially vulnerable to the teratogenic effects of rubella, and anomalies such as patent ductus arteriosus, pulmonary stenosis, and septal defects are frequent sequelae of very early infection, while hepatitis, myocarditis, and encephalitis are commonly seen in the newborn period as the result of more persistent inflammation. Thrombocytopenia, petechiae, hemolytic anemia, jaundice, and hepatosplenomegaly are common signs of the disease, and the expression "blueberry muffin baby" is often used to describe the appearance of the overtly infected infants. The babies tend to be of low birth weight, their organs contain a subnormal number of cells, and there may be radiologic evidence of disturbance of bone growth.

NERVOUS SYSTEM INVOLVEMENT. The neurovirulence of congenital rubella is evident in both nonfatal and fatal forms of the disease. Encephalitis and leptomeningitis have been well documented. Cerebral vasculitis, perivascular calcifications, multifocal necrosis of the brain, and retardation of myelination are features of the process, and the white matter of the cerebral hemispheres and basal ganglia is predominantly affected. Clinical signs of central nervous system infection include lethargy, irritability, hypotonia or spasticity, seizures, and full fontanelles. The cerebrospinal fluid may show a moderate increase in protein and cells, and the virus can be recovered from spinal fluid in many cases. Microcephaly, psychomotor retardation of varying severity, spastic quadriparesis, and sensorineural hearing loss are frequent sequelae of neural involvement, but the extent of the damage may not be fully apparent in the early months of life.

OPHTHALMIC MANIFESTATIONS. Ocular abnormalities are cardinal manifestations of congenital rubella, reflecting both the acute and chronic effects induced by the virus; the eye may harbor live virus for months or years. Infection within the lens characteristically produces unilateral or bilateral pearly nuclear cataract, and this lesion is frequently associated with microphthalmia. Iris hypoplasia, atrophy, synechiae, and vacuolization are common, and complete or partial absence of the iris dilator and focal necrosis of the ciliary body are also rather typical findings. Congenital glaucoma due to incomplete differentiation of the chamber angle also occurs, and transient nonglaucomatous corneal clouding has been described. The most frequent ocular sign of congenital rubella, however, is pigmentary retinopathy caused by a disturbance of pigmentation in the retinal epithelium, with discrete areas of pigment clumping and focal areas of atrophy and depigmentation of varying size and distribution. The pigment mottling and coarse "salt and pepper" changes are often most pronounced in the macular area and just posterior to the equator, and the foveal reflex may be distorted. The retinopathy has minimal, if any, effect on visual functions; it is nonprogressive, and the ERG responses are generally normal. Vision deficits, pendular ocular nystagmus, and strabismus are more commonly due to the cataracts, glaucoma, optic nerve fiber damage, or high refractive error, though vision and ocular motor abnormalities are often a consequence of the encephalomyelitis.

A caution. These damaged and infected infants are capable of disseminating the disease, as the virus is very persistent and may be viable even in the presence of neutralizing antibody.

Congenital Cytomegalovirus Disease

The classic picture of congenital cytomegalovirus infection is one of disseminated or multifocal disease. Hematopoietic tissues and viscera are usually affected, but it is the consequences of central nervous system involvement that are of primary importance in infants who survive.

THE INFECTION AND ITS GENERAL MANIFESTATIONS. Transplacental infection of the embryo or fetus most probably results from the viremia of a primary maternal infection, which is usually subclinical. Hepatitis, jaundice, splenomegaly, hemolytic anemia, thrombocytopenia, pneumonitis, gastroenteritis, and signs of retardation of intrauterine growth are frequent manifestations of extraneural infection in the infant. Systemic symptoms may be relatively benign in some infants, but fulminant infection can result in intrauterine or neonatal death.

A pathognomonic sign of the viral infection is the presence of intranuclear and cytoplasmic inclusion bodies found primarily in epithelial cells in the congenital form of the disease. These characteristic inclusion cells have been demonstrated in every organ, including the nervous system and the eye, and may also be detected in the urine. Hence, an alternative name for the disease is cytomegalic inclusion disease.

NERVOUS SYSTEM INVOLVEMENT. Cytomegalovirus infection of the central nervous system in utero produces an encephalitis of varying severity, and it may progress postnatally. The process may be severe, with extensive necrosis, hemorrhage, and secondary calcifications, but lesser involvement does occur. The distribution of the inflammatory lesions and secondary calcifications is characteristically periventricular, and the region of the lateral ventricles and olfactory tracts is most involved, with relative sparing of the aqueduct and the third and fourth ventricles. This pattern suggests early gestational infection. Microcephaly, maldevelopment of the convolutions, retardation, seizures, blindness, deafness, and spastic paralyses are frequent sequelae. A high percentage of infants with congenital cytomegalovirus disease suffer permanent central nervous system damage, though signs may not be immediately apparent in the neonatal period.

OPHTHALMIC COMPLICATIONS. The usual ocular lesion of congenital cytomegalovirus infection is chorioretinitis. Single or multifocal atrophic and pigmented chorioretinal scars develop. Their distribution is generally peripheral, tending to spare the macula. Perivascular retinal exudates have been described, and anterior uveitis, cataract, optic atrophy, and microphthalmos may develop. Cytomegalovirus has actually been isolated from the aqueous, and inclusion bodies have been demonstrated in the eye.

In addition to ocular infection and inflammation due to intrauterine cytomegalovirus infection, there may be damage to the posterior visual pathways as the result of the encephalomyelitis. Amaurosis, strabismus, and nystagmus are common sequelae.

Congenital Toxoplasmosis

Encephalomyelitis and chorioretinitis are the principal manifestations of congenital toxoplasmosis. Extraneural involvements do occur, and evidence of infection may be found in almost all tissues, including the liver, spleen, lymph nodes, lungs, heart, and skeletal muscle; however, it is the central nervous system and eye that are particularly susceptible to the damaging effects of toxoplasmosis in utero.

THE INFECTION AND ITS GENERAL MANIFESTATIONS. This infection is caused by the intracellular parasite, *Toxoplasma gondii*. The organism is transmitted to the fetus during the parasitemia of a primary maternal infection. Infection in the mother is usually asymptomatic, but infection of the fetus is expressed as disease of varying severity. The familiar form of congenital toxoplasmosis is a generalized infection, often with hepatomegaly, jaundice, anemia, thrombocytopenia, fever, and rash. Signs of the disease may be obvious at birth or may develop some time later. The infection can terminate in fetal or neonatal death, but most infants survive, the majority showing sequelae of the central nervous system infection.

NERVOUS SYSTEM INVOLVEMENT. The cerebral cortex, basal ganglia, paraventricular tissues, ependyma, and meninges are usually involved by rather diffuse inflammation. Areas of necrosis, gliosis, and secondary intracerebral calcifications are common. Clinical manifestations of the central nervous system involvement include microcephaly, hydrocephaly, psychomotor retardation, convulsions, spasticity and paralysis, deafness, and blindness. The spinal fluid often contains cells and increased protein, and the parasite sometimes can be recovered from the spinal fluid. The neural inflammation may be active or inactive at the time of birth, but even after tissue damage stabilizes, live parasites may persist in the brain for years.

OPHTHALMIC INVOLVEMENT. The principal ophthalmic effects of congenital toxoplasmosis are damage to the visual pathways by the meningoencephalitis and damage to the eye by chorioretinitis.

Toxoplasmic chorioretinitis begins with infection and inflammation in the retina; there is secondary involvement of the choroid. The inflammation is usually bilateral, severe, and destructive. There may be single or multiple foci, and macular involvement is common. In the acute stage there is exudation into the vitreous. As the inflammation subsides, atrophic chorioretinal scars form, and these scars tend to be well demarcated by pigment. Viable organisms may persist in the eye, and recurrences and satellite lesions are a feature of toxoplasmic chorioretinitis. Vision loss, optic atrophy, strabismus, nystagmus, retinal detachment, cataract, and glaucoma may result. There is also a tendency toward congenital anomalies of the eye and microphthalmos.

Much of the visual and ocular motor disability may be due primarily to the encephalomyelitis.

Congenital Syphilis

Congenital syphilis is a systemic spirochetal infection that can affect virtually every organ system. It may manifest as early disease in infancy, as late disease after infancy, or as stigmata in the child or adult. Central nervous system and ocular involvement are commonly a feature of late congenital syphilis. Mental deficiency, sensorineural deafness, and vision deficits are principal neural consequences of this congenital disease.

THE INFECTION AND ITS GENERAL MANIFESTATIONS. Syphilis is caused by the motile spirochete, *Treponema pallidum.* Transplacental infection occurs after the first trimester, usually during the latent stage of acquired maternal infection. The infection produces a rather generalized interstitial inflammation in the placenta and in the fetus. Any organ can be affected. Congenital malformations are not a feature of this disease, because fetal infection rarely occurs before the fourth month. Florid infection can result in fetal death, stillbirth, prematurity, or neonatal illness, but often there are no overt signs of infection in the first weeks or months of life. Signs of early congenital syphilis include fever, anemia, and thrombocytopenia, hepatosplenomegaly and lymphadenopathy, pneumonia, restlessness, and failure to thrive. Maculopapular rash and mucocutaneous lesions about the nose, mouth, and genital region develop. Additional signs of early congenital syphilis are snuffles (marked by mucoid, purulent, or hemorrhagic nasal discharge) and osteochondritis and periostitis. Stigmata of early congenital syphilis are depressed nasal bridge (saddle nose deformity), fine scars about the mouth and chin (rhagades), deformity of the permanent teeth (Hutchinson's incisors and mulberry molars), and frontal bossing. The manifestations of congenital infection that appear after infancy reflect mainly the skeletal, central nervous system, and ocular involvement. The classic triad of late congenital syphilis (Hutchinson's triad) consists of nerve deafness, interstitial keratitis, and hutchinsonian incisors. There may also be osteoperiostitis, arthritis, gummas, and visceral and cardiovascular disease in late congenital syphilis. Even when illness subsides, the *T. pallidum* can persist in the tissues for years.

NERVOUS SYSTEM INVOLVEMENT. Meningovascular inflammation and central nervous system damage are relatively frequent effects of congenital infection with *T. pallidum.* There may be signs of meningitis in infancy, but nervous system involvement is not a usual feature of the early form of congenital syphilis; more commonly the neural involvement is a feature of the late form. In some cases, the meningovascular involvement manifests abruptly in prepubertal children as hemiplegia and convulsions. In others, the neurosyphilis becomes apparent in the teens. In many patients, however, the central nervous system involvement does not become manifest until the adult years.

The sequelae of the meningovascular inflammation include low grade hydrocephalus, mental deficiency, seizures, irritability, abnormal behavior, and organic dementia. Neural deafness (resulting from eighth nerve damage) and optic atrophy are significant consequences of the nervous system infection; often the sensorineural damage does not become apparent for years.

OCULAR MANIFESTATIONS. Perivascular infiltration by *T. pallidum* and the establishment of inflammation in the cornea, uvea, retina, and optic nerve are common consequences of congenital syphilis, and the organism can persist in the eye for decades. Most of the ocular manifestations of congenital syphilis are late manifestations of the disease.

A classic sign of congenital syphilis is interstitial keratitis, an inflammation in the parenchyma of the cornea, particularly in the deep stroma. Interstitial keratitis is usually a late manifestation of the disease, developing after age 5 or 6 years, but it can develop at any age. The active inflammation is accompanied by anterior uveitis (iridocyclitis) and intense photophobia. Vascularization and opacification of the cornea develop, and progressive inflammation can lead to blindness in weeks or months.

Retinitis and choroiditis are relatively common signs of congenital syphilis, and they too are usually late manifestations of the disease. In the retina, there can be widespread damage of the neural layers and of the pigment epithelium. In the choroid, the inflammatory foci are primarily in the choriocapillaries. The usual ophthalmoscopic sign of retinal pigment epithelium necrosis, pigment migration clumping, and glial scarring is salt-and-pepper retinopathy. The pigment changes may be fine or coarse, sometimes with bone spicule aggregates and plaques; they are usually more marked peripherally, and they are usually accompanied by arterial attenuation and optic atrophy. There may be larger focal chorioretinal scars. In some cases there is retinal periphlebitis, and vascular occlusions may occur.

Exudative uveitis occurs in some cases. Acute iridocyclitis can be present in the fetus or infant, and it may terminate in occlusion of the pupil by an exudative membrane. There may be exudation into the vitreous, and a picture of pseudoglioma or phthisis may result.

In addition, there may be infiltration in the arachnoidal sheath of the optic nerve, producing optic nerve edema in its acute stage and optic atrophy in its chronic stage.

TUMORS

With the exception of the leukemias and the group of tumors that arise in the renal and suprarenal area, intracranial tumors are the most frequent neoplasms of childhood. It has long been recognized that there is a peak incidence of intracranial tumors in the latter half of the first decade, and in recent years increasing numbers of brain tumors are being recognized and treated in the first years, even in the first weeks of life; undoubtedly some are present at birth. As the many tumors that occur within the brain and its coverings early in life very frequently produce ophthalmic signs and symptoms, they command special attention in a text on pediatric ophthalmology.

In certain ways, intracranial tumors of childhood differ from those of adult life. Whereas the majority of intracranial tumors in adults occur above the tentorium, in children the greater number occur below the tentorium. Also, there is a tendency for the tumors in early life to arise along the central neural axis—that is, within the third or fourth ventricle, the brain stem, hypothalamus, and optic chiasm. With tumors in these regions there may be a paucity of lateralizing signs and subjective complaints. In addition, manifestations of increased intracranial pressure may be delayed because of the ability of the young skull to expand. Delay in diagnosis is a distressingly common problem with tumors in the early years.

Intracranial tumors of childhood also differ from those of later years in the incidence of specific histologic types. In childhood there is a large preponderance of gliomas, whereas three types of tumors so common in adult life, namely pituitary adenomas, meningiomas, and acoustic neurinomas, are infrequent in the early years. Certain tumors that are common to both age groups, particularly craniopharyngiomas, choroid plexus papillomas, optic pathway gliomas, and teratomas, also may show a preponderance in childhood.

In the anterior fossa and chiasm area, the principal tumors of childhood are optic glioma, hypothalamic glioma, and craniopharyngioma. Tumors of the cerebral hemispheres are not common in childhood, but gliomas and some vascular lesions are encountered. In the posterior fossa, the most frequent tumors are cerebellar astrocytomas, medulloblastomas, brain stem gliomas, and ependymomas; hemangioblastomas occur, but infrequently. Intraventricular tumors encountered in the early years are usually gliomas or teratomas; pineal area lesions are an especially important diagnostic consideration in childhood. Tumors of the cranial nerves are limited almost entirely to the neurinomas of von Recklinghausen's disease.

Craniopharyngioma (Rathke's pouch tumor, hypophyseal duct tumor, suprasellar cyst)

During embryonic development of the hypophysis, ectodermal cell rests may come to lie in the region of the hypophyseal stalk and in the anterosuperior region of the anterior lobe of the pituitary gland. A tumor which arises from these displaced squamous cells is a craniopharyngioma, and this mass lesion is the most common intracranial tumor of nonglial origin in childhood.

The craniopharyngioma grows by proliferation of its epithelial cells, by desquamation and accumulation of epithelial debris, and by reactive proliferation of connective tissue. Cyst formation is common, and the cysts usually contain a thick, oily yellow or brown mixture of cellular debris, liquefied end products of epithelial growth, and cholesterol crystals. Calcification of the tumor tissue also is common and is often sufficient to be visible radiologically.

Histologically the craniopharyngioma is a benign tumor. It produces deleterious effects by its growth, particularly by expansion of its cysts and by compression of adjacent structures. The structures most often affected are the cerebrospinal fluid pathways, the pituitary gland, the hypothalamus, and the optic chiasm.

CLINICAL FEATURES. The principal effects of craniopharyngioma are increased intracranial pressure, endocrine disturbances, hypothalamic dysfunction, and vision defects. The clinical signs and symptoms may appear at any age, and they may develop insidiously or abruptly.

Signs and symptoms of increasing intracranial pressure develop when the tumor obstructs the cerebrospinal fluid pathways, producing an internal hydrocephalus. Headache, vomiting, listlessness, and irritability commonly are the presenting symptoms. Objective signs of hydrocephalus and increasing intracranial pressure in these cases include increased head size, separation of the cranial sutures, abducent palsies and papilledema.

When the tumor extends downward into the sella, it compresses the pituitary and produces a variety of disturbances of target gland function. Dwarfing due to reduction of growth hormone is a particularly frequent effect of craniopharyngioma. There may also be hypothyroidism, manifested by weight gain, lack of energy, and delayed skeletal maturation. Signs of gonadotrophic or adrenocorticotrophic disturbances are less likely to occur, but delayed or precocious sexual development may result. In rare instances there is panhypopituitarism with cachexia.

Should the tumor extend into the hypothalamus, diabetes insipidus, autonomic seizures, chronic hypernatremia, adiposogenital dystrophy, drowsiness, and disturbances of temperature and vasomotor regulation may develop, but these manifestations are not common.

In occasional cases, the tumor may even compress a cerebral hemisphere or the brain stem, producing focal neurologic signs.

OPHTHALMIC MANIFESTATIONS. Vision loss is one of the cardinal manifestations of craniopharyngioma. The suprasellar mass usually encroaches on the optic chiasm, and it frequently compresses one or both optic nerves or optic tracts. Visual acuity of one or both eyes may be impaired, and a variety of unilateral or bilateral field defects can develop, depending upon the direction and extent of tumor growth. The field defects tend to be irregular and asymmetric. The range of possible vision defects associated with craniopharyngioma includes central scotomas, bitemporal hemianoptic defects, homonymous hemianoptic defects, concentric depression, and complete blindness. Damage to the visual pathways generally progresses gradually, often insidiously, and a child or parent may be unaware of even severe loss, especially if the defect is asymmetric or predominantly unilateral.

The damage to the anterior visual pathways is usually reflected in the discs as optic atrophy. However, in some cases the discs appear normal, and in others there may be papilledema of increased intracranial pressure rather than the pallor of progressive compression.

Pupillary signs of an afferent conduction defect are commonly present, and can provide valuable objective evidence of the visual pathway lesion when subjective responses are unreliable or when disc signs are absent.

In many cases there is diplopia as the result of unilateral or bilateral abducens paresis secondary to increased intracranial pressure or secondary to direct extension of the tumor. It is not uncommon for diplopia or crossing of the eyes to be the first indication of craniopharyngioma.

Optic Glioma

The optic glioma of childhood is a clinically indolent tumor that in many ways resembles a congenital hamartoma. It usually presents early in life, it tends to grow slowly, and in many cases it is self-limited, ceasing to progress after it has produced symptoms early in childhood.

This lesion arises in the neuroglia of the anterior visual pathway, more frequently in the intra-orbital portion of the optic nerve than in the intracranial portion of the optic nerve or chiasm. Grossly the lesion generally appears as a globular or fusiform enlargement of the optic nerve or chiasm. Histologically the tumor is usually an astrocytoma or spongioblastoma —though it often consists of a mixture of glial cell types in varying proportions—and the cellular pattern is generally benign. Intracellular and extracellular mucosubstance contributes to the mass, and there is often considerable arachnoidal hyperplasia around the tumor.

The primary deleterious effect of the tumor is disruption of visual fibers. The degree of neuronal damage is quite variable, however. In some cases, surprising numbers of normal axons may persist in the presence of extensive mass, while in other instances there is profound loss of vision in the presence of a seemingly small tumor.

By virtue of the location, extent, and growth pattern of the mass, optic glioma can produce a variety of clinical effects in addition to vision loss, including proptosis, increased intracranial pressure, and hypothalamic dysfunction, but as optic glioma is primarily an intrinsic tumor of the visual pathway, the ophthalmic manifestations are considered first.

OPHTHALMIC MANIFESTATIONS. The principal ophthalmic manifestations of optic glioma are vision loss and proptosis. Attendant ophthalmoscopic signs, pupillomotor defects and ocular motor dysfunction also occur.

Because the tumor may arise in any portion of the optic nerve, chiasm, or tract, and extend proximally, distally, or in both directions, a great variety of patterns of vision loss are possible. When the tumor is confined to an optic nerve without involvement of the chiasm, progressive unilateral loss of vision is the rule, and the defect may be any type of central or peripheral depression or contraction. When the tumor is confined to the chiasm, bitemporal hemianoptic field loss is expected, but the defect tends to be irregular and asymmetric, and in fact any type of chiasmal or parachiasmal field defect is possible. Often the defect is complex, reflecting involvement of contiguous portions of the optic nerve, chiasm, and tract.

Regardless of the predominant site of involvement, the vision loss of optic glioma tends to progress slowly, often insidiously, and the impairment may not be clinically apparent in a child until late in the course. Thus it is often an associated sign such as proptosis, amaurotic strabismus, or increased intracranial pressure that is detected first.

The ophthalmoscopic findings with optic glioma are variable, depending on the predominant location and extent of the tumor. Primary optic atrophy due to neuronal damage is the usual finding. However, there may be papilledema consequent to increased intracranial pressure, or congestion of the disc secondary to pressure of tumor in the orbit. Tumor immediately behind the globe may produce distortion or protrusion of the disc and some forward displacement of the posterior pole. Tumor may actually present in the nervehead itself. Sometimes the discs appear normal in the presence of vision loss; in such cases, objective pupillary evidence of an afferent conduction defect (the Marcus Gunn pupillary sign) is invaluable.

Proptosis develops when the glioma involves the optic nerve—particularly the intraorbital portion—either primarily or by extension from the chiasm. In most cases, the globe is displaced directly forward and there is usually resistance to retroplacement of the globe. As a rule, the proptosis is painless, and there is no pulsation or bruit, unless there is a coexistent bony defect of the orbit.

Ocular motility generally is not affected by optic glioma. However, strabismus or nystagmus may develop secondary to progressive loss of vision, and limitation of eye movement may develop in cases of extreme proptosis, extensive orbital mass, or increasing intracranial pressure.

OTHER CLINICAL FEATURES. Optic glioma within the cranium can, by progressive growth and extension, produce obstructive hydrocephalus and increased intracranial pressure, hypothalamic dysfunction, and even pituitary dysfunction.

Increased intracranial pressure is not a frequent complication of intracranial optic glioma, but in some cases signs and symptoms of increased intracranial pressure are the presenting or predominant manifestations of optic glioma in a young child. The more common signs include irritability, nausea, vomiting, increasing head size, separation of the cranial sutures, abducens paresis, and papilledema.

With extension of chiasmal tumor into the hypothalamus, there may be signs of diabetes insipidus, diencephalic seizures, alteration of sexual development, or failure to thrive.

Pituitary dysfunction caused by optic glioma is uncommon, but it may manifest as growth failure, hypothyroidism, or gonadotrophic or adrenocorticotrophic disturbances.

To be mentioned along with the clinical signs of optic glioma are the important radiographic signs of this tumor. Chiasmal glioma commonly produces a boat-, pear-, or J-shaped deformity of the sella, with erosion of the tuberculum sella and anterior clinoids, while optic nerve glioma frequently produces enlargement of the optic canal or its foramina. Although enlargement, asymmetry, or irregularity of the optic canal may be evident on conventional x-rays of the foramina, axial tomograms of the optic canal are a preferred way of determining extension of the tumor into or through the canal.

A special clinical feature of optic glioma—both optic nerve and chiasmal glioma—is its frequent association with Recklinghausen's neurofibromatosis. Many patients with optic glioma have café au lait spots, cutaneous neurofibromas, skeletal deformities, or other stigmata of Recklinghausen's disease, and, conversely, patients with neurofibromatosis frequently develop optic nerve or chiasmal glioma.

Because the natural clinical course of optic glioma is usually one of indolent, often self-limited progression, conservative treatment or no treatment may be the best management. Radiation may or may not alter the growth of the tumor; it is advocated by some clinicians. Surgery rarely, if ever, changes the course of the tumor. Surgical intervention may be necessary to control hydrocephalus and increased intracranial pressure, but the results may be disappointing. Resection of the optic nerve to control progressive and unsightly proptosis of a blind eye is usually done, and the globe can be left in place with little risk of regrowth of tumor from the severed nerve. In general, with glioma of the optic nerve, except for loss of vision, the prognosis is good. The prognosis with intracranial glioma may be less favorable because of complicating hydrocephalus, increased intracranial pressure, and the deleterious effects on the hypothalamus and endocrine functions.

Meningiomas of the Optic Nerve and Orbit

Although meningiomas may develop at various sites throughout the nervous system, consideration is given here only to those that originate in the optic nerve sheaths or arise primarily within the orbit or optic canal. Such tumors are infrequent in childhood, but they present special problems.

The meningioma, arising principally from the arachnoid and attached to the inner side of the dura, generally is a histologically benign tumor, but in some instances the lesion is relentlessly progressive and invasive. When incompletely removed, the tumor tends to recur and extend, and it often fails to respond to irradiation.

Meningioma that develops within the orbit in the early years has a rather poor prognosis. Total loss of vision in the affected eye can rarely be avoided, and there may be recurring problems with infiltrating tumor. Furthermore, the meningioma quite often is a forerunner of central neurofibromatosis.

OPHTHALMIC MANIFESTATIONS. The tumor within the orbit characteristically produces proptosis. As a rule there is no pulsation or pain. There may be varying degrees of limitation of ocular movement.

Vision loss may occur, but even when the nerve is ensheathed with tumor, the visual acuity and field may be deceptively good.

Optic atrophy commonly results, but there may be disc edema.

In addition, there may be x-ray evidence of enlargement of the optic canal, thickening of the orbital wall, or calcifications.

Cerebral Hemisphere Gliomas

Gliomas of the cerebral hemispheres are relatively infrequent tumors in childhood. Usually they are benign astrocytomas, but malignant varieties do occur.

The benign Grade 1 or 2 astrocytoma tends to be a well-demarcated, relatively avascular lesion that is solid or partially cystic. The more malignant Grade 3 to 4 astrocytoma or glioblastoma multiforme generally is a rapidly growing, infiltrative tumor that may show considerable degeneration with hemorrhage and cyst formation.

CLINICAL FEATURES. Important localizing signs of cerebral gliomas are motor and sensory deficits, visual field defects, and impairment of intellectual functions. Hemiparesis, hemianesthesia, seizure phenomenon, and behavior changes are often readily apparent, but evidence of visual field loss, memory impairment, astereognosis, aphasia, and deterioration of judgment and initiative may not be so obvious in a child, particularly in a very young child. In some cases, the effects of increasing intracranial pressure may overshadow the focal signs and symptoms.

OPHTHALMIC MANIFESTATIONS. The most significant ophthalmic effects of cerebral hemisphere gliomas are visual field changes. The loss characteristically is a homonymous hemianoptic defect, the features of which will vary with the site and extent of the lesion. With temporal lobe lesions the defect typically is an upper quadrantanopia. With parietal lesions, the defect commonly is a lower quadrantanopia, or a "visual inattention" or "visual extinction" phenomenon in the homonymous half-fields. Whereas incongruity is frequent with anterior optic radiation involvement, congruity is usual with posterior optic radiation involvement. With an occipital pole glioma there may possibly be a double homonymous hemianopia, resulting in blindness.

Lesions producing deep parieto-occipital involvement may also produce impairment of optokinetic nystagmus.

In addition to the localizing ophthalmic signs, there may well be papilledema, abducent paralysis, and pupillomotor dysfunction consequent to increased intracranial pressure.

Brain Stem Gliomas

Brain stem gliomas are infiltrative tumors that arise from the neuroglial elements in the portion of the brain between the hypothalamus and the upper level of the cervical spinal cord. These tumors are particularly common in the pons and medulla.

Histologically the tumors are usually astrocytomas or mixed gliomas; some contain polar spongioblasts, and some show features of glioblastoma multiforme. Regardless of their histology, in effect they are all malignant and fatal by virtue of their crucial location and relentless progression. They are inoperable, and radiation provides only temporary prolongation of the course.

CLINICAL FEATURES. As the gliomas spread through the brain stem, irregularly infiltrating the cranial nerve nuclei and the ascending and descending pathways connecting the cerebrum and the thalamus with the spinal cord and cerebellum, they typically produce multiple cranial nerve palsies, pyramidal tract dysfunction, and ataxia.

The cranial nerve palsies are usually bilateral, but the involvement is often asymmetric or spotty. Cranial nerves V to IX are most commonly involved. The sixth nerve particularly is frequently affected, producing abduction paresis or paralysis, and crossing of the eyes. The seventh nerve is also frequently involved, producing a peripheral (nuclear type) facial palsy. Other frequent manifestations are reduced corneal sensation, impaired hearing, poor articulation, defective swallowing, palatal and vocal cord paresis, pharyngeal hypesthesia, and protracted vomiting.

Truncal ataxia with an unsteady wide-based gait is a common early sign because of involvement of the cerebellodentate-rubrothalamic tracts. The corticospinal tracts also are generally involved early, producing hyperactive deep tendon reflexes, ankle clonus, and extensor plantar response. Weakness of the spastic type and paralysis of the extremities develop, progressing finally to spastic quadriplegia.

Progression of the tumor to higher levels can produce pathological somnolence, and affected children usually die within a few months of the onset of clinical symptoms.

Obstruction to cerebrospinal fluid flow usually does not develop, but it may occur as a late manifestation. The combination of multiple cranial nerve palsies, pyramidal tract signs, and truncal ataxia in the absence of signs of increased intracranial pressure is almost pathognomonic of infiltrating brain stem glioma.

OPHTHALMOLOGIC FEATURES. The neuro-ophthalmic signs of brain stem glioma are essentially confined to the cranial nerve palsies affecting ocular motility, lid function, and corneal sensation. The development of diplopia, heterotropia or heterophoria, ptosis, faulty lid closure, or corneal hypesthesia in a child must alert one to the possibility of brain stem glioma. These signs may be deceptively insidious in their development.

Internuclear ophthalmoplegia and nystagmus also develop in some cases, but ophthalmoscopic signs of increased intracranial pressure are uncommon.

Cerebellar Astrocytoma

The cerebellar astrocytoma is the most frequent tumor of the posterior fossa in childhood. In most cases it is a benign tumor, though malignant varieties do occur.

The typical benign or Grade 1 cerebellar astrocytoma is a well-demarcated, relatively avascular lesion that arises in the midline and grows into the lateral cerebellar hemisphere. It is usually a well-differentiated glioma with a uniform cellular pattern. The tumor may be solid, but there is a great tendency to cyst formation, with the cysts ranging in size from microcysts to rather large cysts filled with proteinaceous fluid. There is also tendency to calcification.

As a rule, the benign cerebellar astrocytoma is noninvasive and can be removed without difficulty, but in some cases the tumor extends into the brain stem, the fourth ventricle, the cervical cord, or even into the supratentorial region.

CLINICAL FEATURES. Astrocytoma of the cerebellum characteristically produces increased intracranial pressure and cerebellar dysfunction. Unfortunately, however, the signs are often recognized late in the course of the lesion, since the progress of the tumor is often insidious, the signs of cerebellar dysfunction or brain stem compression are often subtle, and periodic remissions of symptoms early in the course are common.

The first indications of the tumor usually are intermittent headache and vomiting. The headaches tend to be aggravated by stooping and straining. The vomiting commonly occurs on arising. With time, gait disturbance, truncal ataxia, clumsiness, dysmetria, weakness, and hypotonia develop. Eventually there may be enlargement of the head, separation of the cranial sutures, papilledema, and sixth nerve palsies. Unchecked, the course is one of progressive deterioration.

OPHTHALMIC MANIFESTATIONS. The usual ophthalmic signs of cerebellar astrocytoma are papilledema and sixth nerve paresis secondary to the increased intracranial pressure. In symptomatic patients, bilateral papilledema is an almost constant sign. Commonly, however, sixth nerve paresis develops before the papilledema, and double vision with or without overt crossing of the eyes is often the presenting complaint that leads to the diagnosis of the posterior fossa tumor.

Localizing ophthalmic signs of cerebellar and brain stem dysfunction also occur with cerebellar astrocytoma. Nystagmus, particularly gaze-evoked nystagmus, is one of the more frequent ocular motor disturbances seen with cerebellar tumor. Other frequent signs are cogwheel eye movements and ocular dysmetria. Cogwheel eye movements are jerky, saccadic pursuit movements; ocular dysmetria is an inaccuracy of refixation characterized by overshoot and dampening oscillations on refixation. Skew deviation, a vertical dissociation of the eyes, also occurs in some cases.

Although the visual pathways are not directly affected by cerebellar tumor, disturbances of vision are not uncommon with cerebellar astrocytoma. As already noted, diplopia is often an early symptom. With increasing intracranial pressure, obscurations—transient episodes of blurring of vision—also may occur. Secondary to papilledema, there may be varying degrees of enlargement of the blind spot and concentric depression of the visual fields. With longstanding papilledema, there may be irreversible damage to the optic nerve fibers and loss of vision due to compression of the visual fibers in the scleral canal.

In addition to these effects of papilledema on visual function, there may be field defects secondary to dilatation of the third ventricle; compression of the chiasm by the third ventricle can produce bitemporal depression, and compression of the optic nerves against the carotid arteries can produce binasal field defects.

Medulloblastoma

Medulloblastoma is a highly malignant tumor of the posterior fossa. It occurs most frequently in the first decade of life, predominantly in males, and it is the second most common tumor of the posterior fossa in childhood.

Arising most probably from embryonal cell rests of primitive epithelium in the region of the roof of the fourth ventricle, the medulloblastoma usually occupies a midline position within the substance of the cerebellum; less often the tumor is located in the cerebellar hemisphere. As a rule, the tumor grows rapidly and is highly invasive. It commonly extends into the fourth ventricle, the aqueduct, the lateral recesses, and the cerebellopontine angle. It also tends to disseminate and metastasize along the meninges; even extracranial metastases may occur.

On the basis of histologic features, two major types of medulloblastoma are described. The so-called "classic" medulloblastoma is densely cellular, with small round to pear-shaped cells arranged in irregular sheets or rosettes. The nuclei are hyperchromatic, the cytoplasm is scant, and the cellular borders are poorly defined. Mitoses may be abundant. There may be spongioblastic and astrocytic differentiation, and oligodendroglia may be found in the tumor. In the second or "desmoplastic" type of medulloblastoma, the cells are arranged in islands demarcated by reticulin-rich fibrous tissue networks. The course of the desmoplastic type may be less fulminant than that of the classic type, but in general the prognosis is poor, especially in children.

CLINICAL MANIFESTATIONS. The predominant clinical effect of medulloblastoma is increased intracranial pressure. Headache, vomiting, enlargement of the head, and visual complaints are common. Often fulminant, the signs and symptoms of increased intracranial pressure may overshadow localizing manifestations related to the location of the tumor, but increasing weakness, unsteadiness of gait, truncal ataxia, and spasticity often develop. There may be tonic seizures. In some cases there is suboccipital pain or tenderness, and torticollis. There may be cranial nerve palsies, paraplegia, or signs of meningitis due to dissemination of the tumor.

OPHTHALMIC MANIFESTATIONS. With increasing intracranial pressure, sixth nerve palsies are common, and children with medulloblastoma may first present to the ophthalmologist with diplopia or sudden onset esotropia. The majority of children with medulloblastoma develop papilledema, and there may be obscurations or loss of vision secondary to compression of the optic nerve fibers. There may also be pupillomotor signs of increased intracranial pressure. Nystagmus and ocular motor signs of brain stem compression are common.

Pinealoma (and other tumors of the pineal region)

Several types of tumor may arise in the region of the pineal body or within the gland itself. The significance of these tumors lies not in their histology but in their crucial location.

It is helpful to recall that the pineal body is situated under the splenium of the corpus callosum, just over the superior colliculi. Fixed to the habenular and caudal commissure by peduncles of glial tissue, it encloses the pineal recess of the third ventricle, and on its ventricular side it is lined by ependymal cells. The body itself is derived embryologically from epithelioid cells and it resembles a gland, but its physiologic functions and purpose are not clear.

The true pinealoma is a tumor of the parenchyma of the gland. Histologically it is characterized by an intermingling of two types of cells in a recurring pattern; large cells with abundant cytoplasm and prominent nucleoli tend to be arranged in sheets and clumps, while small darkly staining cells form scattered aggregates in a vascular stroma. The true pinealoma is a rare lesion, occurring most commonly in adolescent males. As a rule it is a slow growing tumor, but malignant forms may occur.

Nonparenchymatous tumors of the pineal also occur; these are usually teratomas, dermoids or epidermoid cysts. Such tumors may show calcifications.

Other tumors encountered in the pineal region include gliomas, ependymomas, papillomas and ganglioneuromas.

Regardless of histologic type, the clinical effects of these lesions are similar, and they may be considered together.

CLINICAL FEATURES. By virtue of their proximity to the cerebrospinal fluid pathways, pineal tumors characteristically produce increased intracranial pressure. Obstruction of the aqueduct and posterior third ventricle occurs early. Headache, nausea, and vomiting are generally the presenting symptoms. Papilledema is usually present and there may be sixth nerve paralysis.

Weakness, spasticity, and hyperactive deep tendon reflexes may develop, and with involvement of the superior cerebellar peduncle, there may be ataxia.

Signs of depressed gonadal function may develop with parenchymatous tumors of the pineal, while nonparenchymatous lesions, such as gliomas and teratomas that destroy the pineal body, are associated with precocious puberty.

In some cases, there is pathological sleepiness.

Another possible effect of the tumor is deafness secondary to involvement of the inferior colliculi.

Cardinal manifestations of pineal tumor, however, are the neuro-ophthalmic signs of midbrain involvement.

OPHTHALMIC MANIFESTATIONS. Consequent to involvement of the midbrain tegmentum and periaqueductal gray matter, the principal ophthalmic signs of pineal tumor are paralysis of vertical gaze and light-near dissociation of the pupils. The paralysis of vertical gaze involves upward gaze, or both upward and downward gaze, more often than just downward gaze. The pupils tend to be large and poorly reactive to light, with preservation of the near response, but in some instances there may be selective involvement of the near response, complete pupillary rigidity, and even corectopia. Other midbrain signs of pineal tumor are accommodative disturbances, lid retraction, ptosis, nuclear oculomotor paresis, convergence palsy or convergence spasm, and vertical nystagmus or convergence retraction nystagmus. In various combinations, these signs constitute Parinaud's syndrome or the syndrome of the sylvian aqueduct.

Consequent to increased intracranial pressure, papilledema and sixth nerve palsies occur.

The visual pathways are not directly affected by pineal tumor, but there may be field defects secondary to longstanding papilledema or secondary to compression of the chiasm by the dilated third ventricle.

Choroid Plexus Papilloma

Papilloma of the choroid plexus is a relatively rare tumor that occurs almost exclusively in childhood. Arising most commonly in a lateral ventricle, the choroid plexus papilloma is a rather vascular tumor and its histology is that of the choroid plexus. In most instances this tumor is benign, but malignant change may occur.

CLINICAL FEATURES. As a rule, papilloma of the choroid plexus is associated with communicating hydrocephalus, presumably as the result of overproduction of cerebrospinal fluid. Less often the lesion produces obstructive hydrocephalus. In either case, the principal clinical effect is increased intracranial pressure. Focal signs typically are absent, and the absence of focal signs in the presence of increased cerebrospinal fluid protein, xanthochromia, and increased pressure is highly suggestive of intraventricular tumor. Hyperirritability and hyperactivity of the deep tendon reflexes are common. Occasionally seizures develop.

OPHTHALMIC MANIFESTATIONS. With choroid plexus papilloma there is often papilledema. Localizing ophthalmic signs are not a feature of intraventricular tumor.

Ependymoma

Ependymoma is a glial tumor that apparently arises from the fine membrane lining the ventricles of the brain. In childhood this tumor most commonly occurs in the fourth ventricle, producing signs of obstruction of cerebrospinal fluid flow and compression of the brain stem or cerebellar pathway.

Histologically, the ependymoma is a very cellular tumor, sometimes containing cysts and calcium deposits. All variations occur, ranging from mature well-differentiated tumor to wildly anaplastic, highly malignant, and invasive ependymoma.

CLINICAL FEATURES. The clinical signs of ependymoma, particularly of fourth ventricle ependymoma, are predominantly those of increased intracranial pressure. In some cases there is stiffness and spasm of the neck and shoulder muscles, limitation of neck motion, and suboccipital or upper cervical tenderness resulting from extension of the tumor into the upper cervical region.

OPHTHALMIC EFFECTS. As increased intracranial pressure is the predominant effect of ependymoma, papilledema and sixth nerve paresis are the usual ophthalmic signs of this tumor.

HAMARTOMATOSES (PHAKOMATOSES)

By definition, a hamartoma is a tumor mass arising as an anomaly of tissue formation; it is composed of tissue elements normally present in the involved organ or site. Several well-defined clinical syndromes having predominantly neurologic, ocular, and cutaneous manifestations are distinguished by the presence of such lesions, and these conditions collectively are referred to as the hamartomatoses. The major hamartomatoses are the syndromes of Bourneville (tuberous sclerosis), von Recklinghausen (neurofibromatosis), von Hippel-Lindau (angiomatosis of the retina and cerebellum) and Sturge-Weber (encephalofacial angiomatosis). These same disorders traditionally are referred to as the phakomatoses—this term being derived from a Greek word for birthmark or mother spot—because herald lesions of the eye and skin are common to the group.

The classification may be expanded to include the Wyburn-Mason syndrome (p. 543) and other disorders having certain features in common with the four principal hamartomatoses.

Bourneville's Disease (Tuberous Sclerosis)

Pale firm nodular hamartomas of the brain referred to as tubers are the essential lesions of Bourneville's tuberous sclerosis. Epilepsy, mental deficiency, and abnormal behavior are the principal clinical manifestations of the disorder, and distinctive ocular and cutaneous lesions provide important clues to the diagnosis.

Tuberous sclerosis occurs in about 1 per 30,000 of the general population. The disorder may be inherited as an autosomal dominant condition.

NERVOUS SYSTEM LESIONS AND MANIFESTATIONS. The predominant neurologic signs and symptoms are related to the cortical and subependymal tubers. These hamartomas consist of proliferations of glial elements, with disturbance of the normal gray matter architecture. They develop principally in the cerebral hemispheres, often extending through several adjacent convolutions. They also occur in the cerebellum, midbrain, and spinal cord. Some lesions tend to project into the ventricle and may grow to significant size. The lesions frequently undergo cystic degeneration and secondary calcification. Focal neurologic signs and increased intracranial pressure do occur, but the more common manifestations are epilepsy, mental deficiency, and behavior disturbances of varying severity. These signs become apparent in the first two or three years of life. Generalized developmental delay, especially of speech, is common. The children often exhibit stereotyped movements, motor restlessness, and emotional lability; they are prone to outbursts of violence and may be quite difficult to manage. The EEG is often abnormal; hypsarhythmia is common in infants.

Progressive mental and physical deterioration occur in most cases, but the symptomatology and severity of the disorder are quite variable.

CUTANEOUS SIGNS. The distinctive cutaneous signs of tuberous sclerosis are adenoma sebaceum, shagreen patches, and white maculae called mountain ash leaf spots. The adenoma sebaceum is a reddish or yellowish nodular or papular "rash" which usually occurs on the face, primarily in the butterfly distribution over the cheeks and nasolabial fold area. The papules and discrete nodules are composed of hyperplastic connective tissue, sometimes with telangiectatic elements. The shagreen patches are areas in which the skin has a peculiar tan, irregular, and slightly raised leathery or wrinkled appearance; these abnormal plaques occur over the trunk, extremities, and face. The mountain ash leaf spots are due to abnormalities of the melanotic system, and these pale areas are best seen with the Wood's lamp.

Other cutaneous lesions associated with Bourneville's disease are café au lait spots, nevi, and fibromas. Periungual angiofibromas are said to be peculiar to tuberous sclerosis.

OPHTHALMIC MANIFESTATIONS. The primary ocular manifestations of tuberous sclerosis are glial hamartomas of the retina and disc. These lesions are traditionally described as refractile yellowish multinodular or cystic masses resembling unripe mulberries or clumps of tapioca. Frequently, however, the lesions are smooth and flat, or only minimally elevated, and show considerable variability in size. Some are punctate; others approach the size of the disc. The lesions may be single or multiple, and they may occur in any region of the fundus. Histologically the lesions are composed of proliferations of astrocytes or pleomorphic cells, often with areas of cyst formation, calcification or hyalinization. The masses are relatively avascular, though retinal vessels may traverse their surface or course through their depths. These ocular phakomata generally require no treatment, but their presence is of diagnostic importance in the evaluation of patients with seizures, retardation, and behavior disorders.

In some cases there may be papilledema or optic atrophy as signs of the intracranial lesions, especially if hydrocephalus has developed.

The vision, field, pupillomotor, and other ophthalmic signs vary with the site and extent of the neural and ocular lesions, but often the patients are too retarded or uncooperative for precise testing.

OTHER MANIFESTATIONS. In addition to the typical neurologic, ocular, and cutaneous manifestations of tuberous sclerosis, a variety of congenital malformations and hamartomas of other organ systems occur in this disorder. Embryonal tumors and hamartomas of the kidney, polycystic disease of the kidney, rhabdomyomas of the heart, and cystic lesions of the lung and bone are often found in these patients, contributing to the morbidity and mortality of the disorder. Many patients die from the heart and kidney lesions.

Von Recklinghausen's Disease (Neurofibromatosis)

Von Recklinghausen's disease is a complex hereditary disorder characterized primarily by a variety of hamartomas throughout the nervous system, pigmented lesions of the skin, and developmental malformations of the skeleton. Abnormalities of the eye, optic nerve, orbit, and adnexa are important features of the condition. Signs may be apparent at birth, but they frequently develop later in life and progress with age, especially during puberty and pregnancy.

Von Recklinghausen's disease is usually transmitted as a simple autosomal dominant; it occurs in approximately 1 per 3000 live births. Familial evidences of the disorder show great variability and are sometimes subtle.

NERVOUS SYSTEM LESIONS AND MANIFESTATIONS. The characteristic hamartoma of von Recklinghausen's disease is the neurofibroma, a whorl-like proliferation of Schwann cells producing focal or diffuse thickening and tortuosity of affected nerves. Neurofibromas can develop within any organ or tissue; they develop in cranial nerves, the spinal cord, spinal roots, and in the peripheral and autonomic nerves throughout the body. These tumors generally are histologically benign, but they produce disturbances of function, and even death, because of their location and growth pattern. They are often relentlessly progressive, they tend to recur after surgical excision, and they can show a tendency to sarcomatous degeneration in both

adults and children. Specific clinical neurologic and visceral signs vary with the site and extent of the lesions. Seizures, mental deficiency, and abnormal behavior are common; many patients have abnormalities of cranial nerve function.

Other hamartomas and tumors also occur in von Recklinghausen's disease. Gliomas and meningiomas are frequent, and are of special importance with regard to the optic nerve and orbit. Neurolemmomas, psammomas, fibromas, lipomas, sarcomas, and hemangiomas also occur, and pheochromocytomas, paragangliomas, and disturbances of pituitary and adrenal function have been associated with this condition.

CUTANEOUS SIGNS. Important external signs of von Recklinghausen's disease are café au lait spots — flat, coffee-colored areas of increased pigmentation of the skin, of varying size and shape. They occur on any part of the body, frequently in unexposed areas. Café au lait spots do occur in normal persons and in individuals with tuberous sclerosis, but six or more spots of at least 15 millimeters are considered to be indicative of neurofibromatosis. Also typical of this syndrome are multiple discrete cutaneous nodules, as neurofibromas, fibromas, and even angiomas commonly develop in the skin and subcutaneous tissues. Subcutaneous plexiform masses and elephantiasis are frequent, and the skin overlying the masses is often heavily pigmented and brawny.

SKELETAL MANIFESTATIONS. The skeletal abnormalities are usually due to disturbances of development and growth of bone. Congenital absence of bones, especially in the skull and orbit, are common. Overgrowth of bone also occurs; often a limb, an orbit, or one side of the face is larger than its fellow. Vertebral abnormalities, scoliosis, and bowing of long bones are common. In some instances skeletal abnormalities develop secondary to tumors. Interosseous tumors and periosteal neurofibromas occur, and there may be erosions of bone by contiguous tumors. Pathologic fractures, pseudoarthroses and cystic lesions of bone may develop. Sella deformities also occur, often as the result of intracranial hamartomas or secondary hydrocephalus.

OPHTHALMIC MANIFESTATIONS. The

ophthalmic manifestations of von Recklinghausen's disease are numerous and quite variable. Plexiform neuromas commonly develop in the eyelid and periorbital tissues, producing ptosis and deformity of the lid and face. Neurofibromas also develop in the soft tissues within the orbit, and here can produce exophthalmos and deformity of the orbit. Neurofibromas infrequently develop in the conjunctiva, where they appear as smooth fleshy masses. In the cornea, focal or diffuse enlargement of the nerves occurs, and these changes may be detected by slit lamp examination in some cases. Similar enlargement of ciliary nerves may be detected histologically in the globe. In the uveal tract, hypercellularity and hyperpigmentation are characteristic histologic findings, and clinical manifestations of these alterations can be seen in the iris. Iris nodules, focal or diffuse hyperpigmentation of iris stroma, ectropion uveae, and eccentricity of the pupil are associated with neurofibromatosis. On slit lamp examination the iris nodules appear as ball-like excrescences or small plaques in the iris surface and crypts; they may be hyperpigmented or hypopigmented in relation to the iris color. Retinal and optic disc hamartomas, clinically and histologically similar to those of tuberous sclerosis, do occur, but these lesions are infrequent manifestations of von Recklinghausen's disease. Medullated nerve fibers are said to occur with increased frequency in neurofibromatosis.

Intraorbital and intracranial optic gliomas and meningiomas are commonly associated with the disorder. Both tumors can produce exophthalmos, loss of vision and field, optic atrophy, and papilledema, as well as more serious consequences.

Orbital abnormalities are commonly present. There may be alteration of the optic canals and distortion and erosion of the bones due to tumor. There may be congenital absence of orbit bones, sometimes resulting in pulsation of the globe and exophthalmos due to protrusion of brain through the orbital defect.

An additional clinical manifestation is glaucoma. In some cases the glaucoma is explained by developmental anomalies of the chamber angle or by synechiae and neovascularization of the angle, and the congenital type is often seen in association with plexiform neuroma of the lid. In other cases, the mechanism of the glaucoma is not understood, though it may be related to neurofibromatous hypercellularity of the uvea.

Von Hippel-Lindau Disease (Angiomatosis of the Retina and Cerebellum)

Hemangioblastomas of the cerebellum and of the retina are the primary lesions of von Hippel-Lindau disease. These tumors are often accompanied by cysts, angiomas, and tumors of viscera, but skin lesions are not a distinctive feature of this syndrome.

The disorder is inherited as an autosomal dominant trait with incomplete penetrance. Phenotypic expressions of the disorder are variable and often delayed; the retinal hemangioblastomas, unlike congenital angiomas of other syndromes, do not usually appear until the second or third decade, and several years may lapse before signs of the central nervous system lesions develop.

NERVOUS SYSTEM LESIONS AND MANIFESTATIONS. The characteristic nervous system lesions—the cerebellar hemangioblastomas—typically are cystic, and the actual vascular tumor mass is often incorporated in the wall of the cyst as a small mural nodule. Large afferent and efferent vessels are present. The cerebellar lesions may be single or multiple.

The clinical manifestations are due primarily to expansion of the cystic component of the lesion. Classic signs of cerebellar dysfunction, such as ataxia, clumsiness, and nystagmus, are frequent, but commonly the signs of Lindau's disease are those of increased intracranial pressure or hydrocephalus with headache, nausea, vomiting, and papilledema. Fortunately the cerebellar lesions are generally amenable to surgical treatment.

Although the neurologic manifestations of Lindau's disease are almost exclusively cerebellar, hemangiomas may also occur in the medulla, pons, cerebellum, and cord, and syringomyelia is often associated with the medulla lesions.

OPHTHALMIC MANIFESTATIONS. The distinctive retinal lesions of von Hippel-Lindau disease are true hemangioblastomas or hemangioendotheliomas — tumors composed of plexuses of thin-walled capillaries and solid masses of endothelial cells, often with cystic degeneration. Large, dilated, thickened arteries and veins pass to and from the lesions as paired vessels. The actual tumor mass is usually a reddish globular lesion, but some tend to be yellow or gray as a result of exudation and gliosis. As viewed through the ophthalmoscope, these lesions give the appearance of toy balloons in the fundus. The tumors show considerable variation in size; some are minute, while others are larger than the disc. They can develop in any region of the fundus, but they commonly lie temporally, anterior to the equator. They may be single or multiple, unilateral or bilateral. The classic fully developed lesion is preceded by rete mirabile and dilatation of paired arteries and veins. Isolated peripheral retinal angiomas also occur.

Ocular symptoms vary with the site and progression of the lesions, and angiomatosis retinae is a progressive disease. Hemorrhage, retinal detachment, edema, exudation, and gliosis can destroy the eye. Fortunately the results of current therapy are encouraging, and early diagnosis is aided by fluorescein angiography.

OTHER MANIFESTATIONS. Visceral manifestations occur in von Hippel-Lindau disease; these include angiomas of the kidney, pancreas, liver, and spleen. Cysts also commonly occur in these organs, as well as in bone, omentum, ovary, and epididymis. More serious lesions such as hypernephromas, pheochromocytomas, and cystadenomas of abdominal organs occur, and it is important to be aware of the possibility of life-threatening tumors in patients with von Hippel-Lindau syndrome, and in other members of their family.

Sturge-Weber Syndrome
(Encephalofacial Angiomatosis)

The characteristic lesions of the Sturge-Weber syndrome are vascular malformations of the meninges, brain, skin, and eye. A vascular nevus of the face, commonly referred to as a "port-wine stain" or facial nevus flammeus, and leptomeningeal angiomas are essential to the diagnosis. Seizures, mental deficiency, intracerebral calcifications, and glaucoma are principal manifestations of the disorder.

The etiology is not known, but a common primordial derivation of the meningeal, choroidal, and facial vessels may explain the characteristic distribution of these congenital lesions. The condition is rare, and the complete triad of eye, skin, and intracranial lesions apparently has not been reported in more than one member of a family. Genetic transmission of the disorder is not established.

NERVOUS SYSTEM LESIONS AND MANIFESTATIONS. The intracranial vascular anomalies of this syndrome consist of networks of dilated capillaries and venous channels in the leptomeninges. They most commonly occupy the occipitoparietal region, but they may also cover an entire hemisphere and sometimes extend even to the opposite hemisphere or into the brain substance as well. The cerebral cortex underlying the angiomas usually shows atrophy, gliosis, and calcification, and the involved hemisphere is sometimes poorly developed.

Clinical manifestations of the intracranial abnormalities commence early in life and progress as the lesions grow. Intracerebral calcifications usually become radiologically visible after infancy. Seizures, often of the jacksonian type, and mental deficiency of varying severity are present in most cases. Hemiparesis or hemiplegia may develop. Hemorrhage or thrombosis may produce signs abruptly.

CUTANEOUS SIGNS. Nevus flammeus is the distinguishing cutaneous lesion of the syndrome and is present at birth. It consists of dilated vascular channels that manifest clinically as irregular, sometimes elevated, reddish purple lesions of the skin. The upper face, eyelids, and scalp are most commonly affected, and the cutaneous angiomas are usually ipsilateral to the meningeal lesions. Often the facial nevus flammeus follows the distribution of the trigeminal nerve, particularly the ophthalmic division. The nevus rarely crosses the midline, and rarely is it bilateral. The neurologic and ocular complications occur most often in association with vascular nevi of the upper portions of the face.

OPHTHALMIC MANIFESTATIONS. The principal ocular lesions of the Sturge-Weber syndrome are angiomas of the uvea. The choroidal angiomas, or hemangiomas, are generally diffuse and flat; they may impart a dark appearance to the fundus, but the uveal lesions are best demonstrated by fluorescein angiography. Abnormalities such as dilatation and tortuosity of vessels may also be seen in the retina, conjunctiva, and sclera.

The truly serious ocular manifestation of Sturge-Weber disease, however, is glaucoma. Congenital buphthalmos occurs in some cases, whereas signs of glaucoma develop later in other cases. The pathogenesis of the glaucoma is not known; congestion and obstruction due to the uveal vessel abnormalities, as well as hypersecretion of aqueous and developmental anomalies of the angle, have been implicated. Treatment of the glaucoma is often unsatisfactory. Glaucoma, choroidal angioma, and ipsilateral facial nevi involving the lids and conjunctiva often coexist, but each may occur independently.

Hemianopias related to the intracranial lesions may also occur.

NEUROCUTANEOUS SYNDROMES

The neurocutaneous syndromes are a heterogeneous group of disorders having both neurologic and cutaneous manifestations. Frequently there are associated ocular abnormalities.

Within this classification can be included the syndromes referred to as phakomatoses; it is preferable, however, to describe the four classic phakomatoses separately as hamartomatoses.

The neurocutaneous syndromes described here are the Sjögren-Larsson syndrome, the Bloch-Sulzberger syndrome, the syndrome of linear nevus sebaceous of Jadassohn, and the syndrome of xerodermic idiocy of de Sanctis and Cacchione.

Sjögren-Larsson Syndrome

The Sjögren-Larsson syndrome is a clinical triad of congenital ichthyosiform dermatitis, mental deficiency, and spastic paresis of the extremities. Chorioretinal lesions occur in some cases.

The etiology of the disorder is obscure, but it is hereditary and follows an autosomal recessive pattern. Metabolic studies have demonstrated no consistent abnormality.

NEUROLOGIC MANIFESTATIONS. Mental deficiency and spasticity, present from birth, are the principal neurologic signs of this syndrome. The mental deficiency is characteristically mild and stationary, but severe retardation has been reported. The pyramidal spasticity typically is symmetrical and involves the lower extremities more than the upper extremities; the paresis can be incapacitating. Convulsions and speech disorders also occur in some cases.

Pathologically, loss of neurons and gliosis of the central gray matter have been observed, and cortical atrophy has been demonstrated by pneumoencephalography.

CUTANEOUS SIGNS. Children with the Sjögren-Larsson syndrome have abnormal skin from birth. The abnormalities include thickening, scaling, and hyperkeratosis typical of lamellar ichthyosis or ichthyosiform erythroderma. There is usually scaling of the neck, trunk, and extremities. The axilla and other flexural areas are commonly affected, and there is usually desquamation of the palms and soles. The scalp hair, eyebrows, and eyelashes are usually normal, as are the nails.

OTHER MANIFESTATIONS. Additional neuroectodermal findings sometimes associated with the syndrome include defective sweating and sensory defects of the tongue and anterior oral cavity. There may also be abnormal dermatoglyphics and dental and osseous dysplasia.

OPHTHALMIC MANIFESTATIONS. Fundus abnormalities, specifically chorioretinal lesions, occur in about one fourth of described patients.

The chorioretinal lesions of the Sjögren-Larsson syndrome appear to be discrete defects in the retinal pigment epithelium. Sharply circumscribed symmetrical depigmented lesions of varying size have been described in and about the macula. The pathogenesis of the fundus lesions is not known, and their effect on visual functions has not been fully established.

Bloch-Sulzberger Syndrome (Incontinentia Pigmenti)

The principal hallmark of incontinentia pigmenti, or the Bloch-Sulzberger syndrome, is an unusual dermatosis characterized by a variety of erythematous, vesicular, and verrucous lesions and bizarre pigmentations of the skin. Although the term incontinentia pigmenti focuses attention on the cutaneous abnormalities, the dermatosis is just one facet of a rather complex syndrome of multiple ectodermal and mesodermal defects. Dental and skeletal anomalies are common to the syndrome, and the patients frequently have significant ocular and neurologic abnormalities.

This condition is seen almost exclusively in females. It is usually suggested that the disorder is inherited as an X-linked dominant trait, lethal in the male, with variable expressivity in the carrier females. There is a familial component to the disorder; however, the syndrome has only infrequently been reported in siblings, and affected female relatives, including mothers of index cases, often exhibit only minor manifestations of the condition. The etiology is unknown. Fortunately the condition is comparatively rare.

CUTANEOUS MANIFESTATIONS. Four principal types of skin lesions occur in the Bloch-Sulzberger syndrome, and the lesions are often described as occurring in stages, progressing from inflammatory to pigmented types. The various types or stages, however, may coexist, and not all stages occur in each patient. In the first four months of life, numerous vesicles, bullae, or pustules appear on the trunk and extremities, often in clusters with an erythematous base. These vesicular lesions may be associated with a rising eosinophilia, and the bullae often contain a high eosinophil count. The vesicular stage usually clears by age 4 months. Hyperkeratotic verrucous or lichenoid lesions then develop at the sites of previous vesicular lesions or independently of pre-existing inflammatory changes. The verrucous lesions tend to regress in a matter of months, but they may persist for years, especially on the feet. Atrophic changes also may develop, particularly after the verrucous lesions regress. The distinctive cutaneous lesions, however, are irregular pigmentations; streaks, flecks, whorls, and lacy patterns of gray, brown, or slate hue develop on the trunk and extremities within the first few years of life. Although pigmentation may be the initial manifestation of the syndrome, it usually develops after the inflammatory lesions. Micro-

scopically the pigmented areas show an increase in the number of chromatophores bearing melanin in the upper corium, giving rise to the descriptive, but somewhat inaccurate term, incontinentia pigmenti. The pigmentation may persist, but it tends to fade with age.

In addition to the skin lesions, there may be abnormalities of the skin appendages as further evidence of the disorder of the integument. Patchy alopecia and abnormal nails are common.

EXTRADERMATOLOGIC FINDINGS. Developmental defects of bone and teeth are important signs of the syndrome. The skeletal abnormalities include hemivertebrae, hemiatrophy, extra ribs, syndactyly, short extremities, and short stature. The teeth are often imperfect, and there may be congenital absence of certain teeth. Hypodontia, delayed eruption, and conical crown forms of both deciduous and permanent teeth are described.

Cardiovascular and genitourinary anomalies may occur.

NEUROLOGIC MANIFESTATIONS. Microcephaly, mental deficiency, epilepsy, hemiparesis, and spastic tetraplegia have been described in the Bloch-Sulzberger syndrome, but the pathogenesis of the neurologic manifestations is not clear. Few neuropathologic studies have been reported. Described abnormalities include micropolygyria of the cortex, pyramidal hypoplasia, and some areas of atrophy and neuronal loss in the central white matter.

OCULAR ABNORMALITIES. The major ocular lesions associated with incontinentia pigmenti are intraocular, retrolenticular masses and membranes variously described as pseudogliomas, retrolental fibroplasia, and retinal detachments; more completely described cases appear to be examples of retinal dysplasia, falciform folds of the retina, and persistence and hyperplasia of the primary vitreous. In some patients there have been inflammatory signs leading to the diagnosis of uveitis or ophthalmitis. Vasculoproliferative changes of the posterior pole and intraocular hemorrhage have also been described. There may also be microphthalmia, hyaloid remnants, conus, optic atrophy, papillitis, cataracts, keratitis, corneal opacities, blue sclerae, myopia, strabismus, and nystagmus. These abnormalities may occur independently or in various combinations. In many cases vision is defective because of the developmental defects or inflammatory changes. Curiously, pigmentary mottling of the fundus is infrequently described, and only one case of conjunctival pigmentation has been reported. Proliferation and migration of pigment cells has been noted on microscopic examination of intraocular mass lesions, but whether an inflammatory process involving pigment changes comparable to that of the skin plays a role in true evolution of the ocular lesions of incontinentia pigmenti can only be speculated.

Linear Nevus Sebaceous of Jadassohn With Convulsions and Retardation

Neurologic and ocular abnormalities may occur in association with linear nevus sebaceous of Jadassohn to form a rare and probably sporadic neurocutaneous syndrome.

THE CUTANEOUS LESION. Nevus sebaceous is a congenital lesion of the skin characterized by hyperplasia of the sebaceous glands and thickening and hyperkeratosis of the epidermis. Clinically the lesions appear as well-demarcated plaques of firm yellowish orange papules present from birth. They usually involve the scalp and face. A midline lesion of the face extending over the forehead to the tip of the nose is typical, but other areas of the body are also commonly affected. The nevi may become malignant.

Some patients also have large pigmented nevi on the neck, trunk, back and extremities. In addition there may be cutaneous hemangiomas, palatal nevi, or papillomas of the tongue.

NEUROLOGIC FEATURES. Epilepsy, mental retardation, facial paresis, ocular motor paralysis, nystagmus, vision and hearing defects, and EEG abnormalities have been described in association with nevus sebaceous. The pathology of these manifestations has not been established. Asymmetry of the skull and orbits, premature closure of cranial sutures, widening of the sella turcica, and hydrocephalus also occur.

OTHER SIGNS. Other defects reported with this disorder include slanted auricles, hypoplastic dentition, and coarctation of the aorta.

OPHTHALMIC FEATURES. The spectrum of ophthalmic abnormalities reported in association with linear nevus sebaceous includes proptosis, epibulbar lipodermoids, vascularization of the cornea, colobomata of the eyelid, iris, and choroid, antimongoloid fissures, teratomas of the orbit and aberrant lacrimal glands, ocular motor palsy, nystagmus, corectopia, and defective vision.

Xerodermic Idiocy of de Sanctis and Cacchione

Xeroderma pigmentosum, a syndrome of hypersensitivity to sunlight, freckling, and skin cancer, may occur in association with mental deficiency, microcephaly, and hypogonadism to form an unusual neurocutaneous syndrome in children. The condition is inherited as an autosomal recessive trait.

THE CUTANEOUS LESIONS. The skin abnormalities usually appear in infancy or childhood, beginning as erythema after exposure to sunlight. There is then progressive development of small pigmented lesions, resembling freckles, on the exposed parts of the body. These lesions become more pronounced on exposure to sunlight and coalesce to form larger pigmented areas. Finally, pedunculated lesions develop from the pigmented areas, and the lesions later undergo malignant change. Several types of malignancies, including angiosarcomas, fibrosarcomas, lymphomas, and melanomas, develop in these patients. Telangiectasias and angiomas, scaly parchment-like atrophic areas, and cicatricial patches are also often present in the skin.

NEUROLOGIC FEATURES. Mental deficiency, microcephaly, spasticity, cerebellar ataxia, and sensorineural deafness are the common nervous system manifestations of this syndrome. Their pathogenesis is not understood. One pathologic study has shown cerebral and olivopontocerebellar atrophy.

OPHTHALMIC SIGNS. The major ophthalmic signs of this disorder are photophobia and excessive lacrimation early in the course. The conjunctivae become dry and injected, and corneal ulceration and iritis occur. Atrophy of eyelids, loss of cilia, ectropion, entropion, symblepharon, and ankyloblepharon are the final disastrous ocular complications of this syndrome.

DEGENERATIVE DISEASES

The degenerative diseases of the nervous system are a heterogeneous group of disorders in which the outstanding clinical feature is progressive deterioration of neurologic function. With few exceptions these diseases are genetically determined and hereditary. The majority are known or presumed to be the result of inborn errors of metabolism, though other factors including viruses and altered immune responses are implicated in the pathogenesis of some. In many, the etiology remains obscure.

The diversity of etiologic and pathologic processes responsible for these diseases is reflected in their clinical heterogeneity. Many are characterized by extensive damage to the nervous system resulting in incapacitation or death. Others are less devastating, and some involve only selected portions of the nervous system. Often there are extraneural manifestations such as visceral, skeletal, or cutaneous abnormalities. As a general rule, the manifestations appear insidiously in a previously normally functioning individual, but in some instances the degenerative process is apparent at birth and worsens with advancing age. With rare exception, there is no effective treatment, and the course is usually one of relentlessly progressive deterioration. Nevertheless, accurate diagnosis and delineation is essential for purposes of prognostic and genetic counselling, and every effort must be made to expand our knowledge of the pathologic processes with an aim toward developing effective means of treatment and genetic identification.

No one classification of the degenerative diseases is satisfactory. Certain of the disorders can be classified accurately on the basis of well-defined enzyme defects and metabolic aberrations, but for many of the diseases only traditional anatomic or clinicopathologic grouping is possible. The degenerative diseases of principal importance in pediatric ophthalmology are here classified in mixed fashion, with apologies to purists.

Cerebral Storage Diseases

Cerebral storage diseases are genetically determined metabolic disorders in which there is excessive and abnormal accumulation of complex lipids or other substances in cerebral neurons, with attendant deterioration of cerebral functions. Although gray matter degeneration is a major common denominator of these diseases, the neurologic involvement rarely is limited to cerebral gray matter, and in many of these disorders the cerebral involvement is just one expression of a multifaceted disease affecting several systems.

The majority of the cerebral storage diseases are sphingolipidoses, primary disorders of sphingolipid metabolism caused by specific enzyme deficiencies. The sphingolipids constitute a major group of the cerebral lipids; chemically they are fatty acid esters of ceramide, a generic class of compounds containing N-acyl derivatives of the long chain amino alcohol sphingosine or its cogeners. The stored lipid in each of the sphingolipidoses contains the base unit ceramide; the lipids are further differentiated and classified according to their other substituents. Those which contain mono- or oligosaccharides are referred to as glycosphingolipids; the glycosphingolipids in turn are further classified as gangliosides, cerebrosides, and sulfatides. Specific gangliosides accumulate in several of the major cerebral storage diseases (Table 18–10), including in particular Tay-Sachs disease, Sandhoff's disease, and generalized gangliosidosis, whereas in Gaucher's disease there is storage of cerebroside. Aside from these glycosphingolipids, the other major class of sphingolipids that may be involved in cerebral storage processes are the phosphosphingolipids; representative of this group is sphingomyelin, the storage substance of the Niemann-Pick syndromes.

Two other major groups of cerebral lipids (i.e., nonsphingolipids) involved in cerebral storage disease are the glycerophosphatides and the cholesterols.

TABLE 18–10 THE GANGLIOSIDOSES

Designation	Metabolic Abnormality	General Description	Principal Ophthalmic Signs
G_{m1} type I: Generalized Gangliosidosis	Profound deficiency of B-galactosidase (isoenzymes A, B, and C) with abnormal neuronal and visceral accumulation of G_{M1}, and abnormal visceral accumulation of a mucopolysaccharide resembling keratan sulfate.	A neurovisceral storage disease having combined features of neuronal lipidosis and mucopolysaccharidosis; cerebral degeneration combined with visceromegaly and skeletal dysplasia. Rapidly progressive and fatal in infancy.	Macular cherry-red spots in approximately 50% of cases. Corneas clear (one reported exception).
G_{M1} type II: Juvenile Gangliosidosis	Deficiency of B-galactosidase (isoenzymes B and C) with abnormal neuronal, and to a lesser degree, extraneural accumulation of G_{M1}.	A late onset cerebral degeneration, commencing after age 6 months, with minimal, if any, visceromegaly and skeletal changes. Psychomotor deterioration slower than in type I. Death between 3 and 4 years of age.	Normal fundi. Clear corneas.
G_{M2} type I: Tay-Sachs Disease (infantile amaurotic familial idiocy)	Absence of hexosaminidase A with abnormal accumulation of G_{M2} throughout nervous system, leading to neuronal destruction and demyelination.	Progressive deterioration of mental and motor abilities commencing after age 4 to 6 months, resulting in dementia, paralysis, and death by age 3 to 4 years. Definite ethnic predilection—Jews of northeastern European origin.	Classical macular cherry-red spots and optic atrophy. Progressive loss of vision. Deterioration of eye movements.
G_{M2} type II: Sandoff Variant	Profound deficiency of hexosaminidase A and B, with abnormal accumulation of G_{M2} throughout nervous system, and accumulation of globoside in viscera.	Clinically almost indistinguishable from Tay-Sachs except for presence of some degree of hepatosplenomegaly. No ethnic predilection.	Macular cherry-red spots and loss of vision.
G_{M2} type III: Juvenile Variant	Partial deficiency of hexosaminidase A with abnormal accumulation of G_{M2} to a lesser degree than in G_{M2} type I.	Psychomotor regression and ataxia commencing in the second to fifth year of life, with survival possibly into teens.	Optic atrophy and retinal pigmentary degeneration rather than cherry-red spots. Loss of vision as a late effect.

TABLE 18-11   AMAUROTIC FAMILY IDIOCIES

Type	Clinical Characteristics	Metabolic and Pathologic Correlations
Congenital AFI (Norman-Wood)	Evident at birth. Seizures, rigidity, blindness. Death soon after birth (within days). Signs of retinal degeneration and optic atrophy, but not cherry-red spots.	Neuronal lipidosis with marked neuronal degeneration, demyelination, and astrocytic gliosis; brain characteristically small. Some evidence for ganglioside accumulation, but nature of defect is obscure.
Infantile AFI (Tay-Sachs)	Progressive psychomotor deterioration commencing after age 4 to 6 months, leading to dementia, paralysis, blindness and death by age 3 to 4 years. In classic form (Tay-Sachs), no clinical visceromegaly; in variant (Sandoff type), mild visceromegaly. Characteristic macular cherry-red spot and loss of vision (usually with retention of pupillary light response) evident early in course.	In classic form, type I G_{M2} gangliosidosis: absence of hexosaminidase A leading to abnormal neuronal accumulation of G_{M2} with typical membranous cytoplasmic inclusion bodies, progressive neuronal destruction, demyelination, and gliosis. Alternatively, type II (Sandoff variant) G_{M2} gangliosidosis: deficiency of hexosaminidase A and B; in addition to progressive neuronal accumulation of G_{M2} with neuronal destruction, demyelination, and gliosis, an abnormal accumulation of globoside in the viscera.
Late Infantile AFI (Jansky-Bielschowsky)	Intellectual deterioration, seizures, cerebellar ataxia and vision loss commencing between ages 2 and 5 years. Sometimes marked spasticity. Death within 1 to 3 years. Pigmentary retinal degeneration; in some cases, predominantly macular and perimacular, with loss of foveal light reflex and macular pigment alteration, or sometimes the appearance of a yellow-gray zone around a reddish fovea, but not a typical cherry-red spot. ERG subnormal. Disc pale. Pupillary light response decreased.	In most cases, a neurovisceral storage disease characterized by presence of curvilinear bodies, or by presence of ceroid or lipofuscin accumulation; enzyme defect unknown. In some cases, evidence for type II G_{M1} or "juvenile" type G_{M2} lipidosis. (Also, in certain instances, group C Niemann-Pick disease may present as late infantile AFI)
Juvenile AFI (Batten-Mayou-Spielmeyer-Vogt)	Intellectual deterioration, generalized seizures and vision loss commencing between ages 5 and 8 years, sometimes as late as 14 years. Progressive loss of motor function. Fatal within several years. Pigmentary retinal degeneration, commonly peripheral or generalized, resembling "retinitis pigmentosa," with night blindness and peripheral field loss; in some cases, predominantly macular degeneration characterized by macular pigment alteration, beaten-metal appearance, or a pale spot surrounded by reddish areola. Optic atrophy as a late manifestation.	Generally ceroid lipopigment or lipofuscin accumulation in presence of normal sphingolipid profile, with a variety of cytoplasmic inclusions in neurons and glia, including lipofuscin, membranovesicular bodies, multilamellar cytosomes, fingerprint type inclusions, and principal bodies. Specific enzyme defect unknown.* (In some instances, "juvenile" type G_{M2} or type C Niemann-Pick disease may present as juvenile AFI.)
Late Juvenile or Adult AFI (Kuf)	Behavioral disturbances and impairment of intellectual function beginning in late childhood, adolescence or early adult life (age 15 to 25 years). In early stages, psychotic symptoms commonly predominant; subsequently, ataxia and spasticity. Not uncommonly, myoclonic seizures. Despite terminology, vision and fundi usually normal, though macular degeneration evident in some cases.	Diffuse neuronal lipidosis; presence of lipofuscin material and small membranous cytoplasmic bodies. Ganglioside pattern normal. Specific metabolic defect unknown.

*Deficiency of myeloperoxidase activity in white cells of patients with Batten's syndrome has recently been reported.

Also included in the group of disorders characterized by cerebral storage are the mucopolysaccharidoses; these entities are described in detail in Chapter 20 (p. 664). Combining features of both mucopolysaccharidosis and gangliosidosis is the entity referred to as generalized gangliosidosis.

Within the group of disorders classified as cerebral storage diseases is a special subgroup of lipidoses traditionally referred to as the amaurotic familial idiocies. The term amaurotic family idiocy (AFI), originally applied to Tay-Sachs disease, embraces at least five disorders having in common progressive cerebral and retinal degeneration (Table 18–11). The nosology of the group has been based primarily on clinical features, in particular the age of onset, the clinical symptoms, and the duration of the disease. With recent advances in neuropathologic and biochemical delineation, more precise identification of these disorders is becoming possible. Whereas certain of the amaurotic familial idiocies are gangliosidoses, others of the group are characterized by lipopigment storage in the presence of a normal sphingolipid profile.

Tay-Sachs Disease
(G_{M2} Gangliosidosis, Type 1)

Tay-Sachs disease is a genetically determined metabolic disease characterized by neuronal lipidosis with attendant deterioration of psychomotor functions commencing in infancy. It invariably leads to dementia, blindness, paralysis, and death in early childhood. Macular cherry-red spots are a classic sign of the disease.

The disorder is autosomal recessive. It occurs predominantly in Jews of Northeastern European descent.

THE METABOLIC DISORDER AND ITS PATHOLOGY. The metabolic defect in Tay-Sachs disease is absence of ganglioside G_{M2}-hexosaminidase (hexosaminidase A), the enzyme that normally catalyzes cleavage of N-acetyl galactosamine from ganglioside G_{M2}. As a result of this deficiency there is abnormal accumulation of G_{M2} throughout the nervous system, primarily within the ganglion cells, with a greater proportion of the ganglioside being stored in secondary lysosomes termed membranous cytoplasmic bodies (MCB). The progressive accumulation of stored material leads to disintegration of ganglion cells, loss of axons, and degeneration of myelin. In association with the neuronal destruction and demyelination, there is proliferation and lipid loading of glial cells.

Pathologic changes are most striking in the cerebral cortex. On microscopic examination the ganglion cells appear distended or "ballooned"; the cytoplasm is pale or spongy (often vacuolated), and the nuclei are displaced to the periphery. In later stages there is significant loss of ganglion cells, while remaining neurons may lack nuclei and appear "washed out." There is concomitant decrease in the number of cortical axons; some show fusiform swellings termed "torpedos." In advanced cases there is evidence of gliosis; the glial cells, like the neurons, appear distended with lipid staining material. Demyelination is consistently present and may be extensive.

Pathologic changes similar to those of the cerebrum are found in the cerebellum, basal ganglia, brain stem, and cord. Signs of lipid accumulation are also evident in peripheral nerves and throughout the autonomic nervous system. There is some visceral accumulation of G_{M2} in Tay-Sachs disease, particularly in the liver and spleen, but this is not of sufficient degree to produce visceromegaly or significant impairment of function.

The characteristic MCB can be found in the cytoplasm of ganglion cells, axis cylinders, glial cells, and perivascular tissue cells. These discrete bodies are round to oval structures, 0.5 to 2.0μ in diameter. They consist of concentric layers of dense membranes and contain primarily ganglioside, cholesterol, phospholipids, and possibly other glycolipids.

For purposes of diagnosis, the deficiency of hexosaminidase A is measured in tissues, in cultured cells, in plasma, or in serum leukocytes. Prenatal diagnosis is possible by enzyme assay of amniotic fluid. The carrier state can be detected by enzyme assay, as heterozygotes show a partial deficiency of hexosaminidase A activity.

CLINICAL MANIFESTATIONS. Manifestations of Tay-Sachs disease usually appear by age 4 to 6 months. The clinical onset is often insidious, with listlessness, apathy, weakness, irritability, or feeding difficulties. Psychomotor development is retarded. Hypotonia, exaggerated startle reactions, and extensor responses are common early signs. Hypotonia soon gives way to spasticity. Responses to visual stimuli decrease. As the disease progresses, seizures may occur. With time, megalencephaly may develop.

The course is one of rapidly progressive deterioration leading to paralysis, dementia, and blindness. In most cases, there is loss of all voluntary movement by age 2 years. Death occurs by age 3 to 4 years, rarely later.

OPHTHALMIC MANIFESTATIONS. Ophthalmic abnormalities develop in virtually every child with Tay-Sachs disease.

Progressive deterioration of visual function is the rule, and loss of vision commences early. Blindness is usually complete by age 2 years. Much of the vision loss appears to be predominantly of central rather than peripheral origin; the pupil reaction to light often is retained in blind patients, even in terminal stages of the disease, and the ERG usually becomes abnormal only late in the course. The fundi may appear normal early in life, but macular cherry-red spots invariably develop. As a rule, macular changes are evident by the time other signs of neurologic deterioration appear in infancy. Clinically, the classic cherry-red spot appears as a bright to dull red area at the center of the macula, surrounded by a creamy white or yellowish halo. The halo is the result of loss of transparency of the multilayered ganglion cell ring of the macula. The red area is the normal choroidal vascular blush of the transparent macular center, its redness accentuated by the creamy halo. The cherry-red spot is the focal, ophthalmoscopically visible evidence of generalized retinal involvement.

The pathologic changes throughout the retina are similar to those in the brain. There is lipid loading and degeneration of the ganglion cells, and edema of the internuclear layers; the deeper layers tend to be normal. The ganglioside fractions of the retina parallel those of the brain, and it has been demonstrated that hexosaminidase A is absent in the retina. There is also demyelination and degeneration of the optic nerves, chiasm, and tracts. Clinical evidence of optic atrophy may precede or follow the development of the blindness. In addition, there usually is sequential deterioration of ocular motor function; the eye movements regress in reverse order to their normal ontogenetic development.

Generalized Gangliosidosis (G_{M1} Gangliosidosis, Type 1)

Generalized gangliosidosis is a hereditary metabolic storage disease that is rapidly progressive and fatal in infancy. The disease combines features of gangliosidosis and mucopolysaccharidosis. The predominant manifestations are cerebral degeneration, visceromegaly, and skeletal dysplasia. Macular cherry-red spots develop in many cases.

The disorder appears to be inherited as an autosomal recessive condition with no obvious ethnic predilection.

THE METABOLIC DISORDER AND ITS PATHOLOGY. In generalized gangliosidosis there is neuronal lipidosis throughout the cerebral cortex, the brain stem, the spinal cord, and Meissner's plexus. Neuronal cytoplasm is ballooned with storage material, and the cells contain cytoplasmic bodies of spirally wound membranes (membranous cytoplasmic bodies — MCB). The predominant neuronal storage material is the specific ganglioside G_{M1}, and its accumulation may reach tenfold its normal level in gray matter. A glycolipid structurally related to G_{M1} also accumulates in brain tissue. In addition, there is prominent visceral histiocytosis. The predominant visceral storage material is a mucopolysaccharide similar to keratan sulfate. G_{M1} also accumulates in viscera, and it may increase 20 to 50 times its normal level in the liver, but the visceral mucopolysaccharide storage exceeds the visceral ganglioside storage approximately 50-fold. In spite of the massive mucopolysaccharide storage, mucopolysaccharide excretion in urine is normal or only slightly elevated. In addition, peripheral blood lymphocytes and marrow histiocytes show vacuolization, renal glomerular epithelial cells show evidence of cytoplasmic storage, and there may be foamy mononuclear cells in the urine.

The abnormal accumulation of ganglioside G_{M1}, glycolipid, and mucopolysaccharide reflects a fault in their degradation due to deficiency of a β-galactosidase. There is a profound deficiency of the enzyme in tissues of affected infants, and heterozygotes show a partial defect. For clinical purposes, the β-galactosidase deficiency can be measured in leukocytes, in urine, and in cultured skin fibroblasts, and the defect may be detected prenatally by assay of amniotic fluids.

CLINICAL MANIFESTATIONS. Affected infants are abnormal from birth; they show severe psychomotor retardation and morphologic abnormalities. The infants are lethargic, hypoactive, and hypotonic. Their motor strength and coordination are poor, and their reflexes are hyperactive. Their appetite and weight gain are subnormal, and their suck and cry are weak. There may be facial and peripheral edema. Frontal bossing, depressed nasal bridge, low-set large ears, and hirsutism are physical features common to the disease, and many infants have macroglossia. Skeletal deformities are common. There is often expansion of the shafts of the long bones and beaking of the vertebral bodies. The ribs are wide and spatulate, and the hands are broad, with short stubby fingers. Dorsolumbar kyphoscoliosis, stiffness and flexion contractures of the knees and elbows, and "claw hand" deformity develop. Hepatomegaly invariably appears by age 6 months, and splenomegaly develops in the majority of cases. Some infants develop macrocephaly.

The clinical course is one of progressive deterioration, especially rapid after age 1 year. The children become blind, deaf, and decerebrate. They suffer recurrent bronchopneumonia, and they invariably die, usually by age 2 years.

OPHTHALMIC MANIFESTATIONS. Blindness is common as a manifestation of this cerebral degeneration. Cherry-red spots of the maculae are present in approximately one half the patients with generalized gangliosidosis. Strabismus and nystagmus may develop. The corneas are clear in all but one reported instance.

Niemann-Pick Disease (Sphingomyelin Lipidosis)

Niemann-Pick disease is a metabolic disorder characterized by increased tissue content of sphingomyelin. Actually, four major forms of sphingomyelin lipidosis are described, but they are collectively referred to as Niemann-Pick disease. Specific types are designated on the basis of their clinical manifestations, age of onset, and chemical abnormalities. Characteristically the spleen, liver, lymph nodes, marrow, and lung are involved, and lipid-laden foamy cells in these organs are a hallmark of the disease. Frequently the nervous system and eye are affected, and cherry-red spots develop in some cases. All forms of the disease are inherited as an autosomal recessive characteristic.

METABOLIC AND CLINICOPATHOLOGIC CORRELATES. The abnormality common to all forms of Niemann-Pick disease is increased tissue content of sphingomyelin, and in general, the disease process is characterized by progressive infiltration and re-

placement of tissues by masses of foam cells derived from reticuloendothelial, connective tissue, and parenchymal cells. The accumulating lipid, sphingomyelin, is found predominantly in secondary lysosomes in the foam cells. Cholesterol also invariably accumulates in association with the sphingomyelin.

The tissues affected earliest are the spleen, marrow, lymph nodes, and thymus. Infiltration and crowding of the marrow eventually produce some anemia and thrombocytopenia, but bone changes are not usually apparent radiologically. The spleen and liver become enlarged; liver function tests may reflect abnormalities, but clinical jaundice is not common. The lungs are involved in patients of all ages; pulmonary infiltration can be appreciated radiologically as a fine reticular or nodular pattern, but symptoms of dysfunction are not prominent. The heart, gastrointestinal tract, and endocrine glands as well can be infiltrated, and the skin may show a brownish yellow discoloration and thickening.

When the nervous system is involved, the distribution of the lesions tends to be irregular. Both the peripheral and central nervous system can be affected; the cerebral cortex, cerebellum, basal ganglia, brain stem, spinal cord, spinal ganglia, nerve roots, and autonomic ganglia may undergo changes. Ganglion cells become swollen and vacuolated, and they contain membranous cytoplasmic bodies. There may be loss of cells in the cerebral and cerebellar cortex, some loss of myelin, and varying degrees of glial proliferation. Typical foam cells can be found about the leptomeninges and perivascular spaces of the nervous system.

Presumably the disease process results from a defect in catabolism of sphingomyelin, but sphingomyelinase deficiency has been demonstrated in only two forms of the disease. The sphingomyelinase assays can be done on tissue and cultured fibroblasts.

CLINICAL TYPES

Type A, the acute neuronopathic type, is the classic form of the disease in childhood, with severe neurologic and visceral manifestations. Abnormalities become apparent within a few months of birth, and some infants are abnormal even at birth. Hepatosplenomegaly, vomiting, poor feeding, and failure to thrive are common early signs. Within the first year, often by age 6 months, there is evidence of retardation, hypotonia, and flaccidity, with progressive loss of motor and intellectual functions. There is regression to a vegetative state, terminating in death by age 3 or 4 years. Retinal changes resembling a cherry-red spot occur in some cases of this neuronopathic form. In type A, there is severe deficiency of sphingomyelinase.

Type B, a chronic form of the disease, is characterized by reticuloendothelial and visceral involvement, without nervous system involvement. Systemic manifestations develop in infancy or early childhood. The patients may survive 20 years, reasonably healthy and free of neurologic signs. In type B, there is a deficiency of sphingomyelinase, but of less severe degree than in type A.

Type C, a subacute neurovisceral form, is sometimes referred to as the juvenile type. The development of clinical signs of lipidosis is delayed. The children may seem to be normal during early childhood, and the visceral manifestations are not as severe as those of type A. The neurologic manifestations appear between age 2 and 4 years. Spasticity, seizures and myoclonic jerks are common. In older children, the first sign of the disease may be emotional lability, behavior abnormalities, and learning problems. There may be retinal changes. Death usually occurs before age 20 years. In type C, sphingomyelinase is normal or nearly normal.

Type D is a subacute neurovisceral type, similar to type C, but occurring only in persons of Nova Scotian ancestry. Ataxia, dyskinesia, and retardation often are the initial neurologic manifestations. Seizures become a problem as the disease progresses. In type D, sphingomyelinase is probably normal.

An additional type, *type E*, designates adults who show increased tissue levels of sphingomyelin, normal sphingomyelinase, and no clinical neurovisceral manifestations.

OPHTHALMIC MANIFESTATIONS IN SUMMARY. In Niemann-Pick disease there may be macular cherry-red spots in the acute neuronopathic form (type A) and in the subacute neurovisceral form (type C) late in the disease. Sometimes only a grayish haze develops about the macula.

Vertical gaze palsies have been described in patients having clinical features of Niemann-Pick's disease.

Gaucher's Disease
(Glucosyl Ceramide Lipidoses)

Gaucher's disease is a disorder of cerebroside metabolism with accumulation of glucosyl ceramide. Distinctive storage cells, referred to as Gaucher cells, are a hallmark of the disease. Both neuronopathic and non-neuronopathic forms of the disease occur in childhood. The principal extraneural manifestations are hepatosplenomegaly and the presence of Gaucher cells in the marrow. The major neurologic manifestations are progressive spasticity and cranial nerve palsies, and the usual neuronopathic ophthalmic manifestation is paralytic strabismus.

METABOLIC AND PATHOLOGIC FEATURES. The metabolic defect in Gaucher's disease is deficient activity of the catabolic enzyme glucosyl ceramide β-glucosidase. Glucosyl ceramide, a cerebroside normally found outside the nervous system, accumulates to abnormal levels, and the material is stored primarily in Gaucher cells. The Gaucher cells are derived predominantly from reticulum cells, though other cells of phagocytic potential also store the cerebroside; Gaucher cells are most abundant in lymphoid tissues. The accumulating glucosyl appears to be concentrated in secondary lysosomes in the Gaucher cell, and the Gaucher cell cytoplasm has a distinctive fibrillar appearance unlike the foamy appearance of the cells of other storage diseases.

Extraneural tissues regularly affected are the spleen and liver. Engorgement of the spleen by Gaucher cells produces splenomegaly, thrombocytopenia, anemia, and leukopenia of varying severity. Engorgement of the liver produces hepatomegaly and sometimes portal hypertension; jaundice is not usual. The presence of Gaucher cells in bone marrow is a characteristic feature of the disease; pain, fractures, and deformities may develop. Infiltrations in lung alveolar capillaries and in lung lymphatics are common, and pulmonary manifestations such as pneumonitis, respiratory distress, and chronic cough often develop. The lymph nodes, thymus, adrenal, thyroid, and pancreas also are commonly affected.

When the nervous system is involved, the predominant findings are the presence of swollen periadventitial cells, the deposition of glycolipid in periadventitial cells, and the loss of neurons in selected areas. The neuronal loss occurs primarily in the cerebral cortex, in the basal ganglia, and in the brain stem; also usually affected are the large cranial nerve nuclear masses. Sometimes Gaucher cells appear to lie free in brain tissue. There may be some true neuronal cytoplasmic lipid storage. Neuronophagia and variable degrees of demyelination also occur.

CLINICAL TYPES

Type 1 is the chronic non-neuronopathic form. Although it is commonly referred to as the adult form, manifestations may begin in infancy. The common childhood signs are growth failure, hepatosplenomegaly, thrombocytopenia, bone pain, and fractures. There are no neurologic manifestations, and the course is protracted.

Type 2 is the acute neuronopathic form, less accurately referred to as the "infantile" or "cerebral" form. It is complicated by obvious neurologic manifestations, with rapid progression to death in infancy. The children usually are normal for the first months of life but they soon develop hepatosplenomegaly, chronic cough, pulmonary infections, swallowing and feeding difficulties, and evidence of failure to thrive. Neurologic manifestations are usually apparent by age 6 months. Characteristically there are signs of regression of development and progressive cranial nerve and extrapyramidal involvement. Paralytic strabismus, trismus, dysphagia, laryngeal stridor, muscular hypertonicity, and spasticity with hyperextension of the head and rigidity of the neck, retraction of the lips, increased deep tendon reflexes, and pathologic reflexes are common to the disease. Some children develop seizures. Most children become mentally retarded and apathetic. Some develop a peculiar yellow pallor. The disease progresses rapidly, terminating in death before age 2 years; death is usually secondary to anoxia and infection related to the progressive pulmonary involvement.

Type 3 is the subacute neuronopathic form. Often referred to as the juvenile type, this form is characterized by visceral and neural involvement, but the neurologic manifestations are attenuated, the course is protracted, and death is delayed.

OPHTHALMIC SIGNS. Paralytic strabismus due to brain stem involvement is a regular feature of neuronopathic Gaucher's disease. The fundi usually are normal; occasional macular changes have been described, but true cherry-red spots do not develop. Gaucher's cells have been found in the choroid. Corneal clouding has been described in one instance.

Pingueculae — wedge-shaped conjunctival lesions — occur in the chronic non-neuronopathic form.

Krabbe's Disease (Galactosyl Ceramide Lipidosis)

Krabbe's disease is a genetically determined demyelinating disease that is invariably fatal in early childhood. The presence of unique globoid cells in white matter is the distinctive pathologic feature of the disorder, and Krabbe's disease is often referred to as "globoid cell leukodystrophy". Hypertonicity and progressive spastic paralysis are the principal clinical signs of the disease, and there may be cortical blindness and optic atrophy.

Often classified with the leukodystrophies, this lipidosis is better characterized as a cerebral storage disease.

THE METABOLIC DISORDER AND ITS PATHOLOGY. In Krabbe's disease there is a degradative defect in the metabolism of galactocerebroside (galactosyl ceramide). The significant biochemical finding appears to be the deficient activity of galactosyl ceramide β-galactosidase; the deficiency can be measured in serum, in leukocytes, in cultured fibroblasts, in neural tissue, and in viscera.

In the brain there is symmetrical diffuse loss of myelin of the cerebral white matter with considerable loss of myelin lipids, particularly phospholipids and glycolipids, cholesterol, and cerebroside. There is also severe loss of oligodendroglia. In addition there is reactive gliosis in the white matter. The characteristic pathologic finding, however, is the aggregation of globoid inclusion cells in white matter, particularly in perivascular spaces. The globoid cells are of mesodermal origin. Their inclusions are rich in galactosyl ceramide, but there is no great accumulation of galactocerebroside, for as the oligodendroglial cells are lost, production of the cerebroside diminishes. In addition to white matter, the disorder affects the liver, spleen, and kidney, but without producing clinical visceral manifestations.

CLINICAL MANIFESTATIONS. The clinical features are rather constant, and the clinical course can be divided into several stages. Manifestations develop in infancy or early childhood, often at 3 to 6 months of age. Initially there is generalized hyperirritability, hypersensitivity to external stimuli, and stiffness or even rigidity of the extremities. Feeding difficulties, vomiting, seizures, episodic fever, and slight retardation or psychomotor regression are common early signs. There is then rapid progression of the disease with severe motor and mental deterioration. Long tract signs are prominent. Marked hypertonicity with increased deep tendon reflexes, spastic quadriparesis, pseudobulbar palsies, tonic seizures, and generalized convulsions develop. There commonly is loss of vision and hearing. Finally there is progression to a decerebrate state. The neurologic devastation usually is complete in the first year or two of life. The decerebrate terminal stage may last for years, but rarely more than two. Death invariably results, most commonly from bulbar palsy.

OPHTHALMIC MANIFESTATIONS. The initial ophthalmic manifestation of Krabbe's disease is frequently cortical blindness. Optic atrophy develops later in the course of the disease, and the pupil reactions are diminished late in the course. There is sometimes nystagmus.

Fabry's Disease
(Glycosphingolipid Lipidosis)

Fabry's disease, or angiokeratoma corporis diffusum universale, is an X-linked disorder of glycosphingolipid metabolism. Angiectatic lesions of the skin, cerebrovascular abnormalities, peripheral neuropathy, and autonomic symptoms related to lipid deposits throughout the body are the major manifestations of the disease. Vascular lesions of the eye and distinctive opacities of the cornea are characteristic features.

METABOLIC AND PATHOLOGIC FEATURES. The metabolic defect of Fabry's disease is profound deficiency of trihexosyl ceramide galactosyl hydrolase in the plasma and tissue of hemizygous males, and partial deficiency of the enzyme in heterozygous females. Trihexosyl ceramide accumulates in plasma and in most tissues as a result of the enzymatic defect in its catabolism. In addition, another glycolipid accumulates in the kidney and pancreas, and is also present in urinary sediment. The lipid deposits alter the morphology and physiology of affected sites.

Birefringent lipid crystals are deposited in endothelial, perithelial, and smooth muscle cells of blood vessels. The lipid also accumulates in reticuloendothelial cells, connective tissue cells, and myocardial cells, and in epithelial cells of the kidney, cornea, and adrenal glands. In the nervous system, the lipid crystals are found in ganglion cells of the brain and peripheral nervous system, and in the perineural cells of the autonomic nervous system. The vascular changes are prominent throughout the nervous system.

CLINICAL MANIFESTATIONS. Clinical signs of Fabry's disease become apparent in the hemizygous males during childhood or adolescence. Characteristic clusters of angiectasias develop in the skin, oral mucosa, and conjunctiva. Paroxysmal episodes of fever, and severe burning pain in the extremities occur. Paresthesias, peripheral edema, and hypohidrosis are common. Signs of progressive renal involvement, albuminuria, uremia, and hypertension develop. Premature cerebrovascular disease (strokes) and peripheral neuropathy are the outstanding neurologic developments. Death usually results from renal failure, or from cardiovascular or cerebrovascular complications.

There may be attenuated clinical manifestations of the disease in heterozygous females.

OPHTHALMIC MANIFESTATIONS. Ocular signs of Fabry's disease include papilledema and retinal signs of the renal-hypertensive disorder, and orbital and lid edema develop in some patients.

More specific ocular signs of the disease are conjunctival and retinal vascular changes due to deposits of the lipid locally. Aneurysmal dilatations, sausage-like irregularities of vessel caliber, and telangiectasias develop in conjunctiva.

A distinctive corneal epithelial dystrophy related to epithelial lipid deposits characteristically occurs in Fabry's disease. The fine corneal epithelial opacities typically are arranged in radiating lines and whorls. The corneal opacities may become apparent as early as 6 months of age. They are seen both in hemizygous males and in heterozygous carrier females.

Posterior capsular cataracts also have been described.

The Leukodystrophies

The leukodystrophies are white matter degenerations in which there is an inborn error of metabolism that interferes with normal myelination. The term dysmyelination is applied to these diseases to indicate the endogenous disorder of myelin formation, but the exact nature of the defect in each of the leukodystrophies is not clear. In certain of the leukodystrophies there is accumulation of storage material, but whether it represents myelin precursors or metabolites due to an enzyme defect, or simply degeneration products, remains to be determined. Characteristically there is early loss of myelin with varying degrees of reactive gliosis throughout the neuraxis. The usual clinical manifestations are deterioration of motor abilities, progressive spasticity, dementia, and loss of vision. The dysmyelinating leukodystrophies of greatest ophthalmic interest are metachromatic leukodystrophy, Pelizaeus-Merzbacher disease, and spongy sclerosis of Canavan. Krabbe's globoid cell leukodystrophy is better classified as a cerebral storage disease.

Metachromatic Leukodystrophy (Sulfatide Lipidosis)

The term metachromatic leukodystrophy applies to a hereditary derangement of sulfatide metabolism characterized by progressive loss of myelin and accumulation of metachromatic lipids in the white matter of the central and peripheral nervous system. The usual clinical expression of the disorder is motor and mental deterioration with spasticity, paralysis, seizures, dementia, and death in early childhood, although attenuated and adult forms of the disease do occur. Visual disorders and optic atrophy are common features of the disease in childhood.

Metachromatic leukodystrophy is an autosomal recessive disorder.

THE METABOLIC DISORDER AND ITS PATHOLOGY. The basic defect in metachromatic leukodystrophy of childhood is impaired ability to degrade sulfatides due to a deficiency of the enzyme arylsulfatase. A. There is accumulation of metachromatically staining sulfuric acid esters of cerebrosides in the nervous system, with eventual demyelination of white matter in the cerebrum, cerebellum, brain stem, spinal cord, and peripheral nerves. Electron microscopy shows sulfatide-rich inclusions in myelin and in mitochondria of neurons, glial cells, and Schwann cells, but it is not clear whether the myelin disruption is caused by abnormal composition of myelin due to gradual increase in its sulfatide content, or by impaired function of the Schwann cells or oligodendrocytes. There is also accumulation of spherical granular masses of lipid in the periportal macrophages of the liver, in kidney, in pituitary, in gallbladder, and in adrenal medulla. Demonstration of metachromatic lipids in biopsies of peripheral nerves and other tissues, and demonstration of excess sulfatides in urine are useful clinically, and the arylsulfatase A deficiency can be measured in leukocytes, in urine, and in cultured skin fibroblasts. The heterozygote also can be detected by demonstration of arylsulfatase A deficiency in cultured skin fibroblasts.

CLINICAL MANIFESTATIONS. Early psychomotor development is usually normal, but manifestations of the disease become apparent after age 6 months, often in the second year of life. The early signs are impairment of locomotion and other motor activities, and the development of hypotonia, hyporeflexia, and ataxia. A child who has learned to walk will become awkward, and spasticity and paralysis develop. Later, mental regression, speech deterioration, and bulbar and pseudobulbar palsies develop.

The clinical course reflects progressive cerebral, cerebellar, and long tract involvement. The neurologic deterioration progresses without remission to quadriplegia with decorticate, decerebrate, or dystonic postures. Seizures and myoclonus commonly develop. In the final stages of the disease, the children are without volitional movements, speech, or sight. They die within a few years, usually from apnea or pneumonia.

OPHTHALMIC MANIFESTATIONS. Ocular motor disturbances are common. Strabismus secondary to cranial nerve involvement, and nystagmus are frequent early manifestations. Loss of vision is a rather constant feature of the disease. There are sometimes fundus abnormalities. The macular region often appears abnormally gray with an accentuated central red spot; the macular changes however, are indistinct, unlike a fully developed cherry-red spot. Pigmentary abnormalities of the retina also occur, sometimes resembling retinitis pigmentosa. Optic atrophy may develop. The underlying ophthalmic pathologic changes are similar to those of the brain, with sudanophilia and metachromasia in retinal ganglion cells, attenuation of the nerve fiber layer, and clumping of myelin of the optic nerve and of the ciliary nerves.

Pelizaeus - Merzbacher Disease

Pelizaeus-Merzbacher disease is a rare sex-linked recessive leukodystrophy that affects predominantly males. It is characterized by a prolonged course of slowly progressive spasticity, ataxia, and mental deterioration. Peculiar abnormal eye movements referred to as "eye rolling" are a prominent feature of the disease in infancy.

THE DISEASE PROCESS. The etiology of this white matter disease is unknown; no enzyme defect or storage substance has been identified. The pathologic features suggest dysmyelination; there is lack of staining of myelin in the neural axis, with little evidence of myelin breakdown. The cerebrum, basal ganglia, cerebellum, brain stem, and spinal cord are involved, and the disease process tends to be symmetrical. It seems to begin near the walls of the ventricles and extend toward the cortex. Myelin sheaths are affected first; then axis cylinders are destroyed. There is then proliferation of glia secondary to the demyelination, producing increased density of the brain.

GENERAL CLINICAL FEATURES. Manifestations of the disorder develop early in infancy, often within a few days of birth. There is lack of development of head control and failure to thrive. Cerebellar signs develop early, and there is progressive ataxia and dysarthria; grimacing and athetoid movements develop later in childhood. There is progressive spasticity, first of the lower and then of the upper ex-

tremities. By age 3 to 4 years, the children become bedridden and immobile with spastic quadriparesis. Intellectual deterioration is slow, but the children become mentally incompetent by age 6 years. The sensory system is preserved. Duration of the disease is variable; the course tends to be prolonged with remissions. Patients may live 2 to 3 decades or longer.

OPHTHALMIC MANIFESTATIONS. The distinctive ophthalmic manifestation is "eye rolling"—peculiar abnormal arrhythmic eye movements. Eye rolling is noted shortly after birth, but it may disappear with increasing age. Sometimes rotatory movements of the head are associated with the abnormal movements of the eyes.

Optic atrophy commonly develops, but it is a late manifestation in this disease, and useful vision is usually retained.

Canavan's Disease

Canavan's disease, or spongy degeneration of white matter, is an unusual neurologic disorder of childhood that predominantly affects Jews. Progressive megalocephaly, psychomotor deterioration, blindness, and death as the result of demyelination and vacuolation of white matter are principal features of the disease. The disorder is familial and is probably autosomal recessive.

THE DISEASE PROCESS. The etiology of Canavan's disease is unknown, but it appears to be a disorder of myelin metabolism. It is characterized by widespread loss of myelin without loss of axis cylinders. There is extensive spongy vacuolation of white matter throughout the neural axis, particularly in the cerebellum and brain stem. The vacuolations appear to be free of storage material; the spaces are empty to all stains. There is also an increase in glial tissue in the white matter. The process gives the brain a soggy gelatinous appearance, and the size and weight of the brain are increased.

CLINICAL MANIFESTATIONS. Manifestations of the disease develop in infancy, usually between the second and eighteenth months. In the early stages there is a retardation or arrest of psychomotor development. Abilities such as grasping, visual fixation and following, smiling, and cooing may be acquired but are soon lost. Motor activity and tone are diminished, and there is lack of head control. Early hypotonia gives way to spasticity, first in the lower and then the upper extremities. There is progression to spastic quadriparesis. Seizures develop, and there may be signs of autonomic dysfunction. Frequently, megalocephaly and separation of cranial sutures occur owing to the increasing size of the edematous brain and the increasing intracranial pressure. Feeding becomes difficult because of pseudobulbar palsies. The changes are slowly progressive. In the late stages, the children show little response to stimuli, and the subacute deterioration terminates in decerebrate rigidity and death by age 2 to 6 years.

OPHTHALMIC MANIFESTATIONS. Blindness develops early in the course of the disease. Optic atrophy and retinal abnormalities are common. Vacuolation of the ganglion cell layer of the retina occurs, and supposedly this change is detectable by slit lamp examination. Strabismus, roving eye movements, and nystagmus may develop.

Demyelinating Scleroses

The demyelinating scleroses are myelinoclastic diseases. They are characterized by the destruction of presumably normally formed myelin as the result of exogenous agents or abnormal catabolic processes. Although the precise etiology of the myelin destruction and white matter degeneration in the demyelinating scleroses remains obscure, the theories of pathogenesis include viral infection, autoimmune reaction to some component of myelin, or the destructive effect of an enzyme present in blood or cerebrospinal fluid. The pathologic changes in these demyelinating disorders tend to be multifocal and perivascular, and in some there is evidence of inflammation. Those characterized by perivascular inflammation may well be autoimmune disorders. Unlike most of the degenerative diseases, the demyelinating scleroses do not appear to be familial. The principal demyelinating scleroses, also referred to as demyelinizing encephalomyelopathies, are Schilder's disease, multiple sclerosis, and Devic's disease. Other myelinoclastic diseases which may be considered with the scleroses are the disseminated encephalomyelitides that follow infection, the acute necrotizing hemorrhagic leukoencephalitis of Hurst, and Dawson's subacute sclerosing panencephalitis; it is preferable, however, to describe the latter separately, because of the distinctive nature of the disease process (p. 529).

Schilder's Disease

Schilder's disease is a rapidly progressive myelinoclastic disease of unknown etiology that characteristically produces motor paralysis, mental incapacity, blindness, and death within a period of 1 or 2 years.

Fortunately the disease is relatively rare, and it is nonfamilial. It occurs most commonly in childhood, and affects both sexes equally.

Schilder's disease is also referred to as encephalitis periaxialis diffusa, or Schilder's cerebral sclerosis.

PATHOLOGIC FEATURES. The basic pathologic process is primary demyelination with reactive gliosis. Subcortical white matter of the cerebral hemispheres is the predominant area of involvement. Usually the cerebral lesions are well demarcated; they typically extend up to but not beyond arcuate fibers. The myelin sheaths undergo destruction with little damage to the axis cylinders. There is perivascular reaction of varying degree, and the macrophages contain sudanophilic neutral fat products of myelin destruction. Anisomorphic gliosis occurs in response to the process, giving rise to the descriptive term cerebral sclerosis. The cerebellum is less severely involved, and the spinal cord and brain stem are more rarely affected. Lesions also occur in the optic nerves, in the chiasm and optic tracts, and in the visual cortex.

GENERAL CLINICAL MANIFESTATIONS. Clinical manifestations usually commence in the first decade of life; they vary with the site, extent, and progression of the demyelinating lesions. Motor disturbances, vision disturbances, mental deterioration, and personality alterations are common early signs of the disease. With progressive internal capsule involvement there may be monoparesis, hemiparesis, quadriparesis, or decerebrate rigidity.

Dysphasias, agnosias, apraxias, and emotional lability are common. Suprabulbar signs such as sucking, snout, and palmomental reflexes also develop. Cerebellar signs such as nystagmus, tremor, and scanning speech are infrequent. There may be nonspecific changes on EEG, but clinical seizures rarely develop. Often there is increased intracranial pressure with increased cerebrospinal fluid protein and some monocytes, and possibly increased CSF gamma globulin.

The disease progresses relentlessly without remission. The children become spastic, mentally incapacitated, and comatose. Death occurs within 1 to 2 years of onset, often as the result of intercurrent infection.

OPHTHALMIC MANIFESTATIONS. Vision defects are frequent and often early signs of the disease. Cortical blindness and homonymous defects occur with the cortical involvement. Retrobulbar neuritis and chiasmal syndromes may develop. Optic atrophy and central scotomas are common, but disc edema of active neuritis is rarer. There may also be disturbances of cortical gaze functions. Extraocular muscle palsies of stem involvement are less likely to occur.

Multiple Sclerosis

Multiple sclerosis is a demyelinating disease that is relatively rare in childhood, occurring most commonly in early adult life, but it may present in the first or second decade.

Remitting episodes of varied neurologic symptoms giving evidence of multiple sites of neurologic involvement are typical. Vision loss due to optic neuritis is one of the most frequent of these manifestations.

PATHOLOGIC FEATURES. The etiology of multiple sclerosis is unknown, but pathologically the disease is characterized by disseminated areas of demyelination and glial tissue formation in the white matter and, to a lesser extent, in the gray matter of segmental portions of the brain and cord. Plaques may be found principally in the cerebral hemispheres (commonly near the margin of the ventricles), in the basal ganglia, in the pons and medulla, and in the optic nerves, chiasm, and tracts. Early and late lesions are found interspersed. In early lesions the axons may be tortuous and swollen, showing disintegration of their myelin sheaths, but axons persist to a remarkable degree. In older lesions glial proliferation of varying degree is found. Cavity formation does not occur.

GENERAL CLINICAL MANIFESTATIONS. As the lesions are of rather widespread and haphazard distribution, a variety of manifestations of graded severity occur. There may be minimal symptoms such as transient diplopia, limb weakness, sensory disturbance, or unsteadiness. Spastic paraplegia, cerebellar ataxia, intention tremor, numbness and paresthesias, and sphincter disturbances may develop. Emotional instability is common. Although in the chronic remitting form of the disease there may be long periods of complete or relative freedom from symptoms, the usual course over the years is one of progressive disability. The patients eventually may become incapacitated and bedridden; the prognosis generally is unfavorable.

During active stages, there may be an increase in spinal fluid protein with a positive globulin reaction.

OPHTHALMIC MANIFESTATIONS. The principal ophthalmic manifestation of multiple sclerosis is retrobulbar neuritis, and in the younger age group this is the usual manner of presentation of the disease. The neuritis is unilateral more often than bilateral. Typically there is an acute and severe loss of vision, often preceded or accompanied by retrobulbar pain. The vision may rapidly be reduced to only light perception, but the tendency is for recovery; improvement may begin in days or weeks. Recurrences are usual, but periods of remission may last for as long as several years. With recurrent episodes there may be progressive permanent loss of vision.

Ophthalmoscopic signs are variable. During active neuritis the discs usually appear normal, but there may be disc edema or neuroretinal edema. Eventually disc pallor and atrophy may develop. Some patients with multiple sclerosis exhibit sheathing of peripheral retinal vessels, unrelated to the episodes of optic neuritis.

The usual field defect is a central scotoma that tends to be rather dense. Less common are junction scotomas, bitemporal hemianopias, and homonymous hemianopias.

Nystagmus is one of the most frequent manifestations of the disease. It is commonly present in the early stages, and it may remain permanently. The rapid and jerky oscillations may be horizontal, vertical, or mixed.

There may be supranuclear palsies of lateral or of vertical gaze. Frequently there is internuclear ophthalmoplegia; bilateral internuclear ophthalmoplegia is characteristic of multiple sclerosis, whereas unilateral internuclear ophthalmoplegia is usually indicative of vascular disease.

Paralysis of individual extraocular muscles also occurs in multiple sclerosis. Abduction weakness and ptosis are most frequent.

Devic's Disease (Neuromyelitis Optica)

Devic's disease, or neuromyelitis optica, is a demyelinating disease characterized by optic neuritis and transverse myelitis of varying severity. A sudden episode of vision loss and paraplegia, simultaneously or sequentially, in a child or young adult, is typical of the disease.

Neuromyelitis optica occurs sporadically, and its etiology is unknown.

PATHOLOGIC FEATURES. Neuromyelitis optica is a myelinoclastic disorder. There are scattered demyelinating lesions in the brain, in the optic nerves, and in the spinal cord. The process affects predominantly the white matter, but it may also involve the gray matter. There is generally widespread destruction of myelin sheaths and some destruction of axis cylinders, often with perivascular lymphocytosis. Liquefaction and cavity formation are common. Gliosis occurs in varying degrees; glial tissue formation is not common in fulminating cases, but it is present in cases of mild or moderate severity. The pathologic process may be reflected in the spinal fluid with mild pleocytosis, increased fat content, and increased pressure.

CLINICAL MANIFESTATIONS. The predominant clinical manifestations are vision loss and paraplegia. The two may occur simultaneously, but most often the vision loss precedes the paraplegia by an interval of days, weeks, or months.

THE MYELITIS AND PARAPLEGIA. The myelitis can be mild or severe; often the spinal cord is extensively affected. The onset of the paraplegia usually is sudden, and it may be accompanied by some temperature elevation and severe root pain. Generally there is recovery of function, but there may be residual deficits of minor or severe degree, and there may be recurrences of the myelitis with or without recurrences of the optic neuritis. Also, the myelitis can ascend to affect respiration, sometimes resulting in death.

THE OPTIC NEURITIS AND VISION LOSS. The optic neuritis is typically bilateral, affecting both eyes simultaneously, though involvement of one eye may precede that of its fellow by days or weeks. The involvement may be unequal, and in some cases the vision loss is truly unilateral. The vision loss usually develops rapidly and painlessly, and progresses to an extreme degree, sometimes resulting in complete bilateral blindness. Improvement of vision may commence within 1 or several weeks, but it may take months to reach its maximum. Good recovery of vision occurs in many cases, but there may be permanent residua of varying severity, and there may be recurrences of the optic neuritis. In general, the prognosis for vision is only fairly good in Devic's disease.

Ophthalmoscopic findings related to the optic neuritis are variable. During the acute episode there is usually low grade or marked edema of the discs; in some cases the discs appear normal. Later in the process, there may be some pallor of the discs and some narrowing of the vessels, especially in those cases terminating in permanent reduction of vision.

Field defects in Devic's disease are variable. Transient or permanent central scotomas related to the optic neuritis are the most frequent defects, but there may be other defects as a result of the widespread and irregular nature of the foci of demyelination in this disease.

ADDITIONAL OPHTHALMIC MANIFESTATIONS. Extrinsic ocular muscle palsies, conjugate gaze palsies, nystagmus, and pupillary abnormalities may develop in Devic's disease. The extrinsic ocular muscle and conjugate gaze palsies are infrequent; they are usually a sign of brain stem involvement. Nystagmus is infrequent. The pupillary abnormalities are not distinctive; they most often reflect primarily the afferent dysfunction of the optic neuritis, but they may also develop as a sign of efferent dysfunction.

Special Types of Neurodegenerative Diseases and Neuroabiotrophies

Many of the degenerative diseases and neuroabiotrophies require special classification because of the distinctive nature of either the etiology or the clinicopathologic expression of the disease process. Such conditions, to name just a few, are Dawson's disease, a cerebral degeneration related to slow measles virus infection; Leigh's disease, a cerebral degeneration characterized by specific chemical abnormalities reflecting a disturbance of pyruvate metabolism; Wilson's disease, a degenerative process resulting from a disorder of copper metabolism; the Bassen-Kornzweig syndrome, a disorder characterized by abetalipoproteinemia and acanthocytosis; and the Louis-Bar syndrome of ataxia telangiectasia. Traditionally, many of the disorders relegated to this "special" category would be classified separately as exogenous cerebral degenerations, as progressive extrapyramidal syndromes, as spinocerebellar degenerations, and as cranial and peripheral nerve degenerations, the latter group including the abiotrophies commonly referred to as the congenital sensory neuropathies (Tables 18–12 and 18–13).

Dawson's Disease
(Van Bogaert's Disease; Subacute Sclerosing Panencephalitis)

Subacute sclerosing panencephalitis (SSPE), generally classified as a degenerative disease of childhood, is a progressive neurologic disorder caused by a slow measles virus infection of the central nervous system. It is characterized by deterioration of mental and motor abilities. In many children, vision loss and focal retinitis are prominent features of the disease.

PATHOLOGIC FEATURES. The major abnormalities are in the cerebral cortex and in the subcortical white matter. The brain typically shows changes of a chronic inflammatory process, with neuronal degeneration, demyelination, gliosis, and perivascular and leptomeningeal lymphocytic infiltration. A characteristic finding is the presence of eosinophilic inclusion bodies in the nuclei and cytoplasm of both the neurons and glia of the cerebral hemispheres. These inclusion bodies are the type seen in virus diseases, and the measles virus (rubeola) has been recovered from brain tissue of several patients with SSPE. These patients show high levels of measles antibody in serum and in cerebrospinal fluid, and the spinal fluid gamma globulin is often elevated.

CLINICAL MANIFESTATIONS. SSPE usually develops before age 11 years, and it affects boys more often than girls. As a rule, the disease begins with the development of an organic mental syndrome characterized by intellectual decline and personality and behavioral changes. Indifference and blunting of emotions, withdrawal, sleepiness, forgetfulness, and regression of speech commonly are the early signs; some children tend to be irritable and agitated. The onset usually is insidious, but in some cases the disease presents rather suddenly with seizures, motor disturbances, or vision loss.

Subsequently, myoclonus of the head, limbs, and trunk develops, and the EEG shows periodic discharges that are characteristic of, but not pathognomonic for, SSPE. The course is then one of subacute progressive deterioration of mental and motor function over a period of weeks, months, or years. Apraxia, truncal and limb incoordination, choreo-athetoid movements, spatial disorientation, motor aphasia, slurring of speech, and drooling develop. The motor abnormalities become severe and decerebrate rigidity and decorticate postures develop. Terminal bouts of hyperthermia, hypertension, and tachypnea occur. Death is usually attributed to hypothalamic dysfunction with hyperthermia and with vasomotor and cardiovascular collapse.

OPHTHALMIC MANIFESTATIONS. A frequent ocular finding associated with SSPE is focal retinitis. The retinal inflammation usually involves the macular or paramacular region, but peripheral lesions also are described. The lesions usually are bilateral, but commonly one eye is affected before the other. Most often, the retinitis is symptomatic, with loss of vision of varying severity. Ophthalmoscopically the picture is one of active inflammation and edema proceeding to pigmentary changes and chorioretinal scar formation. The macular findings may be not unlike the appearance of vitelliform degeneration or the Spiel-

(Text continued on page 533)

TABLE 18–12 THE EXTRAPYRAMIDAL SYNDROMES: BASAL GANGLIA DEGENERATIONS

Designation	Predominant Pathologic Features	General Clinical Manifestations	Ophthalmic Manifestations
Wilson's Disease	Disorder of copper metabolism with abnormal accumulation of copper affecting principally the brain, liver, kidney, and cornea. Spongy degeneration and gliosis affecting primarily the putamen, globus pallidus, and caudate nucleus, but disease widespread.	Onset usually in second decade. In juveniles (age 7 to 15 years), hepatic disease often the presenting manifestation, preceding the development of generalized muscular rigidity and bulbar signs; sometimes mental changes. In adults, typically tremor of wrists, "wing beating," of shoulders, and dysarthria. Autosomal recessive.	Kayser-Fleischer ring: copper deposition in peripheral region of Descement's membrane of cornea; regularly associated with neurologic form, but not uniformly present in hepatic form. "Sunflower cataract." Nightblinding retinal degeneration (rarely).
Dystonia Musculorum Deformans	Degeneration, demyelinization, and gliosis involving principally the putamen, caudate nucleus, and dentate nucleus.	Age of onset usually 5 to 10 years or later; sometimes commences shortly after birth. In early stages, pes cavus, muscle spasm causing flexion at hip with adduction, and lordosis. Progressive development of involuntary movements involving primarily proximal segments of limbs and trunk, generally sparing the face, fingers, and speech organs. Axial torsion characceristic; also torticollis. Sometimes rigidity and fixed deformities such as kyphosis and scoliosis. In later stages, some evidence of mental deterioration. Course variable: usually progressive, often resulting in incapacitation within 6 to 8 years; less commonly, stationary for years. Dominant inheritance.	Ocular motor abnormalities.

Hallervorden-Spatz Disease	Degeneration of globus pallidus and reticular zone of substantia nigra characterized by rust-brown discoloration (hyperpigmentation) and pseudocalcareous changes.	Onset at about age 10 years. Progressive rigidity, and, to a lesser degree, hyperkinesia, choreoathetosis, and dystonia. Early involvement of speech. Progressive mental deterioration. Death after course of 10 to 20 years. Familial.	Vision impairment. Optic pallor. Pigmentary retinal degeneration.
Huntington's Chorea	Degeneration of corpus striatum with generalized loss of small ganglion cells and reactive gliosis. Diffuse cortical atrophy.	Childhood onset in only small percentage of cases. In adults, hyperkinesis with choreatic movements affecting primarily the face and distal members of the extremities; progressive mental deterioration, dysarthria. Less commonly, rigidity. In children, usually hypokinesia, muscular rigidity, progressive dementia or personality disturbance, seizures, dystonic posturing. Often without choreatic movements. Generally fatal within 15 years of onset; sooner when disease begins in childhood. Autosomal dominant.	Pseudo-ophthalmoplegia, particularly of vertical gaze. Spasmodic twitching of eyelids.
Parkinson's Disease (Paralysis Agitans)	Degeneration of substantia nigra and other pigmented nuclei of extrapyramidal system.	Rarely evident in early years as a juvenile form; more typically a disease of middle and late life. Tremor, muscular rigidity with cogwheel phenomenon, and akinesia dominate the clinical picture. Pseudobulbar signs in advanced stages.	Oculogyric crises. Impairment of voluntary horizontal or vertical gaze. Jerkiness of eye movements. Infrequent blinking, blepharoplegia – or blepharospasm.

TABLE 18–13　THE HEREDITARY ATAXIA SYNDROMES: SPINOCEREBELLAR DEGENERATIONS

Designation	Predominant Pathology	General Clinical Manifestations	Ophthalmic Manifestations
Friedreich's Ataxia	Progressive atrophy of the long ascending and descending tracts of the spinal cord (dorsal columns, spinocerebellar tracts, pyramidal tracts).	Onset in first or second decade. Ataxia of gait, clumsiness of hands, dysarthria, nystagmus. Deep tendon reflexes absent or diminished. Pes cavus. Kyphoscoliosis. Relentlessly progressive course leading to incapacitation within 5 years; death in the third decade or sooner. Dominant or recessive transmission, affecting males more often than females.	Nystagmus universally present. Infrequently, retinal pigmentary degeneration or optic neuritis, or both, with progressive loss of central and peripheral vision. Possibly ophthalmoplegia.
Hereditary Cerebellar Ataxia: Types of Marie and of Sanger-Brown	Cerebellar atrophy without changes in posterior columns and posterior roots.	Onset in childhood in small percentage of cases; typically commences in early adult life (16 to 35 years). Ataxia with spasticity and hyperactive deep tendon reflexes. In contrast to Friedreich type, absence of skeletal deformities. Slowly progressive course. Eventually bulbar signs, mental deterioration, incapacitation. Usually a simple recessive; alternatively dominant or X-linked.	Optic atrophy, loss of vision, concentric contraction of field early in course. Sometimes pigmentary retinal degeneration. Nystagmus not a typical feature. Extraocular muscle palsies. Possibly internal ophthalmoplegia.
Behr's Syndrome		Onset in first decade. Hypertonia of extremities, increased tendon reflexes, mild ataxia, bladder disturbances, mental deterioration.	Progressive optic atrophy. Nystagmus.
Louis-Bar Syndrome	Atrophy of cerebellum without marked changes in spinal cord.	Onset in first decade. Cerebellar ataxia, choreoathetosis, dysarthria, drooling, combined with oculocutaneous telangiectasias, hypogammaglobulinemia and and recurrent sinopulmonary infections. Mental and physical retardation. Incapacitation and death within a few years. Malignancies in significant percentage of cases. Autosomal recessive.	Conjunctival telangiectasias developing at 4 to 6 years of age. Apraxia of gaze without head thrust. Nystagmus. Strabismus.
Marinesco-Sjögren Syndrome	Cortical atrophy of cerebellum.	Onset in early childhood. Marked ataxia, hypotonia, and weakness, more pronounced in legs than in arms. Retarded physical and mental development. Sometimes cranial nerve dysfunction. Occasionally skeletal anomalies, dental anomalies, microcephaly. Autosomal recessive.	Progressive cataractous changes in childhood, often evident by age 2 to 3 years. Possibly vertical gaze impairment, gaze nystagmus, convergence deficiency, strabismus.

meyer-Vogt type of macular degeneration. There may appear to be a hole, a moth-eaten focal lesion, or nonspecific "salt-and-pepper" changes. Hemorrhages and vitreous reaction are not usual with the retinitis of SSPE.

Pathologically the lesions are characterized by edema and neuronal loss. Circumscribed retinal atrophy, macular necrosis with hole formation, thinning and disorganization, and gliosis of the retina have been described. There may be a retinal infiltrate of plasma cells and lymphocytes adjacent to the necrosis. Inclusion bodies in ganglion and bipolar cells of the retina adjacent to areas of necrosis have been identified. The choroid is minimally involved.

In addition there may be disc edema, as the result of the neuroretinal edema or inflammatory involvement of the optic nerve itself. Perivascular lymphocytic infiltration of the optic nerve has been described. There may be papilledema of increased intracranial pressure due to the cerebral edema. Optic pallor and atrophy may develop.

With the cerebral inflammation, there may be cortical blindness or field defects.

Also reported with SSPE are nystagmus, ptosis, and ocular motor palsies, implying stem or cerebellar involvement.

Leigh's Disease
(Subacute Necrotizing Encephalomyelopathy)

Leigh's subacute necrotizing encephalomyelopathy is a fatal hereditary metabolic disease of infancy and childhood. The principal manifestations are hypotonia, periodic acidosis, progressive motor deterioration, and bouts of respiratory embarrassment. Ocular motor palsies, abnormal eye movements, and progressive optic atrophy are prominent signs of the disease.

THE DISEASE PROCESS. The primary metabolic defect and pathogenesis of Leigh's disease are unknown. A variety of biochemical and enzymatic abnormalities have been reported. The presence of lactic acidemia, pyruvic acidemia, and alaninemia in subacute necrotizing encephalomyelopathy indicates a defect in pyruvate metabolism, and treatment with thiamine and lipoic acid has yielded temporary improvement in some cases.

The characteristic pathologic finding in Leigh's disease is symmetrical microcystic degeneration at many levels of the neural axis; there is neuronal loss, demyelination, neovascularization, and glial proliferation. Both white and gray matter can be affected. There is predilection for involvement of basal ganglia, brain stem, spinal cord, cerebellum, and anterior visual pathways. Partial and complete necrosis of cranial nerve nuclei, demyelination of cranial nerves, segmental demyelination of the optic nerve, chiasm, and optic tract, and diminution of the retinal ganglion cell and nerve fiber population have been reported and are of importance with regard to neuro-ophthalmic manifestations of the disease. The mamillary bodies and cerebral cortex are usually spared.

GENERAL CLINICAL MANIFESTATIONS. The predominant clinical manifestations of Leigh's disease are hypotonia, hyporeflexia, and progressive motor deterioration. Signs of the disease appear between ages 2 months and 6 years. The onset is often insidious, with such nonspecific signs as failure to thrive, weakness, and fatigability. There is progressive impairment of muscle tone and loss of deep tendon reflexes, and the hypotonia and weakness become severe. Ataxia of the head, limbs, and trunk develop. Developmental progress ceases. Feeding difficulties, anorexia, weight loss, apathy, and lethargy are common. There may be loss of vision and hearing, and abnormalities of eye movements often develop. Periodic bouts of dyspnea, tachypnea, and peculiar sobbing respirations occur. In general, the clinical course is one of progressive deterioration over a period of several weeks to several years, but the deterioration is often remittent, with temporary improvement of function. Ultimately there is death, usually as the result of respiratory failure.

OPHTHALMIC MANIFESTATIONS. The principal ophthalmic manifestations of Leigh's encephalomyelopathy are abnormal eye movements, ocular motor palsies, and loss of vision. Horizontal and vertical nystagmus, bizarre rolling eye movements, saccadic ocular movements, and dysjunctive eye movements have been reported. Blepharoptosis, strabismus, and even complete external ophthalmoplegia may develop. Progressive optic atrophy and clinical evidence of visual impairment develop in many patients. Loss of the foveal light reflex and diminution of the macular ganglion cell heap may provide an early clue to the anterior visual pathway involvement. There may also be abnormalities of the pupils; it would seem that both afferent and efferent dysfunction can be implicated.

Wilson's Disease (Hepatolenticular Degeneration)

Wilson's disease is a rare hereditary disorder of copper metabolism. Progressive degeneration of the brain, especially of the basal ganglia, and cirrhosis of the liver are the predominant effects of the disorder, and Kayser-Fleischer rings of the corneas are a pathognomonic sign of the disease.

This condition is inherited as an autosomal recessive. It affects primarily young people and it occurs throughout the world.

THE METABOLIC DISORDER AND ITS PATHOLOGY. The precise etiology and pathogenesis of Wilson's disease are obscure but there are several biochemical and pathologic features common to the disorder. A characteristic finding is decreased levels of ceruloplasmin, the specific α_{-2}-globulin to which the majority of serum copper normally is bound. In persons homozygous for Wilson's disease, the ceruloplasmin may be absent, low, or near normal; it is usually less than 25 per cent of normal values. There is also often a deficiency of ceruloplasmin in healthy heterozygous carriers of the disease. The copper content of the serum is usually low, though it may be normal or elevated, and there is usually increased excretion of copper in the urine. There characteristically is increased tissue content of copper, and accumulation of copper in body tissues resulting in dysfunction appears to be progressive with increasing age.

The tissues most affected are the liver, brain, kidney, and cornea; the copper content of these tissues may reach 10- to 100-fold normal levels. In the liver, the copper is deposited in the parenchymal cells, and cirrhosis ensues; the abnormality can be detected by hepatic function tests, by liver biopsy, and by tissue copper determination. In the brain, the copper is deposited primarily in the glial cell, but there is also deterioration of neurons. Copper can be deposited in large quantities in the cerebral cortex, resulting in loss of neurons,

spongy degeneration, and gliosis, but it is the basal ganglia that appear to suffer most. The putamen, globus pallidus, and caudate nucleus become shrunken and discolored. In the eye, the copper deposition occurs in the posterior region of Descemet's membrane.

Reduction of tissue stores of copper and elimination of excess copper from the body are the aims of therapy; the use of BAL or penicillamine, and restriction of copper in the diet are relatively effective measures.

VISCERAL CLINICAL MANIFESTATIONS. Clinical manifestations of Wilson's disease rarely appear before age 6 years. In children the first sign of the disease is often jaundice or hepatomegaly due to cirrhosis. In severe cases there may be esophageal varices and hemorrhages secondary to portal hypertension. Hemolytic anemia, thrombocytopenia, hypersplenism, and splenomegaly are also common manifestations of the disease. There may also be renal manifestations characterized by albuminuria, aminoaciduria, glycosuria, and hypercalcinuria. In severe longstanding disease, there may be osteomalacia and spontaneous fractures due to impaired renal handling of phosphate and calcium.

NEUROLOGIC MANIFESTATIONS. Neurologic manifestations of Wilson's disease can develop in children, but they more commonly develop in young adults. With progressive nervous system involvement there may be disturbances of behavior, personality, and intellect. There may be progressive dementia during the school years, and psychiatric derangement occurs in some cases. The more common and predominant neurologic manifestations of Wilson's disease, however, are motor abnormalities due to pathologic changes in the basal ganglia. Spasticity and muscular rigidity develop. Dysarthria, drooling, dysphagia, and dystonic postures are common, and there may be seizures. In some patients, flapping tremors of the wrists and shoulders are the predominant sign.

OCULAR MANIFESTATIONS. The pathognomonic ocular sign of Wilson's disease is the Kayser-Fleischer (K.F.) ring. The ring is due to deposition of copper in the periphery of Descemet's membrane, particularly in its deepest zone adjacent to the endothelium. On slit lamp examination the deposits are visible as granules of golden brown, greenish brown, or grayish brown hue owing to the reflection and scattering of light. Often the ring is incomplete, and it is best seen superiorly and inferiorly. Sometimes the ring is visible without biomicroscopy, but slit lamp examination is essential to precise description and diagnosis of the corneal ring. Usually the K.F. ring is present when there are other clinical signs of the disease, but it may be absent when the patient is examined, and the absence of the ring does not exclude the diagnosis of Wilson's disease. Every child presenting with liver disease, a movement disorder, or mental changes should be examined for K.F. ring. The corneal ring may diminish with treatment of the disease.

Another ocular sign of Wilson's disease is the Sonnenblumenkatarakt, a cataract like that seen with intraocular copper foreign body. This sign is rare.

It should also be noted here that a complication of treatment of Wilson's disease with penicillamine is optic neuritis; this complication can be reversed with pyridoxine.

Bassen-Kornzweig Syndrome (Abetalipoproteinemia)

The Bassen-Kornzweig syndrome is characterized principally by five major features: abetalipoproteinemia, fat malabsorption, acanthocytosis, atypical retinitis pigmentosa, and progressive ataxic neuropathic disease. This rare disorder is genetically determined and appears to be autosomal recessive.

THE DISEASE PROCESS. The exact pathogenesis of the disease is unknown, and relatively little is known of its pathology. An important feature is inability to form chylomicrons. Affected patients digest glycerides, absorb the resulting monoglycerides and free fatty acids into the intestinal mucosa cells, and reform them into triglycerides, but fail to release chylomicrons. The liver, like the intestinal mucosa, is able to produce and store glycerides but cannot transfer the lipid into the plasma. The serum is deficient in betalipoprotein. Plasma levels of cholesterol are extremely low, and the plasma and tissue phospholipids are unusually low in essential fatty acids. A distinctive pathologic finding in

the jejunum is the presence of lipid droplets in the mucosal cells, a finding related to the defect in removal from this site. In the nervous system, reported pathologic findings include degeneration and demyelination of the anterior columns and of the spinocerebellar tracts and cerebellum, and patchy focal demyelination of peripheral neurons.

The erythrocytes of the peripheral blood have thornlike projections (acanthocytosis).

CLINICAL MANIFESTATIONS. The first signs of the disorder usually are steatorrhea and abdominal distention mimicking the celiac syndrome in an infant or child who appeared normal at birth. The signs of malabsorption generally become less marked with age. Growth failure is usual. In infancy there may be recurrent infections. Cardiac failure of unknown etiology may develop. With time, neurologic manifestations develop, often appearing by age 5 to 10 years and progressing slowly until adulthood. The usual signs are areflexia, proprioceptive defects, progressive cerebellar dysfunction marked by tremors and ataxia, muscle weakness, ophthalmoparesis, Babinski reflexes, and cutaneous sensory defects. Although cerebral abnormalities are not a regular feature of the syndrome, there may be intellectual deficiency and retardation of development. Frequently there is kyphoscoliosis.

The disease may lead to death in early childhood or there may be survival into adulthood.

OPHTHALMIC MANIFESTATIONS. The principal ophthalmic manifestation of abetalipoproteinemia is pigmentary retinal degeneration with progressive impairment of visual function. The changes are age-related. The fundus appearance and vision usually are normal in early childhood, and show progressive deterioration after age 4 to 5 years, often much later. Night blindness is an early symptom. Decreasing visual acuity and field defects, particularly ring scotomas and concentric contraction, develop with advancing age and are generally evident by adolescence. There may be deficiency of color vision.

The fundus changes consist of depigmentation and granular pigment clumping at both the posterior pole and in the periphery, with diminution or loss of the foveal reflex, attenuation of the retinal arterioles, and pallor of the disc. Pathologically, extensive macular atrophy has been demonstrated.

There is some evidence that vitamin A therapy may favorably influence dark adaptation and night vision in this condition.

In addition to the retinal degeneration there may be cataracts, nystagmus, ptosis, and paresis of the extrinsic ocular muscles.

Refsum's Syndrome (Heredopathia Atactica Polyneuritiformis)

The Refsum syndrome is a familial disorder of lipid metabolism characterized by peripheral polyneuropathy, cerebellar ataxia, retinitis pigmentosa, increased cerebrospinal fluid protein without pleocytosis, and in some cases, ichthyosis. The condition is autosomal recessive.

THE DISEASE PROCESS. Metabolically the disorder is characterized by a deficiency of phytanic acid α-hydrolase activity and impaired oxidation of phytanic acid, a C_{20} branched-chain fatty acid. There are increased levels of phytanic acid in the plasma and abnormal accumulations of phytanic acid in tissues, especially in the liver and kidney.

The pathologic picture is one of hypertrophic interstitial polyneuropathy with neuronal muscular atrophy. The peripheral nerves appear swollen and thickened, and on cross section the nerve fibers appear to be ensheathed by concentric lamellae. There is evidence of degeneration and thinning of myelin, wallerian degeneration of nerve fibers, and some regeneration of nerve fibers. Atrophy of the ventral horns of the spinal cord and degeneration of brain stem tracts can be seen.

A significant laboratory finding is the presence of increased spinal fluid protein without pleocytosis.

CLINICAL MANIFESTATIONS. Signs and symptoms of the disease may appear at any age, usually before age 20 years, and often between ages 4 and 8 years. Failing vision, weakness in the extremities, and unsteadiness of gait are the common presenting manifestations. Polyneuritis-like changes produce sensory and motor deficits, areflexia, and sometimes lightning pains; the process generally is symmetrical and tends to be most marked in the lower limbs. Cerebellar signs, namely ataxia, intention tremor, and sometimes nystagmus, develop. Progressive nerve deafness and anosmia are common features. Often there is ECG evidence of cardiac abnormality, particularly conduction defects. In some cases, ichthyosis-like change of the skin develops, ranging in severity from mild hyperkeratosis of the palms and soles to florid ichthyosis involving the trunk. In addition there may be epiphyseal dysplasia, syndactyly, hammer toe, pes cavus, osteochondritis dissecans, or shortness of the fourth metatarsal.

The course usually is one of gradually progressive deterioration, though in some cases the disease runs a relapsing course marked by remissions and exacerbations. Death may result from heart failure or respiratory paralysis.

OPHTHALMIC MANIFESTATIONS. The principal ophthalmic signs and symptoms in the Refsum syndrome are pigmentary retinal degeneration with progressive impairment of night vision and constriction of the visual field. The visual symptoms commonly develop early in childhood. The retinal degeneration is marked by pronounced arterial narrowing, optic atrophy, and pigment clumping; the bone corpuscle pigment aggregates typical of classical retinitis pigmentosa usually are absent. The ERG response is reduced or absent.

There may be vitreous opacities, cataractous changes, cornea guttata, and pupillary abnormalities, namely miosis.

In some cases ophthalmopareses develop. Infrequently there is nystagmus.

Louis-Bar Syndrome (Ataxia Telangiectasia)

Progressive cerebellar atrophy and ataxia, oculocutaneous telangiectasias, and hypogammaglobulinemia with increased susceptibility to sinopulmonary infections are the major manifestations of the Madame Louis-Bar syndrome. Abnormal eye movements are a frequent neuro-ophthalmic sign of the disorder.

Ataxia telangiectasia is inherited as an autosomal recessive condition. It affects both sexes and may occur in several members of a family.

THE NERVOUS SYSTEM PATHOLOGY AND ITS MANIFESTATIONS. The pathologic changes in the nervous system are atrophy of the cerebellar cortex with loss of Purkinje cells, neuronal dystrophy in the medulla and degeneration in the dentate and inferior olivary nuclei, and demyelination in the posterior columns of the spinal cord. There may also be enlargement of the venules in the cerebellar leptomeninges and white matter.

Neurologic manifestations usually commence early in childhood. Ataxia often develops when the child is just learning to walk, and it initially affects primarily stance and gait. The children develop a stooped appearance. Intention tremor and choreic and athetoid movements follow, and worsen with age. Spasticity—especially of the lower extremities—and areflexia develop in some cases. By age 10 or 11 years the cerebellar dysfunction usually is severe and incapacitating. Scanning speech and drooling are common. Sensation, cranial nerve function, and intellect are not impaired, but the children tend to have a dull affect and an equable disposition.

CUTANEOUS SIGNS. A characteristic feature of the syndrome is telangiectasias that develop in the skin of the face, commonly in the butterfly distribution, the ears, the soft palate, the inner surfaces of the elbows and knees, and the dorsum of the hands. There may also be café au lait spots.

OPHTHALMIC MANIFESTATIONS. Disturbances of conjugate eye movements, essentially an apraxia of gaze, occur in ataxia telangiectasia. The children show inability to execute voluntary gaze movements rapidly and smoothly on command; they can achieve full excursions with great effort or during casual gaze. Horizontal and vertical versions are performed in a halting, dyssynergic fashion, without a head thrust. There is difficulty in maintaining eccentric gaze. Rotations of the body may produce sustained contraversive deviation of the eyes, and the optokinetic nystagmus may be absent. Occasionally there is vertical or horizontal nystagmus and subnormal convergence.

A characteristic finding is the presence of telangiectasias in the bulbar conjunctiva; they are usually evident by age 4 to 6 years.

THE IMMUNOLOGIC DEFECT. Hypogammaglobulinemia characterized by deficient or absent 1A gammaglobulin, and deficiency of thymus tissue with paucity of lymphocytes have been demonstrated in this disorder. The patients suffer recurrent sinopulmonary infections which may result in death by age 12 years. Malignancies have also been reported in the Louis-Bar syndrome; the children show a particular predisposition to leukemia, lymphosarcoma, and basal cell carcinoma.

Death occurs as the result of pulmonary disease, malignancy, or general debilitation.

The Riley-Day Syndrome (Familial Dysautonomia)

The Riley-Day syndrome is a complex neurophysiologic disorder characterized by autonomic dysfunction, relative insensitivity to pain, and absence of the fungiform papillae of the tongue.

The disorder is transmitted as an autosomal recessive condition, with predilection for children of Jewish descent.

NEUROPHYSIOLOGIC ABNORMALITIES. The multiple neurologic abnormalities are present from birth. Characteristically there is lability of blood pressure; postural hypotension is an essential feature of the syndrome, and there often is paroxysmal hypertension or hypertension in response to anxiety. Transient skin blotching occurs with eating or excitement. Hyperhidrosis and instability of temperature control are common, and all patients show a deficiency of lacrimation. Reduced sensitivity to pain (or relative indifference to pain) is a constant feature of the syndrome, though there is perception of touch and pinprick. There is deficient taste perception and discrimination, and absence of the fungiform papillae of the tongue is essential to the diagnosis. Some patients also show deficiency of the circumvallate papillae. Emotional lability is a constant feature. Mental ability is usually normal, though some patients are moderately retarded, and many lack facial expression. Hypoactive deep tendon reflexes, poor motor coordination, defective swallowing, and diminished respiratory responses to hypercapnia or hypoxia are additional manifestations.

The basic defect in the Riley-Day syndrome is unknown. Methacholine infusion can, to some degree, correct the taste deficiency, restore the reflexes, produce tearing, and lower the blood pressure. It may also correct the abnormal response to intradermal histamine, as patients with the Riley-Day syndrome characteristically develop little pain or erythema in response to intradermal histamine. Generally, however, the nerve fibers are normal, and cholinesterase is present.

In addition to the neurophysiologic disorders, there may be kyphoscoliosis or hypertelorism, and the patients are often small.

NEURO-OPHTHALMIC MANIFESTATIONS. Two neuro-ophthalmic abnormalities are essential to the Riley-Day syndrome: depressed or absent corneal sensation and defective lacrimation. The eyes of most patients do appear moist on inspection, but there is diminished production of tears in response to irritants, and the response to the Schirmer tear test is subnormal. Also, there is failure to produce overflow tears in response to emotional stimuli. There is, however, plentiful tearing in response to parenteral mecholyl, and the lacrimal glands are histologically normal. Corneal ulceration and opacities of varying severity are common sequelae of the combined effect of defective lacrimation and defective corneal sensitivity. Many patients require treatment with artificial tear preparations.

A variable finding in this syndrome is a pupillary abnormality having features of a tonic pupil; there may be hypersensitivity to 2.5% methacholine, and in some cases there is anisocoria.

The Pinsky-DiGeorge Syndrome (Congenital Familial Sensory Neuropathy with Anhidrosis)

The Pinsky-DiGeorge syndrome is characterized by congenital insensitivity to pain, anhidrosis, recurrent febrile episodes, mental retardation, and defective tearing. Familial incidence of the syndrome has been reported, but the genetic transmission and pathogenesis of the disorder are unknown.

NEUROLOGIC ABNORMALITIES. There is a universal congenital sensory defect characterized by absence of pain perception, absence of physiologic responses to painful stimuli, and impairment of touch and temperature perception. The problem of insensitivity to trauma and pain is com-

pounded by mental retardation, which is a constant feature of the syndrome. Consequently the children suffer chronic sores on pressure points. Self-mutilation is common; the children bite their hands, arms, lips, and tongue. They may develop fractures that can go undetected, resulting in deformities. In addition to the sensory and mental defects, there is absence of sweating to all stimuli; the skin is warm and dry. There is deficiency of lacrimation. There may also be postural hypotension, disturbance of the swallowing reflex, and unexplained bouts of fever.

Neurophysiologic responses to chemical tests are abnormal. There is no axon flare response to intradermal histamine, nor is there sweating in response to intradermal pilocarpine or mecholyl, and thermal and electrical stimuli also fail to produce sweating.

The reason for the neurologic abnormalities is not clear, and pathologic studies have been inconclusive. Normal sweat glands and normal dermal nerve networks have been demonstrated, but in one patient there was absence of Lissauer's tract and absence of small sensory fibers of the dorsal nerve roots. The tongue papillae are normal.

OPHTHALMIC MANIFESTATIONS. The principal ophthalmic manifestations of the Pinsky-DiGeorge syndrome are defective corneal sensation and defective lacrimation. Lacrimation in response to frustration is normal. Mecholyl fails to produce lacrimation.

NEUROMUSCULAR DISORDERS

This section deals only with the disorders of muscle and neuromuscular function that are of principal importance in pediatric ophthalmoneurologic diagnosis. Included are the muscular dystrophies that manifest in childhood, the myotonic syndromes, and myasthenia gravis.

Generalized Familial Muscular Dystrophy of Childhood (Duchenne Pseudohypertrophic Muscular Dystrophy)

Pseudohypertrophic or Duchenne type muscular dystrophy is the most frequent and most severe of the muscular dystrophies. Inherited as a sex-linked recessive disorder affecting predominantly males, the disease is relentlessly progressive and debilitating.

The prominent features are progressive alteration of muscle size and profound weakness of specific muscles. Weakness and wasting typically appear first in the muscles of the pelvic girdle and lumbosacral spine. Involvement of the muscles of the shoulder girdle and the proximal muscles of the limbs follows. Weakness and wasting of the distal muscles of the extremities may be seen later in the course. There may also be involvement of abdominal muscles. Muscles of the face, jaw, larynx, pharynx, and hands generally are spared, but may be affected. Involvement of the extraocular muscles occurs infrequently; in some cases ophthalmoplegia develops.

Certain of the muscles exhibit enlargement or "pseudohypertrophy." Those which most frequently become enlarged are the gastrocnemii, the infraspinati and the deltoids; less commonly the quadriceps, glutii, and triceps are similarly affected. The enlarged muscles possess a firm and resilient quality, but are weak; ultimately they become atrophied and wasted.

The etiology and pathogenesis of these muscle changes are not known. As in other muscular dystrophies, the prominent histologic findings are marked variation in muscle fiber size, central or internal positioning of the nuclei, considerable loss of muscle fibers with an increase of fibrous connective tissue and fat, and homogenization or hyalinization and vacuolation of muscle fibers. Reflecting the myopathic changes, there are changes in the serum enzymes; transaminase, aldolase, and creatine kinase are elevated.

Clinical manifestations commence early, usually before age 6 years. In infancy there may be hypotonia and weakness. Frequently there is delay in walking. A waddling gait due to weakness of the muscles of the pelvis and spine is common. The child may be unable to climb stairs. He may have difficulty holding a heavy object or raising his arms above his head in dressing. There commonly is difficulty in arising from a lying or squatting position.* As the disease and attendant muscle weakness progress, there is difficulty maintaining erect posture. The feet are placed far apart to maintain stability. Lordosis and abdominal protruberance develop. Eventually all power is lost in the knees, shoulders, elbows, and ankles, and the disease renders the child unable to walk. As the patient becomes bedridden, fixed flexion deformities, especially at the elbows and knees, develop. The deep tendon reflexes, preserved early in the course, diminish as the disease progresses.

The course is one of rapid progression without remission. Death generally occurs within 10 to 15 years of the clinical onset; there is rarely survival beyond 20 years. Death is usually due to respiratory or cardiac disease. The patient is especially vulnerable to respiratory infection due to involvement of the respiratory muscles and muscles of deglutition. Disorders of cardiac rhythm, hypertrophy of the heart, and heart failure may occur.

A more benign form of the disease, the Becker variety, characterized by later onset and a more slowly progressive course, has been described.

Facioscapulohumeral Dystrophy of Landouzy and Déjèrine

Facioscapulohumeral dystrophy of Landouzy and Déjèrine is an autosomal dominantly inherited muscular dystrophy that involves predominantly the muscles of the face and shoulder girdle, leading to loss of facial mobility, difficulty in raising the arms above the head, a characteristic forward sloping of the shoulders, and winging of the scapulae. There frequently is weakness of eyelid closure, and this may be noted early. There rarely is weakness of the extraocular or pharyngeal muscles. Late in the disease there may be weakness and atrophy of muscles of the spine and pelvis, and of the tibial and peroneal muscles.

The clinical onset usually is during adolescence, occasionally earlier. The progression generally is very slow, often with plateau periods of significant duration. Although the disease may produce signifi-

---

*The sequence of movements that a child with muscular dystrophy exhibits in arising from the supine position on the floor is referred to as Gower's sign. The child first turns on his side and then stands on both hands and feet. He supports first one knee and then the other with his hands. Shifting his hand upwards ("climbing up his thighs") he eventually extends one hip and then the other, following which he straightens his shoulders and head.

cant disability, it rarely shortens the life span. Cardiac involvement is rare.

Progressive Ophthalmoplegic Dystrophy (Progressive External Ophthalmoplegia [PEO])

Progressive muscular dystrophy involving primarily the extraocular muscles is a not uncommon condition having hereditary features in approximately 50 per cent of cases. Usually the transmission is dominant.

The onset is in childhood or youth, usually before age 30 years, rarely later. The most frequent initial manifestation is ptosis. Progressive weakness of the external ocular muscles develops gradually, often leading to complete ophthalmoplegia. The involvement is usually symmetrical, though involvement of one eye may precede the other, giving rise to diplopia.

Whereas the extraocular muscles exclusively may be affected, there may also be involvement of other muscle groups. The facial muscles, particularly the orbicularis oculi, may become weak. There may be involvement of the muscles of mastication, the muscles of the shoulder girdle, and even the muscles of the limb girdle of the lower extremities. In addition there may be associated abnormalities such as pigmentary degeneration of the retina, cardiac dysfunction, or mental deficiency. Indeed, progressive external ophthalmoplegia may be just one feature of a multifaceted syndrome (see Tables 18–5A and B).

Dystrophia Myotonica (Steinert's Disease)

Dystrophia myotonica is a heredofamilial disorder characterized by progressive muscular wasting and weakness, myotonia, gonadal atrophy, hair loss and cataracts. There may also be mental deficiency and, in some cases, cardiopathy.

Clinical manifestations usually appear during adolescence or adult life, but in some instances the disease presents in infancy or early childhood. Signs of early onset include floppiness, poor sucking and swallowing, delayed motor and intellectual development, and delayed speech.

The muscle wasting tends to proceed symmetrically, often following a given pattern within an affected family. Generally the distal muscles of the extremities and the muscles of the face, jaw, and neck become weak and wasted early in the course. Proximal extremity and axial muscles are affected later, though some children exhibit predominantly proximal muscle involvement. The deep tendon reflexes may be normal or reduced.

The myotonia (delayed muscular relaxation following strong voluntary contraction, or prolonged contraction after mechanical or electrical stimulation) may appear simultaneously with or precede the muscle wasting. The myotonia is most prominent in the hands, tongue, and facial musculature. Inability to relax the grip, delay in opening the eyelids after crying, and stiffening of the limbs, sometimes leading to falls, are typical. The myotonia tends to be aggravated by excitement, fatigue, and cold, while repetition of a given movement seems to enhance relaxation of affected muscles.

Cataracts can be found in most patients examined with the slit lamp. Frequently the opacities are fine subcapsular dots that may appear polychromatic. In more advanced cases there are globular white opacities situated in the anterior and posterior cortex. In some instances the cataractous change takes the form of a star-shaped opacity in the posterior cortex. Although rapid maturation of the cataracts is reported in some patients with dystrophia myotonica, commonly there is little or no apparent change in the lens opacities over many years. In addition to the lenticular opacities, other reported ocular abnormalities in this disease include dystrophic changes of the cornea and "myotonia" of the pupil, and there frequently is involvement of the extraocular muscles leading to weakness of eye movements, ptosis, weakness of lid closure, or myotonia of the lids.

The clinical course of the disease is one of progressive disability, but the patient may survive for many years. Death is commonly the result of an intercurrent illness or respiratory complication during late middle life.

The etiology and pathogenesis of the disease remain obscure. It is a dominant condition with variable expressivity.

Myotonia Congenita (Thomsen's Disease)

Myotonia congenita of Thomsen is a rare hereditary disease characterized by prolonged contraction and delayed relaxation of voluntary muscle (myotonia) and by enlargement of affected muscles. In some cases there is also mental deficiency.

Practically all of the voluntary muscles may be affected by the myotonia. Often those of the arms and legs are most severely involved. Muscles of the pharynx and larynx usually are spared.

The myotonus generally is greatest on the initial muscular contraction and tends to lessen on successive contractions; thus on repetition of voluntary movements, the rigidity response may disappear. Cold, fatigue, and excitement tend to increase the myotonia.

Clinical manifestations of the myotonia usually appear early in childhood. In infancy there may be difficulty nursing due to myotonia of the tongue. Often after an unexpected stimulus such as a loud noise, or even with anger or excitement, there may be generalized rigidity. Falls are common, especially on sudden movement. Difficulty in chewing and tightness of respiratory movement may be noted. Impaired release of the grip is typical; only after many seconds can the hand be disengaged from its grasp.

The principal ophthalmic manifestation of the myotonia is inability to open the eyelids promptly after sudden or forced closure, particularly after crying. Esotropia may occur with contraction of the facial muscles. There may be intermittent diplopia, or transient diplopia on sudden deviation of the eyes.

The muscular hypertrophy of Thomsen's disease affects primarily the muscles of the limbs and trunk. A Herculean appearance may result.

On pathologic examination, affected muscles appear pale but not fatty. Individual muscle fibers may be enlarged to double normal size or more, and there may be some centralization of nuclei. It is unusual to find atrophic fibers.

The etiology of the disease is not known. In most cases the inheritance is dominant; less frequently it is recessive.

Though somewhat disabling, the condition does not shorten life.

Myasthenia Gravis

Myasthenia gravis is a disorder of neuromuscular transmission, character-ized by weakness and excessive fatigability of voluntary muscle.

The cause of the disease is not yet known, but evidence indicates a block in neuromuscular transmission of competitive or acetylcholine inhibitory type. The possibility that it is due to an autoimmune process is currently under investigation. A complement-fixing serum globulin that binds to the A bands of muscle and to the epithelial cells of thymus can be found in approximately 30 per cent of patients. In some cases, thymoma is present.

Muscles most frequently affected — either singly or in combination — are those subserving ocular movement, facial expression, mastication, deglutition, and respiration. Muscles of the neck, trunk, and limbs are less frequently involved.

The most common presenting manifestations are ptosis and diplopia. In some cases involvement is restricted to the extrinsic ocular muscles for long periods, and it is said that when only the extraocular muscles are affected for as long as eighteen months, the likelihood of involvement of other muscles is small.

The ptosis may be unilateral or bilateral. It may occur as an isolated finding or in combination with other signs. Certain features help to distinguish myasthenic ptosis from other types. The weakness is variable. It tends to worsen with fatigue and to improve with rest; thus, it may be minimal or absent on arising in the morning and become increasingly apparent as the day progresses. The levator weakness can often be accentuated by repeated opening of the lids or by prolonged upward gaze. On raising the eye to the primary position from a position of downward gaze, there may be a transient upward twitch of the lid (Cogan's sign) that may be attributed to the rapid recoverability and easy fatigability of myasthenic muscles.

Involvement of the muscles subserving ocular movement follows no constant pattern. There may be isolated or multiple extraocular muscle palsies. There may be total ophthalmoplegia. The ocular muscle involvement may mimic a conjugate gaze palsy, even an internuclear ophthalmoplegia. There may be jerkiness of the eye movements, but true nystagmus is not a regular feature of the disease.

Other common presenting problems are

difficulty in chewing, in swallowing, and in speaking, and tiring of the extremities. In some cases there is respiratory dysfunction, which may be life threatening.

The clinical onset is usually during the second or third decade, but manifestations may appear at any age. In the pediatric age range, the myasthenic states encountered are myasthenia neonatorum, myasthenia congenita, and myasthenia gravis juvenilis.

Myasthenia neonatorum is a transitory myasthenic state that affects approximately 10 per cent of infants born to myasthenic mothers. Signs usually appear within 2 to 72 hours after birth. Generalized weakness, paucity of spontaneous movement, difficulty sucking and swallowing, difficulty breathing, ptosis, and facial weakness are the common manifestations. As a rule, the myasthenic state subsides within 2 to 4 weeks without further problems.

Myasthenia congenita is a persistent neonatal form of the disease that manifests at or soon after birth. Mothers of affected infants rarely, if ever, are myasthenic, but the familial incidence of the disease in siblings is high, and distant family members are sometimes found to be affected. The presenting signs are usually ocular and bulbar, the most frequent being ptosis, extraocular muscle palsies, dysphagia, and weak cry. Generalized weakness and respiratory dysfunction are not common.

Myasthenia gravis juvenilis commences after infancy, its incidence increasing toward adolescence. It affects females more often than males. It may be familial. Signs and symptoms usually develop gradually, rarely abruptly. The most common presenting sign is ptosis. Ophthalmoplegia, difficulty chewing and swallowing, nasal speech, and weakness of the extremities also are frequent manifestations. As a rule, the condition worsens during periods of infection and stress; in some cases respiratory distress severe enough to require tracheotomy or respirator develops.

The response to anticholinesterase drugs is generally marked. Improvement in muscle function following a test dose of Tensilon (edrophonium chloride) or Prostigmin (neostigmine) is diagnostic. For treatment, the drugs most commonly used are Mestinon (pyridostigmine) and Prostigmin.

Thymoma, when present, should be removed. Opinion regarding the usefulness of thymectomy or thymic irradiation in the absence of thymoma varies.

VASCULAR DISORDERS

Vascular lesions and circulatory disturbances are major causes of neuro-ophthalmic morbidity. Although many vascular conditions most commonly become symptomatic in the adult years, several may become apparent in childhood. Vascular disorders of special importance in the pediatric age group are congenital vascular anomalies, particularly congenital arteriovenous malformations and intracranial saccular aneurysms, and certain "vascular syndromes" which may be variously classified as hamartomatoses, phakomatoses, or neurocutaneous syndromes (Table 18–1). Acquired vascular disorders, such as carotid-cavernous fistulas, and carotid arteritis and stroke, may also be seen in the early years. Migraine, the expression of a disturbance of microvascular regulatory systems, also may begin in childhood.

Arteriovenous Malformation

The lesion variously termed arteriovenous malformation, arteriovenous angioma, or arteriovenous aneurysm is a congenital vascular abnormality. Several different types occur. The most common type is the cortical arteriovenous malformation. This lesion is primarily one of the vessels of the pia-arachnoid. The abnormal vascular channels are usually arranged in a roughly wedge-shaped mass with its base on the cortical surface of the hemisphere and its apex projecting inwardly, usually to the subependymal region of the lateral ventricle. The malformation is usually fed by one or more of the major intracranial arteries. Ordinarily, the enlarged feeding arteries ramify into a network of smaller interconnecting arteries; these are intermixed with thin-walled venous channels that collect into enlarged veins which drain into either the longitudinal or transverse sinus, or the galenic system, or both. Characteristically there is an absence of normal capillaries; arterial blood is shunted directly into venous channels.

The most common presenting manifestation of the cortical arteriovenous malformation is spontaneous intracranial hemorrhage that may occur anytime from the newborn period onward. Hemorrhage may occur into the subarachnoid space, into the subdural space, or—as is usually the case—into the cerebral hemisphere. Signs vary with the severity of the hemorrhage and the location of the malformation. Hemiparesis and hemianopia are common. Next to hemorrhage, the most frequent manifestation is seizures. There may also be progressive deterioration of intellect or behavior, chronic headache, bruit, or visible pulsation of scalp veins. In some cases, calcification within or adjacent to the malformation may be seen on x-ray. The principal diagnostic procedure is angiography. Some cases of cortical arteriovenous malformation are successfully treated surgically.

One type of intracranial arteriovenous malformation of particular interest in the pediatric age group is aneurysm of the vein of Galen. In this condition there is direct shunt from the cerebral arterial system into the posterior midline venous drainage of the brain. While variations in this lesion have been described, there is usually a saccular dilatation of the vein of Galen which is continuous with a dilated sinus rectus and torcular. The lesion may produce hydrocephalus, owing to obstruction of the aqueduct of Sylvius by the vascular enlargement. There may be bruit. In some infants, there may be heart failure.

Of special interest in ophthalmology are retinal arteriovenous malformations and congenital malformations of the orbit.

Arteriovenous malformation of the retina is a rare congenital abnormality. It is usually unilateral, and it may involve the entire retina or only part of it. Depending on the extent of the anomaly, the vision may be normal or impaired. There may be associated intracranial and extracranial vascular malformations (Wyburn-Mason syndrome). There may be associated involvement of (1) the orbit and optic nerve, producing proptosis, bruit, and dilatation of conjunctival vessels; (2) the ipsilateral maxilla, pterygoid fossa, and mandible, leading to epistaxis and oral hemorrhage; (3) the ipsilateral basofrontal area and the sylvian fissure, caus-

ing epilepsy, intracranial hemorrhage, hemiplegia, or hemianopia; and (4) the posterior fossa including the rostral midbrain, with cranial nerve or brain stem involvement.

Congenital vascular malformations in the orbit are usually of the venous type. A characteristic sign is intermittent exophthalmos due to intermittent filling and collapse of the malformation with changes in orbital venous pressure.

Intracranial Arterial Aneurysm

Intracranial saccular aneurysm presenting during chilhood is rare. The infrequency of the problem in the early years is something of an enigma, as the lesion is generally thought to arise from a congenital defect in the media of the arterial wall.

The most frequent sites of intracranial saccular aneurysms are (1) the anterior communicating–anterior cerebral artery complex, (2) the internal carotid–posterior communicating artery junction, (3) the bifurcation of the internal carotid artery, and (4) the major early branching of the internal carotid artery.

Clinical manifestations may arise from pressure of the aneurysm on surrounding structures or from hemorrhage due to rupture. In the majority of cases, the initial manifestation is an acute subarachnoid or intracerebral hemorrhage occurring without warning in a previously healthy individual. The onset is often characterized by sudden severe headache, vomiting, mental confusion or loss of consciousness, and sometimes by convulsions. With intracerebral hemorrhage there may be focal signs such as monoplegia, hemiplegia, or aphasia; when hemorrhage is restricted to the subarachnoid space, there may be no lateralizing signs, but only those of meningeal irritation—namely nuchal rigidity and fever—and increased intracranial pressure. With massive hemorrhage, the spinal fluid may be grossly bloody and under increased pressure.

Ophthalmic signs of saccular aneurysm vary with the site and behavior of the lesion. With aneurysms arising from the junction of the carotid artery and the posterior communicating artery, there may be compression of the oculomotor nerve at its entrance into the dura at the posterior aspect of the cavernous sinus. With aneurysms within the cavernous sinus, combined ocular motor palsies are common. Visual defects may occur with carotid aneurysms arising at or near the origin of the ophthalmic artery. By indirect effects consequent to rupture, aneurysm of the middle cerebral artery may produce homonymous hemianopia.

With acute subarachnoid hemorrhage and the associated precipitous rise in intracranial pressure, there may be bleeding into the tissues of the orbit. Superficial retinal and subhyaloid hemorrhages may be seen within hours of the intracranial bleed; they occur most commonly near the disc, but they may be scattered throughout the retina, especially in children. In addition, there may be subconjunctival hemorrhage. Occasionally there is intraorbital hemorrhage that may be extensive enough to produce exophthalmos. Papilledema, not typically present early, may develop later, sometimes days after the acute episode.

Carotid-Cavernous Fistula

The carotid-cavernous fistula is an acquired arteriovenous shunt created by rupture of the internal carotid artery within the cavernous sinus.

The majority of carotid-cavernous fistulas are the result of trauma. The intracavernous portion of the carotid is particularly vulnerable to injury where it is fixed to the surrounding dura in its bony canal at the base of the skull. It may tear with the impact of a head injury or it may be perforated by a bone splinter from a fracture. The artery is also vulnerable to penetrating injury, as may occur with a bullet wound of the head or with a stab wound through the apex of the orbit. The less common spontaneous carotid-cavernous fistulas as a rule occur only in the later years; they are generally attributed to congenital defects in the media, small congenital aneurysms, or atherosclerotic changes.

The rupture, whether of spontaneous or traumatic origin, permits direct flow of arterial blood under high pressure into the cavernous sinus. Arterial blood escaping into the semi-rigid extradural space finds exit through several channels. One of the largest and most accessible channels ante-

riorly is the superior ophthalmic vein which in turn carries the blood into the angular vein, the facial vein, and the external jugular vein. The arterial blood may also exit through the smaller inferior orbital vein, the pterygoid plexus, and the internal jugular vein. Posteriorly, blood may escape through the inferior and superior petrosal sinus into the sigmoid and lateral dural sinus and the internal jugular vein. There may also be arterialization of the sphenoparietal sinus and the sylvian vein. In addition, arterial blood may flow from one cavernous sinus into the other through a system of intracavernous veins.

Should the blood flow from the ruptured carotid artery escape entirely through the cavernous sinus and its various outflow channels, the "hungry" fistula may draw additional blood from other vessels, including the opposite internal carotid artery (by way of the anterior communicating artery and the circle of Willis), the ipsilateral ophthalmic artery, the vertebral-basilar system, and the ipsilateral middle meningeal artery.

The clinical manifestations of carotid-cavernous fistula are principally those of arterialization of the orbit and impairment of normal orbital venous drainage.* Generalized engorgement and congestion develop. The veins of the lids and conjunctiva become dilated and tortuous. Those of the bulbar conjunctiva in particular become quite prominent; they often appear bright red and on close inspection they may seem to pulsate. The lids, conjunctivae, and orbital tissues become swollen. Exophthalmos develops in most cases, and the arterialized vessels generally impart pulsation to the globe. There is usually an associated bruit, and the patient often is aware of a noise in his head; he may also experience headache. There may be limitation of ocular motility either as the result of pronounced exophthalmos and orbital congestion, or as the result of involvement of cranial nerve III, IV, or VI in the cavernous sinus. Fundus changes develop in some cases. There may be visible engorgement of the retinal veins. Rarely, disc edema and retinal hemorrhages develop secondary to venous stasis.

---

*Orbital signs may be inconspicuous, however, if the carotid flow is effectively shunted posteriorly.

As a late effect there may be loss of vision secondary to impairment of retinal circulation. Any immediate loss of vision is most likely due to the initial trauma itself. As a late complication of the exophthalmos, there may be exposure keratopathy.

As a rule, the signs and symptoms develop rapidly, but in some cases they are delayed for weeks or months. Usually the orbital signs appear first on the side of the fistula, but with time they commonly develop on the contralateral side also.

The prognosis is quite variable. Although the patient usually does not die of intracranial hemorrhage, he frequently suffers ophthalmic complications. A variety of techniques aimed toward effecting thrombosis have been devised, but there can be many problems attendant upon treatment of carotid-cavernous fistulas.

Cerebrovascular Occlusive Disease and Stroke in Childhood

Sudden stroke without evidence of intracranial bleed is far less common in childhood than in adult life. The occurrence of cerebrovascular occlusion in the pediatric age group is, however, a well-documented problem and a subject of increasing interest and investigation in recent years.

The majority of cerebrovascular occlusions that occur in childhood are intracranial in location; few involve the extracranial carotid and vertebral circulation. While the most common manifestation is hemiplegia, other signs and symptoms include hemisensory defects, dysphagia, headache, dizziness, seizures, and stupor. The principal ophthalmic sign of stroke in childhood is hemianopia.

Cerebrovascular occlusion in the young patient has been reported in association with intimal ulceration of unknown etiology, with calcification in the media of small arteries, and with aneurysm caused by intramural dissection of blood through a defect in the intima of an intracranial vessel. Occlusion of the carotid lumen has been reported to follow trauma to the carotid artery in the neck and tonsillar areas. Recent study would indicate that carotid arteritis at the base of the skull is of considerable importance as a cause of cerebrovascular occlusion in childhood. Acute inflammation in the outer layers of the carotid artery, the result of local trauma or sepsis, may lead to subsequent intravascular thrombosis. In a significant number of reported cases, there is evidence of existing or recent infection of the ears, throat, nose, or paranasal sinuses.

Whereas underlying disease is always suspect in children who suffer cerebrovascular thrombosis or embolism, in many cases there is no evidence for congenital heart disease, endocarditis, collagen vascular disease, blood dyscrasia, or infection.

The ultimate effect of cerebrovascular occlusion is extremely variable. It depends primarily on the rapidity of occlusion, the collateral circulation, and the maintenance of systemic blood flow.

Migraine

"Migraine is a periodic polysymptomatic expression of a common hereditary disorder that involves the cranial and cerebral microvascular regulatory systems."* The principal clinical manifestations are paroxysmal headache and abnormal visual sensations.

The migraine headache is usually unilateral (hemicrania), intense (often incapacitating), and may last hours or days. It is often accompanied by photophobia, irritability, nausea, vomiting, constipation, or diarrhea. There may be prodromal symptoms such as hunger, feelings of mounting tension, or declining energy. The onset of periodic headaches of migraine may occur during childhood, often at the time of puberty or menarche, or later in life.

The abnormal visual sensations so characteristic of migraine consist of scotomas often associated with impressions of glittering lights or shimmering, silvery wavelike phenomena. The scotoma is usually restricted to one half of the visual fields, and may vary from a scarcely noticeable blind spot to a total hemianopia. The scotoma usually begins next to the macula and expands toward the periphery. The field defect may be outlined by scintillations— "scintillating scotoma"—and in some cases the illuminated or shimmering border takes the form of "fortification figures," so called because their zig-zag configuration

*Welsh, F. B., and Hoyt, W. F.: Clinical Neuro-Ophthalmology. Vol. 2. 3rd ed. Baltimore, The Williams & Wilkins Co., 1969, p. 1654.

bears resemblance to a map of bastions of a fortified town. The scotomas and scintillations of migraine, congruous in the homonymous field, are the result of a disturbance in the visual cortex. These visual symptoms generally last only 15 to 20 minutes; they usually clear completely, but in rare instances there may be a permanent field defect, presumably due to prolonged focal insufficiency of vascular supply in the affected visual cortex. While the visual symptoms precede or accompany headaches and other manifestations of migraine in classic cases, in many patients visual phenomena are the sole indication of migraine.

Other sensory disturbances of cerebral origin that may occur with migraine are paresthesias, numbness, or analgesia. These symptoms are generally transient—lasting from 5 to 20 minutes—and mild, and they usually affect the side opposite the headache. There may be transient aphasia, occasionally associated with agraphia. Some patients experience transient motor disturbances, such as hemiparesis. In rare instances there is alteration or loss of consciousness.

Extracerebral manifestations of migraine may occur. An array of ischemic and hemorrhagic retinal and optic nerve signs have been recorded; these include unilateral vision loss, retinal arteriolar constriction, retinal and vitreous hemorrhages, and ischemic papillitis. Even conjunctival hemorrhage and lid ecchymosis may develop during severe attacks of migraine.

Ophthalmoplegia is a rare but well-documented manifestation of migraine. The onset of ophthalmoplegic migraine is usually before age 10 years; in some cases it appears in infancy. The ophthalmoplegia may include one or more nerves. In most cases there is oculomotor paresis with pupillary involvement. Sixth nerve and fourth nerve involvement is less common. As a rule the ophthalmoplegia is transient, but in some cases the paralysis may be permanent.

Treatment of migraine has been less than satisfactory. The drugs most commonly used are ergotamine tartrate, Cafergot, and Sansert.

ACKNOWLEDGMENTS

Thanks are due Dr. Norman Schatz, Dr. Warren Grover, Dr. Henry Baird, and Dr. William Buchheit for their expert advice and generous assistance in the preparation of this chapter.

REFERENCES

Duke-Elder, S., and Wybar, K. C.: The Anatomy of the Visual System. In Duke-Elder, S. (ed.): System of Ophthalmology. Vol. II. St. Louis, The C. V. Mosby Co., 1961.

Duke-Elder, S.: Congenital Deformities. In Duke-Elder, S. (ed.): System of Ophthalmology. Vol. III. St. Louis, The C. V. Mosby Co., 1963.

Duke-Elder, S., and Wybar, K. C.: Ocular Motility and Strabismus. In Duke-Elder, S. (ed.): System of Ophthalmology. Vol. VI. St. Louis, The C. V. Mosby Co., 1973.

Duke-Elder, S., and Scott, G. I.: Neuro-ophthalmology. In Duke-Elder, S. (ed.): System of Ophthalmology. Vol. XII. St. Louis, The C. V. Mosby Co., 1971.

Harrington, D. O.: The Visual Fields. 2nd ed. St. Louis, The C. V. Mosby Co., 1964.

Holmes, L. B., Moser, H. W., Halldórsson, S., Mack, C., Pant, S. S., and Matzilevich, B.: Mental Retardation, An Atlas of Diseases With Associated Physical Abnormalities. New York, The Macmillan Co., 1972.

Huber, A.: Eye Symptoms in Brain Tumors. 2nd ed. Translated and edited by F. C. Blodi. St. Louis, The C. V. Mosby Co., 1971.

Matson, D. D.: Neurosurgery of Infancy and Childhood. 2nd ed. Springfield, Ill., Charles C Thomas, 1969.

Menkes, J. H.: Textbook of Child Neurology. Philadelphia, Lea & Febiger, 1974.

Nelson, W. E., Vaughan, V. C., and McKay, R. J.: Textbook of Pediatrics. 9th ed. Philadelphia, W. B. Saunders Co., 1969.

Stanbury, J. B., Wyngaarden, J. B., and Fredrickson, D. S.: The Metabolic Basis of Inherited Disease. 3rd ed. New York, McGraw-Hill Book Co., 1972.

Walsh, F. B., and Hoyt, W. F.: Clinical Neuro-ophthalmology. 3rd ed. Baltimore, The Williams and Wilkins Co., 1969.

CHAPTER 19

INBORN ERRORS OF METABOLISM AFFECTING THE EYE

GEORGE L. SPAETH M.D.,
and VICTOR H. AUERBACH, Ph.D.

Introduction

A large number of *genetic disorders* affect directly, or are localized to, the orbit. Many of these are immediately visible to the examining physician or can be discerned with the use of simple instruments such as the ophthalmoscope or the slit lamp. Un-fortunately many of the abnormalities such as aniridia, colobomas, and the like do not, at the present time, lend themselves to *biochemical* analysis. We will restrict ourselves in this chapter to examples of genetic disorders affecting the eye for which there is sufficient biochemical evidence to categorize them as true "inborn errors of metabolism." With further advances of knowledge many disorders which now appear to be due to a "structural" defect will also prove to have a biochemical component dependent upon the genetic makeup of the individual. We will first consider inborn errors of metabolism in general, then the metabolism of the eye with special regard to inborn errors of this organ, and finally inborn errors of metabolism in other organs, the chemical consequences of which affect the eye in a clinically discernible manner.

A. INBORN ERRORS OF METABOLISM ORIGINATING IN THE EYE

Victor H. Auerbach

Biochemical Genetics

An inborn error of metabolism is a clinical disorder due to genetic inability to produce the full complement of a given functioning protein in its "normal" configuration. Most of the functioning proteins that we will consider are enzymes. Either one or two possible types of genetic alterations can give rise to a functional lack of enzyme activity. The first possibility is that a normally constituted enzyme is produced, but that diminished amounts of the enzyme are synthesized. The second possibility is that approximately normal amounts of an enzyme are synthesized, but that the structure of the protein is altered at some critical point. The enzyme can then no longer catalyze the reaction for which it is responsible at a rate sufficient to maintain proper function.

Although it is not our intent to delineate the dogma of biochemical genetics, a very brief overview may be of value to the general reader. For those who wish to pursue this matter in further detail it is suggested that they read some of the general references given at the end of this chapter.

BIOCHEMICAL MECHANISMS OF INHERITANCE. The information required to specify both the amount and the primary structure of all proteins synthesized by the cell is contained in the chromosomal material found in the nucleus of that cell. More specifically, the linear arrangement of purine and pyrimidine bases (adenine, guanine, cytosine, and thymine) on the large polymer desoxyribonucleic acid (DNA) spells out, in a language consisting of words represented by the sequence and nature of bases taken three at a time, the nature of the protein to be synthesized. Since the necessary information is contained in the master blueprint consisting of chromosomal DNA (which remains in the nucleus) and the protein synthesis takes place predominantly in the cytoplasm, a mechanism must exist for transcribing this information into a form which can leave the nucleus and enter the cytoplasm. Such is the function of *messenger ribonucleic acid* (mRNA), which except for the substitution of the sugar ribose for deoxyribose and of the pyrimidine uracil for thymine resembles DNA. The information contained on a given portion of DNA corresponding to one or more peptide chains is *transcribed* to a discrete piece of newly synthesized mRNA, which then passes through the nuclear membrane into the cytoplasm.

Once in the cytoplasm, the information resident on the mRNA is *translated* into the synthesis of a polypeptide structure by the combined action of a number of factors. These factors include ribosomes and specific *transfer ribonucleic acid* (tRNA) to which are attached the activated amino acids which will form the polypeptide chain. The net result is that there is a one-to-one correspondence between the code words on the chromosomal DNA and the order of amino acids in the sequence forming the newly synthesized polypeptide molecule. One or more similar or dissimilar polypeptide chains then arrange themselves to form what is known as an apoenzyme. The apoenzyme, when attached to its specific cofactor or coenzyme, forms the active enzyme molecule (holoenzyme).

Another mechanism operating within the nucleus and controlled by a different but not necessarily distant region of DNA determines how much mRNA will be produced at a given time, thus ultimately regulating how much of a given enzyme will be formed in the corresponding period. Fig-

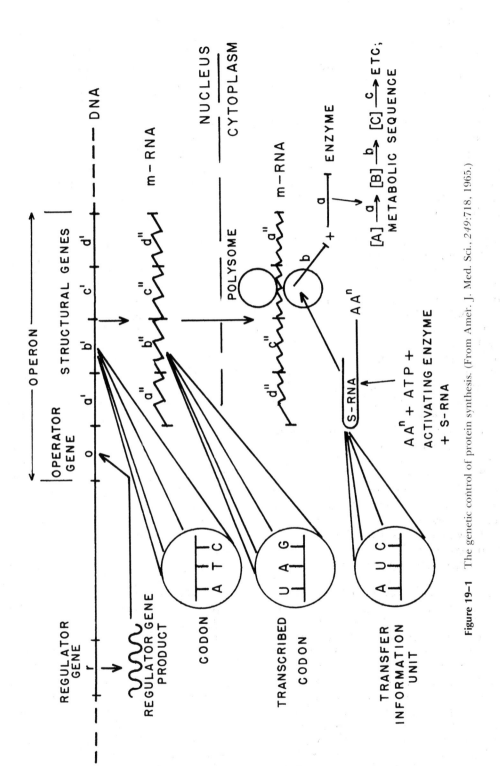

Figure 19–1   The genetic control of protein synthesis. (From Amer. J. Med. Sci. *249*:718, 1965.)

ure 19–1 illustrates the steps between DNA and protein synthesis. Although it is beyond the scope of this chapter to explore these *control* mechanisms, it is important to realize that alterations of DNA structure (mutations) can affect not only the composition of the enzyme produced but quite independently the amount of enzyme synthesized.

Inborn errors of metabolism arise when a specific enzyme reaction cannot proceed at a normal rate, owing to either diminished synthesis of the enzyme or synthesis of an abnormally constituted enzyme. Both events ultimately trace back to a mutation of one form or another in a portion of a DNA molecule. The mutational event may be a new one occurring for the first time in the individual under study or an old one that has been in existence for many generations and hence is *inherited.* The nature of the mutation may be deletion of a piece of the DNA molecule, breaking of the molecule between two bases, or, more commonly, formation of one base from another in situ on the DNA molecule owing to ionizing radiation or the action of a chemical mutagen. Such point mutations (the presence of an inappropriate base in the three-base codeword of the DNA) usually cause the substitution of an inappropriate amino acid at a given point in the structure of the enzyme whose synthesis is "blueprinted" by the mutated position of DNA. If such a substitution of one amino acid for another in the backbone of the protein molecule occurs at or near the site of the molecule which binds to either the substrate or coenzyme, it may affect to a marked degree the ability of the protein to interact with its substrate or coenzyme. If no interaction is possible, the enzyme is functionally dead. If some interaction is still possible, then, depending on the exact nature of the amino acid substitution, an enzyme which can still function, albeit weakly, is produced. It is of interest to note that some such altered but still partially functioning enzymes can be made, to work at a more rapid, and near normal, pace by increasing the cellular concentration of the cofactor whose binding site has been altered. This results in vitamin therapy for a cofactor dependent state such as will be discussed later in connection with homocystinuria.

MODES OF INHERITANCE. A few words now concerning the genetics of the situation are in order. From what has been said previously it should be fairly obvious that for a given biochemical reaction the amount of *functioning enzyme* present in the cell is what determines whether a normal or an abnormal condition will obtain. Many enzymes are present in normal cells in amounts which are orders of magnitude greater than the minimum amount necessary for normal function. Other enzymes are normally present in rate-limiting amounts, i.e., if more enzyme were present, the reaction governed would proceed faster, and, conversely, if less enzyme (or an abnormally structured enzyme) were present, the reaction would proceed at a lower than normal rate. Because most of the reactions so far studied in which inborn errors of metabolism occur are of the type in which an excess of functioning enzyme is normally present, the mode of inheritance most usually observed in conjunction with inborn errors of metabolism is of the *autosomal recessive* type. That is to say, assuming no new mutations, the inheritance pattern is such that each parent has to contribute a defective mutant gene to the offspring. If only one of the pair of corresponding genes is in the mutant form, as is the case in carrier parents, a situation results in which approximately half the enzyme under observation is normally functional. But because this enzyme is present in greater than twofold excess in normal individuals, sufficient enzyme is available, even with a reduction by half, to make detection under ordinary circumstances difficult. In most instances enzyme activity will fall below the threshold required for adequate biochemical integrity only when both genes composing the pair inherited from each parent are similarly defective.

For those enzymes normally present in rate-limiting amounts, a mutation occurring in only one of the pair of parental genes may be sufficient to cause a clinical disorder. This mode of inheritance is called *dominant* and is usually *autosomal.* While few inborn errors of metabolism are inherited in this manner, many of the genetic disorders of man concerned with structural elements are inherited as autosomal dominants, e.g., achondroplasia. It is easy to visualize the situation in which the presence of one half of a structural element (as distinct from a functional catalytic element) in an abnormal form can lead to gross deformities. Many of the structural and genetic abnormalities of the eye are in fact inherited as autosomal dominants (see Chapter 2).

So far we have discussed only the *autosomal* modes of inheritance. As discussed in Chapter 2, there are 46 chromosomes normally present in human somatic cells. Forty-four of these, or 22 pairs, are autosomes. The other pair consists of the sex chromosomes. Normal females have 44 autosomes plus one X chromosome inherited from the mother and another X chromosome inherited from the father. Normal males, like normal females, have 44 autosomes and one X chromosome inherited from the mother, but they have inherited a Y chromosome rather than an X chromosome from their fathers. Aside from the fact that the Y chromosome contains a paucity of genetic information, statistical considerations dictate that most genetic disorders (in the ratio of approximately 22 to 1) should be autosomal in origin. However, many disorders are known to be due to a mutation of the DNA contained on the X chromosome. These disorders are inherited in a *sex-linked* manner. Again, if the reaction is not rate limiting, a female with only one X chromosome in a mutant form will not necessarily have any clinical sequelae. However, the male has only one X chromosome, and if that one is affected, he will manifest the corresponding clinical condition. Rare instances are known in which both X chromosomes in a given female are mutated. In this case, a sex-linked mode of inheritance can affect a female as well as a male. On the other hand, when rate-limiting enzymes are involved, females with only one affected X chromosomal gene can manifest the same symptomatology, though milder than in an affected male. The terms sex-linked recessive and sex-linked dominant have been used to describe these two modes of inheritance.

The Eye and Inborn Errors of Metabolism

Unless specifically stated, it should be assumed that the inborn errors of metabolism to be discussed in the remainder of this chapter are inherited in an autosomal recessive manner. We shall also state at this point that with very few exceptions inborn errors of metabolism *affect* rather than *originate in* the eye. By way of illustration, let us consider two distinctly different inborn errors of metabolism which just happen to be two of the four original "inborn errors of metabolism" delineated by Garrod (1909) when he first coined the term in 1908. Of the four (albinism, alkaptonuria, pentosuria, and cystinuria) the first two markedly affect the eye. The eye in albinism (of the general type or of the ocular type) is devoid of the pigment melanin. This defect can be considered to be due to the lack of activity of the enzyme tyrosinase. The enzyme activity is absent directly within the tissues of the eye itself. The genetic defect is found in the DNA of the nucleus of the orbital tissues. Such is not the case in alkaptonuria. Here the ocular abnormality is the deposition of a melanin-like pigment in the sclera owing to the accumulation in the body tissues as a whole of the polymerized product of a simple normal intermediate of tyrosine metabolism (homogentisic acid). The defect in alkaptonuria is the inability of the *liver* to further degrade homogentisic acid to maleyl-acetoacetic acid, and consequently to carbon dioxide and water. Most of the accumulated homogentisic acid is excreted in the urine, but some slowly accumulates as the polymer in cartilaginous tissues and the sclera. Thus, the ocular manifestations of alkaptonuria are strictly *secondary* to a genetic defect in some other organ system. The same result, as far as the eye is concerned, would obtain in a normal individual in whom large amounts of homogentisic acid were injected daily. In fact, the cataracts of galactosemia can be reproduced in experimental animals who are genetically *normal* by the feeding of large amounts of galactose. The defect in these disorders of metabolism (alkaptonuria and galactosemia) lies not in the eye, but in some other organ, and is only mirrored, as it were, in the eye of the holder.

It should be recognized that there are in excess of 1500 more or less well studied enzymatic reactions and many times that number as yet to be explored in any significant detail. Any enzymatic reaction is potentially capable of being the locus of at least one, and probably more, of the inborn errors of metabolism.

When one discusses inborn errors of metabolism, it is customary to categorize them according to chemical systems. Thus, one speaks of inborn errors of *amino acid* metabolism, or of *carbohydrate* metabolism, or of *lipid* metabolism, and so on. It will not be convenient to use this system when discussing the eye. We will instead look first at intrinsic defects of the eye, all of which involve pigment metabolism, and then at extrinsic defects as they affect different tissues within the orbit, independent of the chemically defined area of metabolism involved.

The number of *possible* inborn errors of metabolism is astronomical, and the number of recognized errors is rapidly expanding. As the result of the process of differentiation the number of possible inborn errors of metabolism that can exist in a given tissue is limited by the extent to which the tissue becomes specialized. Taking the eye as a whole, it would seem a priori that fewer inborn errors due to an intrinsic enzymatic defect should arise in these organs than, say, in liver, in which many more biochemical pathways are patent.

As a matter of present fact, there are extremely few *intrinsic* inborn errors of metabolism pertaining exclusively to the eye. One can definitely speak of ocular albinism as a genetic disorder manifesting as a lack of a given enzymatic activity restricted to the eye. In generalized albinism a similar defect occurs in ocular tissue, but here the same defect occurs in other tissues as well (hair and skin). Similarly, a condition such as xeroderma pigmentosum, which is now known to be due to the genetic inability to synthesize an active form of one of the enzymes responsible for DNA repair, affects the eye simply because parts of this organ, in common with skin, present an outside aspect whose DNA is susceptible to scission by ultraviolet light.

If one examines that function peculiar to the eye, namely, vision (both black and white and color), and asks whether there exist inborn errors of metabolism in this region, one begins to explore uncharted lands. However, since almost all other inborn errors of metabolism so far studied affect the eye in a secondary and almost nonspecific manner (being in reality inborn errors of some other organ or tissue), it behooves us to speculate upon possible errors inherent in the metabolism of the ocular pigments themselves that in one way or another affect vision.

In any discussion of inborn errors of metabolism and the eye one would be remiss not to remember the debt we owe to an acute observer, Thomas Hunt Morgan, for his fundamental discovery that ultimately earned him the Nobel Prize. One part of the many experiments he carried out early in this century depended upon the setting up of genetic models for study of eye color. True, the organism observed was not man, but the lowly fruit fly, *Drosophila melanogaster*. Nevertheless, various defects in a chemical pathway, involving catabolism of the amino acid tryptophan, were clearly established as being inheritable. Specific lesions in the chemical pathway were clearly correlated with visible alterations of the color of the insect's eye. These observations and many which followed, together with similar studies using the mold *Neurospora crassa*, firmly established the now burgeoning field of biochemical genetics. It would be fortunate indeed if we could soon correlate the observable defects in pigmentation of the human eye, which are known to be inherited, with definitive biochemical blocks.

Rod and Cone Vision

There are two major modalities of vision in the human eye. The first involves the retinal rods, is associated with a pigment called visual purple, and is responsible for normal black and white perception at both high and low light intensities. The second involves the retinal cones, in association with three different but only vaguely categorized pigments, and is responsible for normal color perception at relatively high light intensities. There are a number of genetic disorders which result in the loss of one or the other of these modalities, or in partial loss of color vision. Whether any or all of these diseases are inborn errors of metabolism in the sense described earlier in this chapter remains to be seen.

Rod Vision

VITAMIN A METABOLISM. Vitamin A is a long-chain polyunsaturated molecule terminating in an *alcohol* group. After ingestion and absorption the hydroxy group is first oxidized to an aldehyde, then to an acid group. Whatever life-supporting qualities are inherent in vitamin A derive from unknown reactions in which vitamin A *acid* participates (Dowling and Wald, 1960). The intermediate oxidation product, vitamin A aldehyde, in combination with the specific protein, opsin, forms rhodopsin (visual purple). This compound is intimately concerned with the visual process as it occurs in the rods, i.e., black and white vision.

The absorption of light by rhodopsin in the retina initiates a process which ultimately leads to the electrical excitation of the rod and subsequent transmission of an impulse to the brain. The chemical or physiologic steps between the photic excitation of rhodopsin and the electrical excitation of the optic nerve are at present not well understood. Some of the reactions which lead to the formation of rhodopsin from its precursors and the subsequent breakdown of this visual pigment are better understood, although these reactions are not necessarily on the pathway which leads to electrical stimulation.

Before examining some of the known reactions, a few facts must be recognized. Vitamin A alcohol, which we will now call *retinol*, and vitamin A aldehyde, which we will now call *retinaldehyde*, can exist in a number of isomeric configurations, depending upon the arrangement of the double bonds within the molecule.

Whatever form of vitamin A is ingested, or whatever form of retinol is available, it first must be converted, probably by specific enzymes, to 11-*cis*-retinol (one of the isomers). The 11-*cis*-retinol then is oxidized to 11-*cis*-retinaldehyde by a specific dehydrogenase found in the eye. This molecule (11-*cis*-retinaldehyde) combines in the dark with the protein opsin to form rhodopsin. Rhodopsin, when bleached by light, splits to opsin and a different isomer or retinaldehyde (all-*trans*-retinaldehyde). This latter compound must be converted to the 11-*cis*-isomer, either by another enzymatic reaction or after enzymatic reduction to all-*trans*-retinol and subsequent isomerization, before it can again combine with opsin in the dark.

The two systems mentioned above (one leading to neural excitation after light *stimulation*, the other to formation of and to recycling of the visual pigment after *bleaching* by light) are probably independent in part and are depicted in Figure 19–2. A good review of the current state of knowledge concerning the various reactions in which rhodopsin partakes is provided by Bridges (1970).

Both systems are potentially subject to genetic disruption. This could occur at the level of any of the specific enzymes involved or in the formation of the specific protein opsin. If such an error were to occur, it is easy to visualize a disruption of the overall process which could lead to loss of vision. One clue is the association of a partial loss of vision and a chemical event as provided by the night blindness resulting from lack of dietary precursors of retinaldehyde. Prolonged ingestion of a diet deficient in vitamin A and carotinoids results in night blindness. (Carotinoids are precursors of vitamin A which are essentially the backbone of two vitamin A molecules joined together at the site that would normally contain the alcohol group and which are capable of being converted to vitamin A in the intestine.) This symptom occurs after previously stored resources of vitamin A are depleted (a matter of months) and is the first of many pathologic changes that occur. Ultimately, total blindness due to xerophthalmia will ensue, but these changes reflect the more generalized reactions of the whole organism to a lack of vitamin A acid and should not be confused with the temporary impairment of rod vision that follows loss of ability to maintain adequate amounts of retinaldehyde, hence rhodopsin, in the retina.

NYCTALOPIA. In a sense, vitamin A deficiency nyctalopia is an inborn error of metabolism which affects all mankind in the same way that scurvy is an inborn error of metabolism for man and selected other animals. If man possessed the enzymatic

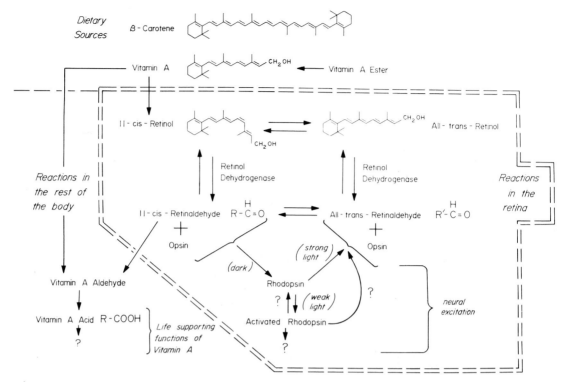

Figure 19–2   Vitamin A metabolism. The precise reactions within the eye that give rise to neural excitation are not known. The figure shows involvement of vitamin A in the metabolism of retinaldehyde, which, in conjunction with the protein opsin, forms rhodopsin.

mechanisms for synthesis of carotinoids he would not be subject to vitamin A deficiency as a species, but certain individuals then could conceivably, on a genetic basis, lose this ability and exhibit retinaldehyde deficiency nyctalopia as an inborn error of metabolism. Once rod vision is compromised, as in vitamin A deficiency, perception occurs only via the cones, i.e., color vision, at increased levels of ambient illumination. Presumably patients with achromatopsia, who lack all forms of color vision (see below), would become totally blind when they were vitamin A deficient.

Night blindness which is not due to vitamin A deficiency but is congenital and genetic in orgin occurs in at least four distinct forms. Essential nyctalopia in which no other ocular findings are abnormal has been extensively studied in large pedigrees. This disorder is transmitted as an autosomal dominant. A sex-linked form of essential nyctalopia and the rarer autosomal recessive form are also known; both are usually associated with myopia. Oguchi's disease, which is inherited as an autosomal recessive, exhibits, in addition to night

blindness, pigmentary changes in the retina (gray or golden color which shifts to normal red only after many hours of adaptation in the dark) and the appearance of an anomalous tissue layer in the retina which seems to contain many pigment granules. In the three forms of essential night blindness and in Oguchi's disease, electroretinograms reveal normal photic waves but absence of the scotopic wave. (See Plate XII – A and B.)

Although nothing more is known at present about the pathophysiology of these four disorders, it is tempting to speculate that an inborn error involving perhaps the specific ocular retinol dehydrogenase or the protein opsin or one of the other known and unknown biochemical reactions involving visual purple is the basis for one or the other of them.

The primary form of retinitis pigmentosa which is inherited as an autosomal recessive (see Chapter 14) first manifests itself as night blindness. In the experiments of Dowling and Wald (1960) which separated the effects of vitamin A aldehyde from vitamin A acid, it was noted that rats

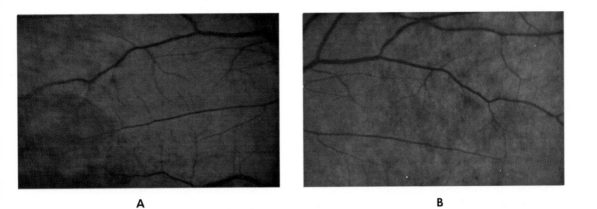

A   B

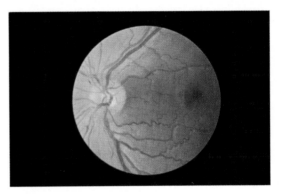

C   D

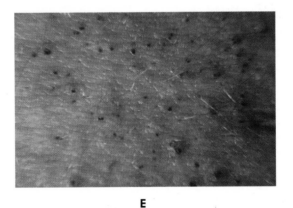

E

Plate XII   *(A)* The fundus of a 12-year-old white boy with Oguchi's disease. The photograph illustrates the shiny metallic appearance of the fundus as normally observed (that is, in the light-adapted state).

(B) Same patient as in *A*, taken after the eye had been patched for 4 hours, demonstrating Mizuo's phenomenon.

(C) Cataract noted in the posterior capsular area of the lens in about 50 per cent of patients with Fabry's disease. Carriers also may show this opacity, which is best seen by means of retro-illumination.

(D) Characteristic retinal vessel tortuosity of a 22-year-old man with Fabry's disease.

(E) Skin lesions, the "angiokeratomas" of Fabry's disease, most prominent in the bathing suit area.

maintained on the acid became night blind but had no other symptoms. The phenomenon was reversible early on (by the administration of the alcohol) but irreversible after sufficient time had elapsed to result in loss of opsin and finally loss of the visual cells themselves. The authors noted the histologic resemblance between the retinal layers from their permanently blind animals and the retinas of humans with retinitis pigmentosa. Perhaps this form of tapetoretinal degeneration is also an inborn error of vitamin A metabolism. Attempts to treat retinitis pigmentosa with vitamin A have failed, however, and illustrate the difficulty of the problem.

Whatever form of nyctalopia may ultimately be shown to be due to the inability to form 11-*cis*-retinaldehyde from vitamin A as a result of the genetic loss of a specific enzyme in the eye, it will not be treatable with vitamin A. Therapy, if possible, must begin at an early age, before histologic changes take place. The proper molecular configuration, that is, the 11-*cis*-retinaldehyde, or other enzymatic product, must be administered, rather than the vitamin A alcohol, which cannot be utilized.

Cone Vision

Partial or complete inability to see and distinguish colors is a phenomenon which has fascinated physicists and physicians alike. Although much is known about the inheritance of "color blindness" and much more has been speculated upon concerning theories of normal and abnormal perception of color, very little solid information is available at present which would establish a pathophysiology for the various entities described. One outstanding exception to this statement is a report by Wald (1964) which establishes the following: normal individuals possess three different *cone pigments*—one sensitive to red light, one to green light, and one to blue light; certain abnormal individuals functionally lack one or the other of these cone pigments.

COLOR BLINDNESS. Let us now recapitulate some of the known forms of color blindness. In general there are four forms with some degree of subdivision within each form. From the Greek roots for first, second, and third (*protos, deuteros,* and *tritos*), signifying the three so-called "primary" colors, red, green, and blue, respectively, and the suffixes "-anopia" to indicate a complete defect and "-anomaly" to signify a partial defect, we obtain the names of the three main forms of "color blindness" and their subdivisions. Thus, protanopia and protanomaly refer to severe forms of red-green color blindness in which the red axis is most affected. These sex-linked recessive conditions each occur in approximately 1 per cent of the male population. Deuteranopia and deuteranomaly refer to severe and less severe forms of red-green color blindness in which the green axis is most affected. These conditions are also inherited in a sex-linked manner and occur in 1 and 5 per cent of the male population, respectively. Tritanopia and tritanomaly affect the ability to see blue light, are inherited as autosomal dominants, and occur in less than 0.1 per cent of the population.

The fourth major form of "color blindness" is achromatopsia, in which no color whatsoever can be perceived and all images are in black and white; hue registers as various shades of gray. Aside from inability to see color secondarily due to a degenerative process, the condition is extremely rare and appears to be inherited as an autosomal recessive trait. There are two types: (a) so-called "rod-monochromatism," in which the defect is associated with a number of pathologic alterations including nystagmus and central scotomas and is probably neural in origin; and (b) so-called "cone-monochromatism," in which the only defect observable is lack of color perception. The latter form is the rarer of the two (1 per 100 million) and is only presumed to be inherited. It is this form which might conceivably be due to an inborn error of metabolism, either of a common precursor of the pigment molecules involved or for a presumed common protein carrier.

Many theories have been formulated as to the number and nature of the pigments responsible for normal color vision. More theories abound to explain what amounts to almost infinite visual discrimination between various hues in the normal individual based upon mechanisms that predicate two or, at most, three primary receptor pigments. In terms of these theories one speaks of the various forms of protan, deuteran, and tritan anomalies as shifts in the axis of perception, i.e., toward the green or red end of the spectrum, or as absences of one or more valences, a term which refers to regions of the spectrum over which each primary pigment can detect and transmit impulses. Much weight is placed upon so-called "neutral points" in the spectra which for affected individuals occur at wavelengths different from those for normal individuals. All these concepts derive from various methods for the detection of color blindness and are extremely useful for diagnosis but unfortunately only confuse and obfuscate a discussion of the pathophysiology of the inability to perceive a color or colors normally. For an excellent discussion of the history of work on color perception the reader is referred to Linksz (1964).

PIGMENTS AND COLOR PERCEPTION. Wald (1964) has cut the Gordian knot of metaphysical speculations concerning color perception and has made measurements of pigments responsible for color perception which could go far in the explanation of both normal and abnormal chromatic vision. By the simple stratagem of dark-adapting the observer's eye to a color other than the one under investigation and then measuring the visual threshold of the fovea as a function of wavelength and luminosity he has obtained action spectra for three distinctly different pigments. After correction of the shape of the spectral curves to take into account the filtering effect of yellowish lenticular tissue and a yellow fovea, the three pigments have the following characteristics: the red-sensitive pigment has broad band absorption with a maximum at 575 nm., the green-sensitive pigment has a maximum absorption at 540 nm. and overlaps much of the red pigment spectrum, and the blue-sensitive pigment has a somewhat sharper spectrum with a maximum at 430 nm. Of the three mechanisms, the red and the green have about the same sensitivity at the cone level (as distinguished from the corneal level, where internal filtering effects have not yet been taken into consideration), while the blue mechanisms appear to be about one half as sensitive. By direct spectral analysis of excited single human cones, Marks et al. (1964) also demonstrated three visual pigments with spectral maxima (570, 535, and 445 nm.) very close to those determined physiologically by Wald. Although Marks and his coworkers felt that their experiments indicated that each pigment was segregated in individual cones, they commented that "the data suggest the possibility that the 'red' receptor may contain red and green pigments coexisting in a single cone."

By comparison of normal action spectra with previously published results on the visual acuity of various color blind individuals as a function of luminosity and wavelength, Wald concluded that "*protanopes* lacked the red-sensitive pigment, and in this sense are literally *red-blind*." He further concluded that *tritanopes* "appear to lack the blue-sensitive pigment, and in that sense are *blue-blind*." *Deuteranopes* are of two classes, one of which "lack the green-sensitive pigment and in this sense are literally *green-blind*." The other "class of *deuteranopes* processes all three color-vision pigments in average proportions, but the red and green mechanisms are fused or confused so as to yield a single sensation." Although nothing is known concerning the biochemistry of these three pigments, one can safely assume that protanopia, one form of deuteranopia, and tritanopia represent inborn errors of metabolism in the classic sense. This would also be true of protanomaly, one form of deuteranomaly, and tritanomaly.

Should the opportunity arise, it would be extremely interesting to use Wald's technique for determining the presence or absence of visual pigment in subjects with pure achromatopsia (cone-monochromatism), although by using a different and perhaps inappropriate technique Weale (1953) claims to have observed two pigments in such individuals. One also wonders about the presence or absence of cone pigments in patients with hemeralopia or day blindness who are said often to be color blind as well. Perhaps rhodopsin is their only visual pigment; it would bleach in strong light and thus would make the patient unable to see; in dim light the rhodopsin would be reconstituted, again permitting vision.

Ocular Pigment and Albinism

One of the first things one notices about a fellow human being is his or her eyes, in particular, the color of the iris. It has long been appreciated that iris color is an inherited characteristic (or more likely a number of characteristics). Brown is obviously dominant over blue, and detailed studies of various pedigrees show a fairly consistent relationship between intermediate shading of the iris and position in the family tree (Fig. 19–3). Iris color follows a regional pattern throughout the world and is obviously the result of long-term genetic inbreeding and segregation. When one looks more closely at an individual iris one usually sees a multiplicity of color specks rather than a uniformity of color; concerning the inheritance of these *patterns* less is known. The situation is further complicated when it is recognized that one may under genetic control have irides of different colors. Thus, in Waardenburg's syndrome, which is inherited as an autosomal dominant and usually consists of deafness, a white forelock, and heterochromia iridis, one may have one brown eye and one blue eye. For other causes of heterochromia iridis the reader is referred to the extensive discussion in Waardenburg, Franceschetti, and Klein (1961). How a genetic defect which is clearly passed on through a number of generations, and therefore is not a somatic mutation of only the eyes, expresses its effect unilaterally is not known. Obviously we are far from a mechanistic answer to such knotty problems.

Perhaps if we knew more about the pigments found in the iris we might be in a better position to discuss the inborn errors of metabolism that produce variations in iris color. At present all that can be said with some certainty is that one of the pigments found in the iris is *melanin*. Depending on the size of the melanin granule, various shades of brown will be seen (Fig. 19–4). The light blue iris that is seen in the absence of melanin or other pigments is not itself due to the presence of a blue pigment but to the scattering, by various small structural elements of the iris, of some of the light incident upon the iris. Since the shorter wavelengths (blue) are scattered by small particles more readily than the longer wavelengths (red), the iris appears blue. Ordinarily the longer wavelengths (red) are transmitted by the "blue" iris and are absorbed in the posterior sur-

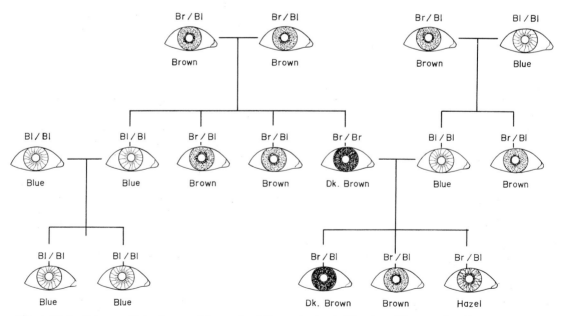

Figure 19–3 Pattern of inheritance of "eye color." Brown is clearly "dominant" in regard to blue. Nevertheless, intermediate grades of shading are common.

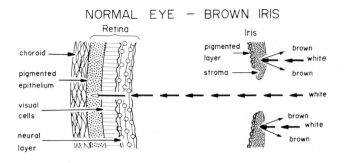

NORMAL EYE — BROWN IRIS

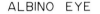

NORMAL EYE — BLUE IRIS

Figure 19–4 Reflection, scattering, absorption, and transmission of light falling on the iris and retina. Three different genotypes are illustrated, representing brown-eyed, blue-eyed, and albino individuals. Refractive changes are omitted for the sake of simplicity.

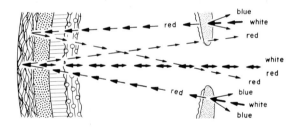

ALBINO EYE

face of the iris by the melanin in the pigmented epithelium directly behind the iris stroma and by the retinal layers including the melanin granules in the pigment epithelium. Thus no light is reflected back and the pupils appear black. Persons with blue eyes lack the ability to form melanin in one ocular tissue (the iris) but form normal amounts of melanin in another (the retinal pigment epithelium). They have an inborn error of metabolism which is remarkably localized. Many other examples of tissue or organ localization of an inborn error of metabolism are known (Auerbach and DiGeorge, 1965).

The reader may not be accustomed to thinking of inborn errors of metabolism

that can affect large segments of the population and may be more at home with the concept when it is applied to a specific disorder that may occur in only 0.1 per cent or less of the population. Nevertheless, if one can demonstrate that a specific chemical reaction is missing in an individual (or in a given tissue of the individual) as a result of his inheritance, then one has made a case for inborn error of metabolism, no matter how rare or frequent the loss may be. If a person with blue eyes does not have brown eyes because he cannot synthesize the brown pigment, he indeed has an inborn error of metabolism. That there is some validity to this hypothesis is illustrated by the fact that in *albinism*, in which the pigment melanin cannot be synthesized from tyrosine anywhere in the eye, the iris is usually blue or blue-gray. This occurs in individuals who, had they not been albinos, would be expected to have brown eyes.

The non-albino with blue eyes illustrates the concept not only that some inborn errors of metabolism can be widespread (another well-defined example is the inheritance of the ABO system of blood groups as correlated with the presence or absence of a specific enzyme, N-acetyl-D-galactose-aminyl transferase) but that there need not be any clinical correlates of a specific inborn error of metabolism. Again, the reader has been preconditioned to think of inborn errors of metabolism only in conjunction with clinical disease states.

Albinism was one of the four disorders Sir Archibald Garrod studied early in this century in order to formulate his now classic concept of inborn errors of metabolism (Garrod, 1909). The phenomenon of albinism is widely distributed in nature and occurs in almost all animal species studied. In man it occurs in at least three forms, each inherited in a different manner. *Generalized albinism* affects the color of the skin, hair, and eyes and is inherited as an autosomal recessive trait. *Ocular albinism*, in which the pigmentary defect is limited to the eye, is transmitted in a sex-linked manner. *Partial albinism* includes only the skin and hair and is inherited as an autosomal dominant trait.

Generalized Albinism

Generalized albinism is much more common than ocular albinism, occurring in about 1 in 20,000 of the average population. In certain groups the gene for generalized albinism is more widespread. In the San Blas Indians of Panama, albinism occurs in almost 1 per cent of the population. Albinism is most certainly not a single condition transmitted by a single pair of mutated genes. This can readily be appreciated from the observation of normally pigmented offspring of two albino parents (Trevor-Roper, 1963). Evidently each parent is homozygous for a different defect and the children, being mixed heterozygotes, can and do synthesize melanin.

Melanin is a large insoluble polymer resulting from the oxidation of the amino acid tyrosine as depicted in Figure 19–5. The first two reactions, the oxidation of tyrosine to 3,4-dihydroxyphenylalanine and its subsequent oxidation to a quinone, are, in man, under the control of a single enzyme called tyrosinase. The subsequent oxidation and polymerization of the quinone to form melanin is thought to occur spontaneously. A similar, if not identical enzyme, found in many fruits and vegetables is responsible for the browning of freshly bruised or cut fruit which results when atmospheric oxygen is made available for the oxidation of tyrosine.

Melanin once formed is contained in organelles called melanosomes which are found in the melanocytes. In albinism the structure of the melanosomes and the melanocytes is normal. The question arises as to whether these structures contain the enzyme tyrosinase. It has now been established by Witkop and his coworkers (1970), using plucked hair bulbs, that there are at least two forms of generalized albinism. In the first type (tyrosinase-negative), the hair bulb, when incubated with tyrosine, cannot form melanin, thus implying a lack of tyrosinase. In the second type (tyrosinase-positive), on the other hand, melanin is formed in vitro by the hair bulb. It is postulated that a defect might occur in a permease which transports tyrosine into the melanosome.

The ocular findings in generalized albinism depend on the type and are listed by Witkop et al. (1970) as follows: tyrosinase-negative—gray to blue iris with little or no visible pigment, red reflex present at all ages and in all races, severe nystagmus, and photophobia with persistent loss of visual acuity; tyrosinase-positive—blue, yellow, or brown pigment which increases with age, especially at the pupillary border of the iris, red reflex in children and in Caucasian but not Negro adults, mild to severe nystagmus, and photophobia with poor visual acuity in childhood which may improve with age.

Yet a third variety of generalized albinism has been observed by the same group (Nance et al., 1970) among the Amish, in whom normal skin pigmentation develops with time. Ocular signs of albinism persist in these individuals into adult life. When tested by the hair bulb reaction, they are

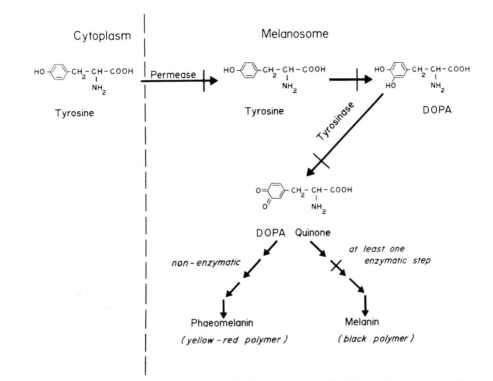

Figure 19–5   The formation of melanin from tyrosine in pigmented cells. At least three separate inborn errors of metabolism exist which can give rise to albinism. One type is due to a lack of permease activity for the transport of tyrosine into the melanosome. A second type is caused by deficient tyrosinase activity; note that this enzyme catalyzes two reactions, that from tyrosine to DOPA and that from DOPA to DOPA quinone. A third variant involves a still unstudied enzyme responsible for one of the many reactions leading from DOPA quinone to melanin.

intermediate between the tyrosinase-positive and tyrosinase-negative forms of albinism. The defect in these persons, designated as ym (yellow mutant), is postulated as occurring on the pathway to melanin after the formation of DOPA quinone, the product of the enzyme tyrosinase. These steps have long been thought to be nonenzymatic. Apparently, there are nonenzymatic reactions which also convert DOPA quinone not to melanin, but to a melanin-like side product called phaeomelanin. Again, an experiment of nature has served to alert us to alternate pathways. Persons with the ym defect, therefore, would be able to make phaeomelanin, but not melanin, in their melanocytes, while tyrosinase-positive persons lacking the melanocyte permease and tyrosine-negative persons lacking melanocyte tyrosinase can make either melanin or phaeomelanin. Witkop et al. (1971) have extended the classification of oculocutaneous albinism and currently include the Hermansky-Pudlak syndrome (albinism with hemor-rhagic diathesis) as a subdivision of the tyrosinase-negative group. Persons with either Chédiak-Higashi syndrome or Cross syndrome (hypopigmentation-microphthalmos) are tyrosinase positive.

Ocular Albinism

The ocular findings in ocular albinism are much the same as those in generalized albinism (Table 19–1). The enzymatic defect must be different, however, since in this case the gene is located on the X chromosome rather than on an autosome. It is conceivable that while the generalized tyrosinase-negative form of albinism may be due to an alteration of structure of the enzyme, depriving it of catalytic function, ocular albinism may be due to a mutation of a controller gene which leads to lack of synthesis of a normally constituted enzyme. Or, the contrary situation might obtain. The female heterozygote for ocular albinism, once ascertained by virtue of her affected son or brother or father, can upon funduscopic examination be seen to

TABLE 19–1 OCULAR MANIFESTATIONS OF GENERALIZED ALBINISM

A. Tyrosinase-negative
   Gray to blue iris
   Little or no visible pigment
   Red reflex
   Nystagmus (severe)
   Photophobia (severe)
   Persistent poor visual acuity

B. Tyrosinase-positive
   Yellow or brown pigment
   Pigment increases with age
   Red reflex in children and Caucasians only
   Nystagmus (mild to severe)
   Photophobia (mild to severe)
   Visual acuity may improve with age

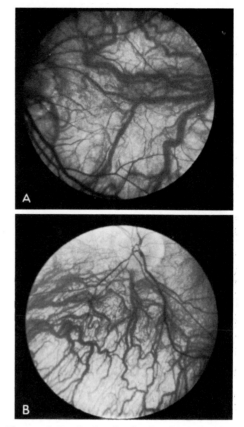

Figure 19–7 Ocular fundus in albinism. Absence of a normal macula is apparent in *A*. In both *A* and *B* the large and tortuous choroidal blood vessels are easily seen; these vessels are not visible when the pigment epithelium of the retina is normal.

have a patchy appearance of the pigmented layer of the fundus, suggesting that certain melanocytes contain tyrosinase while others do not. This would be consistent with Lyon's hypothesis of random X chromosome inactivation in the female. The outward appearance of the eyes in a generalized albino or an ocular albino is shown in Figure 19–6. Figure 19–7 shows the funduscopic picture of an albino.

In the autosomal recessively inherited Chédiak-Higashi syndrome some ocular findings occur which resemble those found in albinism. The defect, however, is not in the formation of melanin, which proceeds normally, but in the morphology of the melanosomes, which are excessively large (Windhorst and Zelckson, 1966). This results in dilution of the color, particularly in the eye in which produces photophobia. Similar structural defects in the granulation of the leukocytes are probably responsible for the susceptibility of patients with this syndrome to recurrent infection and early death.

In the human albino eye two defects are present simultaneously, both of which help explain the severe photophobia typical of such cases. Like the normal blue-eyed individual, the albino has no melanin in his iris. In addition, he lacks melanin in the pigment epithelium layer of the retina as well. As a result, light incident upon the eye passes through the pupil intact and that portion passing through the iris (the red end of the visual spectrum) also

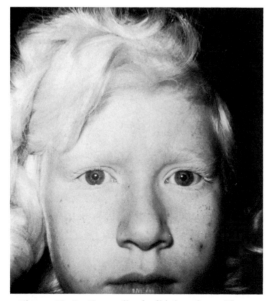

Figure 19–6 Generalized albinism in a 10-year-old girl.

impinges upon the retina. Whereas normally most of the light reaching the retina is absorbed in the pigment epithelium, in the albino it is not. Light is then reflected from the choroidal layer and produces the red pupil and semitransparent iris seen in human albinos.

In the albino rat, with which most people are acquainted, the iris as well as the pupil appears to be red. Presumably the granules in the rat's iris are not of the proper size to scatter blue light. The pupil is red because red light is reflected from the fundus instead of being absorbed by the melanin normally present. In this respect the albino rat resembles the albino human. Observations of albino rodents should not confuse one into thinking that albino humans should also have red eyes; they do not and, as we have seen, most usually have blue irides. Parenthetically, it may also be mentioned that the albino rat and the albino man differ in another important respect. It has been shown in albino rats (Gaudin and Fellman, 1967) that of the two reactions between tyrosine and dihydroxyphenylalanine quinone, the first reaction but not the second can be carried out. This is in contrast to human albinos of the tyrosinase-negative type who cannot carry out the first or both of the two reactions.

B. OTHER INBORN ERRORS OF METABOLISM AFFECTING THE EYE
George L. Spaeth

Having discussed the inheritable disorders involving various pigments found in the eye, one has about exhausted those genetic defects of metabolism that are restricted and intrinsic to the eye. One must now look at more generalized inborn errors of metabolism or those of other organs which secondarily also affect the eye in an easily observable manner. It is important to recognize these disturbances of the eye not only because they cause ocular disease but because they very often are the first easily detectable clues to more generalized symptomatology.

The range of epistemologically and biochemically unrelated diseases which have ocular correlates is beautifully illustrated in the following quotation from Cogan (1966) which represents the summary in toto of his elegant paper.

The eye provides unique opportunities for the detection, during life, of deposits of storage substances and other characteristic changes resulting from inborn metabolic defects. The cornea shows the macromolecular polysaccharides of Hurler's disease, the cystine crystals in cystinosis, and the copper deposits of Wilson's disease. The sclera shows characteristic pigmentation in alcaptonuria. The iris shows the lack of pigmentation in various types of albinism. The lens is cataractous in galactosemia and dislocated in homocystinuria. The vitreous is opacified in familial amyloidosis. The retina shows different and characteristic deposits with the diseases of Tay-Sachs, Neimann-Pick, metachromatic leukodystrophy, and Farber's lipogranulomatosis. The retinal veins show pronounced tortuosity with Fabry's disease. There is some evidence that optic neuropathy occurs in glucose-6-phosphate dehydrogenase deficiency. Curiously, few abnormalities in the eye have been described in subjects with the glycogen storage diseases.

We can do little more than amend and update Cogan's descriptions. Similar listings and discussions of various inborn errors as they affect the eye are found in the general references listed at the end of this chapter (Duke-Elder, 1963; Francois, 1961; Waardenburg et al., 1961) and in several chapters in three recently published books (Graymore and Hsia, 1970; Paulson and Allen, 1970; Sotos and Boggs, 1970; Spaeth, 1971; Tasman, 1971).

Because the retina of the eye is neural tissue, one would expect that many, if not all, of the inborn errors of spingolipid metabolism should have ocular signs and symptoms. In this respect these disorders form a group whose effects are widely generalized, including the eye. Similarly the effects of "albinism" are restricted to the eye, whereas in "generalized albinism" the eye is only one of the sites where genetic observation becomes apparent. Again, with the mucopolysaccharidoses the disorders are generalized in nature and may or may not be evidenced in the eye by cloudiness of the cornea as discussed in Chapter 20. These affectations of the eye, be they restrictive or generalized, should again be considered in a different light than those inborn errors of metabolism such as galactosemia, whose effect on the eye is primarily due to the presence in the circulation of an abnormal concentration of a metabolite formed in another organ.

Prior to passing to this more clinical section of the chapter a few general concepts warrant reintroduction. Frequently confused by those unfamiliar with genetics are the terms "congenital" and "hereditary." "Congenital," of course, refers to the *time* at which an abnormality is noted, and does not indicate causation; something congential is something present *at birth*. "Hereditary" signifies that the condition has been transmitted in the "germ plasma;" as such the term "hereditary" indicates a *method of transmission* and is not concerned with the time of appearance of the characteristic. A child born with white hair would properly be said to have white hair *congenitally*. Members of a family in which, for several generations, white hair had developed at the relatively young age of 35 years, on the other hand, would be thought of as having premature white hair *hereditarily*. It would, of course, be possible, in addition, to have congenital white hair hereditarily. In this chapter, and the Appendix Tables, congenital conditions have not been our subject unless they have also been of a hereditary nature.

Confusion may also be produced when a particular finding is an expression of several different etiologies. For example, a dislocated lens may be due to a deficiency of the enzyme cystathionine synthase (as in the disease "homocystinuria") or the enzyme sulfite oxidase (sulfite oxidase deficiency), or to trauma, and so forth. This single clinical finding, the dislocated lens, can thus be the final (secondary) expression of a number of fundamentally different primary abnormalities. The primary genetic constitution of the individual (the genotype) must not be confused with the actual expression of these genes as modified by each other and by the environment (the phenotype).

Just as one clinical finding can be an expression of a variety of diseases, so one biochemical finding can be a representation of a number of different basic enzyme defects. For example, homocystine occurs in the urine of patients with several different diseases; that is, homocystinuria is not proof that the individual under consideration actually has the disease entity that has come to be called "homocystinuria." He may have a disease in which homocystine in the urine is associated with organic aciduria and vitamin B_{12} deficiency, and in which there is no apparent abnormality of the enzyme cystathionine synthetase (Hollowell et al., 1969). This is not really surprising. Figure 19–8 is a simplified schema of methionine catabolism. Were a block to occur in the catabolic pathway at B (where, indeed, the defect in "homocystinuria" is located), there would be an increase of the compounds whose breakdown is primarily affected, specifically homocysteine and methionine. Were the block at C, there would, in addition, be an excess of cystathionine. Just which compound accumulated and in what concentration would depend on the rate and reversibility of the various reactions, the other metabolic chains linked into the same pathway, and so on. Thus, it can readily been seen that excess methionine could conceivably be a biochemical manifestation of *at least three totally different* entities.

Most enzymes affect more than one site in the body. Consequently, abnormality even of a single enzyme is accompanied by a variety of clinical manifestations. The degree of this "pleiotropism" varies considerably from disease to disease. For example, in cystathionine synthetase deficiency (homocystinuria) mental retardation, malar flush, flapping gait, knock-knees, and a tendency to thrombosis are among the many varied manifestations of the single enzyme abnormality (Laster, 1965). On the other hand, in ocular albinism the clinical expression of disease is limited to the pigment epithelium of the eye.

It may be helpful to discuss in greater detail the most frequently observed ocular changes secondary to biochemical defects

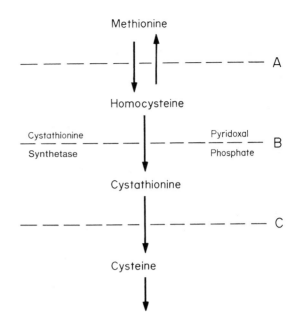

Figure 19–8 Simplified schema of methionine catabolism. Homocystinuria is caused by a block at "B."

occurring elsewhere in the body. Were the matter considered in the most comprehensive manner, this would necessitate the inclusion of *all* hereditary characteristics of normal as well as abnormal, for there almost certainly must be biochemical basis at the root of all truly hereditary states. By the same reasoning, all traits or diseases known to be related to chromosomal function would need to be included. Furthermore, deficiency diseases such as scurvy would demand mention. Such a totally inclusive approach is clearly impractical. To list in tabular form the ocular manifestations of many *diseases* having a biochemical etiology is feasible, however, and has been attempted. The discrete disease entities have not been completely described; this would be an unnecessary duplication of material that is more appropriately presented in texts with a traditional nosological classification (Graymore and Hsia, 1970; Stanbury et al., 1966; Tasman, 1971). It is hoped that the tables at the end of this chapter will help the physician who is confronted by a particular case to identify the primary illness. He may then refer to other sources for more complete information regarding methods of treatment, specific techniques of diagnosis, and so forth.

Data are given in a format that separates entities with purely (or predominantly) ocular findings from those with important systemic abnormalities. These lists are not totally complete, but, hopefully, are fairly comprehensive. Findings are tabulated regionally and alphabetically within subheadings.

In these tables findings that are complications of the major clinical manifestation of the basic disease have not been listed. For example, glaucoma often follows the dislocation of the lens seen in patients with homocystinuria (Spaeth and Barber, 1966). Yet, this glaucoma is not a direct ocular expression of the disease. On the other hand, glaucoma is a major part of Lowe's syndrome (Curtin et al., 1967; Haut and Joannides, 1966). Similarly, the elevation of intraocular pressure seen in Refsum's disease may be due to fat plugging the outflow channels, and as such glaucoma is a relatively direct manifestation of Refsum's disease (Toussaint and Danis, 1971). Even this is, of course, a *secondary* expression of the fundamental defect elsewhere, however, which is an abnormal oxidation of fatty acids (Herndon et al., 1969).

It should not be assumed that because a disease is listed under a particular heading that the finding is invariably present. For example, not all patients with Marfan's syndrome have strabismus, nor do all (or even most) hypoglycemic individuals develop cataracts.

Many inborn errors of metabolism are

associated with mental retardation. Those in which ocular abnormalities are present in addition to the retardation are listed in Table 19–2.

A clinical finding common to remarkably many metabolic diseases is pigmentary degeneration of the retina. A perusal of the list of such entities (Table 19–3) immediately impresses one with the frequency with which "retinitis pigmentosa" is noted

TABLE 19–2 SOME METABOLIC DISEASES WITH OCULAR FINDINGS AND MENTAL RETARDATION

Alpha-amino butyric aciduria
Argininosuccinic acidemia
Ataxia telangiectasia
Congenital tryptophanuria with dwarfism
Cystathioninuria
Fabry's disease
Farber's disease
Galactosemia (transferase defect)
Gaucher's disease
GM_1 gangliosidosis
GM_2 gangliosidoses (Tay-Sachs, Sandhoff, etc.)
Glycinemia
Hartnup disease
Homocystinuria (cystathionine synthetase deficiency)
Hooft's disease
Hunter's syndrome
Hurler's syndrome
Hydroxyprolinemia
Hyperammonemia (carbamyl phosphate synthetase deficiency) (ornithine transcarbamylase deficiency)
Hyperlysinemia
Hyperserotonemia
Idiopathic hypercalcemia
Idiopathic hypoglycemia
Imidazole aminoaciduria
Krabbe's disease
Laurence-Moon-Bardet-Biedl syndrome
Lowe's syndrome
Maple syrup urine disease
Menke's disease
Metachromatic leukodystrophy
Morquio's syndrome
Niemann-Pick disease
Oxalosis
Phenylketonuria
Prolinemia (proline oxidase deficiency)
Riley-Day syndrome
Sanfilippo's syndrome
Sturge-Weber syndrome
Sulfite oxidase deficiency
Tay-Sachs disease
Tuberous sclerosis
Valinemia
Wilson's disease

TABLE 19–3 HEREDITARY PIGMENTARY DEGENERATIONS OF THE FUNDUS OF THE EYE

1. Ocular Disease
     Primary pigmentary retinopathy ("retinitis pigmentosa") and variants
     Retinitis punctate albescens (progressive albipunctate dystrophy)
     Gyrate atrophy
     Choroideremia
     Hyaloideotapetoretinal degeneration of Goldmann-Favre
     Hyaloideoretinal degeneration of Wagner

2. Associated with Metabolic Disease
     Abetalipoproteinemia
     Familial high-density lipoprotein deficiency (Tangier disease)
     Batten's cerebral degeneration with macular changes (juvenile amaurotic familial idiocy)
     Imidazole aminoaciduria
     Hooft's disease
     Refsum's disease
     Hurler's, Hunter's, Sanfilippo's, and Scheie's mucopolysaccharidosis
     Gaucher's disease
3. Associated with Neurologic Disease
     Friedreich's ataxia
     Peroneal muscular atrophy (Charcot-Marie-Tooth disease)
     Myotonic dystrophy
     Ophthalmoplegia and ptosis
     Neuroendocrine dyscrania
     Laurence-Moon-Bardet-Biedl syndrome
     Status dysraphicus
     Pelizaeus-Merzbacher disease
     Hallgren's syndrome
     Cockayne's syndrome
     Werner's syndrome
     Usher's syndrome

in diseases of lipid metabolism and in illnesses in which neurologic signs are preeminent. This connection is an interesting one. Lipids are the basic building block of the nervous system, and neurologic abnormalities are characteristic of lipid disease. Does this suggest that "retinitis pigmentosa" is itself a secondary expression of some as yet unknown defect in lipid metabolism? It would be well worth trying to answer this.

A few of the diseases due to "inborn errors of metabolism" will be discussed in terms of their primary ocular manifestations, stressing differential diagnosis.

Cornea (see Appendix Table C)

Fabry's Disease

The faint, superficial corneal opacity noted in Fabry's disease is of considerable diagnostic aid. This consists of fine curving lines located in the deeper layers of the epithelium which radiate peripherally from a locus approximately 1 mm. below the corneal center (Fig. 19–9). They may spiral into small whorls before reaching the limbus, in some patients being barely visible but in others coating the entire corneal surface with a delicate, gray-white haze (Spaeth and Frost, 1965). Present in approximately 90 per cent of individuals with Fabry's disease, this finding must be sought for with a biomicroscope.

It may be that the corneal changes are invariably present in affected males, though this has not been established with certainty, since there are reports of males in whom no corneal change was noted. Most females who are definite carriers of this disease will have the corneal opacities, but occasionally they are absent in these individuals (Weingeist and Blodi, 1971).

Other ocular findings of Fabry's disease are listed in Table 19–4, Figures 19–10 and 19–11, and Plate XII-C and D. Of these an inconspicuous cataract may be of great diagnostic help (Fig. 19–10). Occurring in about 50 per cent of all patients, both male and female, this subtle change is

TABLE 19–4 OCULAR MANIFESTATIONS OF FABRY'S DISEASE

	Approximate Frequency of Occurrence
Periorbital edema	25%
Superficial, whorled corneal opacities	90%
Dilated, sausage-shaped conjunctival blood vessels	60%
Posterior capsular, spokelike cataract	50%
Dilated retinal veins	50%
Corkscrew retinal blood vessels	50%
Retinal arteriovenous malformation	10%
Macular edema	10%
Papilledema	22%

best appreciated by observing the lens through the direct ophthalmoscope. The pupil must be widely dilated. In such instances a shadow of approximately a dozen branching spokes radiating out from the center of the lens can just be made out. Recently it has been demonstrated that these lines consist of glycolipid deposited along the posterior capsule. The finding may be pathognomonic of Fabry's disease and need be differentiated only from the rare patient in whom the normal posterior suture lines of the lens are visible.

Fabry's disease (angiokeratoma corporis diffusum) is the expression of an abnor-

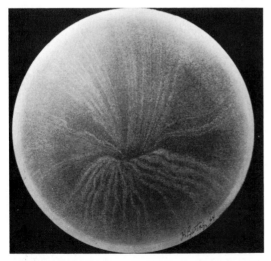

Figure 19–9 Cornea of a 46-year-old woman with no other evidence of Fabry's disease; her son is affected, however.

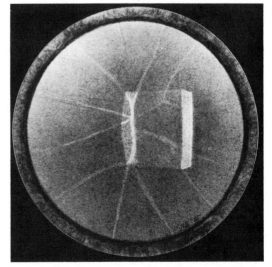

Figure 19–10 Lens of a 6-year-old boy with no signs or symptoms of Fabry's disease; his mother is a definite carrier. The posterior capsular location of the lens opacities can be established by use of the slit lamp.

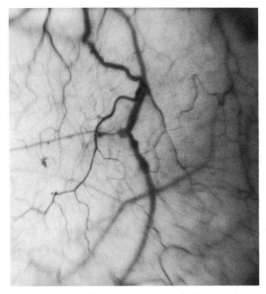

Figure 19–11   Tortuous conjunctival vessels in a 22-year-old man with Fabry's disease. Similar changes are seen in other conditions as well.

TABLE 19–5   CLINICAL FINDINGS IN FABRY'S DISEASE

Youth:
   Burning sensations of extremities
   Severe pain in extremities
Adolescence:
   Fever of unknown origin
   Skin lesions in bathing suit area
Adult:
   Malaise, fatigue
   Blood vessel disease
   Premature death
Genetics:
   Sex-linked recessive
Pathology:
   Excess deposition of ceramide trihexoside
      in many tissues

mality of sphingolipid metabolism that results in excessive storage of ceramide trihexoside (Brady et al., 1967; Sweely and Klionsky, 1963). First described in 1898, it has been the subject of extensive investigation (see reference listing under Fabry's Disease at end of chapter). Recently it has become of special interest because it may represent one of the first diseases of metabolism in which partial reversal of the biochemical abnormalities has been achieved by treating the affected individual with deficient enzyme itself (Mapes et al., 1970).

A diagnosis of Fabry's glycolipid lipidosis can usually be made with reasonable certainty on the basis of the history and physical findings alone (Table 19–5). The inheritance pattern is X-linked recessive (Johnston et al., 1969). However, the characteristic purple angiokeratomas, which are most numerous in the "bathing suit area," are also seen in other conditions; moreover, this dermatologic manifestation may even be absent (Clarke et al., 1971; Kemp, 1967) (Plate XII-E). Histopathologic changes, consisting of PAS-positive, sudanophilic granules in the media of small blood vessels throughout the body are easily seen in biopsy specimens of conjunctiva or rectal mucosa (Frost et al., 1966) (Fig. 19–12).

Deficiency of ceramide trihexosidase establishes the diagnosis with certainty (Brady et al., 1967; Sweely and Klionsky, 1963). Cultured skin fibroblasts may be utilized for this purpose, and antenatal detection is possible (Brady et al., 1971). Furthermore, kidney transplantation has recently been performed on the patient with Fabry's disease (Philipport et al., 1972), with resultant increase in the level of serum ceramide trihexosidase, and decrease in serum lipids to within normal limits. This has been associated with a striking decrease in the acroparesthesia that is so characteristic of this abnormality of sphingolipid metabolism.

Alpha-L-fucosidase deficiency produces a clinical entity that is similar in some ways to Fabry's disease. The dermatologic and histopathologic aspects of the two conditions resemble each other. However, the marked mental and physical retardation that is characteristic of individuals with a deficiency of alpha-L-fucosidase is not a part of Fabry's disease; furthermore, the ocular manifestations so typical of Fabry's disease have not been reported in cases with the other entity, which also resembles to some extent certain of the mucopolysaccharidoses (Patel et al., 1972).

Hypophosphatasia

Hypophosphatasia, a familial disease characterized by abnormalities of the skeleton and subnormal values of serum alkaline phosphatase, has received relatively little mention in the ophthalmologic literature (Brenner et al., 1969). However, cor-

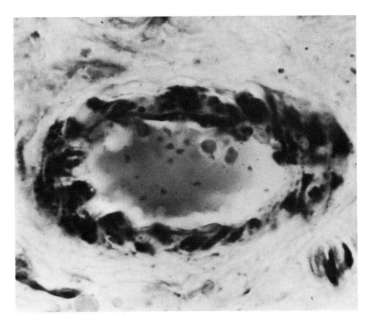

Figure 19–12 Sudan Black stained conjunctival tissue clearly demonstrates the glycolipid material present in the media of small blood vessels (× 1000).

neal epithelial calcification has been described. This may be related to the hypercalcemia which is a frequent correlate of the disease. Other ocular findings include conjunctival calcifications and thin sclerae; lid retraction, proptosis, papilledema, and optic atrophy are probably secondary to the craniostenosis that develops in children owing to premature synostosis. Cataracts have also been mentioned.

The cardinal feature of the disease is inadequate calcification of bone matrix, though the biochemical basis for this is unknown. There is no adequate therapy at the present time.

Diagnosis is based on the demonstration of radiologic and histologic changes in the bone (highly similar to those in rickets) and the finding of phosphoethanolamine in the urine, in addition to decreased serum alkaline phosphatase activity.

Mucolipidoses

Many metabolic diseases due to "inborn errors of metabolism" have opacities of the corneal stroma as part of their clinical expression. This includes the mucopolysaccharidoses (McKusick, 1966), the mucolipidoses (Kenyon and Sensenbrenner, 1971), and the sphingolipidoses (Spaeth, 1971). The mucopolysaccharidoses are more fully discussed in Chapter 20. Corneal haziness is noted in Hurler's, Mor-

quio's, Scheie's, and Maroteaux-Lamy syndromes (Cockayne, 1936; Constantopoulos, 1971; Hurler, 1919; Kenyon et al., 1972; Pfaundler, 1920; Quigley and Goldberg, 1971). Optic atrophy and pigmentary degeneration of the retina have also been described in these disorders of mucopolysaccharide metabolism (Gills et al., 1965).

The mucolipidoses are characterized by storage of both mucopolysaccharides and either sphingolipids or glycolipids (Table 19–6). Several types have been described, and they share clinical features with both the mucopolysaccharidoses and the sphingolipidoses (Kenyon and Sensenbrenner, 1971). In mucolipidosis types I and III, the corneas are grossly clear but with a slit lamp, a ground-glass stromal translucency is apparent, most marked posteriorly and peripherally (Quigley and

TABLE 19–6 MAJOR CLINICAL ASPECTS OF THE MUCOLIPIDOSES; EXPRESSION VARIES WITH ENTITY

Clouding of the corneal stroma
Gargoyle-like facies
Macular cherry-red spot
Mental retardation
Normal mucopolysacchariduria
Skeletal dysplasia
Visceral storage of acid mucopolysaccharide and glycolipids

Goldberg, 1971). Goldberg (1971) has described a mucolipidosis in which both a macular cherry-red spot and corneal clouding are present. This same combination has also been noted in general gangliosidoses (GM type 1). In metachromatic leukodystrophy slight clouding of the corneal stroma has also been described in conjunction with a cherry-red spot (Cogan et al., 1970).

The corneal changes in Fabry's disease are discussed elsewhere in this chapter.

Tangier Disease

Tangier disease is a rare abnormality in which plasma cholesterol and phospholipids are reduced and triglycerides are normal or elevated (see reference listing). It is due to a deficiency or absence of high-density alpha-lipoproteins. The clinical manifestations of the illness are probably due to the storage of cholesterol esters in many tissues throughout the body, especially the reticuloendothelial system. The major ocular manifestation of Tangier disease is a very fine infiltration of the entire corneal stroma. The haziness may be sufficient to be noted without magnification and occurs in approximately 80 per cent of patients (Spaeth, pers. com.). The fine, closely packed dots that can be just resolved with the high power of the biomicroscope do not have the sparkling, multicolored iridescence of the crystals seen in cystinosis or multiple myeloma. They only faintly resemble the changes seen in Fabry's disease, chloroquine keratopathy, or fingerprint lines of the cornea. In Tangier disease the infiltration is predominantly in the posterior third of the corneal stroma, whereas in familial plasma lecithin-cholesterol acyl transferase deficiency the gray dots involve the entire stroma and merge into a soft-edged arcus, with a clear interval immediately adjacent to the limbus.

Exact diagnosis of high-density lipoprotein deficiency (Tangier disease) can be made by determination of lipoprotein fractions, most specifically by immunoelectrophoresis. There is no treatment for the condition.

Plasma Lecithin–Cholesterol Acyl Transferase Deficiency

Deficiency of an enzyme that esterifies cholesterol (lecithin–cholesterol acyl transferase) causes a diffuse corneal haziness in association with an atypical arcus (Gjone and Bergaust, 1969). The entire stroma is involved, and the deposition is resolvable into tiny dots that appear most dense centrally. A clear interval is present immediately adjacent to the limbus. Plasma lecithin-cholesterol acyl transferase deficiency has been reported in three sisters (ages 21 to 35) who appeared to be healthy on gross examination, but who manifested proteinuria, anemia, and the slight corneal haziness just described (Burke and Schubert, 1972).

Cystinosis

Cystinosis, a disease with diffuse aminoacidemia and precipitation of cystine in the tissues, has as one of its most characteristic findings the deposition in the cornea of refractile, iridescent, glistening crystals of cystine (Bürcki, 1941; Seegmiller, 1968). The crystals formed in paraproteinemia (multiple myeloma) are clinically indistinguishable. No other disease known to date produces a similar appearance (Laibson and Damiano, 1969). Peripherally the deposits occupy the entire thickness of the corneal stroma, whereas only the anterior two thirds are affected centrally (Fig. 19–13 A and B). These crystals may also be noted in the conjunctiva or the iris (Wong et al., 1970). They are difficult to demonstrate histologically but show up in a striking fashion when viewed with polarized light, since the crystals are birefringent. Other ocular manifestations of cystinosis include photophobia, which may be the presenting complaint, epiphora, and "red eyes" (Boniuk and Hill, 1966) (Table 19–7). A diffuse, faint mottling of the pigment of the fundus of the eye has also been described; some believe that it is one of the earliest signs of the disease (Seegmiller, 1968). However, a similar mottling may be noted in the eyes of normal children (Kessing, 1971; Spaeth, pers. com.).

The usual form of the disease has its onset in the first year of life and manifests itself by a failure of the child to grow, polyuria, and renal rickets. Death in most instances ensues prior to the age of 10. Various methods of treatment have been proposed but none are entirely satisfactory (Goldman et al., 1970; Mahoney et al., 1970). Cystinosis is inherited in an autosomal recessive pattern.

Wong, Brubaker, and others have re-

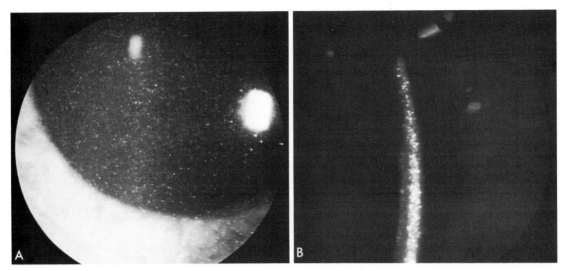

Figure 19–13 *A*, Cornea of an 8-year-old girl with cystinosis, seen in direct illumination. The crystals are too small to see with the naked eye but are readily visible with proper magnification. *B*, Slit beam view of the cornea illustrated in *A*. The refractile, iridescent crystals are scattered throughout the stroma but are most dense in the anterior two thirds.

ported the existence of a different form of the disease, in which the corneal changes are noted in adults. This appears to be a benign disorder, free from the clinical manifestations of childhood cystinosis (Brubaker et al., 1970; Kraus and Lutz, 1971; Leitman et al., 1966; Schneider et al., 1968). The absence of renal tubular or glomerular defects in patients with adult cystinosis has not been explained, and the only symptom of significance may be decreased visual acuity owing to the marked deposition of crystals in the cornea, even to the extent that a keratoplasty becomes necessary.

TABLE 19–7 OCULAR FINDINGS IN CYSTINOSIS

Photophobia (may be first manifestation)
Epiphora (sensation of excess tearing)
Homogeneously dispersed, tinsel-like refractile opacities in the cornea and conjunctiva. Occupy entire thickness of corneal stroma peripherally while centrally only the anterior one third to two thirds is affected. Not present at birth.
Depigmented, patchy, peppery stippling of the far periphery of the fundus. More on the temporal than the nasal side; may be the first ocular finding. Electroretinogram and all other ocular tests normal. Adults show crystals but no fundus changes.

The correct diagnosis of cystinosis is usually suggested by the appearance of the cornea. It can be confirmed by the relatively simple method of conjunctival or rectal biopsy (Holtzapple, 1969), or by the examination of material obtained from the bone marrow.

Cystine is present in all cells of individuals afflicted with cystinosis. It accumulates in cells of the reticuloendothelial system and cornea either because they replicate slowly or because they represent a preferential environment (Hummeler, 1970).

Wilson's Disease

In Wilson's hepatolenticular degeneration, copper is deposited in excess amounts in the liver, brain, kidneys, and cornea. It is interesting that the only pathognomonic sign of Wilson's disease was not noted in the original descriptions of the affliction (1911). The "Kayser-Fleischer" ring may be visible grossly; however, its presence can be definitely excluded only by means of a biomicroscopic examination. The copper deposited in the periphery of the cornea produces a variable effect, sometimes blue, sometimes greenish-brown, and occasionally dark brown. It is most prominent at the superior and inferior aspects of the cornea but may extend 360 degrees, and has been noted in approximately 85 per cent of involved individuals. The granular deposition in Descemet's membrane ends at Schwalbe's line.

Other ocular findings of Wilson's disease include a "sunflower cataract" in about 10 per cent of patients (similar to the cataract seen with intraocular copper-containing foreign bodies) and nystagmus or extraocular muscle palsies in rare cases (Cairns et al., 1969; Stemerling and Oloff, 1922).

It is vitally important to make the diagnosis as soon as possible, even in the "presymptomatic" stages of the disease, because treatment is so effective that when instituted early the tragic clinical course of increasing spasticity, rigidity, and eventual death can be prevented (Sternlieb and Scheinberg, 1968; Warnock, 1967). Diagnosis is based on the deficiency of serum ceruloplasmin (less than 20 mg. per 100 ml.) and the increase in excretion of urinary copper. However, some patients with this disease are known to have had normal ceruloplasmin levels.

Inherited as an autosomal recessive, the disease expresses itself more frequently in males than in females, with the age of onset usually in the second decade of life.

Various methods of treatment are now available and include pyridoxine, penicillamine, potassium sulfide, and a low copper diet (DuBois et al., 1971; Sternlieb and Scheinberg, 1964). BAL has been used in the past but it is more toxic than penicillamine. One case in which the cataract cleared completely on treatment has been reported, but there was no change in the Kayser-Fleischer ring (Cairns et al., 1969). There have been other reports in which the Kayser-Fleischer ring disappeared with treatment (Sussman and Scheinberg, 1969), but the relationship between effectiveness and the appearance of the corneal pigmentation is not a close one (Mitchell and Heller, 1968).

Glaucoma (See Appendix Table F)

Refsum's Disease

Metabolic diseases should come to mind when glaucoma is observed in children. In Refsum's disease, in which night blindness is the pre-eminent ocular symptom, blockage of Schlemm's canal with lipid is apparently responsible for the acute glaucoma that may occasionally be seen (Toussaint and Danis, 1971). Other clinical

TABLE 19–8 CLINICAL ASPECTS OF REFSUM'S DISEASE

Order of Appearance	Occurrence
Autosomal recessive inheritance	
Night blindness and progressively constricted visual fields	Childhood
Anosmia	Childhood
Pes cavus	Childhood
Peripheral neuropathy, sensory and motor	Adolescence
Cerebellar ataxia	Adolescence
Increased cerebrospinal fluid protein; normal cells	Adolescence
Day blindness	Adulthood
Icthyosis	Adulthood
Nerve deafness	Adulthood
ECG changes	Adulthood
Premature death	Adulthood

aspects of Refsum's disease are listed in Table 19–8. The correlation between the biochemical abnormality, which is an excessive accumulation of the long-chain fatty acid, phytanic acid, and the clinical manifestations of the disease is not clear (see reference listing).

Lowe's Syndrome (Fig. 19–14)

Glaucoma is an integral part of the oculocerebrorenal syndrome of Lowe (Table 19–9). In this sex-linked recessive abnormality, affected males manifest cataracts, glaucoma, psychomotor retardation, aminoaciduria, and acidosis in infancy (see reference listing). The carrier state in the female can be recognized by multiple, fine, punctate lens opacities. Almost all have congenital cataract, whereas glaucoma is not always present. In addition, nystagmus, failure to thrive, hypotonia, and osteoporosis may be observed. The lenticular opacities are scattered throughout the entire fetal nucleus and extend into the adult nucleus, two thirds being in the anterior portion of the lens and one third in the posterior. It has been reported that goniotomy may relieve the elevated intraocular pressure, but the fatal termination of the illness must be borne in mind. Moreover, the results of glaucoma surgery are in most instances unsatisfactory, judged even from the limited point of view of control of intraocular pressure. Cataract aspiration may be successful but is often complicated by residual capsular material or corneal clouding. Other forms of renal

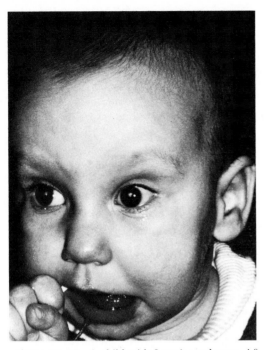

Figure 19–14 A child with Lowe's syndrome. Affected males almost always have congenital cataracts; glaucoma may also develop in early infancy.

TABLE 19–9 OCULAR FINDINGS IN LOWE'S SYNDROME

Congenital Cataract:
   Present in 92% (first sign)
   Bilateral in 90%
   Total in 60%
   Nuclear in 35%
   Zonular in 5%

Glaucoma:
   Present in 56% (unassociated with cataract in 6%)
   Unilateral in 8%
   Of variable type, and accompanied with secondary findings of increased intra-ocular pressure and corneal edema
Convergent or divergent strabismus (almost always)
Nystagmus (almost always)
Miosis (resistant to any pharmacologic agent) in 20%
Iris atrophy in 5%

tubular acidosis must also be considered, especially since some of these may be satisfactorily treated by the administration of sodium bicarbonate. Treatment is also available for other genetic disorders in which mental deficiency is associated with secondary disturbance of renal tubular function, such as galactosemia and Wilson's disease. Other similar entities include nephrogenic diabetes insipidus and phospho-glucoaminoaciduria. There is, however, no effective therapy for Lowe's syndrome.

Elevation of intraocular pressure may be associated with abnormalities of the anterior segment of the eye, such as those seen with microcornea, mesodermal dysgenesis of the iris, Axenfeld's anomaly, or aniridia. In neurofibromatosis, with its well-known "café au lait" spots, glaucoma is usually unilateral.

Sclera (See Appendix Table N)

Alkaptonuria

Alkaptonuria, though one of the four original inborn errors of metabolism described by Garrod in 1908, warrants but brief commentary in a pediatric text. For although this condition, inherited as an autosomal recessive disease, is of great importance historically and biochemically, its manifestations usually do not become apparent until the later years of life, and rarely before the age of 25 years. It is then that the dark brown to slate gray pigmentary changes on the sclera, usually most marked on the temporal aspect of the eye approximately 5 mm. from the limbus, first become apparent. Pigmentation of

DATA FOR FOUR PATIENTS WITH THE OCULOCEREBRORENAL SYNDROMES AT ST. CHRISTOPHER'S HOSPITAL FOR CHILDREN OF PHILADELPHIA

Patients	Age When First Seen (months)	Cataracts	Glaucoma	Ocular Surgery Results
W.B.	10	+	−	Good
R.P.	4	+	+	Fair
J.G.	6	+	+	Poor
P.D.	1½	+	−	Good

Disease	Frequency of Dislocation of the Lens
Homocystinuria (cystathionine synthase deficiency)	Very high
Sulfite oxidase deficiency	Very high
Hyperlysinemia	Moderate
Marfan's syndrome	High
Marchesani syndrome	High
Ehlers-Danlos syndrome	Low

TABLE 19–11 OCULAR MANIFESTATIONS OF THE EHLERS-DANLOS SYNDROME

Angioid streaks	Common
Macular degeneration	Common
Strabismus	Common
Blue sclerae	Uncommon
Thin corneas	Uncommon
Dislocated lenses	Uncommon
Epicanthus	Uncommon
Hypertelorism	Uncommon

other cartilaginous and collagenous structures (ochronosis) also occurs. As with albinism, another disease of abnormal pigment metabolism, alkaptonuria is due to an abnormality in the metabolism of phenylalanine and tyrosine. Owing to the lack of activity of the enzyme homogentisic acid oxidase, homogentisic acid accumulates and is excreted in the urine. When urine containing homogentisic acid is allowed to stand, it gradually turns dark brown, producing the classic sign of the disease, darkly stained diapers. The diagnosis is made by identifying homogentisic acid in urine. There is no effective treatment.

Displaced Lenses (See Appendix Table I)

Abnormal position of the lens of the eye is a sign of several different inborn errors of metabolism (Table 19–10). It is seen in almost every individual with aniridia and is present in the great majority of those with Marfan's syndrome. It is also a characteristic finding of the Marchesani syndrome and is occasionally noted in the Ehlers-Danlos syndrome (Fig. 19–15 and Table 19–11). (See Chapter 20, Part D). Dislocation of the lens is also one of the most prominent findings in diseases of sulfur-containing amino acid metabolism, most specifically homocystinuria and sulfite oxidase deficiency (Mudd, 1967). Furthermore, dislocation of the lens is noted in some individuals with familial hyperlysinemia, a rare abnormality of amino acid metabolism in which spherophakia and lateral rectus palsy have also been observed (Smith et al., 1971).

Though the direction of dislocation of the lens is highly variable, there is a tendency for the lens to move inferiorly in homocystinuria and the Marchesani syndrome, superotemporally in Marfan's syndrome (Table 19–12), and superona-

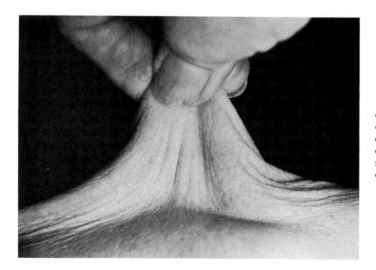

Figure 19–15 Skin near the elbow in elderly woman with Ehlers-Danlos syndrome. The abnormal stretchiness is characteristic. Angioid streaks, macular degeneration, retinal detachment, blue sclerae, and dislocated lenses are typical ocular manifestations.

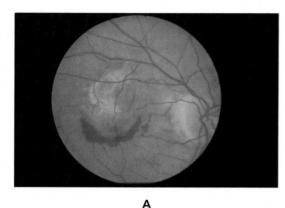

A

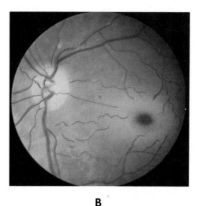

B

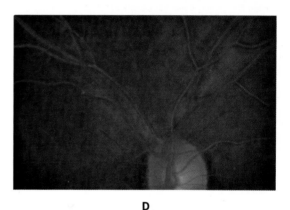

C   **D**

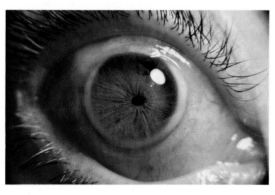

E

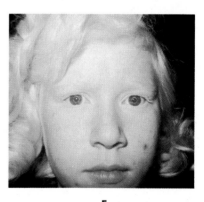

F

Plate XIII   *(A)* The ocular fundus in the case of Ehlers-Danlos syndrome illustrated in Figure 19–15.

(B) Fundus of infant with Tay-Sachs disease. There is optic atrophy, indicating that the disease is in its late stages.

(C) Fundus of 12-year-old with a Batten's cerebral degeneration with macular changes. Mild pigmentary abnormalities are apparent. The electroretinogram is abnormal. There is usually no accumulation of ganglioside in these cases, unlike that shown in *B*.

(D) Lipemia retinalis. The marked fundus changes in this 28-year-old black man with fat-induced hyperlipemia (type I hyperlipoproteinemia) cleared within several days after ingestion of fat was stringently limited.

(E) Arcus senilis. The severe degree of corneal arcus seen here is uncommon even in the elderly. When observed in individuals younger than age 40 years, arcus is an indication of pathologic elevation of serum cholesterol, as occurs in type II hyperlipoproteinemia.

(F) Generalized albinism.

TABLE 19–12 OCULAR FINDINGS IN MARFAN'S SYNDROME AND THE FREQUENCY OF THEIR OCCURRENCE

A. *Globe*		
	Myopia	Usual
	Blue sclerae	Usual
	Megalocornea	Rare
	Keratoconus	Rare
	Microphthalmos	Rare
B. *Iris*		
	Miosis	Usual
	Aniridia	Rare
	Coloboma	Rare
	Heterochromia	Rare
C. *Angle*		
	Prominent iris processes	Usual
	Abnormally deep recess	Usual
	Poorly seen scleral spur	Usual
	Hydrophthalmos	Rare
	Glaucoma in adults	Occasional
D. *Lens*		
	Dislocated	Usual
	Cataract	Rare
	Coloboma	Rare
E. *Retina*		
	Detachment	Frequent
	Pigmentary degeneration	Rare
	Coloboma of macula	Rare
	Coloboma of nerve	Rare

sally in the familial congenital dislocation of the lens. Eyes having traumatic dislocations of the lens usually show other signs of the trauma, and it is frequent for the lens to be hinged inferiorly. Dislocation of the lens may also occur more frequently in syphilitic persons, but the evidence for this has been disputed.

Homocystinuria

Homocystinuria is a disease of methionine metabolism due to a deficiency of the enzyme cystathionine synthetase (Fig. 19–8). (Carson, 1963; Laster, 1965; Waisman et al., 1962). As a consequence the individuals develop excess homocysteine and methionine in blood and other tissues, and excrete pathologically large amounts of homocystine in the urine. The disease can be readily detected by testing the urine with nitroprusside. The false-positive results that occur with this test can be reduced but not eliminated entirely by using Barber's modification (Spaeth and Barber, 1967).

The pathogenesis of the systemic abnormalities has been related to the widespread occurrence throughout the body of vascular thromboses that probably are a function of the elevated homocysteine present in the blood. Numerous infarcts in the brain have been demonstrated and may be responsible for the mental retardation that is found in the majority of cases (Dunn et al., 1966). However, cystathionine is an essential component of brain tissue and has been shown to be deficient in the central nervous system of patients with homocystinuria (Gerritsen and Waisman, 1964).

Cystathionine synthetase deficiency disease is inherited as an autosomal recessive, and has a wide spectrum of symptoms (Finkelstein, 1964; Spaeth and Barber, 1965). Although mental retardation is characteristic, some individuals appear to have entirely normal intellectual abilities (Schimke et al., 1965; Spaeth and Barber, 1965). Furthermore, dislocated lenses are not present in all cases. In the fully affected individuals the disease usually has its onset in early childhood and gradually progresses until the time of death around the age of 20. Fair hair is characteristic with a blotchy appearance to the skin and a malar flush (Fig. 19–16 *A*). The gait is flapping and the knees are knocked (Fig. 19–16 *B*). The fingers are elongated, and a close relationship with Marfan's syndrome has been definitely established (Schimke et al., 1965). Homocystinuria has been named as the second most common metabolic error responsible for mental retardation, the first being phenylketonuria.

Some individuals with homocystinuria respond favorably to large doses of pyridoxine (vitamin B_6) with complete or near complete normalization of biochemical values and a decreased tendency to clot formation (Barber and Spaeth, 1967 and 1969). Other cases are resistant to the effects of pyridoxine, which is the precursor of the coenzyme for cystathionine synthetase (Shih and Efron, 1970). The precise mechanism by which pyridoxine produces the biochemical improvement is not known, however. Raising the concentration of the cofactor may enable the enzyme whose binding site for this cofactor has presumably been altered genetically to function at physiologic rates (Gaull et al., 1969). Management with low methionine

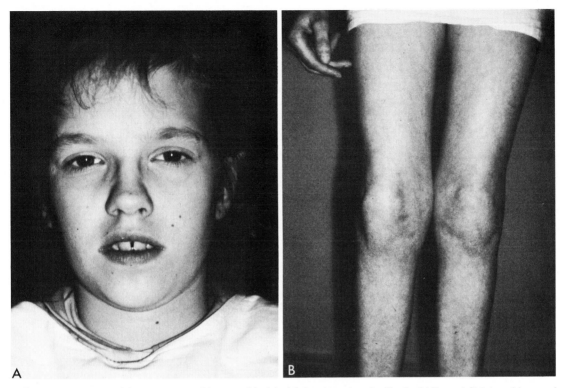

Figure 19–16 *A*, Facial appearance of 7-year-old girl with homocystinuria. She had bilateral dislocated lens and optic atrophy but no glaucoma. *B*, Genu valgum in a girl with homocystinuria.

diet has proved of some help in some cases, but it is not easily accomplished in most homes (Perry, 1966; Perry et al., 1968).

Dislocation of the lens is the most prominent ocular manifestation of homocystinuria (Spaeth and Barber, 1966) (Fig. 19–17). In fact it is not unusual for the affected child to be seen initially because of secondary glaucoma, often produced by the lens having dislocated into the anterior chamber. Displacement of the lens anteriorly appears to be more common than in most other entities associated with ectopia lentis, such as Marfan's syndrome. Whether or not long-term treatment with pyridoxine and/or dietary management will lessen the tendency to progressive dislocation of the lens in patients with homocystinuria is not yet established. Surgery should be undertaken with special caution in these patients, not only because of the well-documented high incidence of complications associated with extraction of a dislocated lens, but also because of the increased tendency of patients with homocystinuria to develop thromboses, which

complicates the anesthesia considerably. When secondary glaucomas occur, they are probably best treated conservatively by repositioning the lens in the posterior chamber or vitreous, and by relieving pupillary block by means of the instillation of cycloplegic agents.

The pathogenesis of optic atrophy in patients with homocystinuria has not been entirely elucidated, but it may well be more an expression of vascular insufficiency of the optic nerve than it is of undetected secondary glaucoma (Spaeth, pers. com.). It is present in approximately 25 per cent of cases (Fig. 19–18).

Other ocular findings associated with homocystinuria are listed in Table 19–13 (Henkind and Ashton, 1965; Martenet et al., 1968; Presley et al., 1969; Spaeth and Barber, 1966; Wilson and Ruiz, 1969).

Sulfite Oxidase Deficiency

Sulfite oxidase deficiency is an extremely rare abnormality of sulfur metabolism in which there is an accumulation of S-sulfocystine, thiosulfate, and sulfite, and a deficiency of sulfate (Mudd et al., 1967). The

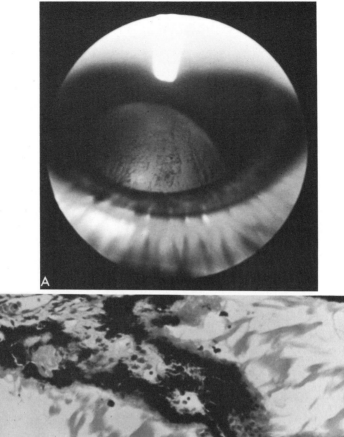

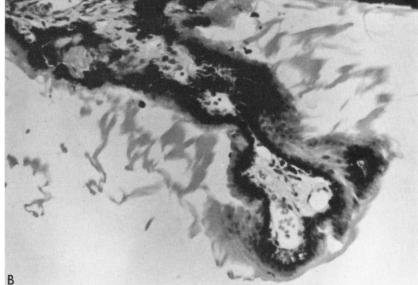

Figure 19–17 *A*, Dislocated cataractous lens in 29-year-old woman with homocystinuria. *B*, Ciliary process and degenerated zonular material from the eye of a girl dying from thrombosis associated with homocystinuria.

abnormality is present at birth and results in death prior to the age of 3. Dislocated lenses, progressive musuclar rigidity, and decerebrate behavior are typical findings. There is no effective treatment.

Cataract (See Appendix Table I)

Galactosemia

Galactosemia necessitates prompt diagnosis. There are at least two genetic dis-

orders which produce galactosemia (Hansen, 1969). In one, activity of the enzyme galactose *kinase* is decreased; in the other, a *transferase* activity (galactose-1-phosphate uridyl transferase) is lacking (Isselbacher et al., 1956) (Fig. 19–19). The first type is relatively benign; the second is extremely debilitating. Both types, if detected early, can have their clinical symptomatology completely aborted simply by the severe restriction of dietary galactose.

The clinical manifestations are directly

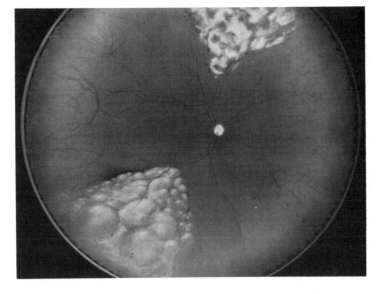

Figure 19–18 Fundus drawing of a patient with homocystinuria; note the optic atrophy, chorioretinal changes, and peripheral cystoid degeneration.

related to the inability to properly utilize ingested galactose. The disease (due to the transferase defect) may be fatal if the diet is not adjusted appropriately (Hansen, 1969). In contrast, if the offending carbohydrate is removed from the diet, most symptoms regress or may even disappear completely. Recent evidence suggests that the incidence of galactosemia is far higher than was previously thought (Shih et al., 1971).

The infant with galactosemia of trans-

TABLE 19–13 OCULAR FINDINGS ASSOCIATED WITH HOMOCYSTINURIA AND THE FREQUENCY OF THEIR OCCURRENCE

Dislocation of lenses	Almost all cases
Myopia	Almost all cases
Peripheral cystoid retinal degeneration	Usual
Optic atrophy	Frequent
Secondary glaucoma	Frequent
White deposits on the ciliary processes and zonular fibers	Uncertain
Congenital cataract	Rare
Papilledema	Rare
Central retinal artery occlusion	Rare
Aniridia	Rare
Coloboma of choroid and optic disc	Rare
Coloboma of iris	Rare
Congenital retinal septum	Rare
Microcornea	Rare
Microphthalmos	Rare

ferase deficiency type usually appears normal at birth but shortly thereafter, associated with the ingestion of the galactose in milk, develops the three most important signs of the disease: cataracts, hepatosplenomegaly, and mental retardation. Diarrhea, dehydration, and death follow. However, it is essential to stress that in many instances the symptoms are much less pronounced, and permanent disability but not death may result. Diagnosis may be made promptly by finding a reducing sugar in the urine, which, when further analyzed, is shown to be galactose. However, since infants with the typical signs of the disease may be placed on parenteral therapy, the usual laboratory findings of galactosuria, aminoaciduria, and albuminuria, may not be present at the time of testing.

The realization that this disease, transmitted by a single autosomal recessive gene, is an expression of the cellular deficiency of the enzyme galactose-1-phosphate uridyl transferase has allowed rapid and specific diagnosis of this condition by means of an analysis of red blood cells. Any infant with nutritional failure, cataracts, hepatosplenomegaly, aminoaciduria, or central nervous system dysfunction must have the appropriate enzyme determination performed immediately. Shih has even suggested that all gravely ill infants should be screened for galactosemia (Shih et al., 1971).

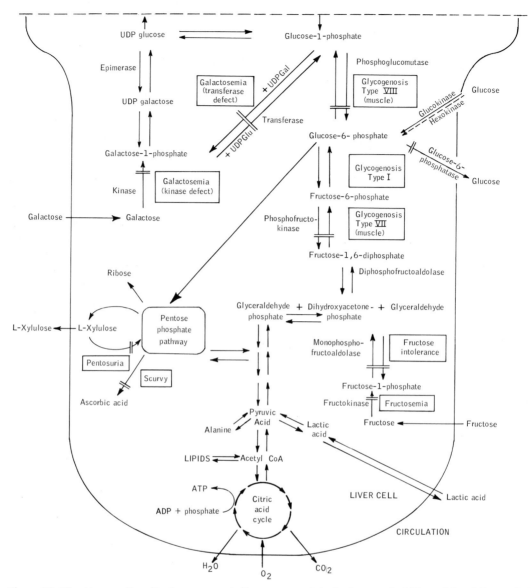

Figure 19–19 Abnormality of galactose metabolism may result in "galactosemia." Two of the different defects responsible for this are shown, one in a kinase enzyme, the other in a transferase. (From Nelson, W. E., Vaughn, V. C., III, and McKay, R. J.: Textbook of Pediatrics. 9th ed. Philadelphia, W. B. Saunders Co., 1969.)

The only significant manifestation of disease due to the kinase defect appears to be the development of a cataract, which may be reversible. The treatment for both types of galactosemia centers around elimination from the diet of galactose. Commercial milk substitutes are now readily available. In the sick infant (with transferase deficiency) symptomatic therapy aimed at correction of the electrolyte and nutritional abnormalities must also be given.

The essential and perhaps only ocular finding is a reversible cataract. The pathophysiology of the lens change probably involves the excessive accumulation within the lens of dulcitol, which is formed by the enzymatic reduction of galactose and is not metabolized further (Dische et al., 1956; Kinoshita, Merola, and Dikmak, 1962; Kinoshita, Merola, Satoh, and Dikmak, 1962). This results in a change in the osmotic balance with a consequent increase in the water drawn into the lens and the subsequent opacification. The first visible change is the development of a posterior lenticonus, which greatly resembles the appearance of an oil droplet. This can be appreciated merely by the use of a penlight in the infant whose pupil has been widely dilated. Also visible in the very early stages of the disease, frequently before two months after birth, are concentric, refractile rings extending from a central whitish opacity in the center of the lens nucleus. Without treatment, the extent and intensity of lenticular opacification progresses until the outer fetal and the deeper layers of the adult nucleus become involved; these lamellar or zonular opacities continue to spread, both eyes being affected to a similar degree. Peripheral spokes appear, and the lens may become totally opaque prior to the age of three months (Fig. 19–20).

When appropriate therapy is instituted the accumulation of dulcitol within the lens apparently ceases, and, indeed, the cataract regresses and may disappear completely, leaving an apparently normal lens. Similar improvement also occurs in the other signs of the disease, with the unfortunate exception of mental retardation, which may persist. This stresses the need for early diagnosis and prompt institution of therapy.

The galactose tolerance test, which has been suggested as a diagnostic method in the past, should *not* be carried out in infants suspected of having galactosemia. This test is definitely not without hazard, and is now unnecessary, since more specific and far safer methods of diagnosis are available, such as that which measures the transferase activity in red cells in vitro.

The role of galactose metabolism in the development of cataracts in individuals who do not have the structural gene mutation responsible for galactosemia is not completely understood (Tedesco and Mellman, 1971). A high-galactose diet can produce cataracts in normal rats (Richter and Duke, 1970; Segal and Bernstein, 1963). Furthermore, there appears to be a wide variation in the degree of enzyme activity in normals. Recently it has been shown that glucose concentration directly effects the metabolism of galactose in galactosemic cells, and it has been suggested that glucose may play a protective role in galactosemia in vivo (Petricciani, 1972). It is, then, entirely possible that the interplay between the amount of ingested galactose and glucose, and the basic level of genetically determined enzyme activity may play a role in the development of cataract to greater extent than has been previously believed.

The younger an individual unable to metabolize galactose properly when faced with a galactose load, the more serious is the damage done. It may then be important to identify carriers so that they may refrain from galactose ingestion during pregnancy.

Glucose-6-Phosphate Dehydrogenase Deficiency

Lenticular opacities also occur in several other diseases of carbohydrate metabolism, specifically glucose-6-phospate de-

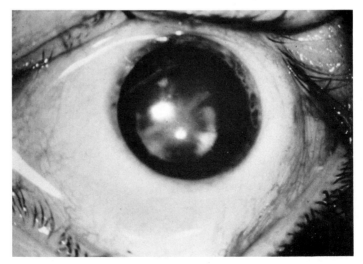

Figure 19–20 Characteristic "oil droplet" cataract in a galactosemic infant. Located centrally in the lens, this defect may clear completely if galactose is eliminated from the diet.

hydrogenase deficiency (Westring and Pisciotta, 1966), hypoglycemia (Scheie et al., 1964), and glycogen storage disease (Schaffer, personal communication). Glucose-6-phosphate dehydrogenase deficiency has come to the attention of physicians since the discovery of "wonder drugs," because the condition becomes manifest in response to certain medications (or the fava bean) (De Lorre and van Gelderen, 1967). Individuals with the enzyme deficiency develop an acute hemolytic anemia after ingestion of certain sulfonamides, antimalarials, phenacetin, and many other drugs. The illness is widely distributed throughout the world, variants being designated by the site of the discovery, but the gene frequency appears to be especially high among Blacks, around 10 per cent. Inherited as a sex-linked trait, glucose-6-phosphate dehydrogenase deficiency results in two populations of red blood cells in female heterozygotes, one being normal and the other being markedly abnormal (Beutler, 1966). The ocular manifestations result primarily from the acute hemolytic anemia and include the retinal changes seen in many severe anemias, that is, retinal hemorrhages and retinal and optic nerve ischemia (Choremis et al., 1960). Cataract has also been reported (Westring and Pisciotta, 1966). Also, vitreous hemorrhage has been noted (Choremis et al., 1960). The diagnosis can be made by a variety of methods of in-vitro assay of dehydrogenase activity in red cells. Treatment consists primarily of avoidance of the fava bean and of the many drugs known to induce the acute hemolytic anemia in affected individuals.

Hypoglycemia

Hypoglycemia, once considered a single entity, is now known to be a sign of a variety of disorders, primarily affecting children. Unlike most adults, infants and children show a marked lowering of blood sugar when more than 24 hours passes without absorption of carbohydrate. Thus, hypoglycemia may occur secondary to inadequate diet or poor intestinal absorption, as with diarrhea. Hypoglycemia may also occur in diseases with defective tubular reabsorption of glucose, as in the de Toni-Fanconi syndrome, or in other con-

TABLE 19–14 OCULAR MANIFESTATIONS OF HYPOGLYCEMIA AND THEIR APPROXIMATE INCIDENCE

Strabismus	10%
Cataract	10%
Nystagmus	5%
Glaucoma	3%
Staring gaze	3%

ditions including hyperinsulinism, galactosemia, and a variety of hepatic abnormalities. Bilateral lamellar cataract occurs in approximately one fifth of patients with "ketotic hypoglycemia" (Grunt and Howard, 1972). It has been observed less frequently in patients with idiopathic hypoglycemia (Merin et al., 1971; Scheie et al., 1964) (Table 19–14). Lens changes are a well-known part of certain conditions (such as Lowe's syndrome, in which a secondary hypoglycemia is present).

Glycogenoses

In the various glycogen deposition diseases ophthalmic aspects have been quite inapparent. However, flat, discrete, drusen-like paramacular yellow spots have been described in type 1 disease (Fine et al., 1968), of which retarded growth, adiposity, enormous abdominal rotundity, pallid skin, and hepatomegaly are the major clinical manifestations. The illnesses of glycogen deposition are of special interest, since the observation by Cori in 1952 that von Gierke's disease was due to a defect in a single tissue enzyme was the first clear demonstration that an inborn error of metabolism was due to an enzyme abnormality.

Optic Atrophy (See Appendix Table L)

Atrophy of the optic nerve is a frequent correlate of diseases due to inborn errors of metabolism. It is most characteristic of the lipid abnormalities, and in such instances may be a reflection of primary disease in the nervous system. On the other hand, the optic atrophy seen in certain illnesses, such as homocystinuria, may be a secondary manifestation of the disease in a similar manner to the ischemia that is due to an abnormal tendency toward intravascular thrombosis.

Abetalipoproteinemia

Abetalipoproteinemia is a rare familial disease characterized by absence of one of the lipoproteins and by abnormally low serum lipids. Bassen and Kornzweig first described the entity in 1950, and noted an atypical retinitis pigmentosa in addition to neuromuscular disturbances similar to those of Friedreich's ataxia and abnormal red cells (acanthocytes) (Bassen and Kornzweig, 1950) (Table 19–15). The primary biochemical lesion appears to be a selective one, affecting the main apoprotein of low-density lipoproteins (Gotto et al., 1971). The defects are not due simply to the lack of circulating beta-lipoprotein, as demonstrated by the failure of intravenous administration of normal plasma to effect lipid metabolism in affected individuals (Lees and Ahrens, 1969). The concurrence of retinitis pigmentosa and lipid abnormality is again noted in this illness.

Ocular manifestations of abetalipoproteinemia (acanthocytosis) include visual loss, night blindness, and scotomatous defects which usually become apparent after adolescence and then continue to progress (Gouras et al., 1971; Jampel and Falls, 1958; Mier et al., 1960). They are probably related to the mottled, pigmentary degeneration of the retina that develops. The macula may also be involved, and optic atrophy becomes apparent as

blindness ensues. Electroretinography indicates decreased rod function. Other ocular signs may also be noted, including partial paresis of the extraocular muscles, exotropia, ptosis, and nystagmus.

There is conflicting evidence regarding the role of vitamin A deficiency in this illness (Gouras et al., 1971; Wolff et al., 1964). The ocular defect does not seem to be directly related to this insufficiency, yet improvement has been noted following the administration of vitamin A, and consequently should probably be recommended. In one patient with this disorder the intravenous administration of cottonseed oil emulsion resulted in marked clinical improvement. Unfortunately, the therapy had to be halted when the patient developed a typical intravenous fat overloading syndrome (DiGeorge et al., 1961).

Metachromatic Leukodystrophy

Common to all the many varieties of *leukodystrophy* is degeneration of the white matter of brain (Moser and Lees, 1966). The fundamental biochemical defects in all these entities may be an abnormality of lipid metabolism (Bargeton, 1963). In *metachromatic leukodystrophy* sulfatide is accumulated in tissues throughout the body owing to a defect in the enzyme responsible for the removal of sulfate from the sulfatide (aryl sulfatase A) (Austin et al., 1964; Austin et al., 1965; Porte et al., 1971). In the myelin sheath this excess lipid apparently replaces the normal molecule, with a resultant loss of the normal function of myelin and its eventual anatomic disintegration (Webster, 1962). There is also a decrease in cerebrosides in patients with metachromatic leukodystrophy, and it may be the imbalance between the ratio of cerebroside and sulfatide that is actually responsible for the observed functional changes (Moser and Lees, 1966).

The clinical manifestations of metachromatic leukodystrophy are listed in Table 19–16. One of the most distinctive aspects of the disease is the apparent normal neonatal period after which there is inexorable retrogression with increasing loss of acquired skills. Optic atrophy is an important, but late, symptom, and the blindness that characterizes the terminal stages is

TABLE 19–15 CLINICAL MANIFESTATIONS OF ABETALIPOPROTEINEMIA

Clinical steatorrhea (first year of life)
Progressive ataxia (ages 2 to 17)
Nystagmus (ages 2 to 17)
Strabismus (adolescent)
Night blindness and retinitis pigmentosa
    (late adolescence)
Laboratory findings:
    Absent beta-lipoproteins
    Acanthocytosis
    Abnormally low plasma cholesterol,
        phospholipid, and triglyceride
    Engorgement of intestinal epithelium
        with triglyceride
    Vitamin A deficiency
Genetics: Autosomal recessive
Pathology: Demyelinization of posterior
            columns and spinocerebellar
            tracts associated with neuronal
            loss of anterior horn cells,
            cerebellar macular level, and
            cerebral cortex

TABLE 19–16 SIGNS AND SYMPTOMS OF METACHROMATIC LEUKODYSTROPHY

Order of Appearance	Age (in years)
Normal development initially	Birth to 1 or 2
Unsteady gait	1 to 2
Mental deterioration (progressive)	$1\frac{1}{2}$ on
Speech impairment	$1\frac{1}{2}$ on
Hypotonia	$1\frac{1}{2}$ to 4
Tetraplegia	2 to 5
Pain in arms and legs	2 to 5
Nystagmus	2 to 5
Generalized rigidity	$2\frac{1}{2}$ to 6
Hypertonic fits	$2\frac{1}{2}$ to 6
Optic atrophy	$2\frac{1}{2}$ to 6
No speech	$2\frac{1}{2}$ to 6
Fever	$2\frac{1}{2}$ to 6
Blindness	3 to 6
Disappearance of pains, fits, and fever	3 to 6
No contact at all with surroundings	3 to 6
Bulbar symptoms	3 to 6
Decerebrate rigidity	3 to 6
Death	3 to 6

more prominent than the optic atrophy itself would suggest.

The ocular manifestations of metachromatic leukodystrophy may be of considerable diagnostic help, especially in those forms of the illness that afflict old individuals, since in these instances vision is lost relatively early in contrast to the infantile variety in which poor sight is not a notable symptom and in which optic atrophy is usually not observed until the illness nears its final stages (Percy and Kaback, 1971). Cogan has described a cherry-red spot in the macula of infants with metachromatic leukodystrophy (Cogan et al., 1970). In other entities with this sign, for example, Tay-Sachs disease, visual loss occurs early in the course of the illness, prior to the development of motor abnormalities.

The ocular histopathologic findings have been described by Cogan et al. (1958). Excess lipid is present in the ganglion cells of the retina, accounting for the occasionally observed cherry red-spot. However, the cells do not show evidence of being damaged by the deposited material, which may explain why vision is lost relatively late in the infantile forms of the disease.

The simplest and most important diagnostic test, which probably should be performed on all individuals with neurologic symptoms in whom a diagnosis is not absolutely definite, is examination of the urine for the presence of metachromatic material (Hagberg, 1963). Various modifications and refinements of technique have made this examination now quite reliably specific for diagnosis of various diseases, including metachromatic leukodystrophy. Deficiency of the enzyme aryl sulfatase A establishes the diagnosis even more conclusively, distinguishing the illness from other forms of leukodystrophy such as Krabbe's disease, Pelizaeus-Merzbacher disease, spongy degeneration, and Schilder's disease, venous blood may be used for this determination (Percy and Brady, 1968). No therapy has proved useful to date.

Krabbe's Disease

Krabbe's infantile diffuse cerebral sclerosis has been thought to be one of the rare inborn errors of metabolism in which the enzymatic abnormality lay in an anabolic rather than a catabolic pathway, the defect being in the enzyme catalyzing the sulfation of cerebroside (Austin et al., 1967). However, more recent evidence suggests that the previous belief was in error and that the actual abnormality is deficient activity of the catabolic enzyme, galactocerebrosidase B (Suzuki and Suzuki, 1971). The clinical manifestations are similar to those of metachromatic leukodystrophy, but the onset of disease is usually within the first six months of life and deterioration is more rapid. Optic atrophy occurs at an earlier age, and nystagmus and early blindness, accounted for by demyelination of both the optic nerve and the optic cortex, are prominent (Nelson et al., 1963). The diagnosis of Krabbe's disease is based on the presence of large multinucleate giant cells (globoid cells) in areas of demyelinization.

Maple Syrup Urine Disease

Optic atrophy has also been reported in maple syrup urine disease, a metabolic abnormality of the degradation of branched-chain amino acids, leucine, isoleucine, and valine (Dancis et al., 1959). This illness is due to a deficiency in the oxidative decarboxylation of the corresponding alpha-keto acids and its outstanding characteristic is a maple syrup odor of the urine. Affected infants usually appear normal at birth but develop neurologic symptoms by the end of the first week. Death may follow promptly, or the patient may live for a decade, in which case severe mental retardation is apparent (Gaull, 1969). The diagnosis is made by demonstrating an elevation in blood and urine of a great excess of branched-chain amino acids and of the corresponding keto acids in the urine, but the odor itself should suggest the entity. Dietary treatment aimed at supplying reduced amounts of the branched-chain amino acid appears to prevent serious complications of the disease, stressing the need for prompt diagnosis in the first week of life (Westall, 1963).

Macular Lesions (See Appendix Table E)

Diseases of sphingolipid metabolism represent a varied, heterogeneous collection of entities virtually unable to be treated. The inability of the body to properly metabolize sphingolipid materials disastrously affects the well-being of the organism; especially upset are the neural systems in which lipid components are basic building blocks. The diversity of ocular manifestations in these illnesses was succinctly described by Cogan and Kuwabara in 1968; more recently these manifestations have been extensively reviewed by Spaeth (1971). A schema of the metabolism is shown in Figure 19–21.

The appearance of a cherry-red spot in the macula of the ocular fundus is an important signal that an inborn error of sphingolipid metabolism may be present. Although a cherry-red spot may be seen in association with retinal edema due to either ischemia or trauma, in these latter instances, the underlying cause for the retinal abnormality is usually readily

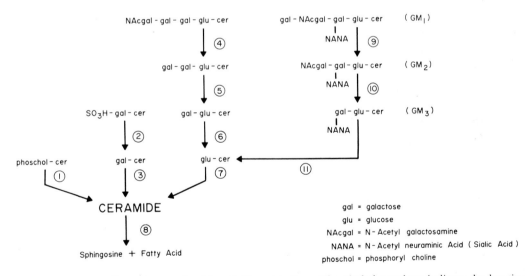

Figure 19–21 Metabolic pathways of sphingolipid metabolism. The circled numbers indicate the location of enzymatic defects responsible for specific diseases:

  1. Sphingomyelinase deficiency   Niemann-Pick disease
  2. Aryl sulfatase A deficiency   Metachromatic leukodystrophy
  3. Galactosyl hydrolase deficiency   Krabbe's leukodystrophy
  4. Hexosaminidase A and B deficiency   Globoside storage disease
  5. Ceramide trihexosidase (alpha-galactosidase)   Fabry's disease
     deficiency
  6. Lactosyl ceramide galactosyl hydrolase deficiency   Lactosyl ceramidosis
  7. Glucocerebrosidase deficiency   Gaucher's disease
  8. (? esterase)   Farber's disease
  9. Beta-galactosidase A, B, and C deficiency   Generalized gangliosidosis
 10. Hexosaminidase A deficiency   Tay-Sachs disease
 11. (?)   Pilz' disease[220]

TABLE 19–17 ILLNESS IN WHICH A MACULAR CHERRY-RED SPOT HAS BEEN NOTED

	Frequency of Occurrence of Sign
Farber's syndrome (ceramide lipidosis)	Uncertain
Goldberg's syndrome (mucolipidosis; uncertain type)	Uncertain
Generalized gangliosidosis (GM$_1$ type 1)	In less than 50% of patients?
Tay-Sachs disease (GM$_2$ type 1)	In all patients
Metachromatic leukodystrophy (sulfatide lipidosis)	In occasional patients
Mucolipidosis type 1	Uncertain
Niemann-Pick disease (sphingomyelin-cholesterol lipidosis type A)	In about 50% of patients

ILLNESSES IN WHICH OCCURRENCE OF A MACULAR LESION RESEMBLING A CHERRY-RED SPOT HAS BEEN REPORTED

Adult Niemann-Pick disease
Gaucher's disease
GM$_2$ type 2 (Sandhoff's disease)
Lactosyl ceramidosis
Sea-blue histiocyte syndrome

apparent. Once these conditions are eliminated, the differential diagnosis involves a number of the lipidoses (Table 19–17).

Tay-Sachs Disease

Tay-Sachs disease is the most commonly recognized disease of sphingolipid metabolism. It occurs primarily in Ashkenazic Jews. Clinical signs in order of appearance are indicated in Table 19–18. Deficiency of hexosaminidase A is the primary enzyme defect (Okada and O'Brien, 1969), but insufficient fructose-1-phosphate aldolase has also been demonstrated (Volk et al., 1964), and apparently results in improper handling of the carbohydrate portion of gangliosides, with the result that they are accumulated in excessive amounts in tissues (Brady, 1969). The cherry-red spot, for example, is due to the presence of ganglioside in the ganglion cells of the macula; since ganglion cells are absent from the fovea, the perifoveolar area ap-

pears a bright, off-white color, whereas the fovea itself stands out as a red spot (Cogan and Kuwabara, 1959; Cotlier, 1971). Optic atrophy is usually not present until after the cherry-red spot has been present for several months (Plate XIII-B).

Because of its relative frequency, the ability to make a prenatal diagnosis of this disease, which is inherited following an autosomal recessive pattern, is of considerable importance (Schneck et al., 1970). While a variety of laboratory studies can be of decided help in the study of the disease, definitive diagnosis is made by identification of the characteristic enzyme defect (Korey et al., 1963; Okada and O'Brien, 1969). Identification of the carrier state of the illness can also be made by appropriate biochemical tests and is of aid in the genetic counseling of the family. No treatment is available.

Generalized Gangliosidosis

Recently it has been possible to subdivide the ganglioside storage diseases much

TABLE 19–18 SIGNS AND SYMPTOMS OF TAY-SACHS DISEASE

Order of Appearance	Time of Onset (in months)*
Exaggerated startle response to sound	1 to 2
Apathy	2
Abnormal SGOT, LDH, F–1–PA**	3
Hypotonia (poor head control, weakness of shoulder girdle)	2 to 4
Poor vision	2 to 3
Cherry-red spot	2 to 3
Mental deterioration	2 to 4
Optic atrophy	3 to 6
Nystagmus	4 to 6
Peripheral cyanosis	4 to 12
Spasticity	6 to 12
Seizures	12 to 24
Abnormal ECG	14 to 18
Megalencephaly	18 to 24
Decerebrate rigidity	24 to 36
Clubbing	30+
Death	24 to 36

*Diagnosis should be apparent between ages 2 and 4 months.
**Serum glutamic oxaloacetic transaminase (SGOT) is elevated, lactic dehydrogenase (LDH) is elevated, fructose-1-phosphate aldolase (F–1–PA) is depressed.

TABLE 19–19 FAMILIAL AMAUROTIC IDIOCIES: THE SPHINGOLIPIDOSES (BY ENZYME DEFECT)

GM$_2$ Gangliosidosis—Type 1 *(Tay-Sachs)* (Infantile amaurotic idiocy)	Absence of hexo-saminidase A
GM$_2$ Gangliosidosis—Type 2 *(Globoside storage disease)* (Sandhoff) (Visceral Tay-Sachs)	Absence of hexo-saminidase A and B
GM$_2$ Gangliosidosis—Type 3 *(Bernheimer-Suzuki-Volk)* (Late infantile amaurotic idiocy) (Bielschowsky-Jansky)	Partial deficiency of hexo-saminidase A
GM$_1$ Gangliosidosis—Type 1 *(Generalized gangliosidosis)* (Landing-O'Brien) (Systemic late infantile amaurotic idiocy)	Absence of beta-galactosidase A, B, C
GM$_1$ Gangliosidosis—Type 2 *(Derry)* (Late infantile amaurotic idiocy)	Absence of beta-galactosidase B and C

Modified from O'Brien, J. S.: Lancet, *II*:805, 1969.)

more clearly, by specific identification of the variety of the stored ganglioside and the associated enzymatic defect (Table 19–19). This table also lists the names most frequently used to describe the various conditions under discussion. A cherry-red spot has also been reported in GM$_1$ type 1 gangliosidosis in which, unlike Tay-Sachs disease, a normally occurring ganglioside accumulates in abnormally excessive amounts (Emery et al., 1971; O'Brien et al., 1965; Suzuki et al., 1968). This cherry-red spot of the macula appears to be present in about 50 per cent of cases of this disease. The major difference between GM$_1$ type 1 gangliosidosis and Tay-Sachs disease (GM$_2$ type 1) is the more generalized involvement in the former, as reflected

in several of the names given to the entity before the biochemical defect was finally unveiled and the "identical" nature of the separately reported illnesses recognized: neurovisceral lipidosis, pseudo-Hurler's disease, and systemic late infantile lipidosis. Not only the neurodegenerative changes that are so typical of the ganglioside storage diseases but also visceromegaly and bony abnormalities are present. The condition becomes manifest at the time of birth, development is grossly retarded, congestive heart failure ensues, and death occurs prior to the age of one year. The ocular manifestations of GM$_1$ type 1 gangliosidosis include the macular redness already mentioned. Most afflicted infants will also have cloudy corneas and optic atrophy; nystagmus and retinal hemorrhages have been reported. The differential diagnosis of generalized gangliosidosis includes the other amaurotic familial idiocies (Tay-Sachs, GM$_2$ type 2 (Sandhoff's disease), GM$_2$ type 3 and so on), the mucopolysaccharidoses, the mucolipidoses, and Niemann-Pick disease.

Batten's Cerebromacular Degeneration

The traditional classification of the sphingolipid diseases is shown in Table 19–20 (Batten, 1903; Bielschowsky, 1914; Collins, 1892; Jansky and Myslivicek, 1918; Kufs, 1925; Mayou, 1904; Norman and Wood, 1941; Sachs, 1896; Spielmeyer, 1906; Tay, 1881; Vogt, 1905). Unfortunately, there is considerable overlap of these entities, both in clinical symptomatology, histopathology, and biochemistry (Table 19–21). Despite the many attempts to organize these illnesses reasonably, no single classification is adequate as yet, for there are inconsistencies in each one (Spaeth, 1970), whether the basis be clini-

TABLE 19–20 THE SPHINGOLIPIDOSES

Eponym	Onset of Disease	Descriptive Name
Tay-Sachs	Birth	Congenital amaurotic familial idiocy
Bielschowsky-Jansky	2 to 5 months	Infantile amaurotic familial idiocy
Batten-Mayou	1 to 3 years	Late infantile amaurotic familial idiocy
Spielmeyer-Vogt	5 to 15 years	Juvenile amaurotic familial idiocy
Kufs	24 to 45 years	Adult amaurotic familial idiocy

TABLE 19–21   PATHOLOGICAL CLASSIFICATION OF SPHINGOLIPIDOSES

Membranous Cytoplasmic Bodies	Curvilinear bodies	Lipofuscin
1. Tay-Sachs	Late infantile amaurotic idiocy	1. Late infantile amaurotic idiocy
2. Systemic late infantile amaurotic idiocy (Landing-O'Brien) 3. Late infantile amaurotic idiocy (Bernheimer-Suzuki-Volk) (Derry)	(Duffy-Gonatas-Zeman)	(Bernheimer-Suzuki-Volk) 2. Juvenile amaurotic idiocy (Batten-Spielmeyer-Vogt)

Modified from O'Brien, J. S.: Lancet, *II*:805, 1969.

cal (Danis et al., 1947; Godtfredsen, 1971), histopathologic (Gonatas et al., 1968) (Table 19–20), or biochemical (O'Brien, 1969; Raine, 1969). From a clinical point of view there seem to be at least two major subgroups, one with a cherry-red spot and the other with an atrophic type of macular degeneration associated with retinal pigmentary changes and an abnormal electroretinogram (Spaeth, pers. com.) (Plate XIII-C). The former tends to afflict younger individuals and the latter an older group (Wolter and Allen, 1964). Cerebromacular degeneration also occurs in the unrelated disease imidazole aminoaciduria (Bessman and Baldwin, 1962).

It is also possible roughly to subdivide the amaurotic familial idiocies on the basis of whether or not there is an accumulation of ganglioside (Donahue et al., 1967; Seitelberger et al., 1967; Zeman and Dyken, 1969). However, there is even overlap in this regard (Zeman and Hoffman, 1962). In the juvenile and adult varieties excess ganglioside is usually not present, whereas the forms in which there is a cherry-red spot usually show deposited ganglioside. The name "Batten's cerebral degeneration with macular changes" has been suggested to replace those entities previously known as "Batten-Mayou" and "Spielmeyer-Vogt" disease. This name has been offered because it underscores the basic findings and gives credit to the original author (Table 19–22). It seems preferable to the others suggested, which include Bielschowsky-Jansky disease, Spielmeyer-Vogt disease, Batten-Mayou disease, juvenile amaurotic familial idiocy, neuronal ceroid-lipfuscinosis, and myoclonic variant of cerebral lipidosis. Instead of ganglioside it appears that lipofuscin is deposited in the neurons. Inherited as an autosomal recessive condition, heterozygotes can be detected by the

azurophilic hypergranulation of the neutrophils or vacuolization of the lymphocytes. The differential diagnosis includes progressive myoclonic epilepsy (Lafora's disease), which also has its onset in early adolescence and which includes myoclonus and convulsions, ataxia, and progressive visual loss as prominent findings (Yanoff and Schwartz, 1965). In myoclonic epilepsy of the Lafora type, however, there are no visible changes in the fundus, that is, there is no optic atrophy, no pigmentary degeneration, and no macular degeneration. A particular intraneuronal inclusion body (the Lafora body) is found in all parts of the central nervous system; in the retina these are noted in the ganglion and the bipolar cells. This disease is also transmit-

TABLE 19–22   CLINICAL MANIFESTATIONS OF BATTEN'S CEREBROMACULAR DEGENERATION

General Signs
  Onset between ages 4 and 6 years
  Progressive cerebellar ataxia, first affecting lower extremities
  Grand mal seizures
  Progressive dementia
  Extrapyramidal signs develop later
  Deterioration may be slow or rapid
  Termination in incessant myoclonic and cerebral fits
Ocular Manifestations
  Visual loss—in all patients, usually early in the disease
  Yellowish atrophy of the optic nerve—in all patients, usually early
  Macular depigmentation—in all patients, early
  Peripheral pigmentary changes—in most patients, later
  Abnormal electroretinogram—in all patients
  Nystagmus—usual
  Posterior cortical cataracts—occasional
  Cherry-red spot—not seen

ted as an autosomal recessive. But the classification of these entities is still clearly very much unsure and will continue to change as new knowledge is added.

Recent investigations by Armstrong et al. have demonstrated a definite deficiency in peroxidase activity in the late infantile and juvenile forms of Batten-Spielmeyer-Vogt syndrome (BSV).

Lipopigments are prominent in BSV and are considered to represent end products of lipid peroxidation. Peroxidase is an enzyme that can hydrolyze peroxides (hydrogen peroxide) and by this means reduce lipid peroxidation. Myeloperoxidase activity was markedly deficient in the white blood cells of four patients with the late infantile and juvenile forms of BSV. Deficient peroxidase activity was found by both histochemical and spectrophotometric methods using two different substrates (benzidine and phenylenediamine).

Other laboratory criteria, such as hypergranulation of the neutrophils, correlated with the peroxidase deficiency. Vacuolated lymphocytes were useful only in the juvenile form. The distinctive accumulation of ceroid in neurons and other cells of patients with this syndrome is attributable to deficient peroxidase activity.

Farber's Disease

Farber's disseminated lipogranulomatosis is due to excessive accumulation of ceramide (Crocker et al., 1967). Respiratory symptoms are prominent in the early months of life, and death is usual before the age of three. Cogan has described the maculas as being distinctly gray with a mild cherry-red center (Cogan et al., 1966). The optic discs show slight atrophy, and the entire fundus has a peppery pigmentation. The differential diagnosis includes the nonlipid cutaneous granulomatous disorders (Letterer-Siwe syndrome), infectious granulomas, and rheumatic conditions. No treatment has been effective.

Niemann-Pick Disease

The appearance of the macula is quite different in the various forms of Niemann-Pick disease. In younger individuals with the more traditional manifestations of this fatal affliction in which there is both visceral and neurologic involvement owing to the deposition of excessive sphingomyelin and cholesterol, a classic cherry-red spot is present in around 50 per cent of cases

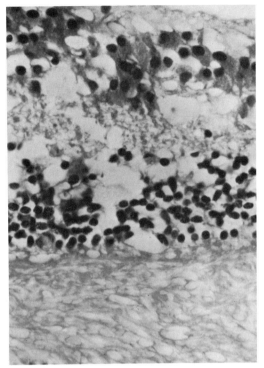

Figure 19–22 The retina in Niemann-Pick disease. (Hematoxylin and eosin stain, ×400) The ganglion cells are distended with lipid material in this area adjacent to the macula.

(Goldstein and Wexler, 1931). On the other hand, in the patient whose disease does not become manifest until adulthood, a ring of crystalloid deposits circling the otherwise normal fovea has been described (Cogan and Federman, 1964).

The histopathologic changes in the retina of the patient with Niemann-Pick disease are quite different from those seen in Tay-Sachs disease (Jansseune et al., 1967; Spaeth, pers. com.). No atrophy of the nerve fiber layer occurs, and though the ganglion cells may be loaded with lipid material, the striking reduction of severely damaged ganglion cells that characterizes Tay-Sachs disease is not apparent (Fig. 19–22). This correlates with the clinical finding as well, since visual loss is a permanent finding in Tay-Sachs disease, whereas in Niemann-Pick disease it is not. Furthermore, optic atrophy is a prominent part of the former disease, whereas in the latter it is absent.

Other than the macular changes there are no other ocular manifestations of Niemann-Pick disease.

The existence and characteristics of the varieties of this illness have become increasingly well-defined (Crocker and

Farber, 1958; Niemann, 1914; Pick, 1927). It is the second most commonly diagnosed sphingolipid disease, and the four subgroups are quite different from each other, though all share the symptom of hepatosplenomegaly and most have central nervous system involvement. The diagnosis should be considered in individuals with enlargement of the liver and spleen, child or adult, especially if a macular lesion is present as well. But a precise diagnosis cannot be made on the basis of clinical evidence alone. Other entities must be considered: cephalin lipidosis (Barr and Hickmans, 1956), Wolman's disease (Wolman et al., 1970), Gaucher's disease (Kampine et al., 1967), lactosyl ceramidosis (Dawson and Stein, 1970), and the ganglioside storage diseases (Spaeth, 1970). Specific diagnosis is made by identification of a deficiency in serum of sphingomyelin cleaving enzyme (Brady et al., 1966).

Gaucher's Disease

Gaucher's disease is due to deficiency of glucocerebroside-cleaving enzyme, as a result of which excess glucocerebroside accumulates in the reticuloendothelial cells of spleen, liver, lymph nodes, and bone marrow and produces the characteristic signs and symptoms of the illness. A macular cherry-red spot has been reported in one patient with Gaucher's disease, but it is certainly not a characteristic finding in this abnormality of sphingolipid metabolism. This case was reported prior to the awareness of the existence of many of the ganglioside-storage diseases. It is quite possible that the correct diagnosis was not in actuality Gaucher's disease, but rather one of the other entities in which a cherry-red spot is a more expected sign.

The usual form of Gaucher's disease is slowly progressive and interferes little with the patient's life. Hematologic changes may develop owing to extensive involvement of the spleen and bone marrow. Brownish deposits on the conjuctiva resembling pingueculas may occur. The more rare infantile form presents a different clinical picture in which neurologic symptoms predominate. Onset is usually in the first year of life, and death usually ensues prior to the first birthday. The sole ocular manifestation is strabismus. Correct diagnosis of Gaucher's disease may be made histopathologically by noting the presence of pathognomonic "Gaucher's cells," which stain strongly with PAS but not with stains used to demonstrate lipids. Demonstration of a deficiency of cerebroside-cleaving enzyme confirms the diagnosis definitely. The carrier state can be identified by the presence of the Gaucher cell, which facilitates genetic counseling. There is no effective therapy.

Lactosyl Ceramidosis

Lesions resembling the cherry-red spot have been reported to occur in entities other than those already discussed (Table 19–17). They are too rare, however, to allow meaningful estimation of the frequency of the finding. Of these, lactosyl ceramidosis is perhaps the most interesting, at least from a historical point of view. Figure 19–21 is a composite picture of the metabolism of the sphingolipids. Many of the steps on this chart have only recently been determined. Diseases were known to exist due to defects in every step of the catabolism of ceramide trihexoside with the exception of one—the degradation of the dihexoside to the monohexoside. Just as it was possible from the nature of the periodic table to predict the existence of still undiscovered elements, so it was postulated that a disease must exist due to a defect in the enzyme (galactosyl hydrolase) responsible for this reaction. In 1970 such a disease was identified in a 3-year old Black girl (Dawson and Stein, 1970). Apparently normal at the time of birth, a course quite similar to that of Tay-Sachs first became apparent at the age of about $2\frac{1}{2}$ years. Mental and neurologic regression was marked by hypotonia, cerebellar ataxia, and then spasticity, without, however, the development of opisthotonos. "Increasing redness" of the maculas was noted. Hepatosplenomegaly was present, as was increased serum acid phosphatase, both being nonspecific findings characteristic of many of the sphingolipid diseases. Foam cells (very large [40 micra] mononuclear cells filled with clear foamy cytoplasm) that are noted in a variety of storage diseases, as indicated in Table 19–23, were present in the bone marrow. Lactosyl ceramide was pathologically elevated in blood and all tissues studied. Lactosyl ceramidase activity (a galactosyl hydrolase) was depressed to less than 20 per cent of normal.

The recognition of lactosyl ceramidosis means that a specific disease entity is now

TABLE 19–23 DISEASES IN WHICH FOAM CELLS ARE PRESENT

Glycogen deposition diseases
Hyperlipoproteinemias
Mucopolysaccharidoses
Sphingolipidoses
Others
Cephalin lipidosis
Tangier disease
Familial lecithin–cholesterol acyl transferase deficiency
Wolman's disease
Urbach's lipoid proteinosis
Histiocytosis X*
Juvenile xanthogranuloma*

*Not hereditary diseases.

known to exist for every step of the catabolism from red cell globoside to the parent lipid, sphingosine (Fig. 19–21). Furthermore, as pointed out by Dawson and Stein, four clinically distinct glycosphingolipidoses (Fabry's disease, Krabbe's leukodystrophy, generalized gangliosidosis, and lactosyl ceramidosis) have now been attributed to specific galactosyl hydrolase deficiencies (Dawson and Stein, 1970). The use of specific substrates allows detection of the diseases and the benefit of genetic counseling.

Sea-blue Histiocyte Syndrome

The syndrome of the sea-blue histiocyte takes its name from the large (20 micra) azure, granulated histiocyte that is the hallmark of the disease. Only two of the nine cases reviewed by Silverstein were children, and the symptomatology varied in intensity, thrombocytopenia, purpura, and anemia seeming to be the most apparent signs (Silverstein et al., 1970). Splenomegaly is the most striking clinical finding, and occasional patients have died owing to progressive liver failure. Increased excretion of mucopolysaccharide in the urine is usual but not invariable. Specific phospholipids and glycosphingolipids are stored in the blue histiocytes (Ardeman, 1972). One of the first patients reported was that of Cogan; he described a macular change in which yellowish-white, scintillating granules surrounded the fovea in a doughnut-shaped pattern (Cogan and Federman, 1964).

Pigmentary Degeneration

Abnormality of the macular area may accompany illnesses in which there is a disturbance of the pigment epithelium of the retina, and such pigmentary degenerations of the fundus of the eye are found in many inborn errors of metabolism, especially those concerned with lipids (Table 19–3). Discussion of these entities is scattered throughout this text, and the reader is referred to the appropriate listing in the index. An entity that deserves specific mention here, however, is alpha-aminobutyric aciduria, in which macular degeneration is associated with mental retardation, deafness, and a neurologic course similar to that of Tay-Sachs disease, with hypotonia changing to spasticity. The diagnosis is made by finding abnormally high levels of alpha-aminobutyric acid in blood and cerebrospinal fluid. Disease of the renal tubules is also present (Martin et al., 1967). It is interesting that this disease resembles in some degree the sphingolipid disorders, though the biochemical defect is apparently in amino acid metabolism.

Hooft's Disease; Imidazole Aciduria

Two conditions in which pigmentary degenerations of the retina are noted are Hooft's disease and imidazole aminoaciduria. Both are characterized by mental retardation. Hooft's disease, in which a tapetoretinal degeneration of the Leber type with an extinguished electroretinogram has been reported, has its onset around the age of two years and has a mixture of clinical and biochemical findings; red skin lesions on the face and limbs, peculiar white nails, and abnormal teeth are the clinical manifestations, and a low level of blood lipids (apparently without a deficiency of beta-lipoproteins) and a generalized aminoaciduria are the major biochemical changes (Hooft et al., 1962).

In imidazole aminoaciduria a more definite abnormality of the macular area is present in association with the pigmentary changes in the periphery. In this regard the disease is similar to Batten's cerebromacular degeneration. Increased amounts of carnosine, anserine, l-methyl histidine, and histidine are excreted in the urine (Bessman and Baldwin, 1962). In this autosomal recessive disease the carriers manifest the imidazole aminoaciduria but do not show the cerebromacular degenerative changes. Warburg has pointed out that the disease must be differentiated from carnosinemia, in which imidazole aminoaciduria with myoclonus, convulsions, and progressive mental retardation also occurs, but without l-methyl histidinuria (Perry et al., 1967; Warburg, 1972).

Oxalosis

In primary hyperoxaluria there is an increased urinary excretion of oxalic and glycolic acid which may eventuate into calcium oxalate nephrolithiasis. Pigmentary retinopathy which is probably secondary to oxalate deposits in the retina and choroid has been described.

Lipemia Retinalis (See Appendix Table E)

Lipemia retinalis is a manifestation of excess triglyceride in the bloodstream (Albrink et al., 1955). Since cholesterol and phospholipid do not contribute to plasma lactescence, it is the triglyceride level that is of most importance in defining this symptom. Lipemia retinalis can usually be noted when plasma triglycerides are in excess of 1000 mg. per 100 ml. but it may be seen in lower concentrations in individuals with heavily pigmented fundi (Plate XIII–D). It is most easily seen in the retinal periphery. The vessels become a creamy orange-yellow, and the normal difference between the lighter-colored arterioles and the darker veins lessens. Near the disc the ves-

sels are more intensely orange, while in the periphery they tend to be whiter. When the triglyceride level is very high, the entire ocular fundus becomes an opalescent, creamy white. Milky streaks or splotches can often be noted beside the vessels. This picture resembles little else and establishes the presence of plasma hyperlipemia; it is an indication for performance of studies necessary to define the underlying disease, which could be diabetes mellitus, chronic renal disease, familial hyperlipoproteinemia, or another entity (Bagdade et al., 1968; Chopra et al., 1971; Gallin et al., 1969; Lees et al., 1970). The fundus abnormalities quickly disappear with elimination of excess triglyceride from the blood.

Hyperlipoproteinemia

Several excellent reports describing the ocular manifestations of lipid diseases have appeared in the past (Blodi, 1962; Cohen, 1921; Dunphy, 1950; Thomas and Smith, 1958). However, the fundamental nature of these disorders, and hence the ability to distinguish accurately among them, has only relatively recently been uncovered (Stanbury et al., 1966). It has brought with it a great increase in the ability to diagnose correctly and to treat effectively. For example, at least five types of hyperlipoproteinemia can be differentiated from each other on the basis of the lipoprotein fractions. While all of them are "hyperlipemias," their biochemical and clinical manifestations are quite distinct (Table 19–24). It is rare for any except type I or type II to

TABLE 19–24 CLINICAL FEATURES OF FAMILIAL HYPERLIPOPROTEINEMIA

Type	Usual Age of Detection	Xanthomas Tendinous	Eruptive	Xanthelasma	Corneal Arcus	Lipemia Retinalis	Vascular Disease	Abdominal Pain	Abnormal Glucose Tolerance	Foam Cells
I	10 years	0	+	0	0	+	0	+	0	+
II	30 years	+	0	+	+	0	+	0	0	0
III	Adulthood	+	0 to +	+	+	+	+	0	+	+
IV	Adulthood	0	0 to +	0	0	+	+	0	+	+
V	Adulthood	0	+	0	0	+	0 to +	+	+	+

Based on table by Stanbury, J. B., Wyngaarden, J. B., and Fredrickson, D. S.: The Metabolic Basis of Inherited Disease. New York, McGraw-Hill Book Co., 1966.

be detected in childhood. Type I disease (familial fat-induced hyperlipemia) is associated primarily with an elevation of serum triglyceride; abdominal pain, eruptive xanthomas, foam cells in the reticuloendothelial system, and lipemia retinalis are cardinal features. None of these are prominent in type II hyperlipoproteinemia (familial hyperbetalipoproteinemia, or familial hypercholesterolemia), in which there is elevation of serum cholesterol but the triglyceride level is normal; clinical features include tendinous xanthomas, xanthelasmas, corneal arcus, and premature death due to vascular disease. Type II is the only one of the hyperlipoproteinemias in which lipemia retinalis does not occur. Fat-induced hyperlipemia appears to be inherited in an autosomal recessive fashion, and the presumed heterozygotes appear normal, whereas type II disease follows the pattern of a strongly penetrant autosomal dominant, and heterozygotes may have definite hypercholesterolemia that is frequently detectable prior to the age of 20 years.

Treatment of type I, fat-induced hyperlipemia consists of limitation of the amount of fat in the diet; prompt improvement can be anticipated by this relatively simple method. Limitation of cholesterol intake, however, is not associated with rapid betterment of type II hyperlipoproteinemia (Fredrickson and Levy, 1970; Lees and Wilson, 1971). Indeed, dietary management may need to be continued for many years before there is any apparent clinical or biochemical improvement. Several reports, however, have suggested that such long-term therapy, especially when combined with one of the chemotherapeutic agents such as cholestyramine or clofibrate, is of significant benefit (Berkowitz, 1971; Fallon and Woods, 1968; Segall et al., 1970; Smith et al., 1972).

The clinical and histopathologic aspects of corneal arcus have been well described (Cogan and Kuwabara, 1959) (Plate XIII-E). However, its relation to systemic disease in the adult is less clearly defined (Andrews, 1962; Bersohn et al., 1969; Hickey et al., 1971; Macaraeg et al., 1968; Rohrenschneider, 1962). It may be fair to generalize that when corneal arcus is present in Whites less than 40 years of age or Blacks less than 30, there is sufficient evidence to justify further study. Since arcus is a reflection of the level of cholesterol, this determination is clearly essential. However, if the exact nature of any underlying disease is to be revealed, it is also necessary to perform an electrophoretic examination of the plasma lipoproteins. Xanthelasmas are also a reflection of excess cholesterol (Pedace and Winkelmann, 1965). Although they are definitely pathologic in youngsters, they are not as closely related to the aging process as is corneal arcus. About one third of all adults with xanthelasma will have pathologically elevated serum cholesterol.

Retinal Hemorrhage (See Appendix Table E)

Ocular S-Hemoglobinopathies

No chapter dealing with metabolic disease would be complete without reference to the sickle cell diseases. Not only are the ophthalmic aspects of these hemoglobinopathies important and varied, but the disorders stand as magnificent models of the nature of inherited illness. In 1949 Pauling described the electrophoretic nature of human hemoglobins. He postulated that sickle cell disease, whose existence and clinical characteristics had been known for over 30 years at that time, was a molecular disease due to an abnormal structure of hemoglobin, commenting further that the charge difference between the normal (hemoglobin A) and the sickle cell (hemoglobin S) was due to loss of two carboxylic residues in hemoglobin S (Pauling et al., 1949). Subsequent investigations by others showed that hemoglobin A was composed of four polypeptide chains, one having 141 residues and the others 146, and the normal sequence of the amino acids composing these chains was unraveled. In 1956 Ingram described the molecular nature of hemoglobin S and observed a substitution of valine in hemoglobin S for glutamic acid in hemoglobin A, thus confirming Pauling's original hypothesis. The abnormal placement of this one amino acid in the polypeptide chain results in a change in the shape of the hemoglobin molecule, altering its physiology and accounting for its tendency to produce "sickling" of the red blood cells, especially if oxygen tension is low. Since the clinical characteristics of hemoglobin S diseases can largely be explained in terms of infarctions caused by sickled cells clogging the vessels, it is possible directly to relate the clinical aspects of the disease to the basic molecular structure of the hemoglobin molecule.

Hemoglobin A is the normal adult hemoglobin; hemoglobin F is the type found in the fetus and hemoglobin S with sickle cell disease. At least 25 other types of hemoglobin due to substitution of one amino acid by another have been identified. The clinical manifestations depend upon the type of hemoglobin and whether the mutational change is expressed in a homo- or heterozygous state. Thus, an individual with AA has no abnormalities; with AS (sickle cell trait), mild disease; with SS (sickle cell disease), more full-blown disease; and with SC, serious disease of a different nature. The ophthalmic aspects of S-hemoglobinopathy are far more diverse than the nonspecific pallor of the optic disc, retinal vein engorgement, and superficial posterior polar retinal hemorrhages seen with anemia of any cause (Kolker, 1966; Markar et al., 1969; Toselli et al., 1969).

The two major ocular manifestations of hemoglobin S are sausage-link-like dilatations of the conjunctival vessels and abnormalities of the fundus of the eye (Condon and Sergeant, 1972; Goodman et al., 1957; Okun, 1969). These are listed with their approximate frequency of incidence in Table 19–25. The Wilmer Eye Institute has provided the bulk of knowledge about the ocular aspects of these diseases (Goldberg, 1971b and 1971c; Paton, 1959; Ryan and Goldberg, 1971; Welch and Goldberg, 1966). A new classification of proliferative sickle cell retinopathy was suggested by Goldberg and Morton in 1971. The first state is apparently peripheral vascular occlusion; this is followed consecutively by arteriolar-venular anastomoses, neovascular proliferation, vitreous hemorrhage, and retinal detachment. Attempts to repair the retinal detachment surgically may cause necrosis of the anterior segment of the globe, but a recent report suggests that surgery can be successful when performed in a hyperbaric chamber (Freilich, 1972). The most characteristic fundus finding in

TABLE 19–25 MAJOR OCULAR MANIFESTATIONS OF THREE HEMOGLOBIN S CONDITIONS, INDICATING APPROXIMATE FREQUENCY OF OCCURRENCE OF THESE ABNORMALITIES*

| | Type of Hemoglobin | | |
	AS	SS	SC
Conjunctival dilatations	5%	100%	100%
Tortuosity of retinal veins	5%	50%	33%
Peripheral obliteration of retinal vessels	10%	33%	75%
Sea-fan sign**	0	0	67%
Black sunburst sign**	5%	50%	33%
Vitreous hemorrhage	0	3%	33%
Retinal detachment	0	0	10%

*Other less frequent and/or less characteristic signs include the following:
1. Angioid streaks
2. Central retinal artery occlusion
3. Central retinal vein occlusion
4. Macular hemorrhage
5. Retinal hemorrhages
6. Refractile retinal deposits
7. Papilledema
8. Optic atrophy
9. Open angle glaucoma

**See text for fuller description.

SC disease is the fan of arteriovenous proliferation (the sea-fan sign). Disc-shaped pigmented chorioretinal scars with feeder vessels (the black sunburst sign) are noted in many forms of the disease, but most typically in sickle cell disease, SS. Other reported signs include those listed in Table 19–25.

Hemoglobin S is of importance not only because of its landmark position in the understanding of the molecular basis of disease, and not only because of the variety and severity of the ocular abnormalities associated with its presence, but also because of the extremely widespread nature of the mutation, which is of remarkably high frequency (40 per cent) in certain areas. The development of an inexpensive and simple diagnostic test is thus of great significance. The method recently described by Greenberg et al. (1972) may supplant the more difficult examination of the blood for sickled cells, or the other previous diagnostic techniques. However, electrophoresis of serum is the most reliable manner of characterizing the exact nature of the patient's hemoglobins. Some hope of effective treatment has been raised by the finding that cyanate increases the survival of red blood cells from patients with hemoglobin S (May et al., 1972).

Familial Bleeding Diseases

The inherited abnormalities of blood clotting may manifest themselves by pathologic change in the eyes and the adnexa (Rubenstein et al., 1966; Wong et al., 1969). This may be a slight subconjunctival or a massive retrobulbar or intraocular hemorrhage. A history of bleeding disease should be sought in all patients about to undergo surgery; occasional patients, however, may be unaware of their underlying disease, and the sometimes catastrophic complication noted in the postoperative period may be the first warning sign of the hematologic disorder.

Lids (See Appendix Table J)

Hartnup Disease

"Hereditary pellagra-like skin rash with temporary cerebellar ataxia, constant renal amino aciduria, and other bizarre biochemical features" (the title of the first report of Hartnup disease) is a précis of the condition known as Hartnup disease (Baron et al., 1956). Named after the 12-year-old boy first diagnosed as having this condition Hartnup disease is a familial illness characterized by abnormal intestinal and renal transport of certain neutral alpha-amino acids (Scriver, 1965). It has been postulated that the neurologic signs of the disorder are due to two mechanisms: (1) because of the abnormality of intestinal transport, amino acids remain in the intestine longer than normal and decompose, and the decomposition products elicit "toxic" effects after they are absorbed; (2) the absorption defect also results in a decreased synthesis of nicotinamide from tryptophan, thus causing a niacin deficiency and "pellagra." The signs of the illness (Table 19–26), inherited as an autosomal recessive trait, respond fairly satisfactorily to prolonged treatment with nicotinamide. Hartnup disease thus stands as another inborn error of metabolism in which vitamin therapy has definitely beneficial effects. The therapeutic mechanism in these conditions, for example, in homocystinuria, are not, however, always as clear as in Hartnup disease.

TABLE 19–26 CLINICAL ASPECTS OF HARTNUP DISEASE

Onset in childhood (ages 1 to 18 years)
Intermittent, red, scaly, pellagra-like rash, appearing after exposure to light
Attacks of cerebellar ataxia
Intermittent emotional instability
Other psychiatric changes, occasionally including delirium
Headache
Nystagmus
Ptosis
Diplopia during attacks
Treatment with nicotinamide beneficial

Visual Loss

Hyperammonemia, Types I and II

At least three disorders in the biosynthesis of urea have ocular manifestations. Hyperammonemias, types I and II, are due to errors at or near the "start" of the urea cycle. The normal steps are as follows: ammonia — carbamyl phosphate — citrulline — argininosuccinic acid — arginine — urea. In hyperammonemia type I, a decrease in the activity of the enzyme carbamyl phosphate synthetase, responsible for the first step of the cycle, results in the accumulation of excess ammonia (Baron et al., 1956). In hyperammonemia type II, the defect is apparently in ornithine transcarbamylase (which catalyzes the next step from carbamyl phosphate to citrulline) as a consequence of which there is, again, an increase in the level of blood and cerebrospinal fluid ammonia (higher even than that seen with hepatic coma) (Levin et al., 1969). The clinical aspects of these entities are indicated in Table 19–27. Type II disease has, to date, been noted only in female infants; it is possible that they represent heterozygotes of a sex-linked disorder, the affected males not surviving the intrauterine period. Restriction of protein

TABLE 19–27 CLINICAL ASPECTS OF HYPERAMMONEMIA

Onset in infancy (females)
Attacks of vomiting, screaming, and confusion followed by lethargy
Ptosis and ataxia between attacks
Mental retardation (atrophy of the cerebral cortex)
Visual loss
Rapid or protracted deterioration

intake has been of some clinical benefit in patients with hyperammonemia.

Argininosuccinic Aciduria

Argininosuccinic aciduria, another disorder of the urea cycle, is a rare abnormality due to a deficiency of argininosuccinic acid-cleaving enzyme. Failure of normal neurologic development, in association with convulsions and friable, tufted hair are the characteristic findings and are noted in early infancy (Allan et al., 1958) (Table 19–28). Marked variability of expression of the clinical findings is common; few cases show all aspects of the disease. For example, in some the hair is normal and in others the ataxia is absent. The grossly retarded children may survive into the teens, and marked limitation of peripheral visual field and cataracts have been noted. Diagnosis is based on finding excess argininosuccinic acid in the urine and cerebral spinal fluid. Probably inherited as an autosomal recessive disease, no treatment has been proved effective.

Specific disease entities have therefore been described for all five steps in the urea cycle. In hyperammonemia types I and II (previously discussed) ptosis and visual loss are the ocular manifestations. These two diseases result from errors in the first and second steps of the cycle. Cataract and visual field loss occur in argininosuccinic aciduria, a disorder of the fourth step. However, abnormality of the eye has not been reported with either of the other two illnesses.

Photogenic Epilepsy

Prolinemia

Prolinemia, an infrequently occurring affliction due to the deficiency of the enzyme proline oxidase, is characterized by

TABLE 19–28 CLINICAL ASPECTS OF ARGININOSUCCINIC ACIDURIA

Apparently normal neonatal period
Onset at about age 1½ years with convulsions (may be earlier)
Curly hair that becomes brittle, frayed, and tufted
Mental retardation
Intermittent ataxia
Limitation of visual field
Cataracts and strabismus (infrequent)

---

nephritis, deafness, renal hypoplasia, prolinemia, and prolinuria (Efron, 1965; Schafer et al., 1962). The ocular manifestations consist of frequent "staring spells" and generalized convulsions, some of which are photogenic. Death due to renal failure occurs in early childhood. No treatment for this condition is known. In one large kindred this type of prolinemia seemed to be inherited as an autosomal recessive while many of the associated clinical findings seemed to segregate as autosomal dominants.

CONCLUSION

One might legitimately ask, "Why devote so much space to diseases that most practicing physicians rarely see, especially when in many instances nothing can be done about them anyhow?" The answer to this is twofold. In the first place, the diseases are of more importance than their numerical volume would indicate, and in the second, it is not correct that they are untreatable. These diseases are of great significance because as examples of altered biochemistry they provide insights into the fundamental nature of human metabolism, which, after all, lies at the root not only of disease but also of health. As such they are an important means of understanding the entire human organism. For example, the great bulk of knowledge regarding the metabolism of sulfur-containing amino acids in humans has evolved from a study of the inborn error of metabolism responsible for the disease homocystinuria. The ramifications of such knowledge spread far beyond learning how to help those few individuals afflicted with the full manifestation of the abnormality. For example, homocysteine plays a role in intravascular thrombosis, and it has even been suggested that an abnormality of homocysteine metabolism may be the fundamental defect in arteriosclerosis.

Increased ability to diagnose correctly the inborn errors of metabolism has been the keystone in the bridge of increased understanding. As clinically similar but biochemically different (or vice versa) entities have gradually been distinguished from each other, the natural histories of the particular disease units have become better defined. The existence of techniques to de-

TABLE 19–29 SELECTED METABOLIC DISEASES WITH OCULAR MANIFESTATIONS

Disease	Deficient Enzyme Activity (or Other Diagnostic Feature)	Prenatal Diagnosis
Argininosuccinic aciduria	Argininosuccinase	Possible
Cystinosis	(Cystine accumulation)	Potentially possible
Fabry's disease	Ceramide trihexoside galactosidase	Possible
Galactosemia—Type I	Galactose-1-phosphate uridyl transferase	Possible
Galactosemia—Type II	Galactokinase	Potentially possible
Gaucher's disease	Beta-glucosidase glucocerebrosidase	Possible
GM$_1$ (generalized) gangliosidosis	Beta-galactosidase A, B, C	Possible
Glucose-6-phosphate dehydrogenase deficiency	Glucose-6-phosphate dehydrogenase	Possible
Glycogen storage disease—Type I	G-6-phosphatase	Possible
GM$_2$ gangliosidosis—Type I (Tay-Sachs)	Hexosaminidase A	Possible
GM$_2$ gangliosidosis—Type II	Hexosaminidase A and B	Possible
Homocystinuria	Cystathionine synthetase	Possible
Hunter's syndrome	Beta-galactosidase	Possible
Hurler's syndrome	Beta-galactosidase	Possible
Hypervalinemia	Valine transaminase	Potentially possible
Juvenile GM$_1$ gangliosidosis	Beta-galactosidase	Potentially possible
Maple syrup urine disease	2-keto-isocaproate decarboxylase	Possible
Marfan's syndrome	(Excess hyaluronic acid production)	Potentially possible
Metachromatic leukodystrophy (2 forms)	Aryl sulfatase A / Aryl sulfatase A and B	Possible / Potentially possible
Morquio's syndrome	Unknown	Potentially possible
Niemann-Pick disease (4 types)	Sphingomyelinase	Possible
Refsum's disease	Phytanic acid alpha-hydroxylase	Possible
Sanfilippo syndrome	Unknown	Potentially possible
Scheie's syndrome	Unknown	Potentially possible
Xeroderma pigmentosum	DNA "repair enzyme"	Possible
Chromosomal diseases (Trisomy 13–15, 18, 21, 22, XYYY, chromosome deletion 18)	(Abnormal number or morphology of chromosomes)	

termine with satisfactory accuracy the activity of individual enzymes has permitted a precision of diagnosis hitherto impossible. It is usually desirable to diagnose these conditions as early in the life of the individual as possible. In this manner therapy can be initiated when it is most essential. This treatment may range from abortion to dietary management to vitamin therapy or even to enzyme replacement. Table 19–29 is a list of a few of the metabolic diseases which affect the eyes; the responsible enzyme deficiency is indicated, and the last column indicates whether or not it is possible to make a diagnosis prior to the time of delivery of the fetus. This ability to make intrauterine diagnosis has proved to be of valuable assistance in genetic counseling of parents, and in deciding upon the wisdom of performing abortion, since it has assured foreknowledge of whether or not the fetus is actually afflicted.

The mother of a child with galactosemia, having witnessed the transformation of her infant from deathly illness to normal health, would be unimpressed by comments regarding the futility of treating diseases due to inborn errors of metabolism. Effective treatment of many of these illnesses, some of which only recently were thought of as completely intractable, is now a reality. Furthermore, those who understand properly the role of the physician realize that he may be of true service even when his effectiveness is limited to offering, compassionately, a realistic prognosis. To be able to advise knowledgeably at times of severe stress is one of the great privileges of caring for patients and is a responsibility to be cherished. It is possible only because of those who have carefully and imaginatively investigated the nature—basic and clinical—of health and disease.

APPENDIX TABLE A   ABNORMALITIES OF THE ANTERIOR CHAMBER

Angle Area
Ocular
Albinism[29, 30, 32–36, 39, 41]
Aniridia[71–77]
Axenfeld's anomaly[82]
Axenfeld's syndrome[82]
Congenital glaucoma[244]
Iridogoniodysgenesis and cataract[444]
Rieger's anomaly[442, 443]

Systemic
Albinism[29, 30, 32–36, 39, 41]
Lowe's syndrome[344–348]
Marfan's syndrome[357]
Mesodermal dysgenesis of iris and cornea[445]
Norrie's disease[408, 409]
Rieger's syndrome[442, 443]
Trisomy 13–15[96, 97, 100, 103, 107]
Trisomy 18[101–103]

APPENDIX TABLE B   ABNORMALITIES OF THE CONJUNCTIVA

Deposits
Systemic
Cystinosis[132–145]
Hypophosphatasia[320]
Icthyosis[321, 322]
Primary familial amyloidosis[50–53]
Inflammation
Systemic
Down's syndrome[105]
Hereditary pseudomembranous conjunctivitis[115]
Icthyosis[321, 322]
Riley-Day syndrome[446–448]
Vitamin A deficiency[470, 473]
Xeroderma pigmentosum[491]
Pigmentation
Ocular
Melanosis[419]
Systemic
Alkaptonuria[42–47]
Down's syndrome[105]

Surface Lesions
Ocular
Hereditary benign intraepithelial dys-keratosis[260a]
Systemic
Gaucher's disease[236–242]
Goldenhar's syndrome[254]
Neurofibromatosis[399]
Tuberous sclerosis[18]
Vitamin A deficiency[470, 473]
Symblepharon
Systemic
Porphyria[421, 422]
Telangiectasia
Systemic
Ataxia-telangiectasia (Louis-Bar)[80, 81]
Congenital tryptophanuria with dwarfism[465]
Fabry's disease[159–168, 170–184]
Osler's disease[435]
S-hemoglobinopathy[54–61, 64–68, 70]
Sturge-Weber syndrome[458]
Vesication
Systemic
Porphyria[421, 422]

APPENDIX TABLE C   ABNORMALITIES OF THE CORNEA

Dry Eye
Ocular
Keratomalacia[470]
Systemic
Porphyria[421, 422]
Riley-Day syndrome[446−448]
Vitamin A deficiency[470, 473]

Opacities
Diffuse
Ocular
Fuchs' dystrophy[123]
Groenouw type 1 (granular)[124]
Groenouw type 2 (macular)[117]
Haab-Dimmer (lattice)[122]
Systemic
Mesodermal dysgenesis[445]

Endothelial
Ocular
Cornea guttata[121]
Peter's anomaly[120]
Posterior embryotoxon[120]
Posterior polymorphous degeneration[121]
Systemic
Mesodermal dysgenesis[445]

Epithelial
Ocular
Aniridia[71−77]
Buckler's annular dystrophy[121]
Fingerprint lines[169]
Keratosis follicularis spinulosa decalvans[146]
Kraupa's epithelial dystrophy[121]
Meesmann's epithelial dystrophy[121, 125]
Schnyder's crystalline dystrophy[121, 127]
Systemic
Cockayne's syndrome[109]
Fabry's disease[159−168]
Farber's disease[186, 187]
Hypophosphatasia[320]

Stromal
Ocular
Central cloudy dystrophy[121]
Congenital dystrophy of the cornea[121]
Cornea farinata[121]
Speckled dystrophy of the cornea[121]
Systemic
Cystinosis[132−145]
Familial plasma lecithin–cholesterol acyl transferase deficiency[338]
Generalized gangliosidosis (GM$_1$ type 1)[15, 209, 218, 234]

Glycogenoses[253]
Goldberg's syndrome (mucolipidosis)[375]
Hurler's syndrome[384, 390]
Hyperlipoproteinemia, types 2 and 3[15, 312]
Icthyosis[321, 322]
Maroteaux-Lamy syndrome[384, 390]
Morquio's syndrome[384, 390]
Osteogenesis imperfecta[390, 411, 412]
Scheie's syndrome[384, 390]
Tangier disease[461−463]
Tay-Sachs disease[15]
Trisomy 18[101, 102, 103]

Pigmentation
Systemic
Alkaptonuria[42−47]
Wilson's disease[482−489]

Size and Shape
Ocular
Familial microcornea[120]
Hereditary anophthalmos[246]
Hereditary cornea plana[120]
Hereditary megalocornea[246]
Keratoconus[121]
Systemic
Chromosome 18 deletion[103, 104, 108]
Pierre Robin syndrome[418]
Treacher Collins syndrome[464]
Trisomy 13–15[96, 97, 100, 101, 103]
Trisomy 18[101−103]

Thinning
Ocular
Congenital anterior staphyloma[120]
Keratoconus[121]
Systemic
Down's syndrome[105]
Ehlers-Danlos syndrome[152−154]
Osteogenesis imperfecta[411−413]
Pseudoxanthoma elasticum[425, 426]

Vascularization
Ocular
Aniridia[71−77]
Systemic
Cockayne's syndrome[109]
Protein deficiency[470]
Riboflavin deficiency[470]
Tuberous sclerosis[18]

Xerosis
Systemic
Vitamin A deficiency[470, 473]
Xeroderma pigmentosum[491]

APPENDIX TABLE D   ABNORMALITIES OF EYE MOVEMENTS

Abnormal Gaze
Ocular
Ocular motor apraxia[409a]
Blinking
Systemic
Pyridoxine dependency[429]
Nystagmus
Ocular
Albinism[29, 30, 32−36, 39, 41]
Systemic
Albinism[29, 30, 32−36, 39, 41]
Apert's syndrome[78]
Behr's syndrome[437]
Charcot-Marie-Tooth syndrome[88]
Chediak-Higashi syndrome[89, 90, 92]
Chromosome 18 deletion[103, 104, 108]
Diabetes mellitus[149]
Down's syndrome[105]
Generalized gangliosidosis[15, 209, 218, 234]
Hartnup disease[258]
Hurler's syndrome[390]
Laurence-Moon-Bardet-Biedl
syndrome[335, 336]
Lenoble-Aubineau syndrome[339]
Systemic
Marfan's syndrome[357, 358]
Menke's disease[360]
Naegeli's syndrome[420]
Refsum's disease[430−434]
Trisomy 18[101−103]
Valinemia[316, 352]
Paresis
Ocular
Albinism[29, 30, 32−36, 39, 41]
Duane's syndrome[158]
External ophthalmoplegia[157]
Marcus Gunn syndrome[355]
Systemic
Albinism[29, 30, 32−36, 39, 41]

Diabetes mellitus[149]
Engelmann's disease[156]
Friedreich's ataxia[187b]
Greig's syndrome[256]
Laurence-Moon-Bardet-Biedl
syndrome[335, 336]
Marie's cerebellar ataxia[359]
Systemic
Neurofibromatosis[18, 399]
Nicotinic acid deficiency[471]
Porphyria[421, 422]
Scurvy[472]
Thiamin deficiency[471]
Staring
Systemic
Glycinemia[250a]
Hyperserotonemia[315]
Prolinemia[423, 424]
Strabismus
Ocular
Duane's syndrome[158]
Systemic
Abetalipoproteinemia[21−28]
Apert's syndrome[78]
Cockayne's syndrome[109]
Crouzon's syndrome[129, 130]
Down's syndrome[105]
Ehlers-Danlos syndrome[152−154]
Systemic
Gaucher's disease[236−242]
Hydroxyprolinemia[449]
Hyperlysinemia[313]
Hypoglycemia[317]
Klippel-Feil syndrome[328a]
Laurence-Moon-Bardet-Biedl
syndrome[335, 336]
Maple syrup urine disease[350, 351, 353]
Marfan's syndrome[357, 358]
Naegeli's syndrome[420]
Riley-Day syndrome[446−448]

APPENDIX TABLE E   ABNORMALITIES OF THE FUNDUS OF THE EYE

Angioid Streaks
Systemic
    Ehlers-Danlos syndrome[152–154]
    Hyperphosphatemia[415]
    Neurofibromatosis[18]
    Paget's disease[415]
    Pseudoxanthoma elasticum[425, 426]
    S-hemoglobinopathy[54–61, 64–68, 70]
    Sturge-Weber syndrome[18, 458]
    Tuberous sclerosis[18]

Atrophy
Ocular
    Central areolar choroidal atrophy[438]
    Choroideremia[436]
    Gyrate atrophy of the choroid[438]
    Myopia[396]
    Primary choroidal sclerosis[438]
    Pseudoinflammatory macular dystrophy[438]
Systemic
    Laurence-Moon-Bardet-Biedl
      syndrome[335, 336]
    Pseudoxanthoma elasticum[425, 426]

Choroidal Angioma
Systemic
    Sturge-Weber syndrome[458]

Deposits
Ocular
    Albipunctate dystrophy[476]
    Doyne's honeycomb dystrophy[440]
    Fundus albipunctatus[476]
    Fundus flavimaculatus[476]
Systemic
    Diabetes mellitus[148]
    Glycogenosis, type 1[252]
    Lipoid proteinosis[342, 343]
    S-hemoglobinopathy[54–61, 64–68, 70]
    Vitamin A deficiency[470, 473]

Hemorrhage
Ocular
    Leber's syndrome[337]
Systemic
    Diabetes mellitus[148]
    Gaucher's disease[236–242]
    Glucose-6-phosphate dehydrogenase
      deficiency[249]
    Porphyria[421, 422]
    S-hemoglobinopathy[54–61, 64–68, 70]
    Thalassemia[69]
    Tuberous sclerosis[18]

Hypopigmentation
Ocular
    Albinism[29, 30, 32–36, 39, 41]
Systemic
    Albinism[29, 30, 32–36, 39, 41]
    Chediak-Higashi syndrome[89, 90, 92]
    Laurence-Moon-Bardet-Biedl
      syndrome[335, 336]
    Porphyria[421, 422]
    Trisomy 18[101–103]

Lipemia Retinalis
Systemic
    Hyperlipoproteinemia, types 1, 3, 4,
      and 5[15, 312]
    Hyperlipoproteinemia, secondary

      (diabetes mellitus, glycogen storage
      disease, idiopathic hypercalcemia)[15]

Macular Lesions
Edema
Systemic
    Fabry's disease[159–168, 170–184]
    Gaucher's disease[236–242]
    Hurler's syndrome[383, 390]
    S-hemoglobinopathy[54–61, 64–68, 70]

Cherry-red Spot
Systemic
    Farber's disease (ceramide lipidosis)[186, 187]
    GM$_1$ type 1 (generalized
      gangliosidosis)[15, 209, 218, 234]
    GM$_2$ type 1 (Tay-Sachs disease)[15, 233]
    Goldberg's syndrome (mucolipidosis)[375]
    Metachromatic leukodystrophy[365]
    Mucolipidosis type 1[372, 376]
    Niemann-Pick disease (sphingomyelin-
      cholesterol lipidosis) type A[401, 403–407]

Resembling Cherry-red Spot
Systemic
    Adult Niemann-Pick disease[402]
    Gaucher's disease[236–242]
    GM$_2$ type (Sandhoff's disease)[15, 225]
    Lactosyl ceramidosis[333]
    Sea-blue histiocyte syndrome[451–453]

Hemorrhagic
Systemic
    Ehlers-Danlos syndrome[152–154]
    Pseudoxanthoma elasticum[425, 426]
    S-hemoglobinopathy[54–61, 64–68, 70]

Pigmentary Degeneration
Ocular
    Central areolar choroidal atrophy[438]
    Cone dysfunction syndrome[449]
    Hereditary macular dystrophies
      (Stargardt, Behr, Haab-Dimmer)[476]
    Pigmentary retinopathies (see Table 19–2)[435a]
    Reticular pigmentary dystrophy (Sjögren)[476]
    Vitelline dystrophy (Best)[84]
Systemic
    Amaurotic familial idiocies (congenital,
      Tay-Sachs, Bielschowsky-Jansky, Kufs)[225]
    Batten's cerebral degeneration with
      macular changes[198, 225]
    Cystathioninuria[131]
    Farber's disease[186, 187]
    Imidazole aminoaciduria[323, 325]
    Lipoid proteinosis[342, 343]
    Menke's disease[360]
    Metachromatic leukodystrophy[365]
    Pigmentary retinopathies (see Table 19–2)
    Porphyria[421, 422]
    Refsum's disease[430–434]

Medullated Nerve fibers
Systemic
    Apert's syndrome[78]
    Crouzon's syndrome[129, 130]

Pigment Deposits
Ocular
    Myopia[396]
    Retinitis pigmentosa (see Table 19–2)[435a]

(Table E continued on following page)

APPENDIX TABLE E   ABNORMALITIES OF THE FUNDUS OF THE EYE *(Continued)*

Systemic
  Porphyria[421, 422]
  S-hemoglobinopathy[54–61, 64–68, 70]
Pigment Mottling
Ocular
  Cone dysfunction syndrome[449]
Systemic
  Abetalipoproteinemia[21–28]
  Batten's cerebral degeneration with
    macular changes[198, 225]
  Bowen's syndrome[85, 86]
  Cystinosis[132–145]
  Ehlers-Danlos syndrome[152–154]
  Generalized gangliosidosis
    (GM$_1$ type 1)[15, 209, 218, 234]
  Homocystinuria[263–282]
Systemic
  Hypophosphatsia[320]
  Isovaleric acidemia[328]
  Pseudoxanthoma elasticum[425, 426]
Retinal Arteriolar Occlusion
Systemic
  Homocystinuria[263–282]
  S-hemoglobinopathy[54–61, 64–68, 70]
Retinal Detachment (or Schisis)
Ocular
  Hyaloideoretinal degeneration (Wagner)[477]
  Hyaloideotapetoretinal degeneration
    (Goldmann-Favre)[477]
  Inferotemporal dialysis[439]
  Retinoschisis[475, 476]
Systemic
  Norrie's disease[408, 409, 477]
  S-hemoglobinopathy[54–61, 64–68, 70]

Retinal Vessel Tortuosity
Systemic
  Angiomatosis retinae[479]
  Cystic fibrosis[131a]
  Engelmann's syndrome[156]
Systemic
  Fabry's disease[159–168, 170–184]
  Hyperlipoproteinemia[15, 312]
  Isovaleric acidemia[328]
  S-hemoglobinopathy[54–61, 64–68, 70]
  Sturge-Weber syndrome[458]
Retinitis Proliferans
Systemic
  Angiomatosis retinae[479]
  Diabetes mellitus[148]
  S-hemoglobinopathy[54–61, 64–68, 70]
  Trisomy 13–15[96, 97, 100, 101, 103]
  Tuberous sclerosis[18]
Tapetal Reflex
Ocular
  Fundus albipunctatus[476]
  Oguchi's disease[436]
  Tapetal-like reflex syndrome[382]
Tumors
  Angiomatosis retinae[479]
  Glycogenosis (type 1)[252]
  Hyperlipoproteinemia[15, 312]
Systemic
  Naegeli's syndrome[420]
  Neurofibromatosis[18, 399]
  Retinoblastoma[441]
  Sturge-Weber syndrome[18, 458]
    Tuberous sclerosis

APPENDIX TABLE F   ABNORMALITIES OF THE INTRAOCULAR PRESSURE

Hypertension
Ocular
  Aniridia[71–77]
  Axenfeld's syndrome[82]
  Congenital glaucoma[244]
  Familial iris hypoplasia[245]
  Peter's anomaly[120]
  Syndrome of microcornea, glaucoma,
    and absent frontal sinuses[371a]
Systemic
  Albinism[29, 30, 32–36, 39, 41]
  Angiomatosis retinae[479]
  Bowen's syndrome[85, 86]
  Chromosome 18 deletion[103, 104, 108]
  Hypoglycemia[317]
  Lowe's syndrome[344–348]

  Mesodermal dysgenesis of iris and
    cornea[445]
  Neurofibromatosis[18, 399]
  Primary familial amyloidosis[50–53]
  Refsum's disease[430–434]
  S-hemoglobinopathy[54–61, 64–68, 70]
Systemic
  Sturge-Weber syndrome[458, 459]
  Trisomy 18[101–103]
  Tuberous sclerosis[18]
Hypotension
Systemic
  Diabetes mellitus[147]
  Myotonic dystrophy[397, 398]
  Osteogenesis imperfecta[411–413]
  Turner's syndrome[466]

APPENDIX TABLE G ABNORMALITIES OF THE IRIS

Absence of Pigment
Systemic
Albinism[29, 30, 32–36, 39, 41]
Chediak-Higashi syndrome[89, 90, 92]
Atrophy
Ocular
Essential iris atrophy[327]
Systemic
Lowe's syndrome[344–348]
Xeroderma pigmentosum[491]
Coloboma
Ocular
Chromosome 13–15 deletion[103, 104, 108]
Systemic
Adrenogenital syndrome (see Chapter 20, Part A)
Albinism[29, 30, 32–36, 39, 41]
Gänsslen's syndrome[235a]
Klinefelter's syndrome (see Chapter 20, Part A)
Laurence-Moon-Bardet-Biedl syndrome[335, 336]
Marfan's syndrome[357, 358]
Norrie's disease[408, 409, 477]
Trisomy 13–15[96, 97, 100, 103, 107]
Trisomy 18[101–103]
Trisomy XYY[106]
Ullrich's syndrome[468]
Weyer's oculovertebral syndrome[427]
Deposit
Systemic
Cystinosis[132–145]
Hyperplasia
Ocular
Flocculi[427]
Persistent pupillary membrane[427]
Systemic
Albinism[29, 30, 32–36, 39, 41]
Hypoplasia
Ocular
Aniridia[71–77]

Familial iris hypoplasia[245, 326]
Mesodermal hypoplasia[326]
Peter's anomaly[120]
Systemic
Marinesco–Sjögren syndrome[359a]
Mesodermal dysgenesis of the iris and cornea[445]
Iritis
Systemic
Gout[255]
Neovascularization
Systemic
Angiomatosis retinae[479]
Diabetes mellitus[147]
Pigment
Ocular
Heterochromia[419]
Melanosis[419]
Systemic
Trisomy 18[101–103]
Waardenburg's syndrome[480]
Pupil
Ocular
Adie's syndrome[28a]
Congenital anisocoria[427]
Congenital microcoria[427]
Corectopia[427]
Systemic
Albinism[29, 30, 32–36, 39, 41]
Diabetes mellitus[149]
Marfan's syndrome[358]
Porphyria[421, 422]
Riley-Day syndrome[446–448]
Trisomy 13–15[96, 97, 100, 103, 107]
Trisomy 18[101–103]
Spots
Systemic
Alkaptonuria[42–47]
Down's syndrome[105]

APPENDIX TABLE H ABNORMALITIES OF THE LACRIMAL SYSTEM

Decreased Tearing
Systemic
Riley–Day syndrome[446–448]
Epiphora
Ocular
Congenital absence of lacrimal puncta[332]
Systemic
Cystinosis[132–145]
Engelmann's disease[156]
Porphyria[421, 422]
Lashes
Ocular
Hereditary distichiasis[341]
Systemic
Menke's disease[360]
Metachromatic leukodystrophy[365]
Werner's syndrome[481]

APPENDIX TABLE I ABNORMALITIES OF THE LENS

Cataract

Ocular

Aniridia[71-77]

Myopia[396]

Systemic

Abetalipoproteinemia[21-28]

Albinism[29, 30, 32-36, 39, 41]

Alport's syndrome[49]

Apert's syndrome[78]

Argininosuccinic aciduria[79]

Cockayne's syndrome[109]

Conradi's syndrome[116]

Crouzon's syndrome[129, 130]

Diabetes mellitus[147]

Down's syndrome[105]

Fabry's disease[159-168, 170-184]

Galactosemia[188-197]

Glucose-6-phosphate dehydrogenase deficiency[249]

Glycogenoses[251]

Homocystinuria[263-282]

Hurler's disease[390]

Hypoglycemia[317]

Hypophosphatasia[320]

Iridogoniodysgenesis and cataract[444]

Laurence-Moon-Bardet-Biedl syndrome[335, 336]

Myotonic dystrophy[397, 398]

Neurofibromatosis[399]

Osteogenesis imperfecta[411-413]

Pierre Robin syndrome[418]

Protein deficiency[470]

Refsum's disease[430-434]

Retinitis pigmentosa (see Table 19-2)

Rothmund's syndrome[450a]

Smith-Lemli-Opitz syndrome[457]

Treacher Collins syndrome[464]

Trisomy 13-15[96, 97, 100, 103, 107]

Trisomy 18[101-103]

Tuberous sclerosis[18]

Vitamin A deficiency[470, 473]

Vitreoretinal dystrophy (Wagner)[474, 477, 478]

Werner's syndrome[481]

Wilson's disease[482-489]

Displaced Lens

Ocular

Aniridia[71-77]

Congenital dislocation[150]

Dominant microspherophakia[151]

Late spontaneous dislocation[151a]

Myopia[396]

Systemic

Ehlers-Danlos syndrome[152-154]

Homocystinuria[263-282]

Hyperlysinemia[313]

Klinefelter's syndrome (see Chapter 20, Part A)

Marchesani's syndrome[354]

Marfan's syndrome[357]

Sulfite oxidase deficiency[460]

APPENDIX TABLE J ABNORMALITIES OF THE LIDS

Deformities

Ocular

Epiblepharon[341]

Hereditary blepharochalasis[341]

Systemic

Crouzon's syndrome[129, 130]

Down's syndrome[105]

Ehlers-Danlos syndrome[152-154]

Franceschetti's syndrome[187a]

Gänsslen's syndrome[235a]

Goldenhar's syndrome[254]

Greig's syndrome[256]

Hypophosphatasia[320]

Neurofibromatosis[399]

Porphyria[421, 422]

Primary familial amyloidosis[50-53]

Treacher Collins syndrome[464]

Trisomy 13-15[96, 97, 100, 101, 103]

Waardenburg's syndrome[480]

Ectropion

Systemic

Icthyosis[321, 322]

Porphyria[421, 422]

Ptosis

Ocular

Hereditary ptosis[341]

Marcus Gunn syndrome[355]

Systemic

Apert's syndrome[78]

Congenital ptosis[341]

Engelmann's syndrome[156]

Fabry's disease[159-168, 170-184]

Hartnup disease[258]

Hurler's disease[384, 390]

Hyperammonemia[486,487]

Laurence-Moon-Bardet-Biedl syndrome[335, 336]

Neurofibromatosis[18, 399]

Porphyria[421, 422]

Primary familial amyloidosis[50-53]

Trisomy 18[101-103]

APPENDIX TABLE K NEUROLOGIC
ABNORMALITIES

Headache
Systemic
  Hyperammonemia[486, 487]
Photogenic Epilepsy
Systemic
  Prolinemia[423, 424]
Visual Loss
Systemic
  Argininosuccinic aciduria[79]
  Progressive myoclonic epilepsy —
    Lafora type[488]

APPENDIX TABLE L ABNORMALITIES OF THE OPTIC NERVE

Atrophy
Systemic
  Abetalipoproteinemia[21−28]
  Albinism[29, 30, 32−36, 39, 41]
  Apert's syndrome[78]
  Batten's cerebral degeneration with
    macular changes[198, 225]
  Behr's syndrome[476]
  Charcot-Marie-Tooth syndrome[88]
  Chromosomal 18 deletion[103, 104, 108]
  Cockayne's syndrome[109]
  Congenital amaurotic familial idiocy[225]
  Crouzon's syndrome[129, 130]
  Diabetes mellitus[149]
  Engelmann's disease[156]
  Generalized gangliosidosis
    (GM$_1$ type 1)[15, 209, 218, 234]
  Glucose-6-phosphate dehydrogenase
    deficiency[249]
  Homocystinuria[263−282]
  Hurler's syndrome[383, 390]
  Hypophosphatasia[320]
  Krabbe's disease[329, 330, 331]

  Kufs' disease[214]
  Laurence-Moon-Bardet-Biedl
    syndrome[335, 336]
  Leber's hereditary optic atrophy[410]
  Maple syrup urine disease[350, 351, 353]
  Menke's disease[360]
  Metachromatic leukodystrophy[365]
  Morgagni's syndrome[371b]
  Naegeli's syndrome[420]
  Neurofibromatosis[399]
  Osteopetrosis[414]
  Refsum's disease[430−434]
  S-hemoglobinopathy[54−61, 64−68, 70]
  Tay-Sachs disease (G$_{M2}$ type 1
    gangliosidosis)[15]
  Trisomy 13−15[96, 97, 100, 101, 103]
  Tuberous sclerosis[18]
Edema
Systemic
  Engelmann's disease[156]
  Fabry's disease[159−168]
  Maroteaux-Lamy syndrome[384, 390]
  Osteopetrosis[414]
  Porphyria[421, 422]

APPENDIX TABLE M PHOTOPHOBIA

Ocular
  Albinism[29, 30, 32−36, 39, 41]
  Cone dysfunction syndrome[449]
  Congenital glaucoma[244]
  Keratosis follicularis spinulosa
    decalvans[146]
Systemic
  Albinism[29, 30, 32−36, 39, 41]
  Chediak-Higashi syndrome[89, 90, 92]
  Cockayne's syndrome[109]
  Cystinosis[132−145]
  Down's syndrome[105]
  Lowe's syndrome[344−348]
  Menke's disease[360]
  Phenylketonuria[417]
  Porphyria[421, 422]
  Tryptophanemia[465]
  Xeroderma pigmentosum[491]

APPENDIX TABLE N   ABNORMALITIES OF THE SCLERA

Blue Sclerae (Thin Sclerae)
Ocular
   Keratoconus[121]
Systemic
   Crouzon's syndrome[129, 130]
   Ehlers-Danlos syndrome[152-154]
   Hypophosphatasia[320]
   Marfan's syndrome[356, 357]
   Osteogenesis imperfecta[411-413]
   Pseudo-pseudohypoparathyroidism
      (see Chapter 20, Part A)
   Trisomy 18[101-103]

Pigmentation
Ocular
   Melanosis[419]
Systemic
   Alkaptonuria[42-47]
   Gaucher's disease[236-242]
Scleritis
Systemic
   Gout[255]
Sclerocornea
Systemic
   Trisomy 18[101-103]
Scleromalacia
Systemic
   Porphyria[421, 422]

APPENDIX TABLE O   ABNORMALITIES OF THE SKIN

Depigmentation
Systemic
   Albinism[29, 30, 32-36, 39, 41]
   Chediak-Higashi syndrome[89, 90, 92]
   Xeroderma pigmentosum[491]
Deposits
Systemic
   Amyloidosis[50-53]
   Lipoid proteinosis[342, 343]
Dermatitis
Systemic
   Cockayne's syndrome[109]
   Hartnup disease[258]
Flushing
Systemic
   Homocystinuria[263-282]
   Hyperserotonemia[315]
Pigmentation
Systemic
   Ataxia-telangiectasia[80, 81]

   Gaucher's disease[236-242]
   Neurofibromatosis[399]
   Porphyria[421, 422]
   Xeroderma pigmentosum[491]
Scaling
Systemic
   Icthyosis[321, 322]
Telangiectasia
Systemic
   Fabry's disease[159-168, 170-184]
   Osler's disease[435]
Tumors
Systemic
   Neurofibromatosis[399]
   Xeroderma pigmentosum[491]
Xanthelasma
Systemic
   Hyperlipoproteinemia, types 2 and 3[15]
Xanthomas
Systemic
   Hyperlipoproteinemia, types 1, 3, 4, and 5[15]

APPENDIX TABLE P   ABNORMALITIES OF THE VITREOUS

Opacities
Ocular
   Familial exudative vitreoretinopathy[474, 477]
   Hyaloideoretinal degenerations[477]
Systemic
   Norrie's disease[408, 409, 477]
   Primary familial amyloidosis[50-53]
   Tuberous sclerosis[18]
Hemorrhage
Systemic
   Diabetes mellitus[148]
   S-hemoglobinopathy[54-61, 64-68, 70]
   Thalassemia[69]

REFERENCES

General References

1. Armstrong, D., Dimmitt, S., and VanWormer, D.: Studies in Batten Disease. Arch. Neurol., *30*:144–152, February, 1974.

1a. Auerbach, V. H., and Di George, A. M.: Genetic mechanisms producing multiple enzyme defects; a review of unexplained cases and a new hypothesis. Amer. J. Med. Sci., *249*:718, 1965.

2. Auerbach, V. H., and DiGeorge, A. M.: Inborn errors of metabolism. In Nelson, W. E., Vaughan, V. C., III, and McKay, R. J. (eds.): Textbook of Pediatrics. 9th ed. Philadelphia, W. B. Saunders Co., 1969.

3. Bondy, P. K. (ed.): Duncan's Diseases of Metabolism. 6th ed. Vol. 1. Philadelphia, W. B. Saunders Co., 1969.

4. Cogan, D. G.: Ocular correlates of inborn metabolic defects. Canad. Med. Assoc. J., *95*:1055, 1966.

5. Cogan, D. G., and Kuwabara, T.: The sphingolipidoses and the eye. Arch. Ophthal., *79*:437, 1968.

6. Dowling, J. E., and Wald, G.: The biological function of vitamin A acid. Proc. Nat. Acad. Sci., *46*:587, 1960.

7. Duke-Elder, S.: Congenital deformities. *In* Duke-Elder, S. (ed.): System of Ophthalmology. Vol. 3, Part 2. St. Louis, The C. V. Mosby Co., 1963.

8. François, J.: Heredity in Ophthalmology. St. Louis, The C. V. Mosby Co., 1961.

9. Garrod, A. E.: Inborn Errors of Metabolism. London, Oxford University Press, 1909.

10. Graymore, C. N., and Hsia, D. Y-Y.: Inborn errors of metabolism affecting the eye. *In* Graymore, C. N. (ed.): Biochemistry of the Eye. London, Academic Press, 1970.

11. Harris, H.: The Principles of Human Biochemical Genetics. New York, American Elsevier, 1970.

12. Paulson, G., and Allen, N.: The nervous system. *In* Goodman, R. M. (ed.): Genetic Disorders of Man. Boston, Little, Brown and Co., 1970.

13. Sotos, J. F., and Boggs, D. E.: Disorders of metabolism. *In* Goodman, R. M. (ed.): Genetic Disorders of Man. Boston, Little, Brown and Co., 1970.

14. Spaeth, G. L.: Personal observation.

15. Spaeth, G. L.: Ocular manifestations of the lipidoses. *In* Tasman, W. (ed.): Retinal Diseases in Children. New York, Harper and Row, 1971, pp. 127–206.

16. Stanbury, J. B., Wyngaarden, J. B., and Fredrickson, D. S. (eds.): The Metabolic Basis of Inherited Disease. 2nd ed. New York, McGraw-Hill Book Co., 1966.

17. Stern, C.: Principles of Human Genetics. 2nd ed. San Francisco, W. H. Freeman, 1960.

18. Tasman, W.: Retinal Diseases in Children. New York, Harper and Row, 1971, pp. 71–104.

19. Volk, B. W., and Aronson, S. M.: Sphingolipids, Sphingolipidoses, and Allied Disorders. New York, Plenum Press, 1972.

20. Waardenburg, P. J., Franceschetti, A., and Klein, D.: Genetics and Ophthalmology, Springfield, Illinois, Charles C Thomas, 1961.

A-Beta-Lipoproteinemia

21. Bassen, F. A., and Kornzweig, A. L.: Malformation of the erythrocytes in a case of atypical retinitis pigmentosa. Blood, 5:381, 1950.

22. DiGeorge, A. M., Mabry, G. G., and Auerbach, V.: A specific disorder of lipid transport (acanthrocytosis): Treatment with intravenous lipids. Amer. J. Dis. Child., *102*:580, 1961.

23. Gotto, A. M., et al.: On the protein defect in A-beta-lipoproteinemia. New Eng. J. Med., *284(15)*:813, April, 1971.

24. Gouras, P., Carr, R. E., and Gunkel, R. D.: Retinitis pigmentosa in a-beta-lipoproteinemia: effects of vitamin A. Invest. Ophthal., *10(10)*:784, October, 1971.

25. Jampel, R. S., and Falls, H. F.: Atypical retinitis pigmentosa, acanthrocytosis, and heredodegenerative neuromuscular disease. Arch. Ophthal., *59*:818, 1958.

26. Lees, R. S., and Ahrens, E. H., Jr.: Fat transport in a-beta-lipoproteinemia: The effects of repeated infusions of β-lipoprotein-rich plasma. New Eng. J. Med., *280*:1261, June 5, 1969.

27. Mier, M., Schwartz, S. O., and Boshes, B.: Acanthrocytosis, pigmentary degeneration of the retina, and ataxia neuropathy: A genetically determined syndrome with associated metabolic disorder. Blood, *16*:1586, 1960.

28. Wolff, O. H., Lloyd, J. K., and Tonks, E. L.: A-beta-lipoproteinaemia with special reference to the visual defect. Exper. Eye. Res., *3*:439, 1964.

Adie's Syndrome

28a. Adie, W.: Complete and incomplete forms of the benign disorder characterized by tonic pupils and absent tendon reflexes. Brit. J. Ophthal., *16*:449, 1932.

Albinism

29. Edmunds, R. T.: Vision of albinos. Arch. Ophthal., *47*:755, 1949.

30. Falls, H.: Albinism. J. Amer. Acad. Ophthal., 57:324, 1953.

31. Gaudin, D., and Fellman, J. H.: The biosynthesis of DOPA in albino skin. Biochim. Biophys. Acta, *141*:64, 1967.

32. Hales, R. H.: Albinism with Axenfeld's syndrome. Rocky Mt. Med. J., *65*:51, February, 1968.

33. Johnson, G. J., Gillan, J. G., and Pearce, W. G.: Ocular albinism in Newfoundland. Canad. J. Ophthal., *6*:237, October, 1971.

34. Kraushar, M. F.: Albinism. Ann. Ophthal., *2*:865, December, 1970.

35. Logan, L. J., Rapaport, S. I., and Maher, I.: Albinism and abnormal platelet function. New Eng. J. Med., *284(24)*:1340, June, 1971.

36. Muniz, F. J., Fradera, J., Maldonado, N., and Perez, S. E.: Albinism, bleeding tendency and abnormal pigmented cells in the bone marrow. A case report. Tex. Rep. Biol. Med., *28(1–2)*:167, 1970.

37. Nance, W. E., Jackson, C. E., and Witkop, C. J., Jr.: Amish albinism: A distinctive autosomal recessive phenotype. Amer. J. Hum. Gen., *22*:579, 1970.

38. Trevor-Roper, P. D.: Marriage of the complete albinos with normally pigmented offspring. Proc. Roy. Soc. Med., *56*:21, 1963.

39. Wallner, A.: Albinism. Report of an unusual family. Amer. J. Ophthal., *33*:785, 1950.

40. Witkop, C. J., Jr., Nance, W. E., Rawls, R. F., and White, J. G.: Autosomal recessive oculocutaneous albinism in man; evidence for genetic heterogeneity. Amer. J. Hum. Gen., 22:55, 1970.

41. Witkop, C. J., Jr., White, J. G., Nance, W. E., Jackson, C. E., and Desnick, S.: Classification of albinism in man. Birth Defects, Original Article Series, 7:13, 1971.

Alkaptonuria

42. Bunim, J. J.: Alkaptonuria. Clinical staff conference at the National Institutes of Health. Ann. Intern. Med., 47:1210, 1957.

43. Garrod, A. E.: The Croonian lectures on inborn errors of metabolism. Lecture II. Alkaptonuria. Lancet, II:73, 1908.

44. Knox, W. E.: Sir Archibald Garrod's 'Inborn Errors of Metabolism.' II. Alkaptonuria. Amer. J. Hum. Gen., 10:95, 1958.

45. Osler, W.: Ochronosis. Lancet, I:10, 1904.

46. Virchow, R.: Ein Fall von Allgemeiner Ochronose der Knorpel und Knorpelähnlichen Theile. Arch. Path. Anat., 37:212, 1866.

47. Von Sallman, L.: Über die Augenpigmentierung bei Endogener Ochronose. Zeit. Augen., 60:164, 1926.

Alpha-Amino-Butyric Aciduria

48. Martin, I., Martin, J. J., Guazzi, G. C., Lowenthal, A., and Maniewshi, J.: New oculo-oto-cerebro-renal syndrome. Lancet I:1112, 1967.

Alport's Syndrome

49. Schatz, H.: Alport's syndrome in a Negro kindred. Amer. J. Ophthal., 71(6):1236, 1971.

Amyloidosis

50. Barth, W. F. (Moderator). Primary amyloidosis. Combined clinical staff conference, Clinical Center, National Institutes of Health. Ann. Intern. Med., 69(4):787, October, 1968.

51. Brownstein, M. H., Elliott, R., and Helwig, E. B.: Ophthalmologic aspects of amyloidosis. Amer. J. Ophthal., 69:423, March, 1970.

52. Kaufman, H. E.: Primary familial amyloidosis. Arch. Ophthal., 60(6):1036, 1958.

53. Ts'o, M. O. M., and Bettman, J. W.: Occlusion of choriocapillaris in primary nonfamilial amyloidosis. Arch. Ophthal., 86(3):281, September, 1971.

Anemia

54. Condon, P. I., and Serjeant, G. R.: Ocular findings in homozygous sickle cell anemia in Jamaica. Amer. J. Ophthal., 73(4):533, April, 1972.

55. Fink, A. I.: Vascular fine structure changes in the bulbar conjunctiva associated with sickle-cell disease. Amer. J. Ophthal., 69:563, April, 1970.

56. Freilich, D. B.: Further studies on the use of hyperbaric oxygen chamber in the treatment of retinal detachment in patients with sickle-cell disease. Paper presented at the A. M. A. Convention, Section on Ophthalmology, June 20th, 1972.

57. Goldberg, M. F.: Classification and pathogenesis of proliferative sickle retinopathy. Amer. J. Ophthal., 71(3):649, March, 1971a.

58. Goldberg, M. F.: Natural history of untreated proliferative sickle retinopathy. Arch. Ophthal., 85(4):428, April, 1971b.

59. Goldberg, M. F.: Treatment of proliferative sickle retinopathy. Trans. Amer. Acad. Ophthal. Otolaryng., 75(3):532, May-June, 1971c.

60. Goodman, G., von Sallmann, L., and Holland, M. G.: Ocular manifestations of sickle-cell disease. Arch. Ophthal., 58:655, November, 1957.

61. Greenberg, M. S., Harvey, H. A., and Morgan, C.: A simple and inexpensive screening test for sickle hemoglobin. New Eng. J. Med., 286(21):1143, May, 1972.

62. Kolker, A.: Ocular manifestations of hematologic disease. In Brown, E. B., and Moore, C. B. (eds.) Progress in Hematology. Vol. V. New York, Grune and Stratton, 1966, pp. 354–389.

63. Markar, M. A. M., Peiris, J. B., DeSilva, G. U., and Prematilleka, N.: Retinopathy in megaloblastic anaemias. Trans. Roy. Soc. Trop. Med. Hyg., 63:398, 1969.

64. May, A., Bellingham, A. J., Hurhns, E. R., and Beaven, G. H.: Effect of cyanate on sickling. Lancet, I(7752):658, March, 1972.

65. Okun, E.: Development of sickle cell retinopathy. Docum. Ophthal., 26:574, 1969.

66. Paton, D.: Angioid streaks and sickle cell anemia. Arch. Ophthal., 62:852, November, 1959.

67. Pauling, L., Itano, H. A., Singer, S. J., and Wells, I. C.: Sickle cell anemia, a molecular disease. Science, 110:543, 1949.

68. Ryan, S. J., and Goldberg, M. F.: Anterior segment ischemia following scleral buckling in sickle cell hemoglobinopathy. Amer. J. Ophthal., 72(1):35, July, 1971.

69. Toselli, C., Bertoni, G., Alessio, L., and Mannucci, P. M.: High incidence of thalassaemia in patients with intraocular haemorrhages. Ophthalmologica (Basel), 157(5):343, 1969.

70. Welch, R. B., and Goldberg, M. F.: Sickle-cell hemoglobin and its relation to fundus abnormality. Arch. Ophthal., 75:353, March, 1966.

Aniridia

71. Blanck, M. F.: A case of familial aniridia. Arch. Ophthal. (Paris), 31(3):209, 1971.

72. Callahan, A.: Aniridia with ectopia lentis and secondary glaucoma: Genetic, pathologic, and surgical considerations. Amer. J. Ophthal., 32(6):28, June—Part II, 1949.

73. DiGeorge, A. M., and Harley, R. D.: The association of aniridia, Wilms' tumor, and genital abnormalities. Arch. Ophthal., 75:796, June, 1966.

74. Flanagan, J. C., and DiGeorge, A. M.: Sporadic aniridia and Wilms' tumor. Amer. J. Ophthal., 67:558, April, 1969.

75. Fraumeni, J. F., Jr.: The aniridia-Wilms' tumor syndrome. Birth Defects, Original Article Series, 5(2):198, 1969.

76. Horvath, L., and Pajor, R.: Rezessive Vererbungsform der Aniridie. Klin. Mbl. Augenheilk., 156:573, April, 1970.

77. Jesberg, D. O.: Aniridia with retinal lipid deposits. Arch. Ophthal., 68:331, September, 1962.

Apert's Syndrome

78. Mann, I.: A theory of the embryology of oxycephaly. Trans. Ophthal. Soc. U. K., 55:279, 1935.

Argininosuccinic Aciduria

79. Allan, J. D., Cusworth, D. C., Dent, C. E., and Wilson, V. K.: A disease, probably hereditary, characterized by severe mental deficiency and constant gross abnormality of amino acid metabolism. Lancet, *1*:182, 1958.

Ataxia–Telangiectasia

80. Harley, R. D., et al: Ataxia-telangiectasia. Arch. Ophthal., *77(5)*:582, May, 1967.

81. Karpati, G., Eisen, A. H., Andermann, F., Bacal, H. L., and Robb, P.: Ataxia-telangiectasia. Amer. J. Dis. Child., *110*:51, 1965.

Axenfeld's Syndrome

82. Sugar, S.: Juvenile glaucoma with Axenfeld's syndrome. Amer. J. Ophthal., *59*:1012, 1965.

Behr's Syndrome

83. Franceschetti, A.: Le syndrome de Behr, ses rapports avec la maladie de Leber et les hérédoataxies. Ophthalmologica, *107*:17, 1944.

Best's Vitelline Dystrophy

84. Duke-Elder, S. and Dobree, J.: Diseases of the retina. *In* Duke-Elder, S. (ed.): System of Ophthalmology. Vol. 10. St. Louis, The C. V. Mosby Co., 1967, p. 632.

Bowen's Syndrome

85. Bowen, P., Lee, C. S. N., Zellweger, H., and Lindenberg, R.: A familial syndrome of multiple congenital defects. Bull. Johns Hopkins Hosp., *114*:401, 1964.

86. Punnett, H. H., and Kirkpatrick, J. A., Jr.: A syndrome of ocular abnormalities, calcification of cartilage, and failure to thrive. J. Pediat., *73(4)*:602, 1968.

Cephalin-Lipidosis

87. Baar, H. S., and Hickmans, E. M.: Cephalin-lipidosis. A new disorder of lipid metabolism. Acta. Med. Scand., *155*:49, 1956.

Charcot-Marie-Tooth Atrophy

88. Walsh, F. B.: Clinical Neuro-ophthalmology. 2nd ed. Baltimore, Williams and Wilkins Co., 1957, p. 763.

Chediak-Higashi Syndrome

89. Kanfer, J. N., Blume, R. S., Yankee, R. A., and Wolff, S. M.: Alteration of sphingolipid metabolism in leukocytes from patients with the Chediak-Higashi syndrome. New Eng. J. Med., *279(8)*:410, 1968.

90. Kritzler, R. A., et al.: Chediak-Higashi syndrome. Cytologic and serum lipid observations in a case and family. Amer. J. Med., *36*:583, April, 1964.

91. Windhorst, D. B., and Zelckson, A. S.: The pigmentary anomaly of the Chediak-Higashi syndrome. Clin. Res., *14*:279, 1966.

92. Wolff, S., et al.: The Chediak-Higashi syndrome: studies of host defenses. Ann. Intern. Med., *76*:293, 1972.

Cholesterol Ester Deficiency

93. Burke, J. A., and Schubert, W. K.: Deficient activity of hepatic acid lipase in cholesterol ester storage disease. Science, *176(4032)*:309, April, 1972.

94. Gjone, E., and Bergaust, B.: Corneal opacity in familial plasma cholesterol ester deficiency. Acta Ophthal., *47(1)*:222, 1969.

Chromosome Diseases

95. Appelmans, M.: Complete bilateral coloboma in a case of Klinefelter-Albright-Reifenstein syndrome due to chromosomal anomaly XXY. Bull. Soc. Belg. Ophtal., *140*:456, 1965.

96. Apple, D. J., Holden, J. D., and Stallworth, B.: Ocular pathology of Patau's syndrome with an unbalanced D/D translocation (trisomy D). Amer. J. Ophthal., *70*:383, September, 1970.

97. Bilchik, R. C., Zackai, E. H., Smith, M. E., and Williams, J. D.: Anomalies with ring D chromosome. Amer. J. Ophthal., *73(1)*:83, January, 1972.

98. Cagianut, B., and Theiler, K.: Bilateral colobomas of iris and choroid. Arch. Ophthal., *83*:141, February, 1970.

99. Collier, M., and Chami, M.: J. François comments on ophthalmological manifestations in Klinefelter's syndrome. Survey Ophthal., *15(5)*:346, March–April, 1971.

100. François, J., Nestens, A., and Carpentier, G.: Microphtalmie et trisomie D. Bull. Soc. Belg. Ophtal., *137*:294, 1964.

101. Ginsberg, J., Perrin, E. V., and Sueoka, W. T.: Ocular manifestations of trisomy 18. Amer. J. Ophthal., *66*:59, July, 1968.

102. Ginsberg, J., et al.: Ocular pathology of trisomy 18. Ann. Ophthal., *3*:273, March, 1971.

103. Keith, C. G.: The ocular findings in the trisomy syndromes. Proc. Roy. Soc. Med., *61*:251, 1968.

104. Levenson, J. E., Crandall, B. F., and Sparkes, R. S.: Partial deletion syndromes of chromosome 18. Ann. Ophthal., *756*, July, 1971.

105. Lowe, R. F.: The eyes in mongolism. Brit. J. Ophthal., *33*:131, 1949.

106. Schwinger, E., and Wiebusch, D.: Iris und Aderhautkolobom bei XYY-Syndrom. Klin. Mbl. Augenheilk., *156*:873, June, 1970.

107. Yanoff, M., Frayer, W. C., and Scheie, H.: Ocular findings in a patient with 13–15 trisomy. Arch. Ophthal., *70*:372, 1963.

108. Yanoff, M., Rorke, L. B., and Niederer, B. S.: Ocular and cerebral abnormalities in chromosome 18 deletion defect. Amer. J. Ophthal., *70*:391, September, 1970.

Cockayne's Syndrome

109. Coles, W. H.: Ocular manifestations of Cockayne's syndrome. Amer. J. Ophthal., *67(5)*:762, May, 1969.

Color Vision

110. Bridges, C. D. B.: Biochemistry of vision. *In* Graymore, C. N. (ed.): Biochemistry of the Eye, London, Academic Press, 1970.

111. Linksz, A.: An Essay on Color Vision and Clinical Color-Vision Tests. New York, Grune and Stratton, 1964.

112. Marks, W. B., Dobelle, W. H., and MacNichol, E. F., Jr.: Visual pigments of single primate cones. Science, *143*:1181, 1964.

113. Wald, G.: The receptors of human color vision. Science, *145*:1007, 1964.

114. Weale, R. A.: Cone monochromatism. J. Physiol., *121*:548, 1953.

Congenital Syndromes

115. Duke-Elder, S. and Leigh, A. Diseases of the outer eye. *In* Duke-Elder, S. (ed.): System of Ophthalmology. Vol. 8, Part 2, St. Louis, The C. V. Mosby Co., 1965, p. 95.

Conradi Syndrome

116. Viallefont, H., and Costeau, J.: La maladie con-

génitale des epiphyses pointillées et ses manifestations ophtalmologiques. Arch. Ophtal.
(Paris), *29(6, 7)*:575, 1969.

Corneal Dystrophies and Malformations

117. Blum, J.-D.: Relations entre les dégénéres-
cences hérédofamiliales et les opacités
congénitales de la cornée (étude clinique et
généalogique). Ophthalmologica, *109*:123,
1945.

118. Bourquin, J. B., Babel, J., and Klein, D.: Nouvel
arbre généalogique de dystrophie cornéenne
granuleuse (Groenouw I). J. Genet. Hum.,
3:137, 1954.

119. Brav, A.: Familial nodular degeneration of the
cornea. Arch. Ophthal., *14*:985, 1935.

120. Duke-Elder, S.: Congenital deformities. *In*
Duke-Elder, S. (ed.): System of Ophthalmology. Vol. 3, Part 2. St. Louis, The C. V.
Mosby Co., 1963, pp. 503, 505–508, 512, 515,
519–521, 535.

121. Duke-Elder, S., and Leigh, A.: Diseases of the
outer eye. *In* Duke-Elder, S. (ed.): System of
Ophthalmology. Vol. 8, Part 2. St. Louis, The
C. V. Mosby Co., 1965, pp. 865, 869, 921,
924, 945, 947–950, 952–956, 964–976.

122. François, J.: Heredity in Ophthalmology, St.
Louis, The C. V. Mosby Co., 1961, p. 305–
309.

123. Fuchs, E.: Dystrophia epithelialis corneae. von
Graefe's Arch. Ophthal., 76:478, 1910.

124. Groenouw, A.: Knötchenförmige Horn-
hauttrübungen (noduli corneae). Arch.
Augenheilk., *21*:281, 1890.

125. Meesmann, A., and Wilke, F.: Clinical and anatomic study of hitherto unknown dominant
hereditary corneal dystrophy. Ophthalmologica, *98*:311, 1940.

126. Mortelmans, L.: Forme familiale de la dystrophie cornéenne de Fuchs. Ophthalmologica,
123:88, 1952.

127. Schnyder, W. F.: Mitteilung über einen neuen
Typus von familiarer Hornhauterkrankung.
Schweiz. Med. Wschr., *59*:559, 1929.

128. Vogt, A.: Lehrbuch und Atlas der Spaltlampen
Mikroskopie des Lebenden Auges. Vol. 1.
Berlin, Springer, Verlag, 1930, pp. 106–107.

Crouzon's Syndrome

129. Crouzon, O.: Dysostose cranio-faciale hérédi-
taire. Bull. Mém. Soc. Med. Hôp. Paris,
33:545, 1912.

130. Greig, D. M.: Oxycephaly. Edinburgh Med. J.,
33:189, 280, 357; 1926.

Cystathioninuria

131. Frimpter, G. W.: Cystathioninuria. New Eng. J.
Med., *268(7)*: 333, February, 1963.

Cystic Fibrosis

131a. Spalter, H. F.: Cystic fibrosis and the eye. J.
Pediat. Ophthal., *8* :6, 1971.

Cystinosis

132. Boniuk, M., and Hill, L. L.: Ocular manifestations of de Toni-Fanconi syndrome with cystine storage diseases. Southern Med. J., *59*:33,
January, 1966.

133. Brubaker, R. F., Wong, V. G., Schulman, J. D.,
Seegmiller, J. E., and Kowabara, T.: Benign
cystinosis. The Clinical, biochemical, and
morphologic findings in a family with 2 affected siblings. Amer. J. Med., *49*:546, October, 1970.

134. Bürcki, E.: Uber die cystinkrankheit im Klien-
kindesalter unter Besonderer Berücksich-
tigung des Augenbefundus. Ophthalmologica, *101*:257, 1941.

135. Goldman, H., Scriver, C. R., and Aaron, K.: Use
of dithiothreitol to correct cystine storage in
cultured cystinotic fibroblasts. Lancet, *1*:811,
April 18, 1970.

136. Holtzapple, P. G., Genel, M. Yakovac, W. C.,
Hummeler, K., and Segal, S.: Diagnosis of
cystinosis by rectal biopsy. New Eng. J. Med.,
281:143, July 17, 1969.

137. Hummeler, K., Zajac, B. A., Genel, M. Holtzapple, P. G., and Segal, S.: Human cystinosis:
Intracellular deposition of cystine. Science,
168:859, May 15, 1970.

138. Kessing, S.: Infantile cystinosis. Acta Ophthal.,
(3):491, 1971.

139. Kraus, E., and Lutz, P.: Ocular cystine deposits
in an adult. Arch. Ophthal., *85(6)*:690, June,
1971.

140. Laibson, P. R., and Damiano, Z.: X-ray and electron diffraction of ocular and bone marrow
crystals in paraproteinemia. Science, *163*:581,
1969.

141. Leitman, P. S., Frazier, P. D., Wong, V. G., Shot-
ton, D., and Seegmiller, J. E.: Adult cystinosis—a benign disorder. Amer. J. Med.,
40:511, April, 1966.

142. Mahoney, C. P., Striker, G. E., Hickman, R. O.,
Manning, G. B., and Marchioro, T. L.: Renal
transplantation for childhood cystinosis. New
Eng. J. Med., *283(8)*:397, August 20, 1970.

143. Schneider, J. A., Wong, V., Bradley, K., and
Seegmiller, J. E.: Biochemical comparisons of
the adult and childhood forms of cystinosis.
New Eng. J. Med., *279(23)*:1253, December 5,
1968.

144. Seegmiller, J. E. (Moderator): Cystinosis. Combined clinical staff conference at the National
Institutes of Health. Ann. Intern Med.,
68:883, April, 1968.

145. Wong, V. G., Schulman, J. D., and Seegmiller, J.
E.: Conjunctival biopsy for the biochemical
diagnosis of cystinosis. Amer. J. Ophthal.,
70:278, August, 1970.

Dermatological Syndromes

146. Duke-Elder, S., and Leigh, A.: Diseases of the
outer eye. *In* Duke-Elder, S. (ed.): System of
Ophthalmology. Vol. 8, Part 2. St. Louis, The
C. V. Mosby Co., 1965, p. 557.

Diabetes Mellitus

147. Duke-Elder, S.: Diseases of the lens and vitreous, glaucoma, and hypotony. *In* Duke-Elder,
S. (ed.): System of Ophthalmology. Vol. 11.
St. Louis, The C. V. Mosby Co., 1969, pp. 166
and 673.

148. Duke-Elder, S., and Dobree, J.: Diseases of the
retina. *In* Duke-Elder, S. (ed.): System of
Ophthalmology. Vol. 10. St. Louis, The C. V.
Mosby Co., 1967, pp. 408–448.

149. Duke-Elder, S., and Scott, G.: Neuro-
opthalmology. *In* Duke-Elder, S. (ed.): System
of Ophthalmology. Vol. 12. St. Louis, The C.
V. Mosby Co., 1971, pp. 223, 665, 765, 880.

Dislocation of the Lens

150. Jarrett, W. H.: Dislocation of the lens: A study
of 166 hospitalized cases. Arch. Ophthal.,
78(3):289, 1967.

151. Johnson, V., Grayson, M., and Christian, J.: Dominant microspherophakia. Arch. Ophthal., 85(5):534, May, 1971.

151a. Vogt, A.: Lehrbuch und Atlas der Spaltlampemikroscopie des lebenden Auges. Part 2. Linse und Zonula. Berlin, J. Springer Verlag, 1930, p. 751.

Ehlers-Danlos Syndrome

152. Cordier, J., and Algen, B.: Une étiologie nouvelle du syndrome de luxation spontanée des cristallins: la maladie d'Ehlers-Danlos. Bull. Soc. Belg. Ophtal., 100:375, 380; 1952.

153. Green, W. R., Friedman-Kien, A., and Banfield, W.: Angioid streaks in Ehlers-Danlos Syndrome. Arch. Ophthal., 76:197, 1966.

154. Moestrup, B.: Tenuity of cornea with Ehlers-Danlos syndrome. Acta Ophthal., 47:704, 1969.

Endocrine Disorders

155. Clements, D. B.: Adrenogenital syndrome and buphthalmos. Brit. J. Ophthal., 55(4):275, 1971. (For additional references see Chapter 20, Part A.)

Engelmann's Disease

156. Morse, P. H., Walsh, F. B., and McCormick, J. R.: Ocular findings in hereditary diaphyseal dysplasia (Engelmann's disease). Amer. J. Ophthal., 68:100, July, 1969.

Eye Movement Syndromes

157. Duke-Elder, S.: Congenital deformities. In Duke-Elder, S. (ed.): System of Ophthalmology. Vol. 3, Part 2. St. Louis, The C. V. Mosby Co., 1963, pp. 984–989.

158. Walsh, F. B., and Hoyt, W. (eds.): Clinical Neuro-ophthalmology. 3rd ed. Vol. 1. Baltimore, Williams and Wilkins Co., 1969, p. 265.

Fabry's Disease

159. Brady, R. O., Gal, A. E., Bradley, R. M., Martensson, E., Warshaw, A. L., and Laster, L.: Enzymatic defect in Fabry's disease. Ceramidetrihexosidase deficiency. New Eng. J. Med., 276:1163, 1967.

160. Brady, R. O., et al.: Fabry's disease: antenatal detection. Science, 172(3979):174, April, 1971.

161. Christensen, L., Heidensleben, E., and Larsen, H. W.: The value of ocular findings in the diagnosis of angiokeratoma corporis diffusum (Fabry's disease). Acta Ophthal., 48(6):1185, 1970.

162. Clarke, J. T. R., Knaack, J., Crawhall, J. C., et al.: Ceramide trihexosidosis (Fabry's disease) without skin lesions. New Eng. J. Med., 284(5):233, February 4, 1971.

163. Desnick, R. J., Bernlohr, R. W., Simmons, R. L., Najarian, J. S., Sharp, H. L., and Krivit, W.: Enzyme therapy for Fabry's disease. Amer. Soc. Hum. Genet. October 1972, p. 23a.

164. Fabry, J.: Ein Beitrag zur Kenntnis der Purpura haemorrhagica nodularis. Arch. Derm., 43:187, 1898.

165. Font, R., and Fine, B.: Ocular pathology in Fabry's disease. Histochemical and electron microscopic observations. Amer. J. Ophthal., 73(3):419, March, 1972.

166. Fordyce, J. A.: Angiokeratoma of the scrotum. Trans. Amer. Derm. Assoc., 19:5, 1896.

167. Frost, P., Spaeth, G. L., and Tanaka, Y.: Fabry's

disease: glycolipid lipidosis. Arch. Intern. Med., 117:440, 1966.

168. Frost, P., Tanaka, Y., and Spaeth, G. L.: Fabry's disease—glycolipid lipidosis. Histochemical and electron microscopic studies of two cases. Amer. J. Med., 40:618, 1966.

169. Guerry, D., III: Fingerprint-like lines in the cornea. Amer. J. Ophthal., 33:724, 1950.

170. Johnston, A. W., Frost, P., Spaeth, G. L., and Renwick, J. H.: Linkage relationships of the angiokeratoma (Fabry) locus. Ann. Hum. Genet. (London), 32:369, 1969.

171. Kemp, G.: Fabry's disease involving the myocardium and coronary arteries, without skin manifestations. Vasc. Dis., 4:100, 1967.

172. Koch, H.: Augenveranderunger beim angiokeratoma. Deutsch. Ophtal. Ges. Berichte, 55:537, 1949.

173. Mapes, C. A., Anderson, R. L., Sweeley, C. C., Desnick, R. J., and Krivit, W.: Enzyme replacement in Fabry's disease, an inborn error of metabolism. Science, 169:987, September 4, 1970.

174. Mibelli, V.: Di una nuova forma di cheratosi "angiocheratoma." G. Ital. Mal. Vener., 30:285, 1889.

175. Nadler, H. L. (Editorial): Allotransplantation for the treatment of inborn errors of metabolism. Ann. Intern. Med., 77:314, 1972.

176. Patel, V., Watanabe, I., and Zeman, W.: Deficiency of alpha-L-fucosidase. Science, 176(4033):426, April 28, 1972.

177. Philipport, M., Franklin, S. S., Gordon, A., Leeber, D., and Hull, A. R.: Studies on the metabolic control of Fabry's disease through kidney transplantation. In Volk, B. W., and Aronson, S. M.: Sphingolipids, Sphingolipidoses, and Allied Disorders. New York, Plenum Press, 1972, pp. 641–651.

178. Spaeth, G. L., and Frost, P.: Fabry's disease. Its ocular manifestations. Arch. Ophthal., 74:760, December, 1965.

179. Stanbury, J. B., Wyngaarden, J. B., and Fredrickson, D. S.: The Metabolic Basis of Inherited Disease. 2nd ed. New York, McGraw Hill Book Co., 1966, p. 430.

180. Steiner, L., and Vorner, H.: Angiomatosis Miliaris, "Eine idiopathische Gefasserkrankung." Deutsch. Arch. Klin. Med., 96:105, 1909.

181. Sweely, C. C., and Klionsky, B.: Fabry's disease: Classification as a sphingolipidosis and partial characterization of a novel glycolipid. J. Biol. Chem., 238:PC3148, 1963.

182. Weicksel, J.: Angiomatosis bzw. Angiokeratosis universalis (eine sehr seltene Haut- und Gefasserkrankung). Deutsch. Med. Wschr., 51:898, 1925.

183. Weingeist, T. A., and Blodi, F. C.: Fabry's disease: ocular findings in a female carrier. Arch. Ophthal., 85:169, 1971.

184. Wise, D., Wallace, H. J., and Jellinek, E. H.: Angiokeratoma corporus diffusum: A clinical study of eight affected families. Quart. J. Med., 31:177, 1962.

Familial Chronic Granulomatous Disease

185. Martyn, L. J., Lischner, H. W., Pileggi, A. J., and Harley, R. D.: Chorioretinal lesions in

familial chronic granulomatous disease of childhood. Amer. J. Ophthal., *73(3)*:403, March, 1972.

Farber's Lipogranulomatosis

186. Cogan, D. G., Kuwabara, T., Moser, H., and Hazard, G. W.: Retinopathy in a case of Farber's lipogranulomatosis. Arch. Ophthal., *75*:752, 1966.
187. Crocker, A. C., Cohen, J., and Farber, S.: The 'lipogranulomatosis' syndrome; a review, with report of patient showing milder involvement. *In* Aronson, S., and Volk, B. (eds.): Inborn Disorders of Sphingolipid Metabolism. Proceedings of the Third International Symposium on the Cerebral Sphingolipidoses. Oxford, Pergamon Press, 1967, pp. 485–503.

Franceschetti's Syndrome

187a. Franceschetti, A., and Kline, D.: Mandibulofacial dysostosis; new hereditary syndrome. Acta Ophthal., *27*:143, 1949.

Friedreich's Ataxia

187b. Duke-Elder, S., and Scott, G. I.: Neuroophthalmology. *In* Duke-Elder, S. (ed.): System of Ophthalmology. Vol. 12. St. Louis, The C. V. Mosby Co., 1971, p. 789.

Galactosemia

188. Dische, Z., Borenfreund, E., and Zelminis, G.: Proteins and protein synthesis in rat lenses with galactose cataract. Arch. Ophthal., *55*:633, 1956.
189. Hansen, R. G.: Hereditary galactosemia. J.A.M.A., *208*:2077, June 16, 1969.
190. Isselbacher, K. J., Anderson, E. P., Kurahashi, K., and Kalckar, H.: Congenital galactosemia, a single enzymatic block in galactose metabolism. Science, *123*:635, 1956.
191. Kinoshita, J. H., Merola, L. O., and Dikmak, E.: The accumulation of dulcitol and water in rabbit lens incubated with galactose. Biochim. Biophys. Acta, *62*:176, 1962.
192. Kinoshita, J. H., Merola, L. O., Satoh, K., and Dikmak, E.: Osmotic changes caused by the accumulation of dulcitol in the lenses of rats fed with galactose. Nature, *194*:1085, 1962.
193. Petricciani, J. C., et al.: Galactose utilization in galactosemia. Science, *175(4028)*:1368, March, 1972.
194. Richter, C. P., and Duke, J. R.: Cataracts produced in rats by yogurt. Science, *168*:1372, June 12, 1970.
195. Segal, S., and Bernstein, H.: Observations on cataract formation in the newborn offspring of rats fed a high galactose diet. J. Pediat., *62(3)*:363, March, 1963.
196. Shih, V. E., et al.: Galactosemia screening of newborns in Massachusetts. New Eng. J. Med., *284(14)*:753, April, 1971.
197. Tedesco, T. A., and Mellman, W. J.: Galactosemia: evidence for a structural gene mutation. Science, *172(3984)*:727, May, 1971.

Ganglioside Diseases

198. Batten, F. E.: Cerebral degeneration with symmetrical changes in the maculae in two members of a family. Trans. Ophthal. Soc. U.K., *23*:386, 1903.
199. Bernheimer, H., and Seitleberger, F.: Über das Verhalten der Ganglioside im Gehirn bei 2 Fällen von spätinfantiler amaurotischer Idiotie. Wien. Klin. Wschr., *80*:163, March, 1968.

200. Bielschowsky, M.: Über spätinfantile familiare amaurotische Idiotie mit Kleinhirnsymptomen. Deutsch. Z. Nervenheilk., *50*:7, 1914.
201. Brady, R. O.: Tay-Sachs disease. New Eng. J. Med., *281*:1243, November 27, 1969.
202. Cogan, D. G., and Kuwabara, T.: Histochemistry of the retina in Tay-Sachs disease. Arch. Ophthal., *16*:414, 1959.
203. Collins, T.: A rare fatal disease of infancy, with symmetrical changes at the macula lutea. Trans. Ophthal. Soc. U.K., *12*:126, 1892.
204. Cotlier, E.: Tay-Sachs' retina. Arch. Ophthal., *86(3)*:352, September, 1971.
205. Danis, P., Begaux, C., and Decock, G.: Bases ophthalmologiques d'une classification des idiotes amaurotiques (sur la valeur relative d'un groupement d'apres les ages du début et les durées d'evolution clinique). J. Genet. Hum., *6*:91, 1957.
206. Derry, D. M., Fawcett, J. S., Andermann, F., and Wolfe, L. S.: Late infantile systemic lipidosis. Neurology, *18*:340, April, 1968.
207. Donahue, S., Zeman, W., and Watanabe, I.: Electron microscopic observations in Batten's disease. *In* Aronson, S. M., and Volk, B. W. (eds.): Inborn Disorders of Sphingolipid Metabolism. Oxford, Pergamon Press, 1967, pp. 3–22.
208. Duffy, P. E., Kornfeld, M., and Suzuki, K.: Neurovisceral storage disease with curvilinear bodies. J. Neuropath. Exp. Neurol., *27*:351, July, 1968.
209. Emery, J. M., Green, W. R., Wyllie, R. G., and Howell, R. R.: $G_M 1$-gangliosidosis. Arch. Ophthal., *85*:177, Feburary, 1971.
210. Godtfredsen, E.: New aspects of the classification and pathogenesis of lipidoses with neuroophthalmological manifestations. Acta Ophthal., *49(3)*:489, 1971.
211. Gonatas, N. K., Gambetti, P., and Baird, H.: A second type of late infantile amaurotic idiocy with multilamellar cytosomes. J. Neuropath. Exp. Neurol., *27*:371, July, 1968.
212. Jansky, J., and Myslivicek, Z.: Beitrag zur familiaren amaurotischen idiotie. Arch. Psychiat. Nervenkr., *59*:668, 1918.
213. Korey, S. R., Gomez, C. J., Stein, A., Gonatas, J., Suzuki, K., Terry, R. D., and Weiss, M.: Studies in Tay-Sachs disease. I. A. Methods 1. Biochemical. 2. Electron miscroscopic; B. Clinical and pathologic descriptions. II. Ultrastructure of the cerebellum. J. Neuropath. Exp. Neurol., *22*:2, 1963.
214. Kufs, H.: Über eine Spätform der amaurotischen Idiotie und ihre heredofamiliaren Grundlagen. Z. Neurol. Psychiat., *95*:169, 1925.
215. Mayou, M. S.: Cerebral degeneration, with symmetrical changes in the maculae, in three members of a family. Trans. Ophthal. Soc. U.K., *24*:142, 1904.
216. Norman, R. M., and Wood, N.: A congenital form of amaurotic family idiocy. J. Neurol., *4*:175, 1941.
217. O'Brein, J. S.: Five gangliosidoses. Lancet, *II*:805, October 11, 1969.
218. O'Brien, J. S., Stern, M. B., Landing, B. H., O'Brien, J. K., and Donnell, G. N.: Generalized gangliosidosis. Amer. J. Dis. Child., *109*:338, 1965.

219. Okada, S., and O'Brien, J. S.: Tay-Sachs disease: generalized absence of a-beta-D-N-acetylhexosaminidase component. Science, *165*:698, 1969.

220. Pilz, H., Sandhoff, K., and Jatzkewitz, H.: Eine gangliosidstoffwechselstörung mit Anhäufung von Ceramid-Lactosid, Monosialo-Ceramid-Lactosid und Tay-Sachs-Gangliosid im Gehirn. J. Neurochem., *13*:1273, 1966.

221. Raine, D. N.: Tay, Sachs, et al. Lancet, *II*:959, November 1, 1969.

222. Sachs, B.: A family form of idiocy, generally fatal, associated with early blindness (amaurotic family idiocy). J. Nerv. Ment. Dis., *21*:475, 1896.

223. Schneck, L., Friedland, J., Valenti, C., Adachi, M., Amsterdam, D., and Volk, B. W.: Prenatal diagnosis of Tay-Sachs disease. Lancet, *I*:582, March 21, 1970.

224. Seitelberger, F., Jacob, H., and Schnabel, R.: The myoclonic variant of cerebral lipidosis. *In* Aronson, S. M., and Volk, B. W. (eds.): Inborn Disorders of Sphingolipid Metabolism. Oxford, Pergamon Press, 1967, pp. 43–74.

225. Spaeth, G. L.: Classification of amaurotic familial idiocies: A system based on biochemical findings. Proceedings of the XXI International Ophthalmolgical Congress, Mexico D.F., March, 1970, pp. 8–14.

226. Spielmeyer, W.: Über eine besondere Form von familiarer amaurotischer Idiotie. Neurol. Cbl., *25*:51, 1906.

227. Suzuki, K., Suzuki, K., and Chen, G. C.: Morphological, histochemical, and biochemical studies on a case of systemic late infantile lipidosis (generalized gangliosidosis). J. Neuropath. Exp. Neurol., *27(1)*:15, January, 1968.

228. Suzuki, K., et al.: A case of juvenile G_M2-gangliosidosis. Neurology, *19*:304, March, 1969.

229. Tay, W.: Symmetrical changes in the region of the yellow spot in each eye of an infant. Trans. Ophthal. Soc. U.K., *1*:55, 1881.

230. Vogt, H.: Über familiäre amaurotischer Idiotie und verwandte Krankheitsbilder. Mschr. Psychiat. Neurol., *18*:161, 1905.

231. Volk, B. W., Adachi, M., Schneck, L., Saifer, A., and Kleinberg, W.: G -ganglioside variant of systemic late infantile lipidosis. Generalized gangliosidosis. Arch. Path., *87*:393, April, 1969.

232. Volk, B. W., Aronson, S. M., and Saifer, S. M.: Fructose-1-phosphate aldolase deficiency in Tay-Sachs disease. Amer. J. Med., *36*:481, 1964.

233. Wolter, J. R., and Allen, R. J.: Retinal neuropathology of late infantile amaurotic idiocy. Brit. J. Ophthal., *48(5)*:277, May, 1964.

234. Zeman, W., and Dyken, P.: Neuronal ceroidlipofuscinosis (Batten's disease): Relationship to amaurotic family idiocy? Pediatrics, *44*:570, 1969.

235. Zeman, W., and Hoffmann, J.: Juvenile and late forms of amaurotic idiocy in one family. J. Neurol. Neurosurg. Psychiat., *25*:352, 1962.

Gänsslen's Syndrome

235a. Gänsslen, M.: Über Hämolytischen Ikterus. Deutsch. Arch. Klin. Med., *140*:210, 1922.

Gaucher's Disease

236. Brady, R. O., Kanfer, J. N., and Shapiro, D.: Metabolism of glucocerebrosides. II. Evidence of an enzymatic deficiency in Gaucher's disease. Biochem. Biophys. Res. Commun., *18*:221, 1965.

237. Brill, N. E.: Primary splenomegaly. Amer. J. Med., *121*:377, 1901.

238. Danes, B. S., and Bearn, A. G.: Gaucher's disease: A genetic disease detected in skin fibroblast cultures. Science, *161*:1347, 1968.

239. East, T., and Savin, L. H.: A case of Gaucher's disease with biopsy of the typical pingueculae. Brit. J. Ophthal., *24*:611, 1940.

240. Gaucher, P. C. E.: De l'epithelioma primitif de la rate. Hypertrophie idiopathique de la rate, sans leucemie. Theses, Octave Doin, Paris, 1882.

241. Hsia, D. Y., Naylor, J., and Bigler, J. A.: The genetic mechanism of Gaucher's disease. *In* Aronson, S. M., and Volk, B. W. (eds.): Cerebral Sphingolipidoses. New York, Academic Press, 1962, p. 327.

242. Kampine, J. P., Brady, R. O., Kanfer, J. N., Field, M., and Shapiro, D.: Diagnosis of Gaucher's disease and Niemann-Pick disease with small samples of venous blood. Science, *155*:86, 1967.

Glaucoma

243. Barkan, H., and Borley, W. E.: Familial cornea plana, complicated by cataracta nigra and glaucoma. Amer. J. Ophthal., *19*:307, 1936.

244. Duke-Elder, S.: Diseases of the lens and vitreous, glaucoma and hypotony. *In* Duke-Elder, S. (ed.): System of Ophthalmology. Vol. 11. St. Louis, The C. V. Mosby Co., 1969, pp. 632–645.

245. Weatherill, J. R., and Hart, C. T.: Familial hypoplasia of the iris stroma associated with glaucoma. Brit. J. Ophthal., *53(7)*:433, 1969.

Globe Syndromes

246. Duke-Elder, S.: Congenital deformities. *In* Duke-Elder, S. (ed.): System of Ophthalmology. Vol. 3, Part 2. St. Louis, The C. V. Mosby Co., 1963, pp. 416–425, 498–503.

Glucose-6-Phosphate Dehydrogenase Deficiency

247. Beutler, E.: Glucose-6-phosphate dehydrogenase deficiency. *In* Stanbury, J. B., Wyngaarden, J. B., and Fredrickson, D. S.: The Metabolic Basis of Inherited Disease. New York, McGraw-Hill Book Co., 1966, pp. 1060–1089.

248. Blattner, R. J.: Ophthalmic complications of favism. J. Pediat., *57*:794, 1960.

249. Choremis, C., Joannides, T., and Kyriakides, B.: Severe ophthalmological complications following favism. Brit. J. Ophthal., *44*:353, 1960.

250. Westring, D. W., and Pisciotta, A.: Anemia, cataracts, and seizures in patients with glucose-6-phosphate dehydrogenase deficiency. Arch. Intern. Med., *118*:385, 1966.

Glycinemia

250a. Childs, B., Nyhan, W. L., Borden, M., Bard, L., and Cooke, R. E.: Idiopathic hyperglycinemia and hyperglycinuria: a new disorder of amino acid metabolism. Pediatrics, *27*:522, 1961.

Glycogen Storage Disease

251. De Lorre, I., and van Gelderen, H. H.: Liver glycogenesis and cataracts in a mentally deficient child. Arch. Dis. Child., *42*:435, 1967.

252. Fine, R. N., Wilson, W. A., and Donnell, G. N.: Retinal changes in glycogen storage disease. Amer. J. Dis. Child., *115*:328, 1968.

253. Schaffer, D. B.: Ocular changes in patients with glycogen storage disease. Personal communication.

Goldenhar's Syndrome

254. Summitt, R. L.: Familial Goldenhar syndrome. Birth Defects, Original Article Series, *5(2)*:106, 1969.

Gout

255. Paufique, L.: The ocular manifestations of gout. J. Med. Lyon, *46*:843, May 5, 1965.

Grieg's Syndrome

256. Meisenbach, A.: Bilateral paralysis of external rectus muscle in hypertelorism, report of a case with convergent strabismus. Amer. J. Ophthal., *33*:83, 1950.

Hartnup Disease

257. Baron, D. N., Dent, C. E., Harris, H., Hart, E. W., and Jepson, J. B.: Hereditary pellagra-like skin rash with temporary cerebellar ataxia, constant renal amino aciduria, and other bizarre biochemical features. Lancet, *2*:421, 1956.

258. Scriver, C. R.: Hartnup disease. A genetic modification of intestinal and renal transport of a certain neutral alpha-amino-acids. New Eng. J. Med., *273*:530, 1965.

Hemophilia and Related Diseases

259. Rubenstein, R. A., Albert, D. M., and Scheie, H. G.: Ocular complications of hemophilia. Arch. Ophthal., *76*:230, August, 1966.

260. Wong, G. Y., Fisher, L. M., and Geeraets, W. J.: Ocular complications of Factor XIII Deficiency. Amer. J. Ophthal., *67*:346, March, 1969.

Hereditary Benign Intraepithelial Dyskeratosis

260a. Graham, J. B., and Witkop, C. J., Jr.: Hereditary benign intraepithelial dyskeratosis. New Physician, *13*:17, 1964.

Hereditary Hemorrhagic Telangiectasia

261. Davis, D. G., and Smith, J. L.: Retinal involvement in hereditary hemorrhagic telangiectasia. Arch. Ophthal., *85(5)*:618, 1971.

Homocysteinemia

262. McCully, K. S.: Vascular pathology of homocysteinemia: Implications for the pathogenesis of arteriosclerosis. Amer. J. Path., *56*:111, July, 1969.

Homocystinuria

263. Barber, G. W., and Spaeth, G. L.: Pyridoxine therapy in homocystinuria. Lancet, *1*:337, February 11, 1967.

264. Barber, G. W., and Spaeth, G. L.: The successful treatment of homocystinuria with pyridoxine. J. Pediat., *75(3)*:463, September, 1969.

265. Carson, N.: Homocystinuria: A new inborn error of metabolism associated with mental deficiency. Arch. Dis. Child., *38*:425, 1963.

266. Dunn, H. G., Perry, T. L., and Dolman, C. L.: Homocystinuria: a recently discovered cause of mental defect and cerebrovascular thrombosis. Neurology, *16*:407, April, 1966.

267. Finkelstein, J. D.: Homocystinuria due to cystathionine synthetase deficiency: The mode of inheritance. Science, *146*:785, 1964.

268. Gaull, G. E., Rassin, D. K., and Sturman, J. A.: Enzymatic and metabolic studies of homocys-

tinuria: effects of pyridoxine. Neuropäd., *1*:189, 1969.

269. Gerritsen, T., and Waisman, H. A.: Homocystinuria: absence of cystathionine in the brain. Science, *145*:588, 1964.

270. Henkind, P., and Ashton, N.: Ocular pathology in homocystinuria. Trans. Ophthal. Soc. U.K., *85*:21, 1965.

271. Laster, L. (Moderator): Homocystinuria due to cystathionine synthase deficiency. Combined clinical staff conference at the National Institutes of Health. Ann. Intern. Med., *63(6)*:1117, December, 1965.

272. Martenet, A.-C., Curtius, H. C., and Anders, P. W.: Altérations oculaires de l'homocystinurie. I. Les acides aminés de l'humeur aqueuse. Arch. Ophtal. (Paris), *28(3)*:295, 1968.

273. Perry, T. L.: Early diagnosis and treatment of homocystinuria. Pediatrics, *37*:502, March, 1966.

274. Perry, T. L., Hansen, S., Love, D. L., Crawford, L. E., and Tischler, B.: Treatment of homocystinuria with a low-methionine diet, supplemental cystine, and a methyl donor. Lancet, *II*:474, August 31, 1968.

275. Presley, G. D., Stinson, I. N., and Sidbury, J. B., Jr.: Ocular defects associated with homocystinuria. Southern Med. J., *62(8)*:944, 1969.

276. Schimke, R. N., McKusick, V. A., Huang, T., and Pollack, A. D.: Homocystinura: Studies of 20 families with 38 affected members. J.A.M.A., *193(9)*:711, August 30, 1965.

277. Shih, V. E., and Efron, M. L.: Pyridoxine-unresponsive homocystinuria. New Eng. J. Med., *283*:1206, November 26, 1970.

278. Spaeth, G. L., and Barber, G. W.: Homocystinuria in a mentally retarded child and her normal cousin. Trans. Amer. Acad. Ophthal. Otolaryng., *69*:912, September-October, 1965.

279. Spaeth, G. L., and Barber, G. W.: Homocystinuria—Its ocular manifestations. J. Pediat. Ophthal., *3*:42, 1966.

280. Spaeth, G., and Barber, G. W.: Prevalence of homocystinuria among the mentally retarded: evaluation of a specific screening test. Pediatrics, *40(4)*:586, part 1, October, 1967.

281. Waisman, H. A., Gerritsen, T., and Vaughn, J. G.: The identification of homocystine in the urine. Biochem. Biophys. Res. Commun., *9*:493, 1962.

282. Wilson, R. S., and Ruiz, R. S.: Bilateral central retinal artery occlusion in homocystinuria. A case report. Arch. Ophthal., *82(2)*:267, 1969.

Homocystinuria and Organic Aciduria

283. Hollowell, J. G., Jr., Hall, W. K., Coryell, M. E., McPherson, J., Jr., and Hahn, D. A.: Homocystinuria and organic aciduria in a patient with vitamin B_{12} deficiency. Lancet, *II*:1428, December 27, 1969.

Hooft's Disease

284. Hooft, C. P., de Laey, J., Herpol, J., deLoore, F., and Verbeeck, J.: Familial hypolipidaemia and retarded development without steatorrhea. Another inborn error of metabolism. Helv. Paediat. Acta, *12*:1, 1962.

Hydroxyprolinemia

285. Efron, M. L., Bixby, E. M., Palattao, L. G., and Pryles, C. V.: Hydroxyprolinemia associated

with mental deficiency. New Eng. J. Med., *267*:1193, December 6, 1962.

Hyperammonemia I and II

286. Hommes, F. A., deGroot, C. J., Wilmink, C. W., and Jonxis, J. H. P.: Carbamyl-phosphate synthetase deficiency in an infant with severe cerebral damage. Arch. Dis. Child., *44*:688, 1969.

287. Levin, B., Abraham, J. M., Oberholzer, V. G., and Burgess, E. A.: Hyperammonaemia: A deficiency of liver ornithine transcarbamylase. Arch. Dis. Child., *44*:152, 1969.

Hyperlipemia

288. Albrink, M. J., Man, E. B., and Peters, J. P.: The relationship of neutral fat to lactescence of serum. J. Clin. Invest., *34*:147, 1955.

289. Anderson, B., Margolis, G., and Lynn, W. S.: Ocular lesions related to disturbances in fat metabolism. Amer. J. Ophthal., *45*:23, 1958.

290. Andrews, J. S.: The lipids of arcus senilis. Arch. Ophthal., *68*:264, 1962.

291. Bagdade, J, D., Porte, D., and Bierman, E. L.: Hypertriglyceridemia: A metabolic consequence of chronic renal failure. New Eng. J. Med., *279*:181, July 25, 1968.

292. Berkowitz, D.: Long-term treatment of hyperlipidemic patients with clofibrate. J.A.M.A., *218(7)*:1001, November, 1971.

293. Bersohn, I., Politzer, W. M., and Blumsohn, D.: Arcus senilis corneae—its relationship to serum lipids in the South African Bantu. S. Afr. Med. J., *43*:1025, August, 1969.

294. Blodi, F. C.: Ocular manifestations of familial hypercholesterolemia. Trans. Amer. Ophthal. Soc., *60*:304, 1962.

295. Chopra, J. S., Mallick, N. P., and Stone, M. C.: Hyperlipoproteinemias in nephrotic syndrome. Lancet, *I(7694)*:317, February 13, 1971.

296. Cogan, D. G., and Kuwabara, T.: Arcus senilis, its pathology and histochemistry. Arch. Ophthal., *61*:553, 1959.

297. Cohen, M.: Report of a case of lipaemia retinalis with hypotony in diabetic coma. Arch. Ophthal., *50*:247, 1921.

298. Dunphy, E. B.: Ocular conditions associated with idiopathic hyperlipemia. Amer. J. Ophthal., *33*:1579, 1950.

299. Fallon, H. J., and Woods, J. W.: Response of hyperlipoproteinemia to cholestyramine resin. J.A.M.A., *204*:1161, 1968.

300. Fredrickson, D. S., and Levy, R. I.: Treatment of essential hyperlipidaemia. Lancet, *I*:191, January 24, 1970.

301. Gallin, J. I., Kaye, D., and O'Leary, W. M.: Serum lipids in infection. New Eng. J. Med., *281*:1081, November 13, 1969.

302. Hickey, N., Maurer, B., and Mulcahy, R.: Arcus senilis: Its relation to certain attributes and risk factors in patients with coronary heart disease. Ophthal. Dig., May, 1971, p. 48.

303. Lees, R. S., Song, C. S., Levere, R. D., and Kappas, A.: Hyperbeta-lipoproteinemia in acute intermittent porphyria. Preliminary report. New Eng. J. Med., *282*:432, February 19, 1970.

304. Lees, R. S., and Wilson, D. E.: Treatment of hyperlipidemia. New Eng. J. Med., *284(4)*:186, January 28, 1971.

305. Macaraeg, P. V. J., Jr., Lasagna, L., and Snyder, B.: Arcus not so senilis. Ann. Intern. Med., *68*:345, 1968.

306. Pedace, E. J., and Winkelmann, R. K.: Xanthelasma palpebrarum. JAMA, *193*:893, 1965.

307. Rohrenschneider, W.: Die Klinische Bedeutung des Arcus lipoides corneae senilis. Wien. Med. Wschr. *112*:845, 1962.

308. Segall, M. M., Lloyd, J. K., Fosbrooke, A. S., and Wolff, O. H.: Treatment of familial hypercholesterolaemia in children. Lancet, *I*:641, March 28, 1970.

309. Smith, E., and Slater, R.: Lipoproteins and the reversibility of atherosclerosis. Lancet, *I(7755)*:840, April, 1972.

310. Stanbury, J. B., Wyngaarden, J. B., and Fredrickson, D. S.: The Metabolic Basis of Inherited Diseases. New York, McGraw-Hill Book Co., 1966, pp. 429–485.

311. Thomas, P. K., and Smith, E. B.: Ocular manifestations in idiopathic hyperlipaemia and xanthomatosis. Brit. J. Ophthal., *42*:501, 1958.

312. Vinger, P. F., and Sachs, B. A.: Ocular manifestations of hyperlipoproteinemia. Amer. J. Ophthal., *70*:563, October, 1970.

Hyperlysinemia

313. Smith, T. H., Holland, M. G., and Woody, N. C.: Ocular manifestations of familial hyperlysinemia. Trans. Amer. Acad. Ophthal. Otolaryng., *75*:355, 1971.

Hypermethioninemia

314. Perry, T. L.: Hypermethioninemia: A metabolic disorder associated with cirrhosis, islet cell hyperplasia, and renal tubular degeneration. Pediatrics, *36(2)*:236, August, 1965.

Hyperserotonemia

315. Southren, A. L., Warner, R.R.P., Christoff, N. I., and Weiner, H. E.: An unusual neurologic syndrome associated with hyperserotonemia. New Eng. J. Med., *260*:1265, 1959.

Hypervalinemia

316. Wada, Y., Tada, K., Minagawa, A., Yoshida, T., Morikawa, T., and Okamura, T.: Idiopathic hypervalinemia. Tohoku J. Exp. Med., *81*:46, 1963.

Hypoglycemia

317. Grunt, J. A., and Howard, R. O.: Eye findings in children with ketotic hypoglycaemia. Canad. J. Ophthal., *7*:151, April, 1972.

318. Merin, S. and Crawford, J. S.: Hypoglycemia and infantile cataract. Arch. Ophthal., *86(5)*:495, November, 1971.

319. Scheie, H. G., Rubenstein, R. A., and Albert, D.M.: Congenital glaucoma and other ocular abnormalities with idiopathic infantile hypoglycemia. J. Pediat. Ophthal., *I*:45, 1964.

Hypophosphatasia

320. Brenner, R. L., Smith, J. L., Cleveland, W. W., Bejar, R. L., and Lockhart, W. S., Jr.: Eye signs of hypophosphatasia. Arch. Ophthal., *81*:614, May, 1969.

Ichthyosis

321. Jay, B., et al.: Ocular manifestations of ichthyosis. Brit. J. Ophthal., *52*:217, 1968.

322. Sever, R. J., Frost, P., and Weinstein, G.: Eye changes in ichthyosis. JAMA, *206*:2283, 1968.

Imidazole Aciduria

323. Bessman, S. P., and Baldwin, R.: Imidazole aminoaciduria in cerebromacular degeneration. Science, *135*:789, 1962.

324. Perry, T. L., Hansen, B., Tishler, B., Bunting, R., and Berry, K.: Carnosinemia: A new metabolic disorder with neurologic disease and mental defect. New Eng. J. Med., *277*:1219, 1967.

325. Warburg, M.: Diagnosis of Metabolic Eye Diseases. Copenhagen, Munksgaard, 1972, p. 70.

Iris Syndromes

326. Duke-Elder, S.: Congenital deformities. *In* Duke-Elder, S. (ed.): System of Ophthalmology. Vol. 3, Part 2. St. Louis, The C. V. Mosby Co., 1963, p. 565.

327. Duke-Elder, S., and Perkins, E.: Diseases of the uveal tract. *In* Duke-Elder, S. (ed.): System of Ophthalmology. Vol. 9. St. Louis, The C. V. Mosby Co., 1966, p. 686.

Isovaleric Acidemia

328. Budd, M. A., et al.: Isovaleric acidemia. Clinical features of a new genetic defect of leucine metabolism. New Eng. J. Med., *277(7)*:321, August, 1967.

Klippel-Feil Syndrome

328a. Ford, F. R.: Diseases of the Nervous System in Infancy, Childhood and Adolescence. 3rd ed. Springfield, Illinois, Charles C Thomas, 1952, p. 308.

Krabbe's Disease

329. Austin, J., Armstrong, D., Stumpf, D., Kretschmer, L., Mitchell, C., van Zee, G., and Bacchawat, B.: Defective sulfatide synthesis in Krabbe's disease (globoid leukodystrophy). Trans. Amer. Neurol. Assoc., *92*:175, 1967.

330. Nelson, E., Aurebeck, G., Osterberg, K., Berry, J., and Jabbour, J. T.: Ultrastructural and chemical studies on Krabbe's disease. J. Neuropath. Exp. Neurol., *22*:414, July, 1963.

331. Suzuki, Y., and Suzuki, K.: Krabbe's globoid cell leukodystrophy. Deficiency of galactocerebrosidase in serum, leukocytes, and fibroblasts. Science, *171(3966)*:73 January 8, 1971.

Lacrimal Syndromes

332. Duke-Elder, S.: Congenital deformities. *In* Duke-Elder, S. (ed.): System of ophthalmology. Vol. 3, Part 2. St. Louis, The C. V. Mosby Co., 1963, p. 929.

Lactosyl Ceramidosis

333. Dawson, G., and Stein, A. O.: Lactosyl ceramidosis: catabolic enzyme defect of glycosphingolipid metabolism. Science, *170*:556, October 30, 1970.

Lafora's Disease

334. Yanoff, M., and Schwartz, G. A.: The retinal pathology of Lafora's disease: A form of glycoprotein-acid mucopolysaccharide dystrophy. Trans. Amer. Acad. Ophthal. Otolaryng., *69*:701, 1965.

Laurence-Moon-Bardet-Biedl Syndrome

335. Francois, J.: Heredity in Ophthalmology. St. Louis, The C. V. Mosby Co., 1961, p. 692.

336. Macklin, M.: The Laurence-Moon-Biedl syndrome: a genetic study. J. Hered., *27*:97, 1936.

Leber's Syndrome

337. Dekaban, A. S.: Hereditary syndrome of congenital retinal blindness (Leber). Polycystic kidneys and maldevelopment of the brain. Amer. J. Ophthal., *68*:1029, December, 1969.

Lecithin: Cholesterol Acyltransferase Deficiency

338. Norum, K. R., and Gjone, E.: Familial plasma lecithin: cholesterol acyltransferase deficiency. Scand. J. Clin. Lab. Invest., *20*:231, 1967.

Lenoble-Aubineau Syndrome

339. Lenoble, E., and Aubineau, E.: Nystagmus-myoclonie syndrome. Rev. Med. (Paris), *26*:471, 1906.

Lenz Microphthalmia Syndrome

340. Herrmann, J., and Opitz, J. M.: The Lenz microphthalmia syndrome. Birth Defects, Original Article Series, *5(5, II)*:138, 1969.

Lid Syndromes

341. Duke-Elder, S.: Congenital deformities. *In* Duke-Elder, S. (ed.): System of Ophthalmology. Vol. 3. St. Louis, The C. V. Mosby Co., 1963, pp. 857–859, 873, 887.

Lipoid Proteinosis (Urbach-Wiethe)

342. Gordon, H., Gordon, W., and Botha, V.: Lipoid proteinosis in an inbred Namaqualand Community. Lancet, *I*:1032, May 24, 1969.

343. Muirhead, J. F., and Jackson, P.: Lipoid proteinosis (of Urbach-Wiethe). Arch. Ophthal., *69*:174, 1963.

Lowe's Syndrome

344. Curtin, V. T., Joyce, E. E., and Ballin, N.: Ocular pathology in the oculo-cerebrorenal syndrome of Lowe. Amer. J. Ophthal., *64(3)*:533, 1967.

345. Fisher, N. F., Hallett, J., and Carpenter, G.: Oculocerebrorenal syndrome of Lowe. Arch. Ophthal., *77(5)*:642, May, 1967.

346. Haut, J., and Joannides, Z.: A propos de 55 cas de syndrom de Lowe. Arch. Ophthal. (Paris), *26(1)*:21, 1966.

347. Mack, J., Masters, P., and Hockey, A.: Lowe's syndrome. Aust. J. Ment. Ret., *1*:89, 1970.

348. Terslez, E.: Two cases of aminoaciduria, ocular changes, and retarded mental and somatic development (Lowe's syndrome). Acta Pediat., *49*:635, 1960.

Lyell Syndrome

349. Schmidt, J. G. H., and Lischka, G.: On the ophthalmological symptomatology, therapy and prognosis of the Fuchs and Lyell syndromes. Klin. Mbl. Augenheilk., *157*:342, 1970.

Maple Syrup Urine Disease

350. Dancis, J., Levitz, M., Miller, S., and Westall, R. G.: Maple Syrup urine disease. Brit. Med. J., *1*:91, 1959.

351. Gaull, G. E.: Pathogenesis of maple syrup urine disease: Observations during dietary management and treatment of coma by peritoneal dialysis. Biochem. Med., *3*:130, 1969.

352. Waisman, H. A., Gerrotsen, T., Boggs, D. E., Polidora, J. J., and Harlow, H. F.: Mental retardation in monkeys. II. Branched-chain amino-aciduria and ketoaciduria. J. Dis. Child., *104*:488, 1962.

353. Westall, R. G.: Dietary treatment of a child with maple syrup urine disease (branched-chain ketoaciduria). Arch. Dis. Child., *38*:485, 1963.

Marchesani's Syndrome

354. Marchesani, V. O.: Brachydaktylie und ange-

borene Kugellinse als Systemerkrankung. Klin. Mbl. Augenheilk., *103*:392, 1939.

Marcus Gunn (Jaw-Winking) Syndrome

355. Gunn, R. M.: Congenital ptosis with peculiar associated movements of the affected lid. Trans. Ophthal. Soc. U.K., *3*:283, 1883.

Marfan's Syndrome

356. Goldberg, M. F., and Ryan, S. J.: Intercalary staphyloma in Marfan's syndrome. Amer. J. Ophthal., *67*:329, March, 1969.

357. McKusick, V. A.: Heritable Disorders of Connective Tissue. St. Louis, The C. V. Mosby Co., 1966, pp. 38–149.

358. Murdoch, J. L., Walker, B. A., Halpern, B. L., Kuzma, J. W., and McKusick, V. A.: Life expectancy and causes of death in Marfan syndrome. New Eng. J. Med., *286(15)*:804, April, 1972.

Marie's Cerebellar Ataxia

359. Walsh, F., and Hoyt, W. (eds): Clinical Neuro-Ophthalmology. Vol. 1. 3rd ed. Baltimore, Williams and Wilkins Co., 1969, p. 726.

Marinesco-Sjögren Syndrome

359a. Marinesco, G., Draganesco, J., and Vasiliu, D.: Nouvelle maladie familiale charactérisée par une cataracte congénitale et un arrêt du development somato-neuro-physique. Encéphale, *26*:97, 1931.

Menke's Disease

360. Seelenfreund, M. H., Gartner, S., and Vinger, P. F.: The ocular pathology of Menke's disease (Kinky hair disease). Arch. Ophthal., *80(6)*:718, 1968.

Metachromatic Leukodystrophy

361. Austin, J., Armstrong, D., and Shearer, L.: Metachromatic form of diffuse cerebral sclerosis: V. The nature and significance of low sulfatase activity: A controlled study of brain, liver, and kidney in four patients with metachromatic leukodystrophy (MLD). Arch. Neurol., *13*:593, 1965.

362. Austin, J., McAfee, D., Armstrong, O., O'Rourke, M., Shearer, L., and Bacchawat, B.: Abnormal sulfatase activities in two human diseases (metachromatic leucodystrophy and gargoylism). Biochem. J., *93*:15c, 1964.

363. Bargeton, E.: The metachromatic form of leucodystrophy and its relationship to lipidosis and demyelination in other metabolic disorders. *In* Folch-Pi, J., and Bauer, H. J. (eds.) Brain Lipids and Lipoproteins and the Leucodystrophies. New York, Elsevier, 1963, pp. 90–103.

364. Cogan, D. G., Kuwabara, T., and Moser, H.: Metachromatic leukodystrophy. Ophthalmologica, *160*:2, 1970.

365. Cogan, D. G., Kuwabara, T., Richardson, E. P., and Lyon, G.: Histochemistry of the eye in metachromatic leukoencephalopathy. Arch. Ophthal., *60*:397, 1958.

366. Hagberg, B.: Clinical symptoms, signs, and tests in metachromatic leucodystrophy. *In* Folch-Pi, J., and Bauer, H. J. (eds.) Brain Lipids and Lipoproteins and the Leucodystrophies. New York, Elsevier, 1963, pp. 134–146.

367. Moser, H. W., and Lees, M.: Sulfatide lipidosis: Metachromatic leukodystrophy. *In* Stanbury, J. B., Wyngaarden, J. B., and Fredrickson, D.

S. (eds.) The Metabolic Basis of Inherited Disease. 2nd ed. New York, McGraw-Hill Book Co., 1966, pp. 539–564.

368. Percy, A. K., and Brady, R. O.: Metachromatic leukodystrophy: Diagnosis with samples of venous blood. Science, *161*:594, August 9, 1968.

369. Percy, A., and Kaback, M.: Infantile and adult-onset metachromatic leukodystrophy. New Eng. J. Med., *285(14)*:785, September, 1971.

370. Porte, M. T., et al.: Correction of abnormal cerebroside sulfate metabolism in cultured metachromatic leukodystrophy fibroblasts. Science, *172(3989)*:1263, June, 1971.

371. Webster, H. deF: Schwann cell alterations in metachromatic leukodystrophy: Preliminary phase and electron microscopic observations. J. Neuropath. Exp. Neurol., *21*:534, October, 1962.

Microcornea, Glaucoma, and Absent Frontal Sinuses

371a. Holmes, L. B., and Walton, D. S.: Hereditary microcornea, glucoma and absent frontal sinuses: a family study. J. Pediatrics, *74*:968, 1969.

Morgagni's Syndrome

371b. Falconer, M. A., and Prerard, B. E.: Failing vision caused by a bony spike compressing the optic nerve within the optic canal. Report of cases associated with Morgagni's syndrome benefited by operation. Brit. J. Ophthal., *34*:265, 1950.

Mucolipidosis

372. Freitag, F., Blumcke, S., and Spranger, J.: Hepatic ultrastructure in mucolipidosis I (lipomucopolysaccharidosis). Virchow's Arch. (Zellpath.), 7:189, 1971.

373. Goldberg, M. F., et al.: Macular cherry-red spot, corneal clouding, and β-galactosidase deficiency: clinical, biochemical, and electron microscopic study of new autosomal recessive storage disease. Arch. Intern. Med., *128*:387, 1971.

374. Kenyon, K. R., and Sensenbrenner, J. A.: Mucolipidosis II (I-cell disease). Ultrastructural observations of conjunctiva and skin. Invest. Ophthal., *10(8)*:555, August, 1971.

375. Quigley, H. A., and Goldberg, M. F.: Conjunctival ultrastructure in mucolipidosis III (Pseudo-Hurler polydystrophy). Invest. Ophthal., *10(8)*:568, August, 1971.

376. Spranger, J. W., and Weidemann, H. R.: The genetic mucolipidoses. Diagnosis and differential diagnosis. Humangenetik, *9*:113, 1970.

Mucopolysaccharidosis

377. Benson, P. F., Bowser-Riley, F., and Giannelli, F.: β-Galactosidases in fibroblasts: Hurler and Sanfilippo syndromes. New Eng. J. Med., *283*:999, October 29, 1970.

378. Cockayne, E. A.: Gargoylism (chondro-osteodystrophy, hepatosplenomegaly, deafness in two brothers). Proc. Roy. Soc. Med., *30*:104, 1936.

379. Constantopoulos, G., et al.: Heterogeneity of disorders in patients with corneal clouding, normal intellect, and mucopolysaccharidosis. Amer. J. Ophthal., *72(6)*:1106, December, 1971.

380. Dorfman, A., and Lorincz, A. E.: Occurrence of

urinary acid mucopolysaccharides in the Hurler syndrome. Proc. Nat. Acad. Sci., *43*:443, 1957.

381. Fratantoni, J. C., Neufeld, E. F., Uhlendorf, B. W., and Jacobson, C. B.: Intrauterine diagnosis of the Hurler and Hunter syndromes. New Eng. J. Med., *280*:686, March 27, 1969.

382. Gerich, J. E.: Hunter's syndrome: Beta-galactosidase deficiency in skin. New Eng. J. Med., *280*:299, April 10, 1969.

383. Gills, J. P., Hobson, R., Hanley, B., and McKusick, V. A.: Electroretinography and fundus oculi findings in Hurler's disease and allied mucopolysaccharidoses. Arch. Ophthal., *74*:596, November, 1965.

384. Goldberg, M. F., Maumanee, A. E., and McKusick, V. A.: Corneal dystrophies associated with abnormalities of mucopolysaccharide metabolism. Arch. Ophthal., *74*:516, October, 1965.

385. Hunter, C.: A rare disease in two brothers. Proc. Roy. Soc. Med., *10*:104, 1917.

386. Hurler, G. P.: Über einen Typ multipler Abartungen, vorwiegend am Skelettsystem. Z. Kinderheilk., *24*:220, 1919.

387. Kenyon, K. R., Topping, T. M., Green, W. R., and Maumanee, A. E.: Ocular pathology of the Maroteaux-Lamy syndrome (systemic mucopolysaccharidosis type VI). Histologic and ultrastructural report of two cases. Amer. J. Ophthal., *73(5)*:718, May, 1972.

388. Levin, B. Fajerman, J., and Jacoby, N. M.: Mucopolysaccharidosis. Proc. Roy. Soc. Med., *65*:339, April, 1972.

389. MacBrinn, M., Okada, S., Woollacott, M., Patel, V., Ho, M. W., Tappel, A. L., and O'Brien, J. S.: Beta-galactosidase deficiency in the Hurler syndrome. New Eng. J. Med., *281*:338, August 14, 1969.

390. McKusick, V. A.: Heritable Disorders of Connective Tissue. 3rd ed. St. Louis, The C. V. Mosby Co., 1966, p. 389.

391. Pfaundler, M.: Demonstrationen über einen Typus kindlicher Dysostose. Jb. Kinderheilk., *92*:420, 1920.

392. Quigley, H. A., and Goldberg, M. F.: Scheie syndrome and macular corneal dystrophy. Arch. Ophthal., *85(5)*:553, May, 1971.

393. Scheie, H. G., Hambrick, G. W., Jr., and Barness, L. A.: A newly recognized forme fruste of Hurler's disease (gargoylism). Amer. J. Ophthal., *53*:753, 1962.

394. Topping, T. M., et al.: Ultrastructural ocular pathology of Hunter's syndrome. Arch. Ophthal., *86(2)*:164, August, 1971.

395. Wiesmann, U., and Neufeld, E. F.: Scheie and Hurler syndromes: Apparent identity of the biochemical defect. Science, *169*:72, July 3, 1970.

Myopia

396. Duke-Elders, S., and Abrams, D.: Ophthalmic optics and refraction. *In* Duke-Elder, S. (ed.): System of Ophthalmology. Vol. 5. St. Louis, The C. V. Mosby Co., 1970, pp. 301–362.

Myotonia

397. Betten, M., Bilchik, R. C., and Smith, M. E.: Pigmentary retinopathy of myotonic dystrophy. Amer. J. Ophthal., *72(4)*:720, October, 1971.

398. Burian, H. M., and Burns, C. A.: Ocular changes in myotonic dystrophy. Amer. J. Ophthal., *63*:22, January, 1967.

Neurofibromatosis

399. Wheeler, J. M.: Plexiform neurofibromatosis (von Recklinghausen's disease) involving the choroid, ciliary body, and other structures. Amer. J. Ophthal., *20*:368, 1937.

Nevoxanthoendothelioma

400. Newell, F. W.: Nevoxanthoendothelioma with ocular involvement. Arch. Ophthal., *58*:321, September, 1957.

Niemann-Pick Disease

401. Brady, R. O., Kanfer, J. N., Mock, M. B., and Fredrickson, D. S.: The metabolism of sphingomyelin. II. Evidence of an enzymatic deficiency in Niemann-Pick disease. Proc. Nat. Acad. Sci. (U.S.A.,) *55*:366, 1966.

402. Cogan, D. G., and Federman, D. D.: Retinal involvement with reticuloendotheliosis of unclassified type. Arch. Ophthal., *71*:489, 1964.

403. Crocker, A. C., and Farber, S.: Niemann-Pick disease: A review of eighteen patients. Medicine, *37*:1, 1958.

404. Goldstein, I., and Wexler, D.: Niemann-Pick's disease with cherry-red spots in the macula. Arch. Ophthal., *5*:704, May, 1931.

405. Jansseune, H., Philippart, M., and Martin, J. J.: Sur deux observations de maladie de Niemann-Pick. Formes chroniques à participation nerveuse retardée. Acta Med. Belg., *21*:239, 1967.

406. Niemann, A.: Ein unbekanntes Krankheitsbild. Jb. Kinderheilk., *79*:1, 1914.

407. Pick, L.: Über die lipoidzellige Splenohepatomegalie Typus Niemann-Pick als Staffwechselerkrankung. Med. Klin., *23*:1483, 1927.

Norrie's Disease

408. Fradkin, A. H.: Norrie's disease. Congenital progressive oculo-acoustico-cerebral degeneration. Amer. J. Ophthal., *72(5)*:947, November, 1971.

409. Holmes, L. B.: Norrie's disease — retinal malformation, mental retardation and deafness. New Eng. J. Med., *284*:367, February 18, 1971.

Ocular Motor Apraxia

409a. Duke-Elder, S.: Normal and abnormal development. *In* Duke-Elder, S. (ed.): System of Ophthalmology. Vol. 3, Part 2. St. Louis, The C. V. Mosby Co., 1963, p. 1002.

Optic Atrophy

410. Duke-Elder, S., and Scott, G.: Neuro-ophthalmology. *In* Duke-Elder, S. (ed.): System of Ophthalmology. Vol. 12. St. Louis, The C. V. Mosby Co., 1971, pp. 108–116.

Osteogenesis Imperfecta

411. Berggren, L., Wessler, E., and Wennerstrom, J.: Intraocular pressure and excretion of mucopolysaccharides in osteogenesis imperfecta. Acta Ophthal., *47(1)*:122, 1969.

412. Manschot, W. A.: Ocular anomalies in osteogenesis imperfecta. Ophthalmologica, *149*:241, 1965.

413. Stein, R., Lazar, M., and Adam, A.: Brittle cornea. A familial trait associated with blue sclera. Amer. J. Ophthal., *66(1)*:67, 1968.

Osteopetrosis

414. Duke-Elder, S.: Congenital deformities. *In* Duke-Elder, S. (ed.): System of Ophthalmo-

logy. Vol. 3, Part 2. St. Louis, The C. V. Mosby Co., 1963, p. 1068.

Paget's Disease
415. Kristensen, E. B.: Ocular manifestations in Paget's disease (osteitis deformans). Acta Ophthal., *49(5)*:741, 1971.

Pelizaeus-Merzbacher Syndrome
416. Rahn, E. K., Yanoff, M., and Tucker, S.: Neuro-ocular considerations in the Pelizaeus-Merzbacher syndrome. A clinicopathologic study. Amer. J. Ophthal., *66*:1143, December, 1968.

Phenylketonuria
417. Knox, W. E.: Phenylketonuria. *In* Stanbury, J. B., Wyngaarden, J. B., and Fredrickson, D. S.: The Metabolic Basis of Inherited Disease. 2nd ed. New York, McGraw-Hill Book Co., 1966, pp. 258–295.

Pierre Robin Syndrome
418. Smith, J. L., Cavanaugh, J. J., and Stowe, F. C.: Ocular manifestations of the Pierre Robin syndrome. Arch. Ophthal., *63*:984, 1960.

Pigment Disturbance
419. Duke-Elder, S.: Congenital deformities. *In* Duke-Elder, S. (ed.): System of Ophthalmology. Vol. 3, Part 2. St. Louis, The C. V. Mosby Co., 1963, pp. 794, 813.
420. Franceschetti, A., and Jadassohn, W.: A propos de l'incontinentia pigmenti, délimitation de deux syndromes differents figurant sous le même terme. Dermatologica, *108*:1, 1954.

Porphyria
421. Barnes, H. D., and Boshoff, P. H.: Ocular lesions in patients with porphyria. Arch. Ophthal., *48*:567, 1952.
422. Sevel, D., and Burger, D.: Ocular involvement in cutaneous porphyria. A clinical and histological report. Arch. Ophthal., *85(5)*:580, 1971.

Prolinemia
423. Efron, M. L.: Familial hyperprolinemia. New Eng. J. Med., *272*:1243, 1965.
424. Schafer, I. A., Scriver, C. R., and Efron, M. L.: Familial hyperprolinemia, cerebral dysfunction, and renal anomalies occurring in a family with hereditary nephropathy and deafness. New Eng. J. Med., *267*:51, 1962.

Pseudoxanthoma Elasticum
425. Tanenbaum, H. L., and de Margerie, J.: Sudden bilateral loss of central vision in pseudoxanthoma elasticum. Canad. J. Ophthal., *1*:221, 1966.
426. Tiberio, G., Negroni, L., and Meduri, R.: Histological and histochemical study of the superficial temproal artery in the Groenblad-Strandberg-Touraine syndrome. Ann. Ottal., *94(3)*:228, 1968.

Pupil Syndrome
427. Duke-Elder, S.: Congenital deformities. *In* Duke-Elder, S. (ed.): System of Ophthalmology. Vol. 3, Part 2. St. Louis, The C. V. Mosby Co., 1963, pp. 590, 592, 594, 600, 775, 1024–1025.

Pyridoxine Deficiency
428. Hooft, C., Timmermans, J., Snoeck, J., Antener, I., Oyaert, W., and Van den Hende, C.: Methionine malabsorption in a mentally defective child. Lancet, *II*:20, July, 1964.
429. O'Brien, D.: Pyridoxine dependency in two mentally retarded subjects. Clin. Sci., *24*:179, August 19, 1962.

Refsum's Disease
430. Herndon, J. H., Steinberg, D., and Uhlendorf, B. W.: Refsum's disease: defective oxidation of phytanic acid in tissue cultures derived from homozygotes and heterozygotes. New Eng. J. Med., *281*:1034, November 6, 1969.
431. Refsum, S.: Heredoataxie hemeralopica polyneuritiformis—et tidligere ikke beskrevet familiaert syndrom? En forelobig meddelelse. Nord. Med., *28*:2682, 1945.
432. Steinberg, D.: Refsum's disease—a recently characterized lipidosis involving the nervous system. Ann. Intern. Med., *66*:365, 1967.
433. Toussaint, D., and Danis, P.: An ocular pathologic study of Refsum's syndrome. Amer. J. Ophthal., *72(2)*:342, August, 1971.
434. Try, K.: Heredopathia atactica polyneuritiformis (Refsum's disease). The diagnostic value of phytanic acid determination in serum lipids. Europ. Neurol. (Basel), *2(5)*:296, 1969.

Rendu-Osler Disease
435. Duke-Elder, S.: Diseases of the outer eye. *In* Duke-Elder, S. (ed.): System of Ophthalmology. Vol. 8, Part 1. St. Louis, The C. V. Mosby Co., 1965, p. 30.

Retinal Degeneration Syndromes
435a. Carr, R. E.: The night-blinding disorders. Int. Ophthal. Clin., *9*:971, 1969.
436. Duke-Elder, S.: Congenital deformities. *In* Duke-Elder, S. (ed.): System of Ophthalmology. Vol. 3, Part 2. St. Louis, The C. V. Mosby Co., 1963, pp. 619–623, 640–643.
437. Duke-Elder, S., and Dobree, J.: Diseases of the retina. *In* Duke-Elder, S. (ed.): System of Ophthalmology. Vol. 10. St. Louis, The C. V. Mosby Co., 1967, pp. 622–645.
438. Duke-Elder, S., and Perkins, E.: Diseases of the uveal tract. *In* Duke-Elder, S. (ed.): System of Ophthalmology. Vol. 9. St. Louis, The C. V. Mosby Co., 1966, pp. 699–703, 711, 715–719.
439. Leffertstra, L.: Desinsertions at the Ora Serrata. Ophthalmologica, *119*:1, 1950.
440. Walsh, F. B., and Hoyt, W. (eds.): Clinical Neuro-Ophthalmology. Vol. 1. 3rd ed. Baltimore, Williams and Wilkins Co., 1969, p. 892.

Retinoblastoma
441. Duke-Elder, S., and Dobree, J.: Diseases of the retina. *In* Duke-Elder, S. (ed.): System of Ophthalmology. Vol. 10. St. Louis, The C. V. Mosby Co., 1967, pp. 672–727.

Rieger's Syndrome
442. Zauberman, H., and Sira, I. B.: Glaucoma and Rieger's syndrome. Acta Ophthal., *48(1)*:119, 1970.
443. Pearce, W. G., and Kerr, C. B.: Inherited variation in Rieger's malformation. Brit. J. Ophthal., *49*:530, 1965.
444. Henkind, P., and Friedman, A. H.: Iridogoniodysgenesis with cataract. Amer. J. Ophthal., *72*:949, 1971.
445. Duke-Elder, S.: Congenital deformities. *In* Duke-Elder, S. (ed.): System of Ophthalmology. Vol. 3, part 2. St. Louis, The C. V. Mosby Co., 1963, pp. 543–547.

Riley-Day Syndrome
446. Boruchoff, S. A., and Dohlman, C. H.: The Riley-Day syndrome. Ocular manifestations in a 35 year old patient. Amer. J. Ophthal., *63(3)*:523, 1967.

447. Keith, C. G.: Riley-Day syndrome (congenital familial dysautonomia). Brit. J. Ophthal. 49(12):667, 1965.
448. Riley, C. M., Day, R. L., Greeley, D. M., and Langford, W. S.: Central autonomic dysfunction with defective lacrimation: report of five cases. Pediatrics, 3:468, 1949.

Rod and/or Cone Dysfunction Syndromes

449. Goodman, G., Ripps, H., and Siegel, I. M.: Cone dysfunction syndromes. Arch. Ophthal., 70:214, 1963.

Rothmund's Syndrome

450. Carr, R. E., Morton, N. E., and Siegel, I. M.: Achromatopsia in Pingelap Islanders. Study of a genetic isolate. Amer. J. Ophthal., 72(4):746, October, 1971.

Sea-Blue Histiocyte

450a. Thannhauser, S. J.: Werner's syndrome and Rothmund's syndrome. Ann. Intern. Med., 23:559, 1945.
451. Ardeman, S.: Syndrome of the sea-blue histiocyte. Lancet, 1:797, April, 1972.
452. Cogan, D. G., and Federman, D. D.: Retinal involvement with reticuloendotheliosis of unclassified type. Arch. Ophthal., 71:489, April, 1964.
453. Silverstein, M. N., Ellefson, R. D., and Ahern, E. J.: The syndrome of the sea-blue histiocyte. New Eng. J. Med., 282:1, January, 1970.

Skeletal Defects

454. Cordier, J., Tridon, P., Thiriet, M., et al.: Syndrome oculovertebral de Weyers. Rev. Otoneuroophtal., 40(4):204, 1968.
455. Fraser, G. R., et al.: Dysplasia spondyloepiphysaria congenita and related generalized skeletal dysplasias among children with severe visual handicaps. Arch. Dis. Child., 44:490, 1969.

Skull Syndromes

456. Duke-Elder, S.: Congenital deformities. In Duke-Elder, S. (ed.): System of Ophthalmology. Vol. 3, part 2. St. Louis, The C. V. Mosby Co., 1963, pp. 1060–1061.

Smith-Lemli-Opitz Syndrome

457. Cotlier, E., and Rice, P.: Cataracts in the Smith-Lemli-Opitz syndrome. Amer. J. Ophthal., 72(5):955, November, 1971.

Sturge-Weber Syndrome

458. Alexander, G. L., and Norman, R. M.: The Sturge-Weber syndrome. Bristol, John Wright and Sons, 1960.
459. Flage, T., and Harven, I.: Corneal indentation pulse in Sturge-Weber syndrome. Acta Ophthal., 48:1166, 1970.

Sulfite Oxidase Deficiency

460. Mudd, S. H., Irreverre, F., and Laster, L.: Sulfite oxidase deficiency in man: Demonstration of the enzymatic defect. Science, 156(3782):1599, June 23, 1967.

Tangier Disease

461. Clifton-Bligh, P., Nestel, P. J., and Whyte, H. M.: Tangier disease: Report of a case and studies of lipid metabolism. New Eng. J. Med., 286(11):567, March, 1972.
462. Fredrickson, D. S., Altrocchi, P. H., Avioli, L. V., Goodman, D. S., and Goodman, H. C.: Tangier disease. Ann. Intern. Med., 55:1016, 1961.

463. Hoffman, H. N. II, and Fredrickson, D. S.: Tangier disease (familial high density lipoprotein deficiency). Clinical and genetic features in two adults. Amer. J. Med., 39:582, October, 1965.

Treacher Collins Syndrome

464. Harrons, S. H.: Treacher Collins syndrome. Brit. J. Plas. Surg., 3:282, 1951.

Tryptophanuria

465. Tada, K., Ito, H., Wada, Y., and Arakawa, T.: Congenital tryptophanuria with dwarfism. Tohoku J. Exp. Med., 80:118, 1963.

Turner's Syndrome

466. Walsh, Frank, and Hoyt, W. (eds.): Clinical Neuro-Ophthalmology. Vol. 1. Baltimore, Williams and Wilkins Co., 1969, pp. 764–767, 919–922.

Tyrosinemia

467. Vernon, M.: Usher's syndrome—deafness and progressive blindness. Clinical cases, prevention, theory and literature survey. J. Chron. Dis., 22(3):133, 1969.

Ullrich's Syndrome

468. Duke-Elder, S.: Congenital deformities. In Duke-Elder, S. (ed.): System of Ophthalmology. Vol. 3, Part 2. St. Louis, The C. V. Mosby Co., 1963, p. 1115.

Usher's Syndrome

469. DeHaas, E. B., et al: Usher's syndrome. With special reference to heterozygous manifestations. Docum. Ophthal., 28(1):166, 1970.

Vitamin Deficiency Diseases

470. Duke-Elder, S., and Leigh, A.: Diseases of the outer eye. In Duke-Elder, S. (ed.): System of Ophthalmology. Vol. 8, Part 2. St. Louis, The C. V. Mosby Co., 1965, pp. 1113, 1115–1130.
471. Duke-Elder, S., and Scott, G.: Neuroophthalmology. In Duke-Elder, S. (ed.): System of Ophthalmology. Vol. 12. St. Louis, The C. V. Mosby Co., 1971, p. 763.
472. Hood, J., Burns, C. A., and Hodges, R. E.: Sjögren's syndrome in scurvy. New Eng. J. Med., 282:1120, May 14, 1970.
473. McLaren, D. S.: Nutritional aspects of the eye. In Graymore, C. N.: Biochemistry of the Eye. London, Academic Press, 1970, pp. 519–564.

Vitreoretinopathy

474. Criswick, V. G., and Schepens, C. L.: Familial exudative vitreoretinopathy. Amer. J. Ophthal., 68(4):578, 1969.
475. Duke-Elder, S.: Congenital deformities. In Duke-Elder, S. (ed.): System of Ophthalmology. Vol. 3, Part 2. St. Louis, The C. V. Mosby Co., 1963, p. 643.
476. Duke-Elder, S., and Dobree, J.: Diseases of the retina. In Duke-Elder, S. (ed.): System of Ophthalmology. Vol. 10. St. Louis, The C. V. Mosby Co., 1967, pp. 543, 559, 658.
477. Ricci, A.: Les dysplasies hyaloideo rétiniennes congénitales et leur diagnostic différentiel. J. Genet. Hum., 17:1 (Suppl.), 1969.
478. van Balen, A. T. M., and Falger, E.L.F.: Hereditary hyaloideoretinal degeneration and palatoschisis. Arch. Ophthal., 83:152, February, 1970.

Von Hippel-Lindau Disease

479. Welch, R. B.: Von Hippel-Lindau disease: The recognition and treatment of early angioma-

tosis retinae and the use of cryosurgery as an adjunct to therapy. Trans. Amer. Ophthal. Soc., *68*:367, 1971.

Waardenburg's Syndrome

480. Waardenburg, P.: Embryonic fixation syndrome. Amer. J. Hum. Genet., *3*:195, 1951.

Werner's Syndrome

481. Schumacher, K., Rodermund, O. E., and Doepfmer, R.: Das Werner-Syndrom. Arch. Klin. Med., *216(2)*:116, 1969.

Wilson's Disease

482. Cairns, J. E., Williams, H. P., and Walshe, J. M.: "Sunflower cataract" in Wilson's disease. Brit. Med. J., *3*:95, 1969.

483. DuBois, R. S., et al.: Orthotopic liver transplantation for Wilson's disease. Lancet, *1*:505, March, 1971.

484. Mitchell, A. M., and Heller, G. L.: Changes in Kayser-Fleischer ring during treatment of hepatolenticular degeneration. Arch. Ophthal., *80(5)*:622, 1968.

485. Siemerling, E., and Oloff, H.: Pseudosclerosis, corneal ring and bilateral cataract after copper injury. J. Klin. Wsch., *1*:1087, 1922.

486. Sternlieb, I., and Scheinberg, I. H.: Penacillamine therapy for hepatolenticular degeneration. JAMA, *189*:748, September 7, 1964.

487. Sternlieb, I., and Scheinberg, I. H.: Prevention of Wilson's disease in asymptomatic patients. New Eng. J. Med., *278*:352, February, 1968.

488. Sussman, W., and Scheinberg, I. H.: Disappearance of Kayser-Fleischer rings. Effects of penicillamine. Arch. Ophthal, *82*:738, December, 1969.

489. Warnock, C. G.: Presymptomatic Wilson's disease. Lancet, *II(7523)*:990, November, 1967.

Wolman's Disease

490. Wolman, M., Stark, V. V., Gatt, S., and Frenkel, M.: Primary familial xanthomatosis with involvement and calcification of the adrenals. Pediatrics, *28*:742, 1961.

Xeroderma Pigmentosum

491. Duke-Elder, S.: Diseases of the outer eye. *In* Duke-Elder, S. (ed.): System of Ophthalmology. Vol. 8, Part 1. St. Louis, The C. V. Mosby Co., 1965, p. 551.

CHAPTER 20

OCULAR CHANGES IN PEDIATRIC SYSTEMIC DISORDERS

A. OCULAR MANIFESTATIONS IN ENDOCRINE DISORDERS

George L. Spaeth, M.D.

A hormone is a substance released into the bloodstream from specialized cells and carried to other cells which are responsive to it. This classic definition first proposed by Starling is still valid. It does not imply complete specificity of action, for even within single cells individual hormones usually have more than one fundamental action. Furthermore, hormones may act quite differently in different cells or tissues or organisms.

The eye is not the major site of receptors for any hormone yet isolated. It does not closely resemble an organ such as the adrenal gland, which is responsive to, and in a sense even controlled by, the hormone adrenal corticotropin. Yet many of the various hormones do affect the eye, either directly (as an expression of one or more

nonspecific actions) or indirectly (secondary to a biochemical alteration evoked by the hormone in a receptor organ elsewhere) (Radnot, 1961). A list of hormones (with standard abbreviations) may be found in Table 20–1.

Disease may occur when hormones are present in abnormally large or small amounts. Disease may also result when, for any of a variety of reasons, a hormone acts abnormally. Because hormones are components of an intricately integrated system of interreactions, their activity depends on the nature and concentration of other substances such as enzymes, coenzymes, and metal ions. Consequently, the biological effectiveness of a hormone is not a function simply of its concentration in the bloodstream. An organism may suffer from an

622

TABLE 20–1

Hormone	Abbreviation	Major Source
Follicle-stimulating hormone	FSH	Anterior pituitary
Luteinizing hormone	LH	Anterior pituitary
Prolactin	LTH	Anterior pituitary
Growth hormone	GH	Anterior pituitary
Thyrotropin	TSH	Anterior pituitary
Corticotropin	ACTH	Anterior pituitary
Exophthalmos-producing substance	EPS	Anterior pituitary
Melanocyte-stimulating hormone	MSH	Intermediate lobe of pituitary
Vasopressin	GRF	Posterior pituitary or hypothalamus
Oxytocin	GRF	Posterior pituitary or hypothalamus
Melatonin	GRF	Posterior pituitary or hypothalamus
Growth hormone-releasing factor	GRF	Posterior pituitary or hypothalamus
Long-acting thyroid-stimulating hormone	LATS	? Hypothalamus
Corticotropin-releasing factor	CRF	Hypothalamus
Thyrotropin-releasing factor	TRF	Hypothalamus
Luteinizing hormone-releasing factor	LRF	Hypothalamus
Corticotropin-releasing factor	CRF	Posterior pituitary
Calcitonin	TCT	Thyroid
Thyroxin	T-4	Thyroid
Triiodothyronine	T-3	Thyroid
Parathyroid hormone	PTH	Parathyroid gland
Adrenal androgen		Adrenal cortex
Glucocorticoids		Adrenal cortex
Mineralocorticoids		Adrenal cortex
Norepinephrine		Adrenal medulla
Epinephrine		Adrenal medulla
Testosterone		Testes
Estrogen		Ovary
Progesterone		Corpus luteum
Relaxin		Corpus luteum
Insulin		Beta cells of pancreas
Glucagon		Alpha cells of pancreas
Erythropoietin		Kidney
Renin		Kidney
Secretin		Gut
Cholecystokinin		Gut
Gastrin		Stomach
Angiotensin		Liver
Acetylcholine		Autonomic nervous system

actual biological insufficiency even though the level of hormone circulating in the blood is excessively high.

BASIC PRINCIPLES OF ENDOCRINOLOGY

Four general theories of hormone action have been proposed: (1) alteration of membranes, (2) effect on enzymes, (3) action on genes, and (4) release of ions or other small molecules (Rasmussen, 1968). Involved in the basic metabolic life of the cell and consequently of the organism, hormones are remarkably potent; physiologic effects may be evoked by concentrations between 10^{-7} and 10^{-12} M. There-

fore, we should anticipate that non-physiologic hormonal concentrations, whether due to endocrinologic abnormality or medical manipulation, should cause widespread alterations in the body, including the eye.

In clinical practice hormones are used in three major ways: they may be utilized as diagnostic tools to clarify a metabolic defect; they may be used in physiologic amounts (usually small) to replace specific deficiencies; or they may be given as pharmacologic agents (usually in large doses) to produce effects quite different from the normal role of the hormone. Most often hormones are utilized in this third manner. And it is in this capacity that they may produce "side-effects" which may be more serious than the abnormality they were intended to correct. In ophthalmology it is especially important to recall the undesirable "side-effects" of hormones when they are used in a pharmacologic manner, to treat either ocular disease or more generalized disorders elsewhere in the body.

This chapter will deal with each endocrine organ in turn; the ocular manifestations of endocrine disease will be discussed. In some instances, such as disorders of the pituitary gland, ophthalmic disease is not due to specific hormonal abnormality, but rather to something else, such as pressure on the optic nerve.

However, before proceeding further, it is important to review the basic organization of the endocrine system. The stability of the body, termed "milieu organique intérieur" by Claude Bernard, is maintained by the autonomic and the endocrine systems. These are highly interdependent; separation between them is quite artificial. For example, an autonomic neural stimulus (preganglionic fiber to the adrenal medulla) causes the release of a neurohumor (acetylcholine) which causes the release of a hormone (epinephrine) which is then widely circulated throughout the body,

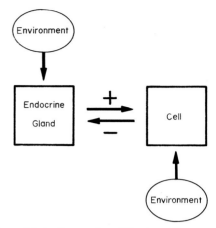

Figure 20–2 External modification of hormone action. Environmental factors influence the secretion of hormone and the manner in which the hormone acts at a cellular level. Thus, measurement of the level of hormone stimulator (such as TSH) or even of circulating hormone itself is not always an accurate indication of actual biological activity.

producing many diverse effects. By and large, however, the autonomic system is concerned with rapid, total adjustments to environmental change, whereas the endocrine system concerns itself with adjustments that are more gradual. Essential to both systems is the concept of "feedback control." In most cases this is a "negative" type of system, as illustrated in Figure 20–1. "A" stimulates "B"; "B" inhibits "A." When "A" increases its stimulation of "B," usually by increasing its concentration, "B" responds by inhibiting the activity of "A" until once again a balance of power is reached. Positive feedback systems also occur in the body but are less common; here, increased concentration of "A" leads to increased production of "B" which itself stimulates "A" to increase its concentration even further, and so on.

In organisms many other factors impinge on the system. Certain stimuli cause the endocrine gland to increase or decrease its production of hormone. Others may affect the responsive cell itself (Fig. 20–2). Perhaps the most interesting example is that of the hypothalamus-hypophysis-adrenal gland cell system diagramed in Figure 20–3. Feedback systems, usually negative, exist between the endocrine gland and the hypothalamus and hypophysis. Furthermore, external stimuli modify the system at every step; for example, central nervous system activity con-

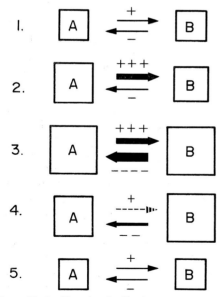

Figure 20–1 Negative feedback regulation of hormonal secretion. Gland "A" secretes a hormone that stimulates organ "B," which responds by elaboration of a hormone that inhibits secretion by A. Increase in amount of hormone elaborated by A is followed by increase in B's activity and a return to the previous equilibrium of step #1 (see text).

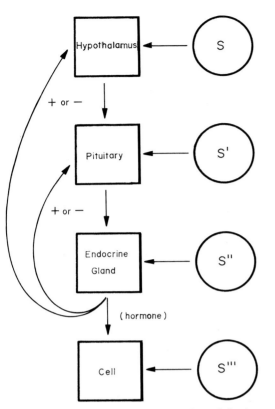

Figure 20–3 Schematic representation of the hypothalamic-hypophyseal-adrenal system. Different environmental stimuli (indicated as S, S', S", and S''') modify the system at every step. For example, central nervous system activity affects the hypothalamus, other hormones alter the functional state of the pituitary gland, and dietary components influence the secretion of hormones by the endocrine gland.

tinually alters the functional state of the hypothalamus.

Endocrinologic abnormalities can be considered primary or secondary. For example, nodules of the thyroid can apparently become autonomous; free from the feedback control of the pituitary, they secrete excessive amounts of thyroid hormone, producing a primary thyrotoxicosis. Such disease is not associated with the elevated levels of thyroid-stimulating hormone that are characteristic of secondary forms of thyrotoxicosis in which the prime offender is the hypophysis.

HYPOTHALAMUS

The hypothalamus is of supreme importance, because it serves as the integrative center for the autonomic and the endocrine systems; it is therefore appropriate to

consider it first even though there is little evidence of specific ocular disease related to hypothalamic malfunction. Regulation of intraocular pressure, however, may be effected by hypothalamic activity. Von Sallmann (1959), following work by others, found that stimulation of the dorsal hypothalamus in cats evoked an elevation of intraocular pressure independent of change in blood pressure or other measured parameters. Von Weinstein believes that dysfunction of the hypothalamus is the initial phase of glaucomatous disease (1963). Brand's finding that intraocular pressure is frequently low in diseases of the central nervous system is also intriguing, but secondary effects such as hypotonicity of the extraocular muscles could explain this (Brand, 1967).

The role of the adrenal gland must also be remembered. Although reports are not entirely consistent, it does appear that adrenalectomized animals show low intraocular pressure, perhaps owing to decreased production of aqueous. Such animals manifest little rise of intraocular pressure in response to water loading (Linnér and Wistrand, 1963). In contrast, intraocular pressure has been reported to be elevated in patients with adrenal overactivity (Bayer and Neuner, 1967). Others have noted changes in intraocular pressure in association with abnormality in the area of the hypothalamus (Follman et al., 1967), though not all reports are in agreement (Chiriceanu et al., 1968). Several studies suggest a neurohumoral effect on intraocular pressure, but the data are sparse and the findings require further documentation (Henkind et al., to be published; Podos et al., 1971; Spaeth and Vacharat, 1972; Thomas, 1968). Conceivably such effects could be involved in the type of glaucoma most commonly found in adults, chronic open angle glaucoma. This illness is rare in children, however, and it seems unlikely that hormones play a role in the pathogenesis of infantile glaucoma, which can be effectively relieved in many cases by the minor alteration in the anatomy of the anterior chamber angle produced by goniotomy.

PITUITARY GLAND

The hypophysis, or pituitary gland, serves with the hypothalamus as the integrator of neuroendocrine function. Ocular manifestations of disease of the pituitary are thus diverse. Changes elsewhere in the body, for example, the skin or the breasts, are usually, but not invariably, manifestations of abnormal activity in one or more of the endocrine glands regulated by the hypophysis and are not a function of the pituitary itself. Visual symptoms, in contrast, are often the direct result of compression by the pituitary of the optic tract, optic chiasm, or optic nerves.

Pituitary tumors constitute about 30 per cent of all intracranial new growths (Jackson, 1965). Chromophobe adenomas account for the great majority of these (about 85 per cent) and have been occasionally noted in children (Henderson, 1939). They are more common in individuals with parathyroid or islet cell adenomas. Essentially nonsecretory in nature, they produce disease by pressing on surrounding structures.

Chromophobe Adenoma

Productive of a number of ophthalmic abnormalities, the classic visual sign of the chromophobe adenoma is bitemporal visual field loss (Table 20–2) (Chamlin et al., 1955). Other types of field defect occur depending on the location of the chiasm (in the great majority of cases the chiasm lies directly over or slightly posterior to the

TABLE 20–2 OCULAR SIGNS OF CHROMOPHOBE ADENOMAS OF THE PITUITARY GLAND

Finding	Incidence (%)
Visual field defects	
Bitemporal hemianopsia	80
Blindness (one eye) and temporal loss (other eye)	10
Homonymous hemianopsia	6
Inferior altitudinal loss (one eye) and temporal loss (other eye)	2
Central scotoma	2
Decreased visual acuity (unilateral or bilateral)	80
Pallor of the optic discs	60
Atrophy of the optic discs	20
Extraocular muscle palsies	5
Gross pupillary changes	1
Fifth nerve involvement	1
Papilledema	1
Proptosis	Rare
Venous engorgement of the eye	Rare

covering of the fossa in which the hypophysis rests), the size of the tumor, the direction in which the tumor grows (for example, acidophil adenomas tend to grow anteriorly owing to the concentration of acidophils in the anterior portion of the pituitary), and the nature of the surrounding structures (calcified internal carotids and the like).

No one has better described the pathophysiology of visual field loss caused by pituitary tumors than George DeSchweinitz in his Bowman Lecture in 1923. Though temporal loss must always be specifically searched for, its absence must not be considered indicative of normalcy of the pituitary area, nor should the presence of scotomatous defects eliminate suspicion of the sellar area. Unfortunately, patients with unilateral central visual loss and optic atrophy are still not always considered as potential harborers of pituitary tumors, and preventable visual loss is incorrectly attributed to "retrobulbar neuritis" (Asbury, 1965; Schlezinger and Thompson, 1967). Visual field examination must be carefully done with small enough test objects to uncover small defects; in most instances these will be found in the superior temporal quadrant. Because of the wide range of normal values found with color fields and the difficulty of performing perimetry with colored test objects, it is best to rely predominantly on white test objects. Color fields serve mainly as a check, as pointed out by DeSchweinitz. The most important determinant of accurate visual field testing is not the type of instrument employed, nor even the method used, but the person doing the testing. Visual acuity is reduced in almost all cases with pituitary tumors, usually bilaterally. This reduction need not be great; it is characteristically more advanced in one eye (Table 20–2).

Benedict (1920) described in meticulous detail the characteristic appearance of the optic disc. He believed that a "peculiar waxy pallor of the nerve without shrinkage is seen so often that it has become practically a diagnostic feature." This pallor is not due to atrophy, except in far advanced cases, and there is little loss of tissue. Unlike the optic atrophy of "toxic neuritis," in which vision fails and shrinkage of the nerve and pallor follow together, in chiasmal disease the pallor precedes loss of visual acuity, and loss of nerve substance occurs later. This is in contrast to open angle glaucoma, in which the degree of cupping should always exceed the amount of pallor. Mooney (1952) stated that pallor of the optic nerve head was more marked in cases having compression anterior to the chiasm.

Involvement of other cranial nerves by chiasmal tumors is uncommon but does occur (Table 20–2).

Diagnosis of chromophobe adenoma necessitates intelligent interpretation and integration of the results of visual field examination, ophthalmoscopy, endocrinologic survey, and radiologic investigation. Treatment is necessary when there is definite evidence of progressive loss of visual function. Some centers now favor radiologic rather than surgical attempts to extirpate the gland.

Basophil Adenoma

Basophil adenomas are rare, particularly in children. The presence of adrenocorticism, especially when associated with intense skin pigmentation, should bring to mind the possibility that primary disease may be in the hypothalamus, with excess elaboration of corticotropin-releasing factor, causing excessive production of ACTH and consequent adrenal overactivity. Adrenalectomy in these cases may make matters worse by removing the inhibiting effect of adrenal corticoids on the hypothalamus with consequent sudden increase in size of the basophil adenoma. These tumors are associated with extraocular muscle palsies in almost one fourth of the cases; also, pituitary apoplexy is not uncommon in Cushing's syndrome (Rovit and Duane, 1968).

Acromegaly

Acidophilic cells of the hypophysis produce growth hormone. When hypersecretion of growth hormone occurs after puberty, the characteristic changes of acromegaly follow. Less frequently, excess growth hormone secretion occurs in children, causing true gigantism. The ocular manifestations of both are similar. Visual field defects are less common than with chromophobe adenomas, as would be expected in view of the small size of most acidophilic tumors. Bitemporal hemianop-

sia is present in only about half of affected individuals (Spaeth, in prep.). On the other hand, glaucoma may be more frequent than in the general population (Howard and English, 1965). However, section of the hypophyseal stalks (producing severe panhypopituitarism) has been noted to be without effect on the intraocular pressure of eyes with diabetic retinopathy (Lee and Field, 1966), suggesting that pituitary hormones probably do not play a primary role in the maintenance of intraocular pressure. Angioid streaks have been reported by Howard (1963) in one case. In addition, the ocular manifestations of diabetes mellitus may be present. Treatment is not highly satisfactory; it may be advisable to try irradiation before resorting to surgical removal of the hypophysis, but not all concur with this (Pearson et al., 1970). Others have noted clinical improvement following treatment with chlorpromazine; its mechanism of action may be suppression of growth hormone via the hypothalamus (Kolodny et al., 1971).

Craniopharyngioma

The most important differentiation in youngsters must be the distinction between craniopharyngiomas and the other causes of an enlarged sella turcica (Nelson et al., 1969). Craniopharyngiomas, arising from cells related to Rathke's pouch, are not secreting tumors. They are usually suprasellar rather than intrasellar and consequently produce a different pattern of visual field defects than do pituitary adenomas. Craniopharyngiomas cause loss of the *inferior* temporal rather than the superior temporal field in their early stages. This loss progresses to a complete temporal loss and is associated with optic atrophy in most cases. Since the tumors are slow-growing, they may be present for years without causing progressive loss of visual function. The presence of calcification within the tumor in 85 per cent of the cases aids the radiologist in his diagnosis. Air studies, however, are essential for proper management of cases. Because the tumors usually have solid extensions into the hypothalamic area, complete excision is rarely possible. Compression of the hypothalamus causes diabetes insipidus, retarded sexual development, infantilism, obesity, and other metabolic disturbances.

TABLE 20–3 OCULAR SIGNS IN FRÖHLICH'S SYNDROME

Decreased visual acuity
Headaches
Impaired vision in the dark (poor dark adaptation)
Optic atrophy or papilledema
Chiasmal type visual field defects

Pressure on the hypophysis results in growth and sexual retardation. Obstruction of the third ventricle may cause signs of increased intracranial pressure.

HYPOPITUITARISM

Hypopituitarism may be associated with ocular signs. Decreased hypophyseal function follows compression of the hypothalamic area by expanding masses such as chromophobe adenomas, craniopharyngiomas, and intracranial aneurysms. In these cases the ocular signs are in line with those already discussed (Table 20–3).

Fröhlich's Syndrome

Fröhlich's syndrome may also be noted in these cases. Fröhlich's original patient had a cyst in the hypothalamic area, with consequent headaches, vomiting, loss of vision, destruction of the dorsum sellae, obesity, and sexual retardation (Fröhlich, 1901). Papilledema is present in those cases with increased intracranial pressure.

Hypopituitarism secondary to encephalitis may produce a similar picture except for the lack of signs indicating a pituitary-area expanding mass. Landau and Bromberg (1955) have noted that such individuals may have impaired dark-adaptation with consequent poor night vision.

Laurence-Moon-Bardet-Biedl Syndrome

Differential diagnosis in these cases must include obesity of adolescence (Warkany and Di George, 1957) and the Laurence-Moon-Bardet-Biedl syndrome (Table 20–4). The full expression of the Laurence-Moon-Bardet-Biedl syndrome involves obesity of the Fröhlich type, polydactyly, mental deficiency, hypogenitalism, and tapetoretinal degeneration (Bardet, 1920; Biedl, 1922; Laurence and Moon, 1866). Usually having an autosomal recessive pattern of inheritance, the abnormality can affect males or females of all races. Although the exact pathogenesis is not known (Ornsteen, 1932), a chromosomal abnormality of the XXY type has been found in individuals with mental retardation, retinitis pigmentosa, sexual retardation, and skeletal defects (not polydactyly). A deficiency of germ cells in the majority of the seminiferous tubules was thought to be a primary effect of the XXY sex chromosome complement. Perhaps the most conspicuous ocular manifestation in these patients is the night blindness that is almost invariably present (Ehrenfeld et al.,

TABLE 20–4 DIFFERENTIAL DIAGNOSIS OF FRÖHLICH'S SYNDROME, OBESITY OF ADOLESCENCE, AND LAURENCE-MOON-BARDET-BIEDL SYNDROME

	Fröhlich's Syndrome	Obesity of Adolescence	Laurence-Moon-Bardet-Biedl Syndrome
Onset of symptoms	Any age	About 8 years	Birth
Obesity	Moderate	Moderate to excessive	Marked
Genital development	Delayed	Boys: Slow	Delayed
		Girls: Normal	
Development of secondary sex characteristics	Delayed	Boys: Slow	Delayed
		Girls: Normal	
Skin	Dry, scaly	Moist, perspiration increased	Moist
Skeleton	Slender	Heavy	Heavy, polydactylism
Headaches, vomiting	Present	Absent	Absent
Ocular fundi	Papilledema or optic atrophy	Normal	Retinitis pigmentosa, optic atrophy
Mentality	Usually normal	Usually normal	Retarded
Family history	Usually negative	Often familial	Often familial

Modified from Warkany, J., and DiGeorge, A. M.: *In* Nelson et al.: Textbook of Pediatrics. 6th ed. Philadelphia, W. B. Saunders Co., 1957.

TABLE 20–5 OCULAR SIGNS IN THE LAURENCE-MOON-BARDET-BIEDL SYNDROME

Finding	Incidence
Night blindness	Always
Abnormal electroretinogram	Almost always
Diffuse, widely scattered pigmentation of the fundus	Usual
Nystagmus	Frequent
Yellow, waxy optic atropy	Frequent
Narrowed retinal vessels	Frequent
Bone-corpuscular pigmentary changes	Unusual
Cataract	Unusual
Strabismus	Unusual
Keratoconus	Unusual
Internal ophthalmoplegia	Unusual

1970). Also prominent is nystagmus, probably secondary to abnormality of the macula. The optic discs may appear quite normal but are often of the yellow, waxy type seen in retinitis pigmentosa. When optic atrophy is marked there is also often severe generalized chorioretinal atrophy similar to that seen in choroideremia (Walsh, 1957). The retinal vessels are usually narrowed. Pigmentary changes of the bone-corpuscular type are not common but may be present, especially later in life; more frequently, there is scattered, pepper-and-salt type pigmentation widely distributed over the fundus; in some cases this is concentrated in the macular area. Marked pigmentary changes are present in only about 15 per cent of affected individuals. The electroretinogram almost always shows an extinguished or diminished response, even in cases in which no definite retinal abnormalities are seen (Mazzantini and Ioli Spada, 1964). Other abnormalities include cataracts, refractile white spots on the retina, strabismus, keratoconus, and internal ophthalmoplegia (Table 20–5).

Posterior Pituitary Abnormality

The hypothalamus, the hypothalamic-neurohypophyseal tracts, and the neurohypophysis (posterior pituitary) form a secretory unit productive of at least two hormones, oxytocin and vasopressin. Oxytocin is involved with uterine contraction and milk let-down, whereas the major effect of vasopressin is antidiuresis. Abnormality of these hormones is not known to cause ocular disease. However, diabetes insipidus, the consequence of insufficient activity of vasopressin, is found in conditions which themselves have ocular manifestations. Diabetes insipidus may be associated with acute or chronic infections, tumors in the area of the hypothalamus, and head trauma. It is an integral part of the Hand-Schüller-Christian syndrome, which has exophthalmos and small xanthomatous skin lesions on the lids as additional ocular findings.

PINEAL GLAND

The pineal gland is involved in circadian rhythms, especially those mediated by light, but its complete function is not understood. Nor is a totally satisfactory explanation for the sexual precocity that affects boys with pinealomas apparent. The ocular manifestations of tumors of the pineal gland are important and include abnormalities of the pupil (similar to those described by Argyll Robertson), vertical conjugate palsy, and third and fourth cranial nerve palsies. This syndrome is highly characteristic of space-taking lesions in the region of the midbrain or pineal gland. Papilledema occurs early in the development of tumors in this area.

THYROID GLAND

Hypothyroidism

Hypothyroidism is the most common endocrine disorder in children. (Table 20–6) The majority of such cases are congenital, usually caused by agenesis or dysgenesis of the gland or by defective production of hormone (as seen in the offspring of women receiving antithyroid medica-

TABLE 20–6 CLINICAL MANIFESTATIONS OF HYPOTHYROIDISM

Physical and mental lethargy
Decreased peripheral circulation
Slow pulse
Diminished muscle tone
Retarded physical and mental growth
Retarded bone development (epiphyseal dysgenesis)
Subcutaneous edema
Coarse thick skin
Coarse dry hair

TABLE 20–7   OCULAR MANIFESTATIONS OF HYPOTHYROIDISM

Edema of the margin of the upper lid
Nystagmus
Exophthalmos
Myotonia of the orbicularis oculi
Uveal effusion

tion while pregnant), but some are acquired after birth (Carswell, 1970; DiGeorge, 1969). Ocular signs are not an important part of childhood (or adult) hypothyroidism (Table 20–7). Edema of the pretarsal portion of the upper lid has recently been reported as a reliable sign of hypothyroidism, but this requires confirmation (Katz, 1970). Myotonia of the orbicularis oculi has been reported (Sisson et al., 1962), as has uveal effusion (Richardson and Walsh, 1969). Perhaps the most important sign in children is nystagmus (Schulman and Crawford, 1969). In this regard, youngsters with nystagmus should have appropriate laboratory studies so that necessary therapy can be promptly instituted if hypothyroidism is actually present. Hypercholesterolemia is an early sign of myxedema (Fowler et al., 1970). However, xanthelasmas, which are sometimes a sign of hypercholesterolemia, are seen in both hypo- and hyperthyroidism (Martinez-Rovira, 1968). Cutaneous manifestations consist of thickened, dry, scaly skin with little exocrine secretion. Scalp hair is coarse, brittle, and scanty.

Hyperthyroidism

Hyperthyroidism is not common in children (Hoyles et al., 1959); the younger the age, the less likely it is to occur. When present, however, it is quite similar to the adult type of disease; symptoms tend to be less prominent in young people, and progressive or malignant exophthalmos is extremely uncommon (Wilkins, 1965).

Systemic symptoms of hyperthyroidism include tremor, tachycardia, large pulse pressure, flushing of the cheeks, cardiac enlargement, accelerated growth and development, loss of weight, vomiting or diarrhea, and enlargement of the thyroid gland. The presence of a goiter is often the first observed symptom in children.

The ocular symptoms and signs of hyperthyroidism are prominent and impor-

tant (Table 20–8) (Day and Carroll, 1962; Haddad, 1967; Hedges and Scheie, 1955; Henderson, 1969; Hugonnier, 1965). Decreased blinking is not usually observed in children, but an appearance of staring is characteristic. Ophthalmic manifestations are of such significance that a classification of Graves' disease in terms of the severity of ocular findings has been suggested by the American Thyroid Association (Table 20–9) (Werner, 1969).

In the practice of ophthalmology "endocrine exophthalmos" is a frequent and often baffling problem. As knowledge of the entity has accumulated it has become apparent that hyperthyroidism is by no means an invariable accompaniment of exophthalmos (Michaelson and Young, 1970). The exophthalmos may be present when the patient is in the hypothyroid, hyperthyroid, or euthyroid state. Furthermore, it is frequently difficult to determine with certainty into which of these categories an individual patient falls, for there is not always agreement between the various clinical findings and the diagnostic procedures. Several classifications have been suggested to resolve this dilemma: for example, exophthalmos was termed "thyrotoxic" when present in patients with active clinical hyperthyroidism and was

TABLE 20–8   OCULAR MANIFESTATIONS OF HYPERTHYROIDISM

Symptoms
    Foreign body sensation
    "Soreness" or "fullness"
    Redness
    Fatigue
    Tearing
    Dry eyes
    Double vision
    Photophobia

Signs
    Lid retraction (stare)
    Exophthalmos
    Lid lag
    Lid edema and periorbital swelling
    Limitation of extraocular muscles
    Conjunctival congestion or edema
    Corneal lesion (erosion, ulceration, necrosis)
    Palpable lacrimal gland or extraocular muscle
    Optic atrophy
    Visual field loss (arcuate or central scotomas
                   or peripheral loss)
    Papilledema, papillitis or retrobulbar neuritis
    Elevated intraocular pressure or upward gaze
    Glaucoma (?)

TABLE 20–9 EYE CHANGES IN GRAVES' DISEASE

Stage	Findings
0	No signs or symptoms
1	Only signs (no symptoms)
2	Soft tissue involvement
3	Proptosis
4	Extraocular muscle involvement
5	Corneal involvement
6	Sight loss

Stages 0 to 1 are "noninfiltrative"; Stages 2 to 6 are "infiltrative."

Werner, S. C.: Classification of the eye changes of Graves' disease. J. Clin. Endocr., *29*:982, 1969.

typified by relatively mild exophthalmos, lid lag and widening of the palpebral fissure, absence of congestion, normal vision, and relief following measures designed to decrease the activity of the thyroid gland. On the other hand, "thyrotropic" exophthalmos, thought to be a response to the secretion of TSH, was characterized by more actual proptosis, congestion, occurrence of visual loss, presence *or absence* of the other typical ocular signs of hyperthyroidism, and exacerbation following thyroidectomy. The dividing lines between these conditions are so crooked and so overlapping that the usefulness of such a classification has been challenged. In fact, the precise mechanism for "endocrine exophthalmos" is still not fully comprehended and continues to evoke heated controversy.

It has already been mentioned that some believe that the exophthalmos is due to excess activity of thyrotropin (TSH). Another hypothesis is that it is the result of a hormone similar to TSH, perhaps originating in the anterior pituitary gland and productive of exophthalmos when injected into appropriate experimental animals (Dobyns et al., 1961). Termed exophthalmos-producing substance (EPS), this material has been found in patients with exophthalmos. Other investigators have not been able to confirm these findings and suggest that EPS is not a separate fraction, but rather is TSH itself (Stelzer et al., 1961).

The discovery of a hormone, not of pituitary origin, that increases the activity of the thyroid gland (long-acting thyroid stimulator [LATS]) led to the suggestion that LATS itself was the agent responsible for the exophthalmos. Once again, however, the evidence is not clear-cut (Adams, 1958; Anderson, 1969; Burke, 1969; Depisch et al., 1969; Hall et al., 1970; Hedley et al., 1970; Sellers et al., 1970). The assay for the hormone is complicated and negative results may be falsely negative owing to technical problems. The likelihood, however, is that *not* all cases of "endocrine exophthalmos" are due to excess activity of LATS. There may be a combination of hypophyseal and extrahypophyseal causes (Mertz and Stelzer, 1969). At any rate, at this time there is no clear relation between abnormality of one of the thyroid hormones and the presence of a particular clinical finding.

As the basic physiology related to the thyroid gland becomes better understood, the meaning of the plethora of diagnostic tests will become better appreciated and therapy placed on a more rational footing (Bowden and Clifford, 1969; Hershman and Pittman, 1971; Lawton et al., 1971). Until that time empirical pragmatism is the best rule to direct treatment.

Because of the importance of the ocular manifestations of thyroid disease and the real possibility of irreversible visual loss due to corneal or optic nerve damage, it is important to keep them carefully in mind when considering therapy. Aranow and Day (1965) suggest that when the ocular signs of thyroid disease are active or progressive, the systemic aspects of thyrotoxicosis should be treated only to the extent demanded by the patient's general condition; that is, antithyroid therapy should be minimal. On the other hand, when the eyes do not appear to be threatened, achievement of a euthyroid state by appropriate antithyroid treatment should be vigorous and prompt.

More problematical are those cases in which exophthalmos is progressing in the absence of apparent overactivity of the thyroid gland. Some reports suggest that therapy with thyroid hormone helps in these situations, but the greatest benefit is to be expected from the use of corticosteroids, whether systemically or intraorbitally (Cant, 1969). Surgical decompression is infrequently needed in children, since progressive, sight-threatening exophthalmos is rare. Needle aspiration of the orbit has proved effective in some cases and may eliminate the need for surgical procedures and may facilitate tarsorrhaphy (Haddad, 1968). Guanethidine (5 per cent topically) is of limited value in relieving the "hyperthyroid" aspect of exophthalmos, that is, the excess sensitivity of Müller's muscle to sympathetic stimulation with consequent widening of the palpebral fissure (Asregadoo, 1970; Martin and Jay, 1962). Guanethidine may cause conjunctival congestion and pupillary miosis, and its effect is neither universal nor long-lasting (Bowden and Rose, 1969).

Local disease of the thyroid gland, such as Hashimoto's or Riedel's thyroiditis, is very rare in children. Ocular manifestations of these diseases occur but are less striking than in other entities such as "Graves' disease" (Arnott and Greaves, 1965; Mason and Walsh, 1963). However, unilateral exophthalmos is not rare in children, and the differential diagnosis of this condition must always be kept in mind (Pohjola, 1964) (Table 20–10).

To make the proper diagnosis and to institute the appropriate therapy of thyroid disease are demanding and difficult procedures. The ophthalmologist, the internist or pediatrician, and the clinical pathologist must combine forces if the patient is to receive optimal care. Both diagnosis and management demand integration of data from many sources, and values are frequently borderline or even in conflict with other determinations. Clinical wisdom in high degree becomes a prerequisite to successful therapy.

PARATHYROID GLAND

Abnormalities of the eyes are found in association with both hyperparathyroidism and hypoparathyroidism. In addition, two conditions resembling hypoparathyroidism also have ocular manifestations of importance; these two entities—pseudohypoparathyroidism and pseudo-pseudo-hypoparathyroidism—will be discussed in this section.

The primary role of the parathyroid gland appears to be to assist in the control of calcium metabolism (DiGeorge, 1969). The blood level of calcium and phosphate is regulated primarily by gastrointestinal absorption, renal excretion, and osseous turnover of calcium. The parathyroid gland provides additional homeostatic regulation, especially when there are gross dietary abnormalities, bone destruction, overabundant or insufficient supply of vitamin D, or other major maladjustment. Two hormones involved in accomplishing this homeostasis are *parathyroid hormone* (PTH), manufactured by the parathyroid gland itself, and *calcitonin*, manufactured by cells located within the thyroid gland. The polypeptide calcitonin was identified in 1961 and has been synthesized. PTH is a small polypeptide hormone, the existence of which has been known for much longer. The two hormones act in a manner analogous to insulin and glucagon. Parathyroid hormone is the primary agent; it causes release of calcium and phosphorus from bone, increased reabsorption of calcium in renal tubule, and increased renal excretion of phosphate. The hypercalcemia produced by this stimulates secretion of calcitonin which tends to return the calcium back to normocalcemic levels. Thus, a feedback system is developed. Unlike the thyroid or the adrenal gland the activity of the parathyroid is not under the control of another gland but responds directly to the level of the metabolites it regulates; hypocalcemia stimulates and hypercalcemia inhibits secretion.

Through its control of calcium metabo-

TABLE 20–10 DIFFERENTIAL DIAGNOSIS OF UNILATERAL EXOPHTHALMOS IN CHILDREN

Orbital asymmetry
Relaxation of rectus muscles
Myopia
Buphthalmos (congenital glaucoma)
Hemangioma
Rhabdomyosarcoma
Meningioma
Glioma
Retinoblastoma
Other tumor (primary or metastatic)
Dermoid cyst
Neurofibromatosis
Histiocytosis
Abscesses
Granulomas
Encephalocele
Mucocele
Craniostenosis
Aneurysms
Pseudotumor
Endocrine exophthalmos

lism the parathyroid gland affects many vital functions of the organism, including the structure of bone, regulation of neuromuscular activity, conduction of cardiac electrical impulses, and the coagulation of the blood. In addition, there are other less well known effects of PTH; for example, PTH appears to have a direct effect on the respiration of mitochondria.

Hyperparathyroidism

Overactivity of the parathyroid gland results in hypercalcemia and hypophosphatemia. Clinically apparent alterations are due primarily to the excess calcium and not to the deficient phosphate (Table 20–11). A variety of other conditions may also produce hypercalcemia and consequently have remarkably similar clinical symptomatology (Table 20–12).

Hyperparathyroidism is very uncommon in children; when it occurs in infants it may be associated with failure to thrive, mental retardation, convulsions, and even blindness. In older children the clinical manifestations are more similar to those in adults (Table 20–11). Diagnosis is based primarily on the concurrent finding of hypercalcemia and hypophosphatemia, but there must be additional confirmatory data (Raisz, 1971). Treatment consists of removal of any parathyroid adenoma

TABLE 20–11   CLINICAL MANIFESTATIONS OF HYPERPARATHYROIDISM

A. Acute hypercalcemia
  1. Anorexia, nausea, and vomiting
  2. Dehydration and azotemia
  3. Somnolence and confusion
  4. Electrocardiographic changes
B. Chronic hypercalcemia and hypercalciuria
  1. Weakness and hypotonia
  2. Failure, depression, and psychosis
  3. Recurrent renal stones, polyuria and polydipsia, renal failure
  4. Dyspepsia, constipation
  5. Calcification of cornea and conjunctiva
  6. Pseudogout
  7. Neonatal hypocalcemia of offspring
C. Increased bone resorption
  1. Osteitis fibrosa cystica
  2. Generalized demineralization
  3. Secondary increase in bone formation (elevated alkaline phosphatase)

Modified from Raisz, L.: Current concepts: The diagnosis of hyperparathyroidism (or what to do until the immunoassay comes). New Eng. J. Med., *285*:1006, 1971.

TABLE 12–12   CAUSES OF HYPERCALCEMIA

Hyperparathyroid disease
Other causes:
  Neoplastic disease
  Sarcoidosis
  Milk-alkali syndrome
  Acute osteoporosis of disuse
  Thyrotoxicosis
  Vitamin D intoxication
  Idiopathic hypercalcemia of infancy
  Hypophosphatasia

found at the time of surgery, or subtotal parathyroidectomy if there is generalized hyperplasia (DiGeorge, 1969).

The ocular signs of hyperparathyroidism are calcification of the cornea and conjunctiva and are probably related solely to the hypercalcemia. As such they are of no specific diagnostic help. Furthermore, the same signs may be found in conditions in which there is neither hyperparathyroidism nor hypercalcemia. "Band keratopathy" may be the result of long-standing ocular inflammation; it may be secondary to trauma or in rare instances it is unassociated with any other apparent abnormality (Duke-Elder, 1965). In children, uveitis secondary to Still's disease is an important cause of band keratopathy. This corneal lesion has a characteristic appearance; it starts with a mild haziness at the level of Bowman's membrane, consisting of a multitude of gray dots in which there are round gaps. This becomes increasingly dense until the area of the cornea exposed between the lids takes on a dull white, granular appearance. Closer examination discloses that this is usually located subepithelially. Although the clinical appearance of the band keratopathy does not allow specific diagnosis and indicates nothing more definite than the presence of hypercalcemia or chronic ocular disease, the appearance of the deposited crystals when examined microscopically may be of more diagnostic value. Berkow, Fine, and Zimmerman (1968) have noted that the calcium deposited in the cornea of patients with hyperparathyroidism is located intracellularly as hydroxyapatite, whereas in band keratopathy without hypercalcemia the calcium is extracellular, confined to the subepithelial zone and Bowman's membrane, and takes the shape of spherules of tiny crystals in concentric circles.

When the corneal opacity becomes so dense that visual ability is hampered, it may be removed by a variety of methods, perhaps the simplest of which is the scrubbing of the anterior surface of the cornea with the chelating agent disodium ethylenediaminetetraacetic acid, 1.0 per cent; anesthesia and removal of the epithelium prior to this treatment can be accomplished by instilling cocaine 4 per cent.

IDIOPATHIC HYPERCALCEMIA OF INFANCY. This is an unusual disease resulting from vitamin D intoxication or possibly an unusual sensitivity to this vitamin. Mild forms may recover but severe forms of the disease show dwarfism, elfin facies, mental retardation, hypertension, craniostenosis, and osteosclerosis. Harley et al. described a case with a serum calcium of 13.9 mg. per 100 ml., increased thickening of the skull base, and bilateral optic atrophy resulting from narrowing of the optic foramina. Strabismus and papilledema have been mentioned.

Ocular changes in idiopathic hypercalcemia include the following:
Convergent strabismus
Optic atrophy secondary to reduced size of optic foramina
Prominent epicanthal folds
Nystagmus
Osteosclerosis of orbital bones
Pupillary changes
Hypertensive retinopathy
Lenticular opacities
Calcium deposition in cornea

Hypoparathyroidism

Underactivity of the parathyroid gland occurs more frequently than overactivity, though both are relatively uncommon. The most important biochemical derangement is a decrease in the level of calcium, associated with elevation of phosphorus. The clinical aspects of the disease are primarily those of hypocalcemia (Table 20–13). Hypocalcemia may be present during the first week of life in the newborn infant, but it is not known whether the parathyroid gland plays a causal role in this tetany of the newborn. Other forms of hypocalcemia occur in infancy in which parathyroid activity is definitely reduced (Table 20–14) (DiGeorge, 1969). Congenital transient hypoparathyroidism is probably a temporary alteration in the newborn

TABLE 20–13 CLINICAL MANIFESTATIONS OF HYPOPARATHYROIDISM

Finding	Approximate Incidence
A. Neuromuscular	
1. Muscular pain and cramps	Usual
2. Positive Chvostek sign	Usual
3. Punctate calcification of basal ganglion	Frequent
4. Irritability	Frequent
5. Convulsions (similar to grand or petit mal epilepsy)	Fairly often
6. Headache	Occasional
7. Mental retardation	Infrequent
B. Intestinal	
1. Diarrhea	Fairly often
2. Pain	Fairly often
C. Teeth, hair, and skin	
1. Late eruption of teeth	Usual
2. Irregular and incomplete enamel formation	Usual
3. Dry, rough skin; short, thin, lined nails	Frequent
4. Coarse, thin, patchy hair	Frequent
5. Mucocutaneous moniliasis	Fairly often
D. Ocular	
1. Lenticular opacities	Usual
2. Photophobia	Fairly often
3. Chronic blepharospasm	Occasional
4. Conjunctivitis or keratitis	Occasional
5. Papilledema	Fairly often
6. Alopecia of eyebrows	Occasional
7. Ptosis	Occasional
8. Strabismus	Occasional
9. Nystagmus	Occasional

secondary to hypercalcemia in the mother. Congenital permanent hypoparathyroidism is associated with hypoplasia or aplasia of the parathyroid glands and often with other developmental defects. Congenital familial hypoparathyroidism is apparently not associated with other defects, however, and is transmitted in a sex-linked recessive pattern. Idiopathic hypoparathyroidism is more frequent in adults than in children; its cause is unknown, but an autoimmune mechanism may be responsible. Most often hypoparathyroidism is secondary to damage to the parathyroid glands produced by surgical or nonsurgical trauma. The acute hypocalcemia following thyroidectomy with inadvertent removal or trauma of the parathyroid gland is now a well-recognized entity.

"Tetany" is highly suggestive of hypocalcemia and thus of underactivity of the parathyroid glands. However, tetany and the signs that accompany it are not proof

TABLE 20–14 CONDITIONS ASSOCIATED WITH HYPOCALCEMIA

Tetany of the newborn
Hypoparathyroidism
    Congenital transient
    Congenital permanent
    Familial congenital
    Idiopathic
    Postoperative
Renal glomerular insufficiency
Renal tubular disorders
Vitamin D deficiency
Vitamin D resistant rickets
Steatorrhea
Postacidotic hypocalcemia

that hypocalcemia is actually existent. The Chvostek sign (facial twitch elicited by tapping the facial nerve) may occasionally be seen in normal individuals and is expected in the tetany associated with respiratory or metabolic alkalosis (Table 20–15).

Laboratory findings in hypoparathyroidism include a low serum calcium, elevated serum phosphorus, negative urine calcium (Sulkowitch), prolongation of the Q-T interval on the electrocardiogram, and abnormality of the electroencephalogram.

Abnormalities of the eyes are an integral part of the clinical manifestations of hypoparathyroidism (Table 20–13). Most frequent is cataract, which occurs in about two thirds of cases with idiopathic hypoparathyroidism, but most striking is photophobia, especially in children. This marked sensitivity to light is present in about 10 per cent of affected individuals and may be noted in the absence of the less frequently observed corneal epithelial defects and ulcerations that resemble Salzmann's nodular dystrophy (Pohjola, 1962). A misdiagnosis of phlyctenular keratoconjunctivitis may be made because of the intense photophobia and blepharospasm. The corneal disease may improve distinctly when the serum calcium has (owing to appropriate therapy) been returned to normal.

TABLE 20–15 CAUSES OF TETANY

Hypocalcemia (see Table 20–14)
Alkalosis
    Hyperventilation
    Excessive alkali therapy
    Prolonged vomiting with loss of hydrochloric
      acid

The cataract of "tetany" was recognized in 1801. In 1929 Goldmann demonstrated that the most plausible explanation for this lens opacity was the concomitant hypocalcemia. The observation that a similar type of cataract is found in other hypocalcemic states lends support to his experimental studies (von Bahr, 1936). However, changes in all these conditions are complex, and the role of hyperphosphatemia or other known or unknown abnormalities is not established. For example, a zonular type of cataract may occur in patients with chronic renal insufficiency treated with hemodialysis. This has been attributed to the hypocalcemia that is often present (Mauntner, 1972), but Laqua (1972) could not relate the cataract to the serum calcium and postulated that another factor in the uremic condition was primarily responsible. Furthermore, Berlyne, in commenting on the cataract that occurs in patients with chronic renal disease, noted that although hypocalcemia resistant to therapy was present, there was poor correlation between the level of calcium and the development of cataract (Spaeth, in press).

The appearance of the cataract is not such that the trained observer may be sure its bearer is afflicted with hypoparathyroidism, or even with hypocalcemia (Fig. 20–4). A similar appearing cataract occurs in other conditions including hypothyroidism, myotonic dystrophy, and Down's syndrome. Most frequently, tiny punctate opacities sprinkle the anterior and posterior cortex; intermixed with these are iridescent crystalline flakes. The opacities are usually densest near the visual axis; the nucleus is typically clear. The cataract may progress rapidly, especially in association with the acute hypoparathyroidism that follows inadvertent removal of the parathyroid glands at the time of thyroidectomy. It may regress partially as calcium metabolism is restored to normal. Surgical extraction of the cataract may be complicated by the orbicularis spasm characteristic of hypocalcemia.

Papilledema is seen in cases with increased intracranial pressure, a not infrequent aspect of the disease; in this regard the differential diagnosis of symptoms (papilledema, gastrointestinal dysfunction, and convulsions) that suggest an intracranial mass must include hypo-

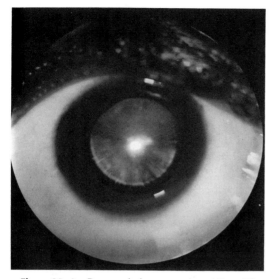

Figure 20–4 Cataract in hypoparathyroidism. The lens changes in this 12-year-old boy are characteristic of hypocalcemia. The slight upward direction of gaze allows the edge of the "zonular cataract" to be seen. With the slit lamp it is possible to visualize spots, flakes, and iridescent crystals in the anterior and posterior cortex, separated from the capsule by a clear area. The nucleus is usually not involved.

parathyroidism. Strabismus has been reported, but uncommonly, and nystagmus or ptosis may also be present but are not characteristic. Alopecia of the eyebrows and eyelids reflects the more generalized epithelial changes.

"Chronic constitutional tetany" has been suggested as a common cause of the cataract (Klotz and Fiks, 1962; Klotz et al., 1963); however, the evidence for this is far from conclusive, and therapy with vitamin D or dihydrotachysterol does not appear to be justified except in investigative settings.

Pseudohypoparathyroidism and Pseudopseudohypoparathyroidism

Pseudohypoparathyroidism was distinguished from true disease of the parathyroid gland in 1942 and its close relative, *pseudo-pseudohypoparathyroidism*, 10 years later; both these contributions were made by Albright et al. (1942, 1952). Since the two variants may occur in the same kinship they probably share similar genetic backgrounds (Bartter, 1966). Pseudohypoparathyroidism was the term employed to describe a syndrome characterized by the biochemical and clinical signs of hypoparathyroidism but resistant to the effects of parathyroid hormone. Additional clinical alterations were also observed (Fig. 20–5 and Table 20–16). The administration of parathyroid hormone in these cases neither corrects the hypocalcemia or hyperphosphatemia nor produces a phosphate diuresis. The disorder apparently represents an inability to respond to parathyroid hormone and not an actual deficiency of PTH. The parathyroid glands are in fact hyperplastic. Pseudo-pseudohypoparathyroidism, in contrast, features clinical aspects similar to pseudohypoparathyroidism, except that the biochemical aspects of hypoparathyroidism are mild or absent (Table 20–16). The characteristic changes are primarily in the skeletal system

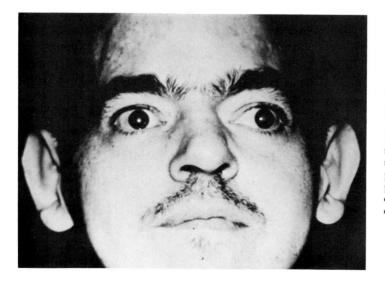

Figure 20–5 Characteristic appearance of pseudohypoparathyroidism. Patients with pseudohypoparathyroidism differ from those with hypoparathyroidism primarily in the failure of the former to respond normally to parathyroid hormone. Mental retardation, a round face, and a stocky physique are also more common in pseudohypoparathyroidism. Cataracts occur in about 25 per cent of such cases.

TABLE 20–16 CLINICAL ASPECTS OF HYPOPARATHYROIDISM, PSEUDOHYPOPARATHYROIDISM, AND PSEUDO-PSEUDOHYPOPARATHYROIDISM

Finding	Incidence		
	Hypoparathyroidism	Pseudo-hypoparathyroidism	Pseudo-pseudo-hypoparathyroidism
Hypocalcemia	All cases	All cases	No
Hyperphosphatemia	All cases	All cases	No
Tetany	Most cases	Most cases	Most cases
Convulsions	Frequent	Frequent	Uncommon
Calcification of the basal ganglion	Common	Common	Absent
Extraskeletal calcification	No	All cases	All cases
Bony dysplasia	No	All cases	All cases
Mental retardation	Infrequent	Frequent	About 50%
Cataracts	60%	About 25%	Not usual
Blue sclerae	?	?	About 25%
Mucocutaneous moniliasis	Common	No	No
Response to PTH	Yes	No	No
Response to Vitamin D	Yes	Yes	No
Inheritance	Varies	Sex-linked recessive	Sex-linked recessive

Modified from Hanno, H., and Weiss, D.: Hypoparathyroidism, pseudohypoparathyroidism, and pseudo-pseudohypoparathyroidism. Arch. Ophthal., 65:238, 1961.

(Table 20–17) and are similar in both pseudo- and pseudo-pseudohypoparathyroidism (Bartter, 1966; Forbes, 1965; Hanno and Weiss, 1961; Klotz et al., 1965).

The type of cataract observed in patients with hypoparathyroidism is also present in patients with pseudohypoparathyroidism, as would be expected, since they are probably both intimately related to hypocalcemia. Cataract has also been reported in pseudo-pseudohypoparathyroidism but is a less common finding; since the two diseases apparently represent a variation in intensity of involvement rather than a totally separate genetic entity, such similarity is not surprising even though hypocalcemia is not characteristic of pseudo-pseudohypoparathyroidism. Of more diagnostic value is the thin and hence

TABLE 20–17 CLINICAL FEATURES PRESENT IN BOTH PSEUDOHYPOPARATHYROIDISM AND PSEUDO-PSEUDOHYPOPARATHYROIDISM (all findings are not present in all cases)

Short stature
Round face
Short digits with shortened metacarpals
Ectopic bone in skin and fascial planes
Bony exostoses
Obesity, often starting in childhood
Hypometabolism
Mental retardation
Diabetic glucose tolerance curve

"blue" sclera noted in cases of pseudo-pseudohypoparathyroidism (Hanno and Weiss, 1961). This has not been reported in other similar conditions.

ADRENAL GLAND

Two different endocrine systems are housed in the adrenal gland. Both are of extreme importance to the well-being of the individual. Coverage in this chapter will be brief, however, since ocular abnormalities are a relatively insignificant part of adrenal gland dysfunction. One exception to this generalization is pheochromocytoma, in which eye signs are frequent and important.

The adrenal cortex secretes four classes of hormones: (1) *glucocorticoids*, which are concerned with regulation of carbohydrate metabolism, to a lesser degree fat and protein metabolism, loss of potassium, and the inflammatory response; the principal hormone is hydrocortisone, which, like the other members of this family, contains 21 carbons; (2) *mineralocorticoids*, which are involved in the maintenance of electrolyte homeostasis, particularly sodium reabsorption in the kidney, and secondarily with blood volume and pressure; the major hormone is the 21-carbon-containing aldosterone; (3) *androgens*, which affect growth, nitrogen retention, and male secondary sex characteristics; the adrenal gland is the source of androgen in the female and of two thirds of the androgens in the male, exceeding the testicular production of these 19-carbon-containing hormones; (4) *estrogens*, which are concerned primarily with female sex characteristics.

The regulation of adrenal cortical hormones is complex (Catt, 1970). Glucocorticoids are primarily controlled by the level of corticotropin (ACTH). Aldosterone, however, is only minimally affected by ACTH, regulation being accomplished by the activation of the renin-angiotensin system; changes in electrolyte concentration, blood volume, blood pressure, or renal blood flow evoke responses in the juxtaglomerular apparatus of the kidney, determining the output of angiotensin and, secondarily, the secretion of aldosterone. Precise measurement of the level of circulating *active* adrenal cortical hormone is still difficult, not only because of the technical problems of the determinations themselves but because of interpretation of the results; the degree of binding of the hormone and other variables make direct extrapolation from the laboratory value to clinical situation invalid. Roughly speaking, the urinary or blood levels of 21-carbon-containing corticosteroids are a measure of glucocorticoid activity, and the 17-ketosteroid content in urine is an index of androgen production. However, the accurate laboratory assessment of endocrinologic activity should usually be undertaken only by an individual skilled in the technique and interpretation of the various determinations now available. This is true of all the endocrinologic disorders, not just those affecting the adrenal gland.

The hormones of the adrenal medulla are the catecholamines, mainly dopamine, norepinephrine, and epinephrine. Not only do these hormones play essential roles in the cardiovascular system, but they are also concerned with carbohydrate metabolism; this is especially true of epinephrine. Assay of the catecholamines is relatively difficult, but an estimation of their production can be made by measurement of the end-product of their catabolism, vanilmandelic acid (VMA), which is excreted in the urine.

Adrenal Cortex

Adrenal cortical insufficiency has many causes (DiGeorge, 1969). The abnormality may be genetically determined, secondary to acute or chronic infection, secondary to corticotropin (ACTH) deficiency, iatrogenic, immunogenic, or idiopathic. Addison's disease refers to chronic adrenal insufficiency due to a destructive lesion of the adrenal gland itself. The symptoms of adrenal insufficiency vary, depending upon the speed of onset and the underlying cause. When the illness is acute, cyanosis, profound hypotension, coma, and death occur in rapid succession. In the chronic forms the symptomatology is more variable (Table 20–18).

Ocular manifestations of adrenal insufficiency are not prominent. In the acute condition the eyes may be sunken and the globes so soft that they resemble those of diabetic coma. Tortuosity and dilatation of the retinal vessels were observed by one author in 50 per cent of patients with Addison's disease (Cerviso et al., 1961), and isolated cases with other findings have also been reported, including choroidal edema, papilledema, and exophthalmos (Cerviso et al., 1961; Wimer and Bunao, 1961) (Table 20–19).

Hyperactivity of the adrenal gland produces different symptoms, depending upon which hormone is oversecreted; there are, then, four major groups of entities: Cushing's syndrome (due to excess hydrocortisone), hyperaldosteronism, the adrenogenital syndromes (due to excess androgen), and feminizing syndromes (due to estrogen-excreting tumors). In

TABLE 20–18 CLINICAL MANIFESTATIONS OF ADRENAL INSUFFICIENCY

Finding	Incidence
Weakness	All
Loss of weight and appetite	All
Dehydration	All
Vomiting, diarrhea, abdominal pain	Almost all
Increased pigmentation of skin	Almost all
Increased pigmentation of mucosa	Almost all
Hypotension	Almost all
Small heart	Almost all
Hypoglycemia	Many
Convulsions	Many

TABLE 20–19 OCULAR FINDINGS IN PATIENTS WITH ADRENAL INSUFFICIENCY

Finding	Incidence
Low intraocular pressure	Most cases
Tortuosity of retinal vessels	About 50%
Choroidal edema	Occasional
Pigmentation of skin of lids	Occasional
Papilledema	Rare
Exophthalmos	Rare

Cushing's syndrome adrenal hyperactivity is frequently but not invariably associated with overproduction of ACTH. In young children malignant adrenal tumors are more frequent than the benign cortical hyperplasia that is typical of the adult. The classic finding is obesity in combination with systemic hypertension (Table 20–20). Treatment has been surgical, with removal of the responsible tumor(s). However, adrenalectomy has been followed by development of pituitary tumor and is not without significant hazard (Rovit and Duane, 1968).

The ocular aspects of Cushing's syndrome have been well discussed by Rovit and Duane. They point out that ocular signs and symptoms of pituitary tumors must be specifically sought in all patients with Cushing's syndrome, especially those having had adrenalectomy, and most particularly if excess pigmentation of the skin signals development of pituitary overactivity. Sufficient evidence is not available to determine whether actual glaucomatous disease is more common in individuals with adrenal cortical hyperfunction. However, there seems little doubt that such hyperfunction does cause slightly higher intraocular pressure, and that adrenalectomy results in a fall in intraocular pressure (Bayer and Neuner, 1967; Neuner and Dardenne, 1968) (Table 20–21).

TABLE 20–20 CLINICAL MANIFESTATIONS OF CUSHING'S SYNDROME

Hypertension
Increased blood volume
Obesity
Weakness
Retarded growth
Osteoporosis
Hirsutism
Acne

TABLE 20–21 OCULAR MANIFESTATIONS OF ADRENAL CORTICAL HYPERACTIVITY

A. Cushing's syndrome
   1. Elevated intraocular pressure
   2. Hypertensive retinopathy
   3. Signs of pituitary tumor
      a. Decreased visual acuity
      b. Visual field loss
      c. Optic atrophy
      d. Headaches
      e. Extraocular muscle palsies
      f. Exophthalmos
B. Hyperaldosteronism
   1. Hypertensive retinopathy
C. Adrenogenital syndromes
   1. Elevated intraocular pressure (?)
D. Feminizing syndromes
   1. Occasional hypertensive retinopathy

Primary excess mineralocorticoid activity is rare in children, though secondary forms of *hyperaldosteronism* may occur in conditions such as the nephrotic syndrome and congestive heart failure. The paramount clinical aspect is always hypertension, and associated with this is a retinopathy indistinguishable from other hypertensive retinopathies and often productive of visual symptoms. Though tetany may be present in some cases with hyperaldosteronism, it is not due to hypocalcemia, and consequently it is unlikely that these individuals would be prone to develop the typical "tetany cataract."

In the various *adrenogenital syndromes* clinical manifestations vary, depending on the constellation of hormonal abnormalities and the sex of the afflicted individual. The major alterations are in the secondary sex characteristics. Specific enzyme defects have now been identified in some instances. No ocular manifestations that could be attributed to the hormonal abnormality have been reported. However, androgens do affect intraocular pressure, and one case has been observed in which the administration of androgens to an individual having had a hypophysectomy caused definite, dose-related, reversible increases in intraocular pressure.* Adrenal tumors that secrete excess estrogen cause *feminization*; hypertension is usual in adults, but no characteristic ocular findings have been reported.

_____

*Personal observation.

Adrenal Medulla

Pheochromocytoma

Pheochromocytoma is a neoplastic growth of chromaffin tissue. Chromaffin cells, a mature type of sympathetic nervous system cell, secrete the two hormones epinephrine and norepinephrine. Though present in the many sympathetic ganglia throughout the body this chromaffin tissue is largely located in the medulla of the adrenal gland, and 90 per cent of pheochromocytomas are found there. The neoplasm produces disease largely owing to the secretion of excessive, variable amounts of epinephrine and norepinephrine, but may in addition encroach upon neighboring structures. Only 3 per cent of these tumors are malignant (Wilkins, 1965).

It is interesting to remember that epinephrine was the first of all hormones to be isolated and chemically defined, this important work being accomplished during the time of the Spanish-American war around the turn of the century. This discovery and the later elucidation of the role of norepinephrine in the sympathetic nervous system form an exciting chapter in the development of medical knowledge. The clinical manifestations of pheochromocytoma are mainly expressions of the effects of epinephrine and norepinephrine. As such they are widespread (Table 20–22). Furthermore, since similar symptoms may be caused by other, unrelated clinical entities, a thorough evalua-

TABLE 20–22 CLINICAL MANIFESTATIONS OF PHEOCHROMOCYTOMA

Finding	Incidence (%)
Hypertension (sustained or intermittent)	Almost 100
Anxiety and nervousness*	90
Visual disturbances	90
Attacks of flushing or pallor	80
Headache	80
Increased sweating	90
Hypermetabolism	35
Increased blood glucose	35
Weight loss	70
Gastrointestinal symptoms**	60
Polyuria and polydipsia	50

*Dizziness, palpitations, dyspnea, substernal pain, weakness.
**Constipation, vomiting, abdominal pain.

TABLE 20–23 DIFFERENTIAL DIAGNOSIS OF THE SIGNS AND SYMPTOMS SEEN IN PHEOCHROMOCYTOMA

A. Hypertension
  1. Renal disease
  2. Coarctation of the aorta
  3. Arteriolar disease
  4. Essential hypertension
  5. Acrodynia
  6. Primary aldosteronism
  7. Cushing's syndrome
B. Hypermetabolism
  1. Thyrotoxicosis
C. Elevated blood glucose
  1. Diabetes mellitus
D. Paroxysmal disturbances; emotional lability
  1. Riley-Day syndrome
  2. Functional hyperventilation
E. Decreased gastrointestinal mobility
  1. Hirschsprung's disease

tion of a patient with any of the individual signs or symptoms is imperative (Table 20–23). Children as young as 1½ years of age may be affected, and males predominate. In some conditions such as thyrotoxicosis there are several findings in common, including hypermetabolism, weight loss, tremulousness, anxiety, and increased respiratory rate. In pheochromocytoma the most serious pathologic effects are due to the systemic hypertension; although the baseline level itself may be consistently elevated, paroxysms of even greater elevation, in association with increased sweating, anxiety, flushing or blanching, and headache, are typical. Especially when such symptoms are present must the physician proceed with necessary diagnostic procedures.

Pheochromocytoma has a definite familial predilection. Furthermore, it occurs more commonly in patients with neurofibromatosis than in the random population.

The administration of a sympathetic blocking agent such as phentolamine (Regitine) usually induces a large fall in systemic blood pressure in the individual whose hypertension is due to a chromaffin cell tumor. If pheochromocytoma is suspected because of other findings, but the patient is not hypertensive, the intravenous injection of histamine phosphate (0.001 to 0.025 mg.) may be considered; this is likely to cause a sudden rise in blood pressure in the person harboring the tumor but tends to produce a decrease in pressure in the normal or emotionally labile individual. Furthermore, the usefulness of the test may be increased by analysis of blood samples taken before and after injection of the histamine to determine whether any change in the level of catecholamines was elicited. The level of catecholamine circulating in the blood or of catecholamine end-product in the urine is also of diagnostic help, but both false positive and false negative results can occur. When a definite clinical diagnosis has been established, treatment consists of surgical removal of the tumor after careful determination of its location (Poole, 1964).

Pheochromocytoma has been discussed in some detail in this text because its ophthalmic aspects are so important (Table 20–24) (Bonamour and Bonnet, 1965; Breffeilh and Robinson, 1965; Norton, 1964). Ninety per cent of affected individuals will have visual disturbances. The eye findings are in no way diagnostic, however, and reflect the intensity of the hypertension. Large deflections in the tonography tracing have been noted and are a reflection of the large pulse pressure that is transmitted to the tonometer; any condition causing a large difference between the systolic and diastolic blood pressures will cause a similar phenomenon. Although it has been stated that there is complete resolution of the ocular abnormalities after the successful removal of the responsible tumor, this is not always so (Norton, 1964). In fact, residual optic atrophy and macular degenerative changes are frequent.

Several aspects of the ocular manifestations of pheochromocytoma are especially

TABLE 20–24 OCULAR MANIFESTATIONS OF PHEOCHROMOCYTOMA

During Active Disease:
  Dilated pupils
  Superficial and deep retinal hemorrhages
  Retinal exudates, dense and extensive
  Retinal arteriolar spasm
  Retinal vessel tortuosity
  Retinal edema
  Papilledema
  Stellate figure of the macula
  Neovascularization of the retina
Following Successful Removal of Tumor:
  Macular scar
  Optic atrophy

interesting. Braley (1952) stated that myelinated nerve fibers are visible in the corneas of patients with active disease, and that these disappear after successful removal of the catecholamine-secreting tumor. Rubey (1969) reported a case in which cotton-wool spots and retinal hemorrhages were noted in the fundus as one of the first signs of definite clinical disease, antedating the onset of hypertension. The association between pheochromocytoma and the "phakomatoses" has been reported by several authors, though the basis for the relationship is not understood (Dono, 1964; Hagler et al., 1971).

THE CARCINOID SYNDROME

Although the carcinoid syndrome is not an abnormality of adrenal function, it is included here because it is an endocrinologic illness affecting the same organ systems as pheochromocytoma, specifically the cardiovascular, the vasomotor, and the gastrointestinal. Owing primarily to excessive secretion of serotonin from neoplastic tissue, the pharmacologic aspects of the carcinoid syndrome appear to involve the catecholamines and the kinin peptides as well. Symptoms consist of episodic flushes, cyanosis, abdominal pain, diarrhea, emesis, hypotension, valvular and endocardial plaques, and congestive heart failure. Yellow-white, intraretinal lesions, in association with tortuosity and widening of the retinal veins, and large venous aneurysmal dilatations have been noted in one case (Young, 1968). Although carcinoid tumors are usually benign, they have been known to metastasize to the choroid and the orbit.

GONADS

Hypofunction of the gonads may be due to a chromosomal abnormality or a number of other causes, such as panhypopituitarism. Several "secondary" types of hypogonadism have already been discussed, specifically the Laurence-Moon-Bardet-Biedl syndrome and pituitary insufficiency.

Turner's Syndrome

Twenty-one years after Turner, in 1939, described a syndrome of sexual infantilism, webbed neck, and cubitus valgus, a chromosome defect was found to be the underlying abnormality. Normal females possess two X chromosomes (XX); this is not the case in patients with Turner's syndrome, in whom there is either complete absence of one X chromosome (XO), so that the total number is only 45, or a mosaic pattern due to mitotic nondisjunction. The most common of the mosaics is the XO/XX type.

The most important clinical manifestation of this fundamental defect is failure of normal sexual development, though a variety of other findings may be present as well (Table 20–25). This condition is not rare, occurring in about 1 in 2599 live-born females (DiGeorge, 1969), and is the underlying problem in about 50 per cent of women with primary amenorrhea. Replacement therapy with estrogens can result in development of the normal female sex characteristics, but because the ovaries themselves are aplastic the affected individuals are sterile. Ocular abnormalities are prominent in Turner's syndrome; there is no particularly characteristic constellation but rather a wide spectrum of findings, many of which are noted only slightly more frequently than in the general population (Table 20–26) (Blervacque et al., 1968; Cordier et al., 1966; Lessell and Forbes, 1966; Royer and Genin, 1963; Thomas et al., 1969).

TABLE 20–25 CLINICAL ASPECTS OF TURNER'S SYNDROME*

Finding	Incidence
Incomplete X chromosomal complement	All
Incomplete female sex characteristics	All
Short, stocky stature	All
Webbing of the neck	Many
Prominent ears	Many
Small mandible	Many
Coarctation of the aorta	Often
Horseshoe kidney	Often
Skeletal abnormalities	Often
Edema of hands and feet	Often
Mental retardation	Occasional

*Signs vary with chromosomal complement; they are more marked in XO than in mosaic individuals.

TABLE 20–26 OCULAR FINDINGS IN TURNER'S SYNDROME

Finding	Incidence
Microcornea	Over 50% of cases
Eccentric pupil	About 50% of cases
Cataract (anterior, axial, embryonal)	About 33% of cases
Epicanthus	About 20% of cases
Color blindness	About 10% of cases
Strabismus	Occasional
Blue sclerae	Occasional
Retinal vessel tortuosity	Occasional
Macular "degeneration" or "aplasia"	Occasional
Retinitis pigmentosa	Infrequent
Posterior embryotoxon	Infrequent
Infantile glaucoma	Infrequent
Uveal coloboma	Infrequent
Nystagmus	Infrequent
Pseudopapillitis	Infrequent
Ptosis	Infrequent
Corneal nebulae	Infrequent
Primary open-angle glaucoma	Infrequent
Optic atrophy	Infrequent

Klinefelter's Syndrome

Hypogonadism in the male due to chromosomal abnormality is known as Klinefelter's syndrome. In contrast to Turner's syndrome, in which absence of an X chromosome causes incomplete expression of female sexuality, in Klinefelter's syndrome the presence of one or more extra X chromosomes suppresses the Y chromosome, with consequent incomplete development of male sex characteristics. Though XXY is the most frequently observed anomaly, other combinations include XXXY, XXXXY, and XXXXYY; mosaics such as XX/XXY or XY/XXXY have also been observed (Turner, 1938). Klinefelter's syndrome is not rare, being noted in about 2 per 1000 live male births. The incidence is higher among the mentally retarded. The major clinical manifestation of this counterpart of Turner's syndrome is incomplete sexual development, though other findings have been recorded (Table 20–27). The eyes are usually normal, but epicanthus and strabismus are not rare. One case was noted to have a dislocated, small lens (Bessière et al., 1962).

Ocular myopathy may occur in individuals who do not have Klinefelter's syndrome but have hypogonadism secondary to the prepubertal castration syndrome (Carton et al., 1964).

TABLE 20–27 CLINICAL MANIFESTATIONS IN KLINEFELTER'S SYNDROME

Finding	Incidence
Extra X chromosome(s)	All
Incomplete expression of male sex characteristics	All
Gynecomastia	Frequent
Mental retardation	Common
Obesity	Occasional
Epicanthus	Uncommon
Strabismus	Uncommon
Hypotonia	Uncommon
Dislocated lens	Uncommon

PANCREAS

Diabetes Mellitus

Clearly central to the pathogenesis of diabetes mellitus is malfunctioning of the pancreas. However, this disease is certainly more than a manifestation of the insulin deficiency classically considered to be due to insufficiency of pancreatic beta cells. Diabetes appears to be a group of diseases which have as their hallmark elevated blood glucose in association with glucose in the urine (Editorial, 1971). It is not a single entity. In the differential diagnosis one must consider not only the conditions listed in Table 20–28 but also the heterogeneity of diabetes itself. It seems quite

TABLE 20–28

A. Differential diagnosis of hyperglycemia
  1. Deficient insulin activity
    a. Abnormal beta cells of pancreas
    b. Abnormal insulin
    c. Excess normal insulin antagonist
    d. Presence of abnormal insulin antagonist
  2. Excess pancreatic hyperglycemic factor
  3. Excess pituitary growth hormone
  4. Excess adrenal cortical hormone
  5. Excess epinephrine
  6. Impaired hepatic glycogen storage
  7. Brain stem lesions
  8. Galactosemia*
B. Differential diagnosis of glycosuria
  1. Diabetes mellitus
  2. Cushing's syndrome
  3. Hyperthyroidism
  4. Fanconi's syndrome
  5. Heavy-metal poisoning
  6. Glomerular nephritis
  7. Acute pancreatitis
  8. Pentosuria*
  9. Galactosemia*

*Excess sugar, not glucose.

likely that several genes are involved in the cluster of conditions with elevated blood sugar and glucosuria; the inheritance pattern is not simply autosomal recessive. Moreover, environmental factors may play a role in the development of the disease.

According to Nelson (1969) there are about 3 million diabetics in the United States, 4 per cent of whom are less than 15 years of age. Furthermore, according to certain surveys, diabetes has now become the most common cause of blindness. Nevertheless, the ocular aspects of diabetes in youngsters are not particularly striking. The usual ocular complications of this disease are apparently related more to duration than to severity of illness. Much controversy exists regarding the pathogenesis of the angiopathy that develops in almost all diabetics within 20 years of the onset of the disease; some authors correlate blood sugar with retinopathy (Szabo, 1970), some with insulin response (Elkeles et al., 1971), and others with growth hormone level (Beaumont et al., 1971; Lundback et al., 1970); still others believe that no definite relationship has been established. Most agree, however, that the incidence of complications increases with increasing duration of disease. Safir found that only 10 per cent of juvenile diabetics with disease less than 5 years manifested diabetic retinopathy, whereas this increased to 80 per cent by 20 years, and to almost 100 per cent 5 years after that (Safir and Rogers, 1970).

Since most youngsters with diabetes have had their disease but a short while, the frequency with which the ocular complications of diabetes are observed is relatively low. Some authors have even stated that diabetic retinopathy is "universally absent" in juvenile diabetics (Soler Sala and Santalo, 1969). This is incorrect, since retinopathic changes have occurred in patients less than 10 years old (Barta and Molnár, 1970). However, it underscores the difference between the young diabetic with recent onset of disease and the adult with illness of less well-defined duration. When the ocular aspects of diabetes become apparent in a young person, the range of expression is as wide as in the adult (Table 20–29) (Dereani and Kolar, 1970; Ferrer, 1964; Grosz and Berki, 1969; Kato, 1964; Labram and Lestradet,

TABLE 20–29 OCULAR MANIFESTATIONS IN CHILDREN WITH DIABETES MELLITUS

Retinal venous dilatations and tortuosity
Retinal arteriolar dilatations and tortuosity
Retinal vessel microaneurysms
Retinal hemorrhages
Slow intraretinal circulation time
Retinal neovascularization
Retinal exudates
Vitreous hemorrhages
Retinitis proliferans
Retinal vein thrombosis
Rubeosis of the iris
Neovascular glaucoma
Iritis
Ocular hypotony (with diabetic coma)
Chronic open-angle glaucoma
Refractive changes
Cranial nerve palsies (especially III and IV)
Pupillary changes
Pseudopapillitis
Papilledema
Lipemia retinalis
Cataract
Anterior reduplication of the lens capsule
Conjunctival blood vessel irregularities
  (caliber, edema, aneurysms)

1966; Lubow and Makley, 1971; Rosen, 1969).

Special mention must be made of the relation between diabetes mellitus and intraocular pressure. Severe ocular hypotony is a well-recognized finding of diabetic coma. On the other hand, ocular hypertension appears to be characteristic of diabetes, including that among juveniles, when cases are not so seriously out of control (Safir et al., 1964; Traisman et al., 1967). There are indications that actual glauco natous disease is also more common in diabetics than in the normal population (Becker, 1971; Hauff, 1970), but dissenting opinions about this have been expressed (Bankes, 1967; Bouzas et al., 1971). There is enough substance in the reports of those who find an interrelationship between diabetes and glaucoma that any patient with one disease should be checked to be sure the other is not also present.

Ophthalmic symptoms may be the initial manifestation of diabetic disease; this is especially the case in adults but is not often so in children. The finding may be as mild as a sudden unexplained change in refractive error or as dramatic as a central retinal vein occlusion or even hemorrhagic glaucoma (Heinrich, 1969). Whenever it is important to establish with certainty the presence or absence of diabetic retinopathy, the greatly increased ability of fluorescein angiography to determine the early vascular changes should be remembered (Norton and Gutman, 1965). This remarkably safe diagnostic procedure allows visualization of changes that cannot be seen with the ophthalmoscope. Fluorescein studies are essential in all cases being considered for photocoagulation treatment of retinopathy. Fluorescein may also be used to visualize the vascular changes in the anterior segment of the eye (Rosen and Lyons, 1969).

The treatment of the ocular complications of diabetes mellitus is becoming more rational as a better understanding of the basic pathologic abnormalities emerges. Beaumont and Hollows suggested a new classification of diabetic retinopathy based on the correlation between the ocular and biochemical findings, and pointed out that certain types of therapy are more likely to succeed in certain types of disease; for example, pituitary ablation has the best chance of success in cases with excess growth hormone (Beaumont and Hollows, 1972). The local treatment of retinopathy with photocoagulation appears to have a place in the therapy of these patients, but the eventual benefit of such treatment is still not established (Beetham et al., 1970; Editorial, 1970; Irvine and Norton, 1971; Krill et al., 1971). Certainly afflicted individuals are best handled in most instances by being referred to one of the centers where such treatment can be given in a controlled manner. Studies of an international scope are under way at present, and it is hoped that they will result in information that will make the therapy of these unfortunate diabetic ocular complications more successful and less hazardous.

Caution must be the rule in interpreting the results of therapy for conditions such as diabetes. For example, one of the oral agents previously considered uniquely able to limit the complications of diabetes has recently been found to be of little help (Knatterud et al., 1971). Hypophysectomy, once promulgated as the solution to diabetic retinopathy, has proved to be of limited value. Long-term prospective studies must be conducted far more extensively before meaningfully accurate evaluations of treatment are possible. This is especially true of heterogenous, slowly evolving diseases, of which diabetes is a classic example.

REFERENCES

Adams, D. D.: The presence of an abnormal thyroid stimulating hormone in the serum of some thyrotoxic patients. J. Clin. Endocr., *18*:699, 1958.

Albright, F., Burnett, C., Smith, P., and Parson, W.: Pseudohypoparathyroidism: an example of Seabright-Bantam syndrome. Endocrinology, *30*:922, 1942.

Albright, F., Forbes, A., and Henneman, P.: Pseudo-pseudohypoparathyroidism. Trans. Assoc. Amer. Physicians, *65*:337, 1952.

Anderson, D. R.: Mechanisms of Graves' disease and endocrine exophthalmos. Amer. J. Ophthal., *68*:46, 1969.

Aranow, H., and Day, R. M.: Management of thyrotoxicosis in patients with ophthalmopathy; antithyroid regimen determined primarily by ocular manifestations. J. Clin. Endocr., *25*:1, 1965.

Arnott, E. J., and Greaves, D. P.: Orbital involvement in Riedel's thyroiditis. Brit. J. Ophthal., *49*:1, 1965.

Asbury, T.: Unilateral scotoma as the presenting sign of pituitary tumor. Amer. J. Ophthal., *59*:510, 1965.

Asregadoo, E. R.: Guanethidine ophthalmic solution 5%. Arch. Ophthal., *84*:21, 1970.

Bankes, J. L. K.: Ocular tension and diabetes mellitus. Brit. J. Ophthal., *51*:557, 1967.

Bardet, G.: Sur un syndrome d'obésité congénitale avec polydactylie et rétinite pigmentaire (contribution à l'étude des formes cliniques de l'obésité hypophysaire). Paris, A. Legrand, 1920.

Barta, L., and Molnár, M.: Time of development of retinopathy in diabetic children. Helv. Paediat. Acta, *25*:242, 1970.

Bartter, Frederick: Pseudohypoparathyroidism and pseudo-pseudohypoparathyroidism. *In* Stanbury, Wyngaarden, and Fredrickson (Eds.): The Metabolic Basis of Inherited Disease. 2nd ed. New York, McGraw-Hill Book Co. 1966, p. 1024.

Bayer, J., and Neuner, H.: Cushing's syndrome and raised intraocular pressure. Deutsch. Med. Wschr., *92*:1791, 1967.

Beaumont, T., and Hollows, F. S.: Classification of diabetic retinopathy with therapeutic implications. Lancet, *1*:419, 1972.

Beaumont, P., Schofield, P. J., Hollows, F. C., Williams, J. F., and Steinbeck, A. W.: Growth hormone, sorbitol, and diabetic capillary disease. Lancet, *1*:579, 1971.

Becker, B.: Diabetes mellitus and primary open-angle glaucoma. Trans. Amer. Acad. Ophthal. Otolaryng., *75*:239, 1971.

Beetham, W. P., Aiello, L. M., Balodimos, M. C., and Koncz, L.: Ruby laser photocoagulation of early diabetic neovascular retinopathy. Preliminary report of a long-term controlled study. Arch. Ophthal., *83*:261, 1970.

Benedict, W.: Early diagnosis of pituitary tumor with ocular phenomena. Amer. J. Ophthal., *3*:571, 1920.

Berkow, J., Fine, B., and Zimmerman, L.: Unusual ocular calcification in hypoparathyroidism. Amer. J. Ophthal., *66*:812, 1968.

Bessière, E., Rivière, J., Leuret, J. Ph., and le Rebeller, Mme.: Sur une association de maladie de Klinefelter et d'anomalies congénitales (camptodactylie, microphakie). Bull. Soc. Ophtal. Fr., *62*:197, 1962.

Biedl, A.: Ein Geschwisterpaar mit adiposogenitaler Dystrophie. Deutsch. Med. Wschr., *48*:1630, 1922.

Blervacque, A., Constantinides, G., and Dufour, D.: Les manifestations ophtalmologiques dans le syndrome de Turner. Bull. Soc. Ophtal. Fr., *68*:589, 1968.

Bonamour, G., and Bonnet, M.: Les signes oculaires des pheochromocytomes. Presse Méd., *55*:3194, 1965.

Bouzas, A. G., Gragoudas, E. S., Balodimos, M. C., Brinegar, C. H., and Aiello, L. M.: Intraocular pressure in diabetes. Arch. Ophthal., *85*:423, 1971.

Bowden, A. N., and Clifford, R. F.: Investigation of endocrine exophthalmos. Proc. Roy. Soc. Med., *62*:13, 1969.

Bowden, A. N., and Rose, F. C.: Dysthyroid eye disease. A trial of guanethidine eye drops. Brit. J. Ophthal., *53*:246, 1969.

Braley, A., cited by D. W. Larson in Walsh, F. B.: Papilledema associated with increased intracranial pressure in Addison's disease. Arch. Ophthal., *47*:86, 1952.

Brand, I.: Über intraokulare Hypotonie als Merkmal einiger Krankheiten des Zentralnervensystems. Klin. Monatsbl. Augenheilk., *150*:813, 1967.

Breffeilh, L. A., and Robinson, J. P.: The ocular manifestations of pheochromocytoma. Southern Med. J., *58*:73, 1965.

Burke, G.: Long acting thyroid stimulator and exophthalmos. Ann. Intern. Med., *70*:1045, 1969.

Cant, J. S.: The treatment of dysthyroid ophthalmopathy with intralesional corticosteroids and local guanethidine. Brit. J. Ophthal., *53*:233, 1969.

Carswell, F., Kerr, M. M., and Hutchison, J. H.: Congenital goitre and hypothyroidism produced by maternal ingestion of iodides. Lancet, *1*:1241, 1970.

Carton, H., Gybels, J., and Brucher, J. M.: Ocular myopathy with pre-pubertal functional castration syndrome. Acta Neurol. Psychiat. Belg., *69*:265, 1964.

Catt, K. J.: The ABC of endocrinology. *V.* Adrenal cortex. Lancet, *1*:1275, 1970.

Cerviso, J. M., Garbino, C., Maggiolo, J., Jourdan de Baylay, E., and Pasquet, N.: Alteraciones oculares en algunas endocrinopatias. An. Fac. Med. Montevideo, *46*:47, 1961.

Chamlin, M., Davidoff, L., and Feiring, E.: Ophthalmologic changes produced by pituitary tumors. Amer. J. Ophthal., *40*:353, 1955.

Chiriceanu, M., Ioanitiu, D., Cuvin-Sarafian, E., and Glavan, I. I.: Considerations on ocular tension alterations in hypophyseal tumors. Oftalmologia (Buc.), *12*:213, 1968.

Cordier, J., Tridon, P., and Reny, A.: Syndrome de Turner et rétinite pigmentaire. J. Genet. Hum., *15*:105, 1966.

Day, R. M., and Carroll, F. D.: Optic nerve involvement associated with thyroid dysfunction. Arch. Ophthal., *67*:289, 1962.

Depisch, D., Hofer, R., and Schatz, H.: Der Einfluss von immunosuppressiver Therapie auf den Long Acting Thyroid Stimulator (LATS) und das klinische Bild bei Patienten mit local isiertem Myxodem und Exophthalmus. Wien. Klin. Wschr., *81*:8, 1969.

Dereani, C., and Kolar, G.: Augenhintergrundveränderungen bei jungen Diabetikern. Klin. Mbl. Augenheilk., *157*:101, 1970.

DeSchweinitz, G.: Concerning certain ocular aspects of pituitary body disorders, mainly exclusive of the usual central and peripheral hemianopic field defects. Trans. Ophthal. Soc. U. K., *43*:12, 1923.

DiGeorge, A. M.: Disorders of the adrenal glands. *In* Nelson, W. E., Vaughn, V. C., and McKay, R. J. (Eds.): Textbook of Pediatrics. 9th ed. Philadelphia, W. B. Saunders Co., 1969, p. 1205.

DiGeorge, A. M.: Disorders of the gonads. *In* Nelson, W. E., Vaughn, V. C., and McKay, R. J. (Eds.): Textbook of Pediatrics. 9th ed. Philadelphia, W. B. Saunders Co., 1969, p. 1224.

DiGeorge, A. M.: Disorders of the parathyroid glands. *In* Nelson, W. E., Vaughan, V. C., and McKay, R. J. (Eds.): Textbook of Pediatrics. 9th ed. Philadelphia, W. B. Saunders Co., 1969, p. 1200.

DiGeorge, A. M.: Disorders of the thyroid gland. *In* Nelson, W. E., Vaughan, V. C., and McKay, R. J. (Eds.): Textbook of Pediatrics. 9th ed. Philadelphia, W. B. Saunders Co., 1969, p. 1187.

Dobyns, B. M., Wright, A., and Wilson, L.: Assay of the exophthalmos-producing substance in the serum of patients with progressive exophthalmos. J. Clin. Endocr., *21*:648, 1961.

Dono, M.: Case of pheochromocytoma with Recklinghausen's disease. Jap. J. Clin. Ophthal., *18*:941, 1964.

Duke-Elder, S. and Leigh, A. G.: Diseases of the outer eye. *In* Duke-Elder, S. (Ed.): System of ophthalmology. Vol. 8, Part 2. St. Louis, The C. V. Mosby Co., 1965, p. 897.

Editorial: Diabetes mellitus: Disease or syndrome? Lancet, *I*:583, 1971.

Editorial: Diabetic retinopathy. Lancet, *II*:1073, 1970.

Ehrenfeld, E. N., Rowe, H., and Auerbach, E.: Laurence-Moon-Bardet-Biedl syndrome in Israel. Amer. J. Ophthal., *70*:524, 1970.

Elkeles, R. S., Wyllie, A. D. H., Lowy, C., Young, J. L., and Fraser, T. R.: Serum insulin, glucose and lipid level among mild diabetics in relation to incidence of vascular complications. Lancet, *I*:880, 1971.

Ferrer, J.: Ocular complications of infantile and juvenile diabetes. Bull. Soc. Ophtal. Fr., *77*:692, 1964.

Follmann, P., Vadász, Z., and Takács, L.: Hypothalmopathie und Glaukom. Klin. Mbl. Augenheilk., *151*:57, 1967.

Forbes, A.: Données récentes sur le pseudohypoparathyroidisme et pseudo-pseudohypoparathyroidisme. Probl. Actuels Endocrinol. Nutr., *6*:111, 1965.

Fowler, P. B. S., Swale, J., and Andrews, H.: Hypercholesterolaemia in borderline hypothyroidism stage of premyxoedema. Lancet, *II*:488, 1970.

Fröhlich, A.: Ein Fall von Tumor der Hypophysis cerebri ohne Akromegalie. Wien. Klin. Rundschau, *15*:883, 1901. (Cited in Nelson, W. E. (Ed.): Textbook of Pediatrics. 6th ed. Philadelphia, W. B. Saunders Co., 1957.)

Goldmann, H.: Experimentelle Tetaniekataract. von Graefes Archiv. f. Ophthal., *122*:146, 1929.

Grant, M.: New treatment of calcific corneal opacities. Arch. Ophthal., *48*:681, 1952.

Grosz, I., and Berki, E.: Coexistence of primary optic nerve atrophy and juvenile diabetes. Acta Med. Acad. Sci. Hungary, *26*:57, 1969.

Haddad, H. M.: Tonography and visual fields in endocrine exophthalmos; report on 29 patients. Amer. J. Ophthal., *64*:63, 1967.

Haddad, H. M.: Needle aspiration of malignant (progressive) endocrine exophthalmos. Arch. Ophthal., *80*:703, 1968.

Hagler, W. S., Hyman, B. N., and Waters, W. C., III: Von Hippel's angiomatosis retinae and pheochromocytoma. Trans. Amer. Acad. Ophthal. Otolaryng., *75*:1022, 1971.

Hall, R., Kirkham, K., Doniach, D., and Kabir, D. E.: Ophthalmic Graves' disease; diagnosis and pathogenesis. Lancet, *I*:375, 1970.

Hanno, H., and Weiss, D.: Hypoparathyroidism, pseudohypoparathyroidism, and pseudo-pseudohypoparathyroidism. Arch. Ophthal., *65*:238, 1961.

Hanno, H., and Weiss, D.: Pseudohypoparathyroidism: report of two new cases. Arch. Ophthal., *65*:221, 1961.

Harley, R. D., DiGeorge, A. M., Mabry, C. C., and Apt, L.: Idiopathic hypercalcemia of infancy, optic atrophy and other ocular changes. Trans. Amer. Acad. Ophthal. and Otolaryng., *69*:879, 1965.

Hauff, D.: Glaukom und Diabetes. Ophthalmologica, *160*:391, 1970.

Hedges, T. R., and Scheie, H. G.: Visual field defects in exophthalmos associated with thyroid disease. Arch. Ophthal., *54*:885, 1955.

Hedley, A. J., Ross, I. P., and Crooks, J.: L.A.T.S. and Graves' disease. Lancet, *II*:468, 1970.

Heinrich, P.: Augenhintergrundveränderungen als Frühsymptom von Diabetes mellitus. Klin. Mbl. Augenheilk., *154*:716, 1969.

Henderson, J. W.: Eye changes with thyroid disease. Postgrad. Med., *45*:96, 1969.

Henderson, W.: The pituitary adenomata. A follow-up study of the surgical results in 338 cases (Dr. Harvey Cushing's series). Brit. J. Surg., *26*:811, 1939.

Henkind, P., Leitman, M., and Weitzman, E.: The diurnal curve in man: new observations. Invest. Ophthal., to be published.

Hershman, J. M., and Pittman, J. A., Jr.: Control of thyrotropin secretion in man. New Eng. J. Med., *285*:997, 1971.

Howard, G.: Angioid streaks in acromegaly. Amer. J. Ophthal., *56*:137, 1963.

Howard, G., and English, F.: Occurrence of glaucoma in acromegalics. Arch. Ophthal., *73*:765, 1965.

Hoyles, A. B., Kennedy, R. L. J., Beahrs, O. H., and Woolner, L. B.: Exophthalmic goiter in children. J. Clin. Endocr., *19*:138, 1959.

Hugonnier, R.: "Ocular paralysis" in Graves' disease. J. Med. Lyon, *46*:859, 1965.

Irvine, A. R., and Norton, E. W. D.: Photocoagulation for diabetic retinopathy. Amer. J. Ophthal., *71*:437, 1971.

Jackson, H.: Management of pituitary tumours. Proc. Roy. Soc. Med., *57*:471, 1965.

Kato, K.: Studies on the retinal changes and cataract in juvenile diabetes. Acta Soc. Ophthal. Jap., *68*:1815, 1964.

Katz, M.: Edema of the margin of the upper eyelid

(pretarsal) in hypothyroidism. New Eng. J. Med., *282*:514, 1970.

Klotz, H., and Fiks, Mme.: Les anomalies du cristallin (cataractes) dans la tétanie chronique constitutionelle et dans l'hypoparathyroidisme partiel méconnu. Probl. Actuels Endocrinol. Nutr., *6*:245, 1962.

Klotz, H., Tomkiewics, S., and Benhamou, R.: A propos de 14 cas de pseudo-pseudohypoparathyroidisme. Probl. Actuels Endocrinol. Nutr., *6*:142, 1965.

Klotz, H., Witchitz, S., and Kleinman, Mme.: The NA$_2$, EDTA-induced hypocalcaemia test: A test for functional exploration of the parathyroid. Ann. Endocr. (Paris). *24*:1068, 1963.

Knatterud, G. L., et al.: Effects of hypoglycemic agents on vascular complications in patients with adult-onset diabetes. *LV*. A preliminary report on Phenformin results. J.A.M.A., *217*:777, 1971.

Kolodny, H., Sherman, L., Singh, A., Kim, S., and Benjamin, F.: Acromegaly treated with chlorpromazine. New Eng. J. Med., *284*:819, 1971.

Krill, A. E., Archer, D. B., Newell, F. B., and Chishti, M. I.: Photocoagulation in diabetic retinopathy. Amer. J. Ophthal., *72*:299, 1971.

Labram, C., and Lestradet, H.: Development in five years of the state of the vascular field of the bulbar conjunctiva in juvenile diabetes mellitus. Diabetes, *14*:203, 1966.

Landau, J., and Bromberg, Y. M.: Impaired scotopic vision in adiposo-genital dystrophy. Brit. J. Ophthal., *39*:155, 1955. (Cited in Geeraets, W. J.: Ocular Syndromes. Philadelphia, Lea and Febiger, 1965.)

Laqua, H.: Kataract bei chronischer Niereninsuffizienz und Dialysebehandlung. Klin. Mbl. Augenheilk., *160*:346, 1972.

Laurence, J. Z., and Moon, R. C.: Four cases of "retinitis pigmentosa" occurring in the same family and accompanied by general imperfections of development. Ophthal. Rev., *2*:32, 1866.

Lawton, N. F., Ekins, R. P., and Nabarro, J. D. N.: Failure of pituitary response to thyrotrophin-releasing hormone in euthyroid Graves' disease. Lancet, *II*:14, 1971.

Lee, P. F., and Field, R.: Hypophyseal stalk section and intraocular pressure. Amer. J. Ophthal., *62*:11, 1966.

Lessell, S., and Forbes, A. P.: Eye signs in Turner's syndrome. Arch. Ophthal., *76*:211, 1966.

Linnér, E., and Wistrand, P.: Adrenal cortex and aqueous humour dynamics. Exp. Eye Res., *2*:148, 1963.

Lubow, M., and Makley, T. A., Jr.: Pseudopapilledema of juvenile diabetes mellitus. Arch. Ophthal., *85*:417, 1971.

Lundbaek, K., Christensen, N. J., Jensen, V. A., Johansen, K., Olsen, T. S., Hansen, A. P., Ørskov, H., and Østerby, R.: Diabetes, diabetic angiopathy, and growth hormone. Lancet, *II*:131, 1970.

Martin, B., and Jay, B.: Use of guanethidine eye drops in dysthyroid lid retraction. Proc. Roy. Soc. Med., *62*:18, 1962.

Martinez-Rovira, G. R.: Xanthelasma in association with hyperthyroidism. J.A.M.A., *206*:1081, 1968.

Mason, R. E., and Walsh, F. B.: Exophthalmos in hypothyroidism due to Hashimoto's thyroiditis. Bull. Johns Hopkins Hosp., *112*:323, 1963.

Mauntner, W.: Hämodialysebehandlung und Verän-derungen am vorderen und mittleren Augenabschnitt. Klin. Mbl. Augenheilk., *160*:350, 1972.

Mazzantini, L., and Ioli Spada, G.: Electroretinogram in patients with the Laurence-Moon-Bardet-Biedl syndrome. Bull. Oculist, *43*:786, 1964.

Mertz, D. P., and Stelzer, M.: Zur pathogenetischen Bedeutung hypophysärer Faktoren bei der endokrinen Ophthalmopathie. Deutsch. Med. Wschr., *1*:27, 1969.

Michaelson, E. D., and Young, R. L.: Hypothyroidism with Graves' disease. J.A.M.A., *211*:1351, 1970.

Mooney, A.: Perimetry and angiography in the diagnosis of lesions in the pituitary region. Trans. Ophthal. Soc. U. K., *72*:49, 1952.

Nelson, W. E.: Diabetes mellitus. *In* Nelson, W. E., Vaughn, V. C., and McKay, R. J. (Eds.): Textbook of Pediatrics. 9th ed. Philadelphia, W. B. Saunders Co., 1969, p. 1155.

Nelson, W. E., Vaughan, V. C., and McKay, R. J. (Eds.): Textbook of Pediatrics. 9th ed. Philadelphia, W. B. Saunders Co., 1969, p. 1285.

Neuner, H. P., and Dardenne, U.: Augenveränderungen bei Cushing-Syndrom. Klin. Mbl. Augenheilk., *152*:570, 1968.

Norton, E. W. D., and Gutman, F.: Diabetic retinopathy studied by fluorescein angiography. Ophthalmologica, *150*:5, 1965.

Norton, H.: Photographic analysis of the retinopathy accompanying adrenal pheochromocytoma. Amer. J. Ophthal., *57*:967, 1964.

Ornsteen, A. M.: Contribution to pathogenesis and heredity of Laurence-Biedl syndrome (dystrophia adiposogenitalis, retinitis pigmentosa, mental deficiency, and polydactylism). Report of three cases in one family. Amer. J. Med. Sci., *183*:256, 1932.

Pearson, O., Kaufman, B., and Brodkey, J.: Treatment of acromegaly. New Eng. J. Med., *283*:999, 1970.

Podos, S., Krupin, T., and Becker, B.: Effect of small-dose hyperosmotic injections on intraocular pressure of small animals and man when optic nerves are transected and intact. Amer. J. Ophthal., *71*:898, 1971.

Pohjola, S.: Ocular manifestations of idiopathic hypoparathyroidism. Case report and review of literature. Acta Ophthal., *40*:255, 1962.

Pohjola, S.: Unilateral exophthalmos with special reference to endocrine exophthalmos and pseudotumor. Acta Ophthal., *42*:456, 1964.

Poole, A.: Pheochromocytoma. Med. J. Aust., *2*:373, 1964.

Radnot, M.: Endocrine manifestations in ophthalmology. Budapest, Kultsura Publ. Dept., 1961, p. 1.

Raisz, L.: Current concepts: The diagnosis of hyperparathyroidism (or what to do until the immunoassay comes). New Eng. J. Med., *285*:1006, 1971.

Rasmussen, H.: Organization and control of the endocrine system. *In* Williams, R. (Ed.): Textbook of Endocrinology. 4th ed. Philadelphia, W. B. Saunders Co., 1968.

Richardson, J., and Walsh, M.: Uveal effusion as a sign of myxoedema. Brit. J. Ophthal., *53*:557, 1969.

Rosen, E.: The anterior reduplication sign in the diabetic lens. An. Inst. Barraquer, *9*:85, 1969.

Rosen, E., and Lyons, D.: Microhemangiomas at the pupillary border. Demonstrated by fluorescein photography. Amer. J. Ophthal., *67*:846, 1969.

Rovit, R., and Duane, T.: Eye signs in patients with

Cushing's syndrome and pituitary tumors. Arch. Ophthal., *49*:512, 1968.

Royer, J., and Genin, M.: Anomalies du segment antérieur et anomalies congénitales somatiques (présentation de cas cliniques). Bull. Soc. Ophtal. Fr., *63*:235, 1963.

Rubey, F.: Fundusveränderungen bei Phäochromozytom. Klin. Mbl. Augenheilk., *155*:860, 1969.

Safir, A., Paulsen, E. P., and Klayman, J.: Elevated intraocular pressure in diabetic children. Diabetes, *13*:161, 1964.

Safir, A., and Rogers, S. H.: Ocular effects of juvenile-onset diabetes. Amer. J. Ophthal., *69*:387, 1970.

Schlezinger, N., and Thompson, R. A.: Pituitary tumors with central scotomas simulating retrobulbar optic neuritis. Neurology, *17*:782, 1967.

Schulman, J. D., and Crawford, J. D.: Congenital nystagmus and hypothyroidism. New Eng. J. Med., *280*:708, 1969.

Sellers, E. A., Awad, A. G., and Schönbaum, E.: Long-acting thyroid stimulator in Graves' disease. Lancet, *II*:335, 1970.

Sisson, J. C., et al.: Myotonia of the orbicularis oculi with myxoedema. Arch. Intern. Med., *110*:323, 1962.

Soler Sala, J. M., and Santalo, R. M.: Consideraciones sobre el diagnostico de la retinopatia diabetica en la infancia. Arch. Soc. Oftal. Hisp. Amer., *29*:794, 1969.

Spaeth, G. L.: Comments on Berlyne, G. M., et al. in Survey Ophthal., in press.

Spaeth, G.: Ophthalmic and radiologic signs in acromegaly: their relative value in diagnosis and management. In preparation.

Spaeth, G., and Vacharat, N.: Provocative tests and chronic simple glaucoma. I. Effect of atropine on the water-drinking test: intimations of central regulatory control. II. Fluorescein angiography provocative test: a new approach to separation of the normal from the pathological. Brit. J. Ophthal., *56*:205, 1972.

Stelzer, M., Mertz, D. P., and Heinzmann, M.: Exophthalmotroper Faktor (EPF) und Thyreotropes Hormon (TSH) bei endemischem euthyreotem Jodmangelkropf. Schweitz. Med. Wschr., *99*:73, 1969.

Szabo, A. J.: Relationship of diabetic retinopathy to blood-sugar. Lancet, *I*:1402, 1970.

Thomas, R.: Neurohumeral factors in experimental glaucoma. Amer. J. Ophthal., *65*:729, 1968.

Thomas, C., Cordier, J., and Reny, A.: Les manifestations ophtalmologiques du syndrome de Turner. Arch. Ophtal. (Paris), *29*:565, 1969.

Traisman, H. S., Alfano, J. E., Andrews, J., and Gatti, R.: Intraocular pressure in juvenile diabetics. Amer. J. Ophthal., *64*:1149, 1967.

Turner, H. H.: A syndrome of infantilism, congenital webbed neck, and cubitus valgus. Endocrinology, *23*:566, 1938.

von Bahr, G.: Studies on the etiology and pathogenesis of cataract zonularis. Acta Ophthal., Suppl. II, 1936.

von Sallmann, L.: The role of the central nervous system in the regulation of the intraocular pressure. Doc. Ophthal., *13*:93, 1959.

von Weinstein, P.: Moderne Anschauung des Glaukomproblems. Klin. Monatbl. Augenheilk., *142*:642, 1963.

Walsh, F. B.: Papilledema associated with increased intracranial pressure in Addison's disease. Arch. Ophthal., *47*:86, 1952.

Walsh, F. B.: Clinical Neuro-ophthalmology. 2nd ed. Baltimore, Williams and Wilkins Co., 1957, p. 643.

Warkany, J., and DiGeorge, A. M.: The endocrine system. In Nelson, W. E., Vaughan, V. C., and McKay, R. J. (Eds.): Textbook of Pediatrics. 6th ed. Philadelphia, W. B. Saunders Co., 1957, p. 1230.

Werner, S. C.: Classification of the eye changes of Graves' disease. J. Clin. Endocr., *29*:982, 1969.

Wilkins, L.: The diagnosis and treatment of endocrine disorders in childhood and adolescence. 3rd ed. Springfield, Illinois, Charles C. Thomas, 1965, p. 141.

Wilkins, L.: The diagnosis and treatment of endocrine disorders in childhood and adolescence. 3rd ed. Springfield, Illinois, Charles C. Thomas, 1965, p. 445.

Wimer, B. M., and Bunao, R.: Case report of the association of exophthalmos and Addison's disease. Guthrie Clin. Bull. (Sayre), *30*:66, 1961.

Young, L. A.: Carcinoid syndrome—ocular manifestations. J. Natl. Med. Assoc., *60*:8, 1968.

B. OCULAR MANIFESTATIONS IN DISORDERS OF THE BLOOD, BLOOD VESSELS, HEART, AND LUNGS, AND IN THE HISTIOCYTOSIS SYNDROMES

Joseph Calhoun, M.D.

LEUKEMIA

The retinopathy that occurs with the various forms of leukemia has been recognized since the middle of the 19th century. It is not surprising, therefore, that many observations have been made of the fundus lesions in this disease.

Briefly, leukemias are classified into two broad categories—acute and chronic—depending on the course. In addition, these two major divisions are further divided according to the predominant leukocyte type involved. In children, over 95 per cent of leukemias are of the acute lymphocytic type.

Leukemia is capable of involving all structures of the eye, with the exception of the lens and cornea. The disease produces iritis and hypopyon if the neoplastic involvement is in the anterior part of the eye. Heterochromia accompanies the iritis, the lighter-colored iris being on the side of the iritis, but this difference disappears as the iritis is treated. Occasionally, a nodular thickening of the iris can be seen along with iritis, and this probably represents an infiltration of the iris with leukocytes.

Leukemia occasionally presents with proptosis secondary to the orbital mass that may be associated with leukemia. This is said to be more common in children than in adults with leukemia.

The retinopathy of leukemia occurs in a variety of forms, either singly or in combination. Retinal hemorrhages are the most frequent abnormality noted and may assume different formations, depending upon the exact position of the extravasation. The location and therefore the appearance of the hemorrhage have no diagnostic significance. The various sites of bleeding and the clinical appearance are as shown in the table at right.

White centers in the retinal hemorrhages or white lesions adjacent to and part of the hemorrhage may be seen. These white centers are not diagnostic for leukemias but can be seen in other blood diseases. The white component of the hemorrhage is due either to an infiltration with leukemic cells or degeneration of the nerve fibers (Fig. 20–6).

Retinal hemorrhages are usually more frequent in the posterior pole of the eye.

Site of Hemorrhage	Clinical Appearance
Nerve fiber layer	Red, serrated edges
Deeper retinal layers	Small or moderate size, red, round, smooth borders
Subretinal	Round, larger than above, smooth borders
Between vitreous and retina	Large, red, covers retinal vessels, red cells may settle out
In vitreous	Dark spots or irregular clumps, size varies from single cells to masses of cells

Their relation to the clinical course is not a consistent one. There is no correlation between the presence or degree of retinopathy and the prognosis or the course of the leukemic disease. The presence of hemorrhage does not have diagnostic significance, either for the type of leukemia or for the diagnosis of leukemia itself. A similar picture may appear in a wide variety of hematologic disorders. The presence of retinal hemorrhages seems to be related to the degree of anemia, thrombocytopenia, and the number of circulating immature cells. It does not seem to be related to the total white blood cell count.

In addition to the more commonly observed hemorrhagic phenomena, retinal exudates also may be part of the retinopathy of leukemia. They may be either the soft cotton-wool or the hard waxy type. Their presence seems to be related to the

Figure 20–6 Retinopathy in leukemia. There are superficial or flame-shaped hemorrhages with serrated borders temporal to the disc. Nasal to the disc is a large preretinal or subhyaloid hemorrhage obscuring the view of the retinal vessels. Some of the hemorrhages have white centers.

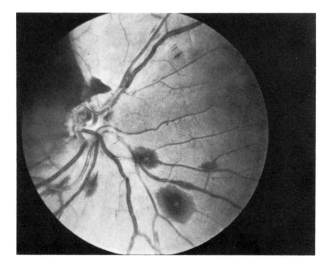

degree of accompanying anemia, usually when the hemoglobin is below 6 to 7 grams per 100 cc. They are not at all characteristic of leukemia but are similar to exudates found in anemia or vascular disease of any cause.

Dilated and tortuous retinal blood vessels are frequently observed in leukemia, but their occurrence is not as marked as the retinal vascular changes in primary or secondary polycythemia. Perivascular sheathing is infrequent. In the absence of any ocular signs of inflammation or evidence of hemoglobinopathy, this uncommon finding is said to be highly suggestive of leukemia and is probably a result of perivascular leukemic infiltrates.

Histologically, the choroid is the ocular structure most frequently involved in leukemia. There is a leukemic infiltration between the vessels, especially the inner layers, which is more extensive in the posterior part of the choroid and gradually fades anteriorly, causing a thickening of the entire choroidal layer. However, the involvement is diffuse, not focal, thereby explaining why choroidal infiltration is rarely appreciated clinically.

Involvement of the central nervous system during the course of the leukemia is a frequent occurrence. This may take one of three forms: (1) leukemic infiltrations of the meninges or brain, (2) intracranial hemorrhage, or (3) infections. The first is the most common of the three and usually presents with symptoms and signs of increased intracranial pressure or meningeal irritation.

Papilledema is usually present. Lumbar puncture is safe and usually reveals increased pressure together with an increased cell count (blasts). Typically, patients with this process are in a hematologic remission, suggesting that the antileukemic agent may not have crossed the blood-brain barrier in a sufficient concentration to prevent proliferation of leukemia cells in the meninges.

Intracranial hemorrhage, the second most common neurologic involvement, usually occurs late in the disease and is accompanied by thrombocytopenia and a rising white cell count. It usually occurs rather suddenly, with a rapid deterioration of the patient's condition. Recovery is uncommon.

Because of the impaired immunity resulting from both the disease and the therapy, it is not surprising that some of the patients develop superimposed infections of the central nervous system, either diffuse or focal. The diagnosis and treatment are similar to those for patients without leukemia.

ANEMIA

Despite the variety of etiologies of anemias in childhood, the retinal picture is remarkably similar in all. Because of the wide variation in the normal choroidal and retinal pigmentation of the fundus, the diagnosis of anemia by color of the fundus alone is unreliable. However, when the anemia is severe enough, there may be a detectable loss of color in the vessel. In the more severe anemias the size of the vessels increases, and the ratio of the size of the arterioles to that of the venules approaches 1:1.

As in leukemia, if the decrease in circulating red blood cells is severe enough, there may be scattered hemorrhages and exudates. These have no special diagnostic significance.

Hemolytic anemia may occur in persons with a hereditary deficiency of erythrocyte glucose-6-phosphate dehydrogenase after exposure to certain drugs, chemicals, and foods. Fava beans may cause a fulminating hemolytic anemia with severe visual loss in some cases. The visual loss occurs as a result of intraocular bleeding or some apparent retrobulbar process of obscure mechanism. An interesting although rare condition involving the hematopoietic system is the Chediak-Higashi syndrome, which is an autosomal recessive disorder of the blood and pigmentary system that usually results in death by age 10. Photophobia is a common symptom and is related to the pigmentary deficiency occurring in the uveal tract. The tendency toward albinism may also be observed in the skin and hair, and there is an intolerance to ultraviolet light. The disease is characterized by the presence of anemia, neutropenia and thrombocytopenia, and giant, greenish-brown cytoplasmic inclusions in the leukocytes, which represent large, abnormal lysosomes. There is an increased susceptibility to infection that leads to pyoderma, sinusitis, and pneumonia. Lymphadenopathy, hepatomegaly, and splenomegaly occur late. A high incidence of lymphoreticular malignancy is seen.

HEMOGLOBINOPATHIES

Among the reported hemoglobinopathies, sickle cell disease containing S hemoglobin is most prevalent with respect to both incidence and ocular complications. The systemic investigations of abnormal hemoglobins was aided significantly by the discovery in 1949 by Pauling and his associates that normal hemoglobin (A) and hemoglobin S could be separated electrophoretically, based upon their different mobility in an electric field.

The globin portion of the hemoglobin molecule is composed of two different halves, each half containing two polypeptide chains of 141 and 146 amino acids per chain. Hemoglobin S and hemoglobin C are different from hemoglobin A only by the substitution of a single amino acid on one of two chains.

The heterozygous state, the sickle trait (SA hemoglobin), is found in about 8.0 per cent of the black population in the United States. The homozygous state or sickle cell disease (SS hemoglobin) occurs in about 1 in 400 or 0.25 per cent of blacks. The combination of hemoglobin S and C (SC disease) is much rarer, found in about 0.1 per cent of the black population.

In general the systemic manifestations are most severe in sickle cell disease, least severe or nonexistent in persons with the sickle trait, and intermediate in severity in SC disease. There are many ophthalmic alterations that may suggest the diagnosis.

The conjunctival sign of sickle disease is reported to be positive in nearly all symptomatic sickle hemoglobinopathies. Symptomatic sickle disease includes SS and SC patients. According to Paton, "The sign consists of multiple short comma-shaped or curlicued capillary segments which often are seemingly isolated from the vascular network, in that the afferent and efferent lumens have become devoid of blood. These transient sites of tightly clumped intravascular erythrocytes are found on the bulbar conjunctiva where it is covered by the lids. They are particularly prevalent (or may be exclusively found) toward the lower fornix." The abnormal segments will decrease in number or disappear from the continued heat of the slit lamp beam.

Ophthalmoscopic changes in patients with sickle hemoglobinopathy (SS, AS, SC, and thalassemia) are many and varied. The "sea-fan sign," when present, is probably characteristic of SC disease. This abnormality is a retinal neovascularization which projects into the vitreous. It was so named by Welch and Goldberg because of the similarity of appearance to the naturally occurring coral. In the eye, sea fans tend to occur between the equator and the ora serrata in any quadrant of the fundus. Surrounding these lesions is an avascular zone, best seen with fluorescein angiography. After intravenous fluorescein injection there is a large leakage of dye into the vitreous (Fig. 20–7). Vitreous hemorrhage, with its sequelae of gliosis, traction, and retinal detachment, is not uncommon in SC disease. In an attempt to forestall these complications, all these lesions should probably be photocoagulated. In the series studied by Welsh and Goldberg, typical sea fans were found in 59 per cent of their SC patients of all ages. Although it is not known at what age sea fans develop in SC disease, patients generally develop vitreous hemorrhage from the sea fans when young or middle-aged adults.

A typical finding in patients with sickle cell disease is the "black sunburst sign," which has been reported to occur with a high incidence in patients suffering from sickle cell (SS) disease. It may be described as a round, darkly pigmented lesion, with serrated or feathery edges, about 1 or 2 disc diameters in size. It is usually located in the mid-periphery or equatorial region. There is an arteriolar feeder vessel leading to the the "black sunburst" peripheral to which the vessel appears occluded. This lesion is found in many SS patients, occasionally in SC patients, and rarely in patients with sickle trait. This sign is therefore highly suggestive of sickle cell disease. As first suggested by Welch and Goldberg, the "black sunburst" may be secondary to an arteriolar infarct. The vascular insult in those patients that develop a "sea fan" may be more

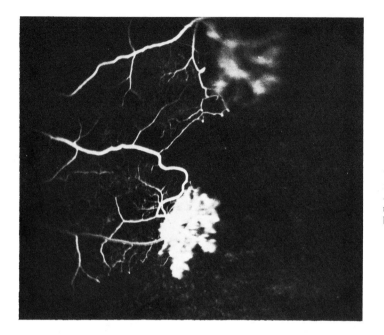

Figure 20–7   By fluorescein angiography the highly vascular nature of the "sea fan" is well shown. Later photographs will show the dye leaking into the vitreous. (From the Retina Service, Wills Eye Hospital; through the courtesy of Dr. Richard Goldberg.)

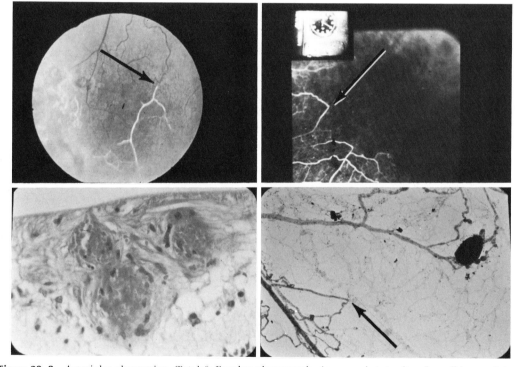

Figure 20–8   Arteriolar obstruction. *Top left*, Fundus photograph. Arrow points to site of possible arteriolar obstruction. White cordlike vessels suggest obstruction. *Top right*, Fluorescein angiogram. Avascular area is distal to the obstruction (arrow). *Bottom left*, Histopathology of retina. The retinal vessels are obstructed by compact sickle erythrocytes within the lumen. *Bottom right*, Trypsin digestion of retina. Distal to abrupt arteriolar obstruction (arrow) the retinal vessels appear acellular. Tortuosity, beading, and microaneurysm of the retinal vessels are adjacent to the acellular capillary bed. (Courtesy of Dr. N. Romayananda, Dr. M. Goldberg, and Dr. R. Green.)

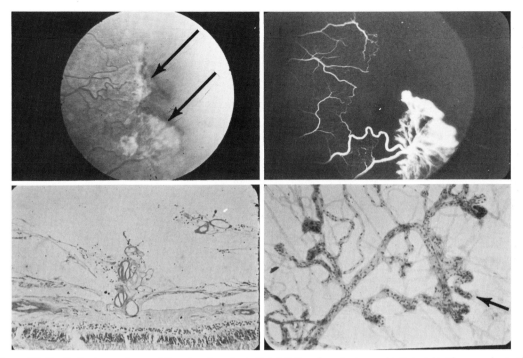

Figure 20–9   Retinal vascular proliferation (sea fan). *Top left,* Fundus photograph. *Top right,* Fluorescein angiogram. *Bottom left,* Histopathology. Proliferation of the retinal vessels extends through the internal limiting membrane into the vitreous cavity. *Bottom right,* Trypsin digestion of retina. Multiple buds of new vessels (arrow) are within acellular capillary bed. (Courtesy of Dr. N. Romayananda, Dr. M. Goldberg, and Dr. R. Green.)

distal, in the capillary bed, thereby stimulating vasoproliferative regeneration from the remaining uninvolved patent capillaries.

There are other fundus changes that occur with about equal frequency in both SC and SS disease, so that they have no differential diagnostic significance. Venous tortuosity is common in either SC or sickle cell disease.

Small yellow or gold, glistening refractile bodies (iridescent deposits) may be found in the peripheral fundus in both sickle cell and SC patients. Their presence in asymptomatic SC disease, even in patients as young as 5 years old, has been emphasized by Levine and Kaplan.

Lesions that have the configuration of the sunburst but are not darkly pigmented and not at the end of an arteriolar feeder vessel are found in either SC or SS disease. Obliteration of the terminal arterioles and venules is frequent in both diseases. In addition to the typical "sea fan," nonspecific neovascularization is found in both SC and sickle cell disease (Figs. 20-8 and 20-9).

According to the study of Romayananda,

Goldberg, and Green, vascular occlusion in the retina appears to be the primary event leading to the development of sickle retinopathy. Histopathologic evidence confirms previous clinical opinion that arteriolar occlusion is followed, in sequence, by arteriolar-venule anastomosis, neovascularization, vitreous hemorrhage, fibrosis and traction, retinal hole formation, and retinal detachment. Preretinal, intraretinal, and subretinal hemorrhages are followed by the development of iridescent deposits and black sunburst lesions in the fundus. Hemosiderosis bulbi was commonly observed in their study (Figs. 20-10 and 20-11).

Angioid streaks have also been found in patients with sickle cell disease. Even in patients with sickle cell trait there may be found in the retina the various abnormalities that are found in SS and SC patients. The incidence, however, is much lower. It can be seen that careful slit lamp and ophthalmoscopic examination may reveal important clues about the presence and occasionally the type of hemoglobinopathy (Table 20-30).

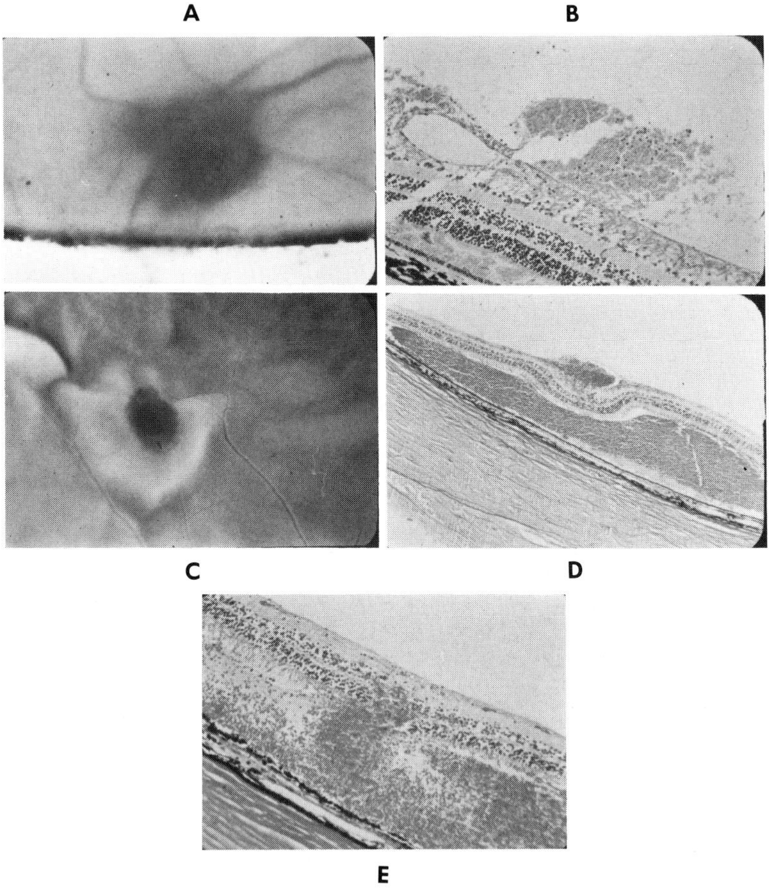

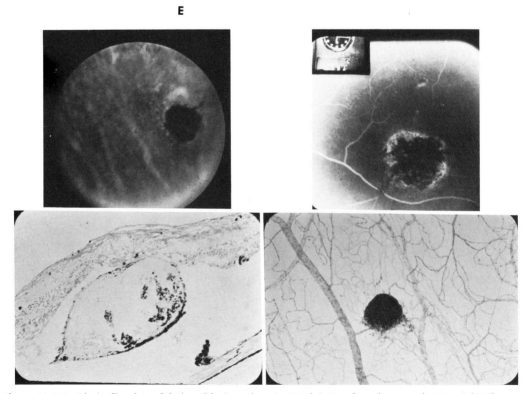

A

B

C

D

E

Figure 20–10 Various types of retinal hemorrhages.

A, Gross specimen. Retinal hemorrhage.

B, Section through the lesion *(A)*. The hemorrhage is superficial to the retina and erupts into the vitreous cavity.

C, Gross specimen. Retinal hemorrhage.

D, Section through the lesion *(C)*. Hemorrhage is superficial to the retina and is localized by the intact internal limiting membrane. The retina is detached by a large subretinal hemorrhage.

E, Section through another level of the lesion *(C)*. Blood in the deeper layers of the retina erupts into the subretinal space. (Courtesy of Dr. N. Romayananda, Dr. M. Goldberg, and Dr. R. Green.)

Figure 20–11 Black disc-shaped lesion (black sunburst). *Top left*, Fundus photograph. *Top right*, Fluorescein angiogram. *Bottom left*, Histopathology of the retina. *Bottom right*, Trypsin digestion of the retina. (Courtesy of Dr. N. Romayananda, Dr. M. Goldberg, and Dr. R. Green.)

TABLE 20–30 RETINAL FINDINGS IN SICKLE HEMOGLOBINOPATHIES

Associated with Increased Viscosity
    Vascular tortuosity
    Central retinal artery occlusion
    Central retinal vein occlusion
    Retinal hemorrhage

Associated with Peripheral Arteriolar Disease
    Peripheral arteriolar occlusion
    Peripheral arteriovenous anastomoses
    Neovascular proliferation
    Vitreous hemorrhage
    Pre-retinal fibrosis
    Retinal holes
    Retinal detachment
    Retinal hemorrhage

Associated with Antecedent Hemorrhage
    Refractile iridescent patches
    Disc-shaped lesions
        Tan—"Salmon patch"
        Black—"Black sunburst"

VASCULAR DISORDERS

Occasionally the detailed examination of the blood vessels of the conjunctiva may reveal clues to the diagnosis of a systemic disease. Mention has already been made of the reliability of the conjunctival signs of Paton in patients with symptomatic sickle hemoglobinopathies.

Ataxia telangiectasia is an autosomal recessive disease characterized by progressive cerebellar ataxia, telangiectasias of the skin and conjunctiva, and recurrent infections of the respiratory tract. The telangiectasias of the bulbar conjunctiva usually develop at 3 to 7 years of age, several years after the ataxia has first manifested itself. The telangiectasias are large, tortuous vessels of the exposed bulbar conjunctiva, most prominent in the canthal area (Fig. 20-12). There is also an ocular motor disturbance consisting of inability to perform voluntary gaze movements in addition to the nystagmus and disturbance in the opticokinetic response. Quite commonly there is an immunologic defect as evidenced by a low level or absence of IgA globulin in the serum, recurrent infections, and defective thymus tissue at autopsy. Death occurs frequently in the second decade from either a sinopulmonary infection or a lymphoreticular malignant condition.

Hereditary hemorrhagic telangiectasia (Rendu-Osler-Weber disease) is characterized by multiple telangiectasias of the skin, especially of the head and arms, and of the mucous membranes. The conjunctival involvement is usually on the palpebral surface, more rarely on the bulbar side. The disease is transmitted as an autosomal dominant disease. Symptoms, usually of hemorrhage from the nose or the gastrointestinal tract, typically begin in middle age. The telangiectasia may be seen, however, at any time of life.

Pulseless disease (Takayasu's syndrome) occurs predominantly in young girls during puberty and up to age 20. It is an arteritis that affects primarily the aortic arch area and its branches. Transient blurring

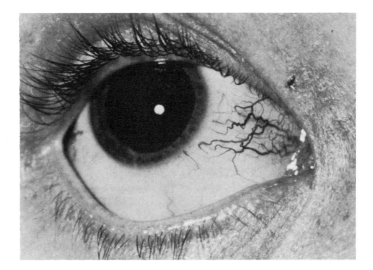

Figure 20–12 Telangiectasias of the bulbar conjunctiva in ataxia telangiectasia. (Courtesy of Dr. R. D. Harley.)

or complete visual loss in one or both eyes as a result of carotid insufficiency is the most constant symptom. Neurologic symptoms include paresthesias of the arms after exercise, syncope, transient paresis, vertigo, and headache. Late changes from chronically reduced ocular blood flow include retinal neovascularization, cataract, vitreous hemorrhage, and hypotony.

HEMORRHAGIC DISORDERS

Hemorrhagic disorders in childhood may be divided into three large groups, depending on the etiologic mechanism: (1) coagulation defects which include the various hemophilias; (2) thrombocytopenic purpuras; (3) nonthrombocytopenic purpuras which include anaphylactoid purpura or the Henoch-Schönlein syndrome.

In the bleeding disorders secondary to coagulation defects, soft tissue bleeding is the rule. Ocular complications are uncommon. There may be peri- or intraorbital or intraocular hemorrhage following minor trauma. Spontaneous ocular or retinal hemorrhages are rare. Occasionally visual loss may result from uncontrolled intraorbital hemorrhage, with resultant pressure on the optic nerve. Retinal hemorrhages in nonspecific patterns are not uncommon in thrombocytopenia from any cause. Much more common are the purpuric lesions in more dependent parts of the body.

Henoch-Schönlein purpura may present to the ophthalmologist as painful facial, scalp, or periorbital edema, typically in a young child. The proper diagnosis can be suggested by the accompanying purpuric skin rash concentrated on the lower extremities, joint pain, abdominal pain with or without melena, or hematuria. If the edema is painful, systemic steroids usually give prompt relief.

HYPERTENSION

Hypertension in children is considerably less common than in adults. In children, hypertension is usually secondary to another disease process and is rarely "essential" or idiopathic. The primary disease is commonly renal. Other causes may be coarcta-

tion of the aorta or an endocrine abnormality such as pheochromocytoma or Cushing's syndrome. The differential diagnosis is complex and outside the scope of this chapter, but it has been reviewed recently by Loggie.

An ophthalmoscopic evaluation of the retinal vascular changes should help to determine the degree of the hypertension as reflected in the retinal arterioles and aid in judging the extent of the arteriolar sclerosis which reflects the permanent vascular damage induced by the hypertension. Although there may be other causes of sclerosis, especially in the adult, the retinal changes are a good indication of the nature of the arteriolar changes throughout the rest of the body. Arteriolar sclerosis is dependent upon the degree of hypertension and its duration. A milder hypertension will require a longer time to produce a given degree of arteriolar sclerosis than will a more marked hypertension.

These changes can be classified as suggested by Kirkendall and Armstrong, modified slightly from that classification first proposed by Keith, Wagener, and Barker and later by Scheie.

Since the hypertensive process in children is often severe, symptoms occur rather early in its course, and the opthalmoscopic changes tend to be different from the retinovascular changes of the hypertensive adult. Frequently the short duration of the disease prior to ophthalmic evaluation precludes the development of

CLASSIFICATION OF RETINAL VASCULAR CHANGES

Grade	Arteriolar Sclerosis	Hypertension
O	None	None
I	Thickening of vessels with slight depression of veins of A-V crossing	Narrowing in terminal branches
II	Definite A-V crossing changes and moderate local sclerosis	Narrowing general and severe, with local constriction
III	Invisibility of veins beneath arteriole and severe local sclerosis with segmentation	Plus hemorrhages and exudates
IV	Plus venous obstruction and arteriolar obliteration	Plus papilledema

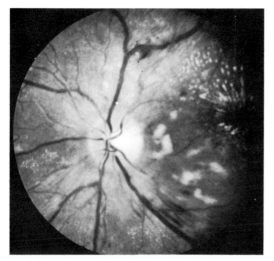

Figure 20–13 Hypertensive retinopathy with narrow arterioles, exudates, and edema radiating out from the macula, the so-called macular star figure.

many of the changes of arteriolar sclerosis. Instead, the picture is frequently one of focal and diffuse constriction of the arterioles, with hemorrhages and exudates in the more severe cases (Fig. 20-13). In mild cases, early hypertensive changes are best seen in the retinal vessels nasal to the disc.

Sometimes, in children with severe hypertension, extensive retinal edema develops which may culminate in retinal detachment. The retinal detachment is similar in appearance to other secondary detachments in that it is smooth and bullous, with an absence of retinal holes or breaks, a shifting subretinal fluid with change of position, and no extension to the ora serrata. If the primary hypertensive disease can be corrected, the retina reattaches spontaneously.

In patients with chronic renal disease the retinopathy may be reversed by a transiently or permanently successful renal transplant. The retinal hemorrhages usually fade away rather quickly after transplant, but cotton-wool patches tend to remain for several weeks. Hard waxy exudates, arteriolar narrowing, and crossing defects generally persist for a much longer time, if not indefinitely. Macular edema, one of the causes of reduced vision in chronic renal disease, can be expected to improve within several weeks following a successful renal transplant.

Children with hypertension may present first to the ophthalmologist because of either unexplained headaches or visual loss. There are many children whose chief complaint is headaches who seek aid from an ophthalmologist. Blood pressure should be determined in these children as a routine part of the examination. In a small, but very rewarding, number of cases, otherwise occult hypertension will be detected and appropriate referral may then be made.

Visual loss in hypertension may either be a result of the ocular involvement by the hypertensive process or by a cerebral mechanism. In the former group, retinal hemorrhage, exudate, edema, or detachment affecting the macular area can be seen ophthalmoscopically and may correlate reasonably well with the visual loss. There remains a small group of hypertensive children in whom visual loss is often severe, yet the retinal changes are not of great enough degree to account for the poor vision. These patients may or may not also manifest signs of encephalopathy such as lethargy, irritability, and headaches. Presumably,cerebral ischemia secondary to the vasospasm involves the optic radiations resulting in a cortical blindness. The visual impairment resolves along with the hypertension.

Occasionally a hypertensive child under treatment with hydralazine hydrochloride (Apresoline) may complain of blurred vision for no apparent reason. This results from a drug-induced paresis of accommodation that converts an otherwise symptomless facultative hyperopia into absolute hyperopia.

CARDIOVASCULAR DISEASE

The diagnosis of certain diseases primarily affecting the heart and great vessels may be suggested by careful ocular examination. Among these defects with ocular signs is *coarctation of the aorta*.

Ophthalmoscopic examination reveals in a significant portion of the cases the rather unique and characteristic findings of corkscrew tortuosity and serpentine pulsation of the arterioles. The tortuosity is unlike the tortuosity often seen as an anomaly in otherwise normal individuals, affecting arteries more than veins. In the tortuosity associated with coarctation, vessels spiral or corkscrew in three dimensions, unlike the flat, two-dimensional tortuous vascular course in the benign anomalous condition (Fig. 20-14). In addition to the peculiar tortuosity there are usually serpentine pulsations. This is manifested by a small lateral shift in the vessel course or by a slight straightening of one of the curves in the vessel as a result of the pressure of the pulse.

In those congenital cardiac defects in children in which there is a right-to-left shunt, the resulting cyanosis may be reflected in the conjunctival and retinal vessels. The external appearance may suggest that of a mild conjunctivitis with darkened and congested vessels. The vessels in the retina may have a similar appearance superimposed on a cyanotic background from the darker blood in the choroid.

Subacute bacterial endocarditis (SBE) may often present a diagnostic problem, the solution to which may be aided by careful examination of the eyes. SBE is usually, if not always, superimposed on pre-existing disease of the cardiac valves. Occasionally the disease is rheumatic cardiovascular disease. Other more common nonrheumatic cardiac lesions are bicuspid aortic valves or aortic stenosis, patent ductus arteriosus, interventricular septal defects, and *tetralogy of Fallot* (Fig. 20-15). In addition to the small petechial hemorrhages in the conjunctiva, there may be

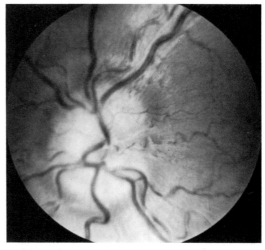

Figure 20–15   Tetralogy of Fallot. Vessels appear dilated, tortuous, and dark-colored, similar to polycythemia. Chronic low-grade papilledema is evident.

lesions in the retina that suggest the diagnosis. Usually the patients have no visual symptoms, but the ophthalmoscopic appearance is in striking contrast. There may be hemorrhages and, less often, exudates. The hemorrhages may be in any depth in the retina, and therefore vary in appearance. Frequently there is a white spot in the center of the hemorrhage, the typical "Roth spot." These white spots may appear without surrounding hemorrhage. Swelling and edema of the nerve head may also be found. The retinal arterial circulation may share in the embolization from the infected cardiac defect. Depending on the localization of the emboli, central or branch arterial occlusion may result.

Pathologically, the white areas in the retina appear to be cellular infiltration, especially in the inner layers. These infiltrations are more numerous histologically than clinically. The choroid is infiltrated extensively, chiefly between the vessels. This pathologic change in the choroid is usually not observed or appreciated clinically.

RETINAL VASCULAR OCCLUSION IN CHILDREN

by

HUNTER STOKES, M.D.

Clinical Assistant Professor of Ophthalmology, Medical University of South Carolina.

Clinical Picture

Occlusion of the central retinal artery in

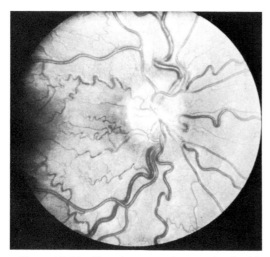

Figure 20–14   Vascular tortuosity associated with coarctation of the aorta. (Courtesy of Dr. R. D. Harley.)

children presents the same clinical picture as that seen in adults. The patient often reports a disturbance of vision in one eye that is painless and usually total. Examination reveals a level of vision in the range of 20/200 to hand motion, occasionally with no light perception. The pupil is usually fixed and dilated. The retina is pale and edematous, with the typical "cherry-red spot" in the macula. The arterioles (and often the venules) show partial collapse, narrowing obliteration, and the typical "box-car" effect owing to stasis of arterial circulation. The disc is usually normal in color and margins are flat. Depending on the cause of the arterial occlusions, obstructive particles lodged in the arterial system may be noted.

The occlusion of the central retinal vein in children also gives a clinical picture similar to that seen in adults, with one important difference. Since the etiology of venous occlusion in the retina in adults is almost always associated with an arteriosclerotic condition, arteriosclerotic retinopathy is a part of the clinical picture, particularly in the posterior pole beyond the area of acute involvement and at the site of arteriovenous crossings in branch occlusions. In children, arteriosclerotic changes are exceedingly rare. The patient with a central vein occlusion may report a sudden loss of vision but more often reports a gradual loss over several weeks, with remissions and exacerbations, and the visual acuity may often be in the range of 20/40 to 20/100, even with a fully developed clinical picture. The disc is elevated and its margins are blurred; the veins are engorged, tortuous and dilated, and surrounded by many hemorrhages. The hemorrhages are usually superficial and flame-shaped but may be deep and round. Preretinal and vitreous hemorrhages have been recorded. There is an absence of spontaneous venous pulsation on the disc.

Etiology

In adults, arteriosclerosis, hypertension, and diabetes mellitus are the most common etiologic considerations in retinal vascular occlusive disorders. These conditions are rarely encountered in children. The most common causes of arterial occlusions in the pediatric age group are included in Table 20–31. As can readily be noted, cardiovascular disorders of childhood must be considered in the etiologic evaluation of these patients. Cardiac disorders of children associated with retinal vascular occlusive phenomena include subacute bacterial endocarditis, mitral valve disease, and cardiac myxoma. Cardiac myxoma is quite uncommon but has been reported as a cause of retinal arterial occlusion in children. It is a potentially lethal condition which can often be surgically corrected if the diagnosis is made early.

Central retinal vein occlusions in children are quite rare and only a few systemic conditions can be incriminated as causative factors. Leukemia, sickle cell disease, and retinal vasculitis must be considered.

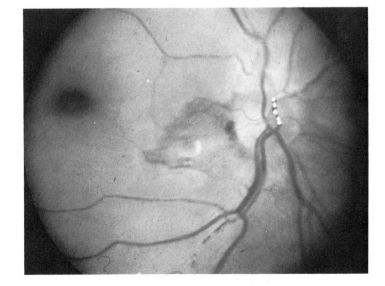

Figure 20–16 Mercury embolism and branch artery occlusion in a young patient. (Courtesy of Dr. Hunter Stokes.)

TABLE 20–31 DIFFERENTIAL DIAGNOSIS IN PRE-ADULT RETINAL ARTERIAL OCCLUSIONS

Diagnosis	Diagnostic Tests
1. Heart disease	
A. Rheumatic	
1. Mitral stenosis with atrial fibrillation	
2. Subacute bacterial endocarditis	
B. Congenital	
1. Secondary polycythemia	CBC with RBC count
C. Post-op open heart surgery	History of recent open heart surgery
2. Hematologic disorders	
A. Leukemia*	CBC with peripheral smear
B. Anemia, familial	CBC, hemoglobin electrophoresis
C. Sickle cell disease*	CBC, hemoglobin electrophoresis
3. Migraine	History, neuro-ophthalmologic exam
4. Arterial obliterative disorders	
A. Raynaud's disease	Bilateral, symmetrical cyanosis in hands; most often in females (ages 15 to 40)
B. Takayasu's disease	Loss of peripheral pulses
	Aorta contrast x-ray makes diagnosis
C. Periarteritis nodosa	Biopsy of skin or muscle
5. Contraceptive pill	History of taking the pill
6. Atrial myxoma	Arteriography of left atrium
	Differentiate from SBE and mitral stenosis
7. Carotid disease	Auscultation, ophthalmodynamometry, arteriogram
A. Congenital aneurysm	Palpation and auscultation of neck, carotid arteriogram, ODM
B. Premature arteriosclerosis	Neck soft-tissue, x-ray, carotid arteriogram, ODM
8. Nephritis with hypertensive attack	BP, urinalysis, BUN
9. Retinal vasculitis*	Clinical picture — retinal edema with hemorrhages — VA returns to normal
10. Dehydration	History, urinalysis, electrolytes

*Also a cause of venous occlusions.

Treatment

The primary responsibility in the care of retinal vascular occlusive disease in children remains with the pediatrician. As in adult retinal occlusive problems, the approach to treatment includes two considerations: (1) prompt attention, diagnosis and treatment of the underlying etiologic condition and (2) awareness of the grave prognosis for return of useful vision in eyes in which these vascular catastrophes have occurred. There is no evidence that the young retina tolerates the insult of a vascular occlusion better or worse than the eye of an older person.

PULMONARY DISEASES

Chronic and severe pulmonary disease may be reflected in changes in the appearance of the retina. In childhood, pulmonary disease of such magnitude is most commonly seen in patients with cystic fibrosis.

Cystic fibrosis is a disease of unknown etiology in which there is widespread dysfunction of all the mucous exocrine glands. The pulmonary involvement is the result of the abnormally thick and viscous secretion in the bronchi and bronchioles. These secretions create increased resistance to the outflow of air, producing an obstructive emphysema. Secondary infection and bronchiectasis aggravate the process.

The earliest recognizable changes on ophthalmoscopic examination are vascular tortuosity and engorgement, more prominent in the veins. As the degree and/or duration of the pulmonary insufficiency increases, the retinal picture may progress to scattered retinal hemorrhages, retinal edema, and edema of the disc (papilledema). These changes are reversible if the pulmonary function can be improved.

It is well known that increased carbon dioxide in the blood will increase cerebral blood flow. The retinal circulation shares in this augmentation. The increased flow is evident as dilation more in the veins than in the arteries, probably because of the thin walls and the lower pressure of the veins.

It has been shown clinically that the presence and degree of retinal changes correlate best with the severity and duration of the respiratory insufficiency, as reflected in chronic carbon dioxide retention. Patients with cystic fibrosis may manifest other ocular abnormalities in addition to those listed here due to chronic respiratory insufficiency.

The organisms most frequently encountered in patients with cystic fibrosis are *Pseudomonas aeruginosa* and *Staphylococcus aureus*. The control of these organisms may require long-term therapy with chloramphenicol when sensitivity testing indicates that the infecting organisms would be susceptible. In roughly one fourth of a series of patients receiving 30 to 60 mg. per kg. per day of chloramphenicol for several months, visual loss became evident. This visual loss was due to an optic neuritis that showed either edema of the nerve head (papillitis) or no abnormal fundus findings (retrobulbar neuritis). Central scotomas were found in those patients with visual loss. The course of optic neuritis is variable. Improvement in central vision may not occur even though chloramphenicol therapy is discontinued (Fig. 20–17). On the other hand, return to normal may occur in spite of the continuation of the drug. Furthermore, if visual improvement occurs when the drug is stopped, it may not deteriorate again even if chloram-

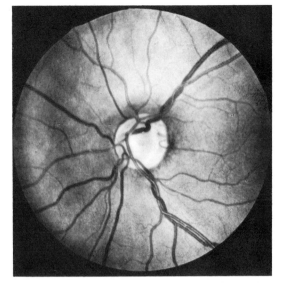

Figure 20–17 Optic atrophy following long-term use of chloramphenicol in a patient with cystic fibrosis. (Courtesy of Dr. R. D. Harley.)

phenicol must be reinstituted later at the same dosage. The role of vitamin therapy for the optic neuritis following chloramphenicol therapy is still undetermined. Optic neuritis has not been seen, however, in patients maintained on less than 30 mg. per kg. per day, suggesting a dose-related effect (Dr. N. N. Huang, personal communication).

It is evident that patients on long-term chloramphenicol therapy should have their visual acuity checked frequently by either the physician or the parents or both. If optic neuritis develops, chloramphenicol should be discontinued if medically possible and replaced with another antibiotic. A therapeutic trial of B vitamins is probably also warranted in the absence of any known specific therapy. The possible value of corticosteroids will have to be carefully weighed against their potential danger. Athough the evidence seems to point rather strongly to chloramphenicol as the significant factor in the causation of optic neuritis in these patients, it would seem wise to test the vision of all patients with cystic fibrosis being treated with antibiotics. Until the mechanism can be determined for the relationship between long-term chloramphenicol therapy for patients with cystic fibrosis and optic neuritis, it is possible that some entirely unrelated factor may be responsible for the optic nerve changes.

In addition to the optic neuritis and the retinal vascular abnormalities, patients with cystic fibrosis occasionally develop unilateral proptosis. It is well established by clinical and x-ray examination that cystic fibrosis patients have an extremely high incidence of sinus disease. A few of these patients are discovered to harbor a mucocele which, after eroding into the orbit, will produce an orbital mass or proptosis. Mucoceles are cysts lined with mucus-secreting respiratory epithelium. The mucocele in children characteristically involves the ethmoid sinus and at times the sphenoid sinus. If they arise from the ethmoid sinuses, the thin medial wall of the orbit will be eroded, producing lateral and forward displacement of the eyeball. Mucoceles from the frontal sinus in children are uncommon. Frontal sinuses normally do not develop to a significant degree until about 6 years of age. The mucocele in adults, however, usually involves the frontal sinus and typically produces a mass in the upper nasal quadrant.

If the mucocele in a patient with cystic fibrosis becomes large enough to produce symptoms, a deviation of the eyes, or a cosmetic deformity, it should be removed.

THE RETICULOENDOTHELIOSES

This category of diseases, also called the histiocytosis syndromes, represents a wide spectrum of clinical manifestations. All, however, are characterized histopathologically by granulomatous infiltrates in which histiocytes are a dominant finding. The etiology of this group of diseases is unknown but it does not appear to be familial or contagious. The histologic appearance does not suggest a neoplastic disease.

Portions of the clinical spectrum have been given the distinction of a separate name, but more recently the interrelationship of these apparently unrelated clinical pictures has been recognized. As a result of this awareness, the more inclusive terms "reticuloendothelioses" or "histiocytosis syndromes" have become more popular.

Single lesions in bone have been called eosinophilic granulomas. These lesions are radiographically lytic, are often painful, and commonly involve the skull, spine, pelvis, and legs. Occasionally there may be a lesion of the orbital bones, resulting in proptosis. Biopsy or curettage of isolated lesions should be undertaken unless the resulting cosmetic or functional defect would be too great. In such cases low doses of radiation should be utilized. Multiple bony lesions can be treated with irradiation and antimetabolites as symptoms warrant.

In addition to bone changes, the more extensive form of the disease includes moderate visceral, skin, and mucous membrane involvement. When diabetes insipidus and exophthalmos are present in patients of this group the term "Hand-

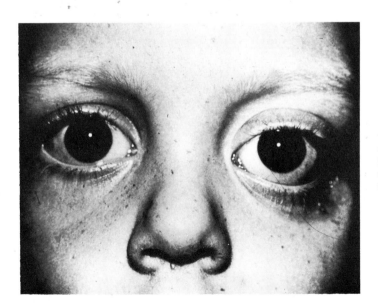

Figure 20–18 Reticuloendotheliosis. There are, in addition to the proptosis, visible skin lesions on the face. Combined with diabetes insipidus, this phase could be called the Hand-Schüller-Christian syndrome.

Schüller-Christian syndrome" could be applied (Fig. 20–18). This particular manifestation of the reticuloendothelioses is, however, uncommon.

The severe end of the spectrum may be called the Letterer-Siwe syndrome. The picture is typically seen in an infant with extensive involvement of the viscera, skin, mucous membrane, and medullary cavity of bone. Osseous lesions may not be evident radiographically. The course is rapidly progressive and generally fatal.

REFERENCES

Allen, D. M., Diamond, L. K., and Howell, D. A.: Anaphylactoid purpura in children (Schönlein-Henoch syndrome). J. Dis. Child., 99:834, 1960.

Allen, R. A., and Straatsma, B. R.: Ocular involvement in leukemia and allied disorders. Arch. Ophthal., 66:68, 1961.

Blattner, R. J.: Ophthalmic complications of favism. J. Pediat., 57:794, 1960.

Bruce, G. M., Benning, C. R., and Spalter, H. F.: Ocular findings in cystic fibrosis of the pancreas. Arch. Ophthal., 63:391, 1960.

Buchannan, W. S., and Ellis, P. P.: Retinal separation in chronic glomerulonephritis. Arch. Ophthal., 71:90, 1964.

Dienst, E. C., and Gartner, S.: Pathologic changes in the eye associated with subacute bacterial endocarditis. Arch. Ophthal., 31:198, 1944.

Duke-Elder, S., and Leigh, A. G.: Diseases of the outer eye. In Duke-Elder, S. (Ed.): System of Ophthalmology. Vol. 8, Part 1. St. Louis, The C. V. Mosby Co., 1965, p. 31.

Ellis, P. P., and Fonken, H. A.: Retinopathies of chronic glomerulonephritis. A study of cases treated with renal transplantation. Arch. Ophthal., 75:36, 1966.

Geeraets, W. J., and Guerry, D.: Angioid streaks and sickle-cell disease. Amer. J. Ophthal., 49:450, 1960.

Harley, R. D., Baird, H. W., and Craven, E. M.: Ataxia-telangiectasia. Report of seven cases. Arch. Ophthal., 77:582, 1967.

Harley, R. D., Huang, N. N., Macri, C. H., and Green, W. R.: Optic neuritis and optic atrophy following chloramphenicol in cystic fibrosis patients. Trans. Amer. Acad. Ophthal. Otolaryng., 74:1011, 1970.

Holt, J. M., and Gordon-Smith, E. C.: Retinal abnormalities in diseases of the blood. Brit. J. Ophthal., 53:145, 1969.

Huang, N. N., Harley, R. D., Promadhattevedi, V., and Sproul, A.: Visual disturbances in cystic fibrosis following chloramphenicol administration. J. Pediat., 68:32, 1966.

Judge, R. D., Currier, R. D., Graire, W. A., and Figley, M. M.: Takayasu's arteritis and the aortic arch syndrome. Amer. J. Med., 32:379, 1962.

Kearney, W. F.: Leukemic hypopyon. Amer. J. Ophthal., 59:495, 1965.

Keith, N. M., Wagener, H. P., and Barker, N. W.: Some different types of essential hypertension; their course and prognosis. Amer. J. Med. Sci., 197:332, 1939.

Kirkendall, W. M., and Armstrong, M. L.: Vascular changes in the eye in the treated and untreated patient with essential hypertension. Amer. J. Cardiol., 9:663, 1962.

Levine, R. A., and Kaplan, A. M:: The ophthalmoscopic findings in C + S disease. Amer. J. Ophthal., 59:37, 1965.

Lieberman, P. H., Jones, C. R., Dargeon, H. W. K., and Begg, C. F.: A reappraisal of eosinophilic granuloma of bone, Hand-Schueller-Christian syndrome and Letterer-Siwe disease. Medicine, 48:375, 1969.

Loggie, J. M. H.: Hypertension in children and adolescents. J. Pediat., 74:331, 1969.

Marshall, R. A.: A review of lesions in the optic fundus in various diseases of the blood. Blood, 7:882, 1959.

Mortada, A.: Orbital lymphoblastomas and acute leukemias in children. Amer. J. Ophthal., 55:327, 1963.

Oberman, H. A.: Idiopathic histiocytosis. A clinicopathologic study of 40 cases and review of the literature on eosinophilic granuloma of bone, Hand-Schueller-Christian disease and Letterer-Siwe disease. Pediatrics, 28:307, 1961.

Paton, D.: The conjunctival sign of sickle cell disease. Arch. Ophthal., 68:627, 1962.

Romayananda, N., Goldberg, M. F., and Green, W. R.: Histopathology of sickle cell retinopathy. Trans. Amer. Acad. Ophthal. Otolaryng. In press.

Rubenstein, R. A., Albert, D. M., and Scheie, H. G.: Ocular complications of hemophilia. Arch. Ophthal., 76:230, 1966.

Scheie, H. G.: Evaluation of ophthalmoscopic changes of hypertension and arteriolar sclerosis. Arch. Ophthal., 49:117, 1953.

Spalter, H. F., and Bruce, G. M.: Ocular changes in pulmonary insufficiency. Trans. Amer. Acad. Ophthal. Otolaryng., 68:661, 1964.

Stool, S., Kertesz, E., Sibinga, M., and Frayer, W.: Exophthalmos due to pyocele of the sinus in children with cystic fibrosis. Trans. Amer. Acad. Ophthal. Otolaryng., 70:811, 1966.

Walker, G. L., and Stanfield, T. F.: Retinal changes associated with coarctation of the aorta. Trans. Amer. Ophthal. Soc., 5:407, 1952.

Welch, R. B., and Goldberg, M. F.: Sickle-cell hemoglobin and its relation to fundus abnormality. Arch. Ophthal., 75:353, 1966.

Zimmerman, A., and Merigan, T. C.: Retrobulbar hemorrhage in a hemophiliac with irreversible loss of vision. Arch. Ophthal., 64:949, 1960.

Retinal Vascular Occlusion in Children

Brenneman, J., and McQuarrie, I.: Practice of Pediatrics. Vol. 4. Hagerstown, Md., W. F. Prior Co., 1970.

Caccamise, W. C., and Okuda, K.: Takayasu's or pulseless disease. Amer. J. Ophthal., 37:784, 1954.

Cohen, M.: Lesions of the fundus in polycythemia, report of cases. Arch. Ophthal., 17:811, 1937.

Delpech, A., Amabric, P., Bardenat, M., and Delpech, J.: Retinal arterial thrombosis and the pill. Rev. Med. Toulouse, 7:375, 1971.

Dienst, E. C., and Gartner, S.: Pathologic changes in the eye associated with subacute bacterial endocarditis. Report of 5 cases with autopsy. Arch. Ophthal., *31*:198, 1944.

Doherty, W. B., and Trubek, M.: Significant hemorrhagic retinal lesions in bacterial endocarditis (Roth's spots). J.A.M.A., *97*:308, 1931.

Dunphy, E. B.: Ocular manifestations of Raynaud's disease. Trans. Amer. Ophthal. Soc., *30*:420, 1932.

Friedenwald, J. S., and Rones, B.: Ocular lesions in septicemia. Arch. Ophthal., *5*:175, 1931.

Gilman, S.: Cerebral disorders after open-heart operations. New Eng. J. Med., *272*:489, 1965.

Goodwin, J. F.: Diagnosis of left atrial myxoma. Lancet, *1*:464, 1963.

Gronwall, A.: On changes in the fundus oculi and persisting injuries to the eye in migraine. Acta Ophthal. (Kobenhavn), *16*:602, 1938.

Hanno, H.: Teen-age central retinal arterial occlusion. Presented at Tenth Annual Clinical Conference of Wills Eye Hospital, 1958.

Hayashi, H.: Study of pulseless disease and typical aortitis. Jap. J. Clin. Ophthal., *25*:797, 1971.

Holt, L. B.: Pediatric Ophthalmology. Philadelphia, Lea and Febiger, 1964.

Hutchinson, E. C., and Stock, J. P. P.: Paroxysmal cerebral ischaemia in rheumatic heart disease. Lancet, *1*:653, 1963.

Lyle, T. K., and Wybar, K.: Retinal vasculitis. Brit. J. Ophthal., *45*:778, 1961.

McEntyre, J. M., Keates, E. U., and Whitely, W. H.: Retinal embolus from extracranial carotid artery aneurysm. Arch. Ophthal., *77*:317, 1967.

Nelson, W. E., Vaughan, V. C., and McKay, R. J. (Eds.): Textbook of Pediatrics. 9th ed. Philadelphia, W. B. Saunders Co., 1969.

Smith, J. L.: Ocular complications of rheumatic fever and rheumatoid arthritis. Amer. J. Ophthal., *43*:575, 1957.

Sugar, H. S., and Franzen, N. A.: Retinal vascular obliteration associated with familial anemia and mesoectodermal dysplasia. J. Pediat. Ophthal., *8*:126, 1971.

Sybers, H. O., and Booke, W. E.: Coronary and retinal embolism from left atrial myxoma. Arch. Path., *91*:179, 1971.

Tasman, W.: Retinal Diseases in Children. New York, Harper and Row, 1971.

Walsh, F. B., and Hoyt, W. F.: Clinical Neuro-ophthalmology. 3rd ed. Baltimore, Williams and Wilkins, 1969, 1181, 1629–1926.

Walter, J. R., and Burchfield, W. J.: Ocular migraine. J. Pediat. Ophthal., *8*:173, 1971.

Wood, P.: An appreciation of mitral stenosis. Part I. Clinical features. Part II. Investigations and results. Brit. J. Med., *1*:1051, 1113; 1954.

C. OCULAR MANIFESTATIONS IN CONNECTIVE TISSUE DISORDERS

The Mucopolysaccharidoses

Lois J. Martyn, M.D.

The conditions generically referred to as the mucopolysaccharidoses are genetically determined metabolic disorders characterized by excessive urinary excretion of acid mucopolysaccharides and abnormal tissue accumulation of mucopolysaccharide substances with a rather distinctive spectrum of clinical manifestations. Affecting primarily the connective tissues, these systemic disorders characteristically produce skeletal deformity with abnormalities in both the bones and joints and typical facies with coarse, often grotesque features that have been likened to those of a gargoyle. Visceromegaly, cardiac disease, respiratory problems, deafness, and mental deficiency occur in certain of these syndromes, and the principal ocular signs of the various mucopolysaccharidoses are progressive corneal clouding and retinal degeneration with attendant deterioration of vision.

Delineation of these conditions began with the clinical descriptions — particularly the classic reports by Hunter and by Hurler — that appeared in the early 1900s. Early pathologic studies showed the presence throughout the body of cells distended with large amounts of deposited material displaying metachromasia; the terms "clear cell" and "gargoyle cell" were applied. Subsequent studies demonstrated the presence of metachromatic granules (Reilly granulations) in circulating polymorphonuclear leukocytes and in bone marrow cells. Clarification of the biochemical nature of the syndromes was advanced in the 1950s by the isolation of specific mucopolysaccharides from tissue and urine of affected patients. By 1965 the presence of cytoplasmic metachromasia in cultured fibroblasts was reported. More recently, it has been shown that the cells in several of the mucopolysaccharidoses have a defect in degradation of mucopolysac-charides and that a diffusable factor produced by normal cells or by cells from different mucopolysaccharidoses corrects this metabolic defect in vitro.

At the present time, six major types of mucopolysaccharidoses can be identified on the basis of their clinical, genetic, and biochemical features. (For a summary, see Table 20–32 at the end of this section.)

MPS I H (HURLER'S SYNDROME)

MPS I H, the Hurler syndrome, is the prototype mucopolysaccharidosis. There is deposition of acid mucopolysaccharide in virtually every system of the body, giving rise to both somatic and visceral abnormalities. The patients develop a characteristic appearance (often unkindly likened to that of a gargoyle) with a dwarfed, deformed body, large head, and grotesque facies. Mental deficiency, hepatosplenomegaly, cardiac lesions, respiratory disease, and early death are usual. Progressive corneal clouding is the rule, and there often is concurrent retinal degeneration.

In MPS I H there is deficiency of α-L-iduronidase accompanied by excessive urinary excretion of both dermatan sulfate and heparan sulfate. The disorder is inherited as an autosomal recessive condition. Occurring in many races, Hurler's disease is probably the most frequent of the mucopolysaccharidoses.

General Features

Manifestations of MPS I H develop in infancy and early childhood, becoming more apparent with increasing age.

In typical patients the head is large and misshapen. Scaphocephaly due to premature closure of the saggital suture is common, and there often is a prominent longitudinal ridge along the saggital suture, the result of hyperostosis. Hypertelorism is usual; it is evident in even mildly affected patients before other signs of the disorder develop.

The facial appearance is markedly abnormal. The features are coarse and the expression is dull. The wide-set eyes are prominent, with cloudy, often large-ap-pearing corneas. The lids tend to be puffy, the brows heavy. The nose is broad, with wide nostrils and a flattened bridge. Often the ears are large and low set. The lips are large and patulous, and they are usually separated, exposing a large protuberant tongue, small, stubby, widely spaced teeth, and hypertrophic gums.

Characteristically there is moderate dwarfism with abnormalities throughout the skeleton. A short neck, kyphoscoliosis, and gibbus are typical, and on x-ray the vertebral bodies, particularly those of the lower dorsal and upper lumbar region, appear wedge-shaped, with an anterior hooklike projection referred to as beaking. The extremities are short, the hands and feet are broad, and the phalanges tend to be short and stubby. On x-ray the tubular bones show expansion of the medullary cavity, with widening of the shaft and thinning of the cortex. The terminal phalangeal bones commonly are hypoplastic.

Abnormalities of joint surfaces combined with changes in the ligaments and tendons contribute to the skeletal deformities. The joints are stiff, and flexion contractures develop. Typically the gait is awkward, the posture semi-crouching. Often the patients walk on their toes. Especially characteristic is clawlike deformity of the hands and feet. Other skeletal abnormalities common to the syndrome are genu valgum, coxa valga, pes planus, and talipes equinovarus.

Thoracic deformity, reflecting both bony and articular abnormalities, is another regular feature of the syndrome. The chest appears large and wide, with flaring of the lower ribs over the abdomen. Expansion of the rib cage is restricted. The ribs are spatulate or saber-shaped, being broad in the blade and narrowing toward the vertebral end. The scapulae and clavicles also are widened.

The abdomen characteristically is protuberant, owing in part to supporting tissue abnormalities and in part to visceromegaly. As a rule, there is marked enlargement of the liver and spleen, although dysfunction generally is minimal. Diastasis recti, and umbilical and inguinal hernias are common.

The skin tends to be thick, and there is generalized hypertrichosis. In younger patients the hair is fine, but with increasing age it becomes coarse and dark. The hirsutism often is especially striking over the arms and legs.

Often there is clinical evidence of cardiac disease. Murmurs, angina, myocardial infarction, and congestive heart failure are common, even in very young patients. Pathologic changes in the heart secondary to mucopolysaccharide accumulation can be extensive. The endocardium, particularly that of the heart valves and cordea tendinae, becomes thickened, and often nodular. Changes occur in the myocardium and pericardium. Engorged cells compromise the lumina of the coronary arteries. The great vessels and peripheral vessels are also affected.

Respiratory problems occur in virtually every patient. Recurrent upper respiratory infections, frequent attacks of bronchitis, and chronic nasal congestion are typical, and the patients almost universally are noisy mouth breathers. Several factors contribute to these conditions. The deformity of the facial and nasal bones is significant. There are abnormalities of the tracheobronchial cartilages and there is deposition of mucopolysaccharide in the lungs. In some cases, there is a mass of adenoid tissue in the nasopharynx that on x-ray appears to narrow or obliterate the air shadow. In addition to the abnormalities of the respiratory passages and lungs, cardiac disease and thoracic deformity may add to the respiratory difficulties, often producing dyspnea.

The predominant neurologic finding is mental deficiency. Although development often is normal in the first year or so, mental retardation becomes evident thereafter, and mental deterioration is likely to be progressive. There may also be motor changes—paralyses, increased tone, and abnormal reflexes. Relative to the neurologic abnormalities, pathologic changes can be found throughout the nervous system. Ballooned nerve cells are found in the cerebral cortex and in the peripheral ganglia, atrophy of the cortex may occur, and the leptomeninges are often thickened with engorged cells. In some cases internal hydrocephalus develops, probably as the result of meningeal involvement. When present, hydrocephalus can contribute to the mental deficiency and macrocephaly.

A special feature in some cases is the presence of leptomeningeal cysts; located most commonly anterior to the sella turcica, the cysts are associated with erosion of the sphenoid body and the anterior clinoids. Aside from the bony changes in the skull associated with arachnoid cysts, there generally is shoe-shaped enlargement of the sella, occurring probably as a primary bony manifestation of mucopolysaccharidosis. The optic foramina may also be enlarged.

Deafness occurs with some frequency in the Hurler syndrome. Its severity is variable and its etiology is not clear. As these patients are prone to middle ear infection consequent to deformity of the nasopharynx, the deafness may be related to recurrent otitis media. Progressive nerve deafness, which in some cases may be secondary to bony abnormalities, is also described. There may be deformity of the ossicles with limitation of motion.

Progressive mental and physical deterioration is the rule. The patients die young, often before age 10 years. Death most frequently is due to cardiac and respiratory disease.

Ophthalmic Features

The principal ocular manifestations of MPS I H are progressive corneal clouding, retinal degeneration, optic atrophy, and vision loss.

The corneal clouding usually becomes clinically apparent before age 3 years, generally before age 1 year; in some cases it may be apparent at birth. The clouding progresses from a generalized haze or steamy appearance to a dense, milky, ground-glass appearance. On slit lamp examination, fine granular noncrystalline opacities can be seen in the corneal stroma, increasing in density from the anterior stroma and subepithelial regions to the posterior stromal layers. On histologic examination, abnormalities can be found in almost all regions of the cornea. The epithelium, particularly the basal layers, may show edema and cytoplasmic vacuolization, with accumulation of metachromatic material in and around the cells. Bowman's membrane shows thinning and fragmentation with infiltration of vacuolated cells beneath the membrane and in the areas of disruption; these cells contain both homogeneous and granular metachromatic material, and Bowman's membrane itself may be permeated by a homogeneous electron-dense material. In the stroma there is swelling, granularity, and vacuolization of corneal corpuscles, with intracellular accumulation of metachromatic material, extracellular deposition of homogeneous metachromatic material, and lamellar separation throughout. Descemet's membrane and the endothelium are usually described as normal, but cytoplasmic vacuolization and metachromatic staining of the endothelium have been reported.

The progressive corneal changes may obscure ophthalmoscopic signs of underlying retinal degeneration and optic atrophy. The electroretinogram, however, can provide objective evidence of retinal dysfunction. The reported fundus abnormalities include retinal pigmentary changes, loss of the foveal reflex, arteriolar attenuation, and optic pallor. Related histologic changes include enlargement and vacuolization of the cells of the nuclear layers of the retina, vacuolization of ganglion cells, and interstitial atrophy of the optic nerve. Thickening of the arachnoid of the optic nerve by an infiltration of small vacuolated cells also has been reported.

In addition to these corneal, retinal, and optic nerve changes, there may be evidence of mucopolysaccharide accumulation in the epithelium of the ciliary body, in the walls of iris capillaries, in the sclera, and in the conjunctiva, and conjunctival biopsy has been recommended as a diagnostic procedure. Glaucoma and megalocornea also have been reported.

The vision loss in MPS I H results primarily from corneal opacification, retinal degeneration, and optic atrophy, independently or in combination. Glaucoma and the effects of cerebral storage and hyderocephalus may also contribute.

As stated in the description of the facies, the eyes tend to be prominent and wide set (hypertelorism), the lids tend to be puffy, the brows are heavy, and the lashes are coarse.

MPS I S
(SCHEIE'S SYNDROME)

The Scheie syndrome is an autosomal recessive mucopolysaccharidosis in which the predominant abnormalities are corneal clouding, stiff joints, carpal tunnel syndrome, and aortic valve disease. The characteristic somatic changes of mucopolysaccharidosis are generally minimal, and intellect is usually normal or nearly normal.

Despite striking clinical differences, the Scheie syndrome is a variant of Hurler's disease. In both syndromes there is excessive urinary excretion of dermatan sulfate and heparan sulfate. By the method of mixed fibroblast culture, both disorders are corrected by Hurler factor, and both conditions show deficiency of the same enzyme, α-L-iduronidase; presumably the two disorders are allelic.

Once thought to be quite distinct from other mucopolysaccharidoses, the Scheie syndrome was originally designated MPS V; on the basis of the recent findings showing its identity with MPS I H, the Scheie syndrome is now designated MPS I S.

General Features

Patients with Scheie type MPS I have somewhat coarse features and a typically broad-mouthed appearance, but they do not develop the grotesque facies characteristic of Hurler's syndrome, nor do they develop the distorted habitus of the Hurler patients. In the Scheie syndrome, stature is normal or nearly normal, although the neck tends to be short and the joints stiff. Limitation of movement usually begins in the first decade. Clawlike deformity of the hand is present, and there may be deformity of the feet. The carpal tunnel syndrome — compression of the median nerve in the carpal tunnel with numbness of the fingers — develops in many patients.

Frequently there is evidence of aortic valve disease, most commonly aortic regurgitation. Involvement of other organs is usually not clinically evident, although some patients have hepatomegaly. Hernias are commonly present. There may be a hearing defect. As a rule, there is hypertrichosis.

Characteristically the intellect is normal or nearly normal, in striking contrast to MPS I H.

The usual x-ray findings in the Scheie syndrome are hypoplastic or cystic changes of the carpal bones and proximal portion of the metacarpals. The tubular bones are well formed. The ribs are spatulate.

Scheie type patients have a relatively normal life span.

Ophthalmic Features

Corneal clouding is a predominant feature of the Scheie syndrome. Developing early in life, often present at birth, the corneal haze tends to be slowly progressive with age, ultimately interfering with vision. The corneal involvement is diffuse, though is some cases the clouding is most dense peripherally. The corneas are described as having a thickened and somewhat edematous appearance, with opacities through all depths of the cornea; dull, ground glass-like changes of the epithelium and increased density of Descemet's membrane are reported.

As vision is often severely affected by the corneal changes, corneal transplants have been performed, but with little success.

Retinal degeneration also occurs in the Scheie syndrome. Progressive night blindness, often commencing in the second or third decade, is a common complaint, and the fields become constricted. In these cases the ERG is abnormal, sometimes almost extinguished, with loss of the scotopic response. Although corneal clouding may obscure the retinal changes, the ERG is diagnostic.

MPS II
(HUNTER'S SYNDROME)

The Hunter syndrome is an x-linked recessive mucopolysaccharidosis that closely resembles the Hurler prototype phenotypically; coarse features, dwarfed habitus, stiff joints, hepatosplenomegaly, cardiac disease, respiratory difficulties, and mental deficit develop. The manifestations of MPS II, however, are less severe than those of MPS I H, and the Hunter syndrome is distinguished clinically by longer survival and by the absence of gross corneal clouding.

As in the Hurler syndrome, there is excessive urinary excretion of both dermatan sulfate and heparan sulfate in the Hunter syndrome, though the pattern of mucopolysacchariduria differs in the two conditions, the proportion of dermatan sulfate to heparan sulfate being approximately 50:50 in MPS II and 70:30 in MPS I.

The enzyme defect in the Hunter syndrome has recently been found to be sulfoiduronate sulfatase deficiency.

At least two presumably allelic forms of MPS II occur, differing in length of survival and in severity of neurologic involvement. MPS II A is characterized by relatively more rapid regression of intellect, and death usually occurs before age 15 years. MPS II B is characterized by slower mental regression, and this form is compatible with survival to 50 years or beyond.

General Features

Appearing normal in early childhood, patients with MPS II gradually develop features typical of "gargoylism" with increasing age. The face becomes coarse. The supraorbital ridges tend to be prominent. The tongue is large, and the teeth widely spaced. With age, the complexion may assume a deep rosy or ruddy appearance.

Characteristically there is dwarfism, with limitation of joint mobility. Lumbar gibbus, however, is not usually present, and there often is not the beaking of the vertebrae so typical of the Hurler syndrome. Kyphoscoliosis may be present. Clawhand deformity is usual. There commonly is pes cavus, often with overlapping of the fifth toe.

The abdomen is protuberant. Hernias commonly are present. As a rule, there is hepatosplenomegaly; dysfunction, however, is minimal even with longstanding or severe visceromegaly.

Cardiac involvement is a regular feature of the syndrome. Cardiomegaly, heart murmurs, and pulmonary hypertension occur with frequency. As in MPS I, congestive heart failure and coronary artery disease are common causes of death.

Respiratory disability is evident in most patients. Upper airway obstruction due to deformity of the larynx and nasopharynx is common. Usually there is chronic congestion with noisy breathing. Upper respiratory infections occur with frequency. Kyphoscoliosis, restriction of chest movement, and abnormalities of perfusion due to parenchymal involvement contribute to the respiratory problems.

Frequently the skin shows ridging or nodular thickening, most commonly on the posterior thorax, extending from the angle of the scapula toward the axillary line. There is usually striking hypertrichosis.

Neurologic manifestations are variable. Mental deterioration is a regular feature of MPS II, progressing more rapidly in MPS II A than in MPS II B. As a rule, the mental defect in the Hunter syndrome is less severe than in the Hurler syndrome.

The shoe-shaped deformity of the sella so characteristic of the mucopolysaccharidoses is evident in MPS II.

Progressive deafness occurs in the Hunter syndrome, and with greater frequency than in the Hurler syndrome.

Ophthalmic Features

In contrast to Hurler's syndrome, macroscopic corneal clouding is not a feature of the Hunter syndrome. However, slight corneal changes may be detected on slit lamp examination of older patients with MPS II, and histologic evidence of abnormal corneal mucopolysaccharide deposition is reported.

The principal ophthalmic manifestation of MPS II is progressive retinal degeneration, with attendant deterioration of vision. Night vision problems and field defects are common, and the disorder may lead to blindness. Retinal pigmentary disturbance—sometimes with perivascular spicule formation—retinal artery attenuation, and optic pallor are the characteristic fundus abnormalities. The ERG is markedly reduced or extinguished.

The reported ocular pathology in MPS II indicates abnormal mucopolysaccharide accumulation in the iris and ciliary body epithelium and in the sclera as well as in the cornea. The corneal abnormalities appear to be confined to the stroma, the epithelium, and the more peripheral areas of Bowman's membrane, leaving the endothelium and Descemet's membrane unaffected. Thickening of the sclera, and foamy distension of the cells of the epithelium of the iris and ciliary body are described.

Histologic changes within the retina include pigment clumping and migration, and paucity of pigment epithelial cells, loss of rods and cones, reduction in the number of ganglion cells, and moderate gliosis of the nerve fiber layer, although mucopolysaccharide deposits are not evident in the retina.

There may be disc edema, suggesting the possibility of increased intracranial pressure in MPS II.

MPS III (SANFILIPPO'S SYNDROME)

Also referred to as polydystrophic oligophrenia, the Sanfilippo syndrome is a mucopolysaccharidosis in which there is severe mental retardation and relatively less severe somatic abnormalities.

Two biochemically different, clinically indistinguishable forms of the syndrome occur; in type A there is deficiency of heparan sulfate sulfatase, while in type B there is deficiency of N-acetyl-α-D-glucosaminidase. There is heparansulfaturia in both forms. The disorder is autosomal recessive.

General Features

The predominant clinical manifestation of MPS III is mental deficiency. Mental retardation generally becomes evident by school age; as a rule, intellect and behavior progressively deteriorate with increasing age. The patients usually have good bodily strength, however, so that management often becomes a problem as they regress.

Somatic abnormalities typical of "gargoylism" tend to be mild or inconspicuous. There is slight coarseness of the facial features; the lips are large, the nose is widened with a depressed bridge, and the teeth are abnormal. There may be hypertrichosis of mild degree.

Dwarfing, joint stiffness, and clawhand deformity are usually evident, but not severe.

Slight to moderate hepatosplenomegaly develops, the abdomen tends to be protuberant, and there may be hernias.

Respiratory difficulties, particularly recurrent respiratory infections and upper airway obstruction with noisy mouth breathing, are common. Cardiac problems, however, do not develop, and the patients may survive into the third or fourth decade.

Ophthalmic Features

Corneal clouding is not a regular feature of MPS III, though microscopic corneal changes were reported in one of Sanfi-lippo's patients.

There may be retinal involvement. Sub-normal ERG responses have been re-corded. Narrowing of the retinal vessels has been noted.

MPS IV
(MORQUIO'S SYNDROME)

Morquio's syndrome, an autosomal re-cessive condition, is a form of spondyloepi-physeal dysplasia characterized by severe dwarfism and skeletal deformity, often combined with extraskeletal abnormalities such as corneal clouding and aortic valve disease.

In this mucopolysaccharidosis there is excessive urinary excretion of keratan sul-fate, predominantly in younger patients. The enzyme defect is N-acetylhexosamine sulfatase deficiency.

General Features

Patients with MPS IV appear normal at birth, and their growth and development are normal in infancy, though x-ray abnor-malities may be present in the first year. In the second or third year of life, awkward gait, retarded growth, knock knees, flat feet, prominent joints, sternal bulging, flaring of the rib cage, and dorsal kyphosis begin to develop. The deformities worsen with age, and growth is severely retarded. Characteristically the patients are strik-ingly dwarfed, and they develop a semi-crouching stance. The joints usually are not stiff, however; some may be hyperex-tensible. The wrists are enlarged and the hands are misshapen. A barrel chest with pigeon breast deformity is common. The neck is short. The facies is abnormal, with a broad mouth, prominent jaw, short nose and widely spaced teeth. The dental enamel is often thin, giving a dull gray ap-pearance to the crowns of the teeth, and giving rise to flaking and fracturing of the enamel and multiple cavities. The skin usually is thickened, inelastic, and loose, particularly over the limbs, and there may be telangiectasia over the face and limbs. In some cases aortic regurgitation is present. There may be increased incidence of inguinal hernias. Sensorineural hearing loss may develop.

Spinal cord and medullary compression is a frequent and major complication of MPS IV, resulting from hypoplasia or aplasia of the odontoid and ligamentous laxity of the vertebral column. The neuro-logic abnormalities range from minimal long tract signs to spastic paraplegia, respiratory paralysis, and death.

A principal radiologic feature of MPS IV is platyspondyly. Flat vertebrae are par-ticularly characteristic of Morquio's syn-drome. The odontoid process is hypoplas-tic or absent. The femoral head becomes flattened and eroded. The long bones are short and poorly tubulated. The carpal centers are small and retarded in develop-ment. The ribs are spatulate. There is bulging of the sternum, and dorsal ky-phosis is also present. Flaring of the ilia may be particularly striking. All the bones become markedly osteoporotic.

Whereas the physical abnormalities of MPS IV are severe, the intellect is normal or only slightly impaired.

Although the prognosis is poor, pri-marily because of atlantoaxial subluxation, survival is variable. In general, the course is one of progressive incapacitation.

Ophthalmic Features

A significant number of patients with MPS IV develop corneal clouding. The corneal changes may not become clinically apparent to the unaided eye for several years, often not before age 10; corneal in-volvement in its early stage may be over-looked unless slit lamp examination is performed, and only by slit lamp examina-tion can the presence of corneal opacities be excluded. The corneal clouding of MPS IV has the appearance of a fine haze rather than of ground glass. Clinically there appears to be homogeneously dif-fuse involvement of the stroma with spar-ing of the epithelium, Bowman's mem-brane, and endothelium. The opacities of the stroma are described as yellowish gray refractile particles, and Descemet's mem-brane may have a slight yellowish hue. Depending on the density of the corneal haze, there may be moderate impairment of vision.

Retinal degeneration is not a feature of MPS IV.

MPS VI
(MAROTEAUX-LAMY SYNDROME)

The Maroteaux-Lamy syndrome is characterized by striking dwarfism accompanied by visceromegaly, cardiac lesions, and progressive corneal clouding, sometimes complicated by hydrocephalus and spinal cord compression. Resembling the prototype mucopolysaccharidosis in many ways, the Maroteaux-Lamy syndrome is distinguished by retention of normal intellect and by its pattern of mucopolysacchariduria—i.e., preponderant excretion of dermatan sulfate. The disorder is inherited as an autosomal recessive trait.

General Features

Manifestations of MPS VI develop in childhood. Retarded growth affecting both the trunk and limbs usually is evident at age 2 or 3 years; the deficiency tends to be severe, with growth seeming to cease in many patients after the age of 7 or 8. Genu valgum, lumbar kyphosis, and anterior sternal protrusion develop. The lower ribs are flared. Restriction of joint movement characteristically is present. Clawhand deformity is usually a feature of MPS VI, and the carpal tunnel syndrome commonly develops. The wrists may be enlarged and prominent. The head appears relatively large, and the neck is short. The facies is suggestive, but not strikingly characteristic of mucopolysaccharidosis, with coarseness of the features. The teeth tend to be stubby and widely spaced. There commonly is mild hypertrichosis.

In patients over 6 years of age there consistently is hepatomegaly; splenomegaly develops in about half the cases, and the abdomen usually is protuberant. Cardiac abnormalities develop, particularly valve lesions similar to those of the Hurler syndrome. Hernias occur with significant frequency. Deafness, probably due in part to recurrent otitis media, is present in some patients.

The principal neurologic complications of MPS VI are communicating hydrocephalus and spinal cord compression. The hydrocephalus most likely results from impaired reabsorption of cerebrospinal fluid secondary to meningeal deposits of mucopolysaccharides. The cord compression with attendant long tract signs—sometimes spastic paraplegia—is the result of atlantoaxial subluxation consequent to hypoplasia of the odontoid process.

Intellectual development is normal in MPS VI, and as a rule there is retention of intelligence, at least until late in the disease.

The radiologic findings include swelling of the diaphyses of the long bones, sometimes with localized constriction of the metaphyses, varus deformity of the upper humerus, irregularity of the epiphyses and metaphyses at the elbows and wrists, and abnormal radiolucencies in the tibial and distal femoral metaphyses. There may be convexity of the superior and inferior margins of the vertebrae, with convexity of the anterior and posterior margins. The odontoid is hypoplastic. The ribs are spatulate, resembling a canoe paddle narrowing toward the vertebral ends. The iliac wings are flared, and the acetabula are small. Involvement of the short bones is variable, but commonly the ends of their shafts are widened and the metacarpal bases are pointed.

Ophthalmic Features

Diffuse corneal clouding, developing usually within the first few years of life, is the principal ocular manifestation of MPS VI. A ground glass haziness develops throughout the stroma, sometimes most dense peripherally.

Histopathologic studies of the eyes of patients with MPS VI have shown the following abnormalities in the corneas; generalized thickening of the cornea; fine cytoplasmic vacuolization of the epithelium; interruption and replacement of Bowman's membrane by accumulation of histiocytes ballooned with foamy cytoplasm; separation of the stromal lamellae by basophilic staining material; swelling of the keratocytes by foamy-appearing cytoplasm; and fine cytoplasmic vacuolization of the endothelium. Deposits of acid mucopolysaccharides have been identified within the basal epithelial cells of the cornea and in the foamy histiocytes in the region of Bowman's membrane, within and without the keratocytes and between the lamellae of the stroma, and also in the corneal endothelium. Similar thickening, histiocyte accumulations, and intra- and

TABLE 20-32 THE MUCOPOLYSACCHARIDOSES*

Designation	General Clinical Features	Ophthalmic Manifestations	Genetics	Excessive Urinary MPS	Metabolic Defect
MPS I H Hurler's Syndrome	Coarse features, moderate dwarfism, stiff joints, gibbus, and clawhand deformity. Protuberant abdomen, hepatosplenomegaly, hernias. Cardiovascular and respiratory disease. Mental retardation. Death usually before age 10 years.	Progressive corneal clouding. Pigmentary retinal degeneration. Optic atrophy.	Homozygous for MPS I H gene	Dermatan sulfate Heparan sulfate	α-L-iduronidase
MPS I S Scheie's Syndrome	Stiff joints, clawhand deformity, carpal tunnel syndrome. Aortic regurgitation. Normal intelligence. Reasonably normal life span.	Progressive corneal clouding. Pigmentary retinal degeneration.	Homozygous for MPS I S gene	Dermatan sulfate Heparan sulfate	α-L-iduronidase
MPS II A Hunter's Syndrome (severe)	Phenotypically similar to MPS I H, but milder. Coarse features, moderate dwarfism, stiff joints. Lack of gibbus. Protuberant abdomen, hepatosplenomegaly. Cardiac disease, respiratory difficulties. Mental deterioration. Nodular skin thickenings. Deafness. Death usually before age 15 years.	Pigmentary retinal degeneration. Corneas clear grossly; minimal microscopic changes.	Hemizygous for X-linked gene	Dermatan sulfate Heparan sulfate	Sulfoiduronate sulfatase deficiency
MPS II B Hunter's Syndrome (mild)	Similar to A, but slower mental regression. Compatible with survival to 30's or 50's.		Hemizygous for X-linked allele for mild form	Dermatan sulfate Heparan sulfate	Sulfoiduronate sulfatase deficiency
MPS III Sanfilippo's Syndrome A MPS III Sanfilippo's Syndrome B	Identical phenotype. Severe mental deficit. Mild somatic and visceral abnormalities.	Clear corneas. Possibly retinal degeneration.	Homozygous for Sanfilippo A gene Homozygous for Sanfilippo B gene	Heparan sulfate Heparan sulfate	Heparan sulfate sulfatase N-acetyl-α-D-glucosaminidase
MPS IV Morquio's Syndrome	Striking dwarfism with distinctive bone changes. Joints not stiff. Semi-crouching stance, dorsal kyphosis, barrel chest, knock knees. Coarse features. Aortic regurgitation. Spinal cord compression; long tract signs. Progressive incapacitation.	Corneal clouding.	Homozygous for Morquio gene	Keratan sulfate	N-acetylhexosamine sulfatase deficiency
MPS V Vacant (formerly Scheie's syndrome)					
MPS VI Maroteaux-Lamy Syndrome	Dwarfism and stiff joints. Normal intellect. Hepatosplenomegaly. Spinal cord compression; long tract signs.	Corneal clouding.	Homozygous for M-L gene	Dermatan sulfate	"Maroteaux-Lamy corrective factor"†
MPS VII β-Glucuronidase Deficiency	Mental and physical retardation. Dysostosis multiplex. Thoracolumbar gibbus. Hepatosplenomegaly.	Corneal clouding reported.	Homozygous for mutant gene at β-glucuronidase locus	Dermatan sulfate	β-glucuronidase deficiency

*After McKusick, V. A.: Heritable Disorders of Connective Tissue. 4th ed. St. Louis, The C. V. Mosby Co., 1972.

extracellular acid mucopolysaccharide deposits have been found in the sclera.

Abnormalities in other portions of the eyes also have been found by histopathologic study. These changes include the presence of vacuolated cells in the trabecular meshwork, in the connective tissue stroma of the ciliary body, and in the choroid, and the presence of acid mucopolysaccharide deposits in the basal portion of the nonpigmented ciliary epithelium and in the stroma of the ciliary body. The retina has been found to be histologically normal, except for a reduction of the ganglion cell population and thinning of the nerve fiber layer in the macular region. In the optic nerve, atrophy of the temporal nerve fiber bundles has been described.

Clinically, retinal degeneration is not a feature of MPS VI. The ERG is normal in these patients.

As hydrocephalus is known to develop in MPS VI, there may be papilledema and sixth nerve paresis.

An interesting finding in some patients with MPS VI is marked tortuosity of the retinal vessels, without papilledema.

MPS VII

MPS VII is a newly described mucopolysaccharidosis in which there is deficiency of β-glucuronidase. Clinical features common to the two reported patients with this disorder are mental and physical retardation, thoracolumbar gibbus, hepatosplenomegaly, and hernias.

Clouding of the corneas evident early in life is described in one patient.

There is evidence for autosomal recessive inheritance.

REFERENCES

Beaudet, A. L., DiFerrante, N., Nichols, B., and Ferry, G. D.: β-glucuronidase deficiency: altered enzyme substrate recognition (abstract). Amer. J. Hum. Genet., 24:25a, 1972.

Beebe, R. T., and Formel, P. F.: Gargoylism: sex-linked transmission in 9 males. Trans. Amer. Clin. Climat. Ass., 66: 199, 1954.

Berliner, M. L.: Lipin keratitis of Hurler's syndrome (gargoylism or dysostosis multiplex); clinical and pathological report. Arch. Ophthal., 22:97, 1939.

Davis, D. B., and Currier, F. P.: Morquio's disease; report of 2 cases. J.A.M.A., 102:2173, 1934.

Dorfman, A., and Matalon, R.: The mucopolysaccharidoses. In Stanbury, J. B., Wyngaarden, J. B., and Fredrickson, D. S. (ed.): The Metabolic Basis of Inherited Disease. 3rd ed. New York, McGraw-Hill-Book Co., 1972, pp. 1218–1272.

Ellis, R. W. B., Sheldon, W., and Capon, N. B.: Gargoylism (chondro-osteo-dystrophy, corneal opacities, hepatosplenomegaly and mental deficiency). Quart. J. Med., 29:119, 1936.

Gills, J. P., Hobson, R., Hanley, W. B., and McKusick, V. A.: Electroretinography and fundus oculi findings in Hurler's disease and allied mucopolysaccharidoses. Arch. Ophthal., 74:596, 1965.

Goldberg, M. F., and Duke, J. R.: Ocular histopathology in Hunter's syndrome; systemic mucopolysaccharidosis, type II. Arch. Ophthal., 77:503, 1967.

Goldberg, M. F., Scott, C. I., and McKusick, V. A.: Hydrocephalus and papilledema in the Maroteaux-Lamy syndrome (mucopolysaccharidosis, type VI). Amer. J. Ophthal., 69:969, 1970.

Gollance, R. B., D'Amico, R. A.: Atypical mucopolysaccharidosis and successful keratoplasty. Amer. J. Ophthal., 64:707, 1967.

Hogan, M. J., and Cordes, F. C.: Lipochondrodystrophy (dysostosis multiplex; Hurler's disease); pathologic changes in the cornea in 3 cases. Arch. Ophthal., 32:287, 1944.

Hooper, J. M. D.: Unusual case of gargoylism. Guy's Hosp. Rep., 101:222, 1952.

Jervis, G. A.: Gargoylism: study of 10 cases with emphasis on the formes frustes. Arch. Neurol. Psychiat., 63:681, 1950.

Kenyon, K. R., Topping, T. M., Green, W. R., and Maumenee, A. E.: Ocular pathology of the Maroteaux-Lamy syndrome; a histologic and ultrastructure report of 2 cases. Amer. J. Ophthal., 73:718, 1972.

Lindsay, S., Reilly, W. A., Gotham, T. J., and Skahen, R.: Gargoylism. II. Study of pathologic lesions and clinical review of 12 cases. Amer. J. Dis. Child., 76:239, 1948.

Mailer, C.: Gargoylism associated with optic atrophy. Canad. J. Ophthal., 4:266, 1969.

McKusick, V. A.: Heritable Disorders of Connective Tissue. 4th ed., St. Louis, The C. V. Mosby Co., 1972.

Meyer, S. J., and Okner, H. B.: Dysostosis multiplex with special reference to ocular findings. Amer. J. Ophthal., 22:713, 1939.

Newell, F. W., and Koistinen, A.: Lipochondrodystrophy (gargoylism): pathologic findings in 5 eyes of 3 patients. Arch. Ophthal., 53:45, 1955.

Quigley, H. A., and Goldberg, M. F.: Scheie syndrome and macular corneal dystrophy; an ultrastructural comparison of conjunctiva and skin. Arch. Ophthal., 85:553, 1971.

Rosen, D. A., Haust, M. D., Yamashita, T., and Bryans, A. M.: Keratoplasty and electron microscopy of the cornea in systemic mucopolysaccharidosis (Hurler's disease). Canad. J. Ophthal., 3:218, 1968.

Sanfilippo, S. J., Podosin, R., Langer, L. O., Jr., and

Good, R. A.: Mental retardation associated with acid mucopolysacchariduria (heparitin sulfate type). J. Pediat., 63:837, 1963.

Scheie, H. G., Hambrick, G. W., Jr., and Barness, L. A.: A newly recognized forme fruste of Hurler's disease (gargoylism). Amer. J. Ophthal., 53:753, 1962.

Sly, W. S., Quinton, B. A., McAlister, W. H., and Rimoin, D. L.: Isolated β-glucuronidase deficiency: clinical report of a new mucopolysaccharidosis. J. Pediat., 82:249, 1973.

Topping, T. M., Kenyon, K. R., Goldberg, M. F., and

Maumanee, A. E.: Ultrastructural ocular pathology of Hunter's syndrome; systemic mucopolysaccharidosis type II. Arch. Ophthal., 86:164, 1971.

Van Pelt, J. F., and Huizinga, J.: Some observations on the genetics of gargoylism. Acta Genet. (Basel), 12:1, 1962.

Von Noorden, G. K., Zellweger, H., and Ponseti, I. V.: Ocular findings in Morquio-Ullrich's disease; with report of 2 cases. Arch. Ophthal., 64:585, 1960.

Wexler, D.: Ocular histology in Hurler's disease (gargoylism). Arch. Ophthal., 46:14, 1951.

The Collagen Diseases

Robison D. Harley, M.D.

Collagen diseases are characterized by connective tissue changes such as edema, mononuclear cell infiltrations, and fibrinoid necrosis. It may be recalled that the fibrous constituents of connective tissue are divided in two primary groups: collagenous and elastic.

The disease entities included in the collagen group are: rheumatoid arthritis, systemic lupus erythematosus, periarteritis nodosa, temporal arteritis, scleroderma, dermatomyositis, Sjögren's syndrome, and relapsing polychondritis. Additional conditions such as Takayasu's arteritis, Buerger's disease, rheumatic fever, and serum sickness may be included also.

RHEUMATOID ARTHRITIS

Rheumatoid arthritis is characterized by an inflammatory involvement of the joints, females are affected three times as often as males. The synovial membrane becomes thickened as a result of edema and cellular infiltration, with ultimate destruction of cartilage and bone leading to ankylosis.

Ocular complications include the occurrence of nongranulomatous uveitis, episcleritis, scleritis, and keratoconjunctivitis sicca. A bizarre change may take place following a necrotizing scleritis with the development of scleromalacia perforans.

Juvenile rheumatoid arthritis or Still's disease has an onset prior to age 10, and is generally less severe than the adult form. Lymphadenopathy, fever, splenomegaly,

and pericarditis occur in Still's disease. Phenylbutazone (Butazolidin) is effective in alleviating pain, while cortisone and chloroquine are useful therapeutic agents in this disease. Ocular complications respond to atropine and cortisone systemically and locally.

Associated cutaneous changes consist of a characteristic transient, erythematous, maculopapular eruption on the extremities and trunk, which may appear prior to arthritic symptoms. A variation of rheumatoid arthritis, Marie-Strumpell disease or rheumatic spondylitis, involves the spine and sacroiliac region. This disease has a higher incidence in men, and it is frequently accompanied by a severe iritis.

LUPUS ERYTHEMATOSUS

Lupus erythematosus is characterized by a generalized but selective fibrinoid necrosis involving the heart, kidney, brain cortex, and multiple arteries of the brain, skin, and eye. Ocular lesions most commonly observed are cytoid bodies, retinal hemorrhages, and low grade papilledema. Embolic petechiae in the retina, perivasculitis, and arterial occlusions have been reported, as well as blepharitis, conjunctivitis, conjunctival scarring, and keratitis. White fluffy areas in the retina (cytoid bodies) and mild edema about the disc also may be observed in periarteritis nodosa, dermatomyositis, and serum sickness. The recognition of lupus erythematosus (LE) cells in the peripheral blood or bone marrow is diagnostic.

Lupus erythematosus embraces a constellation of cutaneous changes in which there is deposition of immunoglobulins at the basement membrane in the skin and alteration of the ground substance in the dermis with or without systemic disease. According to the degree of cutaneous or systemic involvement, LE is subdivided into (1) a discoid or localized form in which lesions are confined to the butterfly area of the face, and (2) a disseminated form in which there may be polysystemic involvement.

The cutaneous manifestations of the localized and disseminated forms are essentially the same, and consist of circumscribed erythematous light-sensitive patches of different size associated with scaling, follicular plugging, and atrophy.

PERIARTERITIS NODOSA (POLYARTERITIS)

Periarteritis nodosa is associated with a vascular inflammation and necrosis manifesting as a variety of systemic disorders. Symptoms are particularly referable to the kidneys, heart, central and peripheral nervous systems, gastrointestinal system, muscles, and skin.

Ocular changes include the presence of cytoid bodies, marked hypertensive retinopathy, retinal separation, episcleritis, and central artery closure. The disease is frequent in childhood, and must be considered when the fundi reveal extensive hypertensive changes. Peripheral corneal degeneration is a serious complication of periarteritis nodosa, but may also be observed in lupus erythematosus and rheumatoid arthritis. Muscle biopsy substantiates the diagnosis.

The cutaneous manifestations, which are present irregularly, depend on the location of the vessel involvement in the skin. Characteristically, they consist of ill-defined painful subcutaneous nodules on the lower extremities, which may become ulcerated. Nonspecific polymorphic skin lesions consisting of erythematous maculopapules, urticaria, and blisters occur, and occasionally break down to form crusts and ulcers.

TEMPORAL ARTERITIS

Temporal arteritis characteristically occurs in older adults and has not been observed in the pediatric age group.

SCLERODERMA

Scleroderma may occur as a generalized or localized disease in which the primary manifestation is the skin involvement. In the generalized form, the onset is associated with fever and an inflammatory induration of the skin followed eventually by atrophy. The patient becomes weak and listless; the joints become stiff, and the skin is so hard and glossy that the face is totally expressionless. Terminal renal failure develops from arteriolar necrosis and thrombosis. The localized form is much less severe, and recovery is possible; however, the localized form may be transformed to the generalized disease.

Ocular signs include skin changes resulting in atrophy with loss of elasticity and lagophthalmos. Cataracts, keratopathy, and partial external ophthalmoplegia have been observed.

DERMATOMYOSITIS

Dermatomyositis occurs as a generalized inflammation and degeneration of muscles involving female children and older adults in a 2 to 1 ratio; it frequently is associated with an underlying neoplasm. Symptoms include skin involvement, myalgia, and generalized weakness. Severe limb contractures may follow.

Ocular manifestations include puffy eyelids, periorbital edema, ocular muscle paralysis, episcleritis, and cytoid bodies in the retina.

SJÖGREN'S SYNDROME

Sjögren's syndrome consists of a deficient lacrimal secretion (keratitis sicca), dry mouth, and frequently polyarthritis, which is most commonly observed in middle-aged women. However, a 9-year-old child has been studied who exhibited the classic syndrome in conjunction with autoimmune disease.

RELAPSING POLYCHONDRITIS

This disease is characterized by recurring attacks of inflammation, involving primarily cartilaginous structures.

The most prominent feature is a recurring episcleritis in which the affected area becomes so thin that scleromalacia perforans may develop. The episcleritis may be unilateral or bilateral; alternating exophthalmos, extraocular muscle paresis, keratitis sicca, and optic neuritis have been recorded as associated ocular features.

Inflammation of the external ear, and tracheal, laryngeal, and rib cartilages are common.

The disease resembles collagen-vascular diseases, and topical steroids improve the episcleritis.

Other Connective Tissue Disorders

EHLERS-DANLOS SYNDROME

Ehlers-Danlos syndrome, which has long been recognized as a hereditary disorder of connective tissue, is characterized by excessive extensibility of the skin. Other manifestations include loose-jointedness, kyphoscoliosis, poor muscle tone, and general friability of tissues, causing the skin to be fragile, brittle, and easily traumatized. Internal changes include dissecting aortic aneurysm, spontaneous rupture of large blood vessels, and carotid-cavernous fistulae. Ocular signs consist of epicanthal folds, blue sclera, dislocated lenses, keratoconus, angioid streaks, choroidal hemorrhages rupturing into the vitreous, and disciform degeneration of the macula.

The condition is inherited as an autosomal dominant of low penetrance.

PSEUDOXANTHOMA ELASTICUM

Pseudoxanthoma elasticum (PXE) is an elastic tissue disorder characterized by cutaneous, ocular and vascular changes, and transmitted as an autosomal recessive trait. It may develop in early childhood, and usually appears before age 30.

The cutaneous manifestations consist of crinkled, yellowish papules arranged in a linear or reticulate pattern, often associated with telangiectasia distributed on the sides of the neck, axillae, clavicular area, and medial aspects of the thighs and abdomen.

Associated abnormalities include vascular disturbances expressed as absent or diminished peripheral pulses, hypertension, and calcification of peripheral vessels.

Ophthalmologic manifestations include angioid streaks of the retina, chorioretinal degeneration, and retinal hemorrhages, especially in the macular area. Angioid streaks appear as wide reddish brown paths streaking out from the optic disc and resembling underlying retinal vessels. The streaks represent cracks in the lamina elastica of Bruch's membrane.

MARFAN'S SYNDROME (ARACHNODACTYLY)

Marfan's syndrome is a congenital anomaly characterized by an abnormal length of the extremities, especially the fingers and toes; subluxation of the lens; and aneurysm of the ascending aorta. Patients tend to be tall and slender, with pronounced kyphosis, scoliosis, and chest deformities. Muscles are flaccid, with joint hyperextensibility. Additional ocular manifestations include cataract, myopia, strabismus, nystagmus, and megalocornea. Other cardiovascular changes include aortic valvular disease and cardiac hypertrophy. Death may occur from rupture of a dissecting aneurysm. The basic defect is the connective tissue, where degeneration of the elastic lamellae appears to be the primary cause. Cutaneous manifestations consist of atrophic striae arranged symmetrically on the trunk and buttocks, and occasionally elastoma perforans and anetoderma. The disease is inherited as an autosomal dominant trait with high penetrance. Older fathers seem to increase the

risk for the development of arachnodactyly.

WEILL-MARCHESANI SYNDROME

This syndrome is characterized by subluxated lenses, spherophakia, myopia, and
possibly glaucoma. In contrast to Marfan's,
short stature, brachycephaly, and stubby
fingers and toes with joint limitation are
typical in this syndrome. Secondary glaucoma from pupillary block of the spherical, subluxated lens may occur as a sudden
complication. Inheritance is autosomal recessive.

AMYLOIDOSIS

Amyloidosis is characterized by an accumulation of amyloid in connective tissue,
clinically manifested as systemic or localized. Secondary (acquired) amyloidosis
may be associated with chronic infections
and takes a typical dark stain with iodine,
but other forms of amyloid disease may
react atypically.

In   hereditary   amyloidosis,   retinal
periarteritis and sheetlike hyaline vitreous
opacities have been described. In primary
nonfamilial systemic amyloidosis, there is
involvement of the conjunctiva and extraocular muscles, which may eventuate in
complete external ophthalmoplegia.

In the localized form of amyloidosis, the
conjunctiva and eyelids become infiltrated.
In systemic amyloidosis, various parts of
the eye, including the conjunctiva, iris, vitreous, and retinal vessels, may become involved. Sheetlike vitreous opacities are important diagnostically.

REFERENCES

Hollenhorst, R. W., and Henderson, J. W.: The ocu-
   lar manifestations of the diffuse collagen diseases.
   Amer. J. Med. Sci., *221*:211, 1951.
McKusick, V. A.: Heritable Disorders of Connective
   Tissue. 3rd ed. St. Louis, The C. V. Mosby Co.,
   1966.
Nelson, W. E., Vaughan, V. C., and McKay, R. J.:
   Textbook of Pediatrics. 9th ed. Philadelphia, W. B.
   Saunders Co.. 1969.
Rucker, C. W., and Ferguson, R. H.: Ocular manifes-
   tations of relapsing polychondritis. Trans. Amer.
   Opthal. Soc., *62*:167, 1964.

D. OCULAR MANIFESTATIONS IN INFECTIOUS DISEASES, MYCOTIC INFECTIONS, PARASITIC INFECTIONS, ALLERGIC STATES, NUTRITIONAL DEFICIENCIES, AND DRUG TOXICITY

Infectious Diseases

Systemic Viral Diseases

David A. Hiles, M.D., and Franklin E. Cignetti, M.D.

Viruses are the smallest known infectious agents to produce disease in their
human hosts. They are living organisms
containing only a single nucleic acid, which
comprises the nucleoid. The nucleic acid,
either deoxyribonucleic or ribonucleic
acid, is the viral genome which conveys
viral heredity and reproductive information to the infected host cell. The nucleoid
is surrounded by a protective protein shell,
or capsid, which protects and stabilizes the
nucleoid against the extracellular environment and acids in viral invasion of the host
cell. The protein is also responsible for
viral antigenicity, which is of importance in
diagnosis and vaccine production. Some
viruses have an additional envelope, fur-
nished by the host cell, that surrounds the

capsid. These constituents, with many variations, make up the virus particle or virion.

Viruses invade the living host cell by adsorption and attachment to a species-specific receptor site on the host cell membrane. Neutralizing antibodies may be effective at this stage. Penetration occurs by phagocytosis or pinocytosis, and the virion is then uncoated by cellular enzymes in a cytoplasmic vacuole. An eclipse phase appears in which viral nucleic acid is liberated and no virus particles are found.

Viruses usually lack the enzyme systems necessary for survival and reproduction, and therefore are obligate intracellular parasites. They depend upon the host cell, under viral direction, to furnish the enzymes, energy, and low molecular weight precursors necessary for replication. The RNA viruses replicate in the cytoplasm of the host cell, while the DNA viruses usually replicate in the nucleus. Oxidative phosphorylation, at the mitochondrial level, serves as the local energy source.

Viral nucleic acid, or genome, serves as the matrix for messenger RNA formation. The DNA viruses transcribe DNA strands into specific messenger RNA, which is translated to synthesize viral enzymes for the production of viral nucleic acids. RNA viruses serve as their own messenger RNA. Capsid protein synthesis takes place simultaneously in the cellular ribosomes. Envelope formation signifies the maturation of the virion. Excretion into the surrounding medium occurs by cell lysis or by diffusion from cell to cell.

Viral disease response in man is usually of a short, violent nature in which the host either survives by the production of antibodies that neutralize the invading virus, or succumbs to the invasion. Vaccines made either of inactivated virus or of live attenuated virus are widely used to stimulate the development of antibodies against the viral coat proteins.

Active antiviral therapy is directed at interfering with the synthesis of viral components or inhibiting viral adsorption, penetration, replication, or release. No agents are available for routine systemic treatment at this time. Topical use of the DNA antilog, 5-iodo-2' deoxyuridine (IDU), has been successful in the treatment of herpes simplex keratitis. Interferon, a naturally occurring cellular protein produced by the host cell, acts as an inhibitor of viral multiplication. It is species-specific, but not virus-specific. Interferon has been used in limited instances to prevent or decrease the severity of viral infections in man.

Systemic viral infections may affect the eye in a specific manner as part of the disease process, as in rubella, or by chance involvement, as in vaccinal inoculation.

Two main classification divisions occur, as determined by the nature of the viral nucleic acid molecule present, either deoxyribonucleic acid (DNA) or ribonucleic acid (RNA). Additional subdivisions are based upon other biological and clinical characteristics.

DNA VIRUSES

Poxviruses

Two disease entities with ocular involvement, variola (smallpox) and vaccinia, occur within this DNA subgroup.

Variola (Smallpox)

Variola, or smallpox, is a highly contagious cutaneous disease with severe systemic manifestations that may become fatal. The disease onset follows a 12- to 13-day incubation period. Fever, headache, and vomiting occur for several days prior to the rash. The fever abates, and the rash presents on the face and upper trunk and spreads down onto the extremities in a regular progression. No new lesions occur within the areas of the older lesions. Cutaneous lesions progress from small deep-seated macules to papules, and then to loculated vesicles in about 4 days. A pustule develops and lasts for several days; it then dries out and forms a crust that falls off in 2 to 4 weeks, leaving a pink scar. Several other clinical modifications of the disease also occur.

Early ocular involvement occurs with the prodromes as a benign catarrhal conjunctivitis or, rarely, as an epithelial keratitis. Pustular conjunctivitis, which is uncommon, is intense and painful, and the phlycten-like lesions progress to necrosis and membrane formation. Limbal lesions may be associated with superficial keratitis, corneal ulceration, and healing by scarring. Hypopyon ulcers and endophthalmitis may occur as late complications in debilitated patients. Congenital corneal leukomas occur as a result of virus passage across the placental barrier. Skin lesions involve the lids in concert with the facial lesions. Secondary infection of the lids may produce gangrene, scarring, trichiasis, and symblepharon. Albinotic spots on the iris follow primary variola iritis. Choroiditis and vitreous opacities are present in many unvaccinated patients. Papillitis and ocular nerve palsies may occur with encephalomyelitis.

The differential diagnosis of variola consists of measles in the initial stage, secondary syphilis in the papular stage, typhus or dengue in the hemorrhagic phase, leukemia due to the preponderence of circulating immature lymphoid elements, and chickenpox.

The diagnosis is confirmed by vesicular stage smears and immunofluorescence tests, and by the presence of cytoplasmic inclusion or Guarnieri bodies. Inoculations of virus onto the chorioallantoic membrane of embryonated eggs distinguishes vaccinia and varicella from variola in 3 days.

Ocular therapy consists of the prevention of secondary bacterial infection. Variola may be prevented by vaccination recommended for endemic areas.

Vaccinia

Vaccinia is a cowpox variant used to induce immunity to variola. The complications of vaccination include ocular involvement, and consist of auto- or cross-inoculation of the eye and adnexa.

Pustular lesions of the eyelid occur 3 days after vaccination in a nonimmune patient. Edema is marked, and preauricular lymph node enlargement is common. Preexisting blepharitis, chronic conjunctivitis, and eczema increase the severity of the lesions. Purulent conjunctivitis associated with ulcerations and membrane formation occur. The process subsides in a week to 10 days, without serious complications. Orbital cellulitis may also develop.

Corneal complications are common, and range from acute but mild superficial keratitis to severe chronic disciform keratitis. Nummular opacification, vascularization,

and abscess formation with perforation may occur with loss of vision or of the eye. Iridocyclitis, central serous retinopathy, and perivasculitis have been noted. Pseudoretinitis pigmentosis, ocular palsy, pupillary disturbances, papillitis, and optic atrophy have followed vaccinial encephalitis.

The diagnosis is confirmed by the inoculation of infected material upon the chorioallantoic membrane of embryonated eggs. Electron microscopy and serologic tests aid in establishing the diagnosis.

Usually no ocular treatment is necessary, although antibiotics may be administered to prevent secondary infection. The corneal lesions might benefit from intensely applied IDU. Interferon administered every half hour inhibits the corneal lesions and aids the healing process. Vaccine-immune globulin given topically and intramuscularly reinforces immunity. However, VIG may result in larger and more persistent corneal scarring. Lamellar keratoplasty may be performed for abscess formation or late stromal opacity removal.

Herpes Viruses

This group includes the virus of herpes simplex, discussed in Chapter 12, and the B herpes subgroup, composed of the varicella-herpes zoster complex and cytomegalic inclusion disease.

Varicella

Varicella (chickenpox) is a benign, highly contagious disease of childhood occurring mainly in the 2- to 10-year age group). Its virus is morphologically identical to herpes simplex virus, and it also produces intranuclear inclusion bodies.

The disease is thought to be transmitted by direct contact, most probably via the respiratory route. A cutaneous eruption, associated with fever and malaise, occurs in successive crops of macular, papular, and vesicular stages in 3 to 4 days. The vesicle deflates and crusting remains for a week, leaving an unscarred depigmented area upon the skin. Superinfection produces scarring.

Uncommon ocular lesions occur on the eyelids and conjunctiva; these are generally benign. Corneal lesions consist of a superficial keratitis or a direct corneal vesicle that develops into disciform keratitis or a descemetocele. Other rare corneal lesions may occur as much as 1 to 2 months later in the course of the disease; these pass through the typical cutaneous varicella phases. An ulcer may develop and resolve spontaneously, with minimal scarring. Iridocyclitis may accompany corneal involvement or exist as a separate entity which is self-limited and mild. Motor and optic nerve involvement occur in association with encephalitis.

There is no treatment for the disease. The ocular complications are best handled by bland ointments for comfort, antibiotics for superinfection, and atropine for iridocyclitis.

Herpes Zoster

This entity has an acute onset of a unilateral cutaneous vesicular eruption that is segmentally distributed over the course of a sensory nerve. It is uncommon and mild in children, and follows a 1- to 3-week incubation period. It is nonepidemic and nonfatal, and occurs more frequently in debilitated persons or in those harboring malignancies, metabolic disease, infection, or neurologic disease. Trauma, sunburn, heavy metal intoxication, and steroids may also precipitate zoster. The virus of both varicella and zoster appear to be the same. Children who have recovered from a zoster infection are resistant to varicella, and vice-versa. A child with zoster may infect another child who in 2 weeks will develop the generalized vesicular eruption of varicella. The virus may remain dormant for many years, until an external insult excites a typical zoster eruption.

The disease is characterized by pain or abnormal sensations in the affected area, followed by the appearance of the cutaneous lesions. These lesions are originally erythematous oval or round plaques which rapidly become vesicles. Their clear fluid becomes cloudy, and a pustule develops within a week. The pustules dry, crust, and drop off in 2 to 3 weeks, leaving a pigmented or depigmented skin area associated with abnormal sensations or anesthesia. Systemic signs of fever, malaise, headache, and adenopathy are more common in children.

Ophthalmic zoster occurs with involvement of the first division of the trigeminal nerve, and lesions appear upon the scalp, forehead, upper eyelid, and nose. The ocular complications consist of conjunctivitis, keratitis, scleritis, endophthalmitis, and optic neuritis. Conjunctivitis is rare, but consists of the same vesicopapular lesions as those of the skin. Scarring is common. Epithelial keratitis supercedes the characteristic stromal opacities, which are 1 to 2 mm. in diameter. These lesions and assorted epithelial lesions may resolve, but more commonly a few areas of stromal scarring remain. Disciform keratitis, closely resembling herpes simplex keratitis, may also be noted. Decreased corneal sensation may remain, depending upon the degree of damage to the cells of the gasserian ganglion supplying the cornea. Neuroparalytic keratitis with disastrous sequelae may also prevail.

Iridocyclitis, either rare primary, or more commonly secondary to keratitis, may be present. Secondary glaucoma, hypotony, and hypopyon exist with a diffuse exudative iridocyclitis. Localized herpetic lesions of the iris, ciliary body, and choroid, associated with pain and severe intraocular reaction, occur only rarely. Pupillary dysfunction may follow third nerve involvement or local disease processes. Optic neuritis, optic atrophy, and cranial nerve involvement may also be present.

The treatment of zoster is symptomatic. Relief of pain, topical antibiotics for superinfection, and atropine for iridocyclitis are recommended. Tarsorrhaphy for intractable ulceration of neuroparalytic keratitis may be necessary.

Cytomegalovirus

Cytomegalic inclusion disease is caused by a species-specific virus widely found in the animal kingdom. It is a DNA virus morphologically identical to that of herpes simplex.

The route of acquired infection is unknown. The disease is most probably congenitally acquired in newborn infants as a result of a primary infection of the mother during pregnancy. It is, however, most commonly asymptomatic at birth, with only viral excretion noted. The more severe forms consist of prematurity, low birth weight, jaundice, hepatosplenomegaly, hepatitis, thrombocytopenia, purpura, pneumonitis, and CNS disorders.

The neurologic abnormalities consist of mental retardation, microcephaly, convulsions, and motor disturbances, and many infants surviving the disease exhibit these latter findings. Mild diffuse peripheral chorioretinitis associated with periventricular cerebral calcification and optic atrophy suggests cytomegalovirus infection. Perivascular infiltrates have also been noted.

Inapparent infection during childhood is common, and the virus may be recovered from the urine, gastric washings, adenoidal tissue, and salivary glands of healthy children.

The disease is confirmed by the presence of cytomegalic cells with intranuclear inclusions found in the urinary sediment of infected infants. A high titer of neutralizing antibody in the first few months of life suggests congenital disease. A complement fixation test is a useful confirmatory test following the first year of life. The differential diagnosis consists of toxoplasmosis, rubella, syphilis, and Coxsackie B virus. No treatment is known.

RNA VIRUSES

Enterovirus

The enteroviruses are members of a large family of picornaviruses. The enteroviruses, which primarily inhabit the alimentary tract of man, include the polio virus, Coxsackie viruses, and ECHO (enteric cytopathogenic human orphan) viruses. The commonest clinical expression of infection by an enterovirus is an acute, self-limited, febrile illness without distinctive features, occurring during the summer months and mainly affecting children. Ocular involvement by these pathogens is rare.

Poliomyelitis

This is an acute viral infection characterized by varying degrees of neuronal injury, with special localization in the anterior horns and the motor nuclei of the brain stem. There is a wide range of clinical manifestations, from inapparent infection to flaccid paralysis of many muscle groups. Death may occur from asphyxia and in-

volvement of vital centers in the brain stem. The patients are described, on a clinical basis, as having spinal, bulbar, cerebellar, encephalitis, or meningeal polio. The bulbar type is most likely to involve the eye, but any of the clinical types may exhibit some ocular signs. Based on a review of ocular abnormalities in poliomyelitis by Murray and Walsh (1954), it appears that the most frequent eye symptom is diplopia, with or without demonstrable muscle palsies, and that nystagmus is the most common ocular sign. Murray and Walsh also note that the muscle palsies are not isolated but are usually associated with other evidences of brain stem involvement. The sixth nerve is involved most frequently, followed by the third and, rarely, the fourth. Other ocular signs and symptoms include papilledema, transient loss of vision, visual agnosia, seventh nerve palsy, and pupillary abnormalities, including Horner's syndrome and nystagmus. Optic neuritis has been reported, but no pathologic examination has revealed damage to the visual cortex, visual pathways, or optic nerves. An important prognostic note for the ophthalmologist is that if the patient survives there is little likelihood of any residual ocular disability. Treatment is symptomatic.

Coxsackie Viruses

These viruses are separated into two groups. Group A characteristically causes flaccid paralysis as a result of the extensive necrosis of skeletal muscle. Group B viruses cause tremors, spasticity, and paralysis with varying degrees of focal myositis, as well as encephalomyelitis, myocarditis, hepatitis, pancreatitis, necrosis of brown fat, and less regularly, lesions of other organs. Twenty-four Coxsackie viruses of group A and 6 of group B have been recognized, each being antigenically distinct. No natural reservoir of infection other than man has been found, although flies, dogs, and possibly cockroaches are able to transport these agents. The virus can produce aseptic meningitis and other neurologic disorders, including paralysis, encephalitis, ataxia, and infectious neuronitis.

In the above disorders, the eye may be involved secondarily with muscle palsies or papilledema, both of which are usually transitory and rare. Primary ocular involvement does occur with Coxsackie virus, group A, type 5 or 16, in association with hand, foot, and mouth disease. This disease is characterized by vesicular and ulcerative lesions in the mouth, maculopapular rash, and vesicles on the hands and feet. In rare instances, a severe keratoconjunctivitis may develop, characterized by a profuse, slimy discharge and a superficial corneal pannus. Limbal, phlyctenule-like lesions may develop which then ulcerate, or a pseudomembranous conjunctivitis may occur. Treatment is symptomatic.

ECHO Viruses

Although slight antigenic relations with other enteroviruses have been found, the ECHO (enteric cytopathogenic human orphan) viruses appear to be distinct entities. They do, however, produce clinical disorders which closely mimic the Coxsackie viruses, and it is expected that similar ocular changes occur.

Paramyxovirus

These medium-sized viruses have receptors for mucin and are therefore able to agglutinate red blood cells. This feature is more variable in the paramyxovirus than in the orthomyxovirus, an influenza disease group. The paramyxo-virus also contains an enzyme, neuroaminidase, which elutes the virus from the red blood cells.

Mumps

Mumps is a common contagious disease characterized by salivary gland involvement. Whether the virus enters the glands from the mouth and a viremia follows with secondary infection of the brain, pancreas, testes, and ovaries or whether it enters the respiratory tract followed by a viremia and organ involvement secondarily is unknown. The incubation period averages 18 to 21 days, and a prodromal period of malaise, anorexia, fever, and headache follows. Rapid enlargement of one or both parotid or other salivary glands occurs, and is associated with pain and fever.

The ocular complications include dacryocystis, dacryoadenitis, episcleritis,

conjunctivitis, keratitis, iridocyclitis, and optic neuritis. Conjunctivitis with a mild discharge is common. Edema and some conjunctival hemorrhages may occur which herald a diffuse episcleritis. A late complication of dacryoadenitis is a keratitis sicca syndrome. A rare unilateral interstitial keratitis with severe visual loss, but with complete recovery hastened by steroid treatment, is found only with mumps. No other specific treatment is known for mumps ocular disease.

Meningitis or encephalitis may occur with mumps to produce the ocular signs of bilateral optic neuritis, with good prognosis for recovery. Optic atrophy is rare, as are involvements of the extraocular muscles and pupillary responses.

Rubella

Rubella is an acute infectious disease characterized by an incubation period of 16 to 18 days followed by a rash. It is preceded by post auricular and suboccipital adenopathy. The rash, a bright red maculopapular eruption which starts on the cheeks and spreads to the trunk and extremities, clears in 3 days. A positive diagnosis of the disease is made by tissue culture techniques and a specific hemagglutination-inhibiting antibody titer.

The ocular findings in acquired rubella consist of a mild catarrhal or follicular conjunctivitis and, rarely, a mild superficial keratitis. An associated encephalitis may produce optic neuritis or nerve palsies.

Congenital rubella takes on considerable significance because of the teratogenic affects of the intrauterine infection. A wide variety of organ systems are involved, which produce early abortion, prematurity, cardiac malformations, deafness, dental anomalies, retardation of growth and mental retardation, microcephaly, bony defects, thrombocytopenia, purpura, hepatosplenomegaly, and jaundice. The earlier the viremia occurs in the pregnancy, the greater is the teratogenic affect. These patients harbor and excrete the virus for long periods. Virus has been recovered from the throat 18 months after birth, from the lens 35 months after birth, and in urine 29 years following congenital rubella infection. The viral effect appears to retard the replication of the fetal cell, delaying normal organogenesis of early gestation. Late gestational disease produces inflammatory responses.

The ocular complications of the congenital rubella syndrome are the results of virus invasion of tissue. Transient or permanent cloudy corneas, unassociated with glaucoma, result from viral involvement of the endothelium, which may delay the elaboration of Descemet's membrane. Other cases of cloudy cornea are associated with congenital glaucoma, which may be based upon fetal angle anomalies. Cataract formation occurs during the second to eleventh week of gestation, when the maximum lenticular blood supply exists. Histopathologically, nuclei are retained in the lens fibers, and areas of necrosis and liquefaction occur in the cortex. The iris stroma is atrophic; the dilator is hypoplastic or absent. There is necrosis of the pigment epithelium of the iris and ciliary body. Subclinical chronic inflammatory uveitis is found in the late fetal and early neonatal periods, and this may account for some of the severe reactions that occur following surgical interventions. Choroidal cellular infiltration also is present. The retinal pigment epithelium is disturbed and presents the clinical picture of irregular pigment spots over the posterior pole. This defect appears to be progressive and may reduce visual acuity in some patients. Microphthalmos or microcornea, or both, occur frequently. Nystagmus, strabismus, and high myopic or hypermetropic refractive errors are also common with the syndrome.

The altered fetal immune response in the rubella syndrome appears to dictate the course of the disease. Early in gestation, there is no fetal immune mechanism to prevent viral cellular organizational disruption. In later gestation, the presence of the virus slows cellular replication and normal tissue growth and development. An inflammatory response, without marked clinical signs, develops as a late immune system attempts a defense response to viral presence.

Immunity is best acquired from the natural disease. Vaccination with live attenuated virus produces immunity, but some feel that it is not of the same lasting quality as that conferred by the natural disease.

Measles

Measles, or rubeola, is an acute, highly infectious disease characterized by a maculopapular rash. The incubation period is 10 days, and is followed by a prodromal period with fever, runny nose, cough, buccal mucosal Koplik spots, and conjunctivitis. The rash occurs 14 days after exposure; it starts at the hairline and mastoid region, and spreads to the face, trunk, and extremities. The papules are slightly raised, soft, red, and isolated, but they may become confluent. The rash fades to a brownish color in 3 to 4 days and then disappears.

The conjunctivitis of prodromal measles lasts 1 to 3 days and is characterized by injection, mucopurulent discharge, palpebral papules, occasional Koplik spots, and swelling of the plica semilunaris. Corneal lesions consist of benign superficial keratitis or epithelial erosions which produce the typical photophobia of measles patients. Corneal ulceration with perforation may occur if secondary infection supervenes; this complication takes place most commonly in debilitated populations. Uncommon neuro-ophthalmologic complications are associated with measles encephalitis. Papilledema and optic neuritis may produce central scotomas which usually disappear; however, total blindness may occur. Accommodative and other rare benign oculomotor palsies are also found.

Diagnosis is accomplished by immunofluorescence and serologic tests, with the hemagglutination test being the most sensitive.

Ocular treatment of uncomplicated measles is unnecessary. Prevention of secondary infection with appropriate antibiotics in specific types of patients, however, is recommended. A live attenuated vaccine can be highly effective for measles prevention.

Chlamydia

The chlamydia are made up of the psittacosis-lymphogranuloma venereum-trachoma group of organisms which have some of the characteristics of both bacteria and viruses. Two species have been recognized: *Chlamydia psittaci* and *Chlamydia trachomatis*. The *C. trachomatis* species has been further subdivided into three groups of strains which cause the clinical entities known as trachoma, inclusion conjunctivitis, and lymphogranuloma venereum. Reiter's syndrome has also been included in this section because of the possible etiologic role that chlamydia have been shown to play in some of these cases.

Trachoma

Trachoma is a disease which still accounts for a large proportion of the blindness in the world. It is generally found in populations that have low levels of personal hygiene associated with desert-like conditions. In the United States, trachoma is found at low incidence levels in the Indian populations of the southwest; there are, however, sporadic cases in other areas of the United States. It is generally felt that trachoma is a disease of the family unit, and infection usually occurs in preschool life by transfer from parents or siblings. It may also be transferred from one school child to another through sharing of cosmetic appliances or through close physical contact sports. The essential clinical features of the childhood disease are as follows: usually insidious onset, minimal exudate and inflammation, minimal or absent bulbar hyperemia, few eye complaints, rare preauricular adenopathy, minimal pseudoptosis, follicles involving the upper tarsal conjunctiva, extension of limbal vessels and infiltration anterior to these vessels (incipient pannus), minimal epithelial keratitis, infrequent limbal follicles or their cicatricial remains (Herbert's pits), common follicles occurring on the semilunar folds, and common spontaneous healing.

The diagnosis of trachoma is still primarily a clinical one, and in mild childhood disease the findings are likely to be considered as a case of folliculosis or "follicular" conjunctivitis, unless there is a high index of suspicion. Unfortunately the laboratory findings are usually not diagnostic. In the United States it is rare to find Giemsa stain inclusion bodies in the conjunctival smears from children or adults. Flourescein antibody studies are often more helpful but are rarely available. Follicles involving the upper tarsus, and an incipient pannus combined with conjunctival scrapings that show a neutrophilic exudate, plasma cells, degenerating germinal center cells (follicle cells), and Leber cells (macrophages), should make the physician highly suspicious that he is dealing with trachoma in a young child. In the adult or older pediatric age group, the same findings are also associated with inclusion conjunctivitis, but this has a more acute onset, and inclusions are often demonstrated in the conjunctival scrapings. The sequelae of trachoma in the United States today are minimal.

The treatment of choice for the child over 7 or 8 years of age is tetracycline, 250 mg. 4 times a day for 3 weeks. For younger children, triple sulfa is used because of the deleterious tooth staining properties of tetracycline in developing teeth.

Inclusion Conjunctivitis

Inclusion conjunctivitis is a chlamydial infection that involves both ends of the pediatric age spectrum. In the newborn, inclusion blennorrhea is probably the most common cause of ophthalmia neonatorum, and is a benign disease in that visual loss has never been documented. It is transmitted passively from the infected cervical discharge of the mother as the child passes through the birth canal. The signs of infection usually occur between the fifth to twelfth day of life, as opposed to silver nitrate chemical conjunctivitis, which occurs almost immediately, or bacterial conjunctivitis, which usually occurs within the first 48 hours. The infection presents as a purulent papillary conjunctivitis (as opposed to the follicular conjunctivitis of the adult) and frequently develops pseudomembranes or true membranes that cannot clinically be differentiated from true gonococcal ophthalmia. Such cases often develop a micropannus and conjunctival scars that are comparable to other types of conjunctivitis which produce membranes. The diagnosis is made by conjunctival scrapings, which show polymorphonuclear leukocyte exudates and usually numerous Giemsa-positive intracytoplasmic inclusion bodies within the epithelial cells. Gram stain and bacterial culture should be included in the diagnostic evaluation to insure that there is not an associated gonococcal or other superimposed bacterial infection. Treatment is usually rapid and effective with sodium sulfacetamide (10%) ointment or tetracycline (1%) in oil or ointment applied 4 times daily for 7 to 10 days.

There is a relative paucity of inclusion conjunctivitis infections following the immediate newborn period. A second peak incidence is seen, however, in the late adolescent or early adult years. In this period, conjunctival infection usually begins with a mucopurulent discharge of relatively acute onset, 5 to 7 days following sexual contact or finger to eye contact in an individual with an infected genital tract. The infection is most often unilateral because of finger to eye transmission, but it can involve both eyes initially. These patients have a history of redness and irritation with a mucopurulent discharge that sticks the eyelids together in the morning. The conjunctiva has a moderate to marked papillary reaction, with an underlying follicular response. The follicles are usually more prominent on the inferior tarsus and inferior fornix, but a few appear on the upper tarsus. There is moderate bulbar conjunctival injection. The cornea often shows a micropannus (pannus less than 1 to 2 mm.) superiorly, and a superior keratitis. A palpable, slightly tender preauricular node occurs on the involved side. If untreated, the disease runs its course over a 6- to 12-month period, without sequelae except for residual micropannus. Conjunctival scrapings reveal a polymorphonuclear leukocyte response in the early stages, but later this becomes a mixed poly- and mononuclear response. Frequently, intracytoplasmic inclusion bodies are found on Giemsa staining, but these are less numerous than in the newborn disease and are more difficult to find as the disease progresses. Frequently a second scraping 2 days after the first, or a short course of topical steroids enhances the recovery of inclusion bodies on cytologic smear. Other cells that may be present and that are helpful in confirming the diagnosis include plasma cells, Leber cells, multinucleated giant cells, and, occasionally, follicle cells. Treatment with tetracycline, 1 gram per day in divided doses for 3 weeks, is usually effective. Occasionally a second course with tetracycline is necessary if the disease recurs. An important point to remember in the evaluation and treatment of the adult cases of inclusion conjunctivitis is the venereal transmission of this disease and the possibility of other concomitant venereal infections.

Lymphogranuloma Venereum

The majority of children with lymphogranuloma venereum acquire the disease by direct transmission either from sexual abuse by an infected adult or from sexual activity among themselves. The agent usually enters the body through a minor abrasion on the penis or vulva; rarely is the primary lesion at other sites. Enlargement of the inguinal lymph nodes is the most prominent manifestation. The site of the primary lesion determines the extent and location of the lymphadenitis. The lymphadenopathy is chronic, and the involved nodes are tender and often painful. They suppurate frequently, form draining sinuses, and the nodes become matted together into adjacent tissues.

Lymphogranuloma is one of the possible causes of Parinaud's ocular glandular syndrome. It is manifested by a follicular or granulomatous conjunctivitis associated with regional nonsuppurative lymphadenopathy of the preauricular, submaxillary, cervical, and subclavicular nodes. Other forms of ocular involvement, usually unilateral, include a chronic lid edema, simple purulent conjunctivitis, chronic follicular conjunctivitis, superficial, marginal, or interstitial keratitis, episcleritis, uveitis, peripapillary edema, tortuosity of the retinal vessels, and retinal hemorrhages. Diagnosis, apart from the typical clinical appearance of the genital involvement, is made by compliment fixation titers of 1:32 or greater. Tetracycline is the treatment of choice in older children, and sulfonamides in younger children.

Reiter's Syndrome

Reiter's syndrome is most commonly a disease of young men. It occasionally occurs in women and is quite rare in children. The etiology is unknown, but it has been related to bacillary dysentery and previous sexual intercourse. The diagnosis is made clinically by a classic triad of arthritis, conjunctivitis, and urethritis. Lockie and Hunder reviewed the literature in 1971 and found only 20 cases in children; they added 1 case, and noted that all the children had the classic triad. Fifteen of the 21 cases had had diarrhea preceding other symptoms or occurring early in the course of the disease; malaise, anorexia, nausea, fever, and weight loss were also described. Conjunctivitis was the most common initial symptom, but there was no consistent order in which the findings developed. All three major symptoms usually occurred within a 1- to 2-week period. The duration of the initial attack averaged slightly over 3 months. Conjunctivitis was bilateral in all cases and ranged in severity from mild to severe with blepharospasm and photophobia. Iritis and keratitis has been commonly reported, and scarring of the cornea has occurred. Urethral discharge is generally scant in children. The arthritis was generally the most prolonged symptom, varying from mild to severe; the joints of the lower extremities were involved in all cases. A few reported cases have had recurrences. Because of the association in some instances of Reiter's syndrome with Shigella infections, stool cultures for this organism should be obtained and appropriate treatment given if necessary. Schacter et al. (1966) have found chlamydial agents in the affected joints of some adult patients. In some older children, the possibility of venereal transmission of chlamydial infections must be considered as one of the etiologic possibilities in the diagnostic evaluation.

Rickettsia

The Rickettsiae are micro-organisms that commonly inhabit the alimentary canal of certain insects (lice, fleas, mites, and ticks) and may be associated with disease in man. Biologically, the Rickettsiae have some of the characteristics of bacteria and viruses, and are classified in an intermediate position. The rickettsial diseases of man may be separated into four groups on the basis of their clinical characteristics, insect vectors, etiologic agent, and epidemiology, as follows: lice-borne typhus group of epidemic and murine typhus; mite-borne group of scrub typhus; tick-borne spotted fever group as in Rocky Mountain spotted fever and Mediterranean fever; and somewhat unrelated organism responsible for Q fever.

Rocky Mountain Spotted Fever

Rocky Mountain spotted fever has an extremely low incidence rate (527 cases reported in 1972) but causes more disability than any of the other rickettsial diseases in the United States. The name would imply that it occurs only in the western United States, but in fact it occurs most commonly in the southeastern Atlantic coastal states. The basic pathologic change is in the small vessels, and the most diverse and extensive lesions are found in Rocky Mountain spotted fever. There is a generalized vasculitis marked by swelling, proliferation, and degeneration of endothelial cells, with extravasation of blood elements and necrosis of arterial muscle cells. Partial or complete thrombosis of the small vessels occurs throughout the body, with symptoms related to the specific organs involved in the process.

The ocular signs of Rocky Mountain spotted fever are usually inconspicuous, but may include conjunctivitis, retinal hemorrhages, and anterior uveitis.

Other Rickettsial Diseases

Other members of the rickettsial group are almost nonexistent in the United States. The signs in these may be more prominent and might include optic neuritis and keratitis as well as the conjunctivitis, retinal hemorrhages, and uveitis seen in Rocky Mountain spotted fever.

Treatment for any disease of this group is tetracycline, 40 mg. per kg. daily in 4 divided doses over a period of 7 to 14 days.

REYE'S SYNDROME

This disease complex of unknown etiology is being included here since there has been some suspected evidence of a virus etiology.

Reye's syndrome is a childhood encephalopathy associated with a fatty metamorphosis of the viscera. The ocular findings include dilated pupils which fail to react or react sluggishly to light stimulus, cortical blindness, and papilledema. Treatment is solely supportive and a fatal outcome results in 50 to 80 per cent of cases within 7 days.

ACKNOWLEDGMENTS

This work was supported in part by grants to the Fight for Sight Children's Eye Clinic of the Eye and Ear Hospital of Pittsburgh by Fight for Sight, Inc., New York, New York.

REFERENCES

Cherubini, T. D., and Spaeth, G. L.: Anterior non-granulomatous uveitis associated with Rocky Mountain spotted fever. Arch. Ophthal., 81:363, 1969.

Debré, R., Celers, J., and Netter, R.: Introduction, in Debré, R., and Celers, J. (eds.): Clinical Virology. Philadelphia, W. B. Saunders Co., 1970.

Dekking, F.: Smallpox: Clinical aspects, diagnosis, and treatment. In Debré, R., and Celers, J. (eds.): Clinical Virology. Philadelphia, W. B. Saunders Co., 1970.

Duke-Elder, S.: Diseases of the Outer Eye. In System of Ophthalmology. Vol. VIII. St. Louis, The C. V. Mosby Co., 1965.

Duke-Elder, S.: Diseases of the Uveal Tract. In System of Ophthalmology. Vol. IX. St. Louis, The C. V. Mosby Co., 1966.

Duke-Elder, S.: Neuro-ophthalmology. In System of Ophthalmology. Vol. XII. St. Louis, The C. V. Mosby Co., 1971.

Fetterman, G. H.: New laboratory aids in clinical diagnosis of inclusion disease of infancy. Amer. J. Clin. Path., 22:424, 1952.

Fulginiti, V. A., Winograd, L. A., and Jackson, M.: Therapy of experimental vaccinal keratitis. Arch. Ophthal., 74:739, 1965.

Jawetz, E., Melnick, J. L., and Adelberg, E. A.: General properties of viruses, In Medical Microbiology. Los Altos, Calif., Lange Medical Publications, 1972.

Lockie, G. N., and Hunder, G. G.: Reiter's syndrome in children. A case report and review. Arthritis Rheum., 14:767, 1971.

Massey, James Y., Hampton, Roy F., and Bornhofen, John H.: Ocular manifestations of Reye syndrome. Arch. Ophthal., 91:441, 1974.

Melnick, J. L., and McCombs, R. M.: Classification and nomenclature of animal viruses, Progr. Med. Virol., 8:400, 1966.

Mordhorst, C. H., and Dawson, C. R.: Sequelae of neonatal inclusion conjunctivitis and associated disease in parents. Amer. J. Ophthal., 71:861, 1971.

Murray, R. E., and Walsh, F. B.: Ocular abnormalities in poliomyelitis and their pathogenesis. Can. Med. Assoc. J., 70:141, 1954.

Nelson, W. E., Vaughan, V. C., III, and McKay, J. R.: Textbook of Pediatrics. 9th ed. Philadelphia, W. B. Saunders Co., 1969.

Schacter, J., Barnes, M. C., and Jones, J. P., Sr.,: Isolation of Bedsoniae from the joints of patients with Reiter's syndrome. Proc. Soc. Exp. Biol. Med., 122:283, 1966.

Thygeson, P., and Dawson, C. R.: Trachoma and follicular conjunctivitis in children. Arch. Ophthal., 75:3, 1966.

Thygeson, P.: Historical review of oculogenital disease. Amer. J. Ophthal., 71:975, 1971.

Wang, S. P., and Grayston, J. T.: Immunologic relationship between genital TRIC, lymphogranuloma venereum, and related organisms in a new microtiter indirect immunofluorescence test. Amer. J. Ophthal., 70:367, 1970.

Wolff, S. M.: The ocular manifestations of congenital rubella. J. Pediatr. Ophthal., 10:101, 1973.

Systemic Bacterial Diseases
Guy H. Chan, M.D.

STREPTOCOCCUS

Scarlet Fever

Along with the systemic effects of fever and rash caused by streptococcus toxin, the eyes of children between ages 2 to 8 years may show effects ranging from mild catarrhal conjunctivitis to severe corneal ulceration and perforation. Uveitis, pigmentary retinal changes, and optic neuritis may also occur.

Erysipelas

Beta hemolytic streptococcus causes acute inflammation of the skin and subcutaneous tissue. The child sick with fever and toxemia may have diffuse dermatitis affecting the eyelids and face. Severe swelling of the eyelids can lead to abscess and gangrene. Optic atrophy may result.

Treatment

Systemic penicillin is effective within 36 hours.

STAPHYLOCOCCUS

The common pathogenic type is *Staphylococcus aureus.* In the newborn, this organism is one of the many causes of ophthalmia neonatorum. Effective management and treatment prevents epidemics within the nursery. Sensitivity testing determines the antibiotics of choice. Penicillin G, nafcillin, oxacillin, methicillin, and cephalothin are effective antistaphylococcal agents. Lincomycin and vancomycin are also excellent.

MENINGOCOCCUS

Neisseria meningitidis causes petechial hemorrhages in the conjunctiva. Papilledema, retinal hemorrhages, and exudates may occur.

Sulfonamides and penicillin are effective antibiotics.

GONORRHEA

Sanguinous, purulent conjunctival discharge accumulating in abundance under the eyelids of a 1- to 3-day-old newborn is highly suspicious of gonococcal conjunctivitis (ophthalmia neonatorum). Corneal ulceration, perforation, and panophthalmitis can result.

Instillation of 1% silver nitrate into the conjunctival sac of newborns as prophylaxis, and penicillin in adequate dosage have been proved effective.

PNEUMONIA

The organism is pneumococcus, which may cause conjunctivitis in the newborn (ophthalmia neonatorum), corneal ulcers, and infection of the lacrimal sac. Blurring of optic discs without visual loss has been mentioned.

Penicillin is effective.

DIPHTHERIA

The diphtheria bacillus, *Corynebacterium diphtheriae*, causes paralysis of accommodation, which occurs early in the illness and can remain permanently. Both eyes lack accommodation, but pupils remain reactive to light stimulation. Other neuro-ophthalmological affections are ptosis and external ophthalmoplegia—either partial (fourth and sixth nerve palsy) or complete. The optic nerve

is not involved. Membranous or pseudomembranous conjunctivitis may vary from a mild, suppurative stage to a cicatricial stage. The cornea can be affected secondarily from pressure, toxin, and lack of nutrition. Early keratitis can progress to ulceration, necrosis, and perforation.

Vigorous treatment consists of penicillin, specific diphtheria antitoxin, and supportive care.

WHOOPING COUGH

Pertussis bacillus, the cause of whooping cough, may affect the eyes with a variety of symptoms ranging from mild conjunctival hemorrhage to severe cortical blindness. Temporary blindness, papilledema, choroiditis, retinal ischemia, and ocular muscle palsies have been described.

Treatment consists of tetracycline and supportive measures.

TYPHOID FEVER

Ocular complications resulting from the typhoid bacillus (*Salmonella typhosa*) may include uveitis, retinal hemorrhages, choroiditis, hypopyon, panophthalmitis, papilledema, optic neuritis, ocular muscle palsies, conjugate gaze paralysis, orbital vein thrombosis, and orbital abscesses.

Herpetic lesions of the cornea developing after injection of typhoid vaccine have been reported.

Management should include chloramphenicol, symptomatic support, good nursing care, and isolation precautions.

INFLUENZA

The influenza bacillus may cause conjunctivitis. Sulfacetamide has been tried for the eye, but therapy is not specific.

BRUCELLOSIS

The causative organisms are the *Brucella abortus* and *Brucella suis* bacilli. The ocular lesions associated with systemic brucellosis are granulomatous uveitis, nummular keratitis, corneal ulcerations, retinal hemorrhage, optic neuritis, optic atrophy, papilledema, chorioretinitis, ocular muscle palsies, dacryocystitis, and panophthalmitis.

Treatment includes aureomycin, streptomycin, sulfadiazine, and tetracycline.

TETANUS

The exotoxin of tetanus bacillus causes generalized and local muscle twitching. In the eye, lids spasm (blepharospasm) is common. Oculomotor spasm or paresis may be associated with the many systemic manifestations of tetany.

Therapy consists of antitoxin as prophylaxis, sedatives to reduce muscle spasms, and selective use of penicillin and broad-spectrum antibiotics.

ANTHRAX

Anthrax bacilli affect the eyelids as pustules. Infection of the globe and conjunctiva can result in panophthalmitis and phlebitis of ophthalmic veins. Neuritis and severe swollen eyelids may be followed by optic atrophy.

Sulfonamides, penicillin, and tetracycline should be administered in adequate dosage.

SYPHILIS

Treponema pallidum affects the eye and the nervous system. Clinically, the eye manifestations are in two forms, the congenital and the acquired.

The ocular signs in congenital syphilis are bilateral interstitial keratitis, which is visible at age 6 years, choroiditis, retinitis, optic neuritis, and optic atrophy. Uveitis, complicated cataracts, and glaucoma may also be present.

In acquired syphilis, primary chancre may be found on the eyelids as well as on other parts of the body.

The treatment of choice is penicillin. Atropine and local steroids are helpful in treating active interstitial keratitis.

TUBERCULOSIS

Direct invasion of the eye structures by tubercle bacilli is not common. Allergy to tuberculin protein is found clinically as phlyctenules of the conjunctiva and cornea. The nodules, which are commonly found near the limbus, are associated with blepharospasm, severe photophobia, and itching.

The cornea may be affected by keratitis, ulcers, vascularization, perforation, leukoma, and pannus formation.

Tuberculous lesions affecting other parts of the body may involve the eyelid, lacrimal sac, regional lymph nodes (oculoglandular or Parinaud's syndrome), uvea (uveitis), lens (cataract), retina (retinitis), optic nerve (optic atrophy), and cranial nerves (third and sixth nerve palsy).

Ocular allergic manifestations are effectively treated with local steroids. Systemic active disease is managed by antituberculous therapy of streptomycin, isonicotinic acid hydrazide (INH) and para-aminosalicylic acid (PAS).

LEPROSY

Loss of eyebrows and lashes is the early noticeable clinical sign in ocular leprosy. *Mycobacterium leprae* affects the eye as superficial punctate keratitis, mild chronic iritis, and nodules of the skin of eyelids and of the episclera, sclera, cornea, uvea, and retina. Facial or seventh nerve paresis leads to complications of poor lid closure, paralytic ectropion, exposure keratitis, and corneal ulceration. Dacryocystitis may also occur.

Ocular therapy consists of management of lagophthalmos by tarsorraphy, iritis with atropine and steroids, and cataract by extraction.

Systemic treatment of leprosy has been the use of diaminodiphenylsulfone and its derivatives.

GLANDERS

The bacillus *Maleomyces mallei* affects the eye as dacryocystitis, corneal ulcers, and panophthalmitis.

The ultimate course is fatal. Therapy

TABLE 20–33 OCULAR MANIFESTATIONS OF INFECTIOUS DISEASES IN CHILDREN

Disease	Causative Agent	Ocular Manifestations	Treatment Recommended*
Scarlet Fever	Streptococcus.	Conjunctivitis, corneal ulceration and perforation, uveitis, retinal pigmentary changes, optic neuritis.	*Ocular:* Local antibiotics.
Erysipelas	Beta hemolytic streptococcus.	Lid edema, severe abscess, gangrene optic atrophy.	*Systemic:* Isolation. Hot compress. Penicillin.
Staphylococcus (Ophthalmia Neonatorum)	*Staphylococcus aureus.*	Conjunctivitis.	Isolation. Antibiotics sensitive to organism.
Meningococcus	*Neisseria meningitidis.*	Papilledema, retinal hemorrhages, retinal exudates.	Sulfonamides. Penicillin.
Gonorrhea (Ophthalmia Neonatorum)	*Neisseria gonorrhoeae.*	Conjunctivitis (sanguinous purulent), corneal ulceration and perforation, panophthalmitis.	Prophylaxis. Silver Nitrate (1%). Penicillin (ocular and systemic).
Pneumonia	Pneumococcus.	Conjunctivitis, corneal ulcers, dacryocystitis, blurred optic discs.	Local and systemic antibiotics.
Whooping Cough	Pertussis bacillus.	Conjunctival hemorrhage, cortical blindness, papilledema, choroiditis, retinal ischemia, ocular muscle palsies.	Tetracycline.
Typhoid Fever	*Salmonella typhosa.*	Uveitis (iritis, choroiditis), hypopyon, panophthalmitis, orbital abscesses, orbital vein thrombosis, retinal hemorrhages, papilledema, optic neuritis, ocular muscle palsies, conjugate gaze paralysis.	*Ocular:* Atropine and antibiotics. *Systemic*:* Chloramphenicol.
	Typhoid vaccine.	Herpes of cornea.	
Diphtheria	*Corynebacterium diphtheriae.*	Paralysis of accommodation, fourth and sixth nerve palsies, complete external ophthalmoplegia, membranous or pseudomembranous conjunctivitis, keratitis, corneal ulceration.	*Ocular:* Antibiotics of choice. *Systemic*:* Penicillin. Diphtheria antitoxin.
H. Influenza	Influenza bacillus.	Conjunctivitis.	*Ocular:* Sulfacetamide. *Systemic*:* No specific therapy.
Brucellosis	*Brucella abortus* and *Brucella suis* bacilli.	Corneal ulcerations, nummular keratitis, granulomatous uveitis, choreoretinitis, retinal hemorrhage, optic neuritis, optic atrophy, papilledema, ocular muscle palsies, dacryocystitis, panophthalmitis.	*Ocular:* Local antibiotics. Atropine. *Systemic*:* Aureomycin. Sulfadiazine. Tetracycline. Streptomycin.
Tetanus	B. tetanus.	Blepharospasm, ocular muscle palsy.	Penicillin. Sedatives to reduce muscle spasm. Antitoxin for prophylaxis.

*The effective dosages for systemic drugs administered to children at various age groups can be found in Gellis and Kagan: Current Pediatric Therapy.

TABLE 20–33 OCULAR MANIFESTATIONS OF INFECTIOUS DISEASES IN CHILDREN (Continued)

Disease	Causative Agent	Ocular Manifestations	Treatment Recommended*
Anthrax	Anthrax bacilli or spores.	Pustules of eyelids, conjunctivitis, pan-ophthalmitis, ophthalmic phlebitis, optic atrophy.	Local and systemic antibiotics (sulfonamides, penicillin, tetracycline).
Syphilis	*Treponema pallidum.*	*Congenital syphilis:* Bilateral interstitial keratitis, choroiditis, retinitis (salt-and-pepper fundus), optic neuritis, optic atrophy, uveitis, complicated cataract, glaucoma. *Acquired syphilis:* Primary chancre on the eyelids.	*Systemic*:* Penicillin.
Tuberculosis	*Mycobacterium tuberculosis.*	Keratitis, corneal ulcers, vascularization, leukoma, phlyctenular pannus, tuberculous lesions affecting eyelid, lacrimal sac, conjunctiva, and cornea, oculoglandular (Parinaud's) syndrome, uveitis, retinitis, cataract, optic atrophy, third and sixth nerve palsies.	*Systemic*:* Rest, diet, hygiene, and appropriate drugs. Streptomycin. Isonicotinic acid hydrazide (INH). Para-aminosalicylic acid (PAS).
	Allergic reaction to tuberculin protein.	Phlyctenules of the conjunctiva and cornea (photophobia, blepharospasm, itching).	*Ocular:* Local steroid for allergic manifestations.
Leprosy	*Mycobacterium leprae.*	Superficial punctate keratitis, iritis, nodular thickening of eyelids, episclera, sclera, cornea, iris, choroid, and retina, loss of eyebrows and lashes, lagophthalmos, exposure keratitis, corneal ulceration, seventh nerve paresis (epiphoria and paralytic ectropion), dacryocystitis.	*Ocular:* Atropine and steroid for iritis. Tarsorraphy for lagophthalmos. *Systemic*:* Diaminodiphenylsulfone.
Glanders	*Malleomyces mallei.*	Dacryocystitis, corneal ulcers, panophthalmitis.	*Ocular:* Antibiotics of choice. *Systemic*:* Supportive measures.
Tularemia	*Pasteurella tularensis.*	Severe conjunctivitis, parotid and submaxillary swelling, optic neuritis, corneal ulceration and perforation, limbal pannus, conjunctival ulcers.	*Ocular:* Antibiotics of choice. *Systemic*:* Streptomycin, aureomycin, chloramphenicol.
Yaws	*Treponema pertenue.*	Granulomas of eyelids and brows, catarrhal conjunctivitis, keratitis, iritis, cicatricial ectropion, lagophthalmos, corneal complications.	Penicillin.
Relapsing Fever	*Borrelia recurrentis.*	Edema of eyelids, iridocyclitis, vitreous opacities, optic neuritis, conjunctivitis, superficial keratitis.	*Ocular:* Atropine steroids. *Systemic*:* Aureomycin, penicillin.
Leptospirosis (Weil's Disease)	*Leptospira icterohaemorrhagiae.*	Conjunctivitis, choroidal and retinal orbital hemorrhages, iridocyclitis, myositis.	*Ocular:* No specific treatment. *Systemic*:* Local antibiotics and steroids of choice.
Rat-bite Fever	*Spirillum minus.*	Lid edema	Penicillin. Supportive therapy.

consists of local antibiotics for eye infection and systemic supportive measures.

TULAREMIA

Pasteurella tularensis causes glandular swelling of the parotid and submaxillary glands, severe conjunctivitis and ulcerations, corneal ulceration and perforation, limbal nodules and pannus, and optic neuritis. Severe forms can be fatal.

Streptomycin, aureomycin, and chloramphenicol are recommended for treatment.

YAWS

Treponema pertenue is carried by flies and affects children.

The eye involvement includes granulomas of the lids and brows, catarrhal conjunctivitis, keratitis, iritis, cicatricial ectropion, and lagophthalmos which can lead to corneal complications.

Penicillin in adequate dosage is effective.

RELAPSING FEVER

Ocular involvement by *Borrelia recurrentis* includes lid edema, conjunctivitis, superficial keratitis, iridocyclitis, vitreous opacities, and optic neuritis.

Aureomycin and penicillin are recommended as effective treatment.

WEIL'S DISEASE (LEPTOSPIROSIS)

The organism is *Leptospira icterohemorrhagiae*, transmitted by rat.

Conjunctivitis, hemorrhage in the choroid, retina, optic nerve, and orbit, iridocyclitis, and myositis of ocular muscles have been described.

Penicillin and streptomycin have been suggested, even though the treatment is not specific.

RAT-BITE FEVER

Spirillum minus is transmitted to man by rat bites, and the eye may be affected as lid edema.

Penicillin and supportive therapy are recommended.

DISEASES OF UNCERTAIN ETIOLOGY

Reiter's Syndrome

This disease consists of a nonspecific conjunctivitis, urethritis, and polyarthritis which occurs typically in young men. The syndrome resembles gonorrhea, but no specific organisms can be identified. An anterior uveitis may also be present. The prognosis for complete recovery from all the symptoms is good.

Uveoparotid Fever (Heerfordt's Disease)

This diagnostic entity was so labeled prior to its recognition as part of the symptom complex of sarcoidosis consisting of uveitis and parotitis.

Infectious Mononucleosis

Characteristically a disease of teenagers, infectious mononucleosis begins with fever, sore throat, lymphadenopathy, and a positive heterophil antibody test. Splenomegaly with a tendency toward rupture is a complication to be considered. Various ocular changes such as episcleritis, uveitis, nystagmus, papilledema, and facial palsy have been described. Isolated third nerve palsy has been reported in 2 cases.

REFERENCES

Ellis, P. P., and Smith, D. L.: Handbook of Ocular Therapeutics. St. Louis, The C. V. Mosby Co., 1969.

Gellis, S., and Kagan, B.: Current Pediatric Therapy. Philadelphia, W. B. Saunders Co., 1971.

Toronto Hospital for Sick Children: The Eye In Childhood. Chicago, Year Book Medical Publishers, 1967.

Mycotic Infections

Robison D. Harley, M.D.

BLASTOMYCOSIS

Blastomycosis is a chronic granulomatous infection caused by the yeastlike fungus Blastomyces. The systemic infection is often fatal and may involve the skin, eyes, lungs, abdominal organs, and central nervous system.

Ocular involvement includes keratitis with hypopyon, iris nodules and iridocyclitis, severe lid infections, conjunctivitis, uveitis, and lacrimal duct obstruction. The histopathologic picture is similar to tuberculosis and must be differentiated by a demonstration of organisms.

Stilbamidine, 2-hydroxystilbamidine, and amphotericin B constitute the preferred treatment.

CRYPTOCOCCOSIS

Human infection by *Cryptococcus neoformans (Torula histolytica)* generally manifests as a fatal meningitis. The fungus has a predilection for the central nervous system including the optic nerve and retina. Iridocyclitis and secondary glaucoma have been reported. Amphotericin B may be successful.

COCCIDIOIDOMYCOSIS

Coccidioidomycosis (*C. imitis*), occurring chiefly in the western United States, has rarely been proved to involve the eye. Iridocyclitis and choroiditis have occurred in which the organisms were recovered from the involved tissue.

LEPTOTRICHOSIS

The leptotrichia are widely distributed in nature, but their mode of transmission as well as their role as a pathogen is uncertain.

Characteristically, a unilateral conjunctivitis develops, particularly in children, and is associated with lymphadenopathy. The lesion appears as a small yellow or gray area on top of the markedly thickened conjunctiva that results from follicular enlargement.

The organism has been identified as an etiologic agent in Parinaud's oculoglandular syndrome, which occurs as an acute unilateral conjunctivitis complicated by regional adenopathy. However, a number of conditions may be classed with Parinaud's oculoglandular syndrome, including cat-scratch fever, syphilis, tuberculosis, tularemia, lymphogranuloma venereum, and glanders.

The treatment consists of topical and systemic antibiotics.

HISTOPLASMOSIS

Histoplasmosis (*H. capsulatum*) is considered one of the commonest causes for uveitis in the United States, especially east of the Mississippi. Although ocular lesions have never been proved, the presumptive evidence for their occurrence is strong. Lesions can be produced experimentally.

Typical lesions consist of discrete, atrophic, lightly pigmented focal lesions in the posterior pole of the eye, accompanied by hemorrhagic macular lesions.

Systemic infection, which usually occurs in children, is characterized by widespread lesions in the reticuloendothelial system, affecting the lungs, liver, lymph nodes, and bone matter.

The histoplasmin cutaneous test may be useful diagnostically.

MUCORMYCOSIS

Mucor occurs everywhere as a saprophyte, but human infection is rare. When it does occur, it is a rapidly fatal disease in the presence of coexisting diabetes mellitus.

Ocular involvement generally proceeds from a gross paranasal sinus infection, characterized by a vascular thrombosis, which spreads to the orbit, producing proptosis, ophthalmoplegia, and meningoencephalitis. Panophthalmitis has been reported. Treatment is usually complicated by the frequent presence of advanced diabetes mellitus, and the prognosis is grave.

CANDIDIASIS (MONILIASIS)

Candida albicans is a yeastlike organism that commonly affects the mouths of newborns from the vulvovaginitis of the mother.

Ocular involvement includes lid lesions, blepharoconjunctivitis, keratitis, corneal ulcers, chorioretinitis, and dacryocystitis. Amphotericin B is the treatment of choice, but preferably under the direction of the pediatrician.

ASPERGILLOSIS

Aspergillosis due to *Aspergillus fumigatus* may be associated with severe iridocyclitis, corneal ulcers, vitreous abscess, and panophthalmitis. Endogenous infections resulting in destruction of the eye have been reported. A generalized mycotic infection involves the uveal tract, central nervous system, and other organs.

ACTINOMYCOSIS (STREPTOTHRICOSIS, LUMPY JAW)

Actinomyces produces a local or generalized infection which may involve the face, neck, lungs, or abdomen. The typical nodular lesion, often preceded by trauma, exhibits a central caseation and is surrounded by a chronic granulomatous reaction.

The eyelids may be involved with an indolent nodule lesion having a purulent discharge. Conjunctivitis and uveitis have been described. Endogenous infections resembling sympathetic disease or the Vogt-Koyanagi syndrome are less common.

The conjunctivitis is often associated with a mycotic canaliculitis. Actually, a very stubborn conjunctivitis persists until the yellow concretions in the lacrimal canaliculus have been sufficiently curetted and removed. The primary symptom may be lacrimation, and a swelling over the lower canaliculi can be palpated. Iodine (1%) and penicillin applied locally following removal of the canalicular concretions are effective. Fungicidals such as iodochlorhydroxyquinoline (Vioform) and penicillin are useful for the more generalized infection.

TRICHOPHYTON (RINGWORM)

Fungus infection by the Trichophyton organisms characteristically involves the superficial skin, producing ever-widening circles in the skin with associated lymphadenopathy. Eyelid involvement is generally secondary to spread from adjacent structures. Loss of eyebrows and eyelashes is associated with a folliculitis. Allergic conjunctivitis from the Trichophyton fungus has been described. Treatment with ammoniated mercury and the fungicide Tinactin is indicated.

Ocular Parasitosis (Systemic Protozoan and Metazoan Diseases)

Robison D. Harley, M.D.

TOXOPLASMOSIS

Toxoplasma gondii is the cause of a protozoan disease found throughout the world with frequent and serious ocular involvement. The disease occurs in the congenital and adult forms.

The congenital disease is derived from a mother who appears symptom free and clinically healthy although serologically positive. Following the birth of a child with congenital toxoplasmosis, it is exceedingly rare that subsequent siblings become infected. Transmission to man appears to be by ingestion of raw meat or through contact with domestic animals (particularly cats) that excrete the parasites in the feces.

The typical ocular lesion is a large healed chorioretinal scar with heavy pigmented borders and having a predilection for the macular area. Lesions may be unilateral or bilateral. The affected infant often exhibits intracranial calcification, and convulsions and retardation are not uncommon. Prematurity, low birth weight, microcephaly, and failure to thrive are also frequent manifestations of the disease. Strabismus and nystagmus may develop secondarily.

While the diagnosis can be ascertained clinically, the Sabin-Feldman dye test assures the diagnosis. The direct fluorescent antibody test also provides an accurate, rapid diagnosis. Treatment with pyrimethamine (Daraprim) and sulfonamide is effective, but serious side effects may occur (see Chapter 11). Adult toxoplasmosis has been studied in infected laboratory workers and may be manifested as an acute febrile illness with lymphadenopathy. It is rarely serious unless the central nervous system is involved. Ocular lesions are uncommon in the acquired form.

MALARIA

The malarial parasite is a protozoan (Plasmodium) and occurs in three species transmitted by the bite of the Anopheles mosquito. Ocular complications are rare even in endemic areas, but iritis, dendritic keratitis, retinal hemorrhages, and optic neuritis have been reported. Dendritic keratitis has occurred even in the presence of asymptomatic malaria, and clears promptly with appropriate malarial therapy and treatment of the dendritic lesions on the cornea. In former days, when quinine sulfate was used therapeutically, optic nerve complications were common.

AMEBIASIS

The protozoan *Entamoeba histolytica* is a cause of chronic dysentery, which may be complicated by abscesses of the liver and brain. Ocular complications include iridocyclitis and a central choroiditis which has been preceded by a macular cyst and hemorrhages frequently occurring bilaterally. The identification of *E. histolytica* cysts in the stool is diagnostic.

LEISHMANIASIS

Leishmania donovani is a protozoan transmitted by the fly which causes kala-azar or Oriental sore. Ocular complications include a chronic suppurative granuloma of the face and eyelids, a severe conjunctivitis, and an ulcerative keratitis.

ONCHOCERCIASIS

The *Onchocerca volvulus* is a filarial worm inhabiting the subcutaneous tissue. It is transmitted to man by the bloodsucking black fly (genus Simulium); a part of the life cycle of the filaria takes place in the fly. The disease is found in restricted areas of Central America and in East and West Africa. Characteristically, a large female and a small male worm are encased in skin tumors about the scalp and pelvic girdle, with secondary lichenification, excoriation, and hyperpigmentation. Countless microfilaria are produced which migrate throughout the body and penetrate the eye.

Microfilaria invade all the ocular tissues and produce iridocyclitis, severe keratitis, chorioretinal lesions, and partial optic atrophy (Figs. 20–19 and 20–20). Microfilaria can be recognized by slit lamp microscopy in the anterior chamber. Marked visual loss is common in endemic areas.

LOAIASIS

Loaiasis results from infection with the filarial worm *Loa loa*, which inhabits the subcutaneous tissue of man and is transmitted by the bloodsucking flies (genus Chrysops). Large, subcutaneous nodules known as Calabar swellings may develop suddenly about the eyelids, causing moderate discomfort. The most dramatic event is the appearance of the adult worm, which travels beneath the conjunctiva, being especially attracted by warmth. Upon stim-

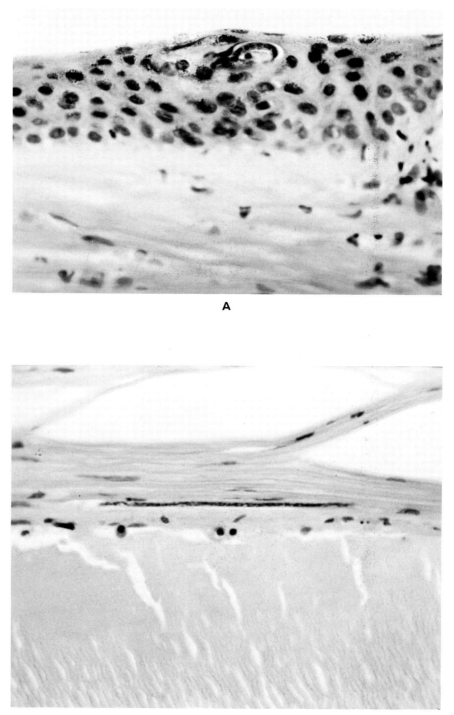

Figure 20–19 Onchocerciasis. *A*, Microfilaria in corneal epithelium (Hematoxylin and eosin, ×485). AFIP acc. 65–2708. *B*, Microfilaria close to Descemet's membrane. AFIP acc. 65–2028. (Courtesy of Eleanor Paul, M.S., and Dr. Lorenz Zimmerman.)

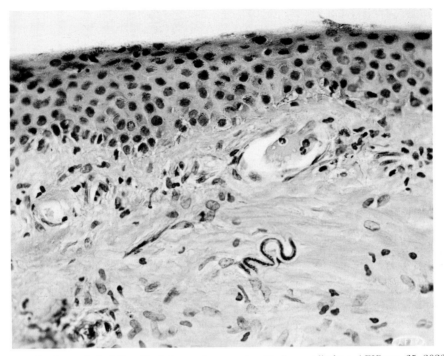

Figure 20–20   Onchocerciasis. Microfilaria beneath corneal epithelium at limbus. AFIP acc. 65–2023. (Courtesy of Eleanor Paul, M.S., and Dr. Lorenz Zimmerman.)

ulation the worm may disappear rapidly in the retrobulbar tissues and can be most elusive when one attempts to extract the little creature.

WUCHERERIASIS

Wuchereria bancrofti (Filaria bancrofti) occurs throughout the tropical world, especially in southern Asia and the Pacific Islands. Transmission occurs via the mosquito. The mature filaria inhabits and blocks the lymphatics, causing gross, deforming enlargements of the legs, genitalia, breasts, and sometimes the eyelids. Ocular complications include iridocyclitis resulting from the intraocular presence of the worm. Microfilaria can be identified from the peripheral circulation at night.

ECHINOCOCCOSIS (HYDATID CYST DISEASE)

Taenia echinococcus is the natural intestinal inhabitant of the dog, but the larval stage may become parasitic for man. Hydatid cysts consist of a collection of larvae

with their surrounding tissue reaction, and occur about the eye, especially the orbit. In countries where the sheep dog is used, hydatid cyst of the orbit is a common cause of unilateral proptosis in children and young adults. The cyst can be excised surgically (Figs. 20–21 and 20–22).

CYSTICERCOSIS

Cysticercus cellulosae is the larval stage of the large pork tapeworm, *Taenia solium.* Man acquires cysticercosis by ingesting the eggs in contaminated food. The eye is involved by the presence of subconjunctival cysts or intraocular penetration. Penetration usually remains subretinal, but the worm may proceed to the vitreous, where it has been observed moving. There is generally no reaction except for a high eosinophilia which lasts until the parasite dies. Surgical excision is the preferred treatment.

TRICHINOSIS

Trichinella spiralis is a small round worm commonly found in pigs of North

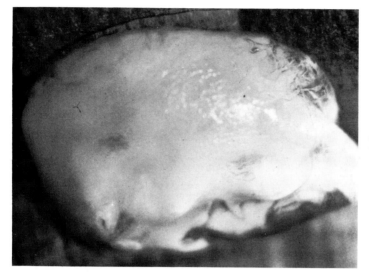

Figure 20–21 Echinococcosis. Hydatid cyst removed from orbit of 15-year-old Tunisian girl. (Courtesy of Dr. William Spencer.)

America. It is transferred to man by consumption of uncooked pork containing encysted larvae. The larvae develop into mature adult worms, at which time the fertilized female discharges hundreds of young larvae which enter the general circulation but have a predilection for striated muscle and frequently the extraocular muscles. As the larvae encyst in the extraocular muscles, pain on ocular movement and conjunctival chemosis and orbital edema develop to a marked degree. Eosinophilia is pronounced, and the flocculation test is positive.

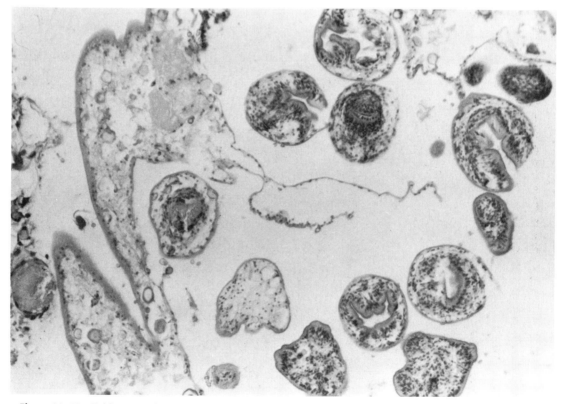

Figure 20–22 Echinococcosis. Ruptured hydatid cyst showing multiple viable scolices. (Courtesy of Dr. William Spencer.)

THELAZIASIS CALIFORNIENSIS

Thelazia is a genus of small, thin nematodes which commonly inhabit the lacrimal glands and tear ducts of animals. At least one species is found in the western United States, but other species of Thelazia are found in the Far East. Although known as "eye worms" in dogs, horses, and cattle, human infestation has been recorded in which the worm moves freely in the conjunctival sac, resulting in irritation, lacrimation, and pain until removed.

OCULAR MYIASIS

Conjunctival and lid infestation of human beings and animals by fly larvae occurs commonly in the tropics. At least three species of flies have been identified. The flies are frequently attracted by filth and fetid smells to localized areas about the nose and eyes, where they deposit their eggs. The larvae burrow into the ocular tissues with symptoms of itching, burning, and lacrimation. The inflammatory reaction, necrosis, and local destruction may become severe.

Enlarged, engorged larvae must be mechanically removed from the conjunctival sac, lids, and adjacent structures after they have been paralyzed with cocaine (10%). In one instance, the larva of the fly *Dermatobia hominis* was excised from a boy's lid, where it resembled and was mistaken for a large chalazion.

DEMODEX FOLLICULORUM

Demodex folliculorum is a mite, 0.08 × 0.04 mm. in size, which parasitizes man with a special preference for the base of the eyelashes. Blepharitis with itching is a common symptom. Demodex may also be associated with pityriasis folliculorum and one type of acne rosacea. Mites are infrequent in children, but are commonly found after age 20. Diagnosis may be sus-

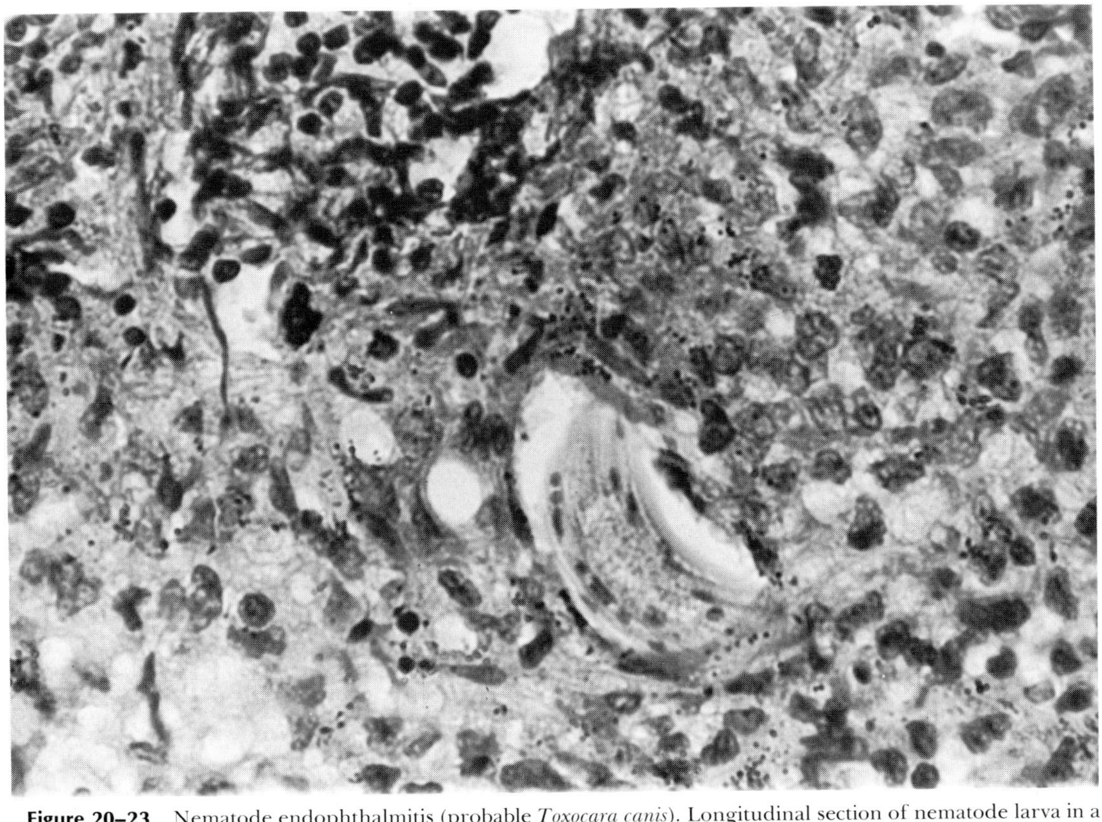

Figure 20–23   Nematode endophthalmitis (probable *Toxocara canis*). Longitudinal section of nematode larva in a vitreoretinal granuloma (Hematoxylin and eosin, ×640). (Courtesy of Dr. Merlyn Rodriguez.)

pected by the finding of fine debris on the lid margin and at the base of the eyelashes. The organism can be demonstrated by removing four lashes from each lid and then covering them with a drop of peanut oil; more than 6 mites from 16 lashes is diagnostic. Sodium sulphacetamide ointment (10%) is effective.

TOXOCARIASIS

Toxocara is a common intestinal parasite of dogs, especially puppies, and also cats. The ova expelled in the feces of puppies are resistant to drying, and frequently contaminate the play areas of children. Fingers in the mouth or eating dirt facilitates transmission. Ocular infestation occurs in children aged 3 to 15, and is manifested as a localized white elevated granuloma in the macular or temporal area. There is usually minimal reaction or pigmentary proliferation about the lesion. Iridocyclitis, endophthalmitis, and retinal detachment occur in some instances.

An eosinophilia is frequently present during the active invasive stage of the nematode larvae. Skin and serologic tests are too nonspecific to be helpful. Ocular toxocariasis may be difficult to differentiate from retinoblastoma, especially in the presence of massive retinal detachment or a severe inflammatory reaction of the vitreous (see Fig. 20–23).

REFERENCES

Conant, N. F., et al. (eds.): Manual of Clinical Mycology. 3rd ed. Philadelphia, W. B. Saunders Co., 1971.

Coston, T. O.: Demodex folliculorum blepharitis. Trans. Amer. Ophthal. Soc., 65:361, 1967.

Duke-Elder, S.: Diseases of the Outer Eye, Part 1. *In* Systems of Ophthalmology. Vol. VIII. St. Louis, The C. V. Mosby Co., 1966, p. 385.

Duke-Elder, S.: Diseases of the Uveal Tract. *In* Systems of Ophthalmology. Vol. IX. St. Louis, The C. V. Mosby Co., 1966, p. 383.

Harley, R. D.: Ocular myiasis (ophthalmomyiasis). Amer. J. Ophthal., 26:742, 1943.

Harley, R. D., and Kaiser, R. F.: Dendritic keratitis associated with chronic malaria. Amer. J. Ophthal., 28:1309, 1945.

Harley, R. D., and Wedding, E. S.: Uveitis, meningitis, poliosis, dysacousia and vitiligo. Report of a case due to actinomyces. Amer. J. Ophthal., 29:524, 1946.

Harley, R. D., and Mishler, J. E.: Endogenous uveitis from Aspergillis. Trans. Amer. Acad. Ophthal. and Otolaryngol., 63:264, 1959.

Irvine, W. C., and Irvine, A. R., Jr.: Nematode endophthalmitis: Toxicara canis. Amer. J. Ophthal., 47:185, 1959.

Somerset, E. J.: Ophthalmology in the Tropics. London, Bailliere, Tindall and Cox, 1962, pp. 106–149.

Verhoeff, F.: Mycosis of the choroids following cataract extraction, and metastatic choroiditis of the other eye, producing the clinical picture of sympathetic uveitis. Arch. Ophthal., 53:517, 1924.

Wilder, H. C.: Nematode endophthalmitis. Trans. Amer. Acad. Ophthal. and Otolaryngol., 55:99, 1950.

Allergic States

Leonard S. Girsh, M.D., and Harry Salem, Ph.D.

The original definition of allergy by von Pirquet (1906) is described by Duke-Elder as an altered or heightened capacity to react to foreign substances, resulting in injury to the body. This hypersensitivity is regarded as an exaggeration of the normal defense mechanisms. Over the years, allergy has become a focal point for the convergence of many disciplines, including immunology, endocrinology, microbiology, physiology, and pharmacology.

The tissues affected by the allergy are called the shock organs, although the common denominator in the shock organ is probably the capillary and venule. The eye tissues are also capable of becoming shock tissues and of giving rise to allergic manifestations. The foreign substances that produce allergic symptoms are called allergens. Allergens are numerous and are classified by the manner in which they gain access to the body. Like other allergic conditions, ocular allergy may be caused by inhalants, ingestants, contactants, injectants, and bacteria. The eye and its adnexa also provide an environment in which a wide spectrum of immunologic reactions may occur, including anaphylaxis,

Arthus reaction, and delayed hypersensitivity. It is postulated that autoimmune mechanisms are operative against lens and uveal antigens, as in phacogenic uveitis and sympathetic ophthalmia, and against the lacrimal glands in Sjögren's syndrome.

HYPERSENSITIVITY — IMMEDIATE AND DELAYED

In general, hypersensitivity reactions are apparent within a few minutes after adequate exposure to the antigen (Figs. 20–24 and 20–25). They are usually associated with the presence of circulating reaginic (gamma E variety) antibodies in the blood plasma, although these may not be demonstrable in every case. The present evidence suggests that the antigen-antibody reactions involve the release of at least four distinct chemical mediators — histamine, serotonin (of questionable significance in humans), bradykinin, and SRS-A. These have the potential for producing smooth-muscle contraction and local increase of vascular permeability. Included in the group of immediate hypersensitivity reactions are the various manifestations of anaphylaxis and the atopic diseases. Anaphylaxis, serum sickness, and the Arthus reaction are readily induced experimentally in susceptible individuals by adequate exposure to antigen. They are usually associated with precipitating antibodies of the gamma G

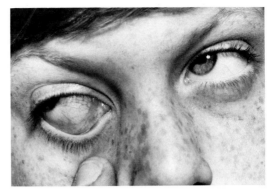

Figure 20–25 Close-up details of positive ophthalmic mucosal test, right eye, to ragweed pollen. Negative test to grass (timothy) in left eye serves as control. The scleral conjunctival inflammation greater than 1 cm. band is seen radiating from small amount of dry pollen, now moistened by the conjunctival mucus.

variety of immunoglobulins in the serum, and heredity does not appear to be a factor. In the atopic diseases, such as hay fever, bronchial asthma, urticaria, infantile eczema, and atopic dermatitis, heredity plays a major role. The antibody present in the serum of these naturally hypersensitive individuals is also known as atopic reagin.

Delayed hypersensitivity reactions usually occur 12 to 24 or more hours after contact with the allergen. Circulating antibodies are not demonstrable in the blood plasma. The sensitization appears to be a property of the cells themselves, and these cellular reactions can occur in the absence of blood vessels and smooth muscles. These conditions can be induced by surface contact (contact dermatitis) and by bacterial sensitization induced by infection.

The antibodies IgA and IgE are the current focus of much basic and clinical research. IgE is now considered to be the reagin-containing immunoglobin or antibody so important in hay fever and asthma. It is present in serum in a concentration of only 100 to 200 ng. (nanogram) per ml., which is about 1/70,000 the level of IgG. Nevertheless, IgE concentrates on the membrane of basophils and mast cells, and renders them susceptible to degranulation on contact with antigen.

It has been estimated that approximately 20 per cent of children under 14 years of age suffer from one or more of the major allergies, and in over 50 per cent of

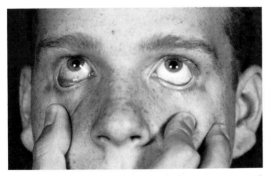

Figure 20–24 Positive ophthalmic test to ragweed pollen (*left*) visible in conjunctival sac. Vascular congestion of scleral conjunctiva is evident.

Negative control (*right*) to oak.

In this patient the ophthalmic mucosal testing correlated better with clinical history than skin testing. Oak was positive on skin testing; however, the history and ophthalmic mucosal testing were negative.

TABLE 20–34 OCULAR MANIFESTATIONS OF ALLERGIC REACTIONS

Condition	Etiology	Signs and Symptoms	Differential Diagnosis	Symptomatic Treatment
Conjunctivitis (Acute, Atopic, or Allergic)	Airborne allergens. Foreign protein ingestion.	Bilateral marked hyperemia and edema. Severe itching, burning, and photophobia. Profuse tearing (serous or mucopurulent). Marked eosinophilia in purulent conjunctivitis. Stringy discharge.	Conjunctival smear containing eosinophils differentiates against epidemic keratoconjunctivitis. Epinephrine (0.1%) blanches allergic condition more than infectious. Provocative skin and ophthalmic testing.	1. Oral antihistaminics. 2. Epinephrine HCl (0.1%) drops. 3. Steroid ophthalmic drops. 4. Irrigation of conjunctival sac. 5. Topical antihistaminic ophthalmic drops. (Local use not recommended because of sensitizing action.)
Conjunctivitis (Chronic, Atopic, or Allergic)	Airborne allergens, molds, bacteria, house dust.	Conjunctivae pale. Edema. Watery or mucoid stringy discharge. Prolonged photophobia. Itching, burning, dryness. Papillary or cobblestone appearance on palpebral conjunctiva.	Mucous and epithelial scrapings contain eosinophils. Less inflammation and irritation than acute form.	1. Same as in acute condition. 2. Desensitization.
Conjunctivitis (Vernal or Vernal Catarrh)	Contributory role: 1. Allergens (tree and grass pollen). 2. Seasonal physical factors, e.g., heat, sunlight.	Photophobia. Lacrimation. Burning. Itching. *Bilateral limbal:* Trantas' dots. Keratitis (superficial punctate). *Palpebral:* Hyperemia. Marked cobblestone conjunctival thickening of upper lid.	Seasonal (spring and summer). Children (especially boys) are more susceptible.	1. Corticosteroid ophthalmic drops, antibiotics. 2. Improves during puberty; uncommon in adults.
Contact Dermatitis of Eyelids	Contactants (poison ivy, oleoresin, cosmetics, chemicals, drugs, pollen, infections).	Itching, burning, redness, thickening, swelling, and papular formation. Unilateral or bilateral vesiculation and eczematous eruption. Weeping.	Usually begins in medial portion of upper lid. Common in females because of use of cosmetics. Positive patch testing when symptom-free for suspected contactant allergen.	1. Discontinue all use of cosmetics. 2. Wet saline compresses. 3. Topical steroids in ointment applied sparingly to skin q3h.
Blepharitis Marginalis	Seborrhea. Staphylococcus.	Scaly dermatitis (ulcerative).		1. Seborrheic treatment. 2. Staphylococcus vaccine or toxoid.
Allergic Edema of Eyelids — Angioedema, Urticaria	*Food* Fresh fruit (strawberries, melons), fish, seafood, nuts. *Drugs* Penicillin, (tetanus) antitoxins. *Insect bites* Bee, wasp, mosquito, gnat.	Accumulation of fluid in loose tissue of lid.	Intradermal testing for suspected allergy to food, drug, insect, or atmospheric mold; or, less commonly, to pollen or other inhalants (cat, dog, or horse dander). Staphylococcal infections from insect bites.	1. Avoidance of offending allergens. 2. Systemic sympathomimetic amine epinephrine (1 – 1000) 0.2 cc. q3h p.r.n. for the older child. 3. Systemic antihistaminics such as Benadryl and hydroxyzine. 4. Systemic corticosteroids. 5. Desensitization.

the adult allergies, the initial symptoms were apparent before the age of 15. Ocular complications often accompany the three major allergies of children — infantile eczema, hay fever (Figs. 20–24 and 20–25), and asthma.

Although the incidence of eye allergy in children may not be high, it must be considered in the differential diagnosis of any inflammatory reaction of the eye.

Table 20–34 summarizes the ocular changes observed in the allergic state.

PHARMACOLOGY OF DRUGS USED IN ALLERGIC CONDITIONS

The pharmacological classes of drugs that are used in the treatment of allergic conditions include the sympathomimetic and vasoconstrictor agents, the antihistaminic agents, and the corticosteroids. These can be used individually or in combination, and can be administered orally or topically.

The sympathomimetic amines with

TABLE 20–34 OCULAR MANIFESTATIONS OF ALLERGIC REACTIONS (*Continued*)

Condition	Etiology	Signs and Symptoms	Differential Diagnosis	Symptomatic Treatment
Conjunctivitis (Phlyctenular-kerato; Micro-bio-allergic)	Antigens (tubercle bacilli).	Nodules on or near cornea. Enlarged blood vessels. Lacrimation. Photophobia.	Children are more susceptible when especially undernourished with low resistance. Seasonal.	1. Antihistaminics. 2. Steroids. 3. Improved nutrition.
Microbioallergic Keratitis	Staphylococcus.	Superficial corneal ulcers, blepharitis.	Isolation of organism.	Topical chemotherapeutic or antibiotic agent.
Interstitial Keratitis	*Treponema pallidum.*	Severe pain. Photophobia. Lacrimation. Spasm of lids. Diffuse corneal haze. Characteristic "salmon patch" in acute stage. Interstitial ghost vessels in chronic and old cases.	Rule out leprosy and tuberculosis. Do not confuse pannus seen in trachoma.	1. Systemic *vs. Treponema pallidum.* 2. Topical steroids. 3. Atropine.
Corneal Allergy	Food (chocolate, cola drinks, strawberries, peanuts, butter, eggs, wheat, cheese, melons).	Photophobia. Lacrimation. Pain. Superficial keratitis.	Intradermal allergy testing.	1. Avoidance of allergen. 2. Topical corticosteroid ophthalmic drops.
Scleral Allergy	Rheumatoid arthritis.	Photophobia, pain and inflammation. Episcleritis and scleritis characteristic of rheumatoid disease.	Episcleral inflammation is segmental. Absence of exudate.	Treatment of rheumatoid arthritis. Topical steroids.
Allergic Uveitis	Bacterial allergy (streptococcus, pneumococcus, gonococcus). Anti-serum. Pollen. Food. Drug.	Acute iritis. Photophobia, lacrimation, pain, decreased visual acuity, posterior synechia, secondary glaucoma, cataracts.	Conjunctivitis and glaucoma. Intradermal allergy testing.	Atropine, systemic topical, and/or subtenon's steroid. Therapeutic trial of desensitization with test and clinically positive allergens.
Endophthalmitis Phacoanaphylactica	Lens protein.	Lens inflammation.	Positive intradermal reaction to lens protein. (Risk involved in testing.)	Atropine, steroids, and aspiration or extraction of lens material.
Sympathetic Ophthalmia	Injury to uveal pigment.	Inflammation and visual impairment.	Injury in one eye results in inflammation in other eye within 6 weeks or even years after injury.	Topical, systemic, and subtenon's steroid. Treatment may be prolonged months or even years.
Allergic Dermato-conjunctivitis	Ophthalmic drugs (atropine, mercurials, sulfas, neomycin, penicillin, pilocarpine, tetracaine, vehicle, preservative, methylmethacrylate and its polymers).	Marked swelling of conjunctivitis and lid chemosis. Lid redness. Intense itching. Photophobia. Papillary proliferation of inner lid. Skin and eyelid eczema.	Conjunctival eosinophilia. Patch testing of skin for suspected contactant drug or drugs. Positive patch test, performed when symptom free with appropriate precautions and dilution.	Steroids. Antibiotics. Avoidance of allergen.

alpha-adrenergic receptor activity cause marked vasoconstriction and blanching when applied topically to nasal mucosal and conjunctival surfaces. The imidazolines also produce vasoconstriction by alpha adrenergic receptor stimulation and are reported to have a longer duration of activity. More recently, topically applied prostaglandins E_1 and E_2 were shown to decrease nasal airway resistance in man. Although their clinical usefulness in nasal congestion remains to be investigated, their topical use as an ocular decongestant should also be considered.

The vasoconstrictors exert their antiallergic effects by preventing the inflammatory response that results from the release of histamine, slow-reacting substance, and other mediators. Until recently, the ability of sympathomimetics to inhibit the anaphylactic histamine release has not been given due attention, even though in 1936 Schild reported that adrenalin was able to produce a significant reduction in the amount of histamine released from actively sensitized guinea pig lung by antigen. Assem (1971) suggests that the antianaphylactic activity of sympathomimetic amines is due to stimulation of beta-adrenergic receptors, i.e, it is mediated via the adenylcyclase system.

The use of antihistaminic drugs is based on their ability to antagonize many of the pharmacological effects of histamine. Most antihistaminic agents also potentiate the action of epinephrine and other adrenergic compounds. Thus, most preparations used in allergic conditions will contain both an antihistaminic* and a sympathomimetic agent. Because of the central stimulating properties of the sympathomimetic, the use of such a combination also reduces the sedative effect of the antihistamine.

The use of steroids in allergic conditions is based on their well-defined clinical anti-inflammatory activity. Although their

---

*Note: Caution must be exercised in the use of antihistaminic preparations locally because of their sensitizing capacity. This is not the case when they are taken orally.

mechanism of action has not been clearly delineated, it appears that the steroids inhibit the formation or storage of histamine. Systemic corticosteroids should be administered to children with caution, since they may cause adrenal insufficiency and growth suppression. Prolonged use of topical corticosteroids may induce ocular complications such as glaucoma and dendritic keratopathy.

Currently, clinical investigations are in progress to determine the therapeutic potential of chromolyn sodium.

REFERENCES

Assem, E. S.: Inhibition of allergic reactions by beta-adrenergic stimulants. Postgrad. Med. J., 47:Suppl.: 31–33, 1971.

Salem, H., and Aviado, D. M.: Topical nasal decongestant preparations available in the United States. Rev. Allerg., 25:271–277, 1971.

Schild, H. O.: Histamine release and anaphylactic shock in isolated lungs of guinea pigs. Quart. J. Exp. Physiol., 26:165, 1936.

Weinswig, M. H.: Antihistamines. In Handbook of Non-Prescription Drugs, A.Ph.A., Washington, D. C., 1971, pp. 17–18.

Nutritional Deficiency Disorders

Guy H. Chan, Jr., M.D.

The deleterious effect of malnutrition on vision is well known and is seen in all age groups, but most commonly in children. Visual defects may be related to the state of nutrition during early childhood and may also be influenced by the mother's nutrition during pregnancy.

Normal growth and development requires a diet that includes adequate amounts of protein, essential amino acids, carbohydrates, fats, minerals, and vitamins. Generally speaking, deficiency states can occur if there is a significant disturbance in the intake, absorption, and utilization of essential foods.

This section is devoted to a discussion of the ocular manifestations of nutritional deficiency diseases that are found in children. It is well known that to elicit meaningful eye symptoms from a child can be difficult; more can be gained by astute observations of available clinical signs.

Awareness of the eye changes that occur in the early and late stages of nutritional deficiency diseases would hopefully alert the pediatrician and ophthalmologist to make an early diagnosis, initiate appropriate therapy, and thus prevent reversible disease from drifting into catastrophic sequelae.

Deficiencies of vitamin A, the vitamin B complex, vitamin C (ascorbic acid), vitamin D, and protein have been incriminated as the causative factors in nutritional diseases associated with ocular manifestations (see Table 20–35).

VITAMIN A DEFICIENCY

Eye Manifestations	Systemic Manifestations
I. Anterior segment (conjunctiva and cornea)	Retardation of mental and physical growth. Apathy.

TABLE 20–35 OCULAR MANIFESTATIONS OF MALNUTRITION

Anatomy	Pathology	Vitamin Deficiency								Protein Deficiency
			B Complex							
		A	B_1 (Thiamine)	B_2 (Riboflavin)	Niacin (Nicotinic Acid)	B_6 (Pyridoxine)	C	D		
Lids	Hyperkeratosis of skin and mucous membrane.	+								
	Angular blepharoconjuctivitis.			+		+				
	Hemorrhage.							+		
Conjunctiva	Wrinkling.	+								
	Xerosis.	++								
	Bitot's spots.	++								
	Pigmentation.	+								
	Hemorrhage.						+			
Cornea	Keratomalacia or softening.	+								
	Vascularization.			++						
	Epithelial keratitis.			++						
	Ulceration.	+		+						
	Hypopyon.			+						
	Xerosis.	+								
	Leukoma.	+								
	Polymorphic superficial keratopathy.									+
Anterior Chamber	Hemorrhage.						+			
Iris	Hemorrhage.						+			
Lens	Lamellar cataract.							±		
Fundus	Macular stippling.	+								
	Macular pallor.	+								
	Optic atrophy.	+			+					
	Optic neuritis.			+						
	Retinal Hemorrhage						+			
Orbit	Hemorrhage.						+			
	Proptosis.						+			
Vision	Night blindness (nyctalopia).	+		+						
	Nutritional amblyopia.		+							
	Photophobia.	+								

(+) Indicates presence of correlation.
(±) Indicates equivocal presence of correlation.

a. Epithelial xerosis or nutritional xeroph-thalmia, Bitot's spots (in mild stage)
   Dry, scaly skin. Follicular hyperkeratosis. Keratinization of mucous membranes.
b. Keratomalacia (in severe stage)
II. Posterior segment (retina)
  a. Night blindness (nyctalopia)—an early symptom

Definitions

Xerosis is a degenerative condition characterized by dryness of the conjunctiva or cornea. Its presence can be an early sign of vitamin A deficiency.

Keratomalacia is a late stage of vitamin A deficiency that is characterized by desiccation and necrosis of the cornea. (See Plate XIV C.)

Night Blindness is the inability of the patient to make normal adaptation to darkness. It can be the earliest symptom in vitamin A deficiency.

Vitamin A deficiency in children may be caused by dietary lack, interference with absorption or storage, or rapid loss of

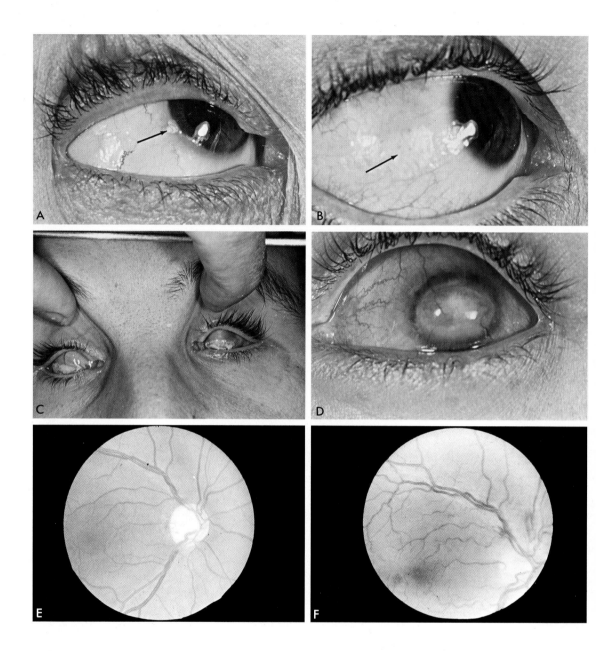

PLATE XIV

(A) and (B) Bitot's spot in vitamin A deficiency. (A) Small triangular white elevated patch (arrow) located near the temporal limbus. (B) Large patch of white foamy material (arrow) can be seen in the interpalpebral temporal bulbar conjunctiva. (C) Keratomalacia. In vitamin A deficiency, dryness of cornea (xerosis) and total bilateral corneal opacification are causes for poor vision. (D) Xerophthalmia. In severe nutritional deficiency, in addition to opacification and vascularization of the cornea, necrosis (keratomalacia) and staphyloma may develop. (E) Optic atrophy following optic neuritis from chloramphenicol in cystic fibrosis. (F) Child with cystic fibrosis has resolving optic neuritis showing dilated veins and retinal hemorrhage in the fundus.

the vitamin from the body. Diseases that interfere with absorption or storage are celiac syndrome, sprue, cystic fibrosis, ulcerative colitis, and cirrhosis of the liver; interference may also result from operations on the pancreas, operations that bypass the duodenum, congenital partial obstructions of the jejunum, and obstructions of the bile ducts. Loss of vitamin A has been reported during infections such as pneumonia, scarlet fever, rheumatic fever, and mild respiratory infections in children.

Eye Manifestations

In vitamin A deficiency, lesions have been noted in the anterior and posterior segments of the eye. In the former, the epithelium of the conjunctiva and cornea undergoes keratinization; in the latter, there is interference with regeneration of visual pigments and specifically with the resynthesis of rhodopsin.

Anterior Segment (Conjunctiva and Cornea)

CLINICAL FEATURES. A child afflicted with vitamin A deficiency may have clinically visible lesions in the conjunctiva and cornea. The clinician should search for the following diagnostic clues:

Conjunctiva

1. *Xerosis.* The bulbar conjunctiva appears dry and lusterless; it is easily wrinkled, forming concentric folds around the limbus.

2. *Bitot's spots.* In some cases, white triangular elevated patches can be seen temporally on the bulbar conjunctiva; these patches are usually located within the lid aperture and are frequently covered by foamy material (Plate XIV *A* and *B*).

3. *Pigmentation.* Melanin material exhibiting a yellowish or gray color may be observed in the lower bulbar conjunctiva, lower fornix, semilunar folds, upper lid, and fornix.

Cornea

In the mild stage of involvement, there is loss of normal luster, with drying and reduced corneal sensitivity. Patchy areas resembling Bitot's spots of the conjunctiva can also be seen on the corneal surface near the limbus (xerophthalmia).

As the disease progresses, the cornea becomes progressively duller and dryer. In the severe stages, infiltrates are formed and the peripheral cornea becomes vascularized. Epithelial erosion, ulceration, infection, and ultimately perforation may develop.

Keratomalacia, the late stage of vitamin A deficiency, is characterized by desiccation and necrosis of the cornea.

Posterior Segment (Retina)

CLINICAL FEATURES. The clinician should become suspicious of vitamin A deficiency if an active child shows more than usual awkwardness in dim surroundings. In patients with night blindness (nyctalopia), vision is adequate in moderate lighting, but poor in dim illumination such as in a movie theater. The eye becomes incapable of adapting to lower light intensities and the visual field may become constricted. Night blindness also occurs as a hereditary and congenital defect, in pigmentary degenerations of the retina, and with the retinal changes found in Oguchi's disease.

Uyemura's syndrome. This is a condition characterized by epithelial xerosis, profound night blindness, and a thick cloud of small white round spots scattered in the equator or the peripheral retina.

Systemic Manifestations

The effects of vitamin A deficiency on other organs are keratinization of mucous membranes and skin, defective tooth enamel, faulty epiphyseal bone formation, and retarded growth. The deleterious effect on the integrity of the epithelial structures increases the susceptibility of these tissues to pyogenic infections.

Diagnostic Aids

1. *Dark adaptation tests* may be helpful as an adjunct to the diagnosis. Under standardized conditions, if response to dim light is poor, the test is considered positive. However, routine clinical use of this test is limited in children.

2. *Blood levels of vitamin A.* Undetectable

or low value (<20 mcg./100 ml.) of plasma level of vitamin A or carotene may reflect inadequate intake of storage.

Therapy

In mild stages, changes in the outer eye, defective dark adaptation, and retinal white spots will disappear on early and adequate supply of vitamin A.

In advanced cases, more vigorous therapy is required and prognosis is poor.

Systemic Therapy

Adequate dosages of vitamin A or carotene can be supplied by oral or intramuscular routes.

ORAL. *Dietetic measures.* Children respond better than adults to special diet. Good natural sources of vitamin A are found in green vegetables, cow's milk, butter, cod liver oil, and halibut liver oil.

Vitamin A therapy. 1. Infants and young children—10,000 to 20,000 U.S.P.U. of vitamin A daily for 7 to 10 days.

2. Older children and adults—25,000 to 50,000 U.S.P.U. daily. If after 2 months of treatment satisfactory response is not evident, investigate for poor absorption,

other complications, or causes not related to vitamin A deficiency. For prevention, 2500 I.U. daily has been recommended as a minimum maintenance dose.

Intramuscular. Vitamin A, 100,000 I.U. in a single injection, can arrest the disease.

Ocular Therapy

Medical. Instillation of oily drops and cod liver oil, and wearing of protective glasses or goggles are palliative measures that may lessen the drying effect on cornea and conjunctiva.

Surgical. Complications of keratomalacia may respond to corneal surgery.

VITAMIN B COMPLEX DEFICIENCY

Eye Manifestations	Systemic Manifestations
Angular blepharokerato-conjunctivitis	Beriberi
Corneal vascularization	Pellegra
Corneal epithelial dystrophy, or keratitis	Cheilosis
Leukoma, ulceration	Stomatitis
Optic neuritis, atrophy	Dermatitis
Night blindness	
Nutritional amblyopia	

The vitamin B complex is composed of several water-soluble substances (thiamine,

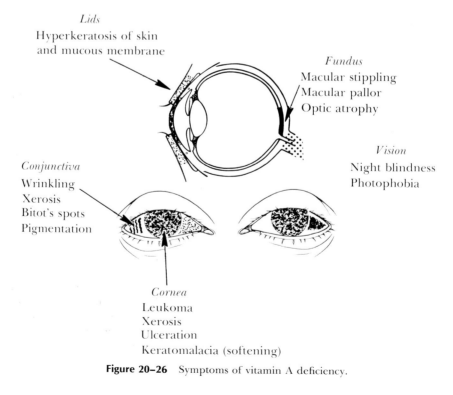

Lids
Hyperkeratosis of skin and mucous membrane

Fundus
Macular stippling
Macular pallor
Optic atrophy

Vision
Night blindness
Photophobia

Conjunctiva
Wrinkling
Xerosis
Bitot's spots
Pigmentation

Cornea
Leukoma
Xerosis
Ulceration
Keratomalacia (softening)

Figure 20–26   Symptoms of vitamin A deficiency.

riboflavin, nicotinic acid, pantothenic acid, pyridoxine, choline, biotin, inositol, *p*-aminobenzoic acid, folic acid, and cyanocobalamin), and it is difficult to relate eye changes to any one of these specific entities.

Clinical Features

Patients afflicted with vitamin B complex deficiency present a multiplicity of complaints. Clinically, one may find a wide spectrum of eye involvement, ranging from mild symptoms of photophobia, lacrimation, and circumcorneal injection to severe corneal vascularization, optic neuritis, atrophy, night blindness, and nutritional amblyopia.

Corneal Vascularization

Corneal vascularization caused by deficiency in riboflavin has been documented in animals, but in humans, convincing evidence has been lacking. In true riboflavin deficiency, the vascularization of the cornea involves all the quadrants—the clear corneal substance is invaded by capillary vessels from the limbus in all directions—whereas in trachoma, only the superior limbus is characteristically affected.

Corneal Epithelial Dystrophy

Clinically, this appears as a form of superficial keratitis. The corneal epithelium

has discrete grayish white dots arranged in patterns of double lines transversing the cornea at the lower pupillary level. Central scotomas have been reported in about 50 per cent of the cases. Frequently the corneal lesion is associated with nutritional amblyopia; however, the exact cause of corneal lesion is still controversial.

Therapy

Treatment with vitamin B complex and riboflavin (Table 20–37) has been found effective in the early stages of the disorder.

VITAMIN C (ASCORBIC ACID) DEFICIENCY

Eye Manifestations	Systemic Manifestation
Hemorrhagic tendency, affecting lids, conjunctiva, orbit, anterior chamber, iris, and retina	Scurvy
Delayed healing of corneal ulcers and wounds	

Vitamin C deficiency affects the eye as a hemorrhagic diathesis. The sites of hemorrhage are found in the lids, conjunctiva, anterior chamber, iris, and retina. Bleeding into the skin of lids appears as petechial hemorrhage. Intraorbital hemorrhage in infantile scurvy manifests clinically

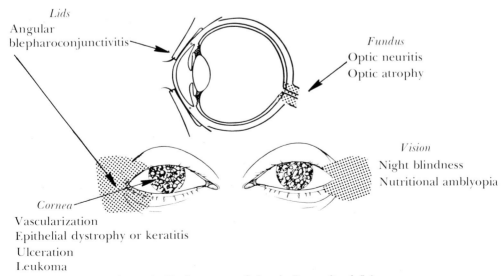

Lids
Angular blepharoconjunctivitis

Fundus
Optic neuritis
Optic atrophy

Vision
Night blindness
Nutritional amblyopia

Cornea
Vascularization
Epithelial dystrophy or keratitis
Ulceration
Leukoma

Figure 20–27 Symptoms of vitamin B complex deficiency.

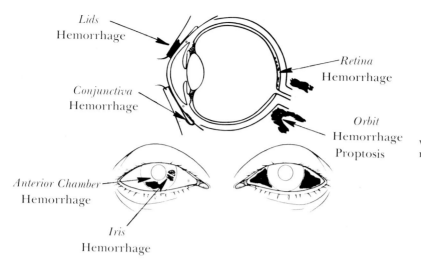

Figure 20–28   Symptoms of vitamin C deficiency ("hemorrhagic diathesis").

as spontaneous proptosis. In a series of several hundred cases of infantile scurvy, 12 per cent were found to have intraorbital hemorrhages.

Therapy

Dietary and synthetic sources of Vitamin C may be tried (Table 20–37).

VITAMIN D DEFICIENCY

Although eye signs caused by vitamin D deficiency are rare, lamellar cataract has been mentioned in Duke-Elder. In children with rickets and in adults with osteomalacia, the lens should be searched for opacities that may be responsible for diminution in vision.

Therapy

Vitamin D therapy is employed primarily for the prevention and cure of sys-

temic involvement (rickets, osteomalacia, and parathyroid deficiency).

Vitamin D intoxications. It is of special interest to note that large doses of vitamin D (150,000 to 160,000 I.U. daily) have led to eye disturbances, clinically manifested as photophobia and calcific deposits in the conjunctiva and cornea. Improvement was noted by withdrawal of the vitamin.

PROTEIN DEFICIENCY

Eye Manifestations	Systemic Manifestations
Chemosis, swelling of lids and face	Kwashiorkor (also known as hypoproteinemia, 3rd degree malnutrition (Gómez), and pluri-deficiency syndrome)
Polymorphic superficial keratopathy	
Xerosis, keratomalacia	
Dull, lusterless cornea	
Pallid conjunctiva	

Protein deficiency is seen endemically in tropical and subtropical countries where malnutrition commonly occurs, and elsewhere in times of famine. Young children

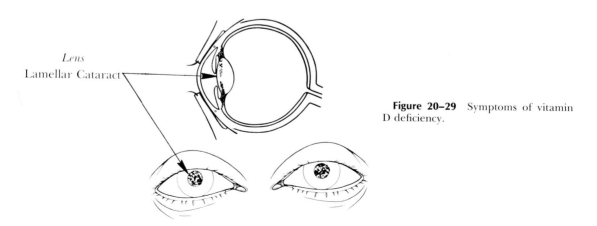

Figure 20–29   Symptoms of vitamin D deficiency.

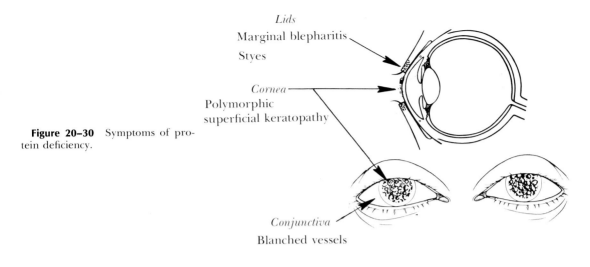

Lids
Marginal blepharitis
Styes

Cornea
Polymorphic
superficial keratopathy

Figure 20–30 Symptoms of protein deficiency.

Conjunctiva
Blanched vessels

TABLE 20–36 CORRELATION OF NUTRITIONAL DEFICIENCIES WITH OCULAR AND SYSTEMIC MANIFESTATIONS

Nutritional Factor	Eye Involvement	Systemic and Other Manifestations
Vitamin A	Xerosis (nutritional xerophthalmia, Bitot's spots). Keratomalacia (corneal softening). Night blindness (nyctalopia).	Faulty epiphyseal bone formation defective tooth enamel, keratinization of mucous membranes and skin (hyperkeratosis), retarded growth.
Vitamin B Complex Thiamine (B_1)	Accommodative fatigue. Nutritional amblyopia.	Beriberi, Wernicke's syndrome, nystagmus, ophthalmoplegia, peripheral polyneuropathy (ptosis, ocular muscle palsy).
Riboflavin (B_2)	Ariboflavinosis (photophobia, blurred vision, burning and itching of eyes, corneal vascularization).	Cheilosis, angular stomatitis, dermatitis.
Niacin (nicotinamide; nicotinic acid)	Conjunctivitis, optic neuritis, optic atrophy, ocular proptosis.	Pellagra (dermatitis, glossitis, gastrointestinal and nervous system dysfunction), mental deterioration, diarrhea, stomatitis, glossitis.
Pyridoxine (B_6)	Angular Blepharoconjunctivitis.	Seborrhea-like skin lesions, nerve inflammation; epileptic form with convulsions in infants; anemias.
Vitamin C (ascorbic acid)	Hemorrhagic diathesis (lids, orbit, conjunctiva, anterior chamber, iris, retina). Delayed healing of corneal ulcers and wounds.	Scurvy (irritability, slow growth, susceptibility to infection, poor wound healing, hemorrhages, loose teeth, gingivitis).
Vitamin D	Lamellar cataract.	Rickets (skeletal deformities, dental anomalies).
Protein (amino acid)	Polymorphic superficial keratopathy.	Kwashiorkor (protein malnutrition).

TABLE 20–37   REMEDIES FOR NUTRITIONAL DEFICIENCIES

Nutritional Factor	Principal Sources	Daily Allowances*	Usual Therapeutic Dose*
Vitamin A	Fish liver oils, liver, eggs, milk, butter, vitamin A-fortified margarine, green leafy vegetables, or yellow vegetables.	Adults: 5000 to 8000 I.U. Children: 1500 to 5000 I.U.	Adults: Up to 100,000 I.U./day Children: Avoid large doses.
Vitamin B complex Thiamine (B₁)	Yeast, whole grains, meat (especially pork and liver), nuts, egg yolk, legumes, potatoes, most vegetables.	All ages: 1 to 2 mg.	Adults: 5 to 30 mg./day Children: Not established.
Riboflavin (B₂)	Milk, cheese, liver, egg white, beef, muscle meats.	Not well established.	Adults: 10 to 30 mg./day (oral and parenteral) Children: Dosage not established.
Niacin (nicotinamide; nicotinic acid)	Yeast, liver, peanuts, wheat germ.	All ages: Niacinamide 300 to 1000 mg.	Adults: 100 to 1000 mg./day Children: Dosage not established.
Pyridoxine (B₆)	Yeast, liver, muscle meats, whole grain cereals, fish, vegetables, molasses.	Not established. 1.5 to 2.0 mg.	Adults: 25 to 100 mg./day Children: Up to 10 mg./day
Vitamin C (ascorbic acid)	Citrus fruits, tomatoes, potatoes, cabbage, green pepper; synthetic ascorbic acid.	Adults: 70 mg. Children: 30 to 80 mg.	Adults: 100 to 500 mg./day Children: 30 to 80 mg./day
Vitamin D	Butter, eggs, liver, milk, sunshine, fish liver oil; synthetic calciferol (D₂)	Adults and children: 400 I.U.	Adults: Calciferol (D₂): 50,000 to 1,000,000 I.U./day Children: 20,000 to 50,000 I.U./day
Protein (amino acid)	Pork, beef, chicken, fish, soy beans, milk	Adequate protein intake is 11 to 14 per cent of total calories	

*One I.U. is equivalent to 1 U.S.P.U.

are particularly prone to severe protein deficiency (kwashiorkor), even though they may be getting an adequate supply of calories, such as on a rice or a maize diet. Basically, essential amino acids are not in adequate supply for growth, and nitrogen equilibrium is not maintained.

Clinical Features

Children in conditions of starvation or protein deficiency appear morbid, and are more susceptible to a large number of diseases. The starved child appears dull and listless. The conjunctival vessels may appear blanched, giving rise to a porcelain-like appearance of the sclera. The incidence of marginal blepharitis and styes is increased. The hair may lose its pigment and appear bleached, but returns to normal color with adequate diet.

Polymorphic Superficial Keratopathy

The corneal lesions observed in protein deficiency consist of patches of degenerative changes in the epithelial cells, associated with round or oval zones of infiltration in the subepithelial tissues. Ulceration may occur, but usually does not penetrate Bowman's membrane.

Xerosis and keratomalacia have been described in young children with kwashiorkor. However, in these cases, vitamin deficiencies may also be contributing factors. The corneal manifestations become more evident in the terminal stages.

Other instances of eye involvement, such as subconjunctival hemorrhage, faulty dark adaptation, night blindness, optic atrophy, and increased myopia, are thought to be related to protein deficiency, but deficiency in other nutrients can also be a contributory factor. In general, it is difficult to attribute the ocular lesions to protein deficiency alone.

Therapy

Unless an adequate diet (see Table 20–37) containing the essential amino acids (lysin, tryptophan, pnenylalanine, leucine, isoleucine, threonine, methionine, valine, histidine, and arginine) can be instituted, children suffering from protein deficiency frequently die. Survivors may develop cirrhosis of the liver and suffer the ocular sequelae of severe starvation or protein deficiency.

REFERENCES

Best & Taylor,: Physiological Basis of Medical practice. 4th ed., Williams and Wilkins, 1945, p. 639.

Cockrum, W. M., Lynch, H. D., Slaughter, H. C., and Austin, E. W.: Styes; role of nutrition in etiology and treatment. J. Indiana Med. Ass., 41:489, 1948.

Davidson, S.: The Principles of Medicine. E. and S. Livingstone, Ltd. Duke-Elder: System of Ophthalmology. Vol. II. St. Louis, The C. V. Mosby Co., 1961, p. 1422.

Duke-Elder, S.: System of Ophthalmology. Vol. VII. Henry Kemton, London, 1962, p. 243.

Duke-Elder, S.: System of Ophthalmology. Vol. VIII, Part 2, St. Louis, The C. V. Mosby Co., 1965, p. 1111.

Duke-Elder, S.: System of Ophthalmology. Vol. IV. St. Louis, The C. V. Mosby Co., 1968, p. 589.

El Sheikh, M.: Vitamin deficiencies in relation to the eye. Brit. J. Ophthal., 44:406–414, 1960.

Eckardt, R. E., and Johnson, L. V.: Nutritional cataract and relation of galactose to appearance of senile suture line in rats. Arch. Ophthal., 21:315–327, 1939.

Fraser, J. D.: Ocular disturbances associated with malnutrition. Trans. Ophthal. Soc. U.K., 66:96, 1946.

Gómez, F., Galvan, R. R., Frenk, S., Cravioto-Muñoz, J., Chávez, R., and Váquez, J.: Mortality in second and third degree malnutrition. J. Trop. Pediat., 2:77, 1956.

Harley, R. D.: Exophthalmos in the newborn from vitamin C deficiency. Amer. J. Ophthal., 26:1314, 1943.

Harley, R. D.: Ocular changes in idiopathic hypercalcemia. Trans. Amer. Acad. and Oto., 69:879, 1965.

Irinoda, K., and Sato, S.: Contribution to the ocular manifestation of riboflavin deficiency. Tohoku J. Exp. Med., 61:92, 1954.

Jayle, G.: Night Vision. Springfield, Ill., Charles C Thomas, 1959.

Keys, A.: Caloric undernutrition and starvation, with notes on protein deficiency. J.A.M.A., 138:500, Sept.-Oct., 1948.

Liebman, S. D., and Gellis, S. S.: The Pediatrician's Ophthalmology. St. Louis, The C. V. Mosby Co., 1966.

Masuda, K., and Aoyama, J.: Endemic occurrence of ariboflavinosis and pellagra. Tohoku J. Exp. Med., 55:1, 1951. (Shibi-Gatchaki).

McLaren, D. S.: Malnutrition and the Eye, New York, Academic Press, 1963.

McLaren, D. S.: Nutrition Today, Vol. 3, No. 1, March, 1968.

Merck Manual. 11th ed. Rahway, N.J., Merck & Co., 1966, p. 264.

Nelson, W. E., et al.; Textbook of Pediatrics. 9th ed. W. B. Saunders, 1969.

Oomen, H. A. P. C.: Xerophthalmia in presence of Kwashiorkor. Brit. J. Nutrition, 8:307, 1954.

Orent-Keiles, E., Robinson, A., and McCollum, E. V.: Effects of sodium deprivation on animal organism. Amer. J. Physiol., 119:651, 1937.

Pillat, A., and King, G.: An inquiry into the origin of the abnormal pigmentation of the skin and conjunctiva in cases of keratomalacia in adults. Brit. J. Ophth., 13:506–512, 1929.

Shapland, C. D.: Trans. Ophthal. Soc. U.K., 66:77, 1946.

Spies, T. D.: Some recent advances in nutrition. J.A.M.A., 167:675–790, 1958.

Toronto Hospital for Sick Children: The Eye in Childhood. Chicago, Year Book Medical Publishers, 1967, p. 450.

Turtz, C. A., and Turtz, A. I.: Vitamin A intoxication. Am. J. Ophth., 50:165–166, 1960.

Venkataswamy, G.: Angular conjunctivitis and riboflavine deficiency. J. All India Ophthal. Soc., 8:33–41, 1960.

Venkataswamy, G.: Malnutritional blindness in India. J. Indian. Med. Ass., 47:67, July 16, 1966.

Venkataswamy, G.: Ocular manifestations of vitamin B-complex deficiency. Brit. J. Ophthal., 51:749, 1967.

Venkataswamy, G.: Ocular manifestations of vitamin A deficiency. Brit. J. Ophthal., 51:854, 1967.

Whol, M. G., and Goodhart, R. S.: Modern Nutrition in Health and Disease. 4th ed. Philadelphia, Lea & Febiger, 1968, p. 1025.

Wolback, S. B., and Howe, P. R.: Tissue changes following deprivation of fat-soluble A vitamin. J. Exper. Med., 42:753–777, 1925.

Yudkin, J.: Nutritional deficiency. In Sorsby, H. (ed.): Systemic Ophthalmology. St. Louis, The C. V. Mosby Co., 1958, pp. 287–301.

Drug-Induced Ocular Side Effects

Guy H. Chan, Jr., M.D.

The purpose of this section is to assist busy pediatricians and ophthalmologists in recognizing quickly those drugs that affect the eye. Using Table 20–38, the clinician can select on the vertical column anatomical structures of the eye that have the lesions. On the horizontal column, the drugs that induce the lesions can be iden-

TABLE 20–38 OCULAR SIDE EFFECTS AND DRUGS ADMINISTERED IN PEDIATRIC OPHTHALMOLOGY

Eye Pathology	Arsenic Compound (Atoxyl)	Atropine	Chloramphenicol	Chloroquine	Epinephrine	Ethambutol	Glucocorticosteroids	Indomethacin	Iodine	Mercury	Isoniazid	Lead poisoning	Neomycin	Penicillamine	Phenothiazines (Chloropromazine)	Phospholine Iodine	Plasmocid	Progesteronal steroids	Quinine	Smallpox Vaccine	Spray talc	Sulfonamides	Triparanol	Vitamin D
LIDS: (FACE) Ptosis												+												
Contact Dermatitis																						+		
Pigmentation			+												+									
Vaccinia																				+				
CONJUNCTIVA: Pigmentation				+											+									
Allergy		+											+											
Conjunctivitis																				+				
CORNEA: Keratopathy				+				+							+									+
Thinning, slow healing							+																	
Herpes Simplex							+																	
Mycosis							+																	
Pigmentation															+									
Edema																			+		+			
SCLERA: Pigmentation															+									
INTRAOCULAR PRESSURE: Glaucoma							+																	
IRIS: Cyst																+								
CILIARY BODY: Accommodative Weakness			+																					
LENS: Cataract				±			+								+	+			±				+	
RETINA: Retinopathy				+				+																
Edema									+										+	+				

(+) Indicates presence of ocular side effects.
(±) Indicates questionable presence of ocular side effect.

tified. For descriptive details, original articles are listed in the references.

REFERENCES

Becker, B., and Mills, D. W.: Corticosteroids and intraocular pressure. Arch. Ophthal., 70:500–507, 1963.

Bernstein, H. N.: Some iatrogenic ocular diseases from systemically administered drugs, Int. Ophthal. Clin., 10:553, Fall, 1970.

Boet, D. J.: Toxic effects of phenothiazine on the eye. Dr. W. Junk N. V., 1970.

Goldmann, H.: Cortisone glaucoma, Arch. Ophthal. 68:621–626, 1962.

Grant, W. M.: Toxicology of the Eye. Springfield, Ill., Charles C Thomas, 1962.

TABLE 20–38 OCULAR SIDE EFFECTS AND DRUGS ADMINISTERED IN PEDIATRIC OPHTHALMOLOGY (Continued)

Eye Pathology		Arsenic Compound (Atoxyl)	Atropine	Chloramphenicol	Chloroquine	Epinephrine	Ethambutol	Glucocorticosteroids	Indomethacin	Iodine	Mercury	Isoniazid	Lead poisoning	Neomycin	Penicillamine	Phenothiazines (Chlorpromazine)	Phospholine Iodine	Plasmocid	Progesteronal steroids	Quinine	Smallpox Vaccine	Spray talc	Sulfonamides	Triparanol	Vitamin D
RETINA: (cont.)	Vascular Thrombosis										+								+						
	Pigment Migration			+					+	+						+									
	Degeneration															+								+	
	Detachment																+								
	Pigment Stippling												+												
MACULA:	Pigment Ring (Bulls Eye)				+											±									
	Pigmentary Disturbance								+				+												
	Edema								+																
	Atrophy																								
OPTIC NERVE:	Papilledema							+					+												
	Optic Neuritis			+			+					+				+				+	±		+		
	Optic Atrophy	+		+	+															+					
	Pigment Stippling												+												
EXTRA OCULAR MUSCLES:	Strabismus												+												
	Paresis																		+						
VISION:	Amblyopia								+													+			
	Transient Myopia																						+		
VISUAL FIELDS:	Defects	+			+				+							+									
COLOR VISION:	Anomalies	+																							
ORBIT:	Exophthalmos																		+						

Harley, R. D.: Optic neuritis and optic atrophy following chloramphenicol in cystic fibrosis patients, Trans. Amer. Acad. Ophthal. Otolaryngol., 74:1101, 1970.

Hobbs, H. E., Eadie, S. P., and Somerville, F.: Ocular lesions after treatment with chloroquine, Brit. J. Ophthal., 45:284–297, 1961.

Macri, F.: Pharmacology and toxicology of ophthalmic drugs, Arch. Ophthal., 84:532, 1970.

Meier-Ruge, W.: Drug-induced retinopathy. Ophthalmologica Additamentum. 158:561–573, 1969.

Oglesby, R. B., Black, R. L., von Sallmann, L., and Bunim, J. J.: Cataracts in patients with rheumatic diseases treated with corticosteroids. Arch. Ophthal. 66:625–630, 1961.

Okun, E., Gouras, P., Bernstein, H., and von Sallmann, L.: Chloroquine retinopathy. A report of 8 cases with ERG and dark-adaptation findings. Arch. Ophthal., 69:5971, 1963.

Sonkin, N.: Stippling of the retina. A new physical sign in the early diagnosis of lead poisoning. New Eng. J. Med. 269:779–780, 1963.

E. OCULAR AND ASSOCIATED DENTAL CHANGES IN PEDIATRIC SYNDROMES

Kenneth C. Troutman, D.D.S.

Disease, Syndrome, or Condition	Eye Involvement	Dental/Oral Involvement
Albers-Schönberg Disease	Cranial nerve palsies with optic atrophy.	Enamel hypoplasia.
Albright's Hereditary Osteodystrophy	Peripheral lenticular opacities, blue sclera, strabismus.	Dental aplasia (missing teeth), delayed eruption.
Apert's Syndrome	Exophthalmos, exotropia, optic atrophy, and cataracts.	Crowded dentition, high arched palate, clefts (25% of cases), Prominent mandible.
Cornelia de Lange Syndrome	Long curly eyelashes, bushy eyebrows, synophrys, strabismus, myopia, and optic atrophy.	High arched palate, widely spaced teeth, enamel hypoplasia.
Down's Syndrome	Brushfield spots, strabismus, keratoconus, cataract, epicanthus, and mongoloid slant to palpebral fissures.	Congenitally missing teeth, peg-shaped (pointed) teeth, microdontia, delayed eruption of dentition, periodontal disease, and periodontal bone loss, underdeveloped maxilla and malocclusion, deep fissured tongue.
Ectodermal Dysplasia	Tear deficiency leading to keratoconjunctivitis, photophobia, and cataracts.	Congenitally missing teeth, microdontia, peg-shaped (pointed) teeth – particularly canines, widely spaced dentition.
Goltz's Syndrome	Strabismus, colobomas of the iris and choroid, and/or microphthalmos.	Microdontia, peg-shaped incisors, enamel hypoplasia, papillomas of the lips.
Hallermann-Streiff Syndrome	Bilateral microphthalmos, congenital cataracts which may spontaneously resorb, nystagmus, strabismus, blue sclera.	High arched palate, hypodontia, congenitally missing teeth, severe enamel hypoplasia, natal teeth, supernumerary teeth, hyperplasia of mandible.
Hypercalcemia (Hyperparathyroidism)	Band-shaped keratopathy.	Microdontia, widely spaced dentition, Generalized osteopetrosis of the bones of the skull, missing lamina dura, congenitally missing teeth, malposed teeth due to giant cell tumors.
Hypoparathyroidism	Bilateral cataracts.	Dental aplasia or enamel aplasia related to the onset of the condition, delayed eruption, external resorption and/or blunting of the roots of teeth (upper bicuspids most frequent), thickening of lamina dura.

Disease, Syndrome, or Condition	Eye Involvement	Dental/Oral Involvement
Hypothyroidism	Swollen, droopy eyelids; corneal opacities and optic neuritis rare.	Missing teeth.
Incontinentia Pigmenti	Strabismus, PHPV, corneal opacities and cataracts.	Congenitally missing lateral incisors.
Lowe's Syndrome	Bilateral congenital cataracts and glaucoma.	Absence of lamina dura around the teeth—compatable with dental changes in rickets.
Mucopolysaccharidosis (MPS I and MPS II)	Corneal clouding in MPS I. Slight or absent in MPS II.	Microdontia, peg-shaped incisors and canines, widely spaced teeth, high palate, enamel hypoplasia, large tongue, open bite.
Oculo-Dental-Digital Dysplasia	Microphthalmos, congenital glaucoma, and iris anomalies.	Wide mandibular ridge, enamel hypoplasia (primary dentition), microdontia (lateral incisors), high arched palate with occasional cleft palate.
Oral-Facial-Digital Syndrome	Lateral placement of inner canthi.	Cleft palate (alone), malposed teeth, midline notch (pseudo cleft) of the upper lip, lobulated tongue, malposed teeth, supernumerary teeth, dental aplasia (lower incisors), enamel hypoplasia, congenitally missing teeth.
Osteogenesis Imperfecta (Dentinogenesis Imperfecta)	Blue sclera, keratoconus, anterior segment defects.	Translucent bluish-gray or yellow-orange color to the dentition due to faulty junction between the dentin and the enamel layers. Small pulp chambers—sometimes completely obliterated.
Pierre Robin Syndrome	Congenital glaucoma, cataracts, myopia, esotropia retinal detachment, and microphthalmos.	Micrognathia, cleft palate (alone).
Popliteal Web Syndrome	Cutaneous webs between eyelids.	Clefts of the lip and palate, lip pits, enamel hypoplasia, heavy webbed bonds in the buccal mucosa, micrognathia.
Prematurity	Myopia of prematurity, cataracts, vitreous haze, strabismus, pupillary membrane and possibly retrolental fibroplasia with oxygen therapy.	Enamel hypoplasia (neonatal line) depending upon the degree and the duration of difficulty following birth.
Rickets	Ocular changes rare, lacrimation and papilledema associated with tetany described.	Absence or decrease in lamina dura around teeth, enlarged pulp chambers and pulp canals.
Rieger's Syndrome	Iris hypoplasia with synechia, glaucoma, partial aniridia, and corneal opacity.	Hypodontia, congenitally missing maxillary incisors, anodontia.
Rubella Syndrome	Retinopathy, cataracts, microphthalmos, iris hypoplasia, strabismus, nystagmus.	Enamel hypoplasia, microdontia, screwdriver shaped incisors (primary dentition).
Sjögren-Larsson Syndrome	Chorioretinal pigmentary changes.	Widely spaced dentition, enamel hypoplasia.

(Table continued on following page)

Disease, Syndrome or Condition	Eye Involvement	Dental/Oral Involvement
Sturge-Weber Disease	Glaucoma, buphthalmos, choroidal angiomas.	Port-wine staining of the buccal mucosa, clefts of the lip and palate, gingival enlargement associated with seizure medication.
Treacher-Collins Syndrome (Franceschetti)	Lid coloboma, microphthalmos and antimongoloid slanting of lids.	Micrognathia, crowded dentition, high arched palate, cleft lip and/or palate.
Trisomy 13	Microphthalmos, corneal opacity, cataract, iris coloboma, and retinal dysplasia.	Cleft lip and palate (frequently bilateral).
Trisomy 18	Corneal opacities, blepharoptosis, and epicanthal folds.	Micrognathia, crowed dentition with large cuspids, enamel hypoplasia.

F. OCULAR-GENITOURINARY MANIFESTATIONS OF DISEASES

Alan B. Gruskin, M.D.

The following compilation provides a concise table of the numerous pediatric disease entities which have in common clinical observations involving both the eye and genitourinary systems. In each of these diseases, the various physical and laboratory abnormalities are reported as pertains to the ocular findings and genitourinary manifestations. This information has been obtained from ophthalmologists, nephrologists, literature reviews, and the author's personal observation at St. Christopher's Hospital for Children.

Disease	Eye Findings	Genitourinary Manifestations
Aarskog Syndrome	Hypertelorism; ptosis.	Scrotal overriding at base of penis; cryptorchidism.
Acral—Renal Syndrome	Macular coloboma; atypical medullated fibers; pigmentary macular changes.	Absent kidney; bilateral hypoplastic kidneys; ureteral abnormalities.
Acrocephalosyndactyly; Absent Digits; Cranial Defects Syndrome	Widely spaced eyes; shallow orbits; hypoplastic supraoptic ridge.	Cryptorchidism.
Acromegaloid Features; Hypertelorism; Pectus Carinatum Syndrome	Widely spaced eyes; epicanthal fold.	Hypogonadism; cryptorchidism.
Acute Glomerulonephritis	Eyelid edema; encephalopathy with unilateral or bilateral abducens palsy; diminished vision secondary to either hypertensive retinopathy or cortical blindness.	Any acute glomerulitis; classically post streptococcal; red cell casts; proteinuria; normal or reduced renal function.
Alkaptonuria and Ochronosis	Pigmentation of sclera, conjunctiva, cornea.	Black urine after adding Benedict's solution, or after standing.
Allergic Antitoxin	Optic neuritis; optic atrophy; swollen lids and conjunctiva.	Proteinuria; nephrotic syndrome; hematuria.

Disease	Eye Findings	Genitourinary Manifestations
Alport's Syndrome (Familial Nephropathy With Deafness)	Cataracts; nystagmus; anterior or posterior lenticonus or both; microspherophakia.	Hematuria; proteinuria; chronic renal failure.
Amyloidosis	Tumors of lid and conjunctiva; vitreous opacities; periorbital ecchymosis; retinal periarteritis.	Amyloid deposition; proteinuria; renal insufficiency; nephrotic syndrome; renal vein thrombosis.
Aniridia, Congenital Sporadic	Cataracts; glaucoma; retinal atrophy; ptosis; dislocated lens; microphthalmia.	Wilms' tumor; unilateral aplastic kidney; cryptorchidism; hypoplastic kidney; double renal artery; hypospadias.
Anophthalmia, Polyploidy, and Multiple Congenital Abnormalities	Anophthalmia.	Crossed fused renal ectopia.
Anterior Ocular Cleavage Syndrome with Urinary Anomalies	Posterior embryotoxon, Axenfeld anomaly; Rieger's anomaly; corneal leukoma; anterior synechiae.	Bifid collecting system.
Apert's Syndrome	Shallow orbits with exophthalmos; spontaneous dislocation of eyeball; exposure keratitis; hypertelorism; divergent strabismus; optic atrophy; field defects.	Polycystic kidney; hydronephrosis; bicornuate uterus.
Ataxia—Telangiectasia (Louis—Bar Syndrome)	Telangiectasia of bulbar conjunctiva; strabismus; oculomotor apraxia; nystagmus.	Sexual immaturity; hematuria; ovarian hypoplasia.
Bacterial Endocarditis	Conjunctival petechiae; retinal hemorrhages; Roth spots.	Proteinuria; hematuria; progressive glomerular sclerosis; flank pain.
Basal Cell Nevi; Broad Facies; Rib Anomaly Syndrome	Cataract; iris coloboma; glaucoma; strabismus; epicanthal fold; hypertelorism.	Small genitalia; hypogonadism; cryptorchidism.
Battered Child Syndrome	Traumatic injury.	Traumatic injury; acute tubular necrosis; personal observation.
Beckwith Syndrome	Prominent eyes because of relative infraorbital hypoplasia; eyelid nevus; exophthalmus.	Large kidney; Wilms' tumor; clitoridomegaly; large ovaries; cryptorchidism; renal medullary dysplasia; hydronephrosis; hypospadias.
Behçet's Syndrome	Acute severe iridocyclitis; uveitis; optic neuritis; retinal perivasculitis.	Genital ulceration.
Behr Syndrome	Temporal atrophy of optic nerve; papillomacular bundle atrophy; nystagmus; strabismus.	Vesical sphincter abnormalities.
Berardinelli's Lipodystrophy	Corneal opacities.	Large penis.
Blood Dyscrasia; Coagulation Defects	Retinal hemorrhages; retinal exudates; proptosis; subconjunctival hemorrhages.	Intrarenal bleeding; hematuria; flank pain.
Borjeson-Forssman-Lehman Syndrome	Narrow palpebral fissures	Small penis; undescended and/or small testes.
Carbon Tetrachloride Ingestion	Optic atrophy; conjunctival and retinal hemorrhages; visual field defects.	Hematuria; red blood cell casts; acute renal failure.

(Table continued on following page)

Disease	Eye Findings	Genitourinary Manifestations
Carpenter's Syndrome	Lateral displacement of inner canthi; epicanthal fold; microcornea; corneal opacities.	Generalized aminoaciduria; cryptorchidism; hypogenitalism.
Cat-Eye Syndrome (Small Extra Chromosome)	Coloboma; downward slant of palpebral fissure; microphthalmos.	Unilateral renal agenesis.
Cerebro-Hepato-Renal Syndrome (Zellweger's Syndrome)	Epicanthal fold; cataracts; congenital glaucoma; Brushfield spots; corneal opacity; abnormal optic nerves; nystagmus.	Renal cortical cysts; cryptorchidism; aminoaciduria; proteinuria; polycystic kidneys; enlarged clitoris.
Chédiak-Higashi Syndrome	Ocular albinism with photophobia and nystagmus.	Glycolipid inclusions in renal tubular epithelium cells.
Chotzen's Syndrome	Ptosis; widely spaced orbits.	Cryptorchidism.
Chromosome 4, Deletion Short Arm Syndrome	Strabismus; iris coloboma; ectopic pupil.	Hypospadias; cryptorchidism.
Chromosome 13, Deletion Long Arm and Ring D Syndrome	Microphthalmus; coloboma; cataracts; retinoblastoma.	Cryptorchidism; hypospadias.
Chromosome 18, Deletion Short Arm Syndrome	Tilted optic disc and strabismus.	Small labia and clitoris; small penis and testes; renal tubular acidosis.
Chromosome 21, Deletion Syndrome	Downward slant of palpebral fissure; blepharochalasis; microphthalmia.	Agenesis of the kidney; cryptorchidism; hypospadias.
Chronic Renal Insufficiency	Calcium phosphate problems; band keratopathy; hypertensive retinopathy; reversible retinal detachment; arteriosclerotic changes; macular and retinal edema; uremic amaurosis; exophthalmos; Siegrist's streaks; unequal pupils; Möbius', Graefe's, and Stellwag's signs.	Progressive renal disease of many etiologies.
Cockayne's Syndrome	Retinal pigmentary changes; optic atrophy; cataract; nystagmus.	Glomerular sclerosis; interstitial fibrosis, cryptorchidism.
Cogan's Syndrome	Interstitial keratitis; photophobia; blurred vision.	Syndrome may be associated with periarteritis nodosa with subsequent renal involvement.
Congenital Heart Disease	Dilated tortuous retinal vessels; papilledema.	Proteinuria; nephrotic syndrome.
Congenital Syphilis	Interstitial keratitis with uveitis; retinal pigmentary changes.	Nephrotic syndrome; proteinuria; acute glomerulonephritis secondary to streptococcal infection of syphilitic lesions; proliferative and membranous glomerulopathy.
Cornelia de Lange Syndrome	Bushy eyebrows; synophrys; long eyelashes; myopia; astigmatism; optic atrophy; coloboma of optic disc; proptosis.	Hypoplastic genitalia; cryptorchidism, hypospadias.
Craniopharyngioma	Papilledema; optic atrophy; bitemporal field defects.	Diabetes insipidus (polyuria).
Cri-du-Chat Syndrome (Partial Deletion of Short Arm of Chromosome 5)	Epicanthal fold; strabismus; downward slant of palpebral fissure; optic atrophy; deficient tears; tortuous retinal vessels.	Renal agenesis; cryptorchidism; hypospadias.

Disease	Eye Findings	Genitourinary Manifestations
Cryptophthalmia Syndrome (Fraser's Syndrome)	Extension of forehead skin over eyes; lens either absent, hypoplastic, calcified or displaced; coloboma of lid; microphthalmos.	Cryptorchidism; hypospadias; chordee micropenis; renal agenesis.
Cystic Fibrosis	Dilated veins; mucoceles of sinuses; papilledema; retinal edema.	Defect in formation of free water (CH_2O) and TCH_2O; defect in spermatogenesis.
Cystinosis	Cystine crystals in cornea and conjunctiva; retinal pigmentary changes; photophobia.	Fanconi's syndrome; renal insufficiency.
Cystinuria	Pigmentary retinopathy (penicillamine therapy may cause retinal hemorrhages, optic neuritis and conjunctivitis).	Cystinuria; renal calculi.
Cytomegalic Inclusion Disease	Chorioretinitis; optic atrophy; microphthalmia.	Urinary excretion of virus; intranuclear inclusions in renal tubular cells.
Déjèrine-Roussy Syndrome (Thalamic Hyperesthetic Anesthesia)	Hemianopia.	Bladder dysfunction.
Dermatomyositis	Heliotrope eyelids; periorbital edema; distention of retinal veins with hemorrhages and exudates.	Nephrotic syndrome; proteinuria; basement membrane thickening.
Diabetes Mellitus	Stationary posterior cortical cataracts; suddent mature cataracts; refractive changes; retinopathy.	Glycosuria; albuminuria; Kimmelstiel-Wilson glomerulopathy; chronic renal insufficiency; pyelonephritis; papillary necrosis; nephrotic syndrome.
Diastrophic Nanism	Pectinate strands at root of iris.	Cryptorchidism.
Down's Syndrome (Trisomy 21)	Epicanthal folds; keratoconus; cataracts; Brushfield's spots.	Small penis; cryptorchidism; decreased uric acid clearance; large labia majora.
Dyskeratosis Congenita	Nasolacrimal duct obstruction; ectropion: blepharitis.	Testicular hypoplasia.
Ehlers-Danlos Syndrome	Retinal detachment; epicanthus; ptosis; myopia; blue sclera; keratoconus; ectopic lens; angioid streaks; vitreous hemorrhage; macular degeneration.	Renal vascular hypertension; renal tubular acidosis; ureteropelvic obstruction; essential hypertension.
Fabry's Disease	Radiating corneal opacity; spokelike cataracts; dilated retinal veins; dilated conjunctival blood vessels; periorbital edema.	"Foamy" glomerular and tubular cells; progressive renal insufficiency; proteinuria.
Familial Nephropathy— Retinitis Pigmentosa	Retinitis pigmentosa.	Nephronophthisis.
Familial Nephropathy— Retinitis Pigmentosa, Nephritis, and Chromosomal Abnormalities	Retinitis pigmentosa; nystagmus.	Chronic glomerulonephritis.
Familial Renal Dysplasia and Blindness	Congenital blindness.	Polycystic kidney; medullary sponge kidney.

(Table continued on following page)

Disease	Eye Findings	Genitourinary Manifestations
Familial Renal Dysplasia With Retinal Dysplasia; Mental Retardation With Hyperprolinuria	Retinal dysplasia; blindness.	Dysplastic kidneys with cysts; hyperprolinuria.
Fanconi's Syndrome (Pancytopenia and Multiple Anomalies	Ptosis; nystagmus; strabismus; microphthalmos.	Hypospadias; small penis; small testes; cryptorchidism.
Farber's Lipogranulomatosis	Grayish Opacification of the retina; xanthoma like lesion on conjunctiva; cherry-red macula.	Increased renal content of ceramide and ganglioside.
Frankl-Hochwart Syndrome (Pineal-Neurologic-Ophthalmologic Syndrome)	Concentric field constriction; choked disc; limitation of upward gaze.	Hypogonadism.
Fröhlich's Syndrome (Pituitary Adenoma)	Impaired scotopic vision; bitemporal hemianopia; papilledema; optic atrophy.	Diabetes insipidus; hypogonadism.
Galactosemia	Cataract.	Reducing substance; proteinuria; renal tubular acidosis; aminoaciduria.
Gansslen Syndrome (Familial Hemolytic Icterus)	Iris coloboma, epicanthus; increased interpapillary distance.	Hypogenitalism.
Generalized Gangliosidosis (Caffey's Syndrome)	Cherry-red macula.	Vacuolization in glomerular epithelial cells; possibly increased mucopolysaccharide excretion.
Goltz's Syndrome (Focal Dermal Hypoplasia)	Microphthalmia; strabismus; coloboma.	Females may have hypoplastic external genitalia.
Gonorrhea	Conjunctivitis; keratoconjunctivitis.	Urethritis; balantitis; epididymitis
Gout	Scleritis; episcleritis; band keratopathy; iridocyclitis; tophus formation.	Acute renal insufficiency due to intratubular precipitation of urates, chronic renal insufficiency; renal calculi; urate crystals.
Guillain-Barré Syndrome	Ocular nerve palsies; facial nerve palsy; optic neuritis; papilledema.	Neurogenic bladder.
Hallerman-Streiff Syndrome	Microphthalmia; cataracts; blue sclera; coloboma of optic disc; chorioretinal pigmentation.	Hypogenitalism; cryptorchidism.
Hartnup Disease	Nystagmus; photophobia; strabismus.	Aminoaciduria; increased indole excretion.
Hemochromatosis	Slate-blue retinal pigmentation; changes of diabetes mellitus; iron deposits in sclera, cilia.	Diabetic nephropathy.
Hemolytic Uremic Syndrome	Retinal hemorrhage.	Acute renal insufficiency; hematuria; proteinuria; chronic renal insufficiency.
Henoch-Schönlein Syndrome	Eyelid edema; changes of acute or chronic renal disease.	Hematuria; acute and/or chronic renal insufficiency; proteinuria.
Hereditary Hemorrhagic Telangiectasia and Polycystic Kidney Disease (Osler-Weber-Rendu)	Telangiectasia of conjunctiva or retina or both.	Bilateral polycystic kidneys; hematuria.

Disease	Eye Findings	Genitourinary Manifestations
Histiocytosis X	Papilledema; optic atrophy; exophthalmos (occasionally pulsating); xanthelasma; eyelid swelling; internal ophthalmoplegia; nystagmus.	Diabetes insipidus (may result in hydronephrosis).
Holoprosencephaly and Facial Dysmorphia Syndrome	Hypo- or hypertelorism or both; mono-. syn-, or an-ophthalmia.	Cystic kidney; hydroureter; double ureter; bicornuate ureter; clitoridomegaly; hypospadias; cryptorchidism.
Homocystinuria	Subluxation of lens; myopia; cataracts; glaucoma; cystic retinal degeneration; retinal detachment.	Increased homocystine excretion.
Hunter's Syndrome (Mucopolysaccharidosis II)	Retinal pigmentation; clear cornea.	Increased excretion of dermatan and heparan sulfate.
Hurler's Syndrome (Mucopolysaccharidosis I)	Cloudy cornea; hypertelorism; retinal pigmentation.	Increased excretion of dermatan and heparan sulfate; hydrocele.
Hypercalcemia (undifferentiated)	Cornea and conjunctival crystals; band keratopathy	Nephrocalcinosis; interstitial fibrosis; renal insufficiency; concentrating defect; stones.
Hyperglycinuria	Cataract; microphthalmia.	Hyperglycinuria.
Hyperlysinemia	Subluxation of lens; strabismus.	Lysinuria; cryptorchidism; hypogenitalism.
Hyperparathyroidism	Band keratopathy; osteolysis of the bony orbit.	Acute and chronic renal insufficiency; renal stones; hypercalciuria; renal concentrating defect; renal tubular acidosis.
Hypertelorism — Hypospadias Syndrome (BBB Syndrome — Familial Telecanthus With Associated Anomalies)	Ocular hypertelorism.	Hypospadias, cryptorchidism.
Hypertension (undifferentiated)	Grades I–IV.	Arteriolar thickening and hypertrophy; endarteritis; necrosis; thrombosis; thickened glomerular capillary walls, hyalinization, and necrosis of glomeruli; hypertension may be seen in virtually any disease primarily involving the kidney; prolonged hypertension itself may produce renal insufficiency.
Hypophosphatasia	Optic atrophy; band keratopathy.	Increased phosphoethanolamine excretion.
Hypothyroidism	Strabismus; myxedema of lids; corneal opacities; optic neuritis.	Defect in hydrogen ion excretion; mesangial prominence; intracellular inclusions.
Infantile Hypercalcemia Syndrome	Epicanthal folds; hypertelorism; strabismus.	Renal insufficiency; concentrating defect; nephrocalcinosis; hypercalciuria; undescended testes.
Klinefelter Syndrome	Color blindness.	Small testes; sterility; small penis.
Laurence-Moon-Biedl Syndrome	Retinitis pigmentosa; strabismus; poor night vision; nystagmus; cataracts.	Chronic glomerulonephritis; hypospadias; hypogonadism.

(Table continued on following page)

Disease	Eye Findings	Genitourinary Manifestations
Lead Poisoning	Papilledema; optic neuritis; muscle palsies; optic atrophy.	Hypertension; Fanconi's Syndrome; hematuria; proteinuria; chronic interstitial nephritis.
Leber's Congenital Retinal Blindness	Congenital blindness; pigmentary degeneration.	Polycystic kidneys.
Lenz Microphthalmia Syndrome (X-linked Colobomatous Micro-phthalmos or Anophthalmia)	Coloboma of retina, iris, optic nerve, and ciliary body; microphthalmos; nystagmus; diminished vision; esotropia; Brushfield's spots.	Hypospadias; cryptorchidism; renal insufficiency; renal aplasia.
Leptospirosis	Conjunctivitis; bleeding into choroid, retina, optic nerve; iridocyclitis; myositis of ocular muscles.	Renal failure; bile in the urine.
Leroy's Syndrome	Inner epicanthal fold; corneal opacities.	May be mild increase in mucopolysaccharide excretion.
Lesch-Nyhan Syndrome	Self-inflicted trauma; changes of gout.	Gouty nephropathy.
Leukemia, Lymphoma	Proptosis; visual difficulty; infiltrates of lids; retinal hemorrhage; papilledema; perivascular infiltrates; Roth spots.	Infiltrative lesions resulting in large kidneys; acute renal insufficiency related to hyperuricemia; calculi; nephrotic syndrome.
Lissencephaly Syndrome	Circumlimbal corneal clouding.	Cryptorchidism; unilateral renal agenesis.
Lowe's (Oculo-Cerebro-Renal) Syndrome	Cataracts; glaucoma; miosis; nystagmus; endophthalmos; corneal dystrophy; iris atrophy; strabismus; posterior synechia.	Fanconi's syndrome; renal insufficiency; nephrocalcinosis; cryptorchidism.
Lupus Erythematosus	Depending on course of disease, eye findings similar to those of acute or chronic renal disease; cytoid bodies; choroid infiltrates.	Proteinuria; hematuria; acute glomerulonephritis; chronic renal insufficiency; nephrotic syndrome.
Male Turner's (Noonan's) Syndrome	Epicanthal folds; ptosis.	Hypoplastic penis; cryptorchidism; small testes.
Maple Syrup Urine Disease	Gray optic discs; cortical blindness; irregular ocular movements.	Increased excretion of leucine, isoleucine, valine
Maroteaux-Lamy Syndrome (Mucopolysaccharidosis VI)	Corneal opacities.	Increased excretion of dermatan and heparan sulfate.
Meckel's Syndrome (Dysencephalia Splanchnocystica; Gruber's Syndrome)	Microphthalmia; posterior synechia; cataracts; coloboma.	Polycystic kidney; renal hypoplasia; cryptorchidism.
Meningococcal Infection	Purulent retinitis.	Inappropriate secretion of antidiuretic hormone.
Meningomyelocele-Hydrocephalus Complex	Setting sun sign; papilledema; strabismus; diplegia.	Neurogenic bladder; urinary tract infection.
Metachromatic Leukodystrophy (Sulfatide Lipidosis)	Optic atrophy; nystagmus; cranial nerve palsies.	Lipid deposits in kidney; excretion of sulfatides.
Morquio's Syndrome (Mucopolysaccharidosis IV)	Late corneal clouding.	Increased excretion of keratosulfate.

Disease	Eye Findings	Genitourinary Manifestations
Mumps	Keratitis; optic neuritis; iritis; dacryocystitis.	Orchitis; epididymitis.
Nail Patella (Fong's) Syndrome	Clover leaf pigmentation; keratoconus; microcornea; microphakia; cataracts; ptosis; sclerocornea	Chronic renal insufficiency; proteinuria; hematuria.
Nephrotic Syndrome	Retinal detachment; lipemia retinalis; lid edema; central retinal artery obstruction; cholesterol deposits; xanthelasma.	Nil disease, i.e., idiopathic childhood; many renal diseases involving the glomerulus may be associated with the nephrotic syndrome; proteinuria; hematuria; lipiduria.
Neuroblastoma	Proptosis or ecchymosis of eyelids or both.	Renal compression from adrenal mass; suprarenal calcification.
Niemann-Pick Disease	Cherry-red spot; blindness.	Foam cells in glomeruli.
Norrie's Disease	Bilateral retinal pseudotumor; cataracts; corneal opacities; phthisis bulbi.	Hypogonadism.
Oculocerebral Syndrome With Hypopigmentation	Cloudy corneas; ectropion nystagmus.	Cryptorchidism.
Ophthalmoplegia-Plus Syndrome	External ophthalmoplegia; pigmentary retinal degeneration; bilateral ptosis.	Elevated plasma renin; low serum potassium; hyperaldosteronism; enlarged juxtaglomerular apparatus.
Osteogenesis Imperfecta	Retinal detachment; blue sclera; corneal opacity; keratoconus; megalocornea.	Nephrotic syndrome.
Osteopetrosis (Albers-Schönberg Disease)	Compression of optic nerve; retinal atrophy.	Proximal and distal renal tubular acidosis.
Oxalosis	Oxalate crystals.	Oxalate stones; deposition of crystals in renal parenchymal; renal insufficiency.
Periarteritis Nodosa	Conjunctivitis; hypertensive retinopathy; changes of acute or chronic renal disease.	Proteinuria; hematuria; flank pain; may resemble acute glomerulonephritis without hypertension; renal insufficiency; granuloma.
Phenylketonuria	Cataracts; corneal opacities.	Phenylpyruvic acid excretion increased; positive ferric chloride test.
Pheochromocytoma	Hypertensive retinopathy; papilledema; medullated corneal nerves.	Acute or chronic hypertensive nephropathy
Phocomelia; Flexion Deformities and Facial Anomalies Syndrome	Cloudy cornea; microphthalmia.	Congenital absence of penal foreskin.
Polycythemia	Vascular congestion of retinal and conjunctival vessels; retinal hemorrhage.	Proteinuria; uric acid nephropathy.
Popliteal Web Syndrome	Webs between eyelids.	Cryptorchidism; ambiguous genitalia.
Post Renal Transplantation	Changes of cytomegalic inclusion disease; changes related to acute or chronic renal disease; steroid related changes.	Interstitial round cell infiltration and fibrosis; glomerular scarring; recurrence of original renal disease; chronic rejection.

(Table continued on following page)

Disease	Eye Findings	Genitourinary Manifestations
Potter Syndrome	Hypertelorism.	Renal agenesis.
Prader-Willi Syndrome	Strabismus.	Small penis; cryptorchidism; central diabetes insipidus; nephrogenic diabetes insipidus.
Pseudohypoparathyroidism (Albright's Hereditary Osteodystrophy)	Strabismus; cataracts; hypertelorism; keratitis; papilledema.	Hypogonadism; renal unresponsiveness to parathormone.
Pseudoxanthoma Elasticum	Retinal detachment; retinal hemorrhage; drusen angioid streaks.	Intrarenal bleeding; hypertension.
Psychologic Disease	Blindness; pain; etc.	Various GU complaints; often urinary frequency.
Reese's Retinal Dysplasia	Bilateral retinal dysplasia with persistence of primary vitreous; coloboma; dense sheet behind lens.	Cryptorchidism.
Reiter's Syndrome	Iritis; sterile mucopurulent conjunctivitis or keratitis.	Urethritis; genital ulceration.
Renal Tubular Acidosis, Distal	Scleritis; hemorrhages in conjunctiva and retina.	Hypercalciuria; nephrocalcinosis; renal insufficiency.
Rheumatic Fever	Iridocyclitis.	Hematuria; proteinuria; focal or proliferative glomerulonephritis.
Rheumatoid Arthritis	Band keratopathy; chronic iridocyclitis.	Hematuria; renal insufficiency; proteinuria.
Rickets	Proptosis.	Renal tubular acidosis; phosphaturia; aminoaciduria.
Riley-Day Syndrome (Familial Dysautonomia)	Decreased tear production; myopia.	Ratio of urinary excretion of homovanillic acid to vanillylmandelic acid increased; urinary frequency.
Robert's Syndrome	Colomba of eyelids; cataracts; corneal opacities.	Genital hypertrophy; cryptorchidism.
Rothmund Syndrome (Poikiloderma Congenita)	Corneal dystrophy; cataracts.	Hypogenitalism; cryptorchidism.
Rubella (congenital)	Pigmentary retinopathy; cataracts; microphthalmia; optic atrophy; nystagmus; glaucoma; transient corneal clouding.	Renal artery stenosis; urinary excretion of virus; undescended testes; hypospadias; posterior urethral valves; ureteropelvic obstruction.
Rubinstein-Taybi Syndrome	Downward slant of palpebral fissure; epicanthal fold; strabismus; refraction error; cataracts; coloboma; ptosis.	Cryptorchidism; penile deformities; duplication of kidney; unilateral renal agenesis; posterior urethal valve; nephronopthisis.
Russell-Silver Syndrome	Ptosis.	Cryptorchidism; increased excretion of urinary gonadotropins.
Sarcoid	Iridocyclitis; exudative chorioretinal lesions; band keratopathy.	Granuloma; endothelial and epithelial proliferation; glomerular hyalinization; changes of hypercalcemia.
Scheie's Syndrome (Mucopolysaccharidosis V)	Cornea clouding; retinal pigmentation.	Increased excretion of dermatan sulfate.
Seckel's Syndrome	Downward slant of palpebral fissure; epicanthal folds.	Cryptorchidism; large clitoris; small labia; single cloacal opening.

Disease	Eye Findings	Genitourinary Manifestations
Senior Syndrome	Abnormal ERG (β scotopic wave).	Nephronophthisis.
Sickle Cell Anemia	Retinal hemorrhages; angioid streaks; A–V connections; neovascularization; lipid deposits; venous tortuosity; "sea fan" sign; dystrophic pigmentary changes.	Concentrating defect; papillary necrosis; renal infarcts; chronic renal insufficiency; nephrotic syndrome.
Smith-Lemli-Opitz Syndrome	Ptosis: epicanthal fold; strabismus; cataracts.	Dilated renal calyces; cryptorchidism; hypospadias; occasional glomerulus exhibits thickened basement membrane; unilateral renal dysplasia.
Steinert's Syndrome	Cataract; blepharitis; keratitis sicca.	Testicular atrophy; amenorrhea; dysmenorrhea; ovarian cysts.
Stevens-Johnson Syndrome	Conjunctivitis; keratitis sicca; corneal opacities; pseudomembranes; symblepharon.	Urethritis.
Streptococcal Infections	Erysipelas involving eyelids; orbital cellulitis; iritis; hypertensive changes; optic neuritis; conjunctivitis.	Acute glomerulonephritis.
Sturge-Weber Syndrome	Retinal hemangioma; congenital glaucoma.	Renal hemangioma.
Subacute Necrotizing Encephalomyelitis (Leigh's Syndrome)	Macular degeneration; cortical blindness; irregular eye movements.	Proximal renal tubular acidosis; renal artery stenosis.
Sulfonamide Administration	Acquired ametropia; usually myopia; optic neuritis; conjunctivitis; retinal hemorrhage.	Sulfur crystalluria; obstructive uropathy.
Takayasu's Arteritis (Pulseless Disease)	Visual disturbances; cataracts; retinal and iris neovascularization; retinal detachment; hyperemia of conjunctiva and sclera.	Renal vascular lesions (aneurysms).
Tay-Sachs Disease	Cherry-red macula.	Absence of hexosaminidase in renal tissue.
Thoracic Asphyxiant Dystrophy (Jeune's Syndrome)	Abnormal ERG; retinal pigmentary changes; blindness.	Chronic renal insufficiency; renal tubular acidosis.
Traumatic Injury (Multiple Organ Involvement)	Retinal detachment; intraocular hemorrhage; signs of increased CSF pressure.	Hematuria; flank mass; intrarenal bleeding; renal artery stenosis.
Treacher Collins' Syndrome	Antimongoloid slant; lid coloboma; absent eyelashes; microphthalmia.	Cryptorchidism.
Trisomy 13 Syndrome	Cyclopia; anophthalmos; absent eyebrows; hypotelorism; microphthalmia; coloboma; retinal dysplasia; blepharophimosis; cataracts; posterior pole colobomas.	Cryptorchidism; bicornuate uterus; polycystic kidneys; horseshoe kidney; double collecting system; hypoplastic ovaries.
Trisomy 18 Syndrome	Hypoplastic orbital ridge; ptosis; cataracts; coloboma; microphthalmos.	Cryptorchidism; hypoplastic labia; horseshoe kidney; ectopic kidney; double ureter; multiple renal cysts; obstructive uropathy.

(Table continued on following page)

Disease	Eye Findings	Genitourinary Manifestations
Tuberculosis	Fundal tubercles; blindness; extra-ocular muscle palsies; nystagmus; optic atrophy; papilledema.	Pyuria; flank pain; hematuria; epididymitis; dysuria; distorted calyces.
Tuberous Sclerosis	Astrocytic hamartomas of disc and retina.	Mixed rhabdomyomatous lesions.
Turner's Syndrome (female)	Ptosis; strabismus; cataracts; blue sclera; color blindness.	Horseshoe kidney; idiopathic hypertension; double collecting system; streaked gonads.
Vitamin A Deficiency	Impaired dark adaptation; keratomalacia; xerophthalmia.	Squamous metaplasia of ureters, bladder, and renal pelvis.
Vitamin C Deficiency	Proptosis; hemorrhage into ocular, orbital, or periorbital structures.	Hematuria; generalized aminoaciduria.
Von Hippel-Lindau Syndrome	Retinal angioma.	Renal hemangioma; hypernephroma.
Von Recklinghausen's Disease	Glaucoma; optic nerve gliomas; iris nodules; exophthalmos.	Renal vascular hypertension; renal cysts; involvement of all size renal arteries; renal neurofibromas.
Werner's Syndrome	Cataracts; absence of eyelashes; scanty eyebrows; retinal degeneration.	Hypogonadism; glycosuria.
Wilson's Hepatolenticular Degeneration	Kayser-Fleischer ring; pigmentary retinal changes; night blindness; peripheral white masses; cataracts; hemeralopia; optic atrophy.	Renal tubular acidosis; aminoaciduria; glycosuria; phosphaturia; uricosuria nephrotic syndrome in association with penicillamine therapy.
Xeroderma Pigmentosa	Ectropion; entropion; corneal ulceration; iritis; photophobia; malignant papilloma.	Small external genitalia.
X-linked Uricaciduria	Changes of renal insufficiency or gout or both.	Gouty nephropathy
XXXXY Syndrome	Wide-set eyes; upward slant to sinuses; strabismus; inner epicanthal fold; Brushfield's spots.	Cryptorchidism; hypoplastic scrotum; hypospadias.

REFERENCES

Beard, C., Falls, H. F., Franceschetti, A., Francois, J., Goodman, G., Krill, A. E., and Scheie, H.: Congenital anomalies of the eye. Trans. New Orleans Acad. Ophthalmol. St. Louis, The C. V. Mosby Co., 1968.

Geeraets, W. J.: Ocular Syndromes. Philadelphia, Lea & Febiger, 1965.

Holmes, L. B., Moser, H. W., Halldorsson, S., Mack, C., Pant, S. S., and Matzilevich, B.: Mental Retardation: An Atlas of Diseases with Associated Physical Abnormalities. New York, Macmillan Co., 1972.

McKusick, V. A.: Heritable Disorders of Connective Tissue. 3rd ed. St. Louis, The C. V. Mosby Co., 1966.

Nelson, W. E., Vaughan, V. C., and McKay, R. J.: Textbook of Pediatrics. 9th ed. Philadelphia, W. B. Saunders Co., 1969.

Ophthalmologic Staff of the Hospital for Sick Children: The Eye in Childhood. Chicago, Year Book Medical Publishers, 1967.

Roy, F. H.: Ocular Differential Diagnosis. Philadelphia, Lea & Febiger, 1972.

Smith, D. W.: Recognizable Patterns of Human Malformations. Vol. VII. Major Problems in Clinical Pediatrics. Philadelphia, W. B. Saunders Co., 1970.

Stanbury, J. B., Wyngaarden, J. S., and Fredrickson, D. S.: The Metabolic Basis of Inherited Disease. New York, McGraw-Hill Book Co., 1972.

Strauss, M. B., and Welt, L. G.: Diseases of the Kidney. Boston, Little, Brown & Co., 1971.

Tasman, W.: Retinal Diseases in Children. New York, Harper and Row, 1971.

CHAPTER 21

RADIOLOGIC DIAGNOSIS AND THERAPY IN PEDIATRIC OPHTHALMOLOGY

JOHN A. KIRKPATRICK, M.D.,
and MARIE A. CAPITANIO, M.D.

Radiologic examination of the orbits is a procedure of value in the diagnosis of certain abnormalities of the visual apparatus. By means of appropriate projections the osseous rims and walls of the orbits, the orifices within them, as well as the surrounding structures, i.e., the facial bones and skull, are equally amenable to radiologic examination. Because soft tissues as a whole absorb x-rays to the same degree, the intraorbital structures (the globe, the muscles, the orbital fat) cannot be distinguished, and hence may be evaluated radiographically only if they calcify or produce alterations in the surrounding bone. Osseous alterations may take the form of a change in the configuration or size of the orbit, thinning of its walls, fracture, or overt destruction of bone. Calcifications of any portion of the soft tissues within the orbit will be visible if the amount is large enough (Fig. 21–1). Foreign bodies in the eye will be seen on radiographs of the orbit if their physical make-up and size result in differential absorption of x-rays so that they are more opaque than the structures in which they lie.

Primary diseases of the orbits and their contents are a significant concern; how-ever, there are a multitude of generalized diseases that have ocular manifestations. In the infant and child, they may be the first manifestation of metastatic neuroblastoma or reticuloendotheliosis; they may be related to a syndrome of which the abnormality of the eye is but one part, such as is common in certain intrauterine infections; or they may be a manifestation of complex anomalies that have genetic significance and hence are of great importance to the family.

In this chapter we will be concerned with those radiologic techniques having to do with the visual apparatus and the alterations to be expected in primary abnormalities of the eye, the orbit, and the skull, as well as those that relate to generalized disease, syndromes, or anomalies.

TECHNIQUE

The roentgen examination of the visual apparatus is concerned primarily with the evaluation of the bony vault (the orbit), which houses the eye, and the fissures and foramina through which course the nerves and vessels of the eye. Though the exami-

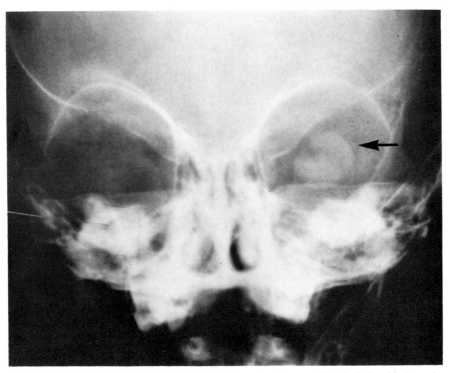

Figure 21–1   Retinoblastoma. Stippled calcification is evident within the left orbit (*arrow*).

nation of the orbits depends in great measure on the clinical findings, it is important that there be a basic "study" to which additional projections are added as indicated. The projections most frequently utilized in the initial examination of the orbit are the posterior-anterior or *Caldwell projection* (nose and forehead against the cassette); the lateral projection of the orbits and facial bones (the side in question against the cassette); an oblique projection of each orbit; and the *Water's projection* (nose and chin against the cassette). Because evaluation of the optic foramina is so important in diseases of the eye, it is likely that appropriate projections for the optic foramina may be included as part of the primary examination.

Depending on the nature of the lesion, it may be desirable to make any one of the projections suitable for stereoscopic viewing, or add body section radiography (tomography). Since there must be no motion of the part being examined between the two exposures necessary for stereoscopy, nor during the relatively long exposure time necessary for tomography (in some instances approximating 1½ seconds), these two examinations may be dif-

ficult to achieve in the infant and young child. Anesthesia, either local or general, may have to be utilized if the examination is critical to diagnosis. The roentgen examination therefore may be coordinated with the ophthalmologic examination of the fundi, necessitating only one period of anesthesia.

One further technique that may be valuable in the young patient is fluoroscopy with the exposure of appropriate spot films. The area of abnormality can often be visualized most successfully by this technique, and with the use of image intensification the radiation levels are quite low.

Special projections are available for visualization of the superior and inferior orbital fissures as well as of the optic canals. There are techniques available for the localization of opaque foreign bodies within the orbit or globe, or both. These include geometric techniques, for example, the Sweet localizer; exposure of the globe in different degrees of elevation and rotation; and examination after placement of a plastic localizer lens in contact with the cornea. Localization of opaque foreign bodies by the *Sweet method* demands precise immobilization of the head, and it is assumed that the average globe measures 24 mm. in diameter (Hartmann and Giles, 1959). The *Comberg technique* utilizes a contact lens with geometric reference points. Again, cooperation of the patient is essential, and the technique is contraindicated in the presence of a laceration of the globe (Seymour and Bane, 1970).

GENERAL CONSIDERATIONS

Abnormalities in Size and Contour of the Orbit

The orbits, being paired structures, are expected to be symmetrical with respect to their size and shape. At all ages their bony margins are well defined. In the infant and child, because of the nature of the growing skull, adaptation to an increase in orbital contents can take place readily and surprisingly rapidly. Depending on the nature of the lesion, there may not be associated deformity of the wings of the sphenoid. From the clinical standpoint, enlargement of the orbit is associated with exophthalmos in most instances.

Symmetrical enlargement of one orbit may be due to enlargement of the globe, as is seen in congenital myopia or buphthalmos. A tumor situated posteriorly in the muscle cone is apt to cause symmetrical enlargement of the orbit because of the more uniform pressure that results from its presence. Evans et al. (1963) note that proptosis was seen in 96 per cent of their patients with retrobulbar optic glioma. Thirty-three per cent of the children who had proptosis due to an orbital optic nerve glioma had enlargement of the bony orbit, and such enlargement was seen in 3 of 18 patients who had ocular extension of a chiasmal glioma to the orbit.

Asymmetrical enlargement of one orbit may result from a variety of lesions that are eccentrically located, such as *hemangioma, dermoid,* or *neurofibroma.* They may also cause local thinning of the orbital wall. Hemangiomas are apt to be found in the superior quadrants of the orbits, dermoids in the superior temporal aspect of the orbit, and neurofibromas in the posterior aspect, where they may be associated with bony defects. Of course, one orbit may be smaller than the other in the presence of microphthalmos (Fig. 21–2).

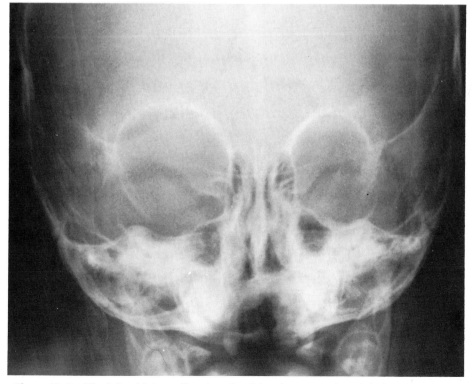

Figure 21–2 The left orbit is smaller than the right; there was microphthalmos on the left.

The wings of the sphenoid are not necessarily distorted in the course of enlargement of the orbit. They are apt to be affected, however, by tumors that are located posteriorly. Long-standing masses in the middle cranial fossa, premature closure of a coronal suture, and hypoplasia of the great wing of the sphenoid are extraorbital lesions that deform the lesser sphenoid wing.

Abnormalities in Size and Contour of the Optic Foramina and Canals

Detection of alterations in the size and shape of the optic foramina is of utmost significance in the study of any infant or child with optic atrophy. The optic foramina (Fig. 21–3) are best seen on oblique projections of the orbits. Several techniques are described, each with some variation having to do with the position of the head, the angle of the x-ray tube, and the relationship of the head to the cassette (Meschan, 1966). No matter which method is utilized, however, it must be reproducible and as comfortable for the patient as possible. Since the maximum diameter of the foramina is more significant than is the configuration, any position which distorts the normal must be avoided. In this connection it is to be noted that enlargement of the orbit is not associated with enlargement of the optic foramina. When there is distortion of the medial walls of the orbit, the optic foramen may in fact be visible on a frontal radiograph. Thus, it is important that the initial or basic studies be reviewed before special projections are added.

The average maximum diameter of the optic foramen increases over the first 5 years of life, being 4 mm. in a newborn infant, 5 mm. at 6 months of age, and 5.5 mm. at 5 years of age (Evans et al., 1963; Kier, 1966). A variation of 1 mm. or more in the size of one of the foramina as compared with its mate raises the question of tumor within the optic foramen or within the optic canal. Variation in the rate of growth of the foramen is significant as well. The optic canal increases from a foramen 2 mm. deep at birth to a true canal 4 to 9 mm. long by 5 years of age. The normal growth of the optic nerve is necessary for development of the optic canal (Evans et al., 1963). Therefore, hypoplasia of the nerve will result in failure of normal development of the canal.

Visualization of the optic canal is usually best obtained by one of the methods of tomography, for which several techniques are available. The examination may be made in the lateral, frontal, or basilar view. The latter results in the visualization of

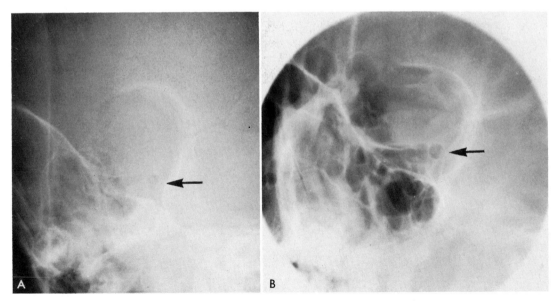

Figure 21–3   Normal optic foramina (*A*) 6 months of age (*arrow*) and (*B*) 13 years of age (*arrow*). The foramen is round, the walls are smooth and the margins are slightly sclerotic.

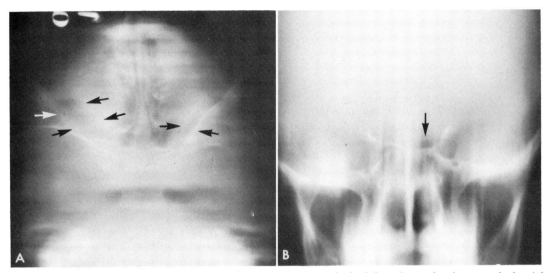

Figure 21–4   Tomography of the skull, a basilar projection, reveals the left optic canal to be normal; the right is irregularly widened secondary to an optic glioma (*A*). Optic glioma may distort the sphenoid bone in the region of the anterior clinoids (*B*), as is visible on frontal tomography of this area.

both canals in their entire length on the same film (Fig. 21–4). Positioning is difficult, since the head must be extended so that the plane of the canals is parallel to the x-ray film. Harwood-Nash (1970) has described a technique utilizing hypocycloidal polytomography, by which one can visualize both canals at the same time. He notes that a difference in width of greater than 1 mm. is abnormal, and in any event a transverse diameter greater than 7 mm. is abnormal. Thus, appreciation of the size and shape of the entire optic canal is important, since a tumor may distort the intracranial portion of the canal and not enlarge the foramen. Conversely, enlargement of the foramen by a tumor of the optic nerve does not necessarily imply significant intracranial extension and hence deformity of the canal.

Destruction of the Bony Portion of the Orbit

Destruction of the wall of the orbit that is not associated with enlargement of that orbit is most suggestive of a malignant or an inflammatory process. Of the primary malignant processes, *rhabdomyosarcoma* is the most frequently encountered. Primary tumors in the nose or nasopharynx may extend to the orbit. Finally, metastatic malignant disease, particularly neuroblastoma and leukemia, is commonly encountered in the pediatric age group. The *reticuloendothelioses* are best not considered malignant in the true sense but may cause

extensive bony destruction. Osteomyelitis of the bones of the orbit is little different from that encountered elsewhere in the skeleton; the clinical findings regularly precede overt bone destruction by 5 to 7 days. Soft tissue swelling, however, is a manifestation of *osteomyelitis* and may be appreciated radiographically as a general increase in density in relation to the involved orbit.

Trauma to the Orbit and its Contents

Fractures of the walls of the orbit are apt to be associated with fractures of the facial bones and skull. Fractures of the orbit may involve the rim of the orbit or its walls, or cause a *blowout-type fracture*. In any instance of trauma it is important to note the presence or absence of an opaque foreign body within the orbit (Freimanis, 1966).

In any fracture of the rim of the orbit, the nature of the fracture and the displacement of fragments must be recognized. Associated soft tissue injury is frequent and air may be visualized within the orbit.

Fractures of the wall of the orbit may be difficult to visualize. However, the fracture lines may extend from the region of the orbit into the base of the skull or into the paranasal sinuses. They may result in damage to structures leading to the orbit, specifically the optic nerve.

A blowout fracture is usually the result of blunt trauma to the eye. Such trauma increases hydrostatic pressure within the

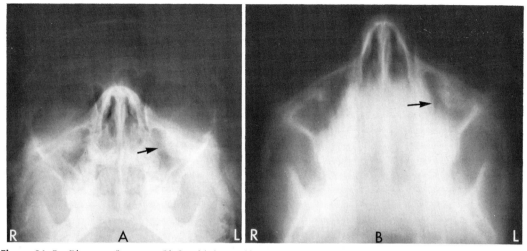

Figure 21–5   Blow-out fracture of left orbit is manifest on the Water's projection by a soft tissue mass in relation to the roof of the maxillary sinus (*A, arrow*). Tomography in the same projection again reveals a mass and, in addition, discontinuity in the bony floor of the orbit (*B, arrow*).

orbit. The resultant pressure displaces outward the thinner portions of the orbital wall, specifically the inferior and medial portions of the wall. Radiographically, spicules of bone are visible medially and inferiorly and there is discontinuity in these portions of the orbit. Thickening of the mucosa and opacity of the adjacent maxillary sinus or the presence of a soft tissue mass in the roof of the adjacent sinus are important radiologic findings (Fig. 21–5). Stereoscopic Water's projections may be of value, but often the diagnosis is best made and the abnormality best defined by tomography of the area in the Water's position. Orbitography utilizing injections of opaque material in the extraconal connective tissues of the orbit may be of value in the identification of fractures by demonstrating the passage of the opaque material through the fractures.

Calcification Within the Orbit

The detection of calcification within the soft tissues of the orbit is of great significance from a diagnostic standpoint. It is necessary that radiographic technique be excellent, since small foci of calcification may not be visible if there is any motion which would blur it. It has been said that calcification occurs within retinoblastoma in approximately 75 per cent of patients (Moss and Bran, 1969). It tends to be stippled in nature (Fig. 21–1). Stippled cal-

cification occurs as well in meningiomas of the sheath of the optic nerve or of the sphenoid bone. This calcification tends to be more posterior in location than that of retinoblastoma. Larger collections of calcification, nodules, or plaquelike areas may be found in the lens and the wall of the globe in some instances of degeneration of the globe (Fig. 21–6). Nodular calcification may be associated with the phakomatoses.

Retinoblastoma

This tumor, which is frequently bilateral, arises within the retina and may extend into the vitreous and hence to other structures within the globe. As noted earlier, calcification within it is common. Direct extension into the optic nerve is said to occur in approximately 27 per cent of patients and may result in seeding of the subarachnoid space and implants over the brain and spinal cord. Distant metastases do occur. The children of a parent cured of retinoblastoma are at risk for development of the tumor.

Therapy consists of surgical enucleation when feasible, although primary radiation therapy has been advocated. If the tumor is large and, after enucleation, tumor remains in the stump of the optic nerve, the orbit, the stump of the optic nerve, and the chiasm are treated. Moss and Bran (1969) suggest 4500 rads in 4 weeks utilizing cobalt-60 therapy. If a tumor should develop

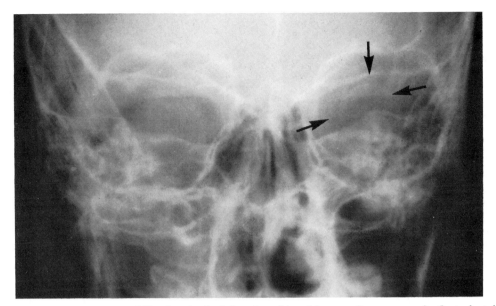

Figure 21–6   Fine granular calcifications in the left retina of boy 14 years of age as a result of retrolental fibroplasia (*arrows*).

in the other eye, irradiation is utilized in order to spare the anterior third of the globe. A single lateral portal is used. Meticulous attention must be given to the definition of the beam and its direction and to immobilization of the patient. In advanced disease, *TEM (triethylenemelamine)* infusion into the internal carotid artery at the same time that external radiation therapy is given has been utilized (Krementz et al., 1966).

Incidentally, bony sarcomas have been reported in patients following irradiation for retinoblastoma. Soloway (1966) has reported the occurrence of three osteosarcomas 12 to 23 years after treatment. In the 22 previously reported cases, there were 3 instances of fibrosarcoma or epithelial tumors and, interestingly, in these cases the radiation dose was less than 8000 rads; in the other 19 it was greater than 8000 rads.

CRANIOFACIAL ABNORMALITIES IN CHILDREN

Sutural Abnormalities of the Skull

One or more of the cranial sutures may close prematurely and as a result cause deformity of the vault and, depending on the suture, deformity of the orbits. The con-

genital form of the disease is of course present at birth; secondary closure does occur and is associated with a variety of postnatal disorders, e.g., *rickets, hypophosphatasia, idiopathic hypercalcemia,* and following successful shunting procedures for the relief of *hydrocephalus* (Duggan et al., 1970). It is the congenital form of *craniosynostosis* that is responsible for the most severe deformity, because closure has occurred during a period when growth of the brain is most rapid. In this situation, growth of the vault is impeded perpendicular to the line of the closed suture; hence, the shape of the vault and the configuration of the orbits will be specific as either relates to any one of the sutures.

On radiographs, the involved suture is seen to be thin, with smooth borders, and to be interrupted by bony bridging that may continue along the line of the sutures and may be seen as sclerosis (Caffey, 1972). When the sagittal suture is closed, the vault is elongated and narrow, and the lateral aspect of the orbits is angulated superiorly (Fig. 21–7). Deformity of the orbits is most marked when one or both coronal sutures are closed. In this instance, the orbit on the involved side is shallow and angled sharply upward laterally (Fig. 21–8). Unilateral closure of a coronal suture may also result in a medial migration of the orbit on the involved side with growth.

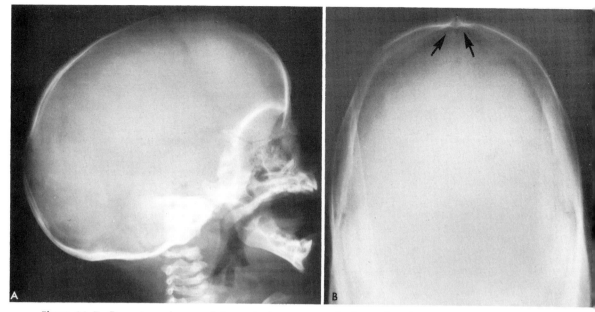

Figure 21–7   Premature closure of the sagittal suture reveals the vault to be elongated and narrow (*A*). The sagittal suture is narrow, bridged, and associated with a build-up of bone along each side of the suture (*B*).

An unusual form of premature closure of the coronal and lambdoid sutures associated with hydrocephalus has been termed *Kleeblattschadel* syndrome, or cloverleaf skull (Smith, 1970). The head is grotesque and the vault becomes trilobed, with bulging in the areas of the sagittal su-ture and the squamosal suture, associated with downward displacement of the ears, severe proptosis, and facial deformities (Fig. 21–9).

Apert's syndrome (acrocephalosyndactyly) is characterized by irregular craniosynostosis which is frequently of the coronal su-

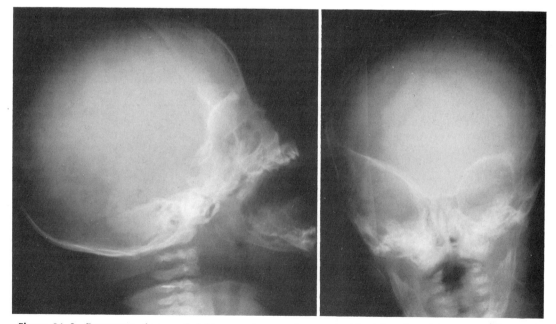

Figure 21–8   Premature closure of right coronal suture has resulted in deformity of the orbit on that side.

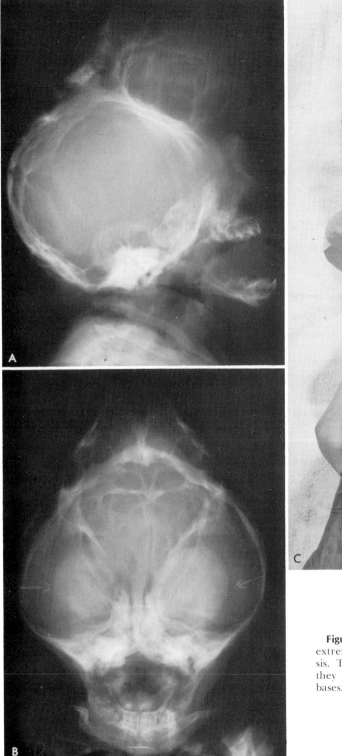

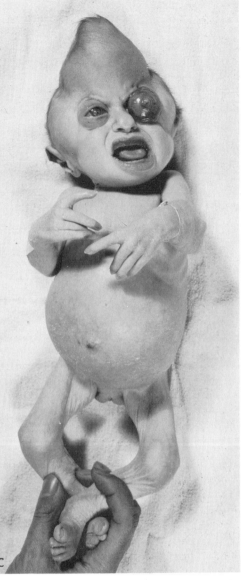

Figure 21–9 Cloverleaf skull. Because of the extremely shallow orbits there is severe proptosis. The globes are visible (*B, arrows*) because they are surrounded by air except at their bases.

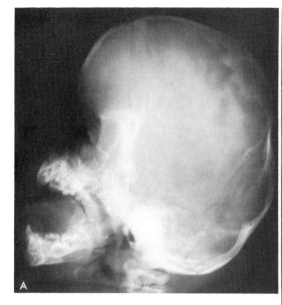
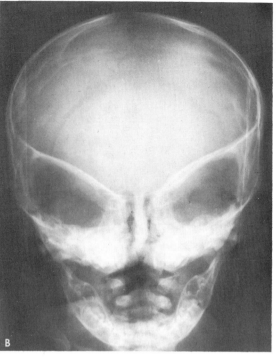

Figure 21–10 Apert's syndrome. The skull is narrow in its anteroposterior dimension; the orbits are shallow; the coronal sutures are closed (*A*). The orbits are angled laterally and superiorly as seen on the frontal projection (*B*).

ture, so that there is pointing of the head anteriorly (Fig. 21–10). It is associated with shallow orbits and hypertelorism. There is osseous or cutaneous syndactyly, most commonly involving the second, third, and fourth digits. *Carpenter's syndrome* is characterized by the same sort of cranial abnormality, brachysyndactyly of the fingers, preaxial polydactyly, syndactyly of the toes, hypogenitalism, obesity, and mental retardation. *Crouzon's disease* (craniofacial dysostosis) is characterized, again, by a similar appearance of the skull and, in addition, a hypoplastic maxilla (Smith, 1970).

Alterations in the Size and Shape of the Vault

Microcephaly results when there is arrest of growth of the brain. Radiologically the sutures are seen to be patent and the vault is relatively symmetrical and round (Caffey, 1967). The bones at the base of the skull and those of the face and the orbits are relatively larger than one would expect as a result of the small size of the vault (Fig. 21–11). *Microcephaly* may occur after injury to the brain, such as that occurring in intrauterine or extrauterine life. Prenatal infections such as those caused by the cytomegalic inclusion disease virus, tox-

oplasmosis, and rubella (Singleton et al., 1966) may be associated with microcephaly. Intracranial calcifications may be present in some instances of cytomegalic inclusion disease and toxoplasmosis (Babbitt et al., 1969; Caffey, 1967); the calcifications tend to be paraventricular in cytomegalic inclusion disease (Fig. 21–12), whereas they tend to be scattered throughout the brain substance in toxoplasmosis (Fig. 21–13). Trauma postnatally as well as certain infections postnatally may result in failure of normal growth of the brain and hence microcephaly.

When the forebrain is defective and the brain is represented by a single solid mass anteriorly, the deformity is classed as one of the arhinencephalies. In *cyclopia*, the eye is single and central. In *cebocephaly* (Fig. 21–14) both eyes are present but the orbits are small and the nose is flattened. Microphthalmos is present, as well as hypotelorism (Nelson et al., 1969).

Enlargement of the vault or *macrocephaly* is usually due to hydrocephalus or a space-taking lesion. True *macrocephaly* or megalencephalon is rare. Congenital hydrocephalus is almost always secondary to an obstructing lesion. The obstruction may be within the ventricular system, at the base

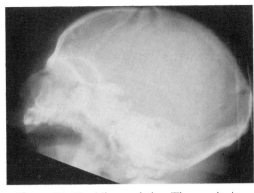
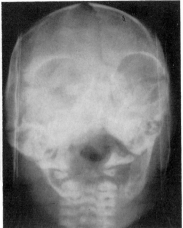

Figure 21–11   Microcephaly. The vault is small in relation to the facial bones and orbits; the sutures are patent.

of the brain, or over its surface. Occasionally, hydrocephalus may result from the formation of an abnormally large amount of cerebral spinal fluid as may be associated with papilloma of the choroid plexus. An obstruction within the ventricular system may occur at the foramen of Monro, the aqueduct of Sylvius, or the foramina of Luschka and Magendie. The

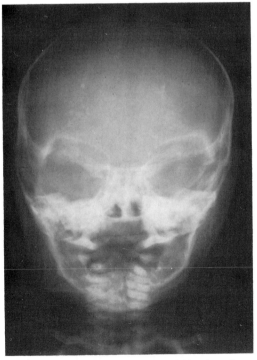

Figure 21–12   Paraventricular calcifications in an infant with cytomegalic inclusion disease.

obstruction in most instances is the result of congenital malformation; it may, however, be secondary to an intrauterine infection which results in gliosis and obstruction of one of the foramina or the aqueduct of Sylvius. The obstruction that occurs at the base of the brain and interferes with the normal circulation of cerebral spinal fluid over the surface of the brain is usually secondary to hemorrhagic phenomena or inflammation.

Radiologically, one expects the vault to be enlarged. If the hydrocephalus is rapidly progressive, the cranial bones will be thinned and the sutures widened. If the enlargement of the ventricular system is but slowly progressive, sutures may not be widened, nor the cranial bones thinned (Murtagh and Kirkpatrick, 1960).

Hydrocephalus is to be expected in the patient with a meningocele. In these instances, early in life, the cranial bones show multiple areas of thinning, separated by bony ridges. This deformity has been called "lacunar skull." Again, if the hydrocephalus is rapidly progressive, in a short period of time one notes disappearance of the bony ridges and thinning of all the cranial bones (Fig. 21–15).

Space-taking lesions may cause enlargement of the vault by virtue of their size alone or because they obstruct the ventricular system. Subdural collections of blood or fluid may result in rapid asymmetrical enlargement of the cranial vault. Tumors involving the cerebral hemisphere may also cause asymmetry of the vault. Those neoplasms beneath the tentorium, specifi-

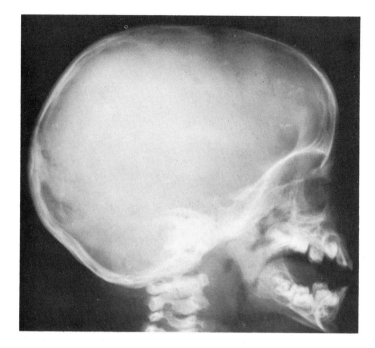

Figure 21–13 Scattered calcifications of the brain in a child of 11 years as a result of toxoplasmosis.

cally those involving the cerebellum, obstruct the fourth ventricle and cause hydrocephalus. In the child, subtentorial lesions are more commonly encountered than are supratentorial ones, specifically medulloblastoma, astrocytoma, and ependymoma. The glioma of the brain stem is not apt to cause enlargement of the vault; the fourth ventricle is displaced rather than obstructed. *Craniopharyngioma* (Fig. 21–16) is associated with destruction of the sella and clinoids, calcification, and increased intracranial pressure, the latter depending on the size of the tumor.

EXTRAORBITAL TUMORS. There is a peculiar association of *Wilms' tumor* with *congenital aniridia*. This was first noted by Miller in a review of 440 cases of Wilms' tumor in which 6 patients were found to have congenital, sporadic aniridia (Miller et al., 1964). Thus, the patient with this form of aniridia is at risk for the development of Wilms' tumor, and in most instances the tumor has become apparent before the age of 2 years. Recently, Fraumeni (1968) has reviewed the charts of 28 patients with aniridia, sporadic and familial, and has found 7 patients who developed Wilms' tumor, 1 of which was a patient with familial aniridia (DiGeorge and Harley, 1965). Wilms' tumor is an intrarenal tumor which is demonstrated best by intravenous urography and which is characterized by distortion of the pelvocalyceal system (Fig. 21–17). This tumor may recur locally and most frequently metastasizes to the lungs (Fraumeni and Glass, 1968).

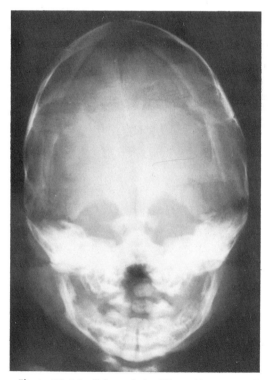

Figure 21–14 Cebocephaly. The orbits are small and there is hypotelorism.

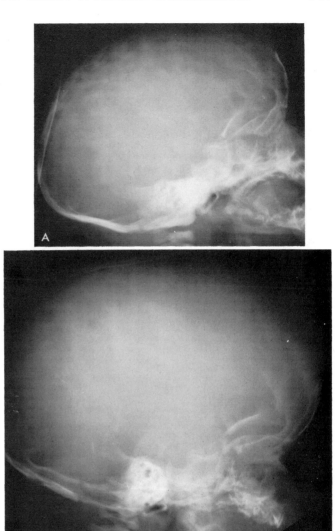

Figure 21–15 Lacunar skull in a newborn infant with a meningomyelocele (*A*). There was rapidly progressive hydrocephalus over the ensuing 6 weeks, resulting in an enlarged vault with thin bones and wide sutures (*B*).

The *neuroblastoma* arises anywhere along the sympathetic chain from the cervical region to the sacrum and from the adrenal medulla. When it arises in relation to the kidney, it results in displacement (Fig. 21–18 *A*). Calcification is common. Skeletal metastases are frequent, and it is said that over 50 per cent of the patients present with metastases. Involvement of the skull and the orbits is not uncommon (Fig. 21–18 *B* and *C*) and thus the patient may present with exophthalmos as a result of the metastases (Hope et al., 1963). An interesting eye sign, opsoclonus, has been described in association with neuroblastoma (Moe et al., 1970). The relationship

is not clear and the opsoclonus may not resolve following treatment of the tumor.

Alterations of the Cranial Vault Associated with Osseous Dysplasias

Osteopetrosis is a dysplasia characterized by bones that are abnormally dense and brittle. The entire skeleton is involved, and although the disease may be present at birth, it is a progressive one in which there is failure of resorption of primary trabeculae of bone and hence may not be manifest until childhood. The bones of the base of the vault are apt to be most severely involved (Fig. 21–19). Progressive thicken-

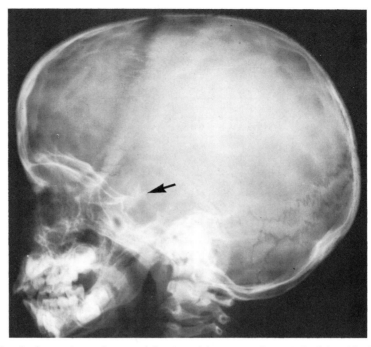

Figure 21–16   Craniopharyngioma. Increased intracranial pressure has resulted in widening of the sutures, particularly the coronal suture. The sella is enlarged and there is suprasellar calcification (*arrow*).

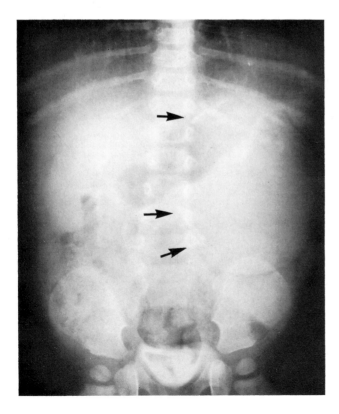

Figure 21–17   Wilms' tumor. There is a large renal mass on the left, and the intravenous urogram demonstrates elongation and deformity of the collecting system (*arrow*).

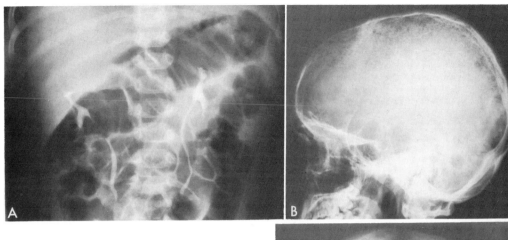

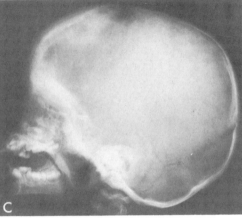

Figure 21–18 Neuroblastoma. The intravenous urogram demonstrates lateral displacement of the right kidney; there is no distortion of the collecting system (*A*). Osseous metastases are characterized by small, scattered areas of destruction of the cranial bones (*B*). Late in the course of the disease, sclerosis may occur as well as destruction, as is seen in the frontal and sphenoid bones (*C*).

ing of the bones results in narrowing of the foramina of the skull, so that optic atrophy may develop with narrowing of the optic canals and foramina. The sutures are patent.

Similar alterations of the optic foramina may be observed in *idiopathic hypercalcemia* (Fig. 21–20) and *craniometaphyseal dysplasia.* Thickening of the bones of the vault may occur in *pyknodysostosis* but this dys-

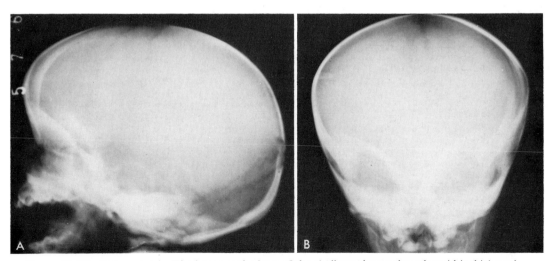

Figure 21–19 Osteopetrosis. The bones at the base of the skull are dense; the sphenoid is thickened.

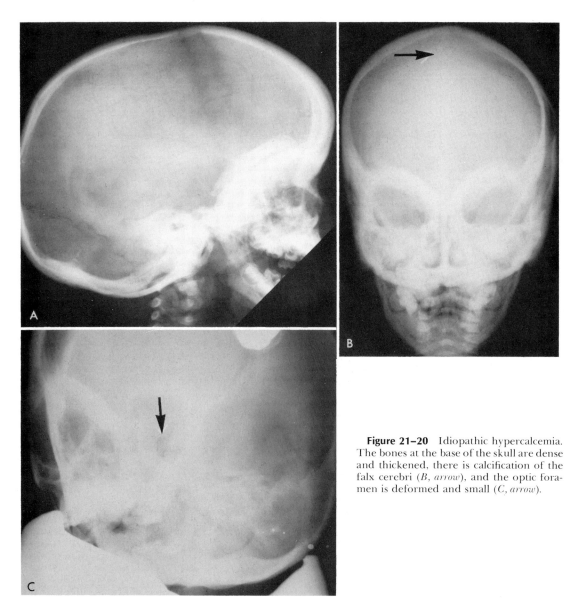

Figure 21–20 Idiopathic hypercalcemia. The bones at the base of the skull are dense and thickened, there is calcification of the falx cerebri (*B, arrow*), and the optic foramen is deformed and small (*C, arrow*).

plasia is associated with the delayed closure of the fontanelles, wide cranial sutures, and absence of the normal angle of the mandible (Schwartz, 1963).

In *osteogenesis imperfecta* there is failure of normal mineralization of the bones of the vault so that the bones are quite thin. The sutures are wide, the fontanelles are quite large in the newborn infant, and there may be numerous intersutural bones (Fig. 21–21). In the tarda form of the disease, the skull may be but minimally involved. Incidentally, the scleras may be blue as a result of their thinness, which

allows the underlying pigment to be apparent. Deafness may be associated but is usually a late manifestation. The entire skeleton is involved and the fragility of the bones is manifest by frequent fracture and subsequent deformity.

Achondroplasia is a generalized dysplasia characterized by dwarfism. Endochondral bone growth is impaired, so that the long bones are most severely affected. The base of the skull is short; however, the bones of the cranial vault continue to grow. The foramen magnum is small. There is bulging of the vault anteriorly in the region of

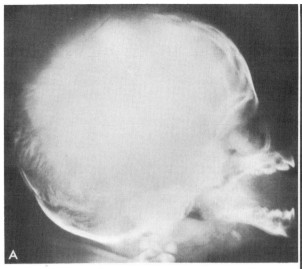

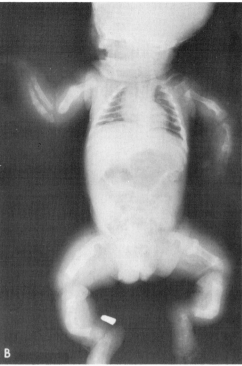

Figure 21–21 Osteogenesis imperfecta. The bones of the vault are thin and intersutural bones are evident in relation to the lambdoid suture (*A*). There are multiple fractures of the long bones, ribs, and spine evident in varying stages of healing and associated with deformities (*B*).

the forehead, and the bridge of the nose is flat (Fig. 21–22). The bones are of normal density and architecture.

The *mucopolysaccharidoses* are a group of disorders, of which Hurler's syndrome is the prototype. There are aberrations to be found in the metabolism of the mucopolysaccharides which make up much of the

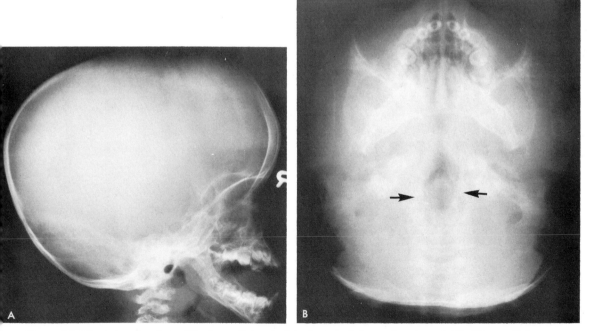

Figure 21–22 Achondroplasia. The base of the skull is short and the vault enlarged (*A*). The small foramen magnum is best seen on the base view (*B, arrows*).

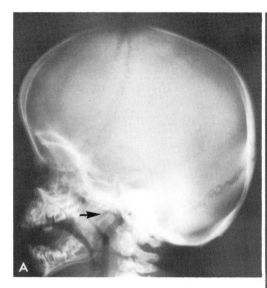

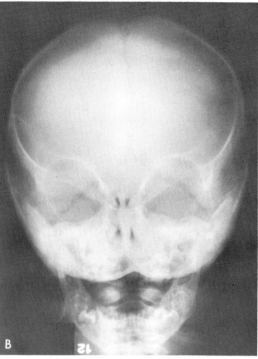

Figure 21–23 Hurler's syndrome. The vault is enlarged and the bones are dense. The articular condyle of the mandible is flat (*A, arrow*). The sella is elongate.

ground substance of connective tissue. The skull is enlarged in its anterior-posterior dimension, most likely because of premature closure of the sagittal suture. The bones are often thick and dense. The sella may be shallow and elongated an-

teriorly beneath the anterior clinoids. The mandible is apt to be short and broad, and there is usually concavity or flattening of the articular surface of the condyle (Fig. 21–23).

In fibrous dysplasia (Fig. 21–24) the os-

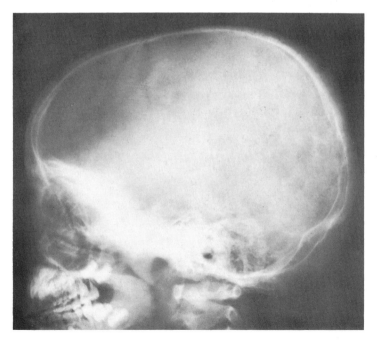

Figure 21–24 Fibrous dysplasia. There are cystlike lucencies in the parietal and occipital bones and marked thickening and opacity of the sphenoid bone.

seous alterations reflect the replacement of normal bone by an abnormal proliferation of fibrous tissue. The bones of the calvarium, when involved, may show areas of expansion that may be cystlike. However, when the bones at the base of the skull are involved the disease is characterized by marked thickening and opacity of the bone, with resultant obliteration of the paranasal sinuses and encroachment on and a decrease in the size of the orbits (Aegerter and Kirkpatrick, 1968; Leeds and Seaman, 1962).

Alterations of the Skull Associated with Hemolytic Anemias

Of the chronic hemolytic anemias, skeletal abnormalities are most marked in Cooley's anemia, less common in sickle cell anemia, and uncommon in spherocytic anemia. Owing to the hyperplasia of the bone marrow, the bones of the skull may be increased in thickness, particularly the frontal and parietal bones. The increase reflects an increase in the width of the diploë in which spicules of bone may be seen to lie perpendicular to the inner table. The outer table, with time, becomes indistinct. When the process is severe, there may be bony encroachment on the paranasal sinuses and enlargement of the facial bones (Fig. 21–25) (Caffey, 1972).

Alterations of the Skull Associated with Endocrine Diseases

The skull in cretinism is apt to be normal in size and configuration (Caffey, 1972). As the result of retarded ossification, the sutures are wider than normal. Intersutural bones are common, particularly in the lambdoid suture. The sella turcica is larger than in the normal individual (Silverman, 1957). In later life, one may note underdevelopment of the paranasal sinuses. The bones of the vault show poor differentiation of the diploetic space (Fig. 21–26).

The skull in *hyperparathyroidism* is expected to be of normal size and shape. The bones are undermineralized. By virtue of bone resorption, the outer table of the cranial bones becomes indistinct and the diploetic bone becomes coarse and granular. There is loss of trabecular detail. The cortex about the tooth sockets in the maxilla and mandible, the lamina dura, very early becomes indistinct and finally disappears as the result of subperiosteal bone resorption (Aegerter and Kirkpatrick, 1968).

In *hypoparathyroidism*, one may see no alterations in the size or shape of the skull. Calcification in the region of the basal ganglia may be evident in chronic hypoparathyroidism. The radiologic examina-

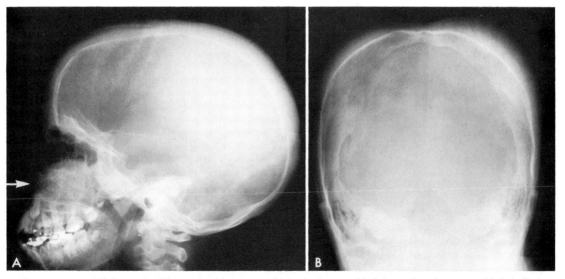

Figure 21–25 Thalassemia. The parietal bones are thick; the inner table is intact but the outer table is indistinct. Perpendicular spicules are seen in the areas of thickening. There is partial bony obliteration of the maxillary sinuses (*A, arrow*).

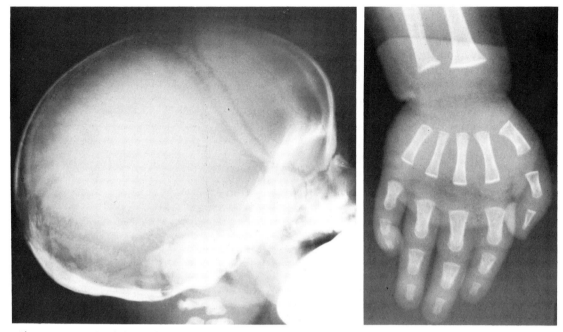

Figure 21–26 Cretinism. The sutures are wide because of lack of ossification; intersutural bones are evident in the lambdoid suture (*A*). The bone age is retarded; two carpal centers should be present at 8 months (*B*).

tion of the skull in pseudohypoparathyroidism and pseudo-pseudohypoparathyroidism is apt to be normal. However, these patients tend to be small, and characteristically there is shortening of the first, fourth, and fifth metacarpals (Aegerter and Kirkpatrick, 1968).

Alterations Associated with Chromosomal Abnormalities

The D-1 trisomy syndrome (*13 trisomy syndrome*) is associated with microcephaly. The forehead may be sloping and the sagittal suture and fontanelles widened. The orbits may be small as a manifestation of microphthalmos, and in some instances intraocular calcifications have been observed (Nelson et al., 1969; Smith, 1970).

In the E trisomy syndrome (18 trisomy syndrome) the vault is apt to be narrow in its biparietal diameter, with a prominent occiput. The mandible is small. Uncommonly, cebocephaly and hydrocephalus, as well as microcephaly, may be encountered (James et al., 1969; Smith, 1970; Warkany et al., 1966).

In the *21 trisomy syndrome* (Down's syndrome) the vault is apt to be somewhat short in its anterior-posterior dimension, and the occiput flattened. There is failure of normal development of the paranasal

sinuses. The nasal bone is small. The intraorbital distance has been shown to be significantly small (Gerald et al., 1965).

Alterations of the Skull Associated with Metastatic Malignant Disease

In the pediatric patient the common malignant diseases that are encountered and which metastasize to the skeleton are neuroblastoma and Ewing's tumor. The pattern of destruction associated with these conditions is identical to that associated with leukemia. There are irregular areas of lucency as a manifestation of bone destruction (Fig. 21–27). The tumor in many instances is confined by the dura, but by virtue of the mass of the tumor associated with bony involvement, increased intracranial pressure may result and the sutures become wide. Apparent widening of the sutures may be the result of bone destruction along the line of the sutures.

A rather specific form of bone destruction is associated with the *reticuloendothelioses* (*Letterer-Siwe disease, Hand-Schüller-Christian disease,* and *eosinophilic granuloma*). The lesions, which vary in size from several millimeters to several centimeters in diameter, tend to be round and sharply defined (Fig. 21–28). The destruction of

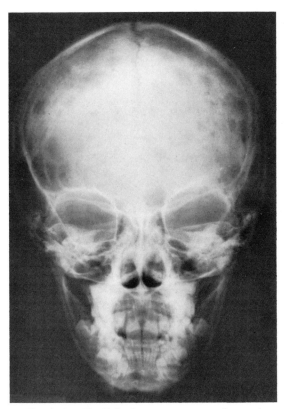

Figure 21–27 Ewing's tumor, metastatic to the skull. There are multiple destructive areas throughout the cranial bones.

the outer table may be slightly larger than that of the inner table of the skull, so that the lesion may appear as a defect within a defect. It is not uncommon for the bones

of the orbit as well as those of the mastoid to be involved, along with the bones of the calvarium. When the mass of soft tissue is great enough, increased intracranial pressure may result with widening of the sutures. There is no sclerosis around the borders of the defects until healing has begun, and then it is most frequent when cortical steroids are utilized in the treatment of the patients (Aegerter and Kirkpatrick, 1968; Caffey, 1972).

Encephaloceles may involve the anterior region of the skull. The basal type of encephalocele is that which occurs along the cribriform plate or through the sphenoid bone. It is rare. The mass of the encephalocele may appear in the nasal cavity, nasopharynx, epipharynx, sphenoid sinus, posterior orbit, or pterygopalatine fossa. It is significant that no external tumor is visible except in those rare instances of herniation so large that they protrude through the mouth or nares.

Pollock et al. (1968) have classified the basal encephalocele as (1) sphenopharyngeal, in which the defect exists in the sphenoid bone and the encephalocele usually extends into the epipharynx; (2) spheno-orbital, in which the encephalocele passes through the superior orbital fissure to lie posterior to the globe, resulting in unilateral exophthalmos; (3) sphenoethmoidal, in which the defect extends through the sphenoid and ethmoid bones, with the

Figure 21–28 Reticuloendotheliosis. There is a sharply circumscribed destructive lesion without surrounding sclerosis in the parietal bone. The lesions are often multiple.

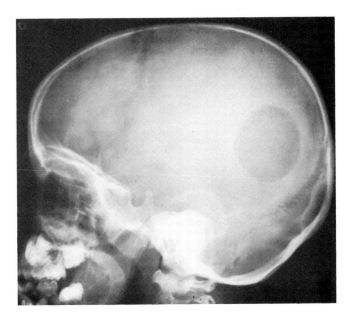

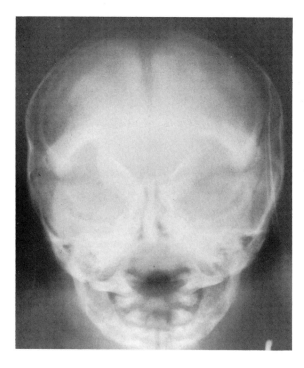

Figure 21–29 Encephalocele. There is a bony defect in the ethmoid area associated with deformity of the medial aspect of the orbits.

mass usually appearing in the posterior nasal cavity; (4) transethmoidal—this type of defect occurs further anteriorly through the lamina cribrosa, with the mass appearing in the anterior nasal cavity; (5) sphenomaxillary—this theoretical type which is listed in most classifications has never been documented clinically or anatomically.

Basal encephaloceles are associated with a broad nasal root, *hypertelorism*, and a wide biparietal diameter of the skull (Fig. 21–29). Associated congenital ocular anomalies have been described (*coloboma of the optic disc, exotropia*), particularly in patients with transsphenoidal encephaloceles. Transsphenoidal encephaloceles usually cause malformation and distortion of the optic nerves, chiasm, and optic tracts.

The roentgen diagnosis of basal encephaloceles rests on the recognition of a bony defect in the base of the skull and evidence of herniation of intracranial contents through this defect. Patients with transsphenoidal encephaloceles may show a sharply circumscribed defect in the floor of the sella that is best seen in the basal view of the skull. In the transethmoidal encephalocele, tomography is necessary to demonstrate the bony defect or defects in the cribriform plate. In any event, the soft tissue mass of the encephalocele may be visible.

Alterations of the Vault Associated with Trauma

Fractures of the bones of the skull are most frequently linear in nature. When associated with increased intracranial pressure they may be diastatic and appear as a defect several millimeters in width. Depressed fractures are associated with displacement of one or more fragments deep to the inner table. The so-called growing fracture or leptomeningeal cyst is the result of a fracture that is associated with injury to the leptomeninges. Over time, the brain or arachnoid (or both) pulsates against the edges of the fracture, causing an enlarging defect in the involved cranial bone (Fig. 21–30). Intracranial bleeding may of course be associated with trauma to the skull and bears little relationship to the presence or absence of a visible fracture. When the blood within the brain or beneath the dura is of sufficient quantity, increased intracranial pressure results (Caffey, 1972).

Miscellaneous Abnormalities of the Skull and Facial Bones

Mucoceles of the ethmoid and frontal sinuses are uncommonly encountered in the pediatric patient (Stool et al., 1966). When seen, one should suspect the presence of underlying chronic respiratory disease, e.g., *cystic fibrosis*. The mucocele

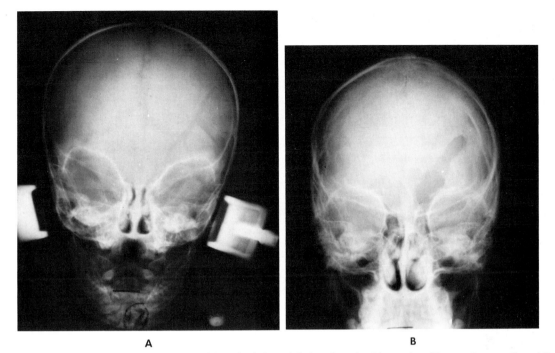

Figure 21–30 A diastatic fracture involving the left occipital and parietal bones is evident at 1 year of age (*A*). A leptomeningeal cyst in the same area was discovered at 3 years of age. The defect persisted unchanged in size after surgical intervention and was still visible at 15 years of age (*B*).

can be defined as an expanding collection of fluid within a paranasal sinus and results in expansion and thinning of the walls of the sinus. When the frontal or ethmoid sinuses are involved, there may be encroachment on the orbit, and exoph-

thalmos may result (Fig. 21–31).

Caffey's disease, infantile cortical hyperostosis, is a self-limited disease of infancy characterized by periosteal new bone formation and adjacent soft tissue swelling. Involvement of the mandible is common;

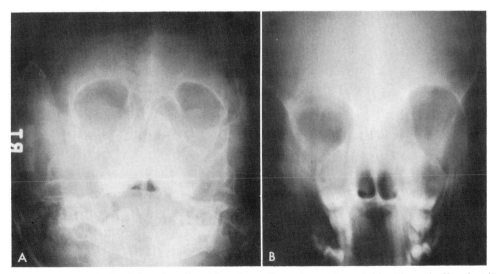

Figure 21–31 Mucocele involving the ethmoid and maxillary sinuses in a child with cystic fibrosis (*A*). The expanded paranasal sinuses with thin walls encroaching on the orbits are best seen by tomography (*B*).

however, an instance characterized by involvement of the lateral and superior margins of the orbits has been described (Galyean et al., 1970). This resulted in bilateral proptosis and increased intraocular tension. The signs and symptoms abated in approximately 4 months.

REFERENCES

Aegerter, E., and Kirkpatrick, L.: Orthopedic Diseases. 3rd ed. Philadelphia, W. B. Saunders Co., 1968.

Babbitt, D. P., Tang, T., Dobbs, J., and Berk, R.: Idiopathic familial cerebrovascular ferrocalcinosis (Fahr's disease) and review of differential diagnosis of intracranial calcification. Amer. J. Roentgen., 105:352, 1969.

Caffey, J.: Pediatric X-Ray Diagnosis. 6th ed. Chicago, Illinois, Year Book Medical Publishers, 1970.

DiGeorge, A., and Harley, R. D.: Aniridia, Wilms' tumor, and associated abnormalities (a new syndrome). Trans. Amer. Ophthal. Soc., 63:64, 1965.

Duggan, C. A., Keener, E. B., and Gay, B. B., Jr.: Secondary craniostenosis. Amer. J. Roentgen., 109:277, 1970.

Ellsworth, R. M.: Treatment of retinoblastoma. Amer. J. Ophthal., 66:49, 1968.

Evans, R. A., Schwartz, J. F., and Chutorian, A. M.: Radiologic diagnosis in pediatric ophthalmology. Radiol. Clin. N. Amer., 1:459, 1963.

Fraumeni, J. F., Jr., and Glass, A.G.: Wilms' tumor and congenital aniridia. J.A.M.A., 206:825, 1968.

Freimanis, A. K.: Fractures of the facial bones. Radiol. Clin. N. Amer., 4:341, 1966.

Galyean, J., and Robertson, W. O.: Caffey's syndrome: Some unusual ocular manifestations. Pediatrics, 45:122, 1970.

Gerald, B. E., and Silverman, F. N.: Normal and abnormal interorbital distances, with special references to mongolism. Amer. J. Roentgen., 95:154, 1965.

Hartmann, E., and Giles, E.: Roentgenologic Diagnosis in Ophthalmology. Philadelphia, J. B. Lippincott, 1959.

Harwood-Nash, D.C.: Axial tomography of the optic canals in children. Radiology, 6:367, 1970.

Hope, J. W., Borns, P. F., and Koop, C. E.: Diagnosis and treatment of neuroblastoma and embryoma of the kidney. Radiol. Clin. N. Amer., 1:593–619, 1963.

Hunt, J. C., and Pugh, D.G.: Skeletal lesions in neurofibromatosis. Amer. J. Roentgen., 76:1, 1961.

James, A. E., Jr., Belcourt, C. L., Atkins, L., and

Janower, M. L.: Trisomy 18. Radiology, 92:37, 1969.

Kier, E. L.: Embryology of the normal optic canal and its anomalies — An anatomic and roentgenographic study. Invest. Radiol. 1:346, 1966.

Krementz, E. T., Schlosser, J. V., and Rumage, J. P.: Combined radiation and regional chemotherapy in the treatment of retinoblastoma. Amer. J. Roentgen., 96:141, 1966.

Leeds, N., and Seaman, W. B.: Fibrous dysplasia of the skull and its differential diagnosis. Amer. J. Roentgen., 78:570, 1962.

Meschan, I.: Roentgen Signs in Clinical Practice. Philadelphia, W. B. Saunders Co., 1966.

Miller, R. W., Fraumeni, J. E., and Manning, M. D.: Excessive occurrence of Wilms' tumor with aniridia, hemihypertrophy and other congenital defects. Abstracts of the Society for Pediatric Research, 1964.

Moe, P. G., and Nellhaus, J.: Infantile polymyoclonia-opsoclonus syndrome and neural crest tumors. Neurology, 20:756, 1970.

Moss, W.T., and Bran, W.N.: Therapeutic Radiology, Rationale, Techniques, Results. St. Louis, Missouri, The C. V. Mosby Co., 1969.

Murtagh, F., and Kirkpatrick J. A.: Diagnostic approach to the infant with an enlarging head. J.A.M.A., 172:538, 1960.

Nelson, W. E., Vaughn, V. C., III, and McKay, R. J.: Textbook of Pediatrics. 9th ed. Philadelphia, W. B. Saunders Co., 1969.

Pollock, J. A., Newton, T. H., and Hoyt, W. F.: Transsphenoidal and transethmoidal encephaloceles. Radiology, 90:442, 1968.

Reese, A. B.: Tumors of the Eye. 2nd ed. New York, Paul B. Hoeber, 1963.

Schwarz, E.: The skull in skeletal dysplasias. Amer. J. Roentgen., 89:928, 1963.

Seymour, E. Q., and Bane, D. B.: A comparison of the accuracy of the Comberg and Sweet techniques for orbital foreign body localization. Radiology, 96:75, 1970.

Silverman, F.: Roentgen standards for size of the pituitary fossa from infancy through adolescence. Amer. J. Roentgen., 78:451, 1957.

Singleton, E. B., Rudolph, A. J., Rosenberg, H. S., and Singer, D. B.: The roentgenographic manifestations of the rubella syndrome in newborn infants. Amer. J. Roentgen., 97:82, 1966.

Smith, D. W.: Recognizable Patterns of Human Malformation. Philadelphia, W. B. Saunders Co., 1970.

Soloway, H. B.: Radiation-induced neoplasms following curative therapy for retinoblastoma. Cancer, 19:1984, 1966.

Stool, S., Kertesz, E., Sibinga, M., and Frayer, W.: Exophthalmos due to pyocele of the sinus in children with cystic fibrosis. Trans. Amer. Acad. of Ophthal. Otolaryng., September-October, 1966, pp. 811–816.

Warkany, J., Passarge, E., and Smith, L. B.: Congenital malformations in autosomal trisomy syndromes. Amer. J. Dis. Child., 112:502, 1966.

CHAPTER 22

CORNEAL AND SCLERAL CONTACT LENSES IN CHILDREN

PHILIP G. SPAETH, M.D.,
and LOUIS S. HEYMAN

The contact lens has been an acceptable therapeutic device for the last several decades and it is apparent that there are many uses for them in children.

REVIEW OF THE LITERATURE

Blaxter (1963) discussed 12 children under 5 years of age and 100 between 5 and 20, including cases of unilateral aphakia, anisometropia, aniridia, and myopia. Ruben (1969) reported on 25 patients (36 eyes) with congenital cataracts, mentioning that no patient had full stereopsis. He also included 18 traumatic unilateral aphakics. These children were fitted with corneal contact lenses, or scleral (haptic) lenses if loss of corneal lenses occurred. Steiner (1961) reported excellent results among 12 children with severe anisometropia. Parks (1967) reported on fitting patients with contacts under general anesthesia and retinoscopy through trial contact lenses. Brady (1969) fitted 32 infants and chil-

dren, finding excellent results in myopic patients and some success with aphakics. Gould (1969) found remarkably good acceptance in infants, with scleral lenses as the choice. Hermann (1968) discussed a pilot program utilizing pinhole contact lenses to see if amblyopia was secondary to aniridia and if it were preventable. Spaeth and O'Neill (1960) discussed the problem of high anisometropia, whether aphakic, myopic, or hyperopic. The vision improved in a large percentage of the cases. Luntz (1969), Coscas (1968), Boudet (1967), and Jackson (1967) have also reported on contact lenses in children.

GENERAL CONSIDERATIONS

The various groups in which contact lenses may be utilized are as follows:
   (1) The unilateral congenital cataract made aphakic by surgery
   (2) The unilateral traumatic cataract made aphakic by surgery

(3) The bilateral congenital cataract made aphakic by surgery
(4) Aniridia
(5) Albinism
(6) High anisometropia
    a. High myopia
    b. Hyperopia
    c. High astigmatism
(7) Early keratoconus

Burian (1962) discusses the optics and fusion in unilateral aphakia. In either group (1) or (2) above, and frequently in (6a), because of the disparate image points, no fusion is possible without contact lenses. Naturally, in group (1), following successful surgery, the inevitable amblyopia must first be managed by routine refraction and aphakic lenses, and in (6a) by refraction and appropriate glasses before contact lenses are worthwhile. Although a high degree of fusion may not be possible, it must be recalled that some degree of peripheral fusion may be sufficient to prevent eyes from becoming tropic. Cataract surgery may be performed in the child as soon as we can be convinced of marked visual impairment. With the more recent utilization of the aspiration technique and superior results, the physician has been enabled to start therapy at an early age with better percentages of success. It is hardly worthwhile to use a lens unless 6/15 or better visual acuity is obtained.

The bilateral congenital cataract usually presents fewer amblyopia problems and is frequently treated simply with aphakic glasses. However, as in the adult, far superior function is possible with contact lenses.

Aniridia is still quite questionable when one considers functional results, but the cosmetic results alone may be well worthwhile (Fig. 22–1).

Albinism is so frequently associated with nystagmus that the use of contact lenses is questionable and of doubtful value in this condition.

The primary use of contact lenses is for children who are simply myopic. There has been no convincing evidence presented that contact lenses decrease the progression of myopia. Baldwin (1969) would seem to agree with this. However, they are a necessity in the unilateral high myope, and far better visual acuity is usually obtained in high astigmatism as opposed to a spectacle correction.

Keratoconus does not usually appear earlier than the teens, and contact lenses are sometimes the only solution for obtaining reasonable visual acuity.

The above conditions have been mainly optical problems. There are, however, pathological conditions for which contact lenses may be considered, such as flush fitting lenses in recalcitrant ulcers, or scleral lenses in advanced keratoconus with incipient hydrops.

Another use which has been reported by Spaeth (Australian Medical Journal, in press) has been in the prevention of exposure keratitis in those cases of unilateral or bilateral ptosis in which levator function is absent and there is absence of Bell's phenomenon and superior rectus muscle function. The results of surgery with a frontalis sling procedure usually produce cosmetic improvement and frequently visual improvement. However, lagophthalmos with corneal exposure, frequently followed by keratitis, corneal opacities, and diminished visual acuity has been seen. The utilization of scleral contact lenses with shelves has the advantage of reducing corneal exposure, thus permitting one to correct the refractive error. In addition, amblyopia can be treated, and the cosmetic

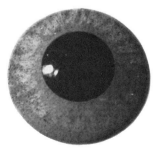 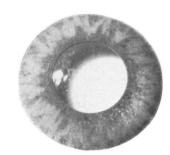

Figure 22–1 Cosmetic corneal contact lenses; left, cosmetic only; right, cosmetic plus functional.

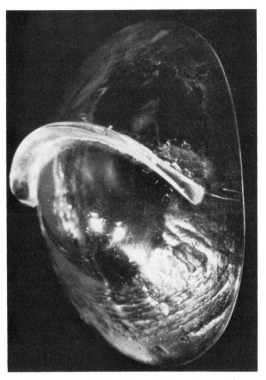

Figure 22–2   Scleral lens with ptosis crutch.

appearance with the lens crutch is quite satisfactory (Fig. 22–2).

Fitting an infant or young child with a contact lens does not necessarily present any unusual fitting problems even though management may vary. Once the determination has been made that the infant or child can benefit from the lens, the fitting proceeds along the same lines as with an adult.

Nakajima, Magatani, and Konyama (1967) comment that they found children 3 to 5 years of age rather difficult to fit due to their egocentricity and failure to appreciate the value of contact lenses, but Girard (1964) reports that young children may be successfully fitted with contact lenses. Parks and Hiles (1967) describe the fitting of an infant within two months after cataract surgery, and Tannehill (1964) states that there seems to be no age restriction. The general consensus of the literature would suggest waiting until the child has the maturity and sufficient dexterity to handle the lens(es) by himself. However, if the condition might adversely affect the development of normal binocularity, or if

amblyopia is a problem, the lens should be fitted at the earliest possible time.

When fitting an infant, up to the age of 3 years, a scleral lens should be used. There is much to recommend this type of lens over a corneal lens. Infants and young children tend to rub their eyes and little can be done effectively to prevent this. All too often the result is a dislocated corneal lens. The parent, whose task it is to handle the lens, cannot always be aware of this development and the result is a lens that is not serving its intended purpose until it is recentered. Recentering can produce its own problems. A parent, trying to recenter a lens on a squirming, rebellious infant or child is quite likely to cause corneal trauma. Lack of finesse on the part of the parent precludes the probability of recentering the lens by manipulation of the lids. Hence a suction cup must be used to remove the lens from its dislocated position; however, a nervous parent can touch more cornea than lens using this method.

None of these problems occurs with a scleral lens. No amount of rubbing can dislodge or dislocate the lens. Even if a suction cup is used for removal the only thing that the suction cup touches is plastic. Insertion is also easier, since the size of the lens permits easier handling by the parent.

MATERIALS AND METHOD FOR THE SCLERAL LENS

The scleral lens is made from a mold of the anterior surface of the eye. Taking a mold of the eye's anterior surface is a brief but deceptively simple process. A poorly centered molding shell, improper eye fixation, undue pressure of the molding shell on the eye or unequal distribution of the molding material can cause subtle distortions to the mold. These distortions will be reproduced in the lens, creating less than the optimum fit.

Best results are obtained with the patient in a supine position and his gaze directed to an overhead target. The eye to be molded must be in a primary position under occlusion. This is established by occluding the patient's eye by hand, enough to obscure vision but permit observation of the eye's position. Deviation is corrected by repositioning the patient's head or relocating the target. A topical anesthetic eases any distress the patient may experience. Success is dependent upon a cooperative and quiescent patient and the young child or infant does not usually fall into this category. Although molds of the eye of an 8-week-old infant without general anesthesia have been reported (Heyman, 1971), practicality does not favor this as the method of choice. Therefore for most children the mold must be taken under general anesthesia deep enough so that the eye will be basically in the primary position and not affected by Bell's phenomenon.

Keratometry is done before the mold is taken. The keratometer, on an instrument stand, is moved into proper position. Cotton-tipped applicators are used to separate the lids, and the cornea is moistened with frequent use of normal saline solution. Care must be taken in separating the lids to avoid exerting pressure on the globe, thereby causing distortion of the keratometer readings.

The molding powder, distributed by Obrig Laboratories, Inc., is premeasured (1.8 grams) in its glass container and is mixed in a bowl with 6 to 7 cc. of distilled water and spatulated to a creamy pastelike state. The spatula is used to place the mixture in a 10-cc. syringe. Some of the material should be lined against the inner surface of the molding shell. This is helpful in obtaining a better riveting effect as gelling takes place. Air is evacuated from the syringe, which is then connected to the shaft of the molding shell.

Working behind the patient's head the technician directs the patient to look downward to his chin. The molding shell is placed under the retracted upper lid. The lid is released and the patient is instructed to look up toward his forehead, the lower lid is retracted, and the molding shell is settled gently on the eye. (If the patient is under general anesthesia, the lids are simply retracted as far as possible in order to insert the molding shell.) Once again the patient's gaze is directed toward his chin; the plunger of the syringe is depressed, which forces some molding compound under the shell over the superior portion of the eye. With the eyes returned to primary position most of the remaining molding compound is injected under the molding shell. Not all is used or needed. Too much may cause undue pressure, leading to distortion of the mold.

The syringe is removed and the technician's finger is used as a brace to support the shaft of the molding shell. It is kept there throughout most of the gelling process. Without this support the shell may shift position, causing an inaccurate mold. During the gelling time the uncovered eye must maintain its focus on the overhead target. Naturally, if the patient is asleep this is not a problem. Tapping the overflow molding compound with a finger determines if gelling is complete. Gelling is not complete if the finger leaves an imprint on the material's surface. Gelling time is approximately 60 to 90 seconds, the molding compound reaching the consistency of the white of a hard-boiled egg.

To remove the shell and its contents, the patient looks toward his chin and the upper lid is retracted while the shaft of the shell is held with the other hand. The lower lid is then retracted while the patient looks toward his forehead. While the patient maintains his upward gaze the margin of the lower lid is used as a lever to break the suction formed between the anterior surface of the eye and the molding compound. With the shell released, the patient looks downward as the shell with adhering mold is simultaneously removed from under the upper lid. Again, if the patient is asleep the lids are simply retracted as widely as possible, upper and lower, to remove the adhering mold. During the removal procedure additional care must be exercised in order to prevent the mold and shell from separating. Without the backing of the shell the mold loses the stability needed to assure accuracy during its reproduction in the permanent model. Any gelled material adherent to the lids is readily removed with a moist cotton-tipped applicator.

A positive, permanent model is made from the negative mold. This must be done within a few moments, since the mold form will shrink and distort as it dries. After the surface of the mold is gently dried with a cotton ball, 5.5 grams of dental stone powder and 8 cc. of water are mixed to a smooth paste. This is slowly spatulated into the negative mold until the entire cavity is filled. Air bubbles are evacuated by means of a vibrator, or tapping the shell gently for a minute or two. The shell, with the casting material in the mold, is inverted and placed on a hard flat surface. It is left in this position until permanent setting takes place, which occurs within 45 minutes to an hour. Before separating the positive model from the negative mold, the back of the model is marked with a line designating the 180-degree or horizontal axis, R or L for right or left eye, N and T for the nasal and temporal sides of the model, and the patient's name.

The positive models are sent to the laboratory, along with all other pertinent information, i.e., prescription, vertex distance, keratometer readings, lens size. This is the method used for making all molded scleral lenses. For the patient with ptosis, instruction regarding the shelf lens must also be given, so that the optics may be decentered superiorly 2 mm. With the lid in place on the shelf, the lens is displaced downward. Without the compensating upward decentration, an excessive amount of induced prism and a superior limbal touch would be present. The plastic used to make the lens is polymethylmethacrylate. Further details for fitting scleral lenses may be found in the text *Corneal and Scleral Lenses* (1967).

CORNEAL LENS TECHNIQUES

Since many present-day contact lens workers have no experience in scleral lens fitting, corneal lenses are the only alternative. Here too, the keratometer readings may have to be taken with the child under general anesthesia. Ketamine is a satisfactory agent for these relatively short procedures.

For corneal lenses accurate keratometry is important and it is advisable to take a few readings using the average as the measurement of reference. However, this accuracy is less critical for a scleral lens. The central posterior curve of the scleral lens vaults the cornea and will be flatter than the keratometer reading, therefore some latitude is acceptable. In addition, it can easily be changed by regrinding.

Retinoscopy (Girard, 1964; Parks and Hiles, 1967) is used to determine the refractive error. Many practitioners (Parks and Hiles, 1967; Sato and Saito, 1959;

Shapiro, 1970) overcorrect the aphakic infants, subscribing to the theory that their world is close at hand and distance acuity can be sacrificed for near point clarity. This is a matter of personal preference and it is possibly far better to bear in mind that the important thing is the equalization of the two eyes, particularly if one eye is aphakic or high myopic.

Initially the fit of the lens should be checked weekly and fitting adjustments carried out as with any other patient. After the optimum fit is achieved, check-up visits are continued at regular intervals. These are determined by the doctor and technician and they should not be scheduled more than 3 months apart.

In fitting a corneal lens, after multiple readings are taken and averaged, a lens based on this measurement is selected from a series of lenses, brought to the operating room, and placed on the eye. Generally the central posterior curve will be steeper than the flattest "K" reading. For the aphakic patient the lens should also have an aphakic correction. This is +25D for rubella syndrome infants and +15D for others (Parks and Hiles, 1967). A study of the fluorescein pattern is made and the lens changed if indicated. After the specifications are established, the lens is ordered and delivered with a minimum of delay. Delivery of the lens constitutes a critical time. The mother is taught how to insert and remove the lens, since it is she who is with the child most of the time. It is natural that she will have anxieties about possibly hurting the child. Careful and detailed instructions will help allay her fears. Written instructions must accompany oral instructions and the parent is taught the fundamentals of hygiene, handling, insertion, removal, and the recentering process in the office, under supervision. If possible, the parent should practice on someone in the office other than the patient, for example, the technician or an individual who wears contact lenses. Great emphasis must be placed on helping the parent(s) gain familiarity and confidence, and extra time may have to be spent with them to ensure their complete understanding. The lens should not be dispensed until the parent has become proficient in performing these tasks.

For the child above 3 years of age, measurements can usually be taken without the use of general anesthesia. Even a mold can be made with the patient under only topical anesthesia. However, either process requires the cooperation of the youngster and, with some, this comes at an earlier age than with others. Gaining the child's confidence may take more than a few office visits. At each visit the child should be allowed to see the equipment and even watch someone having his "K" readings taken. But he definitely should not see the lens being placed on the eye of a new patient. He may be permitted to watch a lens being placed on the eye of an adapted wearer, but not until his confidence has been definitely established. If the child shows any apprehension, the visit is quickly terminated and the child allowed to leave the office. A subsequent visit is scheduled within a few days. Children forget, and too much time between visits necessitates having to rebuild their confidence. No attempt is made to measure the child until his confidence is fully obtained. A child is a patient for a long time and to lose him at the start could mean losing him beyond the point where the lens can be of material benefit. Some practitioners and/or technicians believe that the initial visit(s) should be spent in play with the patient to gain his confidence (Girard, 1964), but Tannehill (1967) asserts the following: "We interview the parents very carefully to determine how cooperative and understanding they are going to be.... In the meantime my office assistant talks to the child alone. The assistant creates a friendly and cheerful atmosphere and establishes the fact that the child has a personal friend in the office. I am completely out of the picture. After she has established a rapport with the child, I come into the picture. I behave very stern, gruff and very quiet. I have found that if you get too friendly with these children, they want to play. I never let them know until it is all over (fit is achieved), that I won't bite them. I think this is the key to the management of small children."

Most children beyond the age of 3 or 4 years can be taught to handle a lens by themselves, although the dexterity is more a result of their maturity than their age. Indeed, they learn to handle the lens so well that they have to be cautioned against putting on a show for their friends, such as taking it off or putting it on while at play.

FOLLOW-UP MANAGEMENT

Fitting procedures are followed according to the normal routine, with check-up visits weekly until the best possible fit is obtained; then the check-ups are gradually spaced to a few visits per year. The probability is that the infant or very young child accepts the lens as part of his body presence. Objective fitting signs, therefore, must be carefully observed, since the infant or very young child cannot articulate his problem. Such signs as excessive blinking, lacrimation, light sensitivity, conjunctival injection, or mucoid discharge should alert one to the possible precipitation of keratitic problems. Obviously fluorescein staining should be checked. Furthermore, the above signs may not always be present while the child is in the office, therefore the parent should be questioned about them.

There seems to be no reason to change the normally practiced wearing schedule, but different attitudes do exist when it comes to infants and young children. Parks and Hiles (1967) suggest that the lens be worn "two hours in the morning and two hours in the afternoon. Within ten days wearing time is increased to three and three hours and, by three weeks the infant is wearing the lens during the entire eight hours he is awake." Shapiro (1970) keeps "a conservative minimum until the first follow-up examination"—one hour on, two hours off, one hour on, for the first week, followed by two hours on, two hours off, and two on during the second week; three hours on, two off, and three on during the third week, then awakening-naptime-awakening-bedtime during the fourth week.

Follow-up keratometry should be standard practice for anyone fitting corneal contact lenses. When fitting an infant or young child this practice takes on added importance. Changes in corneal contour require a change in the lens and special attention must be paid to this possibility. The cornea grows rapidly until the age of 3; thereafter, until the age of 8, the growth is more subtle. At age 8, the cornea has reached its full growth (Davis, 1966). When corneal changes are found, wearing should be stopped and keratometer measurements should be taken each week until they can be duplicated. If the measurements return to their original dimensions the lens must be modified to prevent a recurrence of this induced change. Measurements which stabilize at a contour other than the original require a new lens consistent with the new corneal contour.

CONTRAINDICATIONS AND PROBLEMS

Emotional Factors

It is better to have a one-eyed child or even a poorly visioned child than a neurotic child. Consequently, one must try to work with parents not only technically but emotionally, in order to judge when one should cease the use of one or both contact lenses.

Size of Lens

Corneal lenses are technically easier to produce and to fit and are probably more comfortable. Furthermore, corneal contact lenses are preferable in most cases, since visual results are better and there is less mucous entrapment beneath the lens. However, they are much more easily lost and are frequently handled with more difficulty because of the smallness of size; therefore, scleral lenses may be indicated in an attempt to avoid these problems.

Prescription Changes

Small amounts of continuing refractive change may be ground onto both types of lenses, but changes of more than 0.37 diopter in either direction will probably mean new corneal lenses are necessary. Greater amounts of change can usually be ground on scleral lenses.

Keratitic Problems

The objective fitting signs found during follow-up, and mentioned in the paragraphs above, must be carefully watched for.

Loss of Lens

Corneal lenses must be removed not only for swimming but for ordinary facial bathing.

Corneal Damage

Particularly in children, dust and other foreign particles may be trapped beneath the lenses, although this is much less a problem with scleral lenses. Should corneal problems develop resulting from the lens, immediate medical attention to the cornea is required. The lens must be thoroughly checked before it can be reapplied to the healed cornea. In general, it takes several weeks and on some occasions considerably longer for the cornea to completely heal.

SOFT CONTACT LENSES

Although these have been recently released by the F.D.A., many questions concerning their value are still not adequately answered. (1) It may be that they are better tolerated, which would be an advantage in children. (2) Because of their flexibility, it seems probable that the refractive correction will be harder to obtain and, thus, it is possible that the visual results will not be as good. Of course this is particularly important when amblyopia is a factor. (3) Lenses are difficult to keep clean and a hydrophilic lens may possibly absorb bacteria as well as water, therefore introducing potentially dangerous elements.

Soft contact lenses may be used therapeutically as a corneal protective device in severe drying syndromes. The use of Griffin hydrophilic contact lenses as "corneal bandages" in the treatment of severe drying syndromes such as keratitis sicca, progressive conjunctival scarring (ocular pemphigus), and Stevens-Johnson syndrome has shown gratifying results, according to Gasset and Kaufman (1971).

The use of soft contact lenses for children with aphakia may offer such advantages as facility of tolerance and of measurement when compared to the conventional corneal lenses.

SUMMARY

Contact lenses in children have basically the same uses as in adults—to overcome disparate retinal images and allow fusional ability of various degrees up to third-degree fusion. The increase in visual acuity and depth perception must be of great help in normal learning processes and also in sports and in the individual's adjustment to society. It is significantly rewarding to achieve single binocular vision, correct amblyopia, and prevent heterotropia. Technique and hard work, with the full cooperation of the parent, physician, and technician, are a necessity.

This area remains to be explored, however, and we may find that the new soft lens, more easily tolerated but possibly lacking such good visual qualities, may be a significant improvement.

REFERENCES

Baldwin, W. M., et al.: Effects of contact lens on refractive corneal and axial length changes in young myopes. Amer. J. Optom., *46*:903–999, December, 1969.

Berke, R. M.: Surgical treatment of jaw-winking ptosis. Trans. Ophthal. Soc. Aust., Vol. XXV, 1966, and Trans. Ophthal. Soc. New Zeal., Vol. XIX, 1966, p. 70.

Blaxter, P. L.: The use of contact lenses in infants. Trans. Ophthal. Soc. U. K., *83*:41–50, 1963.

Boudet, R.: Fitting children with contact lenses. Cah. Verres Contact, *13*:9–14, 1967 (French).

Brady, H. R.: Contact lens therapy in infants and children. J. Amer. Osteopath. Assoc., *69*:165–167, October, 1969.

Burian, H. M.: Optics: Fusion in unilateral aphakia in Symposium on Contact Lenses. (Moderator, Elizabeth F. Constantine, M. D.) Trans. Amer. Acad. Ophthal. Otolaryng., May-June, 1962, pp. 285–289.

Corneal and Scleral Lenses. Proceedings of International Congress, St. Louis, The C. V. Mosby Co., 1967, Chapter 42, pp. 33, 337.

Coscas, G., et al.: Optical correction trial of aphake children with contact lenses. Arch. Ophtal., *28*(1): 61–64, 1968 (French).

Davis, H. E.: Contact lenses and the young child. Contacto, *10*:2:27, June, 1966.

Fuchs, E.: Textbook of Ophthalmology. New York and London, D. Appleton and Co., 1905, p. 804.

Gasset, A. R., and Kaufman, H. E.: Hydrophilic lens therapy for severe keratoconjunctivitis sicca and conjunctival scarring. Amer. J. Ophthal., *71*:1185, 1971.

Girard, L. J.: Corneal Contact Lenses. St. Louis, The C. V. Mosby Co., 1964, pp. 113 and 303–304.

Gould, H. L.: Visual rehabilitation of aphakic infants with contact lenses. J. Pediat. Ophthal., *6*:203–206, November, 1969, and personal communication.

Hermann, J. S.: Prophylaxis of amblyopia in aniridia. The role of pinhole contact lenses, J. Pediat. Ophthal., *5*(1): 48–52, February, 1968.

Heyman, L. S.: Flush fitting shell for an eight week old infant, J. Contact Lens Soc. Amer., Vol. 5, No. 1, 1971.

Jackson, W. R., Jr.: Positive effect of contact lens wearing on the growing juvenile myopia; Suddtsch. Optikerztg., *22*(2):75–78, 1967 (German).

Luntz, M. H. (ed.): Proceedings of the First South African International Ophthalmology Symposium. September 1–6, 1968; Symposium on Contact Lenses. Butterworth, 1969, pp. 13–58.

Nakajima, A., Magatani, H., and Konyama, K.: Proceedings of the International Congress on Corneal and Scleral Contact Lenses (Girard, L. J., editor), St. Louis, The C. V. Mosby Co., 1967. Contact Lens Research in Japan, Chapter 30, pp. 259–260.

Parks, M., and Hiles, D.: Management of infantile cataracts. Amer. J. Ophthal., *63*:1:10, January, 1967.

Ruben, M.: Role of contact lenses in aphakia in infants and young children. Proc. Roy. Soc. Med., *62*:696–699, July, 1969.

Sato, T., and Saito, N.: Contact lenses for babies and children. Contacto, December, 1969, pp. 419–424.

Shapiro, A.: Contact lens application in pediatric practice. Contacto, *14*:1:32–34, March, 1970.

Spaeth, P. G.: Australian Medical Journal. Trans. Aust. Coll. Ophthal., Vol. 11, 1970.

Spaeth, P. G., and O'Neill, P. M.: Functional results with contact lenses in unilateral congenital cataracts, high myopia and traumatic cataracts. Amer. J. Ophthal., *49*:3:548, March, 1960.

Steiner, A. A.: Corneal contact lenses; their value in severe anisometropia in children. Eye Ear Nose Throat Monthly, *40*:778–780, 1961.

Tannehill, J. C.: Presentation at the Annual Convention, Contact Lens Society of America, Philadelphia, 1964.

Tannehill, J. C.: Proceedings of the Internatl. Congress on Corneal and Scleral Contact Lenses (Girard, L. J., editor) St. Louis, The C. V. Mosby Co., 1967. Corneal and Scleral Contact Lenses, Chapter 31, p. 267.

Tannehill, J. C.: Personal communication.

CHAPTER 23

ORTHOPTICS AND PLEOPTICS

ADA MOFFITT, B.S.

INTRODUCTION

Orthoptics, meaning "straight eyes," consists of the investigation and treatment of latent and manifest anomalies of the two eyes. The orthoptic investigation includes an accurate determination of visual acuity, an ascertainment and measurement of any muscle imbalance, and tests for the motor and sensory status. The goal of orthoptic treatment is to teach the patient to use his two eyes together correctly and restore comfortable binocular single vision.

The American Orthoptic Council (organized in 1938) is composed of twelve ophthalmologists and four orthoptists. Its functions are to (1) determine the qualifications for candidates who wish to begin orthoptic training, (2) regulate the training and certification of orthoptists, and (3) supervise the practice of orthoptists before and after their certification.

Following the completion of at least 15 months of training, the orthoptist is eligible to take the written, oral, and practical examinations given by the American Orthoptic Council. Upon certification, he or she may become a member of the American Association of Certified Orthoptists. At the present time, there are 411 (active and inactive) members listed in the 1971 Directory. Whether the orthoptist is or is not a member of the Association, he or she functions as a medical auxiliary under the supervision of a sponsoring ophthalmologist.

HISTORY

There have been many doctors and paramedical personnel active in the "history of orthoptics" from the 7th century to the present. Javal was the founder of orthoptics; he found that with the use of the stereoscope, binocular single vision is frequently improved and that squint is an anomaly of binocular vision. Worth (1903) established the second cycle of orthoptics with his fusion theory, classifying binocular vision into three grades, and developed the amblyoscope and the 4 dot test. Miss Mary Maddox (1919) started orthoptic work and in 1930 established the first orthoptic clinic in London—Royal Westminster Ophthalmic Hospital. The first American orthoptic clinic was established (1932) at the Fifth Avenue Hospital, New York, by Dr. Le-Grand Hardy and Miss Elizabeth Stark.

Pleoptics, meaning "full vision," is a systematic method of analysis and treatment of functional amblyopia, especially amblyopia with eccentric fixation. This training was given under the direction of Professor Dr. A. Bangerter in the Pleoptic and Orthoptic School, St. Gall, Switzerland (1947). Professor Curt Cüppers of Giessen, Germany, modified the methods of Professor Bangerter. Pleoptics is now included in the American Orthoptic Council's *Syllabus of Orthoptic Instruction.*

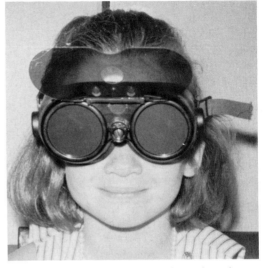

Figure 23–1   Patient being dark adapted.

DETERMINATION OF VISUAL ACUITY

For orthoptic and/or pleoptic investigation, the visual acuity and fixation of the patient's eyes must first be determined. To measure the visual acuity of each eye, total occlusion of the eye (usually the nonfixing eye first, to prevent memorization) by means of a patch, tape, or occluder is essential. The age and intelligence of the patient will be an indication of which chart—picture, "E," numbers, letters—should be used for testing. If the patient is unable to see the 20/200 symbol, bring the acuity chart closer and record the distance. After the visual acuity of each eye is recorded for distance and near reading, bilateral visual acuity is determined. Bilateral viewing provides the examiner with an opportunity to observe the gross fixation of the eyes and to note any unusual position of the head, face, and chin such as occurs with paresis.

Visual acuity of an amblyopic eye for near reading may be the same, slightly poorer, or better than that for distant reading. With nystagmus, visual acuity for near is often disproportionately good. The visual acuity should be taken with single (angular vision) symbols and linear (cortical vision) symbols. An improvement in the visual acuity of either the right or left eye with a pinhole reading indicates the need of a refraction.

If, with the visual acuity testing, amblyopia is detected, the patient should be dark adapted (Fig. 23–1—neutral density filter) for approximately 5 minutes to help determine whether the amblyopia is organic or functional. If functional, the visual acuity reading will be the same or may decrease slightly or improve. If organic amblyopia is present, the visual acuity will markedly decrease. The visual acuity reading of the nonamblyopic eye will become poorer (usually by two lines) than that which was obtained before dark adaptation.

ECCENTRIC FIXATION

Prior to the use of pleoptic instruments, the fixation of an amblyopic eye was grossly determined by the corneal reflection of the examiner's light and the eye movement (or lack of it), with the associated face turn, when the better visioned eye was occluded (marked abduction or adduction of the eye being noted).

At present, the *Visuscope* (Fig. 23–2) or *Projectoscope-modified hand ophthalmoscope* (Fig. 23–3) are widely used to determine the fixation of the functional amblyopic eye. The Visuscope designed by Professor Cüppers has a filter disc containing a diaphragm; in order to determine the eccentric fixation, it contains a black star-shaped figure with seven concentric circles (Fig. 23–4), the distance between each of them being 20′ (i.e., 3 circles equal 1 degree).

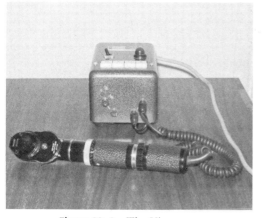

Figure 23–2   The Visuscope.

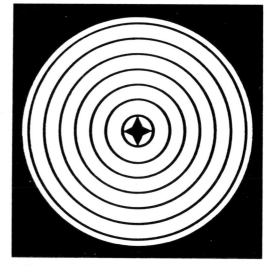

Figure 23–4   Star-shaped figures with concentric circles.

The *Keeler Projectoscope* is provided with a Linksz star graticule with two concentric circles subtending angles of 3 degrees (inner ring) and 5 degrees (outer ring). The intensity of the light (not too bright) and the patient's refractive error may be controlled.

The technique of diagnosing eccentric fixation if essentially the same with both instruments and the pupils must be widely dilated. Both eyes should be checked to ascertain if both eyes have the same type of pattern of fixation. If you are first going to examine the fixing eye, occlude the nonfixing eye (unless latent nystagmus is present). As the patient fixates straight ahead, project the star of the instrument onto his fovea. Ask the patient to look at the star. If

the patient's fixation is central, the fovea will be seen in the center of the star. Now, occlude the fixing eye and project the star of the instrument onto the fovea of the amblyopic eye (Fig. 23–5) as the patient fixates straight ahead. Again ask the patient to look at the star. If the fovea is seen to move immediately away from the star and if the patient has the impression of looking directly at the star, eccentric fixation is present. However, if the fovea should linger in the star and then move

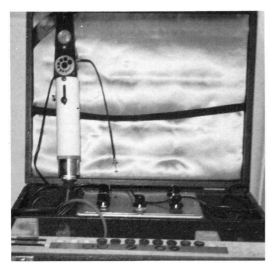

Figure 23–3   The Projectoscope.

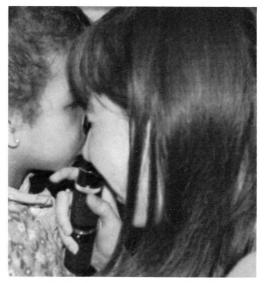

Figure 23–5   Ascertaining the fixation of the right amblyopic eye.

away from the star and if the patient has the impression of looking past the star, eccentric viewing is present. Eccentric fixation and eccentric viewing are both monocular situations but may occasionally be found in both eyes. For reliability, the test should be repeated several times—not necessarily the same day. Another method may be used whereby the patient is first asked to look at the star of the instrument and the examiner then notes where the fovea is in relation to the star. Eccentric fixation may be classified as:

> Parafoveal fixation—fixation near the fovea
> Paramacular fixation—fixation near the macular area (border)
> Peripheral fixation—fixation outside the macular area

At times, eccentric fixation may be inferior or superior to the fovea without an apparent vertical deviation. There may also be paradoxical fixation—the fixation of an esotrope being temporal rather than nasal to the fovea and the fixation of an exotrope being nasal rather than temporal to the fovea.

When proceeding with the examination, if a printed procedure sheet is not available, have a planned routine for the investigation. It will save useless steps and movements—all of which may become irritating to the patient.

If eccentric fixation and/or a diagnosis of poor visual acuity is obtained, the *Hirschberg test* or *Krimsky prism reflex* test is used to estimate the deviation. In the former test, the examiner observes the reflection of the light (which he is holding) on the cornea of the patient's deviated eye. There is a 15-degree deviation when the light reflection is at the pupillary margin, a 30-degree deviation when the light reflection is between the pupillary margin and limbus, and a 45-degree deviation when the light reflection is at the limbus. In the absence of an *angle kappa*, an esotropia exists when the reflection is temporal, an exotropia when the reflection is nasal, a hypertropia when the reflection is inferior, and a hypotropia when the reflection is superior. It may also be computed by using 7^Δ for every 1 mm. of displacement from the center of the cornea.* The Krimsky prism reflex test

---

*$^\Delta$ = prism diopter

utilizes the corneal reflection and adds prisms until the corneal reflections are centered or in the same positions. You place the base of the prism or prisms wherever the reflection is observed (3 o'clock, 9 o'clock, etc.); a vertical deviation as well as a horizontal deviation may be present.

COVER TESTING

When fixation is central and the visual acuity is adequate for a fixation object to be used, a *cover* test may determine the presence of a deviation. In this test, one eye is occluded and the movement or non-movement of the other eye is observed. Using the same size fixation object, the *cover-uncover test* determines the type of deviation present. With this test, one eye is occluded (your thumb may be the cover) and its movement is observed as the occlusion is removed (uncovered); if the eye moves in, out, up, or down to resume fixation, a heterophoria or latent deviation is present (as the other maintains fixation). If the eye does not move in, out, up, or down to resume fixation, a heterotropia or manifest deviation is present. The *alternate cover test with prisms* measures the amount of the deviation, whether latent or manifest. The patient should be seated comfortably approximately 20 feet from and in line with a fixation target—at first, an accommodative symbol should be used; then, a light source. The eyes are alternately occluded, with an even rhythm (not too slow and not too fast), permitting only monocular viewing. As the eye is uncovered, the movement of the eye for refixation is observed. The position from which the eye moves tells one the type of deviation present. In other words, the deviation is diagnosed by what the eye is doing under the cover. For example see opposite page.

Measurement of the Deviation

The intermittence of the deviation is indicated by using parenthesis—E(T), etc. A prime mark following the abbreviation for the deviation denotes the measurement for near—E′, ET′, etc. After the type of deviation is confirmed, proceed to measure the amount of deviation by means of loose

Esophoria — E or S; Esotropia — ET or ST

Exophoria — X; Exotropia — XT

Hyperphoria (right or left) — RH, LH; Hypertropia (right or left) — RHT, LHT Hypophoria (right or left) — R Hypo, L Hypo; Hypotropia (right or left) — only used if fixing eye is hyperphoric or hypertropic

if the eye moves *outward* to resume fixation, it has been *in* under the cover
if the eye moves *inward* to resume fixation, it has been *out* under the cover
if the eye moves *downward* to resume fixation, it has been *up* under the cover
if the eye moves *upward* to resume fixation, it has been *down* under the cover

---

prisms, prism bar, or rotary prism (the latter for small deviations). To offset the length of the examination, estimate the strength of the prism with which to begin. Hold the prism (between the thumb and first finger) in front of the eye (or eyes), with the apex of the prism in the direction of the deviation. Rays of light are bent toward the base of the prism, displacing the image of the fixation object toward its apex. However, it is the custom to speak of the location of the *base* of the prism rather than of the apex. For esophoric or esotropic deviations, the prism should be held *base out* (BO) before the eye. This will displace the image of the object toward the apex of the base out prism and place the image nearer the position of the visual axis of the esophoric or esotropic eye. Increase the strength of the prism and continue the alternate covering until there is no movement; the strength of this last prism is the amount of the deviation. In order to be sure one has measured the full amount of the deviation, use the next stronger prism and there should be a movement of redress in the opposite direction. At times, it will take more than the next prism to obtain a reversal. The deviation is comitant if the prism neutralizes the movement of each eye; if it does not, the deviation is incomitant and the movement of each eye must be tested and measured separately.

With this latter form of testing, one must make sure that the right eye and then the left eye is really fixating. It helps to hold the occluder longer over the nonfixing eye. When the OD fixates, the deviation of the left eye is obtained and when the OS fixates, the deviation of the right eye is obtained. Try to hold the prisms over the deviating eye. The deviation may be in one direction only or it may be in a combination of directions — horizontally and vertically.

The direction of the prism for the esophoria measurement has been previously mentioned. For an exophoria (X) or exotropia (XT), the base of the prism is placed *base in* (BI); for a hyperphoria (H) or hypertropia (HT), the base of the prism is placed *base down* (BD); for a hypophoria (HYPO) or hypotropia, the prism is placed *base up* (BU).

For a thorough evaluation, the deviation should be measured in the primary position — distance and near — with and without glasses, with +3 spheres (at 33 cm.) and in the nine diagnostic positions of gaze. If at all possible, the exotropic and/or exotropic-phoric deviation should be ascertained beyond 20 feet — down a long corridor or looking out a window at a distant target.

DIPLOPIA TESTS, N.P.C. AND N.P.A.

There are many diplopia tests — *Lancaster red-green test, Hess screen test, Maddox rod test, red glass test,* and so on — that may be used to further assist the examiner in an adequate and accurate diagnosis. The Lancaster red-green test and Hess screen test are subjective tests which measure the angle of deviation by virtue of the foveal direction of each eye. The eyes are disassociated by red-green glasses which are worn by the patient. With the Lancaster test, the red-green torch lights are used interchangeably and are projected onto a screen. With the Hess test, the patient has a green torch light and projects his light onto illuminated dots on a screen. With the Lancaster test, the red-colored goggle is always over the right eye. Whichever colored light the examiner projects onto the screen is the color (red or green) used by the fixing eye. The (other colored) light which the patient projects covering the examiner's projected light is the color used by the deviating eye. With the Hess test, the primary deviation is obtained with the red glass goggle over the dominant eye and the secondary deviation is obtained by reversing the goggles. The deviations are recorded on graphs; the esotropia will show crossed diplopia, the exotropia will exhibit uncrossed diplopia, the hypertropia will exhibit vertical diplopia (supra), and the hypotropia will exhibit vertical diplopia (infra). The Maddox rod (red or white) and red glass test are also subjective tests that disassociate the two eyes. With these tests, the patient fixates a light while the Maddox rod or red glass is first placed before one eye, then the other. Since the rod is a series of cylinders, the image of the light is seen as a line perpendicular to the axis of the cylinder. If the line (Maddox rod) or red light (red glass) coincides with the fixation light, it indicates the deviation can be overcome by the patient. However, if the line or red light is displaced from the fixation light, prisms are used until they are fused; this is the angle of deviation. In both tests, since the image of the fixation light falls on retinal elements, the patient will report the projection as follows: the esotrope will see the image displaced nasally or in uncrossed diplopia, the exotrope will see the image displaced temporally or in crossed diplopia, the hypertrope will see the image displaced downward or in vertical (infra) diplopia, and the hypotrope will see it displaced upward or in vertical (supra) diplopia. With these tests, measurements for distant and near vision and the nine diagnostic positions of gaze may be obtained.

The N.P.C. — near point of convergence — is the amount of convergence ability a person can elicit when following an object (pin or colored tip of pen) to the nose; it is not fusional ability. The pin is held in line with the nose and slowly brought toward the nose until the patient reports that he sees "2 pins," and this position is recorded in centimeters. The N.P.C. may be obtained on the exophoric, esophoric, and esotropic patient. With the latter patient, he will report seeing "2 pins" briefly when his deviated eye straightens and then moves outward.

The N.P.A. — near point of accommodation — is the nearest point where print (or symbols) begins to blur when using maximum amount of accommodation. The N.P.A. should be checked for the right eye (OD), the left eye (OS), and then both eyes (OU). It may be recorded in centimeters, age, or diopters by using one of the following instruments: Costenbader accommodometer, R.A.F. near point rule, Foster near point rule, Gulden accommodation rule.

VERSIONS AND DUCTIONS

Versions and ductions, which are usually checked after the visual acuity is obtained, should now be rechecked. Ductions are monocular movements of the one eye in the diagnostic positions of gaze. These movements are examined to check the power of the muscles. Versions (conjugate movements) are parallel movements of the two eyes in the diagnostic positions of gaze and are checked to determine any underaction of a muscle or muscles with the overaction of its yoke muscle or muscles and/or antagonists.

SENSORY TESTING

For testing the sensory status of the two eyes, red-green glasses are used with most of the fusion tests. These glasses are interchangeable which helps to eliminate guesswork. The three character test, Worth 4 dot test, and small single light test may be used at both distance and near to determine fusion, suppression, or diplopia. On the three character test flashlight, the little child is red, the elephant is green, and the ball is white. The ball may be seen as green or red or a combination of the two colors but only three characters may be seen for this gross test of binocular single vision. The Worth 4 dot test has 4 dots (1 colored red, 1 white, and 2 green) in diamond formation. For binocular single vision, 4 dots must be seen; any combination of the two colors are acceptable, i.e., 3 green and 1 red, 2 red and 2 green, and so on. When the single light is used, if the two colors fuse, binocular single vision is present. The following answers may be given for all three of these tests. The images are displaced as with the red glass test.

	Three Character Test	Worth 4 Dot Test	Single Light
SUPPRESSION	Child and ball or elephant and ball	3 green dots or 2 red dots	green light or red light
ESOTROPIA OR UNHARMONIOUS ARC	4 characters seen in uncrossed diplopia	5 dots—3 green and 2 red dots in uncrossed diplopia	2 lights— 1 red and 1 green in uncrossed diplopia
EXOTROPIA OR UNHARMONIOUS ARC	4 characters seen in crossed diplopia	5 dots—3 green and 2 red dots in crossed diplopia	2 lights— 1 red and 1 green in crossed diplopia
EXOTROPIA OR ESOTROPIA HARMONIOUS ARC	Same as BSV	Same as BSV	Same as BSV
HYPERTROPIA	4 characters seen in vertical diplopia	5 dots—3 green and 2 red dots in vertical diplopia	2 lights— 1 red and 1 green in vertical diplopia

Anomalous and Normal Retinal Correspondence

To determine whether *anomalous retinal correspondence* (A.R.C.) is present, i.e., in the esotrope, use base out prisms, increasing the power of the BO prism until the red and green (or white, if the red glass test is used) fuse on the single light; this is the subjective angle of squint. The examiner knows the amount of the deviation previously obtained by the alternate cover test with prisms (the objective angle of squint), and if there isn't any difference between the two angles, A.R.C. is not present. The angle of anomaly is the difference between the objective and subjective angle of squint. If there is a difference, A.R.C. is present. This procedure may be used to determine whether A.R.C. is present in the exotrope (BI prism) and the hypertrope (BD prism).

Normal retinal correspondence (N.R.C.) is present when the two foveas have a common visual direction. Abnormal (or anomalous) retinal correspondence is an anomalous binocular adaptation to strabismus in which (a) the fovea of the fixing eye and a nonfoveal point or element of the deviating eye have acquired a common visual direction, or (b) the two foveas do not have a common visual direction but exhibit two different visual directions.

The Afterimage Test

The afterimage test is a study of the sensorial retinal relationship of the two foveas—N.R.C. and A.R.C. It is determined by using an instrument consisting of a long light filament in the center of which is an opaque fixation square or dot. The latter protects the foveas as the lighted filament is presented first horizontally to the dominant eye and then vertically to the nondominant eye. The principal horizontal and vertical meridians are stimulated by the light. With the *positive* afterimage test, the patient is asked to close his eyes and report what he sees; with the *negative* afterimage test, he is asked to look at a plain wall or screen and report what he sees. Then, he is asked to draw what he has seen. If normal retinal correspondence is present, he will see a plus sign or cross with a space in the center, preventing a complete joining of the lines. An esotrope with abnormal retinal correspondence will see two separate lines (each with a space in the center) in crossed diplopia, i.e., the right eye image will be seen to the left. An exotrope with abnormal retinal correspondence will see two separate lines (each with a space in the center) in uncrossed diplopia, i.e., the right eye image will be seen to the right. A hypertrope with A.R.C. will see two separate lines (each with a space in the center) in supravertical diplopia. The examiner notes central fixation of the eye (Fig. 23–6) before illuminating filament.

Bagolini Striated Glass Test

The Bagolini striated glass (plano glass with striations) test is used for the sensory testing of the two eyes in normal surround-

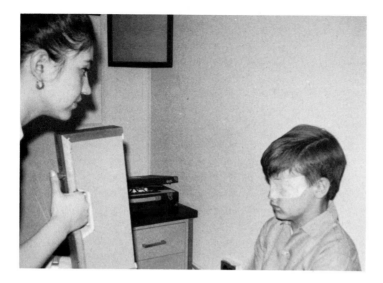

Figure 23–6   The afterimage test.

ings (casual seeing). The patient may be tested for distance and/or near. The glasses are placed before the eyes (in a trial frame), one with the striations at 45 degrees and the other glass with the striations at 135 degrees (Fig. 23–7). The patient

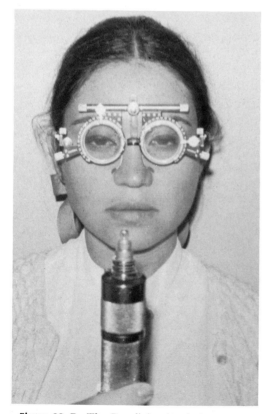

Figure 23–7   The Bagolini striated glass test may be used for convergence exercises.

fixates a light—a penlight at near and a frosted bright light at distance—with the room well illuminated. The patient then reports what he sees. If the two streaks of light pass through the center of the fixation light and form a X, normal retinal correspondence or harmonious anomalous retinal correspondence is present. A cover-uncover test is done and if a deviation is detected, the latter retinal correspondence is present. When one streak of light passes through the center of the fixation light and the other streak is not seen around the fixation light, partial suppression with anomalous retinal correspondence is present. If only one streak of light is seen passing through the center of the fixation light, suppression of the other eye is present. At times, two fixation lights may be seen and this indicates that diplopia is present.

Major Amblyoscopic Testing

Normal retinal correspondence and *anomalous retinal correspondence* may also be determined with the major amblyoscope (Fig. 23–8). In fact, in the office the amblyoscope is one of most important diagnostic and therapeutic instruments. It is a haploscopic instrument consisting of two adjustable eyepieces which provide a separate field of vision for each eye. The *synoptophore, Synoptiscope, orthoptoscope, Troposcope, Clement Clarke major synoptophore* and *oculus synoptophore* are all major amblyoscopes. Each instrument has plus spheres in the eyepieces to relax accommodation to in-

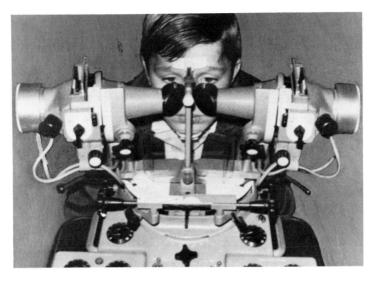

Figure 23-8 Major amblyoscope (Clement Clarke major synoptophore).

finity (O). Inside each tube, there is a mirror which reflects the image of the test slide onto the fovea (and retina) of the eye; at the end (farthest from the eye) of each tube, there is a slide groove and lamp house. A calibrated scale for measuring lateral deviations by means of the horizontal movement of the tubes is on the base; from 0 toward the patient is base in (BI), and from 0 toward the examiner is base out (BO). The calibrated scale for vertical deviations—right hyper (RH), left hyper (LH)—is above and on the side of the tubes facing the examiner. The calibrated scale for the cyclophoria is on the side of the tube—incyclophoria when rotated outward toward the patient, and excyclophoria when rotated inward toward the orthoptist.

FUSION TESTS

There are test slides for the three grades of fusion which also help determine the objective angle of squint, the subjective angle of squint, fusion, and fusional amplitudes. There are also slides for the after-image test, measuring the angle kappa, cyclophoria, and hyperphoria. The Clement Clarke synoptophore has the Haidinger's brush device (Fig. 23-9) used for testing foveal function; it is used in the treatment of eccentric fixation, suppression, and anomalous retinal correspondence. The oculus synoptophore also has a Haidinger's brush attachment.

The three grades of fusion test slides are shown in Figure 23-10. The bottom shows first grade fusion or simultaneous perception slides that have dissimilar figures; the center shows second grade fusion or fusion slides which are similar with a different check mark for each eye; and the top shows third grade fusion or stereoscopic slides which are similar (usually with a check mark for each eye) with a displacement of the figures. All three grades of fusion are in three sizes (Fig. 23-11)—fo-

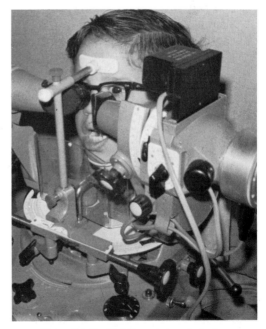

Figure 23-9 Haidinger's brush device.

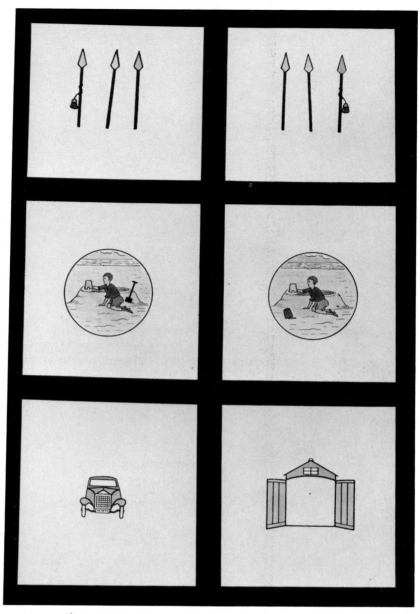

Figure 23–10 The test slides for the three grades of fusion.

veal (*top*), macular (*center*), and peripheral (*bottom*). The size of the test slide selected for use is determined by the age, intelligence, visual acuity of the patient, and, later, the progress of the patient's training; the ultimate goal is improved fusional amplitudes with foveal fusion and stereoscopic slides.

To determine if the patient has fusion and what type of fusion it is, first grade fusion slides are used. There are two methods of testing. With the first method, the

examiner has the patient fixate the targets as he alternately illuminates the targets (alternate cover testing), noting the direction of the eye movement as the eye is uncovered (or illuminated). The examiner then adjusts the arms of the instrument, adding BO (for esotropia), BI (for exotropia), RH (for right hypertropia), or LH (for left hypertropia), etc., as much as is needed to stop the motion of the eyes. This is the objective angle of squint. The patient is now asked if the "lion is in the cage"; if it

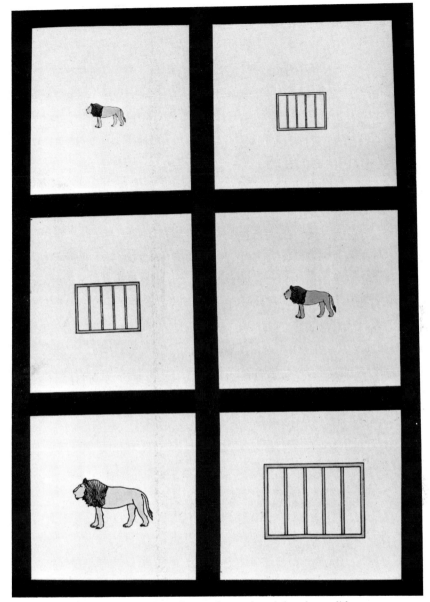

Figure 23–11   Foveal, macular, and peripheral test slides.

is, the subjective angle is equal to that of the objective angle and first grade fusion with normal retinal correspondence is present. Suppression is present if either a portion of the cage and/or lion disappears. If the lion is outside of the cage, the examiner asks the patient to put it inside the cage. After the patient has done so, the examiner in checking, does not use the alternate cover test, since this will break up fusion (if it is present). He uses the cover-uncover test by first illuminating and dark-

ening one eye several times (light control knob) and then repeating the procedure on the other eye. If the illuminated eye continues to fixate as the illumination is presented to the darkened eye and if the latter eye resumes fixation, first grade fusion is present. This frequently happens when testing patients who have accommodation deviations or intermittent phorias-tropias. If, however, as illumination is presented to the darkened eye (observe corneal reflections) it does not resume fixation, note the angle of deviation, since this is the subjective angle. By moving the arms of the instrument the examiner increases the prism measurement until motion of the eye is stopped; this is the objective angle of squint. The difference between the two angles (objective and subjective) is the angle of anomaly. Since the angle of anomaly is not equal to the angle of squint, the anomalous retinal correspondence is unharmonious. If the patient had placed the lion in the cage at 0, the angle of anomaly would have been equal to the angle of squint and the anomalous retinal correspondence would have been harmonious. With the second method of testing, the patient is asked to move the arms of the instrument so that the lion goes into the cage. After the patient has done so, the examiner, using the cover-uncover test, determines if first grade fusion is present. If it isn't, stimulation, flashing, and/or oscillation (with peripheral targets) are used in the endeavor to obtain it. After first grade fusion is obtained, second grade fusion slides are then used—at the objective angle or at any other angle at which the patient may fuse them. However, the latter angle must be checked by the cover-uncover test to ascertain if N.R.C. is still present. The arms of the instruments are then locked with an arm at the same reading on each side of the scale. This allows a smooth even movement of the slides when the horizontal knob is rotated and it also affords a better observation of the corneal reflections. If the patient has an eso deviation, the arms of the instrument will be moved toward the patient until one of the check marks disappears (suppression), two figures are seen (diplopia), or the patient is not aware of break in normal fusion. Record where this break occurs, i.e., 4^Δ BO (on examiner's side of 0—no positive divergence) or 6^Δ BI (on patient's side of 0—divergence adequate). Move the arms slowly away from the patient until the figures are fused; then continue moving the arms in the same direction until suppression, etc., occurs. Record where this break occurs, i.e., 15^Δ BO (low convergence) or 35^Δ BO (adequate convergence). The patient's fusional amplitude may be recorded as 4^Δ BO to 15^Δ BO or 6^Δ BI to 35^Δ BO, the reading from the two break (or suppression) points. For the exo devia-

tion the procedure is reversed, i.e., the arms of the instrument are on the base in (BI divergence) side of the horizontal scale. Frequently, the exo deviation will fuse with less BI anticipated, at 0^Δ or even on the BO (convergence) side of the horizontal scale. The nearness of the instrument stimulates accommodation and hence convergence (instrument convergence). The patient may be able to increase his convergence but when divergence (BI) is attempted, one or both eyes (alternately) may become a marked exo deviation and anomalous retinal correspondence (uncrossed diplopia) may be present. To help this patient, divergence (normal fusion) as well as convergence should be given. The examiner may continue using second grade fusional targets or may proceed to third grade fusion targets. Often, more fusional convergence may be obtained by the exo deviator when third grade fusional targets are used. At times the patient being tested may need an adjustment in the vertical (one figure being too high or low) and/or the cyclophoric scale (one figure tilted).

All the instruments are set for distant readings with orthophoria considered to be zero. One may test the patient under near vision condition by placing minus sphere lenses in the lens wells that are in front of each eyepiece. The angle of convergence is obtained in prism diopters by multiplying the patient's interpupillary distance (PD in cm.) by the amount of lens used (dioptric power), i.e., PD of 6 cm. × 3 (−3.00 sphere used for ⅓ M.) is 18^Δ (BO) of convergence. This angle is considered orthophoria for near on the amblyoscope and thus all readings should be transposed. Transposing an objective and subjective angle of squint reading at 10^Δ BO with a fusional amplitude from 10^Δ BI to 20^Δ BO, the angle of squint would be 8^Δ BI and the fusional amplitude would be 20^Δ BI to 2^Δ BO—poor convergence at 33 cm.

To help stabilize fusion, especially that of the accommodative and nonsurgical divergence excess type deviation, the examiner (after having the patient fuse second grade figures) gradually places minus sphere lenses (−0.50, −1.00, etc.) in the lens wells until the patient is unable to fuse the figures clearly or singularly. With the orthoptoscope, one may make these adjustments and alleviate the changing of

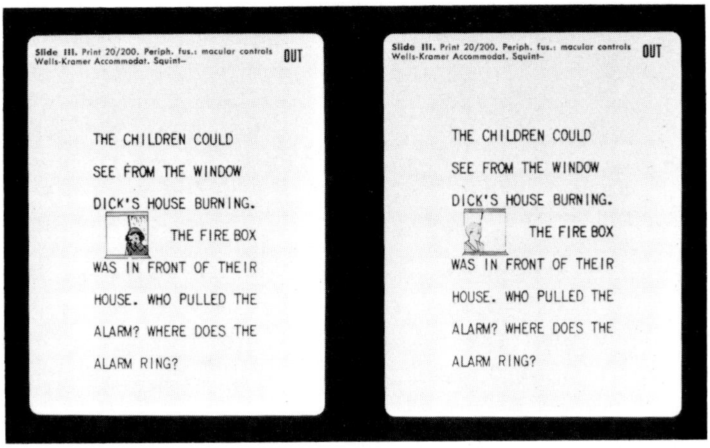

Slide III. Print 20/200. Periph. fus.: macular controls
Wells-Kramer Accommodat. Squint−   OUT

THE CHILDREN COULD

SEE FROM THE WINDOW

DICK'S HOUSE BURNING.

THE FIRE BOX

WAS IN FRONT OF THEIR

HOUSE. WHO PULLED THE

ALARM? WHERE DOES THE

ALARM RING?

Slide III. Print 20/200. Periph. fus.: macular controls
Wells-Kramer Accommodat. Squint−   OUT

THE CHILDREN COULD

SEE FROM THE WINDOW

DICK'S HOUSE BURNING.

THE FIRE BOX

WAS IN FRONT OF THEIR

HOUSE. WHO PULLED THE

ALARM? WHERE DOES THE

ALARM RING?

Figure 23–12 "Fire Story" accommodative test slide.

lenses. "The Fire Story" is a series of accommodative test slides—every other slide consisting of print and figures (Fig. 23–12). These slides may not only be used for orthoptic training but also for pleoptic training. The window (Fig. 23–13) used in conjunction with the Haidinger's brush attachment affords an interesting test target, especially when the patient is asked to place the revolving spokes (or whatever he calls it—few airplane propellors are seen today) in the window.

The angle kappa test slides (one for each eye) consist of a series of figures (animals, numbers, and letters) in a row. Each eye is tested separately. With the arms of the amblyoscope at 0, the test slide is placed before the eye to be tested and the illumination before that eye is increased (darkened over nontested eye). The patient is asked to fixate the central figure (0, dog, or circle with dot) and the examiner observes the corneal reflection of the light; if central, angle kappa is not present. If the light reflection is seen nasally, a positive angle kappa is present. The patient is then asked to look at the other figures until the reflection is central—this is the amount of angle kappa. If the corneal light reflection is seen temporally, a negative angle kappa is present; the patient is asked to look at the other figures until the light reflection is central—this is the amount of the negative angle kappa.

When using the afterimage test slides, each eye is tested separately (the horizontal test target before the dominant eye and the vertical test target before the nondominant eye). With the arms of the instrument (amblyoscope) at 0 and the illumination increased (darkened before the nontested eye) the patient is asked to fixate the dot (or red square) for 10 to 15 seconds—foveal fixation is essential. Then the procedure is repeated for testing of the other eye. When completed, the patient is asked to close his eyes and report what he sees; have the patient also draw it. The position of the space is important, since it indicates the visual direction of the fovea. The replies to this test are the same as with the afterimage instrument.

For testing hyperphoria, the examiner may use the vertical deviation slides or any of the first grade fusion slides. If the pa-

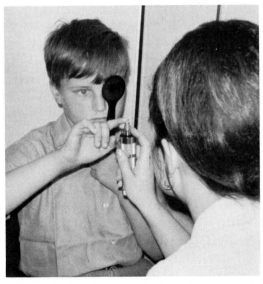

Figure 23–13 Holding fixation with amblyopic eye.

tient states that the test slide figure before his right eye is low (the image being low, the eye is high), the examiner upon doing the cover-uncover test (illumination off and on) will note the patient's right eye moving downward. This is an indication of a right hyperphoria (both vertical scales being at 0). An upward adjustment of the tube before the right eye will even out this vertical displacement. At times, the examiner may in conjunction with the aforesaid vertical adjustment (if deviation large) make a downward adjustment of the tube before the left eye to alleviate the vertical displacement.

When testing cyclophoric deviation, the examiner may use the cyclophoria deviation slides or any of the first grade fusion slides. If the patient states that the test slide figure before his right eye is tilted with the left hand side lower than the right side, incyclophoria is present; if the left hand side is higher than the right hand side, then excyclophoria is present—the tilt of the image is in the opposite direction to the tilt of the eye. An outward adjustment (toward the patient) of the torsional deviation scale will alleviate the tilt for an incyclophoria; an inward adjustment (toward the examiner) will alleviate the tilt for the excyclophoria.

Before completing the examination, the patient should be tested (if fixation and age permit) with one of the *Polaroid tests* such as the House Fly, Animal stereotest, Titmus, and Wirt tests. The patient wears Polaroid glasses. The examiner holds the test which is made of plates with the axes of polarization placed at right angles to each other and slightly displaced. All the tests, except the House Fly, record the stereopsis each plate subtends by seconds of arc.

The Titmus test grades stereopsis from 2000 seconds of arc (Fly) to 40 seconds of arc.

If amblyopia is detected and the fixation of the amblyopic eye is central, the better visioned eye is totally patched, except during treatment sessions. If the patch is worn during sleeping hours, impress upon the parent to check and clean the eye under the patch; also to curl the lashes away from the lids. If the patient will not wear any type of occlusion and there is a hyperopic correction for the good eye, atropine may be used in the aforementioned eye; in conjunction with this, a miotic in the amblyopic eye may be helpful. If glasses are worn, nail polish or some other form of occlusion should be used on the lens on the side of the good eye. He is given monocular exercises such as tracing, cross-outs (large print or symbols), and so forth to do at home. As the visual acuity improves, the size of the reading material decreases.

HOME EXERCISES

When the patient returns, see if he can hold fixation with the amblyopic eye using a red filter over the good eye (Fig. 23–13). If he is briefly successful, this will be part of his home exercises; to practice holding fixation with the nondominant eye for the count of 25, then daily increasing the count to 60 (one minute). This is an essential antisuppression exercise. His home tracings, cross-outs, writing, reading, seed bead articles, and so forth are now done with the red filter over the better visioned or dominant eye. The material used (such as pen, pencil, crayons, beads) should be the same hue as the red filter, i.e., clear red, yellowish red, bluish red.

As the visual acuity of the amblyopic eye improves, tape may be used in place of the patch. The density of the occluding material should be gradually decreased to a slight brush of nail polish before discontinuing it. Although the visual acuity may become equal or nearly so, some form of occlusion should be continued on the better visioned eye or fixing eye if anomalous retinal correspondence is present. This should also apply to all strabismic patients with A.R.C.

On the subsequent office visits, the patient should be taught (if A.R.C. is not present) the awareness of the second image, i.e., uncrossed diplopia for esotropes and crossed diplopia for exotropes, using the red filter over the good eye. Frequently, a vertical prism used over the nonfixing eye will help make the patient aware of diplopia. After the patient has been successful with obtaining and retaining diplopia (either eye fixing) with and without the red filter, he is taught to bring the images together. A rotary or horizontal prism bar may be used if the patient is unable to do it voluntarily.

The office training and home exercises should supplement and aid each other. The willingness and aptitude of the patient to do home exercises are important ingredients for success along with the cooperation of the parent. Suppression is more apt to be eliminated and fusional amplitudes increased on the major amblyopscope when home exercises are undertaken faithfully. To aid the patient, home exercises utilizing the following instruments are given to him; these exercises are first checked in the office and then carefully shown and explained to the patient and/or parent.

The Tibbs binocular trainer has been designed not only to overcome suppression but also to diagnose and treat abnormal retinal correspondence and develop vergence amplitudes. It is a folding wooden portable instrument for near use built on the same principle as the Pigeon-Cantonnet stereoscope. The instrument is placed on a table, with the horizontal scale toward the patient, tilted to one side and forward so that the nondominant eye looks into the mirror which is in the upper portion of the septum. The patient's head must be straight, since the visual line should be perpendicular to the table. Plastic carriers (Fig. 23–14) are held too high; the slot in carrier should be placed over the lower horizontal scale if vertical deviation is not present. Knowing the patient's amount of deviation, the plastic carriers with unlike targets are given to the patient to superimpose. If the patient is unsuccessful, this is given as a home exercise, progressing from peripheral size to foveal size targets. When the patient is successful, fusion (like) targets are used. To increase divergence the plastic carriers (like targets) are moved from the convergence side of the scale to or toward the divergence side of the horizontal scale. Likewise to increase convergence, the plastic carriers (like targets) are moved from the divergence side of the scale (or from 0) to or toward the convergence side of the horizontal scale. The carriers are moved in both directions to improve and increase fusional amplitudes (with the targets fused and both check marks present).

The Cheiroscope consists of an eyepiece,

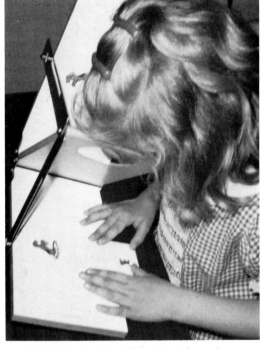

Figure 23–14 The Tibbs binocular trainer.

a drawing board base, and a fixed mirror and picture carrier. The instrument is reversible. It is designed for anti-suppression exercises based on the principle of hand and eye coordination for patients (esotropes or exotropes) who have normal retinal correspondence. The drawing board base is viewed from above through +6.75 spheres, causing relaxation of accommodation. The eyes are dissociated, so that the one eye sees only the picture in the mirror and the other eye sees the hand with the pencil tracing on the drawing board base (Fig. 23–15).

The television trainer (used for anti-suppression exercise) is a screen that fastens in front of the television screen. It may be either a Polaroid television trainer or a red-green television trainer. The former is composed of two polarized sections with axes at 45 degrees from horizontal and perpendicular to each other; polarized glasses are worn. To see one television picture, both eyes must be used correctly together (with head straight). The latter trainer is composed of two sections; one clear red and the other clear green; red-green spectacles are worn. Again, to see one television picture, both eyes must be

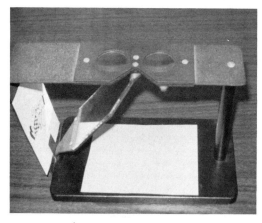

Figure 23–15   Cheiroscope.

used correctly together. At first, the patient is seated in front of the screen at that distance at which his deviation is a tropia-phoria. As suppression is overcome, the patient moves toward or away from the screen, keeping one picture. These trainers may be used by both the esotrope and exotrope.

Another home instrument that will help the patient to overcome suppression and increase his fusional amplitudes is the *stereoscope* (N.R.C. being present). It is also a haploscopic instrument in which the eyepieces are fixed rather than adjustable. There is a shaft (usually calibrated) on which rides the holder for the stereograms. There is a "starter card" which may be set at the far position, intermediate positions, and/or near position, depending upon which the patient wishes to improve— fusional vergences (divergence, convergence) or relative fusional divergence. One of these "starter cards" has two lines—a black horizontal line with numbers from 2 to 9 on it and a red vertical line with letters ranging from a to m. If the patient wishes to improve his fusional divergence at the far position, he notes (using the "starter card") where the red line crosses the black line. If at number 6, he will use the #6 or 6 cm. distance between the constants of the stereogram (Fig. 23–16). After the patient has successfully fused the stereogram, he proceeds with stereogram #7 (7 cm.), #8 (8 cm.), and so on. If a vertical deviation is present (black line above or below the red line) a prism—base up or base down—may be used. If the patient wishes to increase his fusional con-

vergence at the far position, he notes (using the "starter card") at what number the lines bisect and he starts with that numbered stereogram. When successful with it (for example, #9) he proceeds to stereograms at a closer distance, i.e., #8 (8 cm.), #7 (7 cm.), and so on. If the patient wishes to improve either his divergence or convergence at any other distance, he uses the "starter card" at that new distance on the shaft and utilizes the above procedure.

When the patient wishes to increase his relative fusional divergence and/or relative fusional convergence, he notes where the two lines bisect each other on the "starter card" at the far position. Starting with that numbered stereogram, he proceeds to move the holder slowly toward the near position, keeping the figures fused. When successful, the patient returns the holder to the far position and repeats the procedure with the next numbered (higher or lower) stereogram; this is done in sequence. The examiner may check the patient's success with the stereogram by observing his eyes; this can also be done with a cover-uncover test. The examiner may ask the patient to touch first one check mark and then the other check mark on the stereogram. If the patient should touch the right eye check mark with the right hand and then cross over to the left hand figure to

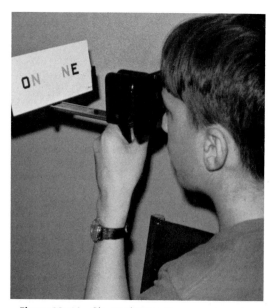

Figure 23–16   Six-centimeter stereogram on stereoscope.

touch the left eye check mark or use his left hand to touch the left eye check mark, fusion is not present.

A horizontal prism bar, rotary prism, or loose prisms may also be used to develop and improve fusional amplitudes. If the deviation is still a tropia for casual seeing, the patient may use the least amount of prism which brings the images together; first with, then without a red filter over one eye. Then, he practices decreasing the amount of prism until his deviation is a phoria without a prism, i.e., numbers 6, 5, 4, 3, 2, 1. When he is successful, the patient is shown how to use prisms to improve his fusional amplitude, especially the one (divergence or convergence) that is low. At times, both may need to be improved. Base out (BO) prism improves convergence (Fig. 23–17 for exophoria) and base in (BI) prism improves divergence (for esophoria). If a light is the fixation target, a red filter (Fig. 23–18) should first be used over one eye to make the patient aware of suppression if it should occur. When print is used for the fixation target, the patient is made aware of suppression by moving the prism in toward the nose; seeing two images as the prism bisects the visual line and then joining them clearly. As the prism is moved out

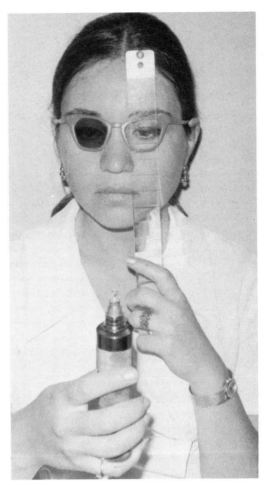

Figure 23–18 Red filter being used in conjunction with light for convergence exercises.

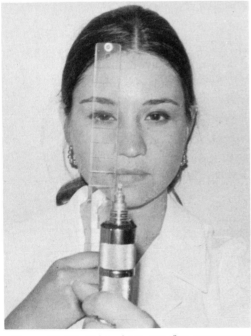

Figure 23–17 Prism base out for convergence exercises.

away from the nose, again two images must be seen as the prism bisects the visual line. The images are joined as the prism is removed. The patient is started on home exercise with the amount of prism with which he is successful and then instructed to increase the amount of prism vergence by daily exercise, keeping the print clear (Fig. 23–19).

Opinions vary as to the amount of divergence and convergence needed for the symptomatic patient. A one to three ratio, or 7^Δ of divergence to 20^Δ of convergence, should be adequate for distance; a one to two ratio, or 18^Δ of divergence to 40^Δ of convergence, should be adequate for near.

For the symptomatic hyperphoric patient, a vertical prism bar or rotary prism may be used to improve his amplitude of vertical vergences; however, this is rarely

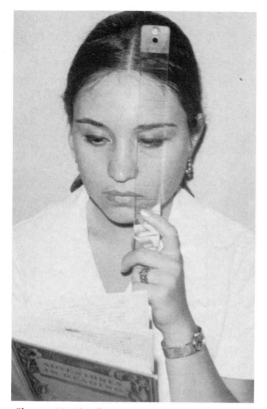

Figure 23–19 Convergence exercises utilizing print.

satisfactory. The positive vertical divergence amplitude is obtained by increasing base down (BD) prism over the right eye or base up (BU) prism over the left eye. The negative vertical divergence amplitude is obtained by increasing base up (BU) prism over the right eye or base down (BD) prism over the left eye. If a right hyperphoria is present, the amplitude of positive vertical divergence would be greater than that of the negative vertical divergence, i.e., amplitude of positive vertical divergence 4^Δ, the amplitude of negative vertical divergence 2^Δ. Here again there is a variance of opinion as to the amount of vertical vergences that are adequate for the comfort of the symptomatic patient. At times, this patient may be helped by increasing his horizontal fusional amplitudes.

Frequently, before prism convergence exercises can be given as a home exercise for near, the N.P.C. (near point of convergence) has to be improved. The objective N.P.C. is improved when any object (star on tongue depressor, pin, pen, and so forth) on which the patient will fixate is slowly brought toward his nose. Sometimes, it is easier for him to bring the object to the tip of his nose; at other times, it is easier for him to bring it to the bridge of his nose. The patient may achieve a better N.P.C. by doing the string exercise. One end of the string (with different colored knots about one inch apart) is held at the nose while the other end is held by the outstretched hand. The patient first fixates the most distant knot, then slowly moves the eyes forward, looking at each knot; if successful, the knot will appear to be in the center of a fuzzy × string. When he can successfully fixate the first knot which is on or close to the nose, the string is removed. Then the patient attempts to hold the eyes in a convergent position, seeing both sides of the nose. The above procedures are repeated until convergence becomes voluntary here (or at any other place in near space). A subjective N.P.C. helps to stabilize fusion at the near point. The patient, using a red filter over one eye, fixates a light which is held in line with the nose and which is moved slowly toward the nose; the eyes converge to keep the light a reddish white. A patient who does not have an adequate N.P.C. (usually less than 7 cm. from the nose) requires exercises.

When the deviation is a phoria (eso or exo), exercises for *physiological* diplopia are taught. A red filter is used over one eye as the patient fixates a distant light. The near light (which he is holding) is seen in crossed diplopia; as the images of the near light fall on temporal retinal elements, they are displaced nasally and seen as one red and one white light. When the patient fixates the near light, the images of the distant light fall on nasal retinal elements and are displaced temporally and seen in uncrossed diplopia (one white light and one red light). After the patient is successful with the red filter and lights, he proceeds to a figure and light (Fig. 23–20). He is next asked to frame different objects at various distances. This he does by using a tongue depressor in place of the near fixation light and objects in the room in place of the distant fixation light. As he fixates an object, the tongue depressor is moved toward or away from the nose, so that the images of the tongue depressor touch or "frame" the object. The size and the distance of the object will determine the correct position of the tongue depressor, i.e., for a large object, the tongue depressor will be close to the nose. The patient now proceeds to bar reading (Fig. 23–21). *Bar readers* may be purchased or made by the orthoptist and/or patient. All the bar readers (utilizing the phenomenon of physiological diplopia) train the patient to be aware of correctly using the two eyes together and/or suppression of the eyes as he clearly "reads through" the two "shadowy" bars. The size of the print varies from large to small type, and the distance may vary (Fig. 23–22).

Many home exercises that stabilize fusion utilize the phenomenon of physiological diplopia. One of these is the "hole in the hand" exercise, which the younger child enjoys doing. Fixating a target (usually for near at first) the patient looks through a tube which is held by one hand close to the eye; the other hand (palm toward the eye) is held near the outer center of the tube. If done successfully, a hole through which the target may be seen appears to be in the center of the hand.

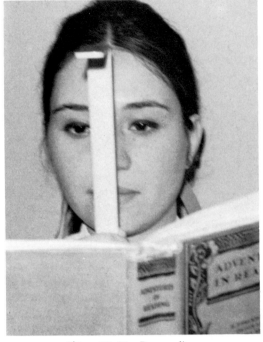

Figure 23–21 Bar reading.

The diploscope is an instrument designed for physiological diplopia exercises with controlled accommodation. The patient looks through a four-holed septum at a card containing three letters—D, O, G—which are printed in the center, with a square of green above the O and a square

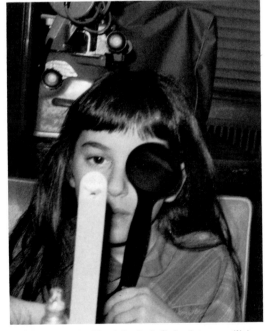

Figure 23–20 Physiological diplopia test utilizing red filter, light, and star stick.

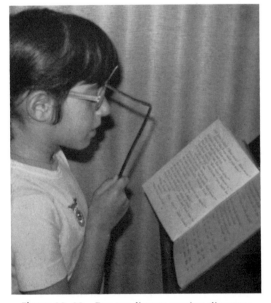

Figure 23–22 Bar reading at varying distances.

of red below the O. The D is seen by the right eye; the O is seen by both eyes; the G is seen by the left eye. If the right eye is suppressed, OG will be seen. If the left eye is suppressed, DO will be seen. This instrument is used to overcome suppression, thus aiding binocular stability. It also teaches the patient to maintain a fixed amount of accommodation to provide clear vision (on the card) as the eyes are converged or diverged for various fixation distances.

The patient with an accommodative deviation should be taught to stabilize fusion, so that through the passage of time the deviation does not become an esotropia or an exotropia. The recognition of physiological diplopia is first taught for a distant target with the glasses. The patient is then asked to do approach exercise (walk toward the distant target) until he is successful with physiological diplopia at near. Then bar framing (at different distances) and bar reading at near is undertaken. When successful with this, the patient attempts to straighten the eyes without glasses as he fixates a distant object (picture, or the like); it will appear "blurry" if the eyes are straight. If the patient should have bifocals, have him look at the object through them, so that he knows what "blurry" is. If he does not have bifocals, you may use plus (8.00 or 9.00) spheres to "blur" the object. Gradually move the glasses up and away from the eyes. If the eyes are straight, the object will appear "blurry." As soon as he is able, he voluntarily blurs without the use of the bifocals or plus spheres. When successful, he clears the object, making sure he sees two images of it, as his eyes deviate inward. Next, he clears (after blurring) the object with his eyes straight. Utilizing physiological diplopia, the patient holds a yellow pencil (or bar) about 7 inches from his nose in line with the object; if the eyes are straight and suppression is not present, two images of the near yellow pencil will be seen. If suppression is present and/or the eyes are not straight, only one yellow pencil will be seen. As he improves, the object is replaced by a chart (which he or the parent has made) of print of decreasing size. When he is successful doing physiological diplopia with the size print equal to that of his distant visual

acuity, he approaches exercises to the near reading position using the preceding procedure. After this has been achieved at the near position, bar framing and then bar reading are given.

The *stereograms*, although difficult to do, are quite rewarding in stabilizing fusion. They too utilize physiological diplopia. When fixating a distant target, the patient is more successful when the card is cut in half; a half is held in each hand (Fig. 23–23). The middle cat (if cat stereogram used) comprising all the components of the two halves will be seen in the space between the two halves. The patient attempting to improve the convergence for near is more successful if he fixates a color-tipped pen approximately 7 inches from the eyes in line with the nose. The stereogram is then held approximately 14 inches from the eyes (in back of the pen); the center of the card being in line

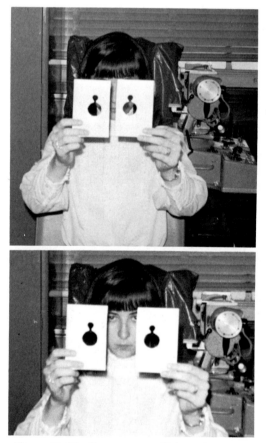

Figure 23–23 Stereogram utilizing physiological diplopia at distance.

with the pen (Fig. 23–24). When a middle (or third) cat is seen in the background with all the components of the two printed cats, the pen is slowly moved toward the nose. When the patient can no longer converge correctly on the pen, he may see two or four cats in the background and one or two pens.

The *Rémy separator* aids in determining the amount of accommodation the patient can exert while convergence is relaxed. The two eyes are dissociated by a separating bar at the end of which are two different transparent figures, placed one for each eye, the distance between each corre-

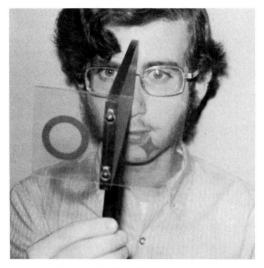

Figure 23–25 Rémy separator.

sponding to the patient's interpupillary distance (Fig. 23–25). Fixating a distant object and looking through the transparent figures, the patient sees the (distant) object singly and a blurred superimposition of the figures, if convergence is relaxed. If the transparencies are not superimposed, accommodation is not relaxed and this hinders relaxation of convergence. The patient then practices voluntary blurring. He holds this blurriness of the transparencies for a few minutes, then attempts to clear them by accommodating but not converging. When successful, the patient replaces the transparent figures with opaque figures. Since the patient cannot see through the latter figures, he must imagine a distant object, i.e., balloon in the sky. The preceding procedure should be repeated with print cards.

The *Orthofusor*, which is for home use, is a small booklike series of plates employing polarization. Polaroid glasses are worn by the patient. This series helps to overcome suppression, obtain single binocular vision, and improve stereopsis. There are three sets: #1 is a beginning set which may be used by patients with either esophoria or exophoria; #2 is a base out series for patients with exophoria; and #3 is a base in series for patients with esophoria. If the patient holds the Orthofusor at different distances from the eyes, the amount of convergence to fuse a specific object varies (according to the dis-

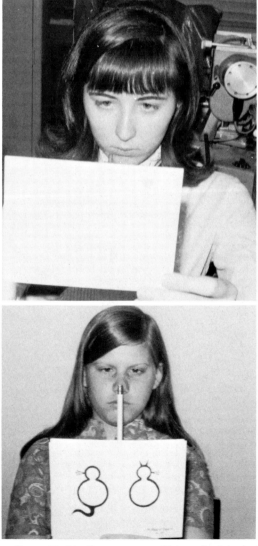

Figure 23–24 Stereograms utilizing physiological diplopia at near.

tance). This also brings about a variance in accommodation. Convergence and accommodation will also change as the patient fixates first a near then a distant object in the vectograph.

After orthoptic exercises have stabilized fusion and helped the patient to use his two eyes together comfortably, the exercises should not be discontinued too soon. In fact, the patient with a convergence insufficiency should practice once weekly until at least his college studies are completed.

Centroptics, meaning "eyes turning to the center," may be used as an adjunct to orthoptics. It utilizes afterimages in the treatment of amblyopia (central fixation), suppression, and fusional problems. The afterimages are obtained by using the Centroscope (Fig. 23–26), which is a rectangular box having a special type bulb and switch handle. One of its four sides has two linear cut-out sections with a black ½ inch wide strip between them. The light is seen through a small round opening in the middle of this black strip. The *Eddy Centroscope* may be held by the examiner, the patient, or the parent, 6 to 12 inches from the eye for about 50 seconds—illuminated first vertically, then horizontally. After the patient perceives a positive afterimage (cross with space), he fixates a symbol about 3 to 4 feet away. He then attempts to perceive

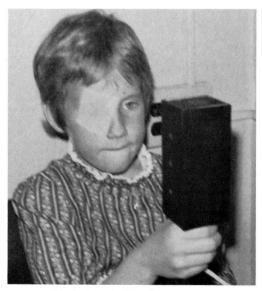

Figure 23–26   The Centroscope.

a negative afterimage with the symbol in the space of the cross. When the patient can recognize the symbols (on a wall) in the space of the cross at 3 feet, he walks away from it, attempting to see the symbol in the space of the cross at 20 feet. The Centroscope is used before the amblyopic (or suppressed) eye until suppression is overcome, vision improves to 20/30, and spatial localization is normal. Then binocular centroptics is instituted. The nondominant eye is patched and the Centroscope is held vertically (illuminated) before the dominant eye; it is then held horizontally (illuminated) before the nondominant eye (dominant eye patched). The positive afterimage is seen with the eyes closed; the negative afterimage is seen with the eyes open.

PLEOPTICS

If the fixation of an amblyopic eye is seen to be eccentric with either the *Visuscope* (Fig. 23–2) or *Projectoscope* (Fig. 23–3), *pleoptic training* is instituted.

Professor Bangerter's technique consists of first dazzling the eccentric area of the retina—obliterating it—and then, with stimulation of the fovea, eliminating the central inhibition scotoma.

Professor Cüppers' technique consists of giving a light stimulus only strong enough to elicit an afterimage, restoring the fovea to predominance, and then reeducating it as the principal visual direction.

During pleoptic therapy, one may use a combination of Bangerter's or Cüppers' methods or use them separately.

All treatment is designed to (a) reestablish central fixation; (b) re-establish the fovea as the seat of the principal visual direction; (c) restore normal visual acuity; and (d) eliminate separation difficulties.

Approximately one month before pleoptic treatment, patch (or use some form of lens occlusion over) the eccentrically fixing eye in children over 5 years of age. For children up to the age of 5, patch the better eye as soon as amblyopia or eccentric fixation is discovered. Continue occlusion during therapy, except for treatment sessions, until fixation becomes unsteady central. When fixation is unsteady

TABLE 23–1 PLEOPTIC INSTRUMENTS

Professor Bangerter's	Professor Cüppers'
Pleoptophor	*Euthyscope*
DAZZLES the peripheral area by protecting macula with a black disc target. Size of target is chosen according to type of fixation; close to fovea—small target and lower illumination. One minute of dazzling. STIMULATES fovea—50 to 100 shots by using ring-shaped target.	AFTERIMAGES (positive and negative) may or may not become apparent after 10 to 30 seconds of flashing, during which a 3- or 5-degree black disc shields the fovea. Prior to this flashing, the fovea is located (green filter used). Patient perceives afterimage by looking straight ahead at wall or screen. The deeper the amblyopia, the more difficult it is to produce afterimage. Positive—round black spot encircled with bright ring. Negative—bright round spot encircled with dark ring.
Localizer	*Light Internal Regulator*
Corrects localization of fovea by means of hand-eye cooperation; locating and touching lights flashing through a perforated designed metal plate.	Permits alternate periods of brightness and darkness —the frequency of which may be regulated. Afterimages more easily appreciated.
Corrector	*Coordinator*
Furtherance of hand and eye cooperation in conjunction with hearing by tracing a line or letter with a metal pointer; buzzer sounds if patient deviates.	Re-educates the visual direction of the fovea by means of Haidinger brushes (a propeller-shaped apparition of polarized light of 3 to 5 degrees, seen only by the macula). Hand and eye cooperation for centering brushes on an object (slide), then touching center of brushes.
Centrophore	*Space Coordinator*
Stabilizes central or near central fixation; varies the size of the interchangeable optotypes and of the Haidinger brushes.	Establishes the awareness of foveal projection in space; uses Haidinger brushes by projection on a screen—propeller to be centered around real objects, i.e., E-hooks. Begin with single optotypes.
Separation-difficulty (E) Trainer	*Visuscope Type "P"*
Overcomes separation difficulties by starting with "E"s widely spaced, then gradually reducing the distance between them.	Rows of E-hooks of different sizes can be projected vertically and/or horizontally on the fundus. Overcomes separation-difficulties.
	Synoptophore with Haidinger brushes
	Provides for binocular examination and binocular training. By placing the Haidinger brushes in front of the amblyopic eye and a test slide (box) in front of the better visioned eye, central or eccentric fixation can be determined. If eccentric, the Haidinger brushes will be seen outside of box.

central, patch the better visioned eye gradually—1 hour, 2 hours, and so on, until total occlusion is achieved. In some cases, patching of the centrally fixing eye in conjunction with a red filter (regular ruby Kodaloid filter) over the eccentrically fixing eye has been effective. As the fixation of the amblyopic eye becomes central, the red filter (Fig. 23–27) is discontinued and the better visioned eye is totally occluded. There are differences of opinion regarding inverse occlusion and the above use of the red filter.

For pleoptic treatment, the inpatient is seen three to four times daily for a week; the outpatient should be seen twice daily for two to three weeks.

Knowing the patient, one can best judge the time—5 to 15 minutes—to be spent with the instrument that creates an after-

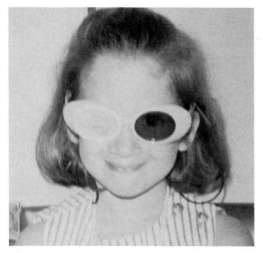

Figure 23–27   Red filter over eccentric fixing eye.

image. The *Keeler Projectoscope* has a Nutt Auto-disc attachment which permits automatically a three-stage treatment: stage 1 — placing of Linksz star on patient's fovea; stage 2 — by pressing trigger, a 3-degree black spot automatically rotates to shield the fovea as a bright light illuminates the retina; stage 3 — a disc of white light automatically replaces the black spot, and releasing of trigger produces a flashing light, causing foveal stimulation. Either the *Euthyscope* or the aforesaid attachment may be used to obtain first a positive afterimage, i.e., a dark dot in a bright circle; then a negative afterimage, i.e., a small light dot in a dark

circle. It is important for the patient to obtain and retain the negative afterimage as another target (such as a symbol, an "E", and so on) may be seen through the light dot.

The flashing on and off of illumination by the Alternator aids the patient in his retention of the afterimage. The short or long periods (whichever preferred) of light and dark may be controlled.

With the *Pleoptophor* (Fig. 23–28), the examiner may obtain a good view of the patient's magnified fundus. The eccentric fixing eye should be dilated and it is most helpful if the centric fixing eye is constricted. There are three different sized carriers to use for (a) near central fixation, (b) unsteady paramacular fixation, and (c) unsteady peripheral fixation. After selecting the size of the carrier needed, the examiner first uses the spot target for dazzling (1 minute) and then the ring target for stimulating the central area with reduced illumination (50 to 100 times). The previous procedure should be done two or three times daily.

On the *Coordinator* (Fig. 23–29), which utilizes the Haidinger brush phenomenon, the patient perceives a "revolving propeller" (or revolving spokes) and attempts to place a pointer in the middle (center) of it. If he is unsuccessful in seeing the center, the Haidinger brush will appear to be a "revolving wheel" — only macular function is present. When the patient is successful in using the fovea (seeing

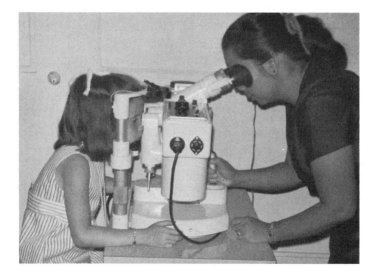

Figure 23–28   The Pleoptophor.

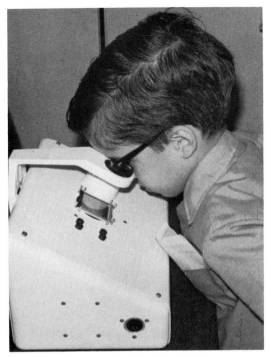

Figure 23–29 The Coordinator.

center), a target (airplane) is placed onto the coordinator and the patient is then asked to point to "where the revolving propeller is." If fixation is central, the revolving propeller will be seen on the propeller of the airplane. If fixation is eccentric, the esotrope should see it nasally and the exotrope should see it temporally; vice versa for paradoxical fixation. There is a diaphragm attachment that may be adjusted to restrict the field.

When the *Haidinger brush* attachment is used on the synoptophore (Fig. 23–9), a blue disc is placed before the centric eye and a target (box, window, or the like) is placed before the eccentric eye. When the patient is successful with placing the "revolving propeller" into the center of the target, the field of vision may be restricted.

When fixation becomes unsteady central and the better visioned eye can be patched, monocular exercises for the poorer visioned eye may be given—first at the office and then for homework. A one-half tape occlusion of the poorer visioned eye (nasal for esotropes and temporal for exotropes) may be used in the office. If glasses are not worn, rubber-framed sunglasses (tinted portion removed) may be used. When monocular exercises such as cross-outs, tracing, reading, and so forth are given, it should be large enough for the patient to see and enjoy doing. As the visual acuity improves, decrease the size of the subject matter (for exercises). The treatment should then continue as for amblyopia with central fixation.

The fixation should be constantly checked and if it has again become eccentric, occlusion of the better visioned eye should be discontinued so as to proceed with inverse occlusion again.

There has been and there will continue to be discussions, debates, and studies as to the usefulness and merits of orthoptics and pleoptics. The reports on the aforesaid usefulness have been (a) favorable, (b) no better than previous methods, or (c) nonfavorable. Orthoptics are particularly useful to promote the development of convergence and fusional amplitudes. The elimination of amblyopia and suppression are essential for successful therapy. Satisfactory results depend on the enthusiastic capabilities of the orthoptist and the cooperative response of the patient.

REFERENCES

Anderson, E. C.: The television trainer in fusion training. Amer. Orthop. J., 7:84–89, 1957.

Binder, H. F.: Orthoptic practice in Europe. Amer. Orthop. J., 9:43–48, 1959.

Binder, H. F., Engel, D., Ede, M. L., and Loon, L.: The red filter treatment of eccentric fixation. Amer. Orthop. J., 13:64–69, 1963.

Brenin, G. M.: Relationship between accommodation and convergence. Trans. Amer. Acad. Ophthal. Otolaryng., 61:375–382, 1957.

Burian, H. M.: Sensorial retinal relationship in concomitant strabismus. Arch. Ophthal., 37:336–368, 504–533, 618–648, 1947.

Burian, H. M.: Adaptive mechanisms. Trans. Amer. Acad. Ophthal. Otolaryng., 57:131–144, 1953.

Burian, H. M.: Syllabus of Orthoptic Instruments. Amer. Orthop. C., 7–13, 17, 19–26, 36–47, 50–60, 1962.

Capobianco, N. M.: Pleoptic treatment of amblyopes with central and eccentric fixation. Amer. Orthop. J., 10:33–53, 1960.

Capobianco, N. M.: The diagnosis and treatment of sensorial anomalies. Amer. Orthop. J., 16: 93–103, 1966.

Cooper, D. L.: The future of orthoptics. Amer. Orthop. J., *19*:143–144, 1969.

Costenbader, F. D.: Principles of treatment. Trans. Amer. Acad. Ophthal. Otolaryng., *57*:163–169, 1953.

Costenbader, F. D.: Principles of treatment. Trans. Amer. Acad. Ophthal. Otolaryng., *61*:390–394, 1957.

Engel, D.: The monocular use of the centroscope, Amer. Orthop. J., *14*:175–177, 1964.

Gibson, G. G., and Harley, R. D.: Strabismus and Associated Sensorimotor Anomalies. 3rd ed. Amer. Acad. Ophthal. Otolaryng., Rochester, Minnesota, 1971.

Jones, B. A.: Orthoptic handling of fusional vergences. Amer. Orthop. J., *15*:21–29, 1965.

Katzin, H. M., and Wilson, G.: Observations on pleoptic diagnosis and treatment. Amer. Orthop. J., *10*:17–27, 1960.

Kramer, M. E.: Centroptics. Amer. Orthop. J., *12*:132–147, 1962.

Krewson, W. E.: Personal communication.

Lancaster, J. E.: The second image in orthoptics. Amer. Orthop. J., *9*:49–54, 1959.

MacLean, F. M.: Bar reading as a home exercise. Amer. Orthop. J., *9*:114–116, 1959.

MacLean, F. M.: Diagnostic orthoptics. Amer. Orthop. J., *9*:10–16, 1959.

MacLean, F. M.: Home orthoptics. Amer. Orthop. J., *20*:118–126, 1970.

Rapoport, A. T.: Orthoptic techniques: Physiological techniques. Amer. Orthop. J., *20*:127–135, 1970.

Sauberli, R.: Pleoptics: Bangerter's method of treatment. Amer. Orthop. J., *11*:109–113, 1961.

Stelzer, A. J.: Nasal occlusion. Amer. Orthop. J., *8*:47–49, 1958.

Swenson, A.: Temporal occlusion in concomitant convergence strabismus. Amer. Orthop. J., *8*:45–47, 1958.

Tibbs, A.: Two new optical instruments: Binocular trainer and physiologic diplopia reader. Amer. Orthop. J., *10*:69–79, 1960.

Walraven, F.: A follow through cheiroscope technique. Amer. Orthop. J., *9*:96–104, 1959.

Wehrheim, D.: Physiologic diplopia as a home exercise. Amer. Orthop. J., *3*:62–65, 1953.

Wilson, G.: The inter-relationship of orthoptics and pleoptics. Amer. Orthop. J., *14*:57–59, 1964.

BROCHURES

Instrument Brochures
Orthoptic Council Brochure

CHAPTER 24

READING DISABILITIES IN CHILDREN (DYSLEXIA)

VIRGINIA T. KEENEY, M.D.

INTRODUCTION

Just a few years ago, ophthalmologists were advised to include in every pediatric eye examination the question "How is the youngster doing in school?" Reading disability might thus have been revealed if parents had been reluctant to verbalize the problem. The question should, of course, continue as a part of the medical history, but it is a rare parent today who doesn't consider a reading difficulty, even if the child's problems only remotely suggest this.

Dyslexia has become a vogueish designation, a sort of umbrella sheltering many reading problems ranging from the frankly retarded to the specific dyssymbolic. It is overly popular and poorly understood by all concerned, including psychologists, educators, parents, and physicians. The problem today is to sort out the few true dyslexic children from the many youngsters whose anxious parents feel their children could be doing better in school.

The concept of dyslexia, however, is not as new as its popularity. Alexia, the loss of a previously acquired ability to read, was first given attention in the literature in 1877. Kussmaul used the term "word blindness," and in 1897 Rudolph Berlin of Stuttgart coined the word "dyslexia." In 1895, James Hinshelwood, eye surgeon of Glasgow, wrote to *Lancet* about visual memory and word blindness. Soon after that publication, a general practitioner, Pringle Morgan, wrote to Hinshelwood citing a case of an intelligent 14-year-old boy who was unable to read. Other cases were reported, and this condition became known as *congenital word blindness.* This became the title of a bound monograph published by Dr. Hinshelwood in 1917, the culmination of his several reports in the literature.

Since then, there has been much discussion, description, and theory but little progress in understanding basic causes. Although the early studies in dyslexia were contributed primarily by ophthalmologists and later by neurologists, there is now extensive literature in psychology, speech therapy, education, behavioral science, psychiatry, audiology, pediatrics, physical therapy, and optometry. A complete review of this literature would exhaust the clinician reader and even reincarnate many exercises which are better left interred.

A quotation from one of Hinshelwood's early reports, in 1900 in *Lancet*, illustrates our lack of progress from that day to this:

His difficulty in learning to read is . . . no doubt due to some defect of his visual memory center which makes it much more difficult for him to retain and store up the visual memories of words. This is the real explanation of the difficulty. It is not owing to any defect of his general intelligence or to any diminution of visual acuity.

Early workers never meant dyslexia or "word blindness" to include the conglomeration of reading disabilities now referred to carelessly as dyslexia. Definitions range from the very simple, such as *difficulty with reading*, to the specific, as *a defect in the verbal interpretation of visual symbols*. A satisfactory definition might be *a familial defective capacity for learning to read in a child with average or superior intelligence, intact senses, and normal motivation*. These definitions refer to primary, developmental, or specific dyslexia and not to dyslexia secondary to any other cause. Neither slow readers nor retarded readers should be included; they are better referred to as children with reading disabilities.

ANATOMIC LOCALIZATION

Although there is certainty that the lesion of alexia or acquired dyslexia is located in or near the dominant angular gyrus, we cannot extrapolate from this that the location is identical in congenital dyslexia. Too little is known about the development of cortical perceptual and intellectual functions. The child's brain has more plastic potential for growth and changes, as well as more potential for problems in how he feels about himself when he is in some way different from other children. Some cortical areas used in visual or reading input are identified.

Brodman's area 17 or the visual registration area is relatively well understood, representing as it does an almost cell-by-cell relationship with percipient cells in the retina. Surrounding it are the visual association areas 18 and 19, which are vague and less well defined.

The angular gyrus is the interpretation center and usually, in some 9 out of 10 cases, is on the opposite side from the dominant hand. It has been said that 60 per cent of school children will learn to read no matter what system or method is used. With these children, the reading skill is acquired almost as easily and naturally as walking or talking. Another 20 per cent will learn with only a modicum of extra help within the classroom situation. This leaves some 20 per cent of the school child population who will experience reading retardation of a severe enough degree to need some kind of special help. Perhaps half these may have severe reading problems which will require tutoring, remedial instruction, or special class participation, or, lacking these, will begin to develop the patterns of frustration and failure that go with inability to read in a world of printed matter. Even among children with severe reading problems, however, only a few will be diagnosed as having a primary development dyslexia, perhaps 1 or 2 per cent, at the most, of the total school-age population.

CLASSIFICATION

There is a strong trend among psychologists, educators, and nonmedical practitioners to include dyslexia as only one of a wide spectrum of reading disabilities and to deprecate efforts to diagnose by cause. Precise diagnosis, however, leads to helpful prognosis, and for this alone, efforts at understanding etiology are necessary. Classification is useful also in organizing mechanisms in diagnosis, so that helpful bits of information are stored in retrievable relationships rather than as a random jumble of uncoordinated facts. Finally, a classification provides an operating basis for analysis of new observations which may delineate previously undescribed lesions and ultimately lead to diagnosis.

A multitude of classifications of dyslexia or reading disabilities have been formulated in various medical specialties, each reflecting the particular interest of its author. The following classification was devised initially by A. H. Keeney in 1967 and later revised to utilize the terms reading disabilities or reading retardations rather than dyslexia to describe the broad spectrum of secondary reading problems as suggested by the National Interdisciplinary Committee for Dyslexia.

Specific Dyslexia

True dyslexia may be described as specific, primary, or developmental. Within the population of children with reading disabilities, there exists a small core of specific cases showing inability to read based on a defect in the visual interpretation of symbols but in the presence of average or superior intellectual potential and with adequate functioning peripheral sensory mechanisms. Findings in this condition will be detailed later.

Secondary Reading Disabilities

SECONDARY TO SLOW MATURATION. These youngsters have been termed "slow bloomers" and show many signs of immaturity, not only in reading but in arithmetic and behavior as well. Their transient deficit is global rather than specific, but the diagnosis is by no means as simple as this may sound. For example, symptoms of immaturity may include mirror writing and transposition of letters which associate with the dyslexic child. They occur as a stage in development and will disappear without remedial therapy. Although the prognosis for adequate reading ability is good, assistance should be given to these children to help them keep up with their work until they "catch on fire" and really learn to read.

SECONDARY TO EMOTIONAL DISTURBANCES. Although emotional disturbances may cause reading disabilities, the latter are not considered primary dyslexia in that the problem is not basically derived from poor interpretation of visual symbols. For example, a schizophrenic child may be unable to exercise his reading ability or other intellectual abilities because he is in poor contact with his en-

vironment, or a depressed child may be blocked from participation in the reading effort. In either case, the resulting reading disability is secondary and not a primary problem with symbol interpretation.

An emotional disturbance secondary to developmental dyslexia, on the other hand, is very common. The frustrations of a bright child subjected to repeated failures and often to the disapproval of those he wants most to please may be expressed in disruptive behavior or emotional disturbances. When true dyslexia is not discovered until early adolescence, differentiation between emotional disturbances and dyslexia regarding which problem is primary may be greatly clouded, and treatment should be directed to both conditions. Attention to the overlay of emotional problems may be necessary before the primary dyslexia can be attacked, but the emotional disturbance that is secondary to congenital or developmental dyslexia will never respond to psychotherapy alone. Lester Jones' saying, "cure the underlying disease, and the symptom will disappear," holds true in relation to dyslexia and emotional disturbances.

SECONDARY TO UNCONTROLLED SEIZURE STATES. Any history of convulsions, unexplained loss of consciousness, or episodic attacks of peculiar behavior should arouse suspicion of the presence of seizure states. Each of such episodes inevitably causes cellular damage and may strike the complexes used in reading. Appropriate analeptic drug therapy is usually effective. Such children should be referred to the neurologist for EEG and neurologic workup.

SECONDARY TO ORGANIC BRAIN DISEASE. These children may have subtle or gross neurologic deficits associated with cortical or subcortical impairments such as brain tumors, cortical atrophy or hypoplasia, porencephalic cysts, and the like. Careful neurologic evaluation, particularly for contralateral disturbances in the extremities or papilledema, may reveal a life-threatening process.

SECONDARY TO ENVIRONMENTAL PROBLEMS. In recent years, lack of stimulation in the home has been recognized as a real barrier to the acquisition of reading ability. Lack of encouragement from illiterate or foreign language-speaking parents, compounded by the problems of poverty, may present serious handicaps. Lack of books or even pencil and paper are common in such environments, and in the early days of the Head Start Program, there were many reports of children who had never seen themselves in a mirror, had never sat down to a table to eat, much less to study, and had little experience with the verbal communication we call conversation. The Head Start and Get Set Programs were federal efforts to help children handicapped by lack of environmental stimulation. Evaluation of these programs is difficult and at present incomplete.

Once the child is attending school, other environmental difficulties may appear such as overcrowded classrooms and harassed and poorly trained teachers with poor class control. Such situations offer little learning opportunity and are synergistic with an inadequate home environment.

Slow Readers

Slow readers are children who are handicapped by a physical defect but are not primary dyslexics. They may be knowledgeable but read slowly because their vision is so poor that they must read one word at a time using high magnification. They may have hypothyroidism or may even be minimally retarded. The slowness will extend not only to reading but to arithmetic and other intellectual skills, such as learning to read music. Their problem is not in interpretation of visual symbols.

Ophthalmologists note a high percentage of visual problems complicating both primary dyslexia and the various reading disabilities. These children require the usual examination for visual function, and correction should be made for any significant defects such as impaired visual acuity or symptomatic problems in motility. It is not true, however, that children with poorly coordinated convergence and accommodation or with a low visual acuity are unable to interpret symbols. A child can read with poor vision or, if blind, by braille.

Children have a great facility for overcoming hyperopia, even 5 or 6 diopters, which the adult doesn't have. Because of the child's great reserve of tonus in the ciliary muscles and the high degree of pliability of the youthful lens, hyperopia that would be disabling in adults may be asymptomatic in children. Therefore, numerical measurements, particularly as derived from instrumental screening devices, have significance only as they relate to specific ocular symptomatology.

Major ophthalmic impediments in sustained reading effort are intermittent heteropia or fatigue heteropia, in which a child tries to maintain binocularity against poor fusional reserve. This represents the type of case reported by Edward Dunlap in New York in which corrective extraocular muscle surgery helps these children to achieve a longer visual or attention span for any task. Significant amounts of uncorrected astigmatism also lead to visual fatigue and impaired school performance.

Alexia

Alexia occurs in older children or adults who because of temporoparietal lobe tumor, trauma, or vascular accident lose their ability to read. The term "acquired dyslexia" is a less accurate term which should be avoided.

Mixed Disabilities

This is probably the largest group of all. Just as tuberculosis and pneumonia may complicate one another, so may reading disabilities overlap. An excellent example of this is in the relationship between primary dyslexia and emotional disorders.

FINDINGS IN DYSLEXIA

The examiner should make an effort to be sure that the child has a reading disability by asking what grade the child is in, looking at his handwriting, and inquiring about reading, spelling, and arithmetic achievements. A record should be kept of the child's reading ability according to a graded reading test or a series of graded reading paragraphs of the examiner's choice (e.g., Durrell, Gray oral reading test).

Primary dyslexia is thought to be congenital, and with careful history usually other members of the family can be found to exhibit symptoms of dyslexia. Hallgren (1950) felt that the mode of inheritance is monohybrid autosomal dominant. It is likely, however, that there is more than one mode of inheritance, since no one mode fits all observations. For example, familiar to all workers are the cases of dyslexic boys with fathers who report their own problems with learning to read which do not fit the mother-to-son inheritance pattern of an X-linked gene; however, the four to one preponderance of boys to girls does not really fit an autosomal dominant genetic pattern.

Many dyslexics are alleged to transpose letters, so that the word "saw" may be interpreted as "was," "on" as "no," or "dog" as "god." Mirror writing is similarly seen. All children with such apparent performance, however, are not dyslexic nor do all dyslexic children show these signs. This probably relates to a child's inconsistency or pattern of laterality in attack for both reading and writing. Mirror-image English letters and words compound any inherently poor pattern of approach from left to right.

The dyslexic child frequently has poor visual memory for language symbols. By repetitive drill, he may learn that C-A-T spells cat only to fail to recognize the word when it is presented again on the following day. For a child with this defect, the "look and tell" or "flash and tell" system of teaching reading by displaying whole words on flash cards for instant identification may be a disaster. Phonetic augmentation of sound to sight may be of conspicuous value to such learners.

Constructional apraxia or the inability to form geometric parts into a whole is concurrent with temporoparietal lobe dysfunctions. This is frequently seen in developmental dyslexia and indeed may be its substrate. It should always be tested for as part of the routine examination. Some simple paper and pencil tests such as asking the child to draw three or four figures, commonly a bicycle, person, clock, and arrows, may be sufficient. More quantitative evaluation of the drawings may be obtained by scoring as in the Meeting House Street School screening test developed by Eric Denhoff of Providence,

Rhode Island. This is available in two forms: one for lay administered screening and one for more complex diagnostic data. Completion ability may be impaired in dyslexic children and the Bender-Gestalt test is an excellent method to elicit this characteristic.

Spelling errors are so frequent and illogical in primary dyslexia as to be pathognomonic, except for the fact that all poor spellers are not dyslexic. The spelling errors in dyslexia may be bizarre, even unrelated to the sound of a dictated word. These persist into adult life, even when reading ability of a fairly useful degree is acquired.

There is frequently defective ability in determining laterality and in orienting a figure in space. These children may be tested by asking them to point out right and left on a doll held in the physician's hands, facing the patient. The test may be made more difficult by turning the doll's back to the patient or, to produce a very high degree of difficulty, by turning the doll upside down.

Hyperactivity or hyperkinesis may complicate dyslexia. These children present a very short attention span which may be only seconds or perhaps a few minutes. If the reading period is 20 minutes and the attention span is 2 minutes, the result in a classroom may be overwhelming futility. Such children are easily distracted and disinhibited, so that they respond by motor activity to every stimulus. If hyperactivity is a problem accompanying dyslexia, the child should be referred to a pediatrician or a neurologist for evaluation and treatment, which might include the institution of therapy with appropriate medications such as dextroamphetamines or Ritalin.

SPECIAL TESTS IN DYSLEXIA

When a complaint of reading disability is elicited, several special tests should be part of the examination. These include recognition of letters, words, and phrases and a quantitation of reading with graded paragraphs. As few tests as possible should be used with children who are often already failure oriented. For example, a child who knows letters and can read a paragraph need not be burdened with test recognition of isolated words. The ophthalmologist should become familiar with a few standardized tests, so that they can be administered with ease in a friendly, encouraging manner. The tests should parallel the practical reading task as closely as possible.

Tests for dominance should be performed and recorded, in part because this is expected by parents. It is well known, however, that although a higher percentage of dyslexic children present ambilaterality or incomplete dominance, many children with these conditions are not dyslexic at all. Many dyslexic children have neither ambilaterality nor "mixed dominance."

Tests of ocular dominance include those that compare functional ability of the two eyes such as visual acuity, retinal rivalry, physiologic diplopia, and the brilliance of afterimages. Muscle balance may be an indicator of the dominant eye, in that the eye maintaining fixation as the other breaks from fusion is usually the dominant eye. An easy office test is preferential sighting, in which the child is given a paper which has a small hole, such as a pinhole, in it. He is asked to look at an object across the room through the peephole as he brings the paper in close to his face. In so doing, he will position the peep hole over the dominant or sighting eye.

Functional lateralization increases with age and is thus partly a matter of maturation. It is possible that ambilaterality in a youngster of age 14 or older bespeaks a degree of central nervous system immaturity, and that perhaps this immaturity is a corollary of the reading problem.

One or two simple pencil and paper tests again are useful for testing for lateralization ability. Drawing an arrow is a rough indicator of lateralization ability. The Bakwin Draw-A-Figure test is helpful in making a rough determination of mental age and may at the same time illustrate constructional apraxia, if that be present. Simply drawing the face of a clock may indicate problems in relating geometric figures when the child is unable to draw a reasonable circle for his age or crowds the numerals on the clock to one side or distributes them in grossly irregular fashion.

Neurologic signs elicited by history, observation, or simple examination suggest the need for referral to the neurologist for a more complete neurologic workup and EEG as indicated. Seizures, disturbances of gait, and supranuclear disturbances of the extraocular muscles are examples of conditions that indicate the need for referral.

In these tests the child should be observed carefully. "Clumsiness" is a most difficult diagnosis but crudeness in handling the pencil may be significant. Hesitancy in attacking the task may indicate such inability that the child can not proceed or wishes to avoid an embarrassing display of his difficulty. The examiner should be acutely aware of the impossibility of properly evaluating a child who has become fatigued. Efforts at evaluation or testing should be postponed to a subsequent visit if it becomes apparent that the child is tired.

Dyslexia occurs in all degrees from mild to severe with a wide range of accompanying symptoms and signs. Furthermore, specific developmental dyslexia should not be regarded as a single disease entity. Just as the type of glaucoma should be specified, so should the type of dyslexia be specified. Several investigators are establishing helpful differentials in this direction.

Elena Boder, a pediatric neurologist, has devised a diagnostic screening procedure based on three characteristic patterns of reading and spelling. For this screening she uses a word recognition inventory supplied by the local school district or the Schiffman list of spelling words. This method seeks not only for the child's errors but for his assets. Dr. Boder divides specific dyslexics into three groups: dysphonetic, dyseidetic, and mixed.

The first group is the dysphonetic, in which the primary deficit is in the letter-sound integration. These children perceive nonphonetically, grasping words as whole configurations. They make semantic substitutions for words, such as "quack-quack" for duck. Infantile articulation or baby talk is often seen in dysphonetic dyslexics at inappropriately advanced ages. Dr. Boder's second group is the dyseidetic, whose reading and spelling are more phonetic. These children are unable to perceive or visualize words as whole configurations, and for them the "look and tell" reading method is impossible. Their misspellings, however, are intelligible, in that by reading them phonetically, the examiner can tell what the child was trying to spell. She feels the youngsters respond well to phonetic and oral instruction. The third group in Dr. Boder's system is the mixed condition, in which characteristics of both the dysphonetic and dyseidetic groups are found. When this is severe, the prognosis is very poor.

THERAPY

Dyslexia is in very much the same state of art as was polio in 1952. Then, as now, when the cause is unknown, treatment was directed toward relief of symptoms rather than toward underlying cause. There are no specifics or curatives to offer, no surgical or medical therapy or even machine-gadgets for these children. As always, the enthusiast, the do-gooder, and all degrees in between enter this therapeutic void with hopeful suggestions. For example, despite the joint statement of the Academies of Pediatrics and Neurology that there is neither theoretical background nor control evidence to support the value of so-called patterning as a therapeutic measure, this technique is still being applied by some enthusiasts.

Carl Rosen reported in 1966 that in normal children time spent in so-called perceptual training is less productive than an equal amount of time spent in reading instruction. In subsequent studies, there have been similar results with children of low reading ability. There are no "smart pills." Help may be offered to the hyperkinetic child through use of one of the behavior-modifying drugs to help him adjust so that he can be receptive to teaching, but no medicine will improve either visual memory or the ability to interpret letters and words.

Highly individualized and personalized special teaching is still the best approach for helping a dyslexic child. Sensory augmentation through visual association and auditory, tactile, and kinesthetic routes

in daily repetitive drill is useful. A teacher trained in remedial reading techniques, fond of her pupils, optimistic, and possessed of the professional's patience is an ideal person to work with these youngsters. All such drills seek visual enhancement or "cross modality transfer."

PROGNOSIS

Prognosis is an important responsibility of the examining physician. The exclusion of specifically treatable disease and use of remedial reading or tutoring at high hourly fees are major decisions that should be made with fullest medical knowledge. Factors affecting the prognosis in dyslexia include its severity, the age at which the diagnosis is made, the performance IQ (which in dyslexic children is always higher than the written IQ), and personality factors, such as motivation, willingness to work, persistence, and self-acceptance. Family attitude and relationships are important in support of the child's own efforts. The availability of remedial reading training is essential.

The severity of the dyslexia may be judged according to such factors as the grades in school versus the age of the child or the presence or absence of specific neurologic findings, such as parietal lobe signs. Following Dr. Broder's groupings, a mixed type of dyslexia is much more severe than either the dysphonetic or the dyseidetic type.

For the secondary reading disabilities the prognosis is dependent upon the underlying cause. The child who is slow in maturing has a very good prognosis, because if there is no neurologic defect, the reading potential should approximate the intelligence potential in time. Problems of ocular motility producing constant or intermittent blurring or double vision while reading can be treated by appropriate ophthalmic or orthoptic techniques.

If a poor or guarded prognosis must be given, care should be taken to shelter the child's self-esteem. A poor prognosis should never be bluntly stated or even hinted at before the physician is absolutely sure of its correctness, and then his wording should be gentle, with an effort to point out positive aspects as well as routes of adjustment.

REFERENCES

Bateman, B.: Mild visual defect and learning problems in partially seeing children. Sight-Saving Rev., *33*:30, No. 1, Spring, 1963.

Bender, L.: Use of the Visual-Motor Gestalt Test in the diagnosis of learning disabilities. J. Spec. Ed., *4*:29, 1970.

Bettman, J. W., Stern, E. L., Whitsell, L. J., and Gofman, H. F.: Cerebral dominance in developmental dyslexia. Arch. Ophthal., *78*:722, December, 1967.

Birch, H. G., and Belmont, L.: Auditory-visual integration in normal and retarded readers. Amer. J. Orthopsychiat., *34*:852, 1964.

Boder, E.: Developmental dyslexia: a diagnostic screening procedure based on three characteristic patterns of reading and spelling. Claremont Reading Conference, 32nd Yearbook, 1968, p. 173.

Cogan, D.: Neurology of the Visual System. Springfield, Ill., Charles C Thomas, 1966, pp. 272, 312f.

Critchley, M.: The Dyslexic Child. Springfield, Ill., Charles C Thomas, 1970.

Denhoff, E., et al.: Measurement of psychoneurological factors contributing to learning efficiency. J. Learning Disabilities, *11*:8, November, 1968.

de Hirsch, K.: Clinical spectrum of reading disabilities: diagnosis and treatment. Bull. N.Y. Acad. Med., Series II, *44*:470, No. 4, April, 1968.

Flower, R. M., Gofman, H. F., and Lawson, L. I. (Eds.): Reading Disorders. Philadelphia, F. A. Davis Co., 1965.

Hallgren, B.: Specific dyslexia: a clinical and genetic study. Acta Psychiat. Neurol. Scand., Supplement 65.

Harstein, J.: Current Concepts in Dyslexia. St. Louis, The C. V. Mosby Co., 1971.

Hinshelwood, J.: Congenital word blindness. Lancet, *1*:1506, May 26, 1900.

Keeney, Arthur H.: Medical diagnostics and counseling in dyslexia. Med. Clin. N. Amer., Vol. 53, No. 5, September, 1969.

Keeney, A. H., and Keeney, V. T.: Dyslexia; Diagnosis and Treatment of Reading Disorders. St. Louis, The C. V. Mosby Co., 1968.

Kenstenbaum, A.: Clinical Methods of Neuro-Ophthalmologic Examination. 2nd ed. New York, Grune & Stratton, 1961.

Money, J. (Ed.): Reading disability: progress and research needs in dyslexia. Baltimore, Johns Hopkins Press, 1962.

Nichtern, S.: Reading disability and the child psychiatrist. Bull. N.Y. Acad. Med., Series II. *44*:488, No. 4, April, 1968.

Pearse, B. H.: Dyslexia. Amer. Ed., April, 1969, p. 10.

Reading Disorders in the United States: Report of the Secretary's (HEW) National Advisory Committee on Dyslexia and Related Reading Disorders, August, 1969.

Rice, D.: learning disabilities: an investigation. J. Learn Dis., *3*:149, 193, 1970.

Robbins, M. P.: Test of the Doman-Delacato rationale with retarded readers. J.A.M.A., *202*:389, October 30, 1967.

Rosen, C. L.: An experimental study of visual perceptual training and reading achievement in first grade. Percept. Motor Skills, *22*:979, 1966.

The Eye and Learning Disabilities. Joint organizational statement of the American Academy of Pediatrics, the American Academy of Ophthalmology and Otolaryngology, and the American Association of Ophthalmology, June, 1971.

CHAPTER 25

EMOTIONAL COMPONENTS IN PEDIATRIC OPHTHALMOLOGY

ROGER D. FREEMAN, M.D.

INTRODUCTION

If I were an ophthalmologist, I might wonder about the relevance of this chapter. Keeping up with one's specialty may seem a major effort without worrying about seemingly unscientific concerns of psychiatrists about the emotional trauma of surgery and the symbolism of visual functions. In addition, the psychiatrist and ophthalmologist do not often come into contact with each other, and have quite different ways of functioning and sources of satisfaction. Nevertheless, child psychiatry has an ever-increasing area of joint concern with ophthalmology, upon which this chapter will focus.

In the last decade there has been a very significant increase in research on the peculiar aspects of development of the blind child. The survival of more children with multiple handicaps (such as in the rubella syndrome) involving slow physical and emotional development means that members of both specialties will be seeing these children. The confusing field of reading problems is one in which a number of specialties and nonmedical professions have been jockeying for a slice of the pie, including ophthalmology, optometry, and psychiatry. As residential and day schools for blind children become less insulated from the rest of the professional community, more help is being sought from child psychiatrists and others regarding behavioral and adjustment problems. The efficiency with which a child utilizes residual vision has also been an area of combined interest. Lastly, the sensitive ophthalmologist (and who would admit to being insensitive?) will be interested in some of the difficulties involved in imparting the diagnosis of blindness, in the sometimes seemingly paradoxical reactions to enucleation of a sightless eye, and the long-term adjustment of patients who have chronic disabilities or repeated surgical procedures.

SCOPE OF THIS CHAPTER

I shall attempt to impart information on two levels: first, a critical and concise summary of research, and second, a practical discussion of the implications of both fact and clinical experience. It will be helpful to begin by looking at some of the different ways in which ophthalmologists and child psychiatrists work, so that one might better understand why there has been so little dialogue between these two groups. A very basic description of the child's ways of thinking and acting will be provided, as well as some more detailed discussion of aspects of development which are especially relevant to the ophthalmologist. Other sections will deal with the general problems of office practice, hospitalization, a variety of special eye problems, and the chapter will conclude with a section on the visually impaired child.

ON MUTUAL ACCUSATIONS

I have previously mentioned some areas of mutual interest. But when one is involved in a team approach to a child, it is impossible to avoid hearing certain criticisms of one field by the other. To the psychiatrist, the surgical specialist seems to be too intently focused upon the mechanical aspects of one area of body functioning, rather than on the total person. There have even been statements regarding the types of personalities of those who choose different medical specialties, from which it might be concluded that most surgeons are in their field because of their need to find socially acceptable outlets for their sadistic impulses. Furthermore, surgeons frequently obtain dramatic results (which we seldom do), see their patients for a relatively brief period of time, and don't really seem to be interested in other aspects of their patients' lives. Thus, although admiring the ophthalmologist's surgical and medical skills, many psychiatrists might view him as a medical technician with tunnel vision when it comes to the human aspects of patient care.

What of the psychiatrist as seen by the ophthalmologist? He seems to do mysterious and probably ineffective things with his patients, and may perhaps upset them more than help them. The psychiatrist frequently makes recommendations which cannot be carried out, which are offered in language which is not easily understood, or which have a "do-gooder" or utopian tone to them. Furthermore, his services cost a great deal of money, he tends to be unavailable, he frequently does not report back to the referring physician, and his treatments seem to take forever. In these ways, he may not seem to be a physician at all! Much of what he describes is unobservable, certainly so when compared with the ocular apparatus.

While most nonpsychiatrist physicians are happy to be rid of the uncomfortable task of dealing with a suicidal or psychotic patient, many will claim that they do not see any of the complications from their medical and surgical efforts which the psychiatrists are so concerned about. The latter would retort that the surgeon usually doesn't ask, and that his contacts with the patient or parent are so structured by virtue of the time allowed and the questions asked that if there were problems they would be unlikely to be brought up.

The psychiatrist, of course, usually has the opportunity to spend long periods of time with his patient and has been trained to listen attentively to him. He may, in fact, specifically educate the patient as to the time-consuming and slow process which therapy entails, so that the psychiatrist usually does not expect rapid response to his ministrations, and his training is supposed to help him deal with the reluctance and resistance which the patient and his family may demonstrate.

In trying to assess these very different ways of functioning of the psychiatrist and ophthalmologist, one can only conclude that the criticisms of each by the other are at least partially valid, although frequently exaggerated. Some suggestions will be made later which may assist the ophthalmologist in working more effectively with his psychiatric colleagues.

CHILD DEVELOPMENT

General Aspects

Ordinarily the child does not come to the physician of his own free will, and one has to deal not only with this kind of resistance but with the complicating factors of dependence upon the parents and their anxious concern (Freud, 1965). Although it might seem presumptuous to instruct another professional about what children are like, there are certain aspects to the ways children think and react which are not sufficiently appreciated.

Dependency

Much has been written about the helplessness of the human infant and the prolonged period of dependency prior to achieving self-sufficiency. Many believe that the human has the advantage of greater flexibility conferred by the absence of stereotyped instinctive mechanisms, yet it is likely that the many years of dependency also allow for greater vulnerability to noxious influences. Recent studies (discussed by Bowlby, 1969) have begun to show that there are built-in mechanisms of behavioral response within both the infant and mother which operate upon each other in a kind of feedback loop, and which have species' survival value.

For human beings, the image of the mother traditionally connotes comfort in time of stress, even in adult life. Speaking more strictly, a permanent inner image of the mother (not subject to disruption by anxiety, anger, or separation) probably does not develop until about age 3. Prior to this time, the normal child begins to initiate gradual separation from the mother through his drive for exploration and satisfaction of curiosity, once sufficient mobility is achieved. Meanwhile, the normal mother takes a certain amount of pride in these beginning steps and rewards rather than discourages them. The development of a separate entity, psychologically, thus takes many years to accomplish, and there may be many temporary setbacks. Unlike physical development, which may not be uniform but does not regress, emotional development is characterized by just such regressions, plateau-like periods, and progressions. Thus, it is reasonable to expect the child to act in a mature, logical fashion at one time and in a rather infantile, difficult manner at another.

The child is usually not proud of his regression to a former level of functioning. Because all of us find it difficult to complete our task in the presence of a crying, anxious child, it is only natural that we exhort him to be more grown up than he can be under the frightening circumstances, and that we may become exasperated and condemnatory of his childish, regressive behavior. Vision provides much security to the sighted child, and its interruption caused by various examination procedures is perhaps even more likely to induce anxiety on the part of the child than something done to another part of the body.

Constructive dependency of the child upon the physician (particularly where the relationship is a prolonged one and involves hospitalization) is probably fostered by truthfulness. Some doctors falsely assure a child that a procedure will not hurt at all rather than acknowledge that it may be frightening and unpleasant.

Thinking

Many studies have been done to elucidate the successive stages in the development of children's thinking. Obviously children are not simply smaller editions of the adult who happen to have less experience and knowledge. Their thought processes differ in a number of *qualitative* ways, and this fact probably accounts for much of the misunderstanding which occurs in the management of children. Logical thinking, as we adults know and practice it, does not develop fully until 9 to 11 years of age. The normal child does not think in a cause-and-effect manner. He has difficulty classifying, generalizing, and discriminating. Things which adults know to be impossible or fanciful are quite possible to the child, whose thinking is more wishful and magical than it is logical.

The young child tends to think that the world centers around himself. We refer to this phenomenon as "egocentrism." Thus, he expects that everyone knows certain things about his feelings, family, and friends which, in fact, they cannot know. He sincerely feels that everyone should cater to him and understand him, yet he shows very limited ability to understand the needs of others. From this standpoint it is quite normal for a child to state that the moon, sun, and stars follow him when he is traveling, rather than recognizing the true relationship.

The child's sense of time is also markedly limited. To be subjected to pain or separation from his parents may be just as intolerable for a few moments as it would be for an adult to have a much more enduring fright.

The concept of an *accidental event* for which no one is "responsible" is difficult for the young child to grasp. For example, the death of a parent may lead to a feeling that he has been abandoned deliberately, or that he did something bad to deserve such treatment. We could then say that the child's thinking is moralistic in situations where no good or bad aspect is involved. (The observant reader will recognize that adults under stress may show precisely the same type of thinking, despite adequate intellectual capacity.)

Because childish thinking is less logical, the rational explanations which are made may have relatively little effect in mitigating anxiety. Most adults who are informed of the facts can persist in cooperating with treatment, in spite of anxiety or discomfort. Thus, they have a relatively strong intellectual process in contrast with their tendency to respond to feelings. The child, however, is just the reverse. He may well know that you are not a monster out to mutilate him, but in the face of the frightening situation his rational processes are relatively ineffective in coping with his emotions. Very often in medical situations the impatience of the professional with the child's fear is partly based upon the mistaken notion that the child should act upon the *intellectual* reassurance given by the doctor.

One of the problems the psychiatrist has in communicating with nonpsychiatric specialists centers around this area just mentioned. We make pleas for psychological preparation of the child for a procedure or for surgery. If this recommendation is carried out, the child usually becomes upset anyway, and the physician's job does not appear to be made much easier. Then it may be said that the psychiatrist had not been helpful and that his recommendations were useless or based upon false premises. In actuality, there is good reason to believe that psychological preparation

makes sense and is useful to a child, but it cannot be expected to significantly alter the behavior *at the time*, so that he becomes tractable. The beneficial effects will be on a longer-term basis.

Along with this relative weakness of rational thinking, it may be seen that the child's sense of security and orientation is more easily disrupted than is the case with an adult. Patching of the eyes, or any other situation which results in a loss of the integrating sense of vision and the testing of reality is quite likely to lead to considerable anxiety. One can sometimes minimize this in hospitalized children by permitting the parents to visit frequently or by arranging to have one of them remain with the child.

Childish vs. "Grown Up" Behavior

It is frequently difficult to strike a balance between the encouragement of reasonable behavior on the one hand and the humiliation of a child for his infantile behavior on the other. The latter is common practice for many doctors and nurses (and parents!) and may result in suppression of emotional reactions by the child. The cost to the child may be some diminution of self-esteem and an impairment of trust and confidence in the child-physician relationship.

Since upset feelings cannot be eliminated in most cases, there is no point in engaging in interminable efforts to reason with the child. If a procedure is necessary, the fear may be accepted, reasonable explanations given, and the work commenced. Afterwards, some reassurance that the child's behavior was not something to be ashamed of may be useful.

Play and Mastery

The child uses play to work out his conflicts and anxieties, to master difficult experiences, to help him identify with different family and occupational roles, and to practice various recently acquired skills.

How does play help the child master painful experiences, such as medical procedures and hospitalizations? Most of us are aware of the following type of situation: a young child goes to the doctor, is examined, and receives an injection. When he returns home he is observed to utilize the syringe (often given to the child by the doctor) to "give a needle" to a sibling, pet, or doll. This common example illustrates (1) repetition of the act, minimizing or eliminating the surprise element; and (2) turning what was passively experienced, and over which the child had no control, into an active experience. The child is now in control; he is the doer. The reader will recognize that the same kind of process takes place in fantasy and daydreams in children and adults: we think over how we could have done things better, come out with the "perfect squelch" when embarrassed, decide how we will do things the next time, or may prepare ourselves for a variety of alternative solutions. These are all potentially healthy and necessary uses of play and fantasy to master anxiety-provoking experiences, either before or after their occurrence, or both.

The practical significance of this process is that the physician can help prevent the miscarriage of mastery attempts by: (1) acknowledging that the child has a right to feel something about the procedure; (2) reducing the "surprise" or overwhelming element by reasonable preparation and telling the truth (to the point necessary); (3) learning of previous situations in which the child has had major upsets and knowing how he tends to react; (4) allowing sufficient physical activity and parent involvement to minimize the feeling of being both attacked and abandoned; and (5) telling parents that certain reactions to procedures (and especially hospitalization) are to be expected.

It is important to remember that the point at which a procedure becomes potentially emotionally harmful for a child cannot be generalized; it will depend upon the age of the child, his stage of development, his family relationships, his past experiences and means of coping with them, and his temperament and preparation.

Danger signs may be rigidly repetitive play over a prolonged period of time (excluding other topics) and a persistently high level of anxiety. This may be accompanied by fearful questioning of the parents about future procedures, failure to be reassured by explanations or answers, sleep disturbance, and regression in one or more areas.

Special Aspects of Child Development Relevant to Ophthalmology

Mother-Infant Attachment Behavior

Numerous scientific investigations have demonstrated the species' survival value of mother-infant behavioral feedback mechanisms. The absence of some of these in the handicapped or blind child may threaten the mutual attachment which is necessary for adequate development.

Spontaneous smiling is present in both blind and sighted infants by about 1 week of age. In the next three months this becomes differentiated so that the child will respond to the configuration of a human face (Bowlby, 1969). The smiling infant evokes a response which is almost essential for the care of the child. Mothers are often observed to peer anxiously into the infant's eyes, to attempt to stimulate a smile, and to be anxious if they cannot. Other aspects of this interaction which will not be considered in detail here involve the infant's discrimination of his mother's voice and different patterns of handling premature and full-term infants by their mothers.

Psychological Significance of the Eyes

It may seem superfluous to point out the importance of vision to those committed to its preservation and improvement. Nevertheless, a brief review may suffice to indicate the factors which may be involved in attitudes and fears about visual or ocular disease.

The sighted individual attaches profound value to the eyes and to the active and passive acts of looking or being looked at. Heaton (1968) mentioned the historical importance of vision and blindness in myths and symbols. Gods, monsters, and extraterrestrial beings are often endowed with only one eye or, conversely, with more than two. The sacrifice of an eye to atone for sin and punishment by blinding are fairly well known. The "evil eye" of witches or others was thought (and still is by some) to be capable of causing (among other things) defects in animals, in unborn babies, and in crops. The power of a glance or stare also finds examples in the legend of Medusa and in the "double whammy" portrayed in "Li'l Abner." Children are told that it is "not nice to stare." The back of the U. S. one-dollar bill has a magical protective eye on it; we say "if looks could kill . . .," emphasizing the aggressive component of looking, and we may be concerned about "peeping Toms" and pornography. Children play many games involving seeing, from the earliest "peek-a-boo" with mother to "hide and seek" and "blind man's buff." Many children (and adults) avert their eyes when guilty, embarrassed, or depressed. And finally, to many people blindness is considered to be the worst affliction, equivalent to death, as if vision were synonymous with life, love, and understanding.

Reactions to Anesthesia

Specific aspects of anesthesia are considered later. In general, the reaction of the child will partly depend upon his stage of development, his view of what is going on, and his life circumstances at the time. Very young children are primarily concerned with separation from the parents and the need to be active rather than restrained; this is probably one source of their difficulty in going to sleep at night. Children who have been in conflict with their parents over sleep are more likely to react adversely to the experience of anesthesia.

As the child develops some independence and is no longer so concerned with security, he becomes more aware of the world around him and of his body. Many workers in this field believe that in the late preschool and early school years, the child is more likely to worry about what will happen to his bodily integrity than about separation.

Even with the best preparation, induction, or explanation, some children *will* be emotionally traumatized (overwhelmed by anxiety which they cannot master) by the anesthetic experience. The interested ophthalmologist can only do his best to defer elective surgery in a few cases, to get help from others when it is indicated, and to assure himself that the child and family have the opportunity to work out these problems thereafter, should they occur and persist. In this, as in all

other areas, the time-honored maxim "primum non nocere" seems most apt.

Sensory Deprivation

A child deprived of his vision may become anxious and uncooperative (Ziskind et al., 1960). His hold on reality is not firm at best, and in the setting of a hospital with strange noises, smells, unpleasant external and internal sensations, and separation from everything and everyone who usually provides security, it should not be astonishing that he may become quite disturbed. This may lead to physical restraint and a compounding of the anxiety. These subjects will be discussed in more detail later, but it is appropriate here to note that these reactions may be anticipated and minimized by planning and preparation, as well as the judicious use of medication.

Despite all efforts, the child who temporarily cannot see may become panicky and believe that he will be permanently blind. Parents of children who had operations for strabismus often used to report, in the days when eye-patching was routine, that their children became extremely agitated. Ziskind and coworkers (1960) described an 8-year-old boy who developed hallucinations and delusions, trembling, and grinding of his teeth after his eyes were patched; these symptoms disappeared abruptly when his better eye was unbandaged; when he closed his eyes a few minutes later, he suffered an immediate but temporary resumption of these symptoms. There was a previous history of sleep disorder in this case.

Linn and coworkers (1953) experimented with preoperative eye-patching of adult cataract patients and found disturbance in 10 of 21; after the operation, 20 showed some pathological behavior, severe in 13 cases. Organic brain disease predisposed to an adverse reaction, and this might well be true of children with special vulnerabilities. Many authorities advise producing situations of sensory isolation only when absolutely necessary (Hospital for Sick Children, 1967; Shipsey et al., 1966).

PROBLEMS OF OFFICE PRACTICE

Whether it is better to separate the child from its parents will depend upon age and the effect the parent has upon the child. In many instances, having the parent present is a reassurance to the child and makes the examination easier. In others, however, it is obvious that parental anxiety is communicated to the child, or that as long as the parent is present, the child will not settle down. The younger the child, the more important it is for the parent to be there.

The question of restraint is not an easy one. Some attention to preparation, the office setting, and approach to the child may obviate the need; once it is done, it is likely to be needed on subsequent occasions. For example, the Hospital for Sick Children (1967) recommends toys in the waiting room, the absence of frightening instruments in the consulting room, and the limitation of children's visits to certain days, so that they can see other children playing, and not have to be squelched because they might upset the adults. A frightened child who is not yet used to the room may be mollified a bit if the parents are talked to first, while he is ignored and permitted to familiarize himself with the setting. Fear is likely to be increased if the room is completely darkened.

The discomfort or fear caused by certain procedures will make it impossible to avoid restraint in some cases. The basic question is whether the ophthalmologist considers it worthwhile to avoid *unnecessary* restraint and force by taking the time to put the child at ease.

As long ago as 1947, Doggart was concerned about these matters. He advised against frightening infants "with dazzling lights and unfamiliar pieces of apparatus" (Doggart, p. 1). He felt that much could be learned from watching the child, playing with him, or from the history rather than a formal examination, and suggested the avoidance of abruptness. Regarding the children's reactions, he said "No one can work happily with children, nor afford comfort to their parents, unless he can learn to look upon childish vagaries with affectionate forbearance" (Doggart, p. 7).

It may be helpful to inquire when and what the child was told about coming, because one may be able to modify punitive parental preparation, or suggest that the child not be lied to. There are quite practical reasons for this, other than the unproven assertion that truthfulness in preparation is "healthier": it will probably make future contacts with the same or other physicians easier. If a major procedure is necessary, the previously established trust will almost certainly stand the doctor in good stead. Many parents bribe children or tell them that they are going somewhere other than to see the physician. The doctor should be tactful in dealing with parents who handle their children in this manner, which is understandable as a means of avoiding unpleasantness, but he should not reinforce this approach.

Preparation of the child by the parent presupposes some knowledge of what will happen. The physician or his nurse should inform the parent of what is anticipated (length of stay, eye-patching, pain, peculiar appearance of the eye, swelling, need for drops, and so forth).

Many doctors do not ask the parents, at the end of a consultation, whether they have any questions or matters they wish to discuss, perhaps assuming that if they do, they will ask. Many people are aware of how busy doctors are, and may be afraid to prolong the interview if they do not know how significant their concern is. An invitation to discussion may help.

HOSPITALIZATION

Preparation and Timing

This subject has been discussed in detail by MacKeith (1953). Shipsey and co-workers (1966) stated that the greatest impact of hospitalization is probably between 4 to 6 years of age, when concern about punishment and mutilation is usually greatest, and again in adolescence, when concern about attractiveness and being different is heightened. It must be admitted, however, that conclusive generalizations based upon research evidence are not yet available.

Vaughan (1957) studied 40 children admitted to the hospital for an eye operation and then followed up for 6 months. Most of them were reported to be confused and frightened upon admission. Many had been told either nothing, very little, or direct lies about what was to happen. These children were given a simple explanation and reassurance. A significant number of those over 4½ years of age were said to benefit from explanations, an opportunity to express their feelings, and the realization that they would be well looked after while in the hospital. It was also pointed out in Vaughan's study that this kind of explanation could be given by the parents, or others, and not necessarily by the physician, whose time is so valuable. However, no control group was employed.

A survey by Kangery (1960) of 50 children hospitalized for at least five days, between the ages of 6 and 10, showed the following: 10 per cent did not know they were to be hospitalized; 30 per cent did not know blood work was to be done; 58 per cent were unaware of the reasons for the latter; 44 per cent did not know they would have to use a bedpan, and some were not told *how* to use it; 38 per cent of children who had x-ray studies did not know that this was a painless procedure. The author recommended simple explanations, perhaps prepared in booklet form, and staff training for child preparation.

Sometimes the question is raised about the optimal length of time intervening between telling the child and the procedure itself. This is of significance because some children "incubate" their anxiety if they have too long to think about it. Frequently parents can give clues about this. The very young child will probably do better with a short period of time; his primary need is to feel protected and trusting. The older child can often use a few days to mentally work over his fantasies and ask questions about areas of concern.

Anesthesia and Continued Awareness

The Hospital for Sick Children (1967) recommends that intravenous induction be used because it is rapid and less upsetting to children than other methods. We have seen children for whom the slow loss of control and feeling of choking associated with inhalation anesthesia seemed to have been traumatic. They became phobic of strange smells and suffered from insomnia.

Williams and Jones (1968) performed a study on six young adult patients and concluded that noxious stimuli did reach the central nervous system of their patients who were under general anesthesia. Preoperative anxiety was said to significantly affect physiological status, and they suspected that high anxiety level "may be more disruptive physiologically than is often recognized" (p. 417).

A recent report (LaScola and Cheek, 1968) suggested that patients may continue to hear while under anesthesia, and that what they hear may be influential later. Some research was done which tends to support this old idea, and the recommendation was made that operating room personnel be cautious about the use of words which may be misinterpreted, especially when using a light plane of anesthesia.

In a way, this caution is an extension of the concept that children (but also adults) may tend to distort or select what they hear, and inappropriately make connections with their other ideas, feelings, and attitudes towards their physical condition. Such distortions are more likely to occur when conscious awareness is partly obtunded, such as before, possibly during, and after anesthesia. The practical importance of this concept is difficult to demonstrate, however, and further evidence is required.

Restraints and Eye-Patching

Shipsey and coworkers (1966) stated that although restraint is obviously necessary at times, it tends to be psychologically disturbing. The child may experience it as an overwhelming attack at a time when he is totally helpless in defending himself. These authors felt that it is best to gain the child's voluntary cooperation, if possible; if not, the parents should not be asked to participate in the restraining procedure unless no alternative is available.

Whether a child generally tends to regard his parent's cooperation in restraining him as worse or more threatening than the parent's acquiescence in having others restrain him, is difficult to determine. Having the parents share in the restraint is standard procedure for many physicians.

Restraint is often practiced unnecessarily or for excessive periods of time. It is known that animals may suffer stress ulcers on a neurogenic basis from physical restraint, so the idea of potential harm is not without some suggestive support. However, the period of time necessary, and the documentation of physical and psychological effects, are not well delineated.

It was previously stated that reduction in sensory input during a time of anxiety, separation, and physiological stress may be productive of mild to severe reactions in children and adults. Mental symptoms occurring in a sample of 88 adults and children with cataracts and detached retina were studied by Ziskind and his coworkers (1960). Symptoms occurred in all the patients with detached retina (who had much longer periods of patching) and in 30 per cent of the cataract cases. Unpatching and moving about against medical advice and against the patient's own apparent wishes for recovery (termed "noncompliance") occurred in 9 of the 10 detached retina patients, and was interpreted as partly due to clouded states of consciousness occurring during, before, or after sleep, or when sleepy during the day. Frightening hallucinatory experiences were reported which could be abolished by unpatching an eye. Factors which seemed to exacerbate such symptoms were greater duration of patching, sensory defects, language problems, and anything tending to reduce coping ability (mental retardation or organic brain syndromes).

Some of the principles described by Weisman and Hackett (1958) for minimizing these reactions may be applicable to older children and adolescents: (1) developing an alliance with the patient, emphasizing areas the doctor and patient can share and which represent security and optimal functioning in the patient's life; (2) providing repeated descriptions of physical surroundings and events; (3) stimulation of other sense modalities. The perceptions of the patient must be given an understandable conceptual framework, because without vision they will tend to seem strange and actually disruptive of reality-testing.

Parent-Child Relationship

There is a plethora of publications about the effects of hospitalization upon the relationship between parent and child. A rather concise review of this field was presented by Work (1956) and a number of innovative programs which have attempted to optimize the hospital experience were described in brief vignettes in the same journal issue that included his article. He cited the resistance to changes in hospital visiting hours and parent rooming-in with young children, attributing them partly to the professional's reluctance to feel that a child might be unhappy in an area for which he has responsibility.

The young child who is separated from his mother tends to go through an identifiable series of phases: (1) *protest*, marked by crying, and lasting from hours to days; (2) a period of varying length marked by *apathy*, as if the child were in a state of *despair*; (3) following prolonged separation, a stage of apparent adjustment or *detachment* develops, which may be regarded by the staff with relief. However, the child may have given up the hope of ever seeing his parents again. Work emphasized that the period of 12 to 36 months of age might be one of maximum vulnerability, when the child has few resources to help him cope with his separation and yet still is very dependent upon his mother. It is of interest that Work singled out eye surgery as the kind of operation that might place more of a strain upon the child than others because it interferes with his maintaining contact with his environment. He also mentioned some situations in which visiting by the mother should be restricted or eliminated: (1) when she cannot cooperate with the hospital and prevents her child from resting, perhaps out of guilt; (2) when the level of the mother's anxiety is judged to play some causative role in the child's illness. A recommendation to restrict visiting should not be made in response to staff irritation, but according to an actual determination of mother-child relationships. Some hospitals, recognizing that some mothers are not able to visit often enough or that some children find the experience of hospitalization too terrifying, have experimented with group therapy to enable the children to act out their feelings.

Vernon and his coworkers (1966) studied 387 children's reactions to hospitalization one week after discharge. They concluded that the combination of illness and hospitalization was generally psychologically upsetting, resulting in increased separation anxiety, sleep disorder, and aggression toward authority. Prior hospitalization and degree of pain involved did not seem to be correlated with severity of response.

Shipsey and his coworkers (1966) agreed that the mother remaining with the child should be encouraged under age 3, but also if possible before the age of 6. Reactions for which the parents should be prepared following hospitalization would include: (1) hyperactivity; (2) regression; and (3) resentment. They pointed out that these reactions might not only be a retaliation by the child for an unpleasant experience, but also a way of releasing anxiety which was not possible during the hospitalization. Prolonged reactions following discharge indicate the need for specialized help.

Vernon and his coworkers completed a comprehensive review of this field and published a book in 1965. They included the possibility that hospitalization might be beneficial to the development of some children.

A study in 1970 by Davenport and Werry has challenged these previous findings with the conclusion that post-hospitalization upset appeared to be an infrequent phenomenon. This report dealt with children admitted for only a very brief time, whose degree of discomfort was minimal. Another study published in the same year (Mattson and Weisberg, 1970) showed that even mild illnesses, treated *at home*, produced irritability and regression in young children.

Until more definitive research is available, it would seem to be wise to follow the recommended course of generally permitting maximum parental involvement with hospitalized children, to prepare children for hospitalization, and to prepare parents for the possibility of reactions after discharge. The latter point should be emphasized, since this is a relatively simple procedure and can avoid much parental misunderstanding. For example, if the parents are told that a young child may regress and temporarily lose a recently-acquired skill (such as toilet-training), or that he may become clinging and excessively dependent or aggressive and hostile for a period of time and that this is fairly normal, they are less likely to become upset and retaliate against the child. If they do not understand what is happening, the child may be subjected to emotional estrangement from his parents for reasons he does not comprehend. A persistent post-hospitalization reaction requires consultation.

Drug Therapy

Along with other modifications in management, previously described, sedation may be necessary to help the child remain calm. It is important to recognize that many children have a need to be active in order to feel in control and to avoid feelings of helplessness. Such children may react paradoxically to tranquilizing medication, since they sense that it is further impairing their efforts to stay in contact with what is going on (Freeman, 1970).

The effective use of sedation or tranquilizers may be aided by telling the verbal child what is happening, why the drug is being given, for how long it will be required, and how long the situation which makes medication necessary is expected to last. The presence of the parents, of a radio, of toys from home, or the help of an occupational therapist may reduce the amount of medication necessary, or make it more tolerable.

It is a matter of conjecture as to whether sedation or tranquilization is better than physical restraint or should be combined with it. My personal opinion is that it would be wise to consider drug use in the child who is uncooperative after other methods have been tried and if restraints are upsetting. The kinds of medication employed have been described in many places (Fish, 1968; Freeman, 1970; Kraft, 1968). Generally, major tranquilizers such as chlorpromazine and thioridazine are more helpful than minor agents (e.g., diazepam, chlordiazepoxide, hydroxyzine).

EYE PROBLEMS

Many, if not all, eye conditions have been tied to psychological factors at one time or another. The early pioneers of psychosomatic medicine were criticized later for trying to invoke specific personality types as directly related to each condition regarded as psychosomatic in origin. Thus, there was the "ulcer personality," the "hypertensive personality," and so forth. We now know that most such constructs are fallacious. Subsequent refinement of the relationships between emotion and disease considered several possible alternatives: (1) The *specificity model* considered that environmental stress evoked a specific unconscious conflict in the individual, which led to anxiety, to regression, and, through the physiological concomitants of that regression, to a specific symptom or disease. (2) The *nonspecific model* postulated that any factor experienced as stressful psychologically would lead to anxiety (common to all) and its physiological by-products; then the physical reaction would depend upon such individual or unique factors as organ susceptibility, rather than the nature of the stress or the psychological state aroused. (3) The *individual response specificity model* pictured a wide range of stressful stimuli evoking emotional reactions specific to that individual, and the symptoms or disease resulting would then be specific to that emotional state, but not to the stimulus. In other words, the arousal pattern would select specific foci of activation. In short, the "choice" of symptom or disease could be described as being based upon (1) unconscious conflict evoked by the stimulus; (2) organ susceptibility (or "somatic compliance"); and (3) specific patterns of emotional arousal, not necessarily based upon unconscious conflict but perhaps having a physiological basis.

These overly concise summations are taken from the excellent review by Kaplan and Kaplan (1967). They concluded that no one model would be likely to fully explain the diverse processes involved, and none had achieved universal acceptance.

In reviewing the literature on psychophysiological eye involvement, the reader cannot avoid some discouragement, for there is relatively little which is well established, and the methodology employed often precludes firm conclusions. For example, the most complete exposition of this field is presented by Schlaegel and Hoyt (1957) entitled *Psychosomatic Ophthalmology*. My impression is that the authors are excessively enthusiastic about emotional factors in many diseases which are not yet well understood. In the history of medicine, many concepts have from time to time been advanced as explanations for a wide variety of conditions. An old example of this was the "focus of infection;" a newer one is the concept of stress.

Shipsey and coworkers (1966) and Weiss and English (1957) pointed out the fears of pain, disfigurement, and blindness which tend to be aroused by eye disease. Someone who already has conflict around visual functions may tend to react especially unfavorably. But these are *secondary* effects, not causes of ophthalmological disorders. Thus, although it is reasonable to suppose that some neuroendocrine mechanism could influence ocular function in disturbed individuals, the mechanisms and their relative importance are poorly understood. Individual cases have been described, however, in which situations known to be stressful to that person have produced or aggravated eye conditions (Wolf and Messier, 1950; Wolff, 1953; Adams et al., 1970).

With this introduction, findings and opinions in a few disorders of ophthalmological interest will now be reviewed.

Strabismus

The idea that a squint may make a child self-conscious seems to require no documentation. Heaton (1968) mentioned that playmates notice this obvious difference and start to tease the afflicted child after the age of approximately 3 years. Talking to a person with strabismus can be discomfiting because one doesn't know which eye to look at. Persons with a squint used to be regarded as dangerous, because of possession of the "evil eye," and many stories attest to the special influences thought to emanate from them. For these and other reasons, the Hospital for Sick Children (1967) asserted that treatment of strabismus should be accomplished before the child develops bad feelings about himself.

In an uncontrolled series of observations, Gibbens (1963) described delinquent girls who became promiscuous after operations to correct squint, as if they were unable to adjust to the change from "ugly duckling" to attractive teenager; he also felt that the operations should be carried out earlier. Similar opinions about the hazards of sudden correction of deformities have been expressed (for example, in obesity). The physician who expects his patient to adjust well after surgery may be disappointed if he doesn't realize that psychological and personality adaptations which have developed over many years may not keep pace with physical changes produced by treatment. (Cardiac surgeons became acutely aware of this when demonstrable hemodynamic improvement did not parallel an increase in exercise tolerance and functional capacity.)

The use of hypnosis in cases of suppression amblyopia was described by Browning and his coworkers (1958). They employed suggestion (without hypnosis) with no success in nineteen children, ages 5 through 15, most of whom would be considered beyond the age for occlusion therapy. Posthypnotic suggestions were given to the nine children who could be successfully hypnotized, and all showed significant post-session immediate gains in near vision after a single treatment. Although there were no true controls, the authors felt that emotional factors in conjunction with ocular factors could be operative. The reported gains were gradually lost. This was attributed to the continued operation of the hypothetical psychogenic factors. I know of no replication of these findings.

The relationship of strabismus to psy-chiatric disorder was demonstrated recently in the important Isle of Wight Study (Rutter et al., 1970), though the exact mechanism was unclear.

Finally, Lipton (1970) has written an interesting paper about the psychological consequences of strabismus from the psychoanalytical point of view. If the strabismus develops, as it often does, at a time when the young child has many developmental tasks to master, then it may lead to mistrust of his own perceptions, mental confusion, and negative reactions from his environment.

In summary, it does appear that the secondary emotional effects of strabismus should be considered in planning surgical or other intervention. The causative influences of emotional factors, if any, are less clear and remain to be satisfactorily elucidated.

Tics and Blepharospasm

Tics or "habit spasms" are usually described as stereotyped, repetitive movements which cease during sleep, may appear as semi-purposive, and may be brought under some temporary voluntary control. They tend to increase in frequency and severity in states of emotional tension and fatigue, and are most common in the face and neck, less so in the lower parts of the body. They are relevant to ophthalmology because the muscles about the eyes are very frequently involved. Excessive blinking is probably most common; it can occur alone or be associated with other tics.

Newell (1969) stated that blepharoclonus (exaggerated reflex blinking) may persist as a tic (unilateral or bilateral), and that this is common in children between the ages of 5 and 10. It may be distressing to parents, and simple reassurance is indicated in most cases.

Other forms of "habit spasm" include repeated nonfunctional activation of the extraocular muscles. Children may begin with a game of rolling the eyes up, or around, or deliberately "looking cross-eyed." Raising of the eyebrows and widening of the palpebral fissures, as if in surprise, may also be seen.

There is much controversy over the

causes and treatment of tics (Yates, 1970). Some attribute them to a maladaptive conditioning process, perhaps superimposed upon an underlying predisposition; others attribute it to a tendency to express bodily tension or conflict through somatic channels. In general, treatment is not very satisfactory. Sources of tension and maladjustment should be ameliorated, if possible. The prognosis is uncertain, but fortunately many seem to improve with time.

Occasionally one sees children who are unable to open their eyes, and the examiner may encounter resistance upon trying to raise the lids. This clinical picture may be associated with conflicts over something the child has seen or wishes to see that upsets him, and management may be appropriately shared with the psychiatrist in the absence of clear ophthalmological disease.

Eyestrain and Headaches

Newell (1969) has stated that severe headaches do not arise from refractive errors, though this idea is common. Headache may be psychogenic or may mimic the headaches of parents, relatives, or others close to the child. It is always worthwhile inquiring about this. Some parents believe that the eyes can be damaged by "strain" or reading in poor light and may focus the child's bodily concern upon this aspect (Hospital for Sick Children, 1967).

Feelings of fatigue and other manifestations thought to be caused by prolonged close work with the eyes were referred to as "asthenopia" in the past (Weiss and English, 1957). The eyes may be blamed for headaches which originate elsewhere. Extraocular muscle imbalance and the presence of tension states may act synergistically to produce or aggravate headaches, probably a result of increased muscle tone in the head and neck regions. These pains are likely to be steady, not very severe, and worse toward the end of the day.

One must consider other organic causes in the differential diagnosis. In a proportion of cases the causative factors will remain unidentified. Exploration of sources of stress may be useful, but invoking psychogenesis by exclusion is hazardous.

Hysterical Amblyopia and Blindness

"Hysteria" is a term much misused in common and technical parlance. Often it simply signifies "psychogenic," or occurring in the absence of physical cause, perhaps with other indications of nervousness, and a dramatic presentation. The personality dynamics assumed by some to be characteristic of this condition will not be discussed here. Most psychiatric texts will provide the interested reader with much further information.

In 1947 Eames studied 193 unselected school children with reading disability and found tubular fields in 9 per cent. One-third of these were diagnosed as "hysteria," and all but one recovered within 12 months.

Schlaegel and Hoyt (1957) gave considerable attention to this subject. Corneal anesthesia, though considered typical of hysteria, is usually not complete. Photophobia is said to be common by both these authors and Newell (1969). Amblyopia is much more common than blindness (5.25 per cent of all patients attending an eye clinic had hysterical tubular fields, according to Schlaegel and Hoyt). There is disagreement about whether this problem is more common in children or in adults (Yasuna, 1963), but there is consensus that it is more frequent in females. Yasuna saw as many cases in children as he did of malignant tumors or intraocular foreign bodies: ". . . hysterical amblyopia is more than a medical curiosity and should be suspected in all instances of amblyopia of unknown etiology" (Yasuna, p. 559).

Tubular fields are usually bilateral; Schlaegel and Hoyt stated that they are inconstant, Yasuna that they are constant; the patients "never complain of poor side vision" (Schlaegel and Hoyt, p. 363). Other organic ophthalmological defects may coexist and cause overlooking of psychogenic cause of impairment of vision. Most authors agree that tubular fields are unique to hysteria. They are usually described as follows: (1) the fields are the same size no matter at what distance they are checked; (2) borders are sharp; (3) shape is circular, without normal temporal widening. It is said that the patient is unlikely to bump into objects, despite his visual "loss." Malingering may be difficult or impossible to differentiate; indifference to the impairment is not necessarily diagnostic of hysteria.

In hysterical blindness, the diagnosis is more difficult because the tubular fields are lacking. Criteria are (1) sudden onset, (2) normal pupillary responses, and (3) normal fundus (in absence of coexisting organic disease). These patients may progress to amblyopia.

Schlaegel and Hoyt also stated that 2 per cent of unselected eye patients had spiral fields, the radii of which contract according to the direction in which the fields are tested. Organic field defects may be difficult to rule out in these patients, whose manifestations are probably related to hysteria (though Yasuna disagrees).

Case Example 1

One of my patients, a 10-year-old girl, developed episodes of blindness with confusion when confronted by upsetting situations. She had never learned to cope with strong feelings in more appropriate ways. As she improved, she complained of episodes of bizarre contraction of the visual fields: a "curtain" moved in from the temporal sides, and reversed its direction after a few minutes. When shown certain cards on psychological testing, her response was that they were "black" and she could see nothing.

Heaton (1968) stated that some children with overanxious, success-oriented parents may develop amblyopia while studying for examinations. Spasm of the near reflex, with complaints of blurring and diplopia, may be associated symptoms (Donaldson and Walsh, 1966).

Friesen and Mann (1966) did a follow-up study of 52 patients, mostly adults. About half had stayed the same or their conditions worsened. The authors felt that the follow-up after a "cure" was often too short. Some of their cases were seen after as much as 31 years. Spasm and weakness of accommodation were described as frequent symptoms in their series.

Malingering is probably relatively uncommon in children (Yasuna). Opticokinetic tests and other ingenious situations have been used to demonstrate the persistence of vision (Grosz and Zimmerman, 1965). Descriptively, the malingerer typically overplays his part, but this cannot be depended upon. The attachment to

reality is weaker in children. Any child who confesses to malingering can be assumed to have serious difficulties which merit investigation.

In summary, there is incomplete agreement about certain aspects of hysterical amblyopia and blindness. The preponderance of opinion in the literature, with which I would concur, favors the following views: (1) a variety of ocular functional peculiarities may be present, among which tubular fields are most common; (2) school-age girls are more likely to present this picture than preschoolers or late adolescents; (3) malingering is rare and difficult to differentiate; (4) incidence is significant; (5) conflicts over impulse expression, often in a setting where appropriate channeling of feelings has not been developed, seem to be present in most cases; (6) prognosis for recovery of vision is fairly good, but symptoms may persist in some, or shift to other areas: (7) psychiatric consultation is usually indicated, though a variety of tricks or uses of suggestion may temporarily lead to abatement; (8) differential diagnosis must consider coexisting organic conditions; and (9) symptoms may be worsened by overresponse to the dramatic presentation.

Glaucoma

Congenital glaucoma can present many problems to the child and family because of its uncertain prognosis, the threat of blindness, and necessarily prolonged contact with medical procedures and treatments (Shipsey et al., 1966). This statement about the emotional *effect* of this condition may be obvious. Assertions about emotional *causes* are less certain. Weiss and English (1957) and Schlaegel and Hoyt (1957) pointed out that attacks of primary glaucoma are said to be precipitated by emotional upsets, presumably via neurohumoral control mechanisms affecting secretion of fluid. (Studies with adults had shown some correlation between glaucoma and personality difficulties, though a small controlled study by Zimet and Berger in 1960 demonstrated more pathological conditions in controls than in glaucoma patients!)

It seems that psychological factors may

aggravate glaucoma to a variable and poorly demonstrated extent. The disease itself may have profound effects which need to be kept in mind, although the recommendation of psychotherapy (as made by Schlaegel and Hoyt, 1957) cannot be supported unless there are independent indications for it.

Miscellaneous Conditions

Chronic and severe headbanging, which may be seen in psychotic, retarded, brain-damaged, or even physically normal children, may produce cataracts and should not be considered a benign habit (Spalter et al., 1970). In some cases aversive conditioning procedures may be necessary (Tate and Baroff, 1966).

Self-injury may involve the eyes or surrounding structures (pulling out of eyelashes, accident-proneness). Suspicion of self-punitive acts should be sufficient indication for further exploration of the problem and referral when appropriate. The rationale for this is that the conditions out of which such acts arise (emotional and environmental) are very likely to continue and to produce further (and possibly more severe) difficulty.

Werner (1952) investigated eye injuries in children. In slightly more than one-third of cases, the child himself caused the damage (whether or not on purpose), and in about one-third, another child was the source. When more than one accident occurs, careful investigation is warranted, just as would be proper with repeated ingestion of toxic substances. (The child who damages another's eye may also be in need of help.)

Solar retinopathy may be an indication of nothing more than misfortune, but older children who are warned of the extreme danger and still stare at an eclipse can be considered self-destructive (Gilkes, 1969).

Self-induced photogenic epilepsy (by means of hand or eye movement) is of significance to the ophthalmologist because such unusual cases may be brought to him (colored glasses may assist in control) and because psychological factors need to be recognized. A series of cases was described by our group (Harley et al., 1967). Contrary to many previous reports,

these were children of normal or close-to-normal intelligence. Follow-up of three of these cases in the past 2 years indicates that the outlook for control of the behavior leading to the seizures is good (perhaps because of maturation of the central nervous system). Two of these three boys received psychotherapy. The possibility of self-induction should be considered in all cases of light-sensitive epilepsy.

Occasionally, cases of children with a succession of different ophthalmological or related conditions over a period of years may turn out to have unrecognized psychological factors as a major contributor to the complex etiological picture (Gilkes, 1969).

DYSLEXIA AND READING RETARDATION

This subject is covered elsewhere in this book. Suffice it to say that there is tremendous confusion and faddism in this field. Differences in etiological views are quite apparent to anyone who reads several books or papers (Money, 1966; Hospital for Sick Children, 1967; Heaton, 1968; Nicholls, 1969; Helveston, 1970; Lawson, 1970). Whether or not there is anything "wrong with the eyes" in reading difficulty is open to question. The last three authors mentioned are ophthalmologists. They reviewed the evidence and felt that reading retardation is not usually within the realm of ophthalmology. Some authors have claimed that there are changes in eye movements, but others argue that these, if present, are results rather than causes.

All sorts of mental conflicts have been thought to be significant in the causation of some or most cases; the evidence is not at all clear. It does seem well demonstrated that reading disability may lead to serious emotional and behavioral consequences, and needs to be taken seriously (Rutter et al., 1970). Generalized anxiety, neurotic fear of success and aggressive activity, and other conflicts may contribute to inhibitions in learning, but whether conflicts over the sexual and/or aggressive components of the act of looking are operative in more than a minority of cases seems questionable at present.

The psychiatrist's role (as well as that

of the ophthalmologist) is to help the patient and his family deal with the component of the problem which lies within his area of competence, as well as guiding them to others for help with additional aspects of the disability. Dogmatic statements seem to be most unwise, as are wholesale applications of any management method (such as psychotherapy or optometric training programs), regardless of theoretical basis or discipline of the professional (Lawson, 1970). The one exception to this would be remedial education, which is felt by most workers to be absolutely essential, regardless of other problems, causes, or treatments.

VISUAL IMPAIRMENT AND BLINDNESS

To prevent visual impairment is the basic *raison d'être* of the ophthalmologist, yet it is in this area, in which he should feel most confident, that trouble frequently arises. There are several points of hazard, which will be separately discussed: (1) withholding or equivocating on the definite diagnosis or prognosis of blindness; (2) problems involving the provision of supportive intervention services for infants and young children; (3) management of the shock of sudden loss of vision; (4) the problem of falsely associating intellectual and behavioral outcome with medical diagnosis.

I would like to make a plea to those who control educational programs to give consideration to these matters. Improvements in practice are sorely needed.

The Problem of Diagnosis

There is sometimes a poor correlation between ophthalmological findings concerning visual acuity and visual function. Some severely impaired children are observed to make surprisingly efficient use of minimal vision, whereas others with partial sight act blind in many respects. Furthermore, it is now well documented that high anxiety levels can interfere with mobility, even to the point of disorientation. Cratty and his coworkers (1968) found that "highly anxious blind individuals will walk significantly slower and will veer about twice as much walking 100 feet

as will the more relaxed blind person" (Cratty, p. 113). Unless he has a chance to see a range of children functioning in settings such as a school, the ophthalmologist may not appreciate this factor (precisely the same point can be made about the efficiency of hearing in the deaf).

Cholden (1958), one of the first psychiatrists to write about his work with ophthalmologists and with the blind, felt strongly about the tendency of many ophthalmologists to avoid telling adults (or the parents of children) the truth about their blindness. This was interpreted as an attempt to hold out hope for eventual recovery of vision, because of a wish to avoid a severe upset. In other instances, he felt that the doctor might imagine that the loss of vision would be a kind of living death. The reason for concern about this approach is that the delay may prevent the patient (or parents) from coming to grips with the loss and going through the necessary period of grief. So long as the reality is avoided, motivation to learn to function as a blind person is lacking (Blank, 1968).

I have no statistics upon which to base a generalization, but I do know that some blind people have emotionally "bypassed" the acceptance of blindness and have learned to function in a pseudo-blind fashion. The lack of coherence between reality and fantasy restricts their functioning in one or more areas and may have serious psychiatric consequences.

Case Example 2

A 19-year-old boy had been blinded at age 12 when his brother and he struggled for possession of a loaded gun. The patient claimed he had "no hard feelings" toward his brother for blinding him. The family was never able to accept the blindness, partly because of guilt over the circumstances which produced it. For months, the boy would visit the doctor's office, where he would be examined and then excluded from the room so that his mother could talk to the physician. She always emerged crying, but he was never told the truth about the prognosis until he insisted upon being told. A later psychotic reaction was ushered in by his breaking his artificial eye. When he began, at long last, to talk about his blindness in the family, and improved, his brother became psychotic. The brother claimed that he was being observed by Martians who had a secret third eye. He insisted his brother was not really blind, but just pretending. Much additional information indicated that the tragedy had never been psychologically dealt with by anyone in the family.

Occasional cases of "delayed visual maturation" are seen in infants who show no sign of visual function, but later develop normally. This picture is not uncommon in some retarded children. Illingworth (1961) has written an interesting paper on this subject. He felt that delayed maturation might be distinguished from blindness by the fact that in the former, roving nystagmus (usually seen in the blind) does not develop by 3 or 4 months of age. The importance of this condition is that in the absence of clear-cut disease indicating blindness, children who act as if they don't see may not be blind, and this possibility must be kept in mind when talking with parents.

In sum, while the diagnosis of blindness needs to be made cautiously in cases in which it might be wrong, when it is certain, the doctor errs in holding out false hope, since a major stumbling block may be placed in the path of rehabilitation. The physician can offer not the hope of vision, but the hope of a full life as a blind person.

Supportive Intervention

Imparting the diagnosis and prognosis needs to be tailored to the individual situation. An excellent and detailed discussion of this process has been provided by Wigglesworth (1969).

When a diagnosis is made at birth or in infancy, the parents need considerable help in digesting the information and getting over their depression. They will have questions, some seemingly silly or repetitive, about possible causes, associated conditions (such as mental retardation), and the future. Being "supportive" means more than sympathy: it entails anticipation of needs, being a good listener, demonstrating that being blind doesn't make the baby repulsive or an outcast, providing contacts with parents who have had similar problems (in selected cases), relating some ideas about agencies which provide help, and showing a willingness to be available to go over things again while the painful truth is being realized. It also means tolerating depression, fear, and perhaps anger directed at physicians, justified or not. If the child has had a period of normal vision, he may also have his own "shock phase" to go through, which adds to the parents' need for help.

In order to develop and maintain mother-child relationships which are so crucial in early life, what the ophthalmologist says and does and the other helping people he can involve all become of crucial importance.

However, there appear to be real limitations in ophthalmological training and practice. A resident in ophthalmology (Simmons, 1966) surveyed 25 ophthalmologists in private practice in Washington, D.C., who were not associated with organizations for the blind, on their attitudes and knowledge about rehabilitation. He concluded that about one-third had an awareness of needs and referred cases to rehabilitation services. One-third seemed receptive to further information, but about one-third had little sensitivity or awareness of what could be done for the blind. Thus, two-thirds were not familiar with existing rehabilitation services.

There is *no excuse* for not being aware of (and referring parents to) the local or regional branches of organizations for the blind, yet it is not rare for the doctor to act as if his obligation is over after he has given the diagnosis and prognosis. Some parents have to find their way to help by means of friends or newspaper articles! Agencies such as the American Foundation for the Blind and the Canadian National Institute for the Blind can provide a wide variety of helpful reading materials to parents and professionals, and are ready to inform them about available rehabilitative facilities.

It would be unreasonable to expect that the ophthalmologist know everything, or be an expert on available resources if he deals with few cases of blindness. But he *should* know the importance of such help (even if it is nonmedical!) and where to find out about it. As MacKeith has said (1961): ". . . ophthalmologists who are asked whether a child can see well must be able not only to test his sight but to give time to the parents' troubles and be aware of their special needs as well as those of their children, or else to enlist the cooperation of a willing paediatrician" (p. 211).

Partially sighted children tend to develop along the lines of sighted children. Congenitally blind children may present a wide variety of developmental deviations which the ophthalmologist may be called upon to see. Only a few can be mentioned here. The interested reader is referred for further details to Norris et al. (1957), MacKeith (1961), Elonen and Zwarensteyn (1964), and Williams (1969).

Mental retardation, brain damage, or psychosis may complicate blindness, but may also be *wrongly diagnosed* because of reversible or preventable developmental deviations, thereby perhaps permanently limiting expectations of the child by parents and school and adding a further stigma. Some of these deviations may include: peculiar sleeping patterns, failure to pass motor and mobility milestones at the expected ages, absent or peculiar speech, primitive eating patterns, excessive passivity and dependency, stereotyped manneristic behavior misleadingly termed "blindisms," and large gaps in general knowledge. There have been a number of reports of successful reversals of these deviations (Williams, 1966; Elonen et al., 1967) in some children. Smith and *her* coworkers (1969) have also pointed out the multiple possible causes of stereotyped behavior in the blind. Brodey (1969) has suggested that some patterns of posture and gait are "normal" but unsightly adaptations to blindness which normal people also develop after being blindfolded for a while.

Those blind children who show deviant development should not be assumed too readily to be retarded or brain-damaged; they require adequate trials of specialized teaching and/or therapy to sort out organic incapacities from reversible developmental peculiarities. This is true even of patients with rubella syndrome, who not infrequently are "late bloomers" after a few years of very slow development. Remember that medical diagnoses are *not* always clearly and directly related to valid predictions of future intelligence and behavior, and that our knowledge and even our diagnostic categories change with time.

Parents need advice about how to stimulate their blind child to smile, move about and explore his world despite painful encounters, and develop hand usage and social skills. Depression interferes with optimal child-rearing, but may be ameliorated when the parents are able to see the results of their assisted efforts. Many do not believe that they can be good parents to these children or that their blind child can develop and be emotionally rewarding to them, until they see it happen. Many agencies for the blind and some residential schools or clinics provide home visitation by experienced workers and courses and groups for parents. The cooperation and interest of the ophthalmologist are usually enthusiastically received by these organizations.

As they grow older, blind children face separation from parents in going to normal or special school. Often they can go to a normal nursery school, and after special training in Braille and mobility, to a regular school. Some children present excessive dependency or social isolation, and psychiatrists or other mental health personnel may be helpful. Parents may need assistance in learning to discipline a blind child. This is usually no serious problem if they have developed a good relationship, but parents who are still overly involved in feelings of pity and resentment may get into major difficulties, especially as adolescence approaches.

Another point of special significance to ophthalmologists has to do with talking with and examining a blind child or adolescent. Newell (1969) has clearly stated: "The physician managing a blind patient must avoid the slightest hint of condescension and learn that the patient's interpretation of his voice and actions are the major factors in reassurance. A person talking to a blind individual should identify himself by name, should not shout, should always give detailed verbal directions and not signals, and should always warn the patient before touching him" (p. 129).

I have found that blind or partially sighted children often have marked fear of the eye examination, some of which can be minimized by following Dr. Newell's excellent advice.

Perhaps my earlier comments about how children think and feel should obviate the necessity to point out that enucleation is *not a benign procedure* psychologically, even though the eye is blind. Some doctors find this hard to understand, particularly in those cases in which the patient complains of pain in the eye. When the same child rejects enucleation as a pleasant solution, this does not necessarily indicate stupidity, stubbornness, craziness, or lack of appreciation for your efforts. It is rather a natural reluctance about losing a part of one's body. Sometimes the concern may be related to a wish for the miraculous restoration of vision at some later time. Some parents may have similar fantasies, or see the procedure as a further mutilation.

SUGGESTIONS FOR DEALING WITH PSYCHIATRISTS

Early in this chapter it was pointed out that psychiatrists and ophthalmologists work in very different ways. If the latter wishes to make the best use of limited psychiatric time, the following might be helpful:

(1) Recognize the way the child psychiatrist works. His day is likely to be filled with hour-long appointments, scheduled far in advance. Since an evaluation usually requires obtaining information from the parents, winning the confidence of the child, and talking with the referring doctor, as well as dictating a report, several hours of work are ordinarily required. He does not operate like a surgeon, who may be able to arrive at a diagnosis quickly and do the necessary studies with little or no patient cooperation. If a child psychiatrist does a complete assessment in less than an hour, I would be suspicious of its validity.

(2) Try hard to give him as much notice as possible, so that the necessary time can be available. "I've got a patient in the hospital I'd like you to see before he goes home tomorrow" is a poor approach except in emergencies.

(3) Specify the problem you wish him to clarify.

(4) Spell out the nature of the eye disorder, the prognosis, special medications, examinations, and hospitalization and surgery in the past and anticipated in the future. Distinguish between procedures which are absolutely necessary and those which are elective.

(5) Provide any information you have about the family and the child's past reactions to separation, medical procedures, etc.

(6) Inform him about what you have told the child and parents about the diagnosis and prognosis.

There are also expectations which you should have of the psychiatrist: he should discuss his findings with you and write a report which is comprehensible; he should provide you with progress reports if he continues to see the case; he must be willing to tell you what he does *not* know or understand.

Indications for referral to a psychiatrist have been mentioned at several points in this chapter. A brief summary will be found in Table 25–1.

SUMMARY

This chapter has discussed the areas of mutual interest and potential conflict

TABLE 25–1   INDICATIONS FOR REFERRAL TO A PSYCHIATRIST

1. Suicidal ruminations, threats, gestures, or attempts.
2. Profound depression which fails to lift soon with sympathetic management.
3. False conviction (or delusion) that something bad is bound to happen (blindness, death, or the like).
4. Severe and persistent regression or loss of previous function and interests, particularly following surgery or hospitalization.
5. Self-punitive behavior, pleasure in pain, martyr-like behavior, accident-proneness.
6. Marked resistance to rehabilitative measures.
7. Evidence of persistent and crippling psychological gain from the illness or disability.
8. Development of severe phobias, fears, compulsions, insomnia.
9. Evidence of incipient or actual psychosis: bizarre behavior, withdrawal, excessive suspiciousness, thought disorder (fragmented and uncompleted thoughts, dissociation of thought content from emotional expression).
10. Consideration of surgery on a patient with previous psychiatric disorder or severe reactions to medical treatment.
11. Loss of physical function without physical cause.
12. Significant parental problems which are unresponsive to general supportive measures.

between ophthalmology and child psychiatry. The two specialties have very different approaches to patients and sources of satisfaction. Although it is unlikely that misunderstandings can be completely eliminated, some suggestions for their amelioration have been attempted.

Behavior disorders in children are quite variable in severity, manifestations, and outcome. The causes are usually multifactorial but far from being fully elucidated. They are probably best understood at present as deriving from interactions among factors including intellectual endowment, temperament, physical and psychological needs, certain central nervous system functions, and environmental (especially family) experiences. It should be obvious that the significance of eye disease and its management may range from trivial and transient to crucial and enduring.

It is the psychiatrist's role to try to understand and influence those factors (among the many) which may be amenable to change in a given situation. He should also be able to assist the ophthalmologist in becoming more aware of the potential psychological effects of his treatment, and in developing ways of dealing with children and their families which minimize emotional trauma and mobilize potential for growth.

Particular needs have been stressed: preparation for hospitalization and surgery; consideration of emotional and family factors in the timing of elective procedures; minimizing sensory deprivation and separation; forthright interpretation of prognosis of permanent blindness; management of reactions to loss of vision as a continuing process, and the need of the blind and their parents for sensitive handling; early supportive intervention services; and caution in making behavioral, intellectual, and educational prognostications.

The role of emotional factors in certain ophthalmic disorders has been discussed, and the diagnosis and management of psychiatric illness presenting as impairment of vision has been outlined. The need for further research to improve knowledge of this area is an obvious conclusion to be drawn from the review of the literature.

REFERENCES

Adams, G. L., Pearlman, J. T., and Sloan, S. H.: Itching, burning eyes. J.A.M.A., *212*:482, 1970.

Blank, H. R.: Reactions to loss of body parts: some research priorities in rehabilitation. New Outlook for the Blind, *62*:137, 1968.

Bowlby, J.: Attachment and Loss: Volume 1. Attachment. New York, Basic Books, 1969.

Brodey, W. M.: Human enhancement: its application to perception. *In*: Proceedings of the National Seminar on Services to Children with Visual Impairment. New York, American Foundation for the Blind, 1969, pp. 17–50.

Browning, C. W., Quinn, L. H., and Crasilneck, H. B.: The use of hypnosis in suppression amblyopia of children. Amer. J. Ophthal., *46*:53, 1958.

Cholden, L. S.: A Psychiatrist Works with Blindness. New York, American Foundation for the Blind, 1958.

Cratty, B. J., Peterson, C., Harris, J., and Schoner, R.: The development of perceptual-motor abilities in blind children and adolescents. New Outlook for the Blind, *62*:111, 1968.

Davenport, H. T., and Werry, J. S.: The effect of general anesthesia, surgery and hospitalization upon the behavior of children. Amer. J. Orthopsychiat., *40*:806, 1970.

Doggart, J. H.: Diseases of Children's Eyes. London, Henry Kimpton, 1947.

Donaldson, D. D., and Walsh, F.: Neuro-ophthalmology in children. *In* Liebman, S. D., and Gellis, S. S. (eds.): The Pediatrician's Ophthalmology. St. Louis, The C. V. Mosby Co., 1966, pp. 179–209.

Eames, T. H.: A study of tubular and spiral fields in hysteria. Amer. J. Ophthal., *30*:610, 1947.

Elonen, A. S., and Zwarensteyn, S. B.: Appraisal of developmental lag in certain blind children. J. Pediat., *65*:599, 1964.

Elonen, A. S., Polzien, M., and Zwarensteyn, S. B.: The "uncommitted" blind child: results of intensive training of children formerly committed to institutions for the retarded. Exceptional Child., *33*:301, 1967.

Fish, B.: Drug use in psychiatric disorders of children. Amer. J. Psychiat., *124 (Suppl. 8)*:31, 1968.

Freeman, R. D.: Use of psychoactive drugs for intellectually handicapped children. *In* Bernstein, N. R. (ed.): Diminished People: Problems and Care of the Mentally Retarded. Boston, Little, Brown, 1970, pp. 277–304.

Freud, A.: Normality and Pathology in Childhood: Assessments of Development. New York, International Universities Press, 1965.

Friesen, H., and Mann, W. A.: Follow-up study of hysterical amblyopia. Amer. J. Ophthal., *62*:1106, 1966.

Gibbens, T. C. N.: The effects of physical ill-health in adolescent delinquents. Proc. Roy. Soc. Med., *56*:1086, 1963.

Gilkes, M. J.: Closing discussion. *In* Gardiner, P., MacKeith, R., and Smith, V. (eds.): Aspects of Developmental and Paediatric Ophthalmology. London, Spastics International Medical Publications/Heinemann, 1969.

Grosz, H. J., and Zimmerman, J.: Experimental analysis of hysterical blindness: a follow-up report and new experimental data. Arch. Gen. Psychiat., *13*:255, 1965.

Harley, R. D., Baird, H. W., and Freeman, R. D.: Self-induced photogenic epilepsy: report of four cases. Arch. Ophthal., *78*:730, 1967.

Heaton, J. M.: The Eye: Phenomenology and Psychology of Function and Disorder. Philadelphia, J. B. Lippincott Co., 1968.

Helveston, E. M.: The ophthalmologist's role in dyslexia. Arch. Ophthal., *83*:132, 1970.

Hospital for Sick Children (Toronto): The Eye in Childhood. Chicago, Year Book Medical Publishers, 1967.

Illingworth, R. S.: Delayed visual maturation. Arch. Dis. Child., *36*:407, 1961.

Kangery, R. H.: Children's answers. Amer. J. Nurs., *60*:1748, 1960.

Kaplan, H. S., and Kaplan, H. I.: Current concepts of psychosomatic medicine. *In* Freedman, A. M., and Kaplan, H. I. (eds.): Comprehensive Textbook of Psychiatry. Baltimore, Williams & Wilkins, 1967, p. 1039.

Kraft, I. A.: The use of psychoactive drugs in the outpatient treatment of psychiatric disorders of childhood. Amer. J. Psychiat., *124*:1401, 1968.

LaScola, R. L., and Cheek, D. B.: Is your anesthetized patient listening? (Report of interview with authors.) J.A.M.A. Med. News, *206*:1004, 1968.

Lawson, L. J.: Reading and learning problems: Ophthalmological management. Illinois Med. J., *137*:623, 1970.

Linn, L., Kahn, R. L., Coles, R., Cohen, J., Marshall, D., and Weinstein, E. A.: Patterns of behavior disturbance following cataract extraction. Amer. J. Psychiat., *110*:281, 1953.

Lipton, E. L.: A study of the psychological effects of strabismus. Psychoanal. Stud. Child, *25*:146, 1970.

MacKeith, R.: Children in hospital: preparation for operation. Lancet, *2*:843, 1953.

MacKeith, R.: Blindness in little children. Cereb. Palsy Bull., *3*:209, 1961.

Mattson, A., and Weisberg, I.: Behavioral reactions to minor illness in preschool children. Pediatrics, *46*:604, 1970.

Money, J.: Reading dysphoitesis. *In* Liebman, S. D., and Gellis, S. S. (eds.): The Pediatrician's Ophthalmology. St. Louis, The C. V. Mosby Co., 1966, p. 274.

Newell, F. W.: Ophthalmology: Principles and Concepts. 2nd ed. St. Louis, The C. V. Mosby Co., 1969.

Nicholls, J. V. V.: Reading disabilities in the young: the ophthalmologist's role. Canad. J. Ophthal., *4*:223, 1969.

Norris, M., Spaulding, P. J., and Brodie, F. H.: Blindness in Children. Chicago, University of Chicago Press, 1957.

Rutter, M., Graham, P., and Yule, W.: A Neuropsychiatric Study in Childhood. Philadelphia, J. B. Lippincott Co., 1970.

Schlaegel, T. F., and Hoyt, M.: Psychosomatic Ophthalmology. Baltimore, Williams & Wilkins, 1957.

Shipsey, M., Gibbons, H., and Jahoda, M. A.: Social and emotional aspects of ophthalmic problems. *In* Liebman, S. D., and Gellis, S. S. (eds.): The Pediatrician's Ophthalmology. St. Louis, The C. V. Mosby Co., 1966, pp. 286–300.

Simmons, R. E.: Current ophthalmological attitudes toward rehabilitation of patients with loss of vision. New Outlook for the Blind, *60*:299, 1966.

Smith, M. A., Chethik, M., and Adelson, E.: Differential assessments of "blindisms." Amer. J. Orthopsychiat., *39*:807, 1969.

Spalter, H. F., Bemporad, J. R., and Sours, J. A.: Cataracts following chronic headbanging: report of two cases. Arch. Ophthal., *83*:182, 1970.

Tate, B. G., and Baroff, G. S.: Aversive control of self-injurious behavior in a psychotic boy. Behav. Res. Ther., *4*:281, 1966.

Vaughan, G. F.: Children in hospital. Lancet, June 1, 1957, p. 1117.

Vernon, D. T. A., Schulman, J. L., and Foley, J. M. Changes in children's behavior after hospitalization: some dimensions of response to their correlates. Amer. J. Dis. Child., *111*:581, 1966.

Vernon, D. T. A., Foley, J. M., Sipowicz, R. R., and Schulman, J. L.: The psychological responses of children to hospitalization and illness: a review of the literature. Springfield, Illinois, Charles C Thomas, 1965.

Weisman, A. D., and Hackett, T. P.: Psychosis after eye surgery: establishment of a specific doctor-patient relation in the prevention and treatment of "black-patch delirium." New Eng. J. Med., *258*:1284, 1958.

Weiss, E., and English, O. S.: Psychosomatic Medicine: A Clinical Study of Psychophysiologic Reactions. 3rd ed. Philadelphia, W. B. Saunders Co., 1957.

Werner, S.: On injuries to the eyes in children. Acta Ophthal., *30*:97, 1952.

Wigglesworth, R.: The conduct of the interview with the handicapped child and his family. *In* Gardiner, P., MacKeith, R., and Smith, V. (eds.): Aspects of Developmental and Paediatric Ophthalmology. London, Spastics International Medical Publications/Heinemann, 1969, p. 106.

Williams, C. E.: A blind idiot who became a normal blind adolescent. Develop. Med. Child Neurol., *8*:166, 1966.

Williams, C. E.: Psychiatric implications of severe visual defect for the child and for the parents. *In* Gardiner, P., MacKeith, R., and Smith, V. (eds.): Aspects of Developmental and Paediatric Ophthalmology. London, Spastics International Medical Publications/Heinemann, 1969, p. 110.

Williams, J. G. L., and Jones, J. R.: Psychophysiological responses to anesthesia and operations. J.A.M.A., *203*:415, 1968.

Wolf, S., and Messier, P. E.: Corneal vascular changes in association with conflict in a patient with phlyctenular keratitis. Proc. Assoc. Res. Nerv. Ment. Dis., *29*:537, 1950.

Wolff, H. G.: Stress and Disease. Springfield, Illinois, Charles C Thomas, 1953.

Work, H. H.: Making hospitalization easier for children. Children, *3*:83, 1956.

Yasuna, E. R.: Hysterical amblyopia in children. Amer. J. Dis. Child., *106*:558, 1963.

Yates, A. J.: Tics. *In* Costello, C. G. (ed.): Symptoms of Psychopathology: A Handbook. New York, John Wiley & Sons, Inc., 1970, p. 320.

Zimet, C. N., and Berger, A. S.: Emotional factors in primary glaucoma: an evaluation of psychological test data. Psychosom. Med., *22*:391, 1960.

Ziskind, E., Jones, H., Filante, W., and Goldberg, J.: Observations on mental symptoms in eye patched patients: hypnagogic symptoms in sensory deprivation. Amer. J. Psychiat., *116*:893, 1960.

CHAPTER 26

DIFFERENTIAL DIAGNOSIS OF LEUKOCORIA

LOV K. SARIN, M.D.,
and JERRY A. SHIELDS, M.D.

INTRODUCTION

A child with leukocoria (white pupil; cat's eye reflex) poses an important diagnostic problem for the ophthalmologist. When evaluating a white pupillary reflex in a child, three diagnostic considerations should immediately come to mind:

1. Retinoblastoma
2. Cataract
3. "Pseudogliomas"

Leukocoria is the most frequent manifestation of retinoblastoma (Fig. 26–1). It is not pathognomonic of retinoblastoma, however, and congenital cataracts and "pseudogliomas" must also be considered.

Cataracts in children, whether congenital, traumatic, or of other cause, may produce leukocoria (Fig. 26–2). The diagnosis can usually be established by the history and clinical examination, and the differentiation from retinoblastoma is not usually difficult.

Certain conditions involving the vitreous and retina, however, may present a greater diagnostic problem. These have been called "pseudogliomas." There is now evidence that the retinoblastoma is of neuronal rather than glial origin, and the term "pseudoglioma" should probably be abandoned. The term pseudoretinoblastoma is perhaps more accurate.

The relative frequency of these conditions producing leukocoria has been determined by Howard and Ellsworth. Of 500 children referred to them with suspected retinoblastoma, almost all of whom had leukocoria in one or both eyes, one of these more benign conditions was subsequently diagnosed in 265 cases. In other words, the white pupillary reflex in more than one-half the children was due to a lesion other than a retinoblastoma.

The diagnosis of retinoblastoma has profound implications. In evaluating a child with leukocoria, therefore, the physician should make every effort to rule out one of these simulating lesions. The following list includes many of the conditions which may simulate retinoblastoma on the basis of producing leuko-

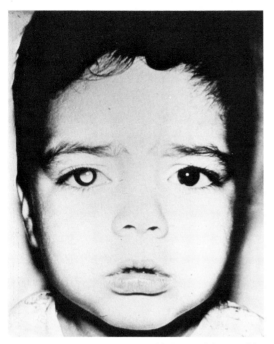

Figure 26–1 Three-year-old boy with a white pupillary reflex in the right eye due to a large retinoblastoma.

coria (some of these commonly produce a white pupillary reflex, whereas others do so only occasionally):

1. Cataracts
2. Persistent hyperplastic primary vitreous
3. Retinopathy of prematurity (retrolental fibroplasia)
4. Coats's disease
5. Larval granulomatosis
6. Chorioretinitis
7. Metastatic retinitis and endophthalmitis
8. Retinal detachment (from any cause)
9. Colobomas
10. Organized vitreous hemorrhage
11. Intraocular foreign body
12. Congenital retinal fold
13. Retinal dysplasia
14. Massive retinal gliosis
15. Congenital retinoschisis
16. Myelinated nerve fibers
17. Medulloepithelioma
18. Norrie's disease
19. High myopia
20. Incontinentia pigmenti
21. Phakomatoses

Since most of these conditions are discussed in other chapters, this section will be concerned only with those features which serve to clinically differentiate them from retinoblastoma.

DIFFERENTIAL DIAGNOSIS

Cataracts

As already mentioned, the diagnosis of cataract in a child is not usually difficult, and the differentiation from retinoblastoma can readily be made.

Persistent Hyperplastic Primary Vitreous

Probably the condition most often confused clinically with retinoblastoma is persistent hyperplastic primary vitreous (PHPV) (Fig. 26–3). Children with

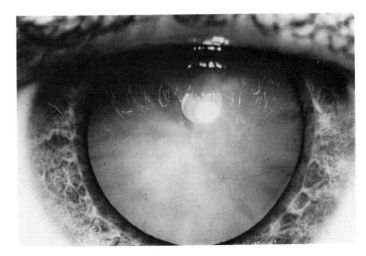

Figure 26–2 Leukocoria in a small child due to a congenital cataract of uncertain cause.

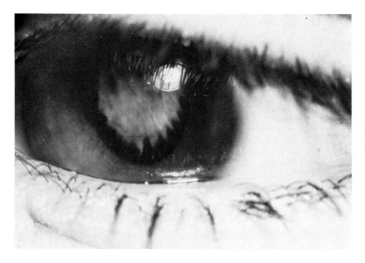

Figure 26–3 Leukocoria due to persistent hyperplastic primary vitreous. Note the elongated ciliary processes being pulled into the retrolental mass.

PHPV invariably have leukocoria, but certain characteristic features are useful in differentiating it from retinoblastoma. PHPV is almost always unilateral and most cases occur in eyes with relative microphthalmos. In cases in which microphthalmos is clinically indiscernible, ultrasound may be useful in determining the size of the eye. Retinoblastoma is bilateral in 30 per cent of cases and invariably occurs in normal-sized eyes. In PHPV, a typical opaque retrolental mass is present, often leading to early opacification of the lens. The retinoblastoma does not present as a retrolental mass unless the entire globe is filled with tumor, and cataractous changes are relatively rare. Characteristic of PHPV is the apparent elongation of the ciliary processes as they become stretched by the contracting retrolental mass. Elongated ciliary processes are not seen in retinoblastoma. PHPV is often associated with hyaloid remnants, particularly persistent hyaloid vessels passing from the optic disc to the lens. X-ray evidence of calcification,

common in retinoblastoma, usually does not occur in PHPV.

Retinopathy of Prematurity (Retrolental Fibroplasia)

Although retinopathy of prematurity (retrolental fibroplasia, RLF) is encountered less frequently than in previous years, it is still a common consideration in the differential diagnosis of retinoblastoma. Certain clinical features, however, are suggestive of this diagnosis. The relationship of this condition to prematurity and oxygen therapy is well known. Retinopathy of prematurity is characterized by vitreoretinal traction. In the early stages there is fibrovascular proliferation particularly in the temporal retinal periphery. This causes traction on the retina posteriorly, resulting in the "dragged disc" appearance. Later the entire retina may become detached and lie as a white vascularized mass in the retrolental area, producing a clinical picture of leukocoria (Fig. 26–4). As in PHPV, contraction of

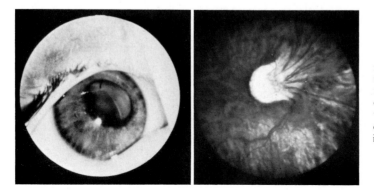

Figure 26–4 *A*, Leukocoria due to retinopathy of prematurity. The detached retina lies as a folded white retrolental mass. *B*, The opposite eye of the same patient is less severely involved. It shows the typical "dragged disc" due to fibrovascular proliferation in the temporal retina.

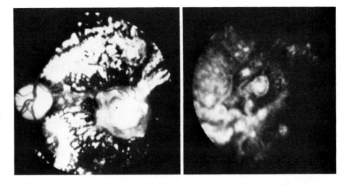

Figure 26–5 *A*, Proliferative mound in the macular region in a patient with Coats' disease. Note the typical deep retinal exudates. *B*, Peripheral to the macular mound in the same eye there are areas of retinal telangiectasia, characterized by saccular dilatations of the retinal vessels.

the retrolental mass may cause elongation of the ciliary processes. In retinoblastoma, in which vitreous traction is not a major consideration, these changes do not occur. Retinopathy of prematurity is more often bilateral and symmetrical.

Coats' Disease

Another condition which may frequently simulate a retinoblastoma is Coats' disease. In most cases, however, differentiation from retinoblastoma should not be difficult. Coats' disease is invariably unilateral and is usually diagnosed at a later age than retinoblastoma. In contrast to retinoblastoma, it is more common in males and has no familial incidence. The two essential features of Coats' disease are telangiectasis of the retinal vessels and deep retinal exudates. The exudates are typically yellow in color and may be found at some distance from the vascular changes (Fig. 26–5). Accumulation of these exudates gradually leads to the large yellow-green bullous retinal detachment

so characteristic of Coats' disease. At this stage, the child may present with a white pupillary reflex (Fig. 26–6). The vascular changes seen with retinoblastoma usually consist of dilated retinal vessels. Rarely, there is neovascularization over the surface of the tumor. Telangiectases and distant exudates are not commonly seen in cases of retinoblastoma. Glistening yellow crystals, representing deposits of cholesterol, are often seen within the exudate of Coats' disease. These are not to be confused with the chalky white calcium depositions seen in necrotic retinoblastomas.

Larval Granulomatosis

During the past 20 years, larval granulomatosis has gained recognition as an important ocular disease in children. A number of ocular parasites are known to cause leukocoria, but the larva of *Toxocara canis* has been most often incriminated. The disease may appear in two forms. In one form there is a localized chorioretinal

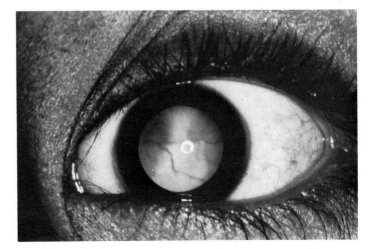

Figure 26–6 More advanced stage of Coats' disease, showing a large bullous retinal detachment due to the accumulation of subretinal exudates.

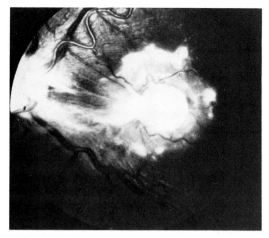

Figure 26–7 Localized chorioretinal granuloma in the macular region, presumably caused by *Toxocara canis.* Note the vitreous traction bands between the disc and macula.

granuloma, often in the posterior pole, with no active inflammation (Fig. 26–7). This form is nonprogressive and should not be confused with retinoblastoma. The second form is characterized by severe inflammation with an intense vitreous reaction. Such cases may simulate a large endophytic retinoblastoma and clinical

differentiation may be especially difficult (Fig. 26–8). In contrast to retinoblastoma, larval granulomatosis is invariably unilateral and the family history is negative. Often there is a history of geophagia or close contact with a dog or a cat.

Chorioretinitis

Inflammations involving the retina and choroid may sometimes produce leukocoria and simulate retinoblastoma. Although a number of conditions may produce a posterior chorioretinitis with vitreous reaction, congenital toxoplasmosis is most often responsible for this clinical picture. As opposed to retinoblastoma, congenital toxoplasmosis is usually bilateral and often associated with jaundice, hepatosplenomegaly, hydrocephalus, and intracerebral calcification. It is characterized by recurrent episodes of inflammation which may vary from mild to severe. Pigmented chorioretinal scars, particularly in the macular region, with satellite lesions are also helpful in the diagnosis. In addition, tests for detecting antibodies against *Toxoplasma gondii,* such as the dye test, complement fixation test, and hemagglu-

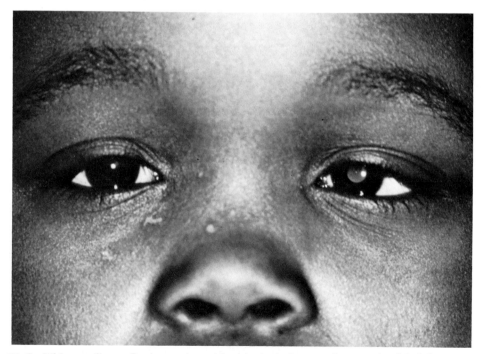

Figure 26–8 White pupillary reflex in a patient with a histologically proved nematode of the left eye, presumably *Toxocara canis.* The eye was enucleated because a retinoblastoma could not be definitely excluded. (Courtesy of Dr. Buford Washington.)

tination test, are available. Cytomegalic inclusion disease may produce a similar clinical picture. Less commonly, peripheral uveitis (pars planitis) may produce white elevated mounds in the peripheral fundus associated with a vitreous reaction. These white exudates may resemble a peripheral retinoblastoma.

In most cases, retinoblastomas do not produce severe inflammation. It has been pointed out, however, that 6 per cent of retinoblastomas present clinically with severe inflammation, and the tumor may be unsuspected for a period of time while the patient is treated for the inflammation. In such cases, the differentiation from retinoblastoma may be extremely difficult, especially if the vitreous haze prevents an adequate view of the fundus.

Metastatic Retinitis and Endophthalmitis

Prior to the days of antibiotic therapy, this was a common cause of a white pupillary reflex simulating retinoblastoma. It was often seen with epidemic cerebrospinal meningitis and sometimes with severe forms of the exanthematous diseases of childhood. Today this condition is quite rare. The presence of meningitis or other concurrent disease is helpful in the diagnosis.

Retinal Detachment (From Any Cause)

Any retinal detachment which occurs in a child can cause a white pupillary reflex and simulate retinoblastoma. A history of trauma or other causes of retinal detachment as well as careful indirect ophthalmoscopy should rule out a retinoblastoma.

Colobomas

Colobomas in the posterior fundus have also been known to cause leukocoria (Fig. 26–9). Indirect ophthalmoscopy will reveal a nonelevated lesion with pigmented margins rather than the elevated tumor seen with retinoblastoma. Nevertheless, on occasions, such eyes have been enucleated because of the mistaken diagnosis of retinoblastoma.

Organized Vitreous Hemorrhage

As a large vitreous hemorrhage undergoes organization, it may assume a yellow-white color and produce leukocoria. There is often a history of trauma or hemorrhagic disease of the newborn. Indirect ophthalmoscopy should localize the lesion within the vitreous cavity, often in an inferior position, and confusion with retinoblastoma should not occur.

Intraocular Foreign Body

Retinal intraocular foreign bodies, particularly vegetable material such as wood, may provoke a severe intraocular inflammatory reaction and produce a white pupillary reflex (Fig. 26–10). A history of antecedent trauma and signs of ocular trauma may establish the diagnosis.

Congenital Retinal Fold

Whether the congenital retinal fold represents a remnant of the primary vitreous or a variant of retrolental fibroplasia is not completely known. The typical appearance of a large vascularized fold of retina, passing from the optic disc to the peripheral retina, will serve to differentiate it from retinoblastoma.

Retinal Dysplasia

This is actually a pathological term which has been inappropriately applied to a clinical condition. It is characterized

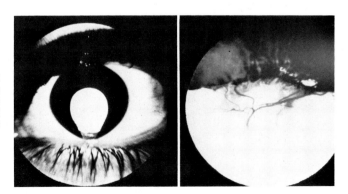

Figure 26–9 *A,* White pupillary reflex in a child with a choroidal coloboma. Note the iris coloboma inferonasally. *B,* Fundus view of the same eye, showing the large choroidal coloboma extending to encompass the optic nerve head.

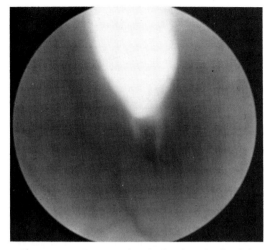

Figure 26–10 Intravitreal foreign body lying against the retina and causing a white pupillary reflex.

by bilateral microphthalmos and malformation of the retina, resulting in leukocoria. In contrast to retinoblastoma, it is often a part of the 13–15 trisomy or other syndromes and is associated with numerous systemic findings such as cerebral agenesis, internal hydrocephalus, cardiac abnormalities, cleft palate, and polydactylism. In addition, bilaterality, microphthalmos, and associated systemic abnormalities will serve to differentiate it from retinoblastoma. In rare instances, however, retinal dysplasia may be unilateral and unassociated with systemic changes.

Massive Retinal Gliosis

There is a rare condition in which the retina becomes gradually replaced by a massive growth of glial tissue, producing a leukocoria. The pathogenesis is uncertain, but it often follows trauma, inflammation, or vascular disease. As in the case of retinoblastoma, x-rays may reveal intraocular calcification. Massive gliosis, however, usually becomes manifest in young adulthood and is not commonly seen in infants.

Congenital Retinoschisis

Congenital retinoschisis may occasionally produce leukocoria. This may occur in two ways: either the inner layer of the retinoschisis may come to lie immediately behind the lens, producing a white reflex,

or a retinal detachment may supervene. The typical dehiscences in the inner layer and the sex-linked recessive mode of inheritance will help to differentiate it from retinoblastoma.

Myelinated Nerve Fibers

Myelinated nerve fibers may occasionally be large enough to produce leukocoria. Their usual location around the optic disc and their typical fibrillated margins should offer little diagnostic problem.

Medulloepithelioma

The medulloepithelioma is a rare tumor which may be either benign or malignant. It appears clinically as a fluffy white mass arising in the ciliary body region. In contrast to retinoblastoma, it is usually located more anteriorly, often invades the anterior chamber early, and sometimes has a cystic appearance.

Norrie's Disease

Norrie's disease is a rare bilateral pseudotumor of the retina, characterized by replacement of the retina and vitreous by vascular scar tissue with proliferation of the pigment epithelium. It differs from retinoblastoma in that it almost always occurs bilaterally and has a sex-linked recessive mode of inheritance.

High Myopia

In rare instances, high myopia may produce leukocoria owing to advanced chorioretinal degeneration. The differentiation from retinoblastoma should offer no problem.

Incontinentia Pigmenti

Incontinentia pigmenti (Bloch-Sulzberger syndrome) has been known to produce a total retinal detachment and leukocoria. It is found almost exclusively in females and is characterized by typical, pigmented, swirling, geographic patterns of the skin. Leukocoria may also result from cataract or PHPV.

Phakomatoses

The retinal lesions of angiomatosis retinae, tuberous sclerosis, and the choroidal hemangioma seen with Sturge-Weber syndrome have been known to produce leukocoria by virtue of their size or, more commonly, by causing a retinal detachment. Their associated skin and systemic abnormalities should serve to differentiate them easily from retinoblastoma.

REFERENCES

Anderson, R. S., and Warburg, M.: Norrie's disease: congenital bilateral pseudotumor of the retina with recessive x-chromosomal inheritance: a preliminary report. Arch. Ophthal., *66*:614, 1961.

Ashton, N.: Larval granulomatosis due to Toxocara. Brit. J. Ophthal., *44*:129, 1960.

Coats, G.: Forms of retinal disease with massive exudation. Roy. Lond. Ophthal. Hosp. Rep., *17*:440, 1907–1908.

Cogan, D. G., and Kuwabara, T.: Ocular pathology of the 13–15 trisomy syndrome. Arch. Ophthal., *72*:246, 1964.

de Buen, S., and Fenton, R. H.: Coloboma of the optic disc mistaken clinically for retinoblastoma. Survey Ophthal., *10*:7, 1965.

Harris, W.: Pseudoglioma due to larval chorioretinal granulomatosis. Brit. J. Ophthal., *45*:144, 1961.

Howard, G. M., and Ellsworth, R. M.: A statistical survey of 500 children. I. Relative frequency of the lesions which simulate retinoblastoma. Amer. J. Ophthal., *60*:610, 1965.

Hunter, W. S., and Zimmerman, L. E.: Unilateral retinal dysplasia. Arch. Ophthal., *74*:23, 1965.

Lewis, P. M.: Eye changes in epidemic cerebrospinal meningitis: a clinical and pathologic study of 200 cases. J. Amer. Ophthal. Soc., *34*:284, 1936.

Manschot, W. A.: Persistent hyperplastic primary vitreous. Arch. Ophthal., *59*:188, 1959.

Manschot, W. A., and de Bruijn, W. C.: Coats' disease: definition and pathogenesis. Brit. J. Ophthal., *51*:145, 1967.

Pruett, R. C., and Schepens, C. L.: Posterior hyperplastic primary vitreous. Amer. J. Ophthal., *69*:535, 1970.

Reese, A. B.: Persistent hyperplastic primary vitreous. Amer. J. Ophthal., *40*:317, 1955.

Reese, A. B.: Telangiectasis of the retina and Coats's disease. Amer. J. Ophthal., *42*:1, 1956.

Reese, A. B.: Tumors of the Eye. 2nd ed. New York, Hoeber Medical Division, Harper and Row, 1963.

Reese, A. B., and Blodi, F. C.: Retinal dysplasia. Amer. J. Ophthal., *33*:23, 1950.

Reese, A. B., King, M. J., and Owens, W. C.: A classification of retrolental fibroplasia. Amer. J. Ophthal., *35*:1333, 1953.

Scott, J. G., Friedmann, A. I., Chitters, M., and Pepler, W. J.: Ocular changes in the Bloch-Sulzberger syndrome (incontinentia pigmenti). Brit. J. Ophthal., *39*:276, 1955.

Stafford, W. R., Yanoff, M., and Parnell, B. L.: Retinoblastomas initially misdiagnosed as primary ocular inflammations. Arch. Ophthal., *82*:771, 773, 1969.

Tasman, W. S.: Retinal Diseases in Children. New York, Harper and Row, 1971.

Treacher Collins, E.: Pseudoglioma. Roy. Lond. Ophthal. Hosp. Rep., *13*:361, 1892.

Ts'o, M. O. M., Zimmerman, L. E., and Fine, B. S.: The nature of retinoblastoma. I. Photoreceptor differentiation: a clinical and histopathologic study. Amer. J. Ophthal., *69*:339, 1970.

Wilder, H. C.: Nematode endophthalmitis. Trans. Amer. Acad. Ophthal., *55*:99, 1950.

Yanoff, M., Davis, R. L., and Zimmerman, L. E.: Massive gliosis of the retina. Int. Ophthal. Clin., *11*:211, 1971.

Zimmerman, L. E., Font, R. L.: Congenital malformations of the eye. J.A.M.A., *196*:684, 1966.

CHAPTER 27

USES OF ELECTRORETINOGRAPHY IN PEDIATRIC OPHTHALMOLOGY

ARNOLD POPKIN, M.D.

Electroretinography has changed from being simply an interesting phenomenon with little practical usefulness to a frequently employed technique with many clinical applications. It may be of great value in the total examination of children for several reasons. First, the patient may be too young for any subjective tests, including visual acuity, visual fields, color vision, or dark adaptometry, and therefore, an objective evaluation of retinal function may be very helpful. In addition, there may be definite evidence of decreased vision with normal or questionable fundi. The ERG may provide objective evidence of abnormal retinal function. In another group of patients, those with definitely abnormal fundi, the ERG may yield additional information to help in the diagnosis, prognosis, and management of the case.

Children who are age 7 or older can usually be tested using topical anesthesia, as in adults. Younger children require either general anesthesia or strong sedation.

PRINCIPLES OF ELECTRORETINOGRAPHY

This section will give only a very brief description of the major principles of electroretinography. Basically, a retinal action potential is produced by light stimulation. The stimulus can be varied in intensity, duration, wavelength, frequency, and other ways. The retinal potential is picked up through a corneal contact lens electrode, of which there are many different types and designs. The potential is then amplified and can be recorded on an inkwriter, displayed on and photographed from a cathode ray oscilloscope, or recorded by a computer or tape. Each ERG laboratory has its own type of apparatus, and very little standardization exists from one laboratory to another. Therefore, each laboratory must determine its own values for normal and abnormal responses.

In addition, the ERG responses depend on the state of adaptation of the eye, pupil size, background illumination, and other factors. These also vary according to the

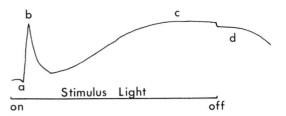

Figure 27–1 Schematic ERG tracing showing small negative a wave, large positive b wave, slow positive c wave, and negative d wave (off-effect) when stimulus light is turned off.

particular technique used in a given laboratory. The exact sequence of test conditions can be changed to emphasize certain aspects of the ERG. Each laboratory tries to control all these variables so that the ERG can be compared accurately from one patient to another, using the same apparatus and test conditions.

The major components of the ERG are the negative a wave followed by the positive b wave. Under certain conditions, a slower c wave and an off-effect can be recorded (Fig. 27–1). These are rarely used for clinical purposes and can be eliminated from further discussion here.

The a and b waves can be separated into two components each by certain techniques. These components are felt to represent photopic and scotopic function (Figs. 27–2A and B). Light adaptation tends to bring out the photopic elements and dark adaptation the scotopic elements. Rapidly flickering stimuli, greater than 30 per second, are a measure of cone function, since rods have a lower critical flicker fusion frequency. Also, different wavelengths produce different types of response. Blue light emphasizes scotopic function, while a deep red stimulus gives a good separation of photopic and scotopic b waves over the course of dark adaptation (Figs. 27–3A and B).

The exact origin of the various waves is still uncertain. It is felt that the a wave is produced mainly by the rods and cones, while the bipolar cells probably contribute most to the b wave. The ganglion cells and optic nerve fibers do not contribute to the ERG. Thus, it is a response due to the external layers of the retina only. This explains the retention of a normal ERG despite severe loss of vision due to glaucoma or optic atrophy.

The ERG is basically a mass response. It is difficult to localize the stimulus to a small discrete retinal area owing to scatter of light by the ocular media plus internal retinal neuronal interaction. Thus, most or all of the retina tends to be stimulated, even if an attempt is made to stimulate only one area such as the macula. This is perhaps the major limiting factor in the clinical usefulness of the ERG at present.

Another problem is related to the number and distribution of rods and cones. One estimate gives about 120 million rods compared to only 7 million cones in each retina. In addition, the most important area of the retina, the macula, contains perhaps only about 200,000 of these 7 million cones. Thus, a destructive macular lesion would leave about 97 per cent of the retinal cones intact. Because of the mass response discussed above, the ERG would be quite normal despite the severe visual handicap. Newer techniques, such as the use of background illumination and computer averaging, show promise for the future in evaluating macular function by the ERG, but these techniques are not yet perfected.

Figure 27–2 *A*, After 4 minutes of dark adaptation. *B*, After 15 minutes of dark adaptation.
  Separation of a and b waves into photopic and scotopic components during the course of dark adaptation. Earlier in dark adaptation, the photopic waves (a_p and b_p) are larger than the scotopic (a_s and b_s), whereas later the reverse is true.

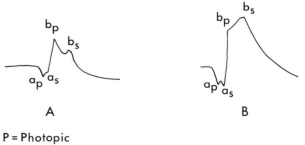

A   B

P = Photopic
S = Scotopic

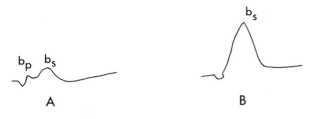

Figure 27–3 *A,* Red stimulus, showing good separation of photopic and scotopic responses in dark adaptation. *B,* Blue stimulus gives only scotopic wave.

P = Photopic
S = Scotopic

CLINICAL APPLICATIONS

A fairly common problem in the practice of ophthalmology is that of a child with decreased vision and normal fundi. The differential diagnosis includes disease of the brain, optic nerve, retina in general, and macula in particular, as well as hysteria or malingering.

Leber's congenital amaurosis is a form of tapetoretinal degeneration in which the vision is greatly diminished at birth or early in life. The disease is inherited as an autosomal recessive. Nystagmus and photophobia are common, and keratoglobus and mental retardation may occur. The fundus may be entirely normal early in the disease. Later, macular changes may occur, as well as pigmentation and vascular narrowing similar to retinitis pigmentosa. The ERG shows greatly reduced or absent photopic and scotopic responses. This proves the presence of widespread retinal dysfunction.

Without the ERG, the diagnosis could easily be missed. Indeed, several retrospective ERG studies of blind children have shown a significant percentage to be due to tapetoretinal degeneration, although the previous diagnosis was different, such as cerebral disease, optic nerve disease, or albinism.

The prognosis of Leber's disease is very poor because both the rods and cones are affected in most or all of the retina.

Congenital retinal dysfunction is a term used by Karpe and Zetterstrom to describe cases with decreased vision, normal fundi, and abnormal ERGs which later improved. They felt the condition was due to retarded development. The prognosis here is better than that of Leber's congenital amaurosis. The exact incidence of this condition is unknown because of the infrequency of ERG testing early in life.

Another cause of poor vision with normal fundi is the *congenital cone dysfunction syndrome.* Other names for this condition include achromatopsia, total color blindness, and rod monochromatism. It is usually inherited as a recessive and may occur in complete or partial forms. In the complete syndrome, the visual acuity is about 20/200, and there is nystagmus, photophobia, and total absence of color discrimination. The partial form shows visual acuity of 20/40 to 20/100, minimal or no nystagmus and photophobia, and only a partial color vision defect. The fundi are usually normal but may show macular abnormalities. The diagnosis of this syndrome is frequently missed, particularly in children who are too young to test color vision or if color vision tests are not performed. The ophthalmologist must be alert to the possibility of this condition and inquire about and test for color vision even though the patient may not mention anything about color blindness. The ERG is usually diagnostic, showing absent photopic responses with normal scotopic responses (Fig. 27–4). This contrasts with the tapetoretinal degenerations, in which both photopic and scotopic responses are reduced or absent.

Correct diagnosis of the cone dysfunction syndrome is important for both prognostic and genetic reasons. The prognosis is relatively good, in that (1) the condition is not progressive, (2) the nystagmus frequently improves with age, (3) the peripheral field remains normal, and (4) most of these children can attend regular schools. This is in contrast to such conditions as retinitis pigmentosa, which may progress to total blindness.

Genetically, the usual recessive mode of inheritance means that each other child

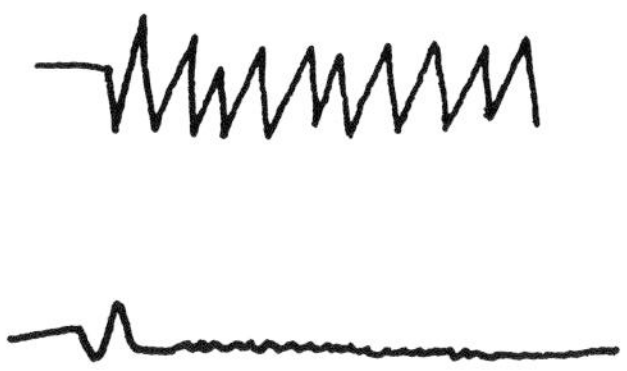

Figure 27–4 Cone dysfunction syndrome. Failure to respond to 30 cycles per second.

of the same parents has a one in four chance of having the disease, but there is very little likelihood that the patient's own children will be affected.

The ERG in the above types of disease may make a definite diagnosis by proving retinal dysfunction. In optic nerve lesions, decreased vision of cerebral origin, and hysteria or malingering the ERG is normal. The ERG not only may make the correct diagnosis but may make further extensive and possibly hazardous tests unnecessary, such as arteriography or pneumoencephalography.

Another use of the ERG is in the evaluation of patients with *albinism.* An albinotic eye shows translucency of the iris on transillumination and great deficiency of pigment in the fundus. There is reduced central vision and nystagmus. There is usually a poor or absent foveal reflex. There is at present some debate over whether or not there is a true histologic hypoplasia of the macula which causes the poor central vision and nystagmus.

Albinism may occur in several forms— complete albinism is usually inherited recessively and ocular albinism is sex-linked. It also may be only partial in the eye. Occasionally, an albinotic fundus can be confused with other types of retinal degeneration, and the poor vision and nystagmus could be confused with either congenital nystagmus or the cone dysfunction syndrome. The correct diagnosis can usually be made by means of a careful history and examination. Color vision tests would help rule out the cone dysfunction syndrome. Transillumination of the iris in both the patient and relatives may help prove the presence of albinism. Finally, the ERG may be helpful. In albinism, the ERG amplitudes are usually normal or even greater than normal. The small macular abnormalities are not enough to diminish the ERG, and increased reflection and scattering of light due to decreased pigmentation of the eye may increase the ERG amplitudes.

Another general area in which the ERG is often useful is in the evaluation of *night blindness.* The most common question that arises is whether there is a progressive retinal degeneration, such as retinitis pigmentosa, choroideremia, or retinitis punctata albescens, or only a stationary condition, such as congenital night blindness.

Congenital night blindness is a stationary condition with normal visual acuity, fundi, and fields. It is apparently due to dysfunction of the rods only, with sparing of the cones. It may be inherited by almost any pattern. The ERG usually shows a decrease or absence of the scotopic components with an essentially normal photopic ERG (Fig. 27–5). This contrasts with the more severe diminution of the ERG seen in most cases of retinitis pigmentosa. However, great care must be taken in interpreting the ERG results for two major reasons: (1) some early cases of retinitis pigmentosa may show loss of only scotopic function, just as in congenital night blindness; and (2) a few cases of stationary congenital night blindness have definitely abnormal photopic responses also. The reason for this is not known at present. The family history may help clarify the situation, but sometimes only the passage of time will tell if the condition is progressive or not.

The ERG may help in another way in the management of the problem of night blindness. By showing objectively a scotopic defect, it can at least prove that a problem does exist. Occasionally, children complain of night blindness which is not believed by the parents, who feel that the child is simply afraid of the dark or may be malingering. If the child is old enough to do dark adaptation testing, this is another objective technique to demonstrate definite night blindness.

In true *retinitis pigmentosa,* the ERG may make the diagnosis before any functional or fundus changes are noted (Fig. 27–6). This may help in genetic counseling and career planning. The ERG may help distinguish primary from secondary retinal

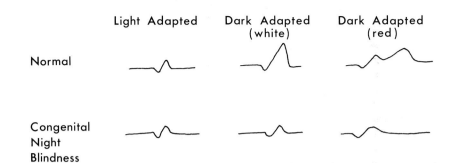

Figure 27–5 Congenital night blindness. ERG shows only a small photopic response to white stimulus even after dark adaptation. With red stimulus, the scotopic b wave is absent.

degeneration, such as may occur in syphilis, trauma, and many febrile illnesses. In primary retinal degeneration, the ERG is usually greatly diminished or even nonrecordable. In the secondary types, the ERG is proportional to the area of retina which is diseased and may be relatively well preserved. Therefore, a fairly good response would rule out primary degeneration. However, the converse is not true; a greatly diminished response does not make the differential diagnosis, because a severe secondary degeneration can also give the same ERG picture.

The ERG may make the diagnosis in the rare type of retinitis pigmentosa in which the typical pigmentation is absent. This condition is called retinitis pigmentosa sine pigmento and is similar to retinitis pigmentosa in almost all other respects. In some cases, the fundus may be almost normal, although usually the vascular narrowing and pallor of the disc are present despite the absence of pigmentation.

In general, the ERG is not of great value in the management of *macular problems*, such as macular degeneration. As explained previously, the ERG is usually quite normal despite a destructive macular lesion. However, some types of macular degeneration are not really localized macular problems but rather only one part of a diffuse retinal degeneration. In these patients, the ERG will be definitely abnormal. There are some families in whom one patient has the typical fundus picture of retinitis pigmentosa and another has a lesion that appears to be only a macular degeneration, Yet, the ERG may look identical, proving widespread retinal disease with different manifestations in the two patients.

In juvenile amaurotic family idiocy

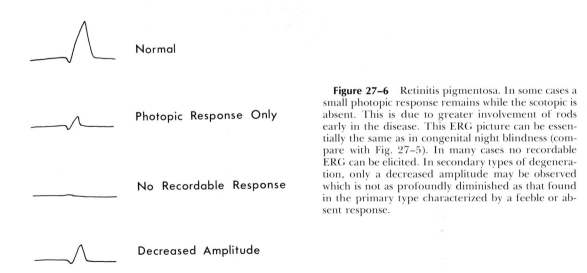

Normal

Photopic Response Only

No Recordable Response

Decreased Amplitude

Figure 27–6 Retinitis pigmentosa. In some cases a small photopic response remains while the scotopic is absent. This is due to greater involvement of rods early in the disease. This ERG picture can be essentially the same as in congenital night blindness (compare with Fig. 27–5). In many cases no recordable ERG can be elicited. In secondary types of degeneration, only a decreased amplitude may be observed which is not as profoundly diminished as that found in the primary type characterized by a feeble or absent response.

(Vogt-Spielmeyer disease), the macula often has a "beaten copper" appearance early in the disease. Later, peripheral changes may also develop, such as pigmentation and narrowed vessels. There is an associated cerebral degeneration. The ERG in this condition is usually decreased and may disappear completely. The pathologic disorder includes not only damage to the optic nerve fibers and ganglion cells, which would not affect the ERG, but also damage to the outer retinal layers. This is in contrast to the infantile form (Tay-Sachs disease), which tends to spare the outer layers, giving a normal ERG despite severe loss of vision.

Visual Evoked Response Technique

One of the most exciting areas of present and future investigation concerns the use of evoked occipital potentials (visual evoked response or VER) in the study of neurological conditions. EEG recordings are made in response to varying types of retinal stimulation, and a computer is needed to help clarify the responses. In humans, scalp electrodes are used, whereas in animals, actual brain electrodes can be inserted, giving a more direct cortical response. The simultaneous recording of the ERG gives added information. Such studies are at present under investigation all over the world, particularly by neurologists and neurophysiologists, but also by ophthalmologists and visual physiologists. Most of these reports are in the EEG or neurology literature, but several can now be found in the ophthalmology journals. This makes it worthwhile for every ophthalmologist to be familiar with the subject.

There are two major aims of this technique: (1) to plot an "objective" visual field by stimulating localized retinal areas and (2) to determine the exact location of lesions of the visual pathway anywhere from the retina to the occipital cortex. An objective visual field test would be especially helpful when dealing with young children as well as uncooperative or comatose patients. Pinpointing a lesion would be useful, for example, in a patient with homonymous hemianopsia, in which several possible sites of lesions could cause similar field defects. It is hoped that characteristic patterns will be found for different locations.

Changes in the evoked occipital response could involve the shape, amplitude, or latency of the waves. Studies to date have not yet defined conclusively the normal and abnormal patterns but are very encouraging for the future.

The VER has also been studied in many other conditions. It may be useful in detecting macular disease not found with the ERG. This is true because of the large cortical area of projection associated with the macula. Amblyopia is another condition which has been studied by this technique.

SUMMARY

The ERG can be helpful in pediatric ophthalmology in many ways. It may prove the presence of retinal dysfunction despite a normal or questionable fundus appearance. It may help make a definitive diagnosis. It may give information of value in prognosis and in genetic counseling. The use of the ERG combined with the VER may be of great future value in the diagnosis of neurological diseases. It must be stressed that the ERG is only one test and must complement a careful history, routine eye examination, and other specialized techniques in order to gain the maximum information.

Finally, the limitations of the ERG must be understood. Although it is an objective test, it still has many limitations and is useless in many conditions. There is good reason to expect that additional technical refinements will overcome many of these problems, so that the ERG will yield even more valuable information in the future.

REFERENCES

Burian, H. M.: Clinical retinography. *In* The Retina. International Ophthalmology Clinics, Vol. 2, No. 1, March, 1962.

Goodman, G., Ripps, H., and Siegel, I.: Electroretinography in infants and children. *In* Diagnostic Procedures in Pediatric Ophthalmology. International Ophthalmology Clinics, Vol. 3, No. 4, December, 1963.

Jacobson, J. H.: Clinical Electroretinography. Springfield, Illinois, Charles C Thomas, 1961.

Jacobson, J. H.: Electroretinography. *In* Pediatric Ophthalmology. Philadelphia, Lea and Febiger, 1964.

CHAPTER 28

THE VISUALLY HANDICAPPED CHILD

REGINA LITTLE LESTER, B. A.

When attempting to present meaningful data about the visually handicapped child, there are two major considerations: First, who are these children by definition; and second, how large a segment of the population do they represent. Although the second question can be dealt with more quickly than the first, the available statistics leave much to be desired.

The National Society for the Prevention of Blindness estimates that in 1969, the *number of* partially seeing children of school age was approximately 100,000. It defines a partially seeing child as one whose best corrected visual acuity falls between 20/70 and 20/200.

The American Printing House for the Blind maintains a national registry of visually handicapped children whose acuity falls between 20/200 and blindness. In 1969, this organization recorded 20,000 children.

The United States Department of Education estimates 63,000 children to be in need of special devices and aids for educational purposes as a result of visual impairment. This seems realistic in view

of the fact that some of the children included in the National Society's statistics would be at the top of the visual acuity scale and may not require special devices.

The question as to the identification of these youngsters and definitive information as to their nonmedical needs is more complex. These data, however, appear in the records of personnel serving them in the fields of *special education, rehabilitation,* and *social service.*

The *eye physician's* role is unique in that, when the child's impairment does respond to surgery or does improve to normal limits with refraction, it is through his skill that the patient maintains his visual status. But when restoration of vision is not immediately possible, it is also his skill that enables him to function as the catalyst for the utilization of any and all services and devices through which the child may realize his optimum potential.

It is with the youngster's need for these services and with the concepts, philosophies, and skills of the professionals in the fields of special education, rehabilitation, and social work that this chapter concerns itself. The ophthalmologist may have to work with the practitioners within any or all of these disciplines in order to bring every available resource to bear on the patient's developmental and educational problems.

THE CHILD WHOSE HANDICAP IS TEMPORARY

If we again refer to the records of the National Society for the Prevention of Blindness, we see that 18 per cent of visual impairment in children results from defects in *muscle function* and about 31 per cent is the result of *anomalies* and *structural defects*. Many of these children, of course, will respond to medical treatment and surgery.

The healing art of the physician must be supplemented by the cooperation of the parents and the child himself. Children respond favorably to frankness. If a child has a detailed outline of what is likely to happen to him in the hospital, the job of coping with this material and the anticipation of events is less traumatic than the fear of the unknown. *Parents* also need to be given information in order that they may help the child understand, because without it, they may transmit their own insecurities to him. This can also be true when treating a child outside the hospital setting. The need to use an eye patch may be far more distressing to the mother than to the wearer. There are many instances of the unwelcome results of withholding important facts. For example, a child who had extensive ophthalmological care proved to be unusually cooperative, but became hysterical following muscle surgery because no one had thought to tell her that both eyes would be bandaged when she awoke.

THE CHILD WHO GAINS OR REGAINS SIGHT

Dr. Valvo gives an interesting report on the behavior patterns of young people who experienced restoration of sight following substantial periods of blindness. These patients suffered periods of depression much as persons who sustain a

visual loss. On the average, it took about a year for them to learn to use their vision efficiently. They had coded their physical surroundings by touch and other *sensory input* and, in a sense, they had to learn to believe what they saw. Much of the *anxiety* which accompanies this adjustment can be cushioned by the understanding of the ophthalmologist and the support of the medical social worker. The parents also need to be acquainted with the situation, since they naturally expect the child to realize instantaneous success with his new-found vision.

THE CHILD WHO IS LOSING SIGHT

Even when a child's vision decreases temporarily, and most certainly if the loss is permanent, he needs to have the facts insofar as he is able to comprehend them. If he is attending school at the time, there are many resources, such as recorded books and special teachers, to help him maintain his normal routine as far as medical management permits.

Accurate information will serve as an

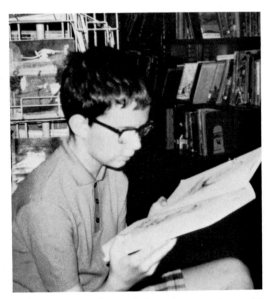

Figure 28–1 Congenital cataract patient with visual acuity of 20/200 reading regular print in grade five. (Photograph taken by Mrs. Bambi Cunningham, Department of Special Education, Delaware County School District, Court House, Media, Pennsylvania.)

impetus for the marshaling of the defenses of the family group and will enable its members to avail themselves of special rehabilitative and supportive services. In situations in which the child's vision fluctuates, as in congenital glaucoma, he may be the victim of considerable anxiety. Psychiatrists indicate that between the ages of 4 and 6, and during the teens, many subconscious fears beset children. The threat of castration and punishment is closely linked to *fear of loss of sight*. It may be necessary for the ophthalmologist to work in concert with a psychiatrist and a medical social worker to help the child through this crisis.

THE CHILD WITH A PERMANENT VISUAL IMPAIRMENT

Without doubt, the child with an impairment that is permanent and irreversible presents to the ophthalmologist the most devastating personal impact. It seems unthinkable that, with all the miracles of medical science at his fingertips, there is no act of his that can change the prognosis. Yet such children, in many respects, represent the best efforts and the most skillful service of the ophthalmologist.

The child's success or failure, and indeed his life style, is in large measure the result of the way in which the physician handles this situation. If he hesitates to tell the parents the facts, their energies and those of the child will be dissipated on concern and conjecture about the unknown, and ultimately will be spent on a useless round of medical shopping. The parents, in the hope that the condition is temporary, will institute stopgap methods for dealing with their own frustrations and the anxieties of the child. The child, in turn, may develop attitudes of dependency and insecurity which will impede his emotional growth. This is the more tragic result, since he needs to get on with the business of refining both a sensory and emotional mechanism which will compensate for his visual loss and enable him to cope with the problems of realizing as much pleasure and productivity as possible from a visually oriented world.

Crucial to the child's successful battle is the understanding of the parents and their total *acceptance* of him as he really is. He is, after all, a person — more like other children than unlike them; capable of love, growth, mischief, and curiosity. In short, he needs to express and develop his personality as does any child. Right at the heart of his chance for success as a human being is the ophthalmologist, with his unique ability to help the child and his parents to understand the extent of the visual loss, the candid facts as to his chances for retaining what vision he has, or the reality of total blindness.

It is true that social workers, psychologists, and psychiatrists can be of great help in offering long-term support and appropriate referral for special services, but they can do nothing unless and until the ophthalmologist paves the way with the solid and unequivocal truth. The professional worker in the field of special education or rehabilitation can attest to the fact that the child and his family who make the best adjustment are the ones with whom the eye physician has dealt in this forthright manner. The youngster who is permitted to exist in an atmosphere of unknown prognosis with uncertain parents, is the one who develops unhealthy attitudes of dependency and helplessness, ultimately producing emotional and physical inertia.

Many times, when the parents finally realize the situation, undesirable behavior patterns have already been established. The doctor who has the courage to state how much the child can see, whether or not the vision is stable, how much he can use his eyes, and how to go about getting special services if they are needed has helped the child take the first positive step toward his successful rehabilitation.

THE ADVENTITIOUSLY HANDICAPPED CHILD

The factor having the most bearing on effective planning for rehabilitation and special education services to the visually handicapped child is the *residual functioning* of his remaining vision. The next most cogent consideration is the age of the child at onset. It is the conviction of most experts that the curriculum and methods for training the adventitiously handicapped child differ greatly from the techniques needed for the training of the congenitally handicapped child.

This dissimilarity is based on the phenomenon of *visual memory*. The usefulness and reliability of visual impression depend, of course, in large part, on the age of the child at the time of visual loss. More will be said later of congenital loss. It suffices to say that the essential difference between the congenitally and the adventitiously handicapped child is the complete lack or limitation of visual orientation and input of visual impression. The child's grasp of three-dimensional concepts, color, and depth are immeasurably enhanced by visual memory. From a counseling and teaching point of view, much effort goes into keeping this memory alive. The child is encouraged to visualize situations and objects too far away for him to see with impaired vision or too remote for him to receive other sensory data. Thus, it is important for him to hold onto visual memories and to build on these experiences. One of the areas in which this is most useful is that of orientation. The adventitiously handicapped child will retain a concept of his relationship to his surroundings, and when he appears to see better than is actually the case, in many instances it is this visual memory bank which is serving him. The child's effective use of this memory bank is strongly affected by the attitudes of parents, friends, and the professional personnel who touch his life.

The extent of *emotional trauma* accompanying the loss of sight is usually relative to whether the loss has been gradual or sudden. The child's coping power will depend upon the degree of acceptance and adjustment the parents are able to achieve. A workable cliché used in the rehabilitation field is that when an individual becomes disabled, he takes his attitudes toward the disability with him. His adjustment will depend upon the extent to which these attitudes can be modified. Certainly, it is natural and generally necessary that a visual loss, particularly a severe one, should be mourned. It is handled by most people, even children, as the death of a loved one is handled — with a point in time when mourning is no longer appropriate. For persons in good emotional health, a return to normal activity is the saving grace. There are always some irreversible changes resulting from an irrevocable loss; just as the loss through death leaves memories that enrich the life experience, so the loss of sight leaves a reservoir to be tapped for the same purpose.

THE CHILD WITH A CONGENITAL ABSENCE OF VISION

What has been said in the foregoing paragraphs is the reverse of the problems of the child born blind or born with an impairment in visual functioning. The one factor common to both groups is parental attitude and acceptance. There are few things as devastating to parents as the knowledge that they have produced a defective child. All the hopes for the perpetuation and fulfillment of their own lives are shattered and there inevitably follows a nagging sense of guilt that in some way they have been punished. Family tension mounts as they focus blame on each other. The unconscious desire to reject the child is in conflict with the certain knowledge that it is their responsibility to love and accept him.

Few, if any, humans can handle this kind of experience successfully without some expert help. The problem is magnified by the fact that there is so much to be done and so little time in which to do it; for if the child is to realize optimum development, his parents will have to initiate the process of adjustment and compensation for him. In order to accomplish this, they need the understanding and knowledge of the ophthalmologist. How much impairment is there? Will the child have any vision? If so, will he keep what he has? Can it be improved? Are there likely to be other impairments such as mental retardation or hearing loss? The answers to these questions are imperative to the parents because they need to know what they have to work with. It will be necessary for the child to have much *sensory stimulation* and input from his environment in order for him to develop a curiosity about the world in which he lives. He will use this to compensate for the lack of sight and to progress as normally as possible.

If there is any vision, he must be encouraged to use it. If not, other ways have to be devised to acquaint him with the three-dimensional world beyond his reach. Above all, he needs to be accepted as a child. He is capable of giving as well as receiving love and he can develop a lively interest in his surroundings if he is made aware of what is out there.

THE TOTALLY BLIND CHILD

The *habilitation of a blind child* begins with the stimulation he receives from his environment. He will not voluntarily reach for toys or other objects. He has to be encouraged to explore. If left to his own devices, he will be very passive and undemanding. Sometimes, to assuage her own guilt feelings, the mother fancies that to keep him in a safe place, such as a playpen or crib, is beneficial to him. If he is a recipient of such over-protection, he will not reach many of the developmental milestones that should be achieved by a blind though otherwise healthy child. It has been said that 85 per cent of all information received by people in our culture is visual. Nowhere does this statement appear to be more accurate than when assessing the problems and developmental lags of these children. Much of what children learn is by imitation and much of this is visual. For example, when a seeing child begins to move about the house, he follows everyone in the family to the bathroom. A blind child does not know the room exists until he is taken there and encouraged to explore. Some children, if kept on baby food too long, will have difficulty learning to chew, and this can then only be accomplished by the child's feeling how the mother's jaws work as she chews. Everything he can learn about his environment will serve to put him more in tune with the world.

He needs to be encouraged to develop *sensory responsiveness.* He may mouth things more than other children do. He needs much more tactual experience than other children. His mother's fear that he might fall and be hurt sometimes prompts her to keep him confined in a safe place, but he will never learn about his world unless he is encouraged to explore it. All

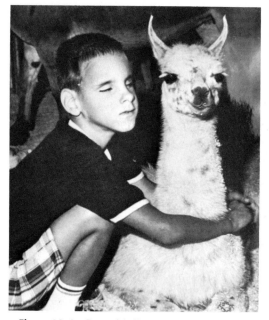

Figure 28–2 Boy with llama. A blind child in the nursery school of this agency is given many and varied experiences, including a trip to the zoo. (Reprinted courtesy of Cleveland Society for the Blind, 1909 East 101st Street, Cleveland, Ohio.)

children fall and hurt themselves in myriad ways and blind children are no exception. "Ring-around-the-rosy" is a good game to teach him about falling down. Sometimes the process of helping him to know about things is a messy one. For example, he needs to handle the food on his plate in order to know where it is coming from and how it gets to the spoon. He will go eventually from finger-feeding to the spoon just as he will progress in other things. Although he should use conventional toys and games, there are some that could have a special meaning and be helpful to him. Finger-painting, even though he can't see it, increases his kinesthetic awareness. Textured things teach him tactual discrimination so valuable in learning to identify articles of clothing and other objects.

Above everything else, he needs to be a part of the family and included in family life. Remember—he can't see a smile, but he learns quickly to identify voices and to interpret tone of voice and body tension. Socializing with every member of the household, especially if there are other youngsters around, will teach him a lot about give and take, as it does all children. If he is not encouraged and stimulated in these ways, the alternative is a nonproductive existence. He will lie in his playpen or crib and rock his body, or bang his head, or develop other mannerisms for lack of environmental stimulation.

The question has often been raised as to whether these children are conscious of a *sensory deprivation* and whether they are not, in a sense, better off than the child who is adventitiously blind. In order for them to become aware of the world in which they live, they have to know that there is a difference between themselves and most other people who inhabit it. Without this awareness, they will not build the skills and defenses needed for coping. The concept of what it is like to have sight is difficult for a blind child to grasp. For example, there were the blind twins who could play hide and seek from each other by the simple means of silence. Their awareness of what having sight means began when they learned they couldn't hide from their mother by the same method. The congenitally blind child faces the emotional impact of his disability the day he has to deal with the fact that there are concepts difficult for him to grasp — like the relative size of a skyscraper — and that it is impossible for him to have all the detailed information that is available to the sighted child because such minutiae are beyond description.

THE CHILD WITH LOW VISION

All the above statements regarding the developmental problems of these children are modified in correlation to the visual functioning of which each is capable, no matter how slight this may be. The happy fact is that very few children are completely without sight; and consequently, only a small number are as sensorially deprived as those discussed in the foregoing section.

In the previously mentioned 1969 registry of the American Printing House for the Blind, only 21 per cent of the children were said to be totally without sight and 79 per cent to have corrected visual acuity ranging from light perception to 20/200. The record yields even more encouraging information: 52 per cent of these children were reading some form of inkprint material. All these children, however, fall within the nationally accepted legal definition of blindness and are therefore eligible for educational facilities and the special services of agencies and schools for the blind.

Until fairly recently, these children have been treated as if they were totally without sight. One of the factors responsible for a change in the method of handling this group of youngsters has been the aroused interest of pediatric ophthalmologists such as Dr. David Hiles of Pittsburgh; and the development of special teaching skills and techniques by educators like Dr. Natalie Barraga. Dr. Hiles states that vision is measurable in the 4-month-old infant. He is, at present, working with members of the staff of special education in the Pittsburgh area toward the development of more reliable ways to assess the visual acuity of children with low vision.

Social workers and teachers are frequently confronted with ophthalmological reports which show the child to be totally blind, when in fact he has *usable functional vision*. Fortunately for these youngsters, the philosophy that a little bit of vision isn't worth evaluating and not much use to them in any case is rapidly becoming extinct. The discipline of rehabilitation counseling can take substantial credit for the change in thinking that has taken place in this regard, for the creed of this professional group holds that one concentrates on what resources an individual possesses, rather than what he has lost or has never had.

A positive approach to the utilization of low vision has begun to produce a measurable body of knowledge which is substantially affecting the delivery of services to children in this category. For one thing, with the growing sophistication in the techniques for teaching mobility, there has come a realization that even light perception can be a very useful tool in orienting an individual to his surroundings. If a child can see a lighted lamp on a desk or an end table or the streetlight outside his bedroom window, his sense of his relationship to space is measurably better than that of a child with no light perception.

In addition to the widely held medical opinion that it does no harm for a low vision patient to use his eyes, there is considerable evidence that their unrestricted use is absolutely necessary for the *maintenance and development of visual functioning.* The special education teachers place considerable emphasis on vision training for all students with any remaining sight, and it is generally believed that the ones having light perception to 8/200 need the most help in this area.

Another observation made by special educators is that the near visual acuity of the low vision child is more germane to the development of good visual functioning for educational purposes than is the distant visual acuity. In low vision children, visual response to stimuli is learned because the visual information is not always reliable and has to be tested and confirmed. In other words, the child must get to know what to look for in order to conceptualize visual impressions. Some ophthalmologists assert that visual acuity is variable according to the mental acuity of the individual. Many special educators agree with the concept of sharpening *visual perception through learning.* Dr.

Barraga maintains that the following steps must occur:

1. Attention
2. Awareness and recognition
3. Response
4. Satisfaction
5. Repetition

She maintains that restriction of any of these hampers visual efficiency. According to her method, visual discrimination takes place with the knowledge that a form exists; then emerge a visual pattern and organization of detail into a recognizable object. The purpose is that if a child can identify an object, he can have meaningful visual experience which will increase his awareness and help him code his environment on his own. The low vision child does not get much satisfaction from seeing. It is possible, however, for his perception to be developed even when the visual patterns are vague and distorted. He then must have stimulation, followed by assurance that his perception is reliable. As a result of this methodology, there are children whose visual acuity was evaluated by the opthalmologist as light or object perception who are now reading, and there is ample evidence to confirm the positive effect of this approach on their total development.

It was previously stated in this chapter that no patient reflects the ophthalmologist's skill more than does the one with a visual handicap. This is especially true with regard to the fitting of *optical aids.* Men like Dr. Gerald Fonda of New York and Dr. Sidney Weiss of Philadelphia have done much to improve the reading skills of these children, particularly as they grow older and the print becomes correspondingly smaller in the school books. The successful fitting of these magnifying devices must be accompanied by adequate follow-up, since the conditions under which the child uses the aid can do much to militate against or build toward its effective use.

A child may make heroic efforts to adjust to the aid with its critical point of focus and its restrictive field, but may be immobilized by the conviction of a teacher that he will lose his precious vision from eyestrain, or he may be discouraged by the school principal's belief that he must wear these glasses at all times. He can also

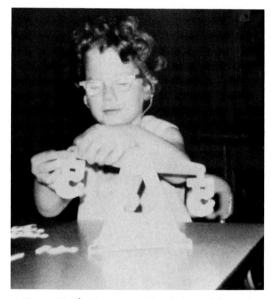

Figure 28–3 Four-year-old rubella child playing with scale. Visual acuity less than 20/200. (Photograph taken by Mrs. Bambi Cunningham, Department of Special Education, Delaware County School District, Court House, Media, Pennsylvania.)

be defeated by inadequate or excessive lighting over his desk at home. These problems, which arise outside the ophthalmologist's office, must be dealt with quickly and in a constructive manner so that the child can be freed to benefit from the optimum use of every modicum of vision he possesses.

THE PARTIALLY SIGHTED CHILD

Children whose visual acuity falls between 20/70 and 20/200 are classified as partially seeing. They do not, as a rule, enjoy the eligibility for special services of agencies for the blind; and, on the other hand, they do not have sufficient vision to drive a car, join the army, or play football. In short, they are neither fish nor fowl, and this confused identity creates many problems for them. Education-wise, they are eligible for special services and equipment. Their needs in this regard may range all the way from large print books to optical aids and special lighting. Certainly, there is no child who needs an understanding ophthalmologist more than does one of these. He is frequently a victim of emotional insecurity and ambivalent feelings because his family, friends, and teachers often try to force him into a pattern of behavior which is incompatible with his visual functioning.

Many times, his ocular disability is not readily apparent to the layman, so that his lack of seeing can be mistaken for stupidity or inattention in school, or snobbishness or indifference if he passes friends on the street and fails to recognize them. Many partially sighted children can see quite well to read if they hold the material close to their eyes. To the adolescent, this can be a source of embarrassment, since it sets him apart from his peers.

The child's dilemma is further compounded by the popular belief of the man in the street that people are either blind or fully sighted. His family tends to believe this also, with the result that he may be over-protected as though he were blind or about to lose his remaining sight; or considered to be somewhat of a fake who uses his poor vision as a dodge for not having a paper route or washing the family car. It is frequently apparent to the ophthalmologist that some intervention is necessary in the best interest of the child, for he has a right to know who and what he is and to develop a realistic self-image.

The fear most frequently voiced by mothers of these children is that they will lose their remaining vision and no one but the ophthalmologist can allay this anxiety. Nor is it wise for the child to develop the habit of relying on his handicap as a crutch. Careful assessment of his visual functioning and an honest effort to answer his questions about his eyes has to be the first step in guiding him toward self-acceptance. The partially seeing child who thinks of himself as blind is in psychological hot water as is the child who denies all deviation from normal and pretends to have 20/20 vision.

THE MULTIPLY HANDICAPPED CHILD

With growing sophistication in the fields of rehabilitation, special education, and social work, the recognition is emerging that *multiply handicapped children* with visual impairment can be helped to realize a measure of satisfaction and achievement. The hard reality of overcrowded and understaffed institutions and the fact that there are not enough resources available to give custodial care to anybody unless absolutely necessary have helped to encourage this recognition. There has been a refinement in the evaluative techniques of psychology and education, as well as medicine, which enables the clinician to be more definitive as to the extent of the involvement stemming from such conditions as congenital rubella, cerebral palsy, and congenital retardation.

One of the difficulties encountered in attempting to develop successful habilitation programs for these children has been the *identification of visual problems*.

In 1960, one of the institutions in Pennsylvania's training school and hospital system for retarded undertook to initiate a program for blind patients. The first survey showed a population of 55 visually handicapped individuals out of the 1500 residents. As the staff became accustomed to making referrals for ophthalmological evaluation, and the eye physician gained experience in working with these patients, the picture changed. By early 1970, the number of patients identified as having severe visual impairment had risen to 300. There is at least one training school in another state which has published the results of a study reflecting similar data.

In view of the foregoing remarks regarding the education of visually handicapped children, the implications are clear enough. If the extent of the child's retardation is in part caused by sensory deprivation, and his visual awareness can be heightened through the methods used to educate visually impaired children, it is likely that his level of functioning will measurably increase. The proof of this is in the fact that one of the children in the Pennsylvania training school, now a young adult, has been returned to the community and is working in a sheltered workshop for the blind. Though not completely self-supporting, he is at least contributing to his own financial maintenance. He is the first blind retarded child to ever leave the institution as "rehabilitated." To find a totally blind child of average intelligence who was committed to an institution for the retarded and who has had many wasted and unproductive years is not an uncommon experience for the practitioner in the field of rehabilitation.

The child with *congenital rubella* represents a great need for good differential evaluation, since problems of hearing impairment or central nervous system damage are in many cases combined with a visual defect. Such a child is frequently described as blind, with no mention of the other disabilities. This is misleading and detrimental to the child's chances for adequate education and social services, since to be effective, any planning for him must take into account the total picture of his liabilities as well as his assets. If a child has a little vision, but is profoundly deaf, then obviously every possible effort must be made to use the residual sight.

Without doubt, one of the most impressive records in work with multiply handicapped youngsters is that of Dr. Louis Cooper of Bellevue Medical Center. Through the work in his clinic for children with congenital rubella syndrome, he has contributed greatly to the understanding of these children and has spearheaded the birth of regional centers for the training and evaluation of *deaf-blind children*, which, strategically placed as they will be, are to serve all 50 states. It must be emphasized, however, that work with the rubella child has been successful only because of the evolution of techniques which deal with the hearing, vision, and brain impairment in combination, and that these methods bear very little, if any, resemblance to the old, established ways of teaching the blind or partially sighted child.

EDUCATIONAL FACILITIES FOR THE VISUALLY HANDICAPPED CHILD

As in every kind of service to human beings, the right educational facility for a child is an individual matter. It must satisfy the expectations of the parents and meet the child's needs as well. In the main, there are two educational systems, and things pro and con can be said of each of them.

The Integrated Program

The first is the *integrated program*, which is a part of the public school system and the only program of special education available to partially sighted children (visual acuity 20/200 to 20/70). It is administered in one of two ways. In some instances, there is a resource room in the school, staffed by a special teacher, where the child goes for the help he requires to modify the effects of his handicapping condition. He attends most classes with his peers, but uses the teacher, the lighting effects, and the equipment of the special room when necessary.

The other method is to have a child attend all regular classes in the public school system. He is visited by an itinerant teacher at regular intervals, who not only assists him with his special problems but acts as consultant to the school faculty. This integrated system is being made increasingly available to blind and low vision children (visual acuity 20/200 or less), and it has many positive aspects. In

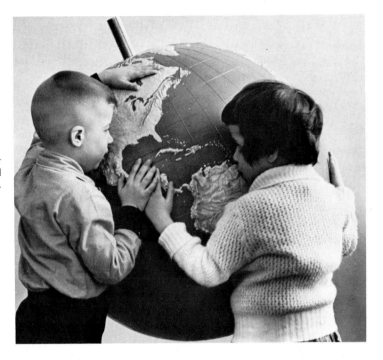

Figure 28–4 Map reading at Lower School, Western Pennsylvania School for the Blind. (Courtesy of Dr. R. D. Harley.)

the first place, the child can live at home, and, if feasible, it is desirable that he do so, since he will then grow up in his own community, where he will probably live, work, marry, and raise a family. If he is accepted by his peers, his social and school life can be a very normal one. If the special education services are adequate, he should be able to compete scholastically according to his innate intelligence and acquired skills, just as does any child.

On the negative side are these factors: Since local school boards are more or less autonomous, much of the policy they set reflects the philosophy of the school officials. As a consequence, the degree of acceptance the child may expect is variable. In one school system, the teachers may

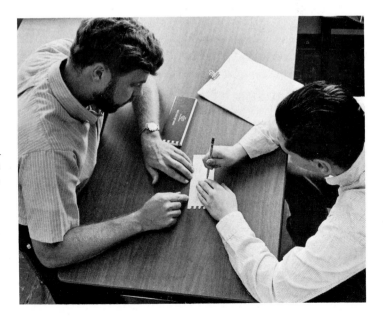

Figure 28–5 Pencil writing in Summer School, Western Pennsylvania School for the Blind. (Charles Martin, Photographer.)

not be thought to have enough time to devote to the special needs of the handicapped child. In another, he may be excluded from all physical education classes or shop training where these restrictions may or may not be realistic. The child who makes it in this system is, generally speaking, one who does not have any secondary handicapping condition, is usually fairly outgoing, and possesses at least a normal amount of aggressiveness. His parents need to be accepting of him and willing to become sufficiently involved to see to it that he gets what he needs.

The Segregated Program

The other method of educating visually handicapped children is one which is available to blind and low vision children — *segregated education* offered through residential or day schools. For many years, the residential schools for the blind were the sole source of education for these youngsters. Originally, the curriculum

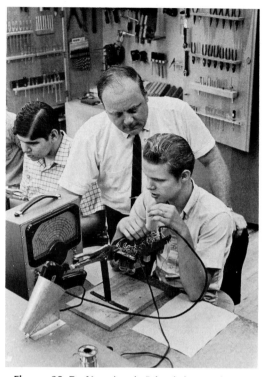

Figure 28–7 Vocational School instruction for electronics, Western Pennsylvania School for the Blind. (Charles Martin, Photographer.)

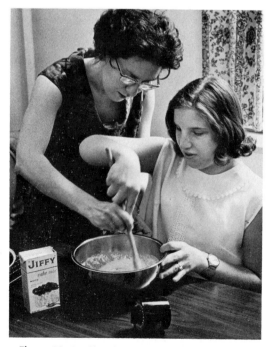

Figure 28–6 Class in Home Economics for cooking instruction, Western Pennsylvania School for the Blind. (Charles Martin, Photographer.)

was restricted; however, by the turn of the century, the picture was beginning to change and for many years these institutions have been accredited schools offering education through the kindergarten, primary, and secondary levels. Their credits are acceptable in any college or university and their graduates have been as successful as have the visually handicapped children graduating from the public school system. In the credit column for the segregated schools, we can place the following items: The classes are small and the teacher is equipped to give a maximum of individual attention to each student. Most of the schools offer intensive training in orientation and mobility (*peripatology*). Almost without exception, the physical education departments are above average and they have excellent programs for helping the child to develop the haptic sense so important to the efficient functioning of blind and low vision people.

On the other hand, their shortcomings

CHART I. LIST OF SPECIAL EDUCATION RESOURCES BY STATE

Alabama

DEPARTMENT OF EDUCATION
64 North Union Street
Montgomery, Alabama   36104

Alaska

DEPARTMENT OF EDUCATION
State Office Building
Juneau, Alaska   99801

Arizona

DIVISION OF SPECIAL EDUCATION
State Capitol
Phoenix, Arizona   85007

Arkansas

DEPARTMENT OF EDUCATION
Division of Instructional Services
Capitol Grounds
Little Rock, Arkansas   72201

California

DEPARTMENT OF EDUCATION
Division of Special Schools and Services
721 Capitol Mall
Sacramento, California   95814

Colorado

DIVISION OF SPECIAL EDUCATION
430 State Office Building
Denver, Colorado   80203

Connecticut

STATE BOARD OF EDUCATION AND
  SERVICES FOR THE BLIND
170 Ridge Road
Wethersfield, Connecticut   06109

Delaware

DEPARTMENT OF PUBLIC INSTRUCTION
P. O. Box 191
Dover, Delaware   19901

District of Columbia

BOARD OF EDUCATION
415 Twelfth Street, N.W.
Washington, D.C.   20004

Florida

DEPARTMENT OF EDUCATION
511 K Street
Tallahassee, Florida   32304

Georgia

DEPARTMENT OF EDUCATION
State Office Building
Atlanta, Georgia   30334

Hawaii

DEPARTMENT OF EDUCATION
Honolulu District Office
1037 South Beretania Street
Honolulu, Hawaii   96814

Idaho

STATE DEPARTMENT OF EDUCATION
Box 1189
Boise, Idaho   83701

Illinois

DEPARTMENT OF SPECIAL EDUCATION
316 South Second Street
Springfield, Illinois   62706

Indiana

DIVISION OF SPECIAL EDUCATION
401 State House
Indianapolis, Indiana   46204

Iowa

DEPARTMENT OF PUBLIC INSTRUCTION
Grimes State Office Building
Des Moines, Iowa   50319

Kansas

DIVISION OF SPECIAL EDUCATION
120 East Tenth Street
Topeka, Kansas   66612

Kentucky

DIVISION OF SPECIAL EDUCATION
State Office Building
Frankfort, Kentucky   40601

Louisiana

DEPARTMENT OF EDUCATION
State Capitol Building
Baton Rouge, Louisiana   70804

Maine

BUREAU OF GUIDANCE, SPECIAL AND
  ADULT EDUCATION
State House
Augusta, Maine   04330

Maryland

DEPARTMENT OF EDUCATION
600 Wyndhurst Avenue
Baltimore, Maryland   21210

Massachusetts

DEPARTMENT OF EDUCATION
182 Tremont Street
Boston, Massachusetts   02111

CHART I. LIST OF SPECIAL EDUCATION RESOURCES BY STATE (Continued)

Michigan

DEPARTMENT OF EDUCATION
Box 20
Lansing, Michigan   48902

Minnesota

DEPARTMENT OF EDUCATION
Centennial Office Building
St. Paul, Minnesota   55101

Mississippi

DEPARTMENT OF EDUCATION
Woolfolk State Office Building
Jackson, Mississippi   39205

Missouri

DEPARTMENT OF EDUCATION
P. O. Box 480
Jefferson City, Missouri   65101

Montana

DIVISION OF SPECIAL EDUCATION
State Capitol Building
Helena, Montana   59601

Nebraska

DEPARTMENT OF EDUCATION
814 Lincoln Building
Tenth and O Streets
Lincoln, Nebraska   68508

Nevada

DEPARTMENT OF EDUCATION
Heroes Memorial Building
Carson City, Nevada   89701

New Hampshire

DEPARTMENT OF EDUCATION
64 North Main Street
Concord, New Hampshire   03301

New Jersey

OFFICE OF SPECIAL EDUCATION
225 West State Street
Trenton, New Jersey   08625

New Mexico

STATE DEPARTMENT OF EDUCATION
P. O. Box 2348
Santa Fe, New Mexico   87501

New York

EDUCATION DEPARTMENT
DIVISION FOR HANDICAPPED CHILDREN
Albany, New York   12224

North Carolina

DEPARTMENT OF PUBLIC INSTRUCTION
P. O. Box 2658
Raleigh, North Carolina   27602

North Dakota

DEPARTMENT OF PUBLIC INSTRUCTION
State Capitol
Bismarck, North Dakota   58501

Ohio

DEPARTMENT OF EDUCATION
DIVISION OF SPECIAL EDUCATION
3201 Alberta Street
Columbus, Ohio   33204

Oklahoma

DIVISION OF SPECIAL EDUCATION
State Capitol Building
Oklahoma City, Oklahoma   73105

Oregon

BOARD OF EDUCATION
313 Public Service Building
Salem, Oregon   97310

Pennsylvania

BUREAU OF SPECIAL EDUCATION
Box 911
Harrisburg, Pennsylvania   17126

Rhode Island

DEPARTMENT OF EDUCATION
1 Washington Avenue
Providence, Rhode Island   02908

South Carolina

DEPARTMENT OF EDUCATION
P. O. Box 1520
Columbia, South Carolina   29202

South Dakota

PUPIL PERSONNEL SERVICES
115 North Grand Street
Pierre, South Dakota   57501

Tennessee

DEPARTMENT OF EDUCATION
134 Cordell Hull Building
Nashville, Tennessee   37219

Texas

TEXAS EDUCATION AGENCY
Capitol Station
Austin, Texas   78711

CHART I. LIST OF SPECIAL EDUCATION RESOURCES BY STATE *(Continued)*

Utah

STATE BOARD OF EDUCATION
136 East South Temple
Salt Lake City, Utah 84114

Vermont

SPECIAL EDUCATION AND PUPIL
 PERSONNEL SERVICES
State Office Building
Montpelier, Vermont 05602

Virginia

STATE BOARD OF EDUCATION
3003 Parkwood Avenue
Richmond, Virginia 23216

Washington

DEPARTMENT OF PUBLIC INSTRUCTION

P. O. Box 537
Olympia, Washington 98501

West Virginia

DEPARTMENT OF EDUCATION
State Capitol Building
Charleston, West Virginia 25305

Wisconsin

DIVISION FOR HANDICAPPED CHILDREN'S
 SERVICE
126 Langdon Street
Madison, Wisconsin 53702

Wyoming

STATE DEPARTMENT OF EDUCATION
State Capitol Building
Cheyenne, Wyoming 82001

---

are that they tend not to develop visual functioning to its optimum, and by the very fact of the institutional living, they tend to create an unreal world for the child, although the better schools recognize this fault and are making efforts to compensate for it. The fact that the child associates exclusively with other blind and visually impaired children can be a mixed blessing. Although it is true that this isolates him from the sighted world in which he must eventually live, it is also true that it exposes him to the competition of other handicapped children with no quarter given. This is the benefit which causes some parents to make use of both systems: to send their child to a residential school long enough for him to acquire haptic and orientation skills, and then transfer him to public school, to what has to be a far more normal climate. The child who is most likely to respond favorably to the segregated system of education is the one whose home does not offer him total acceptance and whose family cannot deal with the special problems which he presents. The child who is withdrawn and insecure can realize some stability from such a setting. If a second handicap is present, the child will receive individual training which would not be available to him to the same degree in the integrated program.

RECREATIONAL AND SOCIAL SERVICES

In concept, much of what has been said about the educational program is also true of *recreational and social services* for the visually handicapped child. There is, as Robert Scott refers to in his book, "The Blindness System." This is a nationwide network of state agencies augmented by a number of private organizations, national and local, offering special services for parents of preschool children through educational and vocational planning for the child in high school. Most of the educational and rehabilitative services are available through state agencies. Many of the agencies for the blind have summer camps, bowling teams, tandem bicycle clubs (with seeing riders from cycling clubs), and other recreational facilities. By and large, these services and facilities are solely for the use of blind and visually impaired people and in this sense, are segregated. If the child is not beset with multiple problems, he can, in many instances, make effective use of the community agencies and organizations serving children with normal vision. There is indeed a growing tendency to meet the needs of the visually handicapped through the resources available to the seeing, and for the staff of the organizations serving only

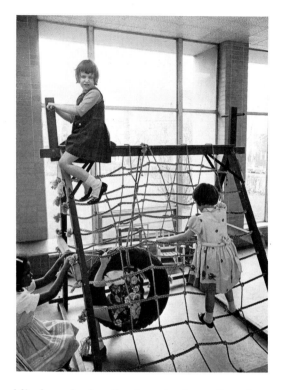

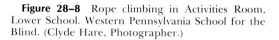

Figure 28–8 Rope climbing in Activities Room, Lower School. Western Pennsylvania School for the Blind. (Clyde Hare, Photographer.)

blind and visually impaired to function as consultants and special resource people. It is true that there are negative aspects to the network of segregated services. Their insularity tends to separate blind persons from the community in which they must live, and some of the regulations would appear to meet the needs of the agencies more adequately than they meet those of the visually impaired person. On the other hand, it is certain that there is contained within the blindness system a body of knowledge and expertise not elsewhere available at the present time.

One very important thing for the oph-

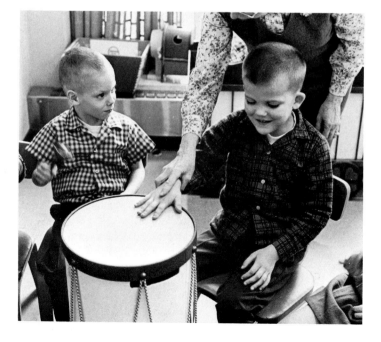

Figure 28–9 Kindergarten students "get rhythm," Western Pennsylvania School for the Blind. (Charles Martin, Photographer.)

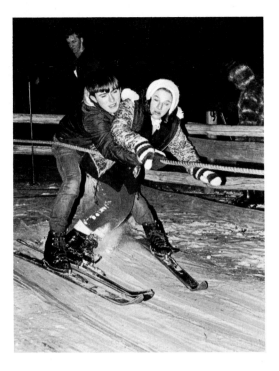

Figure 28–10 Participation in skiing, Western Pennsylvania School for the Blind. (Charles Martin, Photographer.)

thalmologist to know is that special services, other than actual cost for medical care and vocational or college training, are available to all children with a visual loss, regardless of economic circumstances. It would indeed be unfortunate if it were otherwise, since disability is not distributed to the human race according to financial status. The most important decision to be made is what services will best meet the needs of the whole child. His worth as a human being entitles him to the opportunity to go as far as he can in the life experience.

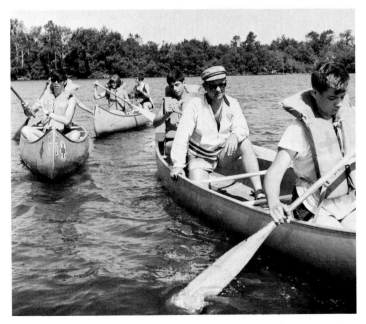

Figure 28–11 Boat handling instruction at Red Cross Training Camp, Western Pennsylvania School for the Blind. (Timothy P. Krikston, Photographer.)

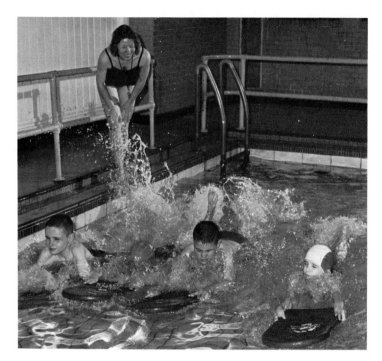

Figure 28–12 Swimming instruction with kickboard at Western Pennsylvania School for the Blind. (Lou Malkin, Photographer.)

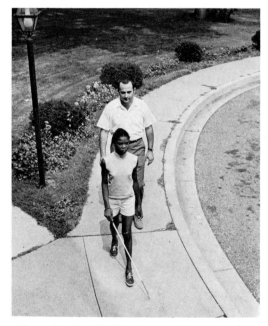

Figure 28–13 Mobility lesson at Summer School, Western Pennsylvania School for the Blind. (Charles Martin, Photographer.)

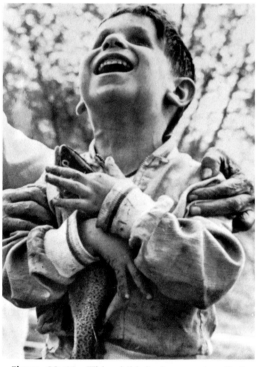

Figure 28–14 This child had never handled a fish and in this photograph had caught his first one. (Reprinted courtesy of the Philadelphia *Evening Bulletin* through the Philadelphia Center for the Blind, 36th and Lancaster Avenue, Philadelphia, Pennsylvania.)

CHART II. LIST OF PUBLIC AGENCIES PROVIDING
PRESCHOOL AND VOCATIONAL COUNSELING SERVICES

Alabama

VOCATIONAL REHABILITATION
2129 East South Boulevard
Montgomery, Alabama 36111

Alaska

OFFICE OF VOCATIONAL REHABILITATION
Pouch F
Alaska Office Building
Juneau, Alaska 99801

Arizona

DIVISION OF REHABILITATION FOR THE
VISUALLY IMPAIRED
Department of Public Welfare
State Office Building
112 North Central Avenue
Phoenix, Arizona 85004

Arkansas

REHABILITATION SERVICES FOR THE
BLIND
900 West Fourth Street
Little Rock, Arkansas 72201

California

DEPARTMENT OF REHABILITATION
714 P Street
Sacramento, California 95814

Colorado

DIVISION OF REHABILITATION
705 State Services Building
Denver, Colorado 80203

Connecticut

BOARD OF EDUCATION AND SERVICES
FOR THE BLIND
170 Ridge Road
Wethersfield, Connecticut 06109

Delaware

DELAWARE COMMISSION FOR THE BLIND
305 West Eighth Street
Wilmington, Delaware 19801

District of Columbia

DEPARTMENT OF VOCATIONAL
REHABILITATION
1331 H Street, N. W.
Washington, D.C. 20005

Florida

DIVISION OF VOCATIONAL
REHABILITATION
Department of Health and Rehabilitation Services
Room 254
725 South Bronough Street
Tallahassee, Florida 32304

Georgia

OFFICE OF REHABILITATION SERVICES
270 State Office Building
Atlanta, Georgia 30334

Hawaii

DIVISION OF VOCATIONAL
REHABILITATION
Department of Social Services
P. O. Box 339
Honolulu, Hawaii 96809

Idaho

IDAHO COMMISSION FOR THE BLIND
State House
Boise, Idaho 83707

Illinois

DIVISION OF VOCATIONAL
REHABILITATION
623 East Adams Street
Springfield, Illinois 62706

Indiana

INDIANA AGENCY FOR THE BLIND
536 West Thirtieth Street
Indianapolis, Indiana 46223

Iowa

COMMISSION FOR THE BLIND
Fourth and Keosauque
Des Moines, Iowa 50309

Kansas

SERVICES FOR THE BLIND
State Department of Social Welfare
State Office Building
Topeka, Kansas 66612

Kentucky

BUREAU OF REHABILITATION SERVICES
State Office Building
High Street
Frankfort, Kentucky 40601

Louisiana

DIVISION FOR THE BLIND
Department of Public Welfare
P. O. Box 44065
Baton Rouge, Louisiana 70804

Maine

DIVISION OF EYE CARE AND SPECIAL
SERVICES
Department of Health and Welfare
State House
Augusta, Maine 04330

CHART II. LIST OF PUBLIC AGENCIES PROVIDING PRESCHOOL AND VOCATIONAL COUNSELING SERVICES *(Continued)*

Maryland

DIVISION OF VOCATIONAL
   REHABILITATION
2100 Guilford Avenue
Baltimore, Maryland   21218

Massachusetts

COMMISSION FOR THE BLIND
39 Boylston Street
Boston, Massachusetts   02116

Michigan

OFFICE OF SERVICES FOR THE BLIND
Department of Social Services
520 Hollister Building
Lansing, Michigan   48913

Minnesota

STATE SERVICES FOR THE BLIND
Department of Public Welfare
Centennial Office Building
St. Paul, Minnesota   55101

Mississippi

VOCATIONAL REHABILITATION FOR
   THE BLIND
528 North State Street
P. O. Box 4872
Jackson, Mississippi   39216

Missouri

BUREAU FOR THE BLIND
Division of Welfare
State Office Building
Jefferson City, Missouri   65101

Montana

DIVISION OF VISUAL SERVICES
State Department of Public Welfare
P. O. Box 1723
Helena, Montana   59601

Nebraska

SERVICES FOR THE VISUALLY IMPAIRED
State Capitol Building
Lincoln, Nebraska   68509

Nevada

SERVICES TO THE BLIND
Department of Health, Welfare, and
   Rehabilitation
311 North Curry Street, Room 113
Carson City, Nevada   89701

New Hampshire

DEPARTMENT OF HEALTH AND WELFARE
State House Annex
Concord, New Hampshire   03301

New Jersey

COMMISSION FOR THE BLIND
1100 Raymond Boulevard
Newark, New Jersey   07102

New Mexico

SERVICES FOR THE BLIND
Social and Rehabilitation Services Division
Department of Health and Social Services
P. O. Box 2348
Santa Fe, New Mexico   87501

New York

COMMISSION FOR THE BLIND AND
   VISUALLY HANDICAPPED
New York State Department of Social Services
1450 Western Avenue
Albany, New York   12203

North Carolina

STATE COMMISSION FOR THE BLIND
410 N. Boylan Avenue
P. O. Box 2658
Raleigh, North Carolina   27602

North Dakota

NORTH DAKOTA DIVISION OF
   VOCATIONAL REHABILITATION
418 East Rosser Avenue
Professional Building
Bismarck, North Dakota   58501

Ohio

BUREAU OF SERVICES FOR THE BLIND
Department of Public Welfare
85 South Washington
Columbus, Ohio   43215

Oklahoma

DIVISION OF REHABILITATION SERVICES
Department of Institutions, Social and
   Rehabilitative Services
P. O. Box 25352
Oklahoma City, Oklahoma   73125

Oregon

STATE COMMISSION FOR THE BLIND
535 S. E. Twelfth Avenue
Portland, Oregon   97214

Pennsylvania

BUREAU OF VISUALLY AND PHYSICALLY
   HANDICAPPED
Office of Family Services
330 Capital Associates Building
P. O. Box 2675
Harrisburg, Pennsylvania   17120

CHART II. LIST OF PUBLIC AGENCIES PROVIDING PRESCHOOL AND VOCATIONAL COUNSELING SERVICES *(Continued)*

Rhode Island

DIVISION OF SERVICES FOR THE BLIND
46 Aborn Street
Providence, Rhode Island   02903

South Carolina

COMMISSION FOR THE BLIND
1400 Main Street
Columbia, South Carolina   29201

South Dakota

SOUTH DAKOTA SERVICE TO THE BLIND
 AND VISUALLY HANDICAPPED
222 East Capitol Avenue
Pierre, South Dakota   57501

Tennessee

SERVICES FOR THE BLIND
Department of Public Welfare
Parkway Towers, Suite 1311
404 James Robertson Parkway
Nashville, Tennessee   37219

Texas

STATE COMMISSION FOR THE BLIND
318 Sam Houston State Office Building
Austin, Texas   78701

Utah

OFFICE OF REHABILITATION SERVICES
1230 University Club Building
136 East South Temple
Salt Lake City, Utah   84111

Vermont

DIVISION FOR THE BLIND AND VISUALLY
 HANDICAPPED
Department of Social Welfare
128 State Street
Montpelier, Vermont   05602

Virginia

VIRGINIA COMMISSION FOR THE VISUALLY
 HANDICAPPED
3003 Parkwood Avenue
Richmond, Virginia   23221

Washington

SERVICES FOR THE BLIND
State Department of Public Assistance
3411 South Alaska Street
Seattle, Washington   98118

West Virginia

DIVISION OF VOCATIONAL
 REHABILITATION
State Capitol Building
Charleston, West Virginia   25305

Wisconsin

DIVISION OF VOCATIONAL
 REHABILITATION
Department of Health and Social Services
1 West Wilson Street, Room 685
Madison, Wisconsin   53702

Wyoming

DIVISION OF VOCATIONAL
 REHABILITATION
State Office Building, Room 305
Cheyenne, Wyoming   82001

CHART III. LIST OF PRIVATE AGENCIES OFFERING SERVICES ON A NATIONWIDE BASIS

American Foundation for the Blind, Inc.
15 West 16th Street
New York, New York   10011

Serves as a national clearinghouse for information about blindness. Promotes the development of educational, rehabilitation and social welfare services.

Conducts and stimulates research to determine the most effective methods of serving visually handicapped persons. Provides professional consultation to governmental and voluntary agencies. Disseminates information on low vision aids and clinics.

Operates a special reference library on blindness and publishes books, monographs, leaflets, and periodicals in conventional print, large type, recorded and braille forms. Develops, manufactures and sells special aids and appliances for use by blind persons.

CHART III. LIST OF PRIVATE AGENCIES OFFERING SERVICES
ON A NATIONWIDE BASIS (Continued)

American Printing House for the Blind, Inc.
1839 Frankfort Avenue
Louisville, Kentucky   40206

National organization for the production of literature and the manufacture of educational aids for the visually handicapped. Provides textbooks and educational aids for all students attending public schools and/or special educational institutions of less than college grade. Publishes braille and talking book editions of the *Reader's Digest*, and a weekly talking book edition of *Newsweek Magazine.*

Publishes braille books, music and magazines; large-type textbooks; talking books and magazines; educational tape recordings. Manufactures special educational aids for blind and visually handicapped persons. Maintains an educational research and development program.

Library of Congress
Division for the Blind and Physically Handicapped
1291 Taylor Street, N. W.
Washington, D.C.   20542

Conducts national program to bring free reading materials of a general nature — classics, current fiction, and non-fiction of the sort available in public libraries — to blind and physically handicapped persons.

Reading materials provided consist of talking books, recorded on microgroove discs and talking book machines; books in braille, large type and on tape. Selects, orders and distributes materials through 42 regional libraries, which function as circulating centers, using the mails to service readers. Materials mailed postage-free.

Provides reference information service on all aspects of blindness and other physical handicaps that affect reading. Conducts national correspondence courses to train sighted persons as braille transcribers and blind persons as braille proofreaders.

National Aid to Visually Handicapped, Inc.
3201 Balboa Street
San Francisco, California

Produces and distributes large-type (18-point) textbooks and leisure reading books to schools, libraries, senior citizen centers, hospitals and individuals on request.

Negotiates to open large-type sections in leading libraries and social centers. Organizes discussion groups for parents of visually handicapped children on coping with effects of the child's impairment.

National Center for Deaf-Blind Youths and Adults
105 Fifth Avenue
New Hyde Park, New York   11040

Serves as a clearinghouse and referral source for persons with combined vision and hearing handicaps.

Coordinates the services of the regional centers for deaf-blind children which provide comprehensive educational and rehabilitative social services.

Conducts an on-going program of public education.

National Society for the Prevention of Blindness, Inc.
70 Madison Avenue
New York, New York   10016

Conducts nationwide prevention of blindness campaigns through mass media and cooperation with medical, educational and industrial and safety organizations.

Sponsors and offers consultation to case-finding programs in glaucoma detection and pre-school children's vision problems.

Supports research on eye disease in hospitals and medical schools and statistical surveys on causes and extent of blindness. Runs public education program including publications, films and legislative activities.

REFERENCES

Barraga, N.: Increased Visual Behavior in Low Vision Children. American Foundation for the Blind, Research Series No. 13, 1964.

Bruner, J. S.: Perceptual readiness. Psych. Rev., *64(2)*:123, March, 1957.

Cholden, L. S.: A Psychiatrist Works with Blindness. American Foundation for the Blind, 1958.

Cooper, L. Z.: Rubella—A Preventable Cause of Birth Defects. National Foundation, March of Dimes, December, 1968.

Cooper, L. Z.: The child with rubella syndrome. New Outlook for the Blind, *63*:10, December, 1969.

Directory of Agencies Serving the Visually Handicapped in the United States. American Foundation for the Blind, 16th ed., 1969.

Fonda, G.: Definition and classification of blindness with respect to ability to use residual vision. New Outlook for the Blind, *55(5)*:169, May, 1961.

Goldberg, M. H., and Swinton, J. R.: Blindness Research: The Expanding Frontiers. A Liberal Studies Perspective. Pennsylvania State University Press, 1969.

Grossman, R.: The Pre-School Child. The Seer of the Pennsylvania Association for the Blind, March, 1970.

Hiles, D. A.: Consideration of Visual Function in Infants and Children. The Seer of the Pennsylvania Association for the Blind, December, 1969.

Hoover, R.: Orientation and travel techniques for the blind. Conference Proceedings of American Association of Workers for the Blind, 1947.

Hoover, R.: The Cane as a Travel Aid. *In* Zahl, P. A. (ed.): Blindness—Modern Approaches to the Unseen Environment. Connecticut, Hafner, 1959.

Kederis, C. J., and Ashcroft, S. C.: The Austin Conference on Utilization of Low Vision. Education of the Visually Handicapped, May, 1970.

Little, R.: Getting the most out of visual aids. New Outlook for the Blind, *59*:4, April, 1965.

National Society for the Prevention of Blindness: 1969 Annual Report.

Ophthalmological Staff of the Hospital for Sick Children, Toronto, Canada: The eye in childhood. The Visually Handicapped Child, 1967.

Salmon, P. J.: Out of the Shadows. National Center for Deaf-Blind Youths and Adults. Regional Demonstration and Research Project, 1962–1969.

Scott, R. A.: The Making of Blind Men: A Study of Adult Socialization. New York, Russell Sage Foundation, 1970.

Shipsey, M., Gibbons, G., and Jahoda, M.: Social and Emotional Aspects on Ophthalmology. Liebman, S. D., and Gellis, S. S. (eds.): The Pediatrician's Ophthalmology. St. Louis, The C. V. Mosby Co., 1966.

United States Office of Education: Statistical Report on Special Needs of Visually Handicapped Children, 1969.

Valvo, A.: The behavior patterns and visual rehabilitation after early and long-lasting blindness. Amer. J. Ophthal., 50th Anniversary Edition, *65(1)*:19, 1968.

Warnick, L.: The effect upon a family of a child with a handicap. New Outlook for the Blind, *63*:10, December, 1969.

Weiss, S.: Aids for partially sighted. Amer. J. Ophthal., *55*:2, February, 1963.

CHAPTER 29

ANESTHESIA IN THE PEDIATRIC PATIENT FOR SURGERY OF THE EYE*

MARTHA HAYDEN DANIS, M.D.

Most surgical procedures in pediatric ophthalmology will require general anesthesia. The patient should be in excellent physical condition because the procedures are usually elective.

Patients for elective endotracheal anesthesia should be free of infection for at least three weeks prior to surgery and have a minimal hemoglobin value of 10 grams or a hematocrit of 32. Although hemorrhage is very rare in pediatric ophthalmology, there is an increased risk for the anemic patient if hypoxia unexpectedly occurs. A rectal temperature greater than 38° C., or 100.4° F. is a contraindication to elective surgery.

*Photographs provided through the courtesy of Bernard Mayer, M.D.

PREANESTHETIC EVALUATION

A knowledge of the anesthetic requirements for a particular surgical procedure is essential for good anesthetic management. However, an important factor in the anesthetic management is the preanesthetic evaluation of the patient undertaken by the anesthesiologist personally. For the pediatric patient it is of inestimable value if the preoperative visit occurs when the patient and parents are together. This visit gives the anesthetist the opportunity to transform himself from a stranger into a friend to the young patient. Questions may be answered and the fears of both relieved. In general, the explanations should be simple, brief, and truthful.

The parents and the older child are

questioned regarding (1) recent upper respiratory infections, (2) loose teeth, (3) previous anesthetics, (4) current and past medications, (5) drug reactions, (6) allergies, (7) wheezing episodes or asthmatic attacks, (8) bleeding tendencies, and (9) any familial history of problems associated with anesthesia.

Prior to emergency surgery, parents should be asked when and what the child last ate. However, regardless of the answer, the anesthetist should assume a possible full stomach and take appropriate measures.

Loose teeth should be carefully evaluated. They may be dislodged spontaneously or during the insertion of an airway or endotracheal tube. The parent and child should be informed of this possibility and the probable removal of the tooth. The tooth will be returned to the patient. If the tooth does become dislodged and cannot

be located, a chest film is taken to rule out aspiration.

All cases for general anesthesia require a recorded history and physical examination. Laboratory tests required prior to anesthesia include a hemoglobin or hematocrit determination, a white cell count, and a urinalysis. Patients with cardiopulmonary or metabolic disturbances require a rather complete pediatric evaluation.

Airway patency should be evaluated prior to sedation. For example, enlarged tonsils and adenoids, nares filled with secretions, or a hypodeveloped mandible may lead to upper airway obstruction after sedation.

In recent years, *echothiopate iodide* (Phospholine iodide) has been used in the treatment of chronic glaucoma and accommodative esotropia. This drug has an inhibitory effect on both true (red cell and brain) and pseudo (plasma and liver) cholinesterase in

TABLE 29–1 PEDIATRIC DISORDERS IN WHICH ANESTHETIC DIFFICULTIES SHOULD BE ANTICIPATED

Disease or Syndrome	Problem

Pierre Robin and Treacher-Collins syndromes
  Down's syndrome (mongolism)
  Hypothyroid
  Hurler's syndrome or gargoylism
  Hunter's syndrome
  Acrocephalosyndactyly (Apert's syndrome)
  Klippel-Feil syndrome
  Torticollis
  Hydrocephalus
  Cervical fusion
	Difficult intubation and upper airway obstruction when unconscious

13–15 Trisomy	Difficult intubation
Encephalo-trigeminal angiomatosis (Sturge-Weber syndrome)	Manipulation of hypopharynx, larynx, and trachea may produce hemorrhage
Lipoid storage disorders (Niemann-Pick disease, Gaucher's disease)	Lymphoid hyperplasia may be marked in the hypopharynx, producing airway obstruction under heavy sedation or postoperatively

Glycogen storage disease
  (Glucose-6-phosphatase deficiency,
  von Gierke's disease)
	Metabolic acidosis may develop in the absence of supplemental glucose; macroglossia may cause difficult intubation

Cystic fibrosis	Ventilatory difficulty with stormy anesthetic course
Familial dysautonomia (Riley-Day syndrome)	Unstable circulatory system
Amyotonia congenita, Dystrophia myotonica	Severe muscle spasm after succinylcholine; hyperpyrexia
Atypical pseudocholinesterase	Prolonged apnea after use of succinylcholine
Myasthenia gravis	Prolonged neuromuscular blockade may occur with muscle relaxants; postoperative depression of respirations and cough reflex
Phenylpyruvic oligophrenia (Phenylketonuria)	Severe hypoglycemic episodes may occur if glucose is withheld for a prolonged period
Acute porphyria	Sensitivity to barbiturates

man in vivo and in vito. The ophthalmic form begins to effect cholinesterase activity within several days. By the third week, profound depression occurs and will persist as long as therapy is continued. After the drug is discontinued, plasma cholinesterase levels return to normal in about three weeks, the red cell cholinesterase in about 120 days. Succinylcholine, a muscle relaxant used to facilitate intubation in many eye patients, is hydrolyzed by pseudocholinesterase. Several cases of prolonged apnea have been reported in patients undergoing eye surgery after the use of succinylcholine. Intubation is accomplished without the aid of the relaxant, succinylcholine, if a patient has been or is on echothiophate therapy.

PREOPERATIVE MEDICATION

Numerous drugs in various combinations have been employed in children for preanesthetic sedation. In our clinic we emphasized the preoperative visit by the anesthesiologist and for the past several years have used a combination of pentobarbital-hydroxyzine-atropine as the premedicant drugs. Emotional upsets regarding anesthesia and surgery rarely occur if the child and parents are calm, cheerful, and confident. We prefer a calm child who will awaken shortly after the surgical procedure and promptly resume oral fluid intake. If heavier medication is required, we add a narcotic drug. Heavy sedation requires

careful observation for longer periods. Even with careful evaluation, there will be an occasional child who is apprehensive or one sedated to the state of unconsciousness and with compromise of the airway.

Of the belladonna derivatives, we prefer atropine for its more effective abolition of vagal reflexes. If halothane is the major anesthetic drug, atropine can be eliminated from the preanesthetic sedation in most patients and be given intravenously in the operating room after the child is asleep, thereby eliminating a "shot."

Atropine as part of the anesthetic regime is not contraindicated in patients with glaucoma; the dosage for premedication is far less than that used for eye drops. The ophthalmologist should be aware that 1 ml. of 1 per cent atropine contains 10 mg. and that one drop in an eye offers 0.6 mg. of atropine for absorption. Patients with Down's syndrome have increased sensitivity of the peripheral cardiovagal receptors and a smaller dose of atropine is usually given to these patients.

Necessary steps are taken to assure that medications which the patient may have been receiving, such as anticonvulsive medications, steroids, and digitalis, incur little interruption in their dose schedule because of the surgery.

Fluid restriction is necessary but should be minimal in the pediatric patient undergoing anesthesia. No solids, milk, or milk products are given for at least 8 hours prior to the induction of anesthesia. Clear liquids are given up to 4 hours prior to in-

TABLE 29–2 PREANESTHETIC MEDICATION

Age in Years	Drugs
0 to 1	Atropine only
1 to 2	Atropine + Pentobarbital
	or
Over 2	Atropine + Pentobarbital + Hydroxyzine

Dosage	
Atropine: 0.02 mg. per kg.	Minimum 0.15 mg.; maximum 0.4 mg.
Hydroxyzine: 1.0 mg. per kg.	Maximum 50 mg.
Pentobarbital: 3.0 to 4.0 mg. per kg.	Maximum 100 mg.
Meperidine: 1.0 to 2.0 mg. per kg.	Maximum 100 mg.
Morphine: 0.05 to 0.10 mg. per kg.	Maximum 10 mg.

Time: 1 to 1¼ hours prior to surgery
Route: Intramuscular

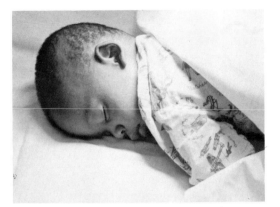

Figure 29–1 Child arrives in operating room asleep.

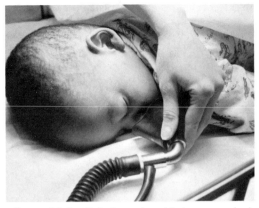

Figure 29–3 Halothane is added to anesthetic mixture and mask is brought closer to face.

duction in infants from newborn to age six months; 6 hours prior to induction from six months to three years; and 8 hours prior to induction in children over three years of age. Children scheduled for afternoon surgery are given clear liquids in the morning 4 to 6 hours prior to the scheduled operating time. (See Figs. 29–1 to 29–7.)

OPERATIVE MANAGEMENT

Many different anesthetic agents and techniques have been utilized for eye surgery in children. The majority of eye procedures in our clinic are managed with halothane-nitrous oxide-oxygen via a non-rebreathing system. These agents provide a smooth induction, satisfactory analgesia, and relaxation for the surgical procedure and a rapid recovery period. Some short procedures can be well managed with a mask or a Water's airway.

Ketamine

Ketamine, a recently approved drug which can be administered intravenously or intramuscularly, produces a peculiar state of unconsciousness with good analgesia. It has been extremely useful in short procedures such as examinations, probings of the lacrimal duct, removal of chalazia, which do not require skeletal muscle relaxation and obtunded pharyngeal and laryngeal reflexes. The drug, however, has two major disadvantages: (1) The recovery period is directly proportional to the amount of ketamine used during the procedure; long procedures with ketamine

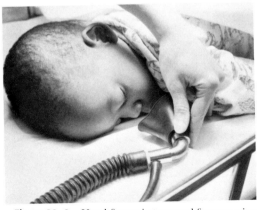

Figure 29–2 Head frame is removed from carrier. Without disturbing patient, high flows of nitrous oxide and oxygen are given through mask.

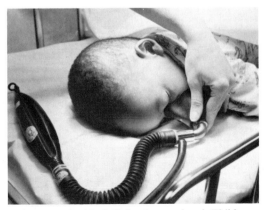

Figure 29–4 Mask fitting is completed. Child may be moved to operating table without waking.

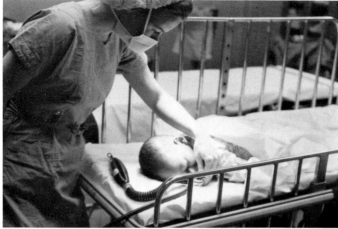

Figure 29-5

Figures 29-5 to 29-7 Successive stages of movement to operating table.

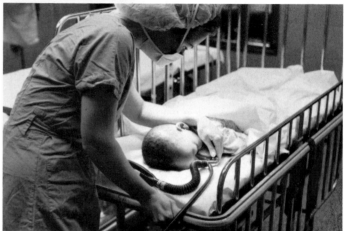

Figure 29-6

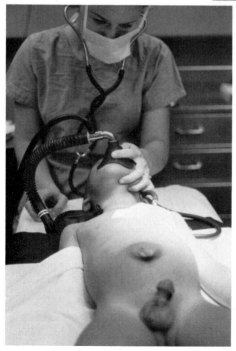

Figure 29-7

will have a prolonged recovery period. (2) Hallucinations are associated with its use in adults but appear to be negligible in children under 14. We have not experienced this problem with this agent in our clinic; we let our patients awaken quietly without stimulation in a quiet recovery room.

Most major eye procedures are best managed with endotracheal anesthesia. The advantages of intubation are (1) the patency of the airway is reasonably assured, (2) secretions can be easily removed from the tracheobronchial tree, (3) positive pressure can be applied without inflating the stomach, and (4) the anesthetist can be situated away from the operative site and still maintain control of the ventilation.

The major complication of endotracheal intubation is postoperative laryngeal or subglottic edema. This may be manifested by hoarseness or croupy cough and stridor and may progress to suprasternal retractions in the recovery room. These patients are placed in humidity tents and/or given dexamethasone intravenously or intramuscularly in doses of 2 to 4 mg. under one year and 4 to 8 mg. in older children. I believe that the safety of endotracheal anesthesia for eye surgery outweighs the complications that may occur from its use in the pediatric patient.

Monitoring in the operating room always consists of a precordial stethoscope. Most patients are also monitored with a blood pressure apparatus and a rectal thermistor probe for continuous measurement of temperature. In recent years there have been many reports in the literature of the occurrence of a sudden, abrupt, unexplained rise in body temperature during the administration of general anesthesia. It is most likely to occur in children over two years of age and in young adults. The mortality is about 70 per cent. This dread complication of general anesthesia can be most easily recognized by the continuous monitoring of the body temperature.

An intravenous route is established in all major procedures and any procedure in the infant.

Patients who come to the operating room asleep are "stolen" from the stretcher by gradually introducing nitrous oxide-halothane-oxygen via a bag and mask. If the patient is awake, he is quietly reassured

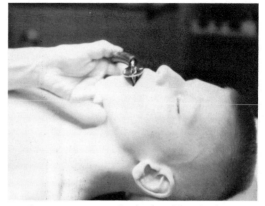

Figure 29–8   Anesthesia via a Water's airway.

and distracted, so that the mask can be lowered gradually to his face. In either instance, a quiet operating room is essential. *Succinylcholine,* 0.5 to 1 mg. per pound of body weight, is given intravenously to facilitate intubation. Nitrous oxide-halothane-oxygen is used for maintenance with assisted or controlled respirations. (See Figs. 29–8 to 29–12.)

In ocular muscle surgery there have been instances in which traction on the rectus muscles, particularly the medial rectus, has produced bradycardia probably due to an oculocardiac reflex. This may be alleviated by the use of adequate atropine preoperatively or with intravenous atropine when it occurs.

In intraocular procedures the possibility of losing the vitreous is of concern to the anesthesiologist. Any coughing, sneezing, straining, or laryngospasm must be pre-

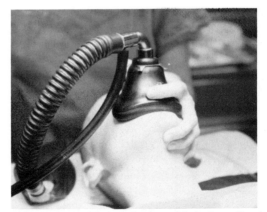

Figure 29–9   Mask induction with Jackson Rees' modification of Ayre's T piece.

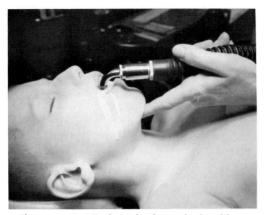

Figure 29–10 Endotracheal anesthesia with anesthetist supporting chin and apparatus.

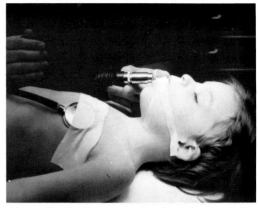

Figure 29–11 Side view of endotracheal anesthesia. Note patient's head in "donut," precordial stethoscope in place, and anesthetist's hand supporting or controlling ventilation.

vented during the induction, maintenance, and extubation. Succinylcholine causes a transient rise in intraocular pressure probably by the contracture of the extraocular muscles. Whether this is a contraindication in glaucoma surgery seems debatable. It has been shown that small doses of gallamine or *d*-tubocurarine infused intravenously 3 or more minutes prior to the dose of succinylcholine will prevent an increase in intraocular pressure. We do not use succinylcholine in penetrating injuries of the globe.

After the surgery is completed, the patient's mouth is suctioned. A catheter is passed through the endotracheal tube if secretions are present. The endotracheal tube is removed when spontaneous respirations are adequate. Rarely do we remove the endotracheal tube prior to the return of pharyngeal and laryngeal reflexes except in intraocular procedures.

Forced duction maneuvers may be altered during the initial phase of succinylcholine injection.

POSTANESTHETIC RECOVERY

After the completion of surgery, all patients are returned to the recovery room for constant observation of ventilation, circulation, and possible anesthetic complications. The patient's vital signs and temperature are monitored. Patients are closely observed for signs and symptoms of laryngeal edema and an increase or decrease in temperature. Appropriate therapy in each case is instituted promptly.

A major hazard of anesthesia during induction and recovery is vomiting with aspiration. If pulmonary aspiration occurs, the patient is placed in Trendelenburg

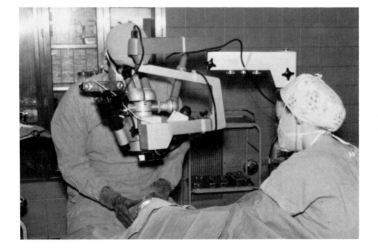

Figure 29–12 Patient draped for surgery, with the surgeon using a microscope.

TABLE 29-3   PEDIATRIC OROTRACHEAL TUBE SPECIFICATIONS

Age	French Size	Internal Diameter (mm.)	Length (cm.)	15-mm. Male Connector Size
Newborn to 1 year	12–18	2.5–4.0	10–12	3–5
1 to 2 years	18–22	4.0–5.5	12–14	5–6
2 to 4 years	22–24	5.5–6.0	14–16	6
4 to 6 years	24–26	6.0–6.5	16–18	7
6 to 8 years	26–28	6.5–7.0	18	7
8 to 10 years	28–30	7.0–7.5	18	8
10 to 12 years	30–32	7.5–8.0	20	8
12 and over	32	8.0	22	8

position and the mouth is suctioned. The trachea is intubated and the patient is ventilated with oxygen. The ability to suction through the endotracheal tube may suffer, but if aspiration of particulate matter is suspected, bronchoscopy is necessary. Systemic steroids seem to decrease the inflammatory reaction when given promptly.

When the patient is fully reacted, has a normal temperature, and his airway can be sustained, he is returned to his ward.

RESUSCITATION

Effective respiration and circulation may cease at any time during the induction, maintenance, and recovery from anesthesia and surgery. Circulatory arrest, for practical purposes, occurs when an effective blood pressure is no longer available to perfuse the myocardium and body tissues adequately. This may occur with asystole, ventricular fibrillation, or arterial hypotension. Cardiac arrest in the operating room in the pediatric ophthalmic patient will almost always be the result of a relative anesthetic overdosage or hypoxia or both. Respiratory arrest may be caused by airway obstruction, central nervous system depression, or neuromuscular paralysis.

The signs of respiratory arrest are cyanosis and apnea. The signs of circulatory arrest are the absence of precordial beats, peripheral pulses, and blood pressure. If circulatory arrest is suspected, one proceeds immediately to oxygenation and external cardiac massage.

Regardless of the cause or type of arrest,

the immediate treatment is (1) to establish an airway and ventilate with oxygen; (2) to restore effective circulation with compression of the heart to empty the ventricles, alternating with periods of relaxation to allow refilling; and (3) to start correction of the hypovolemia, if it exists, and correction of the metabolic acidosis which develops rapidly after cardiac arrest.

Ventilation

Adequate lung inflation for resuscitation may be accomplished by mouth-to-mouth, mouth-to-tube, or bag and mask or tube devices. Needless to say, speed is of utmost importance. Whatever can be done quickly and effectively should be the determining factor. Vomitus and secretions must be aspirated from the oral cavity while the patient's head is extended and the mandible held forward and upward. In the operating room, the airway can probably be best secured by an endotracheal tube. It is rare in the newborn that ventilation other than by endotracheal route can be long maintained because of the gastric distention produced during positive pressure ventilation. The lungs should be inflated rapidly between every four to five cardiac compressions.

External Cardiac Massage

All patients for external cardiac compression should have a rigid board placed underneath them.

Newborn and Small Infants. The midsternum is compressed with superimposed thumbs while the fingers are linked behind the patient for additional support. Lung ventilation by mouth-to-mouth res-

TABLE 29–4   DRUGS FOR RESUSCITATION

Drug	Concentration Used	I.V. Dose	Intracardiac Dose
Sodium Bicarbonate	0.88 mEq./ml.	2.0 to 4.0 mEq./kg.	2.0 mEq./kg.
Epinephrine	1:1000 (1 mg./cc.) diluted to 1:100,000 (0.1 mg./ml.)	0.01 mg./kg.; up to 0.5 mg.	0.005 to 0.010 mg./kg. 0.01 to 0.05 mg./kg.
Isoproterenol	1:5000 (0.2 mg./ml.) or dilute 0.2 mg./ml. to 20 ml.	0.1 ml. (0.02 mg.) 1 to 2 cc. continuous infusion of 0.8 to 1.0 mg. in 250 ml. isotonic solution	0.1 ml. (0.02 mg.) 1 to 2 cc.

piration can be administered by the same operator.

OLDER CHILDREN.   The heel of the left hand is applied over the heel of the right hand over the sternum opposite the fourth interspace. The compression rate in infants is usually about 80 to 100 compressions per minute and in children, approximately 60 to 80 per minute. When the ventilation and cardiac compression are effective, drug therapy should be instituted.

With effective ventilation and cardiac massage, the femoral pulses will become palpable, the pupils will constrict, and the patient's color will improve.

An electrocardiogram for monitoring is attached as quickly as possible after the diagnosis of cardiac arrest is made. If cardiac massage, ventilation with oxygen, and administration of sodium bicarbonate intravenously has not restored an effective circulation, isoproterenol or epinephrine should be injected into the heart.

If the patient is in ventricular fibrillation, external defibrillation can be achieved with shocks of 100 watt-seconds in infants, 200 to 300 watt-seconds in children, and 400 watt-seconds in adults.

The immediate resuscitation must be followed with continuous monitoring of the arterial pressure, electrocardiogram, and blood gases. Successful resuscitation results from coordinated teamwork between the surgical and anesthetic services and each must know how to treat this unfortunate occurrence.

REFERENCES

Bosomworth, P. P., Ziegler, C. H., and Jacoby, J.: The oculocardiac reflex in eye muscle surgery. Anesthesiology, *19*:7, 1958.

Deming, M. V., and Oech, S. R.: Steroid and antihistaminic therapy for post intubation subglottic edema in infants and children. Anesthesiology, *22*:933, 1961.

Gesztes, T.: Prolonged apnea after suxamethonium injection associated with eye drops containing an anticholinesterase agent. Brit. J. Anaesth., *38*:408, 1966.

Harris, W. S., and Goodman, R. M.: Hyperreactivity to atropine in Down's syndrome. New Eng. J. Med., *279*:407, 1968.

Humphreys, J. A., and Holmes, J. H.: Systemic effects produced by echothiophate iodide in treatment of glaucoma. Arch. Ophthal., *69*:737, 1963.

Miller, R. A., Way, W., and Hickey, R.: Inhibition of succinylcholine induced increased intraocular pressure by non-depolarizing muscle relaxants. Anesthesiology, *29*:123, 1968.

Pantuck, E. J.: Echothiophate iodide eye drops and prolonged response to suxamethonium. Brit. J. Anaesth., *38*:406, 1966.

Relton, J. E. S., Creighton, R. E., Johnston, A. E., Pelton, D. A., and Conn, A. W.: Hyperpyrexia in association with general anesthesia in children. Canad. Anaesth. Soc. J., *13*:419, 1966.

Rozen, D. A.: Anaesthesia in ophthalmology. Canad. Anaesth. Soc. J., *9*:545, 1962.

Schwartz, H., and de Roetth, A.: Effect of succinylcholine on intraocular pressure in human beings. Anesthesiology, *19*:112, 1958.

Taylor, T. H. Mulcahy, M., and Nightingale, D. A.: Suxamethonium chloride in intraocular surgery. Brit. J. Anaesth., *40*:113, 1968.

Thaler, M. M., and Stobie, G. H. C.: An improved technic for external cardiac compression in infants and children. New Eng. J. Med., *269*:606, 1963.

Vandam, L. D.: Aspiration of gastric contents in operative period. New Eng. J. Med., *273*:1206, 1965.

OCULAR CHANGES IN SKIN DISORDERS

CHAPTER 30

CARROLL F. BURGOON, JR., M.D.,
and JEAN-PIERRE COLLINS, M.D.

The common embryologic origin of the skin and some structures of the eye from the ectoderm accounts for the many congenital syndromes in which there are parallel eye and cutaneous changes. The skin of the eyelids is anatomically different from other areas of the skin but shares their reactivity, although involvement of the skin of the eyelids frequently results in distinctive changes. Eyebrows and lashes may be involved equally in diseases of the pilar structures of the scalp and beard area but may also be involved alone. The cornea and conjunctiva share with the skin the problems of direct exposure to environmental factors.

In this chapter we take advantage of the presence of cutaneous signs as an aid in evaluation of ocular changes. In many instances, examination of the skin will provide a diagnostic clue when the eye involvement alone may not be diagnostic. Our purpose is to provide a guide for the differential diagnosis of those diseases of the eyes of children in which associated skin diseases may be present. The diseases of the skin are grouped for easy reference according to the anatomic location of the eye involvement (Table 30–1).

CONJUNCTIVA AND CORNEA

The diseases to be discussed are those in which the cornea, alone or in combination with other anatomic sites of the eye, may be involved.

Angiokeratoma Corporis Diffusum

Angiokeratoma corporis diffusum is a systemic disorder inherited as an incomplete recessive, sex-linked trait and is characterized by an extensive deposit of a neutral glycolipid, ceramide trihexoside, in many different cells of the body.

The dermatologic manifestation consists of a diagnostic eruption which appears on the skin and oral mucosa between 7 and 13 years of age and is associated with incapacitating pain in the fingers and toes. The small, bluish-black, maculopapular lesions, which measure 3 to 4 mm. in diameter, are distributed primarily between the knees and the umbilicus. Most affected males die in their early thirties as the result of vascular and renal involvement which results in hypertension and renal failure.

Ophthalmic findings consist of characteristic superficial spokelike corneal opacities,

861

cataracts, and tortuosity and dilatation of retinal vessels.

Anhidrotic Ectodermal Dysplasia

Anhidrotic ectodermal dysplasia, a syndrome genetically transmitted as an incomplete recessive X-linked gene, is characterized by partial or complete absence of sweat glands, hypotrichosis, and hypo- or anodontia.

The dermatologic manifestations in the complete syndrome consist of a distinctive prematurely aged appearance with fine sparse scalp hair, saddle nose, prominent frontal eminence chin, and anodontia. Absence of eccrine sweat glands results in poor heat adaptation.

Ophthalmic manifestations are not the rule, although corneal and lenticular opacities have been reported. Eyebrows may be sparse or absent, but the lashes are usually normal.

Atopic Dermatitis (see Chapter 20)

Atopy is a genetically determined predisposition to develop asthma, hay fever, or atopic dermatitis in the presence of reagin type antibodies (immunoglobulin E).

The cutaneous manifestations of atopic dermatitis depend on the interplay of numerous constitutional and varied precipitating factors. The cutaneous changes may be divided into infantile, childhood, and adult phases, based on variation in cutaneous morphology. The infantile phase usually appears by the second month of life and consists of a papulovesicular eruption involving, in part or entirely, the trunk, extremities, and face. In the childhood and adult phases, there is a characteristic distribution and morphology which consists of lichenified and excoriated patches distributed on the flexural surfaces of the arms, legs, and nuchal area.

Cataracts may be associated with the atopic dermatitis seen in adults, but they occur less commonly in children. The dermatitis precedes the cataract by 10 years. The cataracts are characterized by radiating opacities in the anterior cortex or a dense white plaque in the posterior cortex. They mature rapidly and are usually bilateral. Keratoconus also occurs but is rare. Involvement of the periorbital skin with erythema, scaling, lichenification, and loss of eyebrows may occur.

Congenital Syphilis

Congenital syphilis is a transplacental infection of the fetus caused by *T. pallidum* after the third month of gestation.

Congenital syphilis is divided clinically into three categories: early, late, and stigmata. The skin and mucous membrane involvement in early congenital syphilis consists of papulosquamous lesions similar to those seen in acquired syphilis, although rarely vesiculobullous lesions may occur on the palms and soles. Osteochondritis, splenomegaly, and hepatomegaly are commonly present.

In late congenital syphilis (after 2 years of age) approximately 60 per cent of the patients have a reactive serologic test for syphilis as the only evidence of past infection. The remainder may have skin lesions (gummas) similar to those seen with late acquired syphilis.

The stigmata of congenital syphilis include Hutchinson's triad of eighth nerve deafness, interstitial keratitis, and Hutchinson's teeth. In addition, mulberry molars, Clutton's joint (synovitis of knee joint), saddle nose, characteristic facial changes, scaphoid scapula, and high palatine arch may be present.

The ophthalmic manifestation most commonly seen is interstitial keratitis, which usually appears between age 3 and puberty. In addition, chorioretinitis and optic atrophy may be seen as late evidence of the infection.

Cutis Laxa (Primary Elastolysis)

Cutis laxa is probably a genetically acquired abnormality of elastic tissue characterized by laxity of the skin and underlying connective tissue. The disorder is divided into congenital and acquired forms.

The dermatologic manifestations of the congenital variety are abnormal wrinkling and sagging of the skin in the newborn which produce a senile appearance. In the acquired form, the disorder is localized to one area of the skin.

Ophthalmic involvement is unusual, although eyelid laxity and bilateral corneal dystrophy have been reported.

Dyskeratosis Congenita

Dyskeratosis congenita is a rare, congenital disorder, probably transmitted by a partial sex-limited recessive gene,

TABLE 30–1 OCULAR CHANGES IN SKIN DISEASES

	Cornea	Lens	Periorbital Area (Eyebrows, Lashes, Eyelids)	Conjunctiva, Sclera	Retina
Acne rosacea	+		+	+	
Albinism			+		+
Albright's syndrome				+	+
Allergic contact dermatitis			+	+	
Alopecia areata		+	+		
Alopecia areata universalis		+	+		
Alopecia mucinosa			+		
Angiokeratoma corporis diffusum	+	+			+
Anhidrotic ectodermal dysplasia	+	+			
Atopic dermatitis	+	+	+	+	
Atrichia congenita			+		
Basal cell carcinoma			+	+	
Behçet's syndrome				+	+
Blue nevus of Ota				+	
Bonnet-Dechaume-Blanc syndrome				+	+
Chediak-Higashi syndrome					+
Cockayne's syndrome					+
Congenital syphilis	+				+
Conradi's syndrome		+			
Cornelia de Lange syndrome			+		+
Cutis laxa	+		+		
Diabetes mellitus		+			+
Dinitrophenol		+			
Dyskeratosis congenita	+		+	+	
Dysostosis—Mandibulofacial		+	+		
Eczematous dermatitis				+	
Eczema vaccinatum of Kaposi	+		+	+	
Ehlers-Danlos syndrome				+	+
Epidermolysis bullosa	+		+	+	
Epidermolysis bullosa, dystrophica	+		+	+	
Erythema multiforme	+		+	+	
Familial dysautonomia (Riley-Day syndrome)	+		+		
Focal dermal hypoplasia				+	+
Granulomatous diseases of childhood	+		+	+	+
Hallermann-Streiff syndrome		+	+		
Hereditary hemorrhagic telangiectasia				+	
Hereditary hyperpigmentation			+		
Hydrocystoma			+		
Hypertrichosis lanuginosa			+		
Hypoparathyroidism		+			+
Hypothyroidism			+		
Ichthyosis	+	+	+		
Ichthyosiform erythroderma	+		+		
Incontinentia pigmenti	+	+			
Juvenile melanoma				+	
Juvenile xanthogranuloma				+	+
Kaposi's varicelliform eruption	+		+		
Keratodermia palmaris et plantaris	+		+		
Keratosis decalvans	+			+	
Keratosis follicularis spinulosa	+	+	+		
Keratosis pilaris atrophicans			+		

TABLE 30–1 OCULAR CHANGES IN SKIN DISEASES — *Continued*

	Cornea	Lens	Periorbital Area (Eyebrows, Lashes, Eyelids)	Conjunctiva, Sclera	Retina
Leprosy	+	+	+	+	+
Lipoid proteinosis	+		+	+	
Lobstein's syndrome				+	
Lupus erythematosus			+	+	+
Marchesani's syndrome		+	+		
Marfan's syndrome		+			+
Marinesco-Sjögren syndrome		+			
Melanoacanthoma			+		
Milia			+		
Molluscum contagiosum			+	+	
Mongolism		+	+		
Monilethrix		+	+		
Myotonia dystrophica		+		+	
Oculoauriculovertebral syndrome				+	
Onchocerciasis	+				+
Pachyonychia congenita	+	+			
Pediculosis			+		
Pemphigus foliaceus		+	+		
Periarteritis nodosa				+	+
Piebaldism				+	+
Pili torti			+		
Pityriasis rubra pilaris	+				
Porphyria congenita (erythropoietic)	+		+		
Progeria			+		
Pseudohypoparathyroidism		+			+
Pseudoxanthoma elasticum					+
Psoriasis		+	+	+	
Raynaud's phenomenon					+
Refsum's syndrome					+
Rothmund-Thomson syndrome	+	+	+		
Sarcoidosis			+	+	+
Schönlein-Henoch purpura					+
Seborrheic dermatitis			+	+	
Secondary syphilis			+		
Sjögren-Larsen syndrome					+
Still's disease	+	+			
Sturge-Weber syndrome			+	+	+
Trichoepithelioma			+		
Trichomegaly		+	+		
Trichotillomania			+		
Tuberous sclerosis					+
Turner's syndrome		+			+
Ulerythema ophryogenes			+		
Vitiligo			+		+
von Hippel-Lindau syndrome					+
Vogt-Koyanagi syndrome			+		+
Waardenburg syndrome			+		+
Werner's syndrome	+	+		+	+
Wyburn-Mason syndrome					+
Xeroderma pigmentosum	+		+	+	

which appears to be related to the Fanconi syndrome.

The cutaneous features of this syndrome are characterized by atrophy, pigmentation of the skin, dystrophic nail changes, and leukoplakia. The nail changes usually appear first between the ages of 5 and 13 years, and the pigmentary changes follow in 2 or 3 years. Associated physical changes may include retarded physical and mental growth and blood dyscrasia.

The ocular manifestations may consist of bullous conjunctivitis with minimal scarring of the cornea, ectropion of the lower eyelids, loss of cilia, secondary and chronic blepharitis, and keratinization of the lacrimal puncta.

Epidermolysis Bullosa

Epidermolysis bullosa is made up of a group of genetically transmitted skin diseases characterized by blister formation at the site of trauma. The only point of similarity between the syndromes is the trauma-blister sequence, since the genetic determinants vary and the histologic site of blister formation occurs at different levels of the skin in each. Only the recessively transmitted dystrophic variety is important for this discussion. The cutaneous manifestations consist of large, flaccid bullae which are present at birth and continue to appear throughout life following minor trauma to the skin and mucous membranes. The blisters heal with scarring; involvement on the extremities leads to webbing of the fingers. Squamous cell carcinoma may develop in scarred areas later in life.

Ophthalmic complications occur secondary to cicatricial changes in the conjunctiva and lids.

Erythema Multiforme (Stevens-Johnson Syndrome)

Erythema multiforme is a type of hypersensitivity reaction induced by infectious agents, drugs, or foods and is characterized by mucocutaneous lesions and a systemic reaction.

The cutaneous manifestations consist of macular-urticarial and vesiculobullous lesions, with a predilection for localization on the backs of the hands, the palms, the soles, and the extensor surfaces of the extremities. In 25 per cent of the patients,

mucous membranes are affected, and in some instances this may be the only manifestation. A typical pattern of cutaneous involvement is an urticarial patch with a dusky center and bright red, raised border. Petechiae can be found in most of the lesions on careful inspection. Associated signs and symptoms consist of temperature elevation, malaise, vomiting, myalgia, and arthralgia.

Ocular manifestations include involvement of the eyelids by the inflammatory skin lesions, severe keratoconjunctivitis, corneal scarring, keratinization, and scarring of the conjunctiva. The inferior fornix may be partially obliterated by adhesions and resemble pemphigus. Soft contact lenses may be useful in protecting the cornea and preventing conjunctival adhesions.

Familial Dysautonomia (Riley-Day Syndrome)

Familial dysautonomia (Riley-Day syndrome) is a neurocutaneous disease inherited as a recessive characteristic in Jews, in which there are combined autonomic motor and somatic sensory functional disorders.

The cutaneous manifestations consist of erythematous macular skin lesions measuring 2 to 5 cm. in diameter on the trunk or extremities which appear following emotional upset. Associated findings consist of acrocyanosis, hyperhidrosis, and intermittent hypertension.

The first sign of ophthalmic involvement may consist of an absence of lacrimation, followed by corneal anesthesia. This combination frequently leads to secondary corneal ulceration.

Hereditary Hemorrhagic Telangiectasia (Osler-Rendu-Weber Disease)

Hereditary hemorrhagic telangiectasia is a disorder of blood vessels throughout the body which is transmitted as an autosomal dominant trait.

The cutaneous manifestations may be seen before puberty and consist of thin-walled, ruby-colored papules with ill-defined borders and radiating vessels distributed on the oral mucosa and on the upper half of the body. Associated abnormalities include arteriovenous fistulas, clubbing of the fingers, cyanosis, and polycythemia. Melena and epistaxis are common complications resulting from ruptures of telangiectasia.

Ophthalmic manifestations consist of telangiectatic vascular lesions of the palpebral and bulbar conjunctiva.

Ichthyosis

Ichthyosis is a disease of abnormal keratinization characterized clinically by dry scaly skin. Using clinical, histologic, genetic, and cellular kinetic parameters, a group of distinguishable entities may be differentiated as follows:

1. Ichthyosis vulgaris—Autosomal dominant
2. Congenital ichthyosiform erythroderma—Nonbullous type (psoriatic erythroderma) autosomal dominant with variable expressivity
3. Bullous congenital ichthyosiform erythroderma
4. Lamellar ichthyosis—Autosomal recessive
5. Sex-linked ichthyosis—X-linked trait

Of these, only lamellar ichthyosis and sex-linked ichthyosis may be associated with eye abnormalities (Figs. 30–1 and 30–2).

The characteristic dermatologic manifestation in lamellar and X-linked ichthyosis is present at birth and consists of an erythematous collodion-like membrane covering the skin. In both varieties, the skin changes slowly evolve into brownish, adherent scales which may persist throughout life. In sex-linked ichthyosis, the palms and soles are spared.

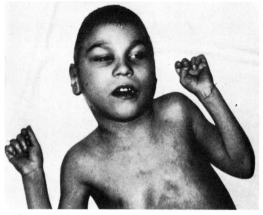

Figure 30–2 Congenital ichthyosis, bilateral cataracts, and severe mental retardation in 6-year-old boy.

The ophthalmic manifestations in both lamellar and sex-linked ichthyosis consist of conjunctivitis and nonspecific corneal erosions due to ectropion. In the sex-linked variety, corneal opacities serve as a distinguishing feature. Bilateral cataracts may develop in the congenital and the vulgaris form of this disorder.

Keratodermia Palmaris et Plantaris

Keratodermia palmaris et plantaris is the result of abnormal keratinization of the palms and soles, a hereditary disorder in which diffuse or focal thickening of the palms and soles occur.

The clinical appearance, various associated defects, and the mode of inheritance serve to differentiate this condition.

The cutaneous manifestations consist of localized or disseminated hyperkeratotic changes of the palms and soles with a tendency toward fissure and secondary infection.

Ophthalmic involvement is most commonly seen in the recessive type of keratoderma and consists of corneal erosions, photophobia, epiphora, conjunctivitis, and corneal opacities.

Ocular Pemphigus (Benign Mucous Membrane Pemphigoid)

Bullous dermatopathies frequently have ocular sequelae. There is a rare form of bilateral conjunctivitis in children occasionally associated with pemphigoid lesions of the nose, throat, and skin, but in

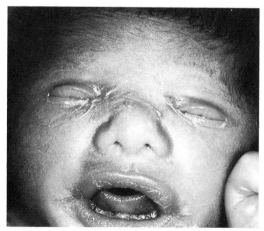

Figure 30–1 Congenital ichthyosis in newborn. (Courtesy of Dr. R. D. Harley.)

general it is solely an ocular problem. It has been referred to as "essential shrinkage of the conjunctiva," and in the chronic form it results in severe cicatrization of the conjunctiva, symblepharon, obliteration of fornices, thick ropy discharge, corneal scarring, and pannus aggravated by xerophthalmia from occlusive scarring of the secretory lacrimal ducts.

Pityriasis Rubra Pilaris

Pityriasis rubra pilaris is a disease of abnormal keratinization of unknown etiology with clinical features which serve to differentiate it from other scaling disorders. It is usually divided into a familial type, having its onset in infancy or childhood, in which an autosomal dominant trait is implicated, and an acquired type, which often begins in middle age and shows no genetic relationship.

The cutaneous manifestation frequently starts insidiously with nonspecific scaling on the scalp and forehead, or with erythema on the face and ears, and with or without thickening of the palms and soles. The typical follicular papules are usually present on the extensor surfaces of the elbows and knees and on the proximal dorsal portions of the phalanges.

Ophthalmic involvement occurs secondary to ectropion and consists of corneal ulcers.

Porphyria Congenita

The porphyrias include several disorders of porphyrin metabolism. Clinically, distinguishable disease may be differentiated on the basis of clinical, genetic, and metabolic parameters. Congenital porphyria is the only abnormality of porphyrin metabolism significant to this discussion.

Congenital porphyria is a rare disease of porphyrin metabolism inherited as an autosomal recessive trait and characterized by the onset of photosensitivity in early life.

The cutaneous manifestation consists of the onset of severe solar hypersensitivity on exposed skin surfaces within the first three years of life. Vesiculobullous lesions appear on exposed areas, rupture, ulcerate, and are followed by severe scarring. Hypertrichosis and erythrodontia are frequently present.

Ophthalmic involvement consists of scarring of the eyelids, ectropion, dystrophic corneal changes, symblepharon, and corneal ulceration.

Rosacea

Rosacea is a clinical syndrome of unknown etiology characterized by recurrent or persistent erythema of the face which may be associated with papules, pustules, and sebaceous hyperplasia in varying degrees. It may rarely occur during adolescence.

The cutaneous changes are characterized by erythema primarily involving the nose, cheeks, forehead, and chin. Inflammatory papulopustules recur within the area of involvement.

Ophthalmic involvement consists of blepharitis, conjunctivitis, and occasionally keratitis with corneal scarring.

Rothmund-Thomson Syndrome

The Rothmund-Thomson syndrome (poikiloderma congenitale) is a rare oculocutaneous syndrome which is probably inherited as a single autosomal recessive gene.

The characteristic cutaneous manifestations appear between the third and sixth months of life and consist of transitory plaques of erythema, which subsequently clear, and combinations of atrophy, telangiectasia, poikiloderma, and hyper- and hypopigmentation. Associated changes consist of ultraviolet hypersensitivity, sparse hair on the scalp, scanty eyebrows and eyelashes, defective dentition, and hypogenitalism.

Ophthalmic involvement consists of bilateral cataracts in 40 per cent of the patients, which become apparent between the ages of 4 and 7. Degenerative corneal changes may also appear (Fig. 30–3).

Wegener's Granulomatosis

This disease, observed in young adults, is characterized by a chronic progressive nasosinusitis leading to complete destruction of superficial and deep structures including the nose, sinuses, orbit, and oral cavity. Inflammatory nodules occur in the lung. A necrotizing glomerulitis develops as a result of a focal vasculitis which usually results in death. Eyelid edema, exophthalmos, nasolacrimal duct obstruction,

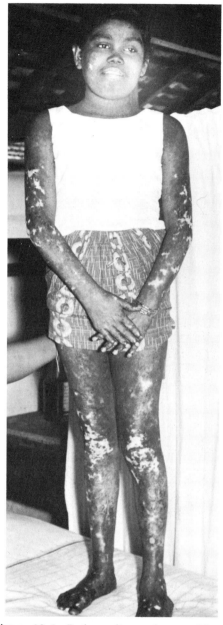

Figure 30–3 Rothmund's syndrome: Bilateral cataracts and numerous areas of depigmentation. (Courtesy of Dr. R. D. Harley.)

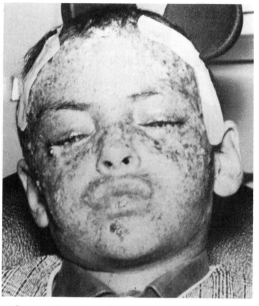

Figure 30–4 Xeroderma pigmentosum. Several areas have undergone malignant changes. (Courtesy of Dr. William Spencer.)

sex linkage and is characterized by unusual defective repair replication of the DNA molecule (Figs. 30–4 and 30–5).

The cutaneous manifestations of this disease are characterized by marked sun sensitivity, photophobia, telangiectasia,

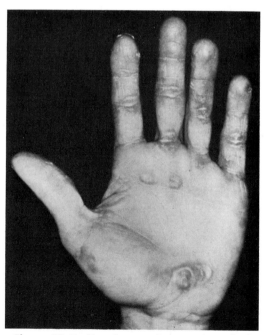

Figure 30–5 Xeroderma pigmentosum of the hand in same boy as in Figure 30–4.

and exposure keratopathy have been described secondary to orbital involvement.

A similar condition known as lethal midline granuloma is difficult to differentiate.

Xeroderma Pigmentosum

Xeroderma pigmentosum is transmitted as an autosomal recessive trait with partial atrophy, and hyperpigmentation on the skin surfaces exposed to the sun. The ultraviolet damage leads to premature aging of the skin, actinic damage, actinic keratoses, and basal cell and squamous cell carcinomas.

The ophthalmic manifestations consist of ectropion, destruction of the lower eyelid, pigmented macules of the conjunctiva, corneal opacities, and carcinoma of the lids and conjunctiva. Corneal ulceration may occur secondary to the ectropion, resulting in severe visual loss.

LENS

Alopecia Areata

Alopecia areata is an inflammatory disease of the hair follicle of unknown etiology that is characterized by a sudden appearance of circumscribed patches of hair loss on the scalp, although the process may become generalized with loss of all body hair, as in alopecia totalis.

Cutaneous manifestations consist of sharply circumscribed nonscarring areas of alopecia with broken-off hairs which may be easily epilated. The early patches are associated with mild inflammation of the skin. Fingernail changes are concurrent in approximately one third of the patients.

Associated ophthalmic involvement consists of loss of eyebrows and eyelashes; cataracts are uncommon complications.

Conradi's Syndrome (Chondrodystrophia Congenita Punctata)

This is a rare congenital disease inherited as an autosomal recessive trait and characterized by stippled foci of calcification in hyaline cartilage and multiple developmental abnormalities.

The cutaneous manifestations consist of patchy erythema and ichthyotic type dryness and scaling which is present at birth. The nails and hair are normal but there may be keratoderma of the palms and soles. Associated developmental defects in the cardiovascular system, disproportionate shortening of the proximal portion of the arms and thighs, short neck, flattened bridge of the nose, and a high arch palate may also be present.

Ophthalmic involvement consists of congenital cataracts, optic atrophy, and hypertelorism.

Diabetes Mellitus

See Chapter 20, Part A.

Drug Reactions

Several drugs are capable of producing changes in the lens and the skin (diametrophenol, triparanol (MER-29), and corticosteroids). Of these, only the latter will be discussed.

Prolonged corticosteroid therapy may be used in the treatment of various systemic diseases in pediatrics and may produce secondary cutaneous and ocular complications. Among the skin manifestations of hypercorticism are the subcutaneous accumulation of fat in the cheeks and over the mid-upper dorsal area, formation of striae distensae, hirsutism, delay in wound healing, proneness to skin infections and increased vascular fragility, and acne.

Ocular complications include the development of subcapsular cataracts and pseudotumor cerebri in patients receiving long-term corticosteroid treatment.

Hallermann-Streiff Syndrome

Hallermann-Streiff syndrome is a rare complex syndrome of developmental origin characterized by parrot facies (craniofacial dysplasia), cutaneous atrophy, and cataracts.

The cutaneous manifestation consists of frontal alopecia on the scalp. Characteristically, loss of hair along cranial suture lines, sparse or absent eyebrows, atrophy of the skin of the face and nose, and prominent vascular markings are also present.

Ophthalmic involvement consists of congenital cataracts, microphthalmos, and congenital glaucoma. Spontaneous absorption of the cataract within the capsules has been observed.

Hypoparathyroidism and Pseudo-Hypoparathyroidism

See Chapter 20, Part A.

Incontinentia Pigmenti

Incontinentia pigmenti is a hereditary disorder of mesenchymal and ectodermal

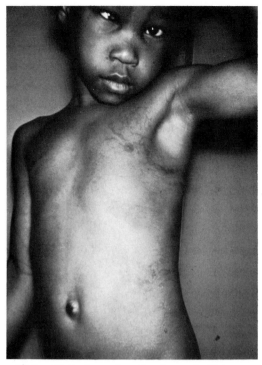

Figure 30–6 Incontinentia pigmenti. Right esotropia associated with persistent hyperplastic primary vitreous. (Courtesy of Dr. R. D. Harley.)

origin that results in neurologic, mental, ocular, osseous, and cutaneous changes. It is transmitted as an autosomal dominant trait which is sex-linked in its transmission, or is due to a sex-linked gene carried on the X chromosome, acting as a dominant gene in females and lethal in the male (Fig. 30–6).

The cutaneous manifestations occur in three stages: vesiculobullous, papular (warty), and pigmentary phases. The duration and sequence of the cutaneous changes are variable. There is an associated eosinophilia during the acute inflammatory stage of cutaneous disease. Associated dental, mental, nervous system, and skeletal defects are also present.

The ocular defects consist of cataract, optic atrophy, strabismus, and persistent hyperplastic primary vitreous.

Marchesani's Syndrome

Marchesani's syndrome is inherited as an autosomal dominant trait and is characterized by short stature, brachydactyly, and spherophakia (small, spherical lens). It is felt to represent a type of mesodermal

hypoplasty in contrast to Marfan's syndrome, although both share the same lens defects.

The cutaneous manifestations consist of small hands with thick palms and short, stubby fingers which restrict flexion and extension, and short stature (average = 148 cm.).

Associated ocular involvement consists of spherophakia, microphakia, myopia, subluxation of the lens, and secondary glaucoma.

Marfan's Syndrome

See Chapter 20, Part C, p. 676.

Marinesco-Sjögren Syndrome

Marinesco-Sjögren syndrome is a rare syndrome inherited as an autosomal recessive trait and characterized by rotary and horizontal nystagmus, dysarthria, mental retardation, retarded growth, skeletal deformities, and cerebellar ataxia which becomes apparent when the child begins to walk.

The cutaneous manifestations of this syndrome consist of very fine, short, sparse hair containing little or no pigment.

The ocular manifestations consist of bilateral cataracts in addition to horizontal or rotary nystagmus.

Mongolism (Down's Syndrome)

See Chapter 2.

Monilethrix

Monilethrix is a developmental defect of the hair shaft which is transmitted as an autosomal dominant trait with high penetrance but variable expressivity. In some instances, there is an associated aminoaciduria.

The cutaneous expression is limited to the skin and is characterized by sparse fragile hairs on the scalp and small erythematous follicular papules. Uniform beading along the shaft of the hair is seen in microscopic examination. The nape of the neck and scalp are the areas most frequently involved, although the changes may be observed in the eyebrows, eyelashes, and pubic and axillary hair.

Associated ophthalmic disease consists of cataracts which have been reported more frequently than in the normal population.

Pachyonychia Congenita

Pachyonychia congenita is an abnormality of keratinization inherited as an autosomal dominant trait which is characterized by abnormalities of the skin, nails, mucous membranes, and eye.

The characteristic cutaneous manifestations consist of thickened fingernails and toenails with a prominent transverse curve which may be present at birth or develop during the first few years of life. Keratoderma of the palms and soles; follicular keratotic lesions on the extremities, buttocks, and nape of the neck; and whitish marks on the mucous membranes of the mouth may also be present.

Associated ophthalmic changes consist of opacities and dyskeratotic changes of the cornea, and occasionally bilateral cataracts.

Pemphigus Foliaceus

Pemphigus foliaceus is a type of acantholytic disease of the epidermis in which the histologic changes are high in the epidermis and differ from those in pemphigus vulgaris and pemphigus vegetans. The cause is unknown, although antibodies to an intracellular substance have been demonstrated regularly.

The cutaneous manifestations initially consist of small, flaccid bullae which rapidly transpose into scaling crusted patches. The clinical appearance and distribution of lesions on the face may simulate lupus erythematosus. Slow but progressive spread eventually produces a generalized exfoliative erythroderma.

Associated ophthalmic disease occurs when the process involves the superciliary region and eyelids. Degeneration of the iris and bilateral cataracts may occur.

Turner's Syndrome

See Chapter 2.

Werner's Syndrome

Werner's syndrome is a rare genodermatosis inherited as an autosomal recessive trait and characterized by premature aging, generalized arteriosclerosis, small stature, hypogonadism, diabetes mellitus, osteoporosis, and a high incidence of sarcomas.

The skin manifestations appear during the second and third decades of life and consist of atrophy of the skin of the extremities, face, and neck, resulting in fixation of the joints (sclerodactyly). Circumscribed hyperkeratoses, callosities, and atrophic ulcers commonly occur over pressure points. Associated changes consist of small stature, hypogonadism, endocrine deficiency, and generalized arteriosclerosis which lead to early death.

Associated ophthalmic findings consist of juvenile cataracts, blue sclerae, retinal changes, retinitis pigmentosa, and degenerative corneal changes.

EYELASHES, EYEBROWS, AND EYELIDS

Developmental abnormalities of the eyelashes are uncommon but may be seen alone or in association with other developmental defects.

Absence of Eyelashes

Partial or total absence of eyelashes may occur as an isolated defect. It is also a characteristic but inconstant feature of several other syndromes, including the following:

1. Anhidrotic ectodermal dysplasia (see under Conjunctiva and Cornea).

2. Mandibulofacial dysostosis (Treacher Collins syndrome). Mandibulofacial dysostosis is an embryologic defect produced by abnormal development of the first branchial arch. It is transmitted as an autosomal dominant trait with wide interfamilial variability.

The cutaneous manifestations consist of a characteristic birdlike facies with abnormal growth of terminal hairs extending in a tonguelike fashion from the temporal areas toward the cheeks. Associated developmental defects include enlarged mouth, high-arched palate, malocclusion, and defective implantation of the teeth. The frontal nasal angle is absent. There is absence or malformation of the auricles, and hypoplasia of the mandibular and malar bones. In addition, there are a variety of skeletal defects in other parts of the body.

The ocular manifestations include an antimongoloid slant, notching of the lower lids, absent or sparse eyelashes over the medial half or two thirds of the lower lids, and occasionally congenital cataracts.

Acquired Dermatoses

The skin of the eyelids is prone to develop irritation from many environmental agents or cosmetics transmitted to them by the fingers. As a consequence of this contact, irritation associated with erythema, edema, eczematization, and pigmentation may be induced. Edema, erythema, and pigmentation may be produced by systemic disease. (See Table 30–2.)

Atrichia Congenita (Total Alopecia)

Total alopecia may appear as an isolated defect usually transmitted as an autosomal recessive trait. Dominant or irregular inheritance has occurred in some families. "Total" loss of hair is relative, for there may be some hairs, although they are extremely few in number. It occurs as an isolated abnormality or with associated defects as in progeria, anhidrotic ectodermal dysplasia, and atrichia with keratin cysts.

Dermatologic manifestations in the isolated variety consist of normal pelage at birth which is shed between the first and sixth months, after which no further growth of hair occurs.

Eyebrows, eyelashes, and body hair may be absent, but usually there are a few hairs in the usual hair-bearing areas.

Cornelia de Lange Syndrome

The Cornelia de Lange syndrome is a rare, developmental abnormality which occurs sporadically and is associated with consanguinity, in which case a recessive gene has been implicated.

Facial and dermatologic manifestations consist of a distinctive masklike expressionless facies with a small nose and depressed bridge of the nose. The lips are thin and the angle of the mouth turned down toward the receding chin. The hairline is low on the neck and forehead, and there is hypertrichosis on the forehead, sides of the face, back, shoulders, and extremities. The skin in general has a marbled appearance. Associated changes include low birth weight, short stature, a distinctive low-pitched growling type cry, and mental retardation.

The ophthalmic manifestations consist of heavy, confluent eyebrows, long curly eyelashes, mild exophthalmos, myopic astigmatism, strabismus, nystagmus, ptosis, optic atrophy, and coloboma of the optic nerve.

Eczematous Dermatitis

Allergic eczematous contact dermatitis is a delayed hypersensitivity reaction occurring 5 to 20 days after sensitization by a contact.

The clinical appearance of the dermatitis varies. In the acute phase, there is erythema, edema, papulovesicles, weeping and crusting, and, in the chronic phase, edema, erythema, and scaling. Among the common causes are perfumes, nail lacquers, eye cosmetics, eyeglass cleaners, and ophthalmic medications (antibiotics, atropine, mercurials). Abnormal conjunctival pigmentation resulting from the use of eyeliner pencils has been described.

TABLE 30–2   EDEMA OF THE EYELIDS

Unilateral	Bilateral
Dacryocystitis	Angioneurotic edema
Chalazion	Cardiac failure
Cavernous sinus thrombosis	Hyper- or hypothyroidism
Trauma (accidental or self-inflicted)	Hypoproteinemia
Insect bite reaction	Anemia
Contact dermatitis	Leukemia
(Allergic or primary irritant)	Renal failure
Erysipelas	Trichinosis
Orbital cellulitis	Filariasis
Myiasis	Onchocercosis
Chance-type lesions (syphilis, anthrax, vaccinia, cat-scratch disease)	
Herpes zoster	
Chronic lymphedema	

Follicular Abnormalities of Keratinization Associated With Atrophy

There is a group of inflammatory diseases of the hair follicle characterized by keratosis pilaris and destruction of the pilar apparatus. They have been differentiated on clinical grounds because of differences in distribution and severity of the inflammatory reaction as follows: ulerythema ophryogenes (keratosis pilaris atrophicans faciei), keratosis pilaris decalvans (follicular ichthyosis).

ULERYTHEMA OPHRYOGENES (KERATOSIS PILARIS ATROPHICANS). This follicular inflammatory reaction which ultimately destroys the hair follicle is present at birth or in early infancy and is characterized by the presence of small horny plugs in the lateral third of the eyebrows. (It is thought to be transmitted as an autosomal dominant trait.)

KERATOSIS PILARIS DECALVANS (SEE ALSO UNDER CONJUNCTIVA AND CORNEA). Keratosis pilaris decalvans may be transmitted as a sex-linked recessive trait. It is characterized by follicular papules which appear on the face in infancy. The process progresses to atrophy of the follicle and scarring alopecia of the scalp and eyebrows. Ophthalmic manifestations consist of loss of eyebrows, photophobia, and corneal opacities with vascularization.

Hypertrichosis Lanuginosa

Hypertrichosis lanuginosa is a rare pilar developmental abnormality in which the fetal pelage persists and grows throughout life instead of being replaced by vellous and terminal hairs. A "dog-face" form, which is transmitted as an autosomal dominant trait, and a "monkey-face" form, of unknown inheritance, may be distinguished clinically.

The dermatologic manifestation of the dog-face type is characterized by excessive hairiness at birth, following which the hair gradually lengthens, until by early childhood the entire skin, excepting palms and soles, is covered by silky hair. Associated defects are developmental and dental abnormalities, deformities of the external ear, and mental retardation.

The monkey-face type is characterized by generalized hypertrichosis, a simian-type facies, with a broad flat nose, thick drooping lips, and prognathism.

The ophthalmic manifestation is primarily an increase in the eyebrow hairs following the general pattern of hypertrichosis.

Hypothyroidism

See Chapter 20, Part A.

Interrelated Congenital Diseases

ICHTHYOSIFORM ERYTHRODERMA. See under Conjunctiva and Cornea.

OCULOVERTEBRAL DYSPLASIA (GOLDENHAR'S SYNDROME). See Chapter 31.

XERODERMA PIGMENTOSUM. See under Conjunctiva and Cornea.

Kaposi's Varicelliform Eruption

Kaposi's varicelliform eruption is a clinical entity caused by a primary type of herpes simplex or vaccinia virus infection superimposed on a pre-existing skin disease.

Dermatologic manifestations consist of crops of vesicles which become umbilicated and may be hemorrhagic on normal skin as well as on areas of previous involvement. The skin lesions are associated with systemic signs and symptoms.

The ophthalmic expression of this type of infection is edema associated with extension of the vesicular lesions to the eyelids. Conjunctivitis, corneal vesicles, and dendritic ulcers may result.

Leprosy

Leprosy is a chronic contagious disease caused by *Mycobacterium leprae* which affects primarily the peripheral nervous system and, secondarily, the skin, mucous membranes of the mouth, upper respiratory tract, reticuloendothelial system, eyes, bones, and testes. In high endemic areas, infection is frequent in childhood.

The clinical manifestations of infection are related to the degree of host resistance to the organism. Leprosy is subclassified accordingly into lepromatous leprosy, in which the degree of resistance of the host is low; tuberculoid leprosy, with high resistance of the host; and borderline or dimorphous leprosy.

In lepromatous leprosy, cutaneous evidence of infection consists of maculopapular, hypopigmented, nonanesthetic lesions which progress into large plaques and nodular lesions scattered in a symmetrical fashion over the entire cutaneous surface.

In tuberculoid leprosy, skin lesions consist of asymmetrically distributed erythematous or hypopigmented macules with well-defined borders and showing some degree of anesthesia.

In borderline leprosy, the clinical lesions intermediate between tuberculoid and lepromatous varieties occur.

Associated ophthalmic findings consist of superficial and deep keratitis, lepromatous nodules of the iris, recurrent attacks of iridocyclitis, and corneal lepromas but rarely chorioretinal lesions. Corneal anesthesia with secondary corneal ulcers results from invasion of the fifth nerve by the lepra bacillus. Involvement of the eyebrows and eyelashes results in thinning and eventual loss of hair.

Lipoid Proteinosis (Hyalinosis Cutis et Mucosae) (Fig. 30–7)

Lipoid proteinosis is an extremely rare metabolic defect probably inherited as an autosomal recessive trait and is characterized by the deposition of hyaline material in the skin and mucous membranes.

Cutaneous manifestations consist of discrete yellowish-white, round, confluent papules on the face, neck, hands, knees, elbows, and feet which appear early in life. Hoarseness is present at birth or develops in the first few years of life. Coincidentally, oral mucosal involvement occurs, as well as infiltrative lesions on the soft palate, anterior pillars, uvula, larynx, and vocal cords.

Ophthalmic manifestations consist of hyaline nodular deposits on the free border of the eyelids with secondary loss of eyelashes. Later, conjunctivitis, corneal deposits, and open angle glaucoma may occur.

Lupus Erythematosus

See Chapter 20.

Molluscum Contagiosum

Molluscum contagiosum is a viral disease of the skin caused by one of the pox group of viruses which grows in the cytoplasm of the epithelial cell.

The cutaneous manifestations consist of well-defined, pearly-appearing papules with umbilicated centers of varying size (3 to 10 mm.). Occasionally, eczematization of the surrounding skin occurs. Lesions may be widely distributed or localized to the eyelids and rarely may involve the conjunctiva and the caruncle.

Piebaldism (Partial Albinism)

Piebaldism is a developmental defect of the melanocytes transmitted as an autosomal dominant trait and characterized by patches of skin totally devoid of pigment.

The cutaneous findings consist of well-defined, white, macular patches, most

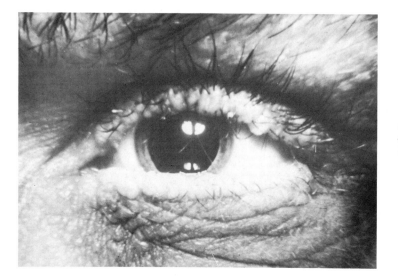

Figure 30–7 Lipoproteinosis showing typical lesions on the eyelids. (Courtesy of Dr. R. D. Harley.)

commonly on the forehead and associated with white forelocks, which are present at birth and remain unchanged throughout life. Other patches may occur on the trunk and/or extremities.

The ophthalmic manifestations consist of the absence of pigment from choroid, photophobia, and nystagmus.

Pigmentation

Hereditary hyperpigmentation of the eyelids may be present as an isolated defect transmitted as an autosomal dominant trait. Melanocytic nevi may involve one or both eyelids.

Hyperpigmentation may be seen secondary to increased melanocyte-stimulating hormones in association with Addison's disease, acromegaly, pregnancy, hyperthyroidism, progestational steroids, pheochromocytoma, Cushing's syndrome, neoplastic disease, lymphomas, and certain diseases of the nervous system.

The application of ophthalmic preparations containing mercurial or silver preparations may produce permanent hyperpigmentation.

Pili Torti

Pili torti is a developmental defect inherited as an autosomal dominant trait in which the affected hairs are flattened and the shaft is twisted 180 degrees off its axis at various points along its length. Some cases may appear sporadically.

The hair is usually normal at birth and is progressively replaced by abnormal hair by the second or third year. The problem becomes manifest when the affected hairs are brushed or combed and break off at the point of the twist in the hair, producing hairs of varying lengths up to 4 to 5 cm. The eyelashes may also be involved in the process.

Progeria (Hutchinson-Gilford Syndrome)

Progeria is a rare syndrome of unknown etiology with retarded physical development and the onset of premature aging commencing in childhood.

The cutaneous manifestations commence during the second year of life and consist of the rapid appearance of age-associated changes of senility. The skin becomes thin, dry, and wrinkled with prominent cutaneous veins and with mottled pigmentation. The nails become thin and brittle. The bald head, birdlike facies, and well-proportioned little body are distinctive features. Advanced generalized arteriosclerosis during adolescence is the rule.

Ophthalmic defects consist of complete absence of eyebrows and eyelashes and occasional microphthalmos.

Psoriasis

Psoriasis is a common genetically determined abnormality of keratinization characterized by altered cellular kinetics that produce abnormal keratinization.

The cutaneous manifestations of psoriasis consist of a typical papulosquamous papule or patch surmounted with a silvery scale. The eruption may be widely distributed; however, lesions appear characteristically over the extensor surfaces of the elbows and knees and on the scalp. Fingernail changes are commonly associated with the cutaneous disease. Associated rheumatoid-like arthritis may occur.

Ophthalmic manifestations consist of blepharitis, conjunctivitis, or keratitis which appear synchronously with the skin lesions. Xerosis, symblepharon, and trichiasis occur uncommonly, and zonular shield-shaped cataracts occur rarely.

Seborrheic Dermatitis

Seborrheic dermatitis is probably a genetically determined structural and functional abnormality which produces an inflammatory reaction of the skin and an oily skin.

The characteristic eruption consists of an erythematous scaling dermatitis with a distribution predisposed to involve the forehead at the hair line, the inter-eyebrow areas, presternal and interscapular areas, the scalp, and intertriginous areas (beneath the breasts, axillary spaces, and the genitocrural fold).

Ophthalmic involvement consists of blepharitis which may be followed by infection and destruction of the lash follicle. Similar changes may be seen in the eyebrows. The blepharitis may be associated with catarrhal conjunctivitis.

Secondary Syphilis

Secondary syphilis is a clinical phase in the dynamic infection caused by *T. pal-*

lidum, which is characterized by constitutional symptoms and skin and mucous membrane lesions. In this stage of infection, the serologic tests for syphilis are always positive.

The cutaneous manifestations consist of generalized maculopapular eruption with characteristic involvement of the palms and soles, oral mucosa, and intertriginous areas (condylomas). Patchy alopecia that produces a moth-eaten appearance may be seen. Associated evidence of systemic infection includes temperature elevation, generalized lymphadenopathy, arthritis, and enlargement of the liver and spleen.

Ophthalmic manifestations of the infection include complete or moth-eaten alopecia of the eyebrows and iridocyclitis.

Trichomegaly

In trichomegaly, the eyelashes and eyebrows may be abnormally large in both diameter and length. The condition may be associated with dwarfism, mental retardation, and pigmentary degeneration of the retina.

Trichotillomania

Trichotillomania consists of the desire to pull or twist hairs of the scalp which results in a patch of partial alopecia.

In some instances, it is a habit, hair pulling or twisting being done while reading, writing, or just before going to sleep. In others, it is part of a psychoneurosis in which there is an uncontrolled compulsion to pull out the hair. The scalp is most frequently involved but eyelashes, eyebrows, or even the cilia of the eyelids may be pulled out.

Tumors of the Eyelids

A wide variety of benign and malignant tumors can appear on the eyelids, the number being limited only by the various components of the skin. The most frequently encountered lesions are trichoepithelioma, hydrocystoma, milia, and vascular nevi (Table 30–3).

BASAL CELL CARCINOMAS. These occur with xeroderma pigmentosum but otherwise are uncommon in children. They consist of dome-shaped, pearly-appearing papules with ectatic vessels over the tumor face. With the passage of time, they slowly enlarge and become centrally crusted.

TABLE 30–3   TUMORS OF THE EYELIDS

Basal and squamous cell carcinomas
Calcifying epithelioma of Malherbe
Trichoepithelioma
Actinic keratoses
Seborrheic keratoses
Sweat gland tumors
Hydrocystoma (usually multiple)
Cysts of Moll's glands (eyelid margins usually solitary)
Sebaceous gland origin
Sebaceous cysts
Milia
Meibomian cysts
Vascular nevi
Angiosarcoma
Pyogenic granuloma
Melanocytic nevi melanoma

Involvement of the conjunctiva and destruction of the lid may occur.

HYDROCYSTOMA (SYRINGOMA). This is a benign tumor which is usually multiple and is produced by malformed sweat ducts and glands. Individual papules are flesh colored or yellowish but sometimes may appear as translucent and cystic.

MILIA. These are pinhead-size epidermal cysts which consist of whitish, well-defined, asymptomatic papules.

TRICHOEPITHELIOMA (EPITHELIOMA ADENOIDES CYSTICUM). This consists of multiple flesh-colored papular lesions with histologic changes suggestive of pilar origin of the tumor.

VASCULAR NEVI. The nevus flammeus is the most commonly seen, though nevus vasculosis and cavernous vascular nevi may also be seen. The importance of nevus flammeus is the possible association with intracranial vascular nevi and glaucoma. The cavernous hemangioma can present problems when it occurs in this area because of progressive increase in size and disturbance of function.

Vitiligo

Vitiligo is an abnormality of pigment production which is probably transmitted by an autosomal dominant gene of variable penetrance.

The cutaneous manifestations consist of spontaneous appearance of completely depigmented patches with hyperpigmented borders. Extension may be rapid or proceed slowly and intermittently for years. Hairs in involved patches of skin may become white or retain their pigment. Associated abnormalities consist of pernicious anemia, hyperthyroidism, and alopecia areata.

The ophthalmic manifestations consist of depigmented patches in the eyebrows and eyelashes. Vitiligo, uveitis, and premature graying of the hair occur in Vogt-Koyanagi's syndrome (see under Uveal Tract and Retina).

Waardenburg's Syndrome

Waardenburg's syndrome consists of a developmental defect in melanocyte development transmitted as an autosomal dominant trait with variable penetrance. It is similar to piebaldism but has other developmental defects of neural crest derivatives.

The cutaneous manifestation is the presence of a white forelock which appears in 17 per cent of the patients affected. A few patients show piebaldism. Perceptive deafness is present in a high percentage (Figs. 30–8 and 30–9).

Ophthalmic manifestations consist of lateral displacement of the medial canthi, dystopia of the lower lacrimal puncta, blepharophimosis, and partial or total heterochromia. The medial third of the eyebrow is hyperplastic, and the brows may be confluent. The nasal root is hypertrophied.

Xeroderma Pigmentosum

Eyelid involvement consists of ectropion and destruction of the lower eyelid. (See also under Conjunctiva and Cornea.)

UVEAL TRACT AND RETINA

Albinism

Albinism is a disorder of pigmentation caused by a defect in the synthesis of tyrosinase in the melanocyte of the skin and eye which is transmitted as an autosomal recessive trait.

The cutaneous manifestation of this disorder consists of complete lack of pigment in the skin and hair. Later in life the light-exposed areas of the skin develop precancerous lesions and finally squamous cell carcinomas.

Associated ophthalmic findings consist of whitish-yellow eyebrows and eyelashes,

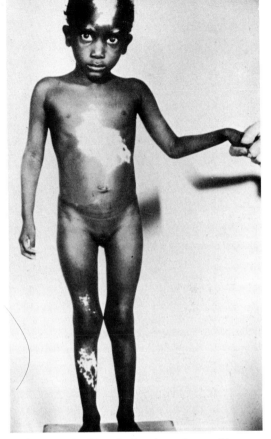

Figure 30–8 Waardenburg's syndrome. (Courtesy of Dr. R. D. Harley.)

pink iris and red pupil, and a characteristic orange-red retina. Errors of refraction, myopic astigmatism, and nystagmus are characteristic features. In the more common incomplete form, hair is yellow or light brown and the iris is light blue or pink, changing to blue or blue-gray.

Albright's Syndrome (Osteodystrophia)

Albright's syndrome is a disease of unknown etiology. It is characterized by association of mono- and polyostotic fibrous dysplasia, hyperpigmented macules, endocrine dysfunction, and osteoma cutis. The full syndrome with precocious puberty occurs only in girls.

The cutaneous manifestations which appear early in life before the age of 2 years consist of large and extensive light brown macular patches with irregular

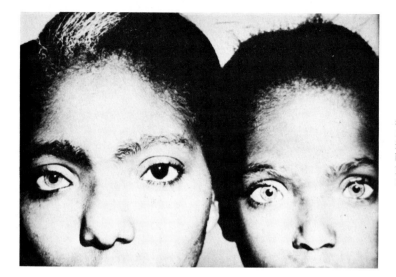

Figure 30–9 Waardenburg's syndrome in mother and daughter. Heterochromia and white forelock in mother; deafness and isochromic blue eyes in daughter. (Courtesy of Drs. R. D. Ohmstead, Di George, and Harley.)

serrated margins, few in number, unilateral, and localized to the trunk and proximal aspects of the lower extremities. Associated findings are the result of bone lesions and consist of aching pain, pathologic fractures, and secondary deformities.

Ophthalmic manifestations are the result of the overgrowth at the base of the skull, with proptosis and compression of the optic nerve resulting in secondary visual field defects.

Allezzandrini's Syndrome

Allezzandrini's syndrome is a rare syndrome of unknown etiology which afflicts adolescents and young adults and consists of unilateral impairment of vision, followed after an interval of months or years by vitiligo and poliosis. Bilateral deafness may also appear.

The ophthalmic finding consists of a degenerative retinopathy.

Behçet's Syndrome

Behçet's syndrome is a chronic, often progressive, inflammatory disease of the mouth, genitalia, and eye and is of unknown etiology. It is most frequently seen in adolescence and middle age but may commence in childhood.

The cutaneous manifestations include the appearance of recurring single or multiple ulcers on the mucous membranes of the mouth and genitalia. The majority of patients later develop skin lesions consisting of nonfollicular pustules on the trunk and extremities and crops of erythema nodosum-like lesions on the lower extremities. Associated systemic involvement includes fever and central nervous system involvement.

Ocular manifestations consist of recurrent uveitis, with or without hypopyon, conjunctivitis, episcleritis, iritis, and retinal vascular lesions. Papilledema and cranial nerve palsies are occasionally seen.

Chediak-Higashi Syndrome

See Chapter 20.

Cockayne's Syndrome

Cockayne's syndrome is an extremely rare syndrome of unknown etiology characterized by cutaneous, neurologic, and skeletal defects which become apparent after the first year of life.

The cutaneous manifestations consist of a light-induced erythematous, maculopapular eruption on the light-exposed areas of the face. In time, the light sensitivity is lost and premature aging of the skin occurs, with the appearance of irregular, macular, hyper- and hypopigmented patches and atrophy. Associated skeletal changes include disproportionately long extremities, large hands and feet, kyphosis, ankylosis, prognathism, and thickened bones of the skull. Neurologic manifestations consist of mental retardation, cerebral atrophy, and neural degeneration. Survival beyond the second decade of life is unusual.

Ophthalmic manifestations are the presence of optic atrophy and pigmentary retinal degeneration which may result in severe visual loss.

Ehler-Danlos Syndrome (Cutis Hyperelasticum)

See Chapter 20.

Granulomatous Disease of Childhood (Chronic)

Chronic granulomatous disease of childhood is a genetically determined abnormality transmitted as an X-linked metabolic defect manifested by inability of the leukocytes to operate the hexose monophosphate shunt during phagocytosis and to oxidize NADH and NADPH.

The characteristic clinical syndrome in affected males consists of chronic suppurative microabscesses, first of the skin and lymph nodes and ultimately of all viscera. A nonspecific eczematous dermatitis may occur around the eyes, mouth, and nose.

Associated ophthalmic findings consist of peripheral conjunctivitis, keratitis, and destructive chorioretinal lesions.

Henoch-Schönlein Purpura (Anaphylactoid Purpura)

Henoch-Schönlein purpura is a nonthrombocytopenic type of purpura produced by a hypersensitivity mechanism that results in vascular damage and produces a syndrome consisting of a skin eruption and gastrointestinal and joint symptoms.

The cutaneous manifestations consist of purpura, urticaria, inflammatory papules, and ill-defined macular erythematous areas which may appear individually or simultaneously. Associated findings are abdominal pain, vomiting and diarrhea, polyarthritis, and nephritis which is often self-limited.

Ophthalmic findings consist of retinal hemorrhages, iritis, and occasional optic neuritis.

Juvenile Melanoma of Spitz (Compound Melanocytoma)

Juvenile melanoma is a benign tumor arising from melanocytes in children with a characteristic clinical picture and a malignant-appearing histologic feature.

The clinical appearance of the lesion is characteristic and consists of a firm, round, red or reddish-brown nodule usually on the face and legs. It grows rapidly at first. The true degree of pigmentation can be demonstrated only by expressing the blood in the tumor by diascopy.

Ophthalmic tumors have occasionally been found involving the conjunctiva and the uveal tract.

Juvenile Xanthogranuloma (JXG) (Nevoxanthoendothelioma)

Juvenile xanthogranuloma is a benign type of localized reactive inflammatory disorder of unknown etiology characterized by cutaneous and occasionally other organ involvement.

The cutaneous manifestations consist of yellowish to reddish-brown papules or nodules which appear during the first six months of life and are irregularly but widely distributed. Spontaneous resolution usually occurs within one year.

Ophthalmic manifestations are not common but the yellowish elevated masses may typically involve the iris and/or ciliary body. Recurrent hyphema is common in JXG.

Pseudoxanthoma Elasticum

See Chapter 20.

Raynaud's Phenomenon

Raynaud's phenomenon consists of episodic constriction of the small arteries or arterioles of the extremities of unknown etiology. It may also be associated with trauma, neurovascular disease, or diffuse connective tissue disease.

The cutaneous manifestations consist of intermittent changes in color of the skin of the extremities with blanching or cyanosis, or both.

Ophthalmic findings may consist of the rare occurrence of retinal angiospasms.

Refsum's Syndrome (Heredopathia Atactica Polyneuritiformis)

Refsum's syndrome is a rare syndrome consisting of cutaneous, ocular, and neurologic manifestations and caused by a disorder of lipid metabolism which is inherited as an autosomal recessive trait.

Cutaneous manifestations consist of

generalized dryness, and scaling similar to ichthyosis develops in childhood. Associated findings which develop slowly and progressively include polyneuritis, weakness, loss of deep tendon reflexes, and nerve deafness.

Ophthalmic findings consist of retinitis pigmentosa and night blindness.

Sarcoidosis

See Chapter 13.

Sjögren-Larsson Syndrome

The Sjögren-Larsson syndrome is transmitted as an autosomal recessive trait and is characterized by mental deficiency, spastic paralysis, and ocular and cutaneous changes. The cutaneous manifestations consist of an ichthyosiform erythroderma, the severity of which may diminish with time, leaving only flexural hyperkeratosis and mild generalized scaling.

The ophthalmic manifestations consist of ectropion, occasional keratitis, cataracts infrequently, and pigmentary degeneration of the retina in 30 per cent of cases.

Tuberous Sclerosis (Epiloia)

See Chapter 18.

Ulcerative Colitis

Ulcerative colitis is a multisystem disease which may have mucocutaneous, joint, and eye involvement in addition to the mucosal lesions of the large bowel.

Cutaneous manifestations may appear in approximately one third of patients and consist of recurrent aphthae, erythema nodosum, and pyoderma gangrenosum. The tender, inflammatory nodules on the lower extremities of erythema nodosum appear in approximately 5 to 10 per cent of patients and usually during the acute phase of the disease. Pyoderma gangrenosum occurs less frequently in either the active or quiescent phase of the disease and consists of a septic, necrotic ulcer on almost any area of the body. Uncommonly, papillary projections on the buccal mucosa, gingiva, palate, and labial surfaces occur. Associated features are perianal abscesses and fistulas, and palmar erythema and clubbing of the fingers.

Ophthalmic manifestations include iritis, uveitis, and episcleritis which are usually seen in association with the devel-

opment of rheumatoid arthritis. The palpebral conjunctiva may be involved in papillomatous changes similar to those seen in the oral mucosa.

Vascular Abnormalities (See also Chapter 18)

There are four syndromes associated with neurologic, ocular, and cutaneous vascular abnormalities.

1. BONNET-DeCHAUME-BLANC SYNDROME. This syndrome consists of vascular nevi of the telangiectatic type on the face, associated with retinal and intracranial angiomatosis.

2. STURGE-WEBER SYNDROME.

3. VON HIPPEL-LINDAU DISEASE. This disease consists of inconstant vascular nevi on the face, hemangioblastomas of the cerebellum, extensive retinal angiomas, hemorrhages, and retinal detachment.

4. WYBURN-MASON SYNDROME. This syndrome consists of telangiectatic vascular nevi of the skin surrounding the affected eye, with midbrain arteriovenous aneurysms and congenital dilated, tortuous retinal vessels.

Vogt-Koyanagi Syndrome (Harada's Disease)

The Vogt-Koyanagi syndrome is a rare disorder of unknown etiology characterized by the appearance of central nervous system, ocular, and cutaneous signs and symptoms appearing in sequence over a period of several months.

The cutaneous manifestations appear within the first three months of the process, which consists of a prodromal episode associated with cephalitis or meningitis, followed within two weeks by bilateral uveitis, often with choroiditis and optic neuritis. As the uveitis begins to subside, vitiligo, poliosis, and alopecia may develop. The pigmentary changes tend to be permanent. Associated findings consist of deafness and/or tinnitus appearing at the time of development of the uveitis. The syndrome is most common in the third and fourth decades, but children and adolescents may be affected.

The ophthalmic findings consist of bilateral uveitis, choroiditis, and optic neuritis which may slowly clear during a lengthy period of time, but extensive visual loss can occur. The poliosis may be limited to the brows and lashes. The relationship of sympathetic ophthalmia to this syndrome is a close one from the viewpoint of the skin and eye involvement. Prognosis for recovery is good with the aid of corticosteroid therapy.

For discussion of Dermatomyositis, Lupus Erythematosus, Periarteritis Nodosa, Relapsing Polychondritis, Rheumatoid Disease, and Scleroderma, see Chapter 20.

REFERENCES

Adams, R. D., and Reed, W. B.: Dermatology in General Practice. Refsum's syndrome, acanthocytosis and Tangier disease. Neurocutaneous diseases. New York, McGraw-Hill Book Co., 1971, p. 1416.

Alezzandrini, A. A.: Manifestation unilaterale de degenerescence tapeto-retinienne, de vitiligo, de poliose, de cheveux blancs et d'hypoacousie. Ophthalmologica, 147:409, 1964.

Allen, D. M., Diamond, L. K., and Howell, D. A.: Anaphylactoid purpura in children (Schönlein-Henoch syndrome). Amer. J. Dis. Child., 99:833, June, 1960.

Amendola, F.: Ocular manifestations of pemphigus foliaceus. Amer. J. Ophthal., 32:35, 1949.

Baer, R. L., and Kopf, A. W.: Clinical and histologic findings of nevus-cell nevi and of juvenile melanoma. Year Book of Dermatology, 1964–1965 Series, pp. 161–163.

Barranco, V. P.: Cutaneous ossification in pseudohypoparathyroidism. Arch. Derm., 104:643, December, 1971.

Beier, F. R., and Lahey, M. E.: Sarcoidosis among children in Utah and Idaho. J. Pediat., 65:350, September, 1964.

Bianchine, J. R., Macoraeg, V. J., Jr., Lasagna, L., et al.: Drugs as etiologic factors in the Stevens-Johnson syndrome. Amer. J. Med., 44:390, 1968.

Blank, H., Eglick, P. G., and Beerman, H.: Nevoxantho-endothelioma with ocular involvement. Pediatrics, 4:349, 1949.

Blodi, F. C., von Allen, M. W., and Yarbrough, J. C.: Duane's syndrome: A brain stem lesion. Arch. Ophthal., 72:171, 1955.

Brady, R. O., Gal, A. E., Bradley, B. S., et al.: Enzymatic defect in Fabry's disease. New Eng. J. Med., 276:1163, No. 1, May, 1967.

Braun-Falco, O.: The pathology of blister formation. Year Book of Dermatology, 1969, pp. 6–42.

Braverman, I. M.: Skin Signs in Systemic Disease. Inflammatory diseases of the bowel. Philadelphia, W. B. Saunders Co., 1970, pp. 329–332.

Brown, C. A.: Incontinentia pigmenti with pseudoglioma. Proc. Roy. Soc. Med., 62:8, January, 1969.

Butterworth, T.: Dermatological aspects of cretinism. Arch. Derm., 70:565, 1954.

Calmettes, L., Deodati, F., Bec, P., et al.: Cutis laxa et dystrophie corneenne. Bull. Soc. Ophthal. Franc. (Paris), 68:820, 1968.

Carr, R. D., Berke, M., and Becker, S. W.: Incidence of atopy in the general population. Arch. Derm., 89:27, 1964.

Chalvignac, A., Pfirsch, F., and Levy, J. P.: Presentation d'un malade atteint d'une "blepharorraphie spontanée." Bull. Soc. Ophthal. Franc., 67:937, 1967.

Champion, R. H., and Wilkinson, D. S.: Textbook of Dermatology. Vol. I. Hereditary hemorrhagic telangiectasia. Philadelphia, F. A. Davis, 1968, pp. 408–410.

Christoferson, L. A., Gustafson, M. B., and Petersen, A. G.: Von Hippel-Lindau's disease. J.A.M.A., 178:126, October 21, 1961.

Cleaver, J. E.: Defective repair replication of DNA in xeroderma pigmentosum. Nature, 218:652, May, 1968.

Cleaver, J. E.: DNA damage and repair in light-sensitive human skin disease. J. Invest. Derm., 54:181, No. 3, 1970.

Clifton, F., and Gordon, W. H.: A case of an adenoma arising in a sweat gland of the upper eyelid. Brit. J. Ophthal., 31:697, 1947.

Comings, D. E., Papazian, C., and Schoene, H. R.: Conradi's disease. J. Pediat., 72:63, No. 1, January, 1968.

Cone, R. B.: A review of Boeck's sarcoid with analysis of twelve cases occurring in children. J. Pediat., 32:629, No. 6, June, 1948.

Connell, H., Churcher, G. M., and Milton-Thompson, G. I.: Stevens-Johnson syndrome associated with Mycoplasma pneumonial infection. Brit. J. Derm., 81:196, 1969.

Costello, M. J., and Buncke, C. M.: Dyskeratosis congenita. Arch. Derm., 73:123, February, 1956.

Curth, H. O., and Warburton, D.: The genetics of incontinentia pigmenti. Arch. Derm., 92:229, September, 1965.

Davenport, D. D.: Ulerythema ophryogenes. Arch. Derm., 89:74, 1964.

Davies, J. H. T.: Seborrheic eczema: An attempt to define the scope of the term. Brit. J. Derm., 64:213, 1952.

Demis, D. J., and Weiner, M. A.: Alopecia universalis, onychodystrophy and total vitiligo. Arch. Derm., 88:195, August, 1963.

DiGeorge, A. M., Harley, R. D., and Olmstead, R.: Waardenburg's syndrome. Trans. Amer. Acad. Ophthal. and Otolaryng., 64:816, 1960.

Duke, B. O. L.: Onchocerciasis. Brit. Med. J., 4:301, 1968.

Duke-Elder, S., and Dobree, J. H.: System of Ophthalmology. Vol. 10. Diseases of the retina. St. Louis, The C. V. Mosby Co., 1967, p. 81.

Duperrat, B., Pringuet, R., and Escande, J. P.: Aphtose de Behçet. Bull. Soc. Franc. Derm. Syph., 74:413, 1967.

Ebling, F. J., and Rook, A.: Textbook of Dermatology. Vol. II. Acquired hypertrichosis lanuginosa. Philadelphia, F. A. Davis Co., 1968, p. 1364.

Eisert, J.: Diabetes and diseases of the skin. Med. Clin. N. Amer., 49:621, 1965.

Eyre, W. G., and Reed, W. B.: Albright's hereditary osteodystrophy with cutaneous bone formation. Arch. Derm., 104:634, December 1971.

Feingold, M., and Gellis, S. S.: Ocular abnormalities associated with first and second arch syndromes. Survey Ophthal., 14:30, No. 1, 1969.

Fellner, M. J.: Manifestations of familial autonomic dysautonomia. Arch. Derm., 89:190, February, 1964.

Findlay, G. H., Scott, F. P., and Cripps, D. J.: Porphyria and lipid proteinosis. Brit. J. Derm., 78:69, 1966.

Fiumara, N. J., and Lessell, S.: Manifestations of late congenital syphilis. Arch. Derm., 102:78, July, 1970.

Francois, J., Bacskulin, J., and Follmann, P.: Manifestations oculaires du syndrome d'Urbach-Wiethe. Ophthalmologica, 155:433, 1968.

Fries, J. H., Borne, S., and Barnes, H. L.: Varicelliform eruption of Kaposi due to vaccinia virus complicating atopic eczema. J. Pediat., 32:532, 1948.

Gifford, R. W., Jr., and Hines, E. A., Jr.: Raynaud's disease among women and girls. Circulation, 16:1012, December, 1957.

Goldberg, A., and Rimington, C.: Diseases of Porphyrin Metabolism. Springfield, Illinois, Charles C Thomas, 1962.

Goltz, R. W., Hult, A. M., Goldfarb, M., and Gorlin, R. J.: Cutis laxa. Arch. Derm., 92:373, October, 1965.

Goltz, R. W., Peterson, W. C., Gorlin, R. J., and Ravits, H. G.: Focal dermal hypoplasia. Arch. Derm., 86:708, December, 1962.

Good, R. A., Quie, P. G., Windhorst, D. B., Page, A. R., et al.: Fatal (chronic) granulomatous disease of childhood: A hereditary defect of leukocyte function. Seminars Hemat., 5:215, 1968.

Gray, H. R., and Helwig, E. B.: Epithelioma adenoides cysticum and solitary trichoepithelioma. Arch. Derm., 87:102, 1963.

Green, W. R., Friedman-Kien, A., and Banfield, W. G.: Angioid streaks in Ehlers-Danlos syndrome. Arch. Ophthal., 76:197, August, 1966.

Greither, A., and Tritsch, H.: Über einen Fall von anhidrotischer ektodermaler Dysplasie mit nahezu vollständiger Alopecie, transgredienten Palmar-Plantar-Keratosen, Macula-Degeneration sowie anderen Augenstörungen, Zahnanomalien und einem Pseudo-Klinefelter-Syndrom. Archiv. f. Klin. Exper. Derma., 216:50, 1963.

Grosfeld, J. C. M., Mighorst, J. A., and Moolhuysen, T. M. G. F.: Argininosuccinic aciduria in monilethrix. Lancet, 10:789, October, 1964.

Grover, W. D., and Harley, R. D.: Early recognition of tuberous sclerosis by funduscopic examination. J. Pediat., 75:991, December, 1969.

Haim, S.: Contribution of ocular symptoms in the diagnosis of Behçet's disease. Arch. Derm., 98:478, November, 1968.

Hanno, H. A., and Weiss, D. I.: Hypoparathyroidism, pseudohypoparathyroidism, and pseudopseudohypoparathyroidism. Arch. Ophthal., 65:238, 1961.

Harley, R. D., and Wedding, E. S.: Syndrome of uveitis, meningoencephalitis, alopecia, poliosis and dysacousia. Amer. J. Ophthal., 29:524, 1946.

Harrison, R., and Okun, M.: Divided nevus. Arch. Derm., 82:235, 1960.

Heijer, A., and Reed, W. B.: Sjögren-Larsson syndrome. Arch. Derm., 92:545, November, 1965.

Hunziker, N.: A propos de l'hyperpigmentation familiale des paupières. J. Genet. Hum., 11:16, 1962.

Hyams, S. W., Dar, H., and Neumann, E.: Blue sclerae and keratoglobus. Brit. J. Ophthal., 53:53, 1969.

Jahr, H. M., and McIntire, M. S.: Piebaldism, of familial white skin spotting (partial albinism). Amer. J. Dis. Child., 88:481, 1954.

Jay, B., Blach, R. K., and Wells, R. S.: Ocular manifestations of ichthyosis. Brit. J. Ophthal., 52:217, 1968.

Jay, B., Blach, R. K., and Wells, R. S.: Eye changes in ichthyosis. J.A.M.A., 208:155, No. 1, April 7, 1969.

Johnson, L. A., and Winkelmann, R. K.: Cutaneous vascular reactivity in atopic children. Arch. Derm., 92:621, December, 1965.

Johnson, W. C.: Vogt-Koyanagi-Harada syndrome. Arch. Derm., 88:146, August, 1963.

Johnson, W. C., Higdon, R. S., and Helwig, E. B.: Alopecia mucinosa. Arch. Derm., 79:395, 1959.

Johnston, A. W., Weller, S. D. V., and Warland, B. J.: Angiokeratoma corporis diffusum. Arch. Dis. Child., 43:73, 1968.

Joseph, H. L.: Pachyonychia congenita. Arch. Derm., 90:594, December, 1964.

Kaldeck, R.: Ocular psoriasis. Arch. Derm., 68:44, 1953.

Keeler, C.: The Cuna moon-child syndrome. Dermato. Tropica, 3:1, 1964.

Kerr, C. B., Wells, R. S., and Cooper, K. E.: Gene effect in carriers of anhidrotic ectodermal dysplasia. J. Med. Genet., 3:169, 1966.

Kersting, D. W., and Rapaport, I. F.: A clinicopathologic study of the skin in mongolism. Arch. Derm., 77:319, March, 1958.

Kim, R., and Winkelmann, R. K.: Follicular mucinosis (alopecia mucinosa). Arch. Derm., 85:490, April, 1962.

Kirby, T. J., Achor, R. W. P., Perry, H. O., et al.: Cataract formation after triparanol therapy. Arch. Ophthal., 68:486, 1962.

Koblenzer, P. J., and Koblenzer, C. S.: Anomalies of the vascular system as they affect the skin. Clin. Pediat., 5:95, No. 2, February, 1966.

Kooij, R.: Sarcoidosis or leprosy? Brit. J. Derm., 76:203, May, 1964.

Lagos, J. C., and Gomez, M. R.: Tuberous sclerosis: Reappraisal of a clinical entity. Mayo Clin. Proc., 42:26, January, 1967.

Lamar, L. M., and Gaethe, G.: Pityriasis rubra pilaris. Arch. Derm., 89:515, 1964.

Lamba, P. A., Shukla, K. N., and Madhavan, M.: Xeroderma pigmentosa with atypical ocular involvement. Canad. J. Ophthal., 4:148, 1969.

Lerner, A. B.: Vitiligo. J. Invest. Derm., 32:285, 1959.

Lieberman, W. J., Schimek, R. A., and Snyder, C. H.: Cockayne's disease. Amer. J. Ophthal., 52:116, 1961.

Lombardo, P. C.: Pseudoxanthoma elasticum. Arch. Derm., 99:370, March, 1969.

Lowenthal, L. J. A., and Prakken, J. R.: Atrichia with papular lesions. Dermatologica, 122:85, 1961.

Martyn, L. J., Lischner, H. W., Pileggi, A. J., and Harley, R. D.: Chorioretinal lesions in familial chronic granulomatous disease of childhood. Amer. J. Ophthal., 73:403, No. 3, March, 1972.

Mashima, Y., and Mevorah, B.: Nevus Ota and nevus Ito in American Negroes. J. Invest. Derm., 36:133, 1961.

McFadden, A. W.: Skin disease in the Cuna Indians. Arch. Derm., *84*:1013, December, 1961.

McGovern, J. P., and Merritt, D. H.: Sarcoidosis in childhood. Adv. Pediat., *8*:97, 1953.

Mehregan, A. H.: Apocrine cystadenoma, a clinicopathologic study with special reference to the pigmented variety. Arch. Derm. (Chicago), *90*:274, September, 1964.

Miller, H. G., and Daley, R.: Clinical aspects of polyarteritis nodosa. Quart. J. Med., *39*:255, 1946.

Monacelli, M., and Nazzaro, P.: Behçet's Disease (Monography). Basel, S. Karger, 1966.

Monnet, P., Paufique, L., Salle, B., et al.: Syndrome familial du type Marinesco-Sjögren. Arch. Franc. Ped., *26*:87, 1969.

Montgomery, H.: Pityriasis rubra pilaris. Dermatopathology, *1*:332, 1967.

Moossy, J.: The neuropathology of Cockayne's syndrome. J. Neur. Exp. Neurol., *26*:654, 1967.

Muller, S. A., and Brunsting, L. A.: Cataracts associated with dermatologic disorders. Arch. Derm., *88*:330, 1963.

Muller, S. A., and Brunsting, L. A.: Cataracts in alopecia areata. Arch. Derm., *88*:202, August, 1963.

Nellhaus, G., Haberland, C., and Hill, B. J.: Sturge-Weber disease with bilateral intracranial calcifications at birth and unusual pathologic findings. Acta Neurol. Scand., *43*:314, 1967.

Nelson, W. E., Vaughn, V. C., and McKay, J.: Textbook of Pediatrics. Degenerative diseases. Philadelphia, W. B. Saunders Co., 1969, pp. 1189–1204.

Oglesby, R. B., Black, R. L., von Sallmann, L., et al.: Cataracts in patients with rheumatic diseases treated with corticosteroids. Arch. Ophthal., *66*:625, 1961.

Pearson, R. W.: Studies on the pathogenesis of epidermolysis bullosa. J. Invest. Derm., *39*:551, 1962.

Perloff, J. K., and Phelps, E. T.: A review of Werner's syndrome with a report of the second autopsied case. Ann. Intern. Med., *48*:1205, 1958.

Petrohelos, M. A.: Werner's syndrome. Amer. J. Ophthal., *56*:941, 1963.

Pillsbury, D. M., Shelley, W. B., and Kligman, A. M.: Dermatology. Trichotillomania. Philadelphia, W. B. Saunders Co., 1956, p. 997.

Pinkus, H.: Vitiligo—What is it? J. Invest. Derm., *32*:281, 1959.

Reed, W. B., Landing, B., Sugarman, G., Cleaver, J. E., et al.: Xeroderma pigmentosum. J.A.M.A., *207*:2073, No. 11, March 17, 1969.

Robinson, R. C. V.: Congenital syphilis. Arch. Derm., *99*:599, May, 1969.

Ronchese, F.: Treatment of pediculosis ciliorum in an infant. New Eng. J. Med., *249*:897, No. 22, November, 1953.

Roper-Hall, M. J.: The ocular aspects of Rosacea. Trans. Ophthal. Soc. U.K., *86*:727, 1966.

Rosen, E.: Atopic cataract. American Lecture Series, Pub. No. 373. Springfield, Illinois, Charles C Thomas, 1959.

Rosen, E.: Fundus in pseudoxanthoma elasticum. Amer. J. Ophthal., *66*:236, 1968.

Rosenberg, P. E., Dana, A. S., Jr., and Changizi, M. H.: Solitary trichoepithelioma occurring on the thigh—Case report. Cutis, *4*:1079, No. 9, September, 1968.

Rovin, S., Dachi, S. F., Borenstein, D. B., et al.:

Mandibulofacial dysostosis, a familial study of five generations. J. Pediat., *65*:215, 1964.

Sagebiel, R. W.: Non-specific inclusions in epidermal cells of keratoacanthoma. J. Invest. Derm., *46*:293, No. 3, 1966.

Saidi, M., and Chagnon, J.: Hernie inguinale, hydrocile, kyste du cordon et manifestations osseuses observées dans le syndrome de Berry-Treacher Collins. Un. Med. Canada, *99*:882, 1970.

Salazar, F. N.: Dermatological manifestations of the Cornelia de Lange syndrome. Arch. Derm., *94*:38, July, 1966.

Scadding, J. G.: Sarcoidosis. London, Eyre and Spottiswoode, 1967.

Schaller, J., Kupfer, C., and Wedgewood, R. J.: Iridocyclitis in juvenile rheumatoid arthritis. Pediatrics, *44*:92, No. 1, July, 1969.

Schnyder, U. W., Franceschetti, A. T., Ceszarovic, B., et al.: La maladie de Meleda Autochtone. Ann. Derm. Syph. *96*:517, 1969.

Schuster, D. S., and Johnson, S. A. M.: Cutaneous manifestations of the Cornelia de Lange syndrome. Arch. Derm., *93*:702, June, 1966.

Sever, R. J., Frost, P., and Weinstein, G.: Eye changes in ichthyosis. J.A.M.A., *206*:2283, No. 10, December 2, 1968.

Simpson, J. A.: Dermatological changes in hypocalcaemia. Brit. J. Derm., *66*:1, January, 1954.

Siskind, W. M.: Pili torti. Arch. Derm., *56*:540, 1947.

Smiley, W. K.: Adult rheumatoid arthritis. Ann. Phys. Med., *10*:157, November, 1969.

Solomons, G., Zellweger, H., Jahnke, P. G., et al.: Four common eye signs in mongolism. Amer. J. Dis. Child., *110*:46, July, 1965.

Spott, D. A., Wood, M. G., and Heaton, C. L.: Melanoacanthoma of the eyelid. Arch. Derm., *105*:898, June, 1972.

Starr, P. A. J.: Oculocutaneous aspects of rosacea. Proc. Roy. Soc. Med., *62*:9, January, 1969.

Sugar, H. S.: The oculoauriculovertebral dysplasia syndrome of Goldenhar. Amer. J. Ophthal., *62*:678, 1966.

Thomson, J., and Forfar, J. O.: Progeria (Hutchinson-Gilford syndrome) Arch. Dis. Child., *25*:224, 1950.

Tillman, W. G.: Alopecia congenita: Report of two families. Brit. Med. J., *2*:428, 1952.

Urbach, F.: Lupus erythematosus. Pediat. Clin. N. Amer., *8*:873, 1961.

Vander Ploeg, D. E., and Stagnone, J. J.: Eyebrow alopecia in secondary syphilis. Arch. Derm., *90*:172, August, 1964.

Vannas, S., and Lapinleimu, J.: Molluscum contagiosum in the skin, caruncle and conjunctiva. Acta Ophthal., *45*:314, 1967.

Varley, R., and Kletz, T.: A case of Kaposi's varicelliform eruption (systemic herpes simplex) with dendritic ulceration of the cornea. Brit. J. Derm., *61*:166, 1949.

Vernier, R. L., Worthen, H. G., Peterson, R. D., et al.: Anaphylactoid purpura. Pediatrics, *27*:181, 1961.

von Gemminger, G., Kierland, R. R., and Opitz, J. M.: Angiokeratoma corporis diffusum (Fabry's disease). Arch. Derm., *91*:206, 1965.

von Noorden, G. K., and Buck, A. A.: Ocular onchocerciasis. Arch. Ophthal., *80*:26, July, 1968.

Waardenburg, P. J.: A new syndrome combining developmental anomalies of the eyelids, eyebrows and nose root with pigmentary defects of the iris and head hair and with congenital deafness. Amer. J. Human Genet., 3:195, No. 3, September, 1951.

Wachtel, J. G.: The ocular pathology of Marfan's syndrome. Arch. Ophthal. (N.Y.), 76:512, October, 1966.

White, J. G.: The Chediak-Higashi syndrome: A possible lysosomal disease. Blood, 28:143, No. 2, August, 1966.

Windhorst, D. B., Zelickson, A. S., and Good, R. A.: A human pigmentary dilution based on a heritable subcellular structural defect — the Chediak-Higashi syndrome. J. Invest. Derm., 50:9, January, 1968.

Wise, D., Wallace, H. J., and Jellinek, E. H.: Angio-

keratoma corporis diffusum. Quart. J. Med., 55: 177, 1962.

Wolter, J. R., and Henderson, J. W.: Ruptures of Descemet's membrane in keratoconus. Amer. J. Ophthal., 63:1689, 1967.

Wyburn-Mason, R.: Arteriovenous aneurysm of midbrain and retina, facial nevi and mental changes. Brain, 66:12, September, 1943.

Zabriskie, J., and Reisman, M.: Marchesani syndrome. J. Pediat., 52:158, 1958.

Zegarelli, E. V., and Kutscher, A. H.: Oral "pyoderma." Amer. J. Digest. Dis., New Series 7:281, No. 3, 1962.

Zuckerman, B. D.: Conjunctival pigmentation due to cosmetics. Amer. J. Ophthal., 62:672, 1966.

OCULAR MANIFESTATIONS OF SKELETAL DISORDERS

ROBERT A. SARGENT, M.D.

A number of hereditary skeletal disorders may be observed in the skull and orbit. These changes may affect the eye directly or indirectly despite the relative insulation of the surrounding tissues.

Altered separation of the orbits, shallowness of the orbits, extraocular muscle defects, and bony impingement about the optic foramen may result from skeletal disturbances and deformities with varying effects on the ocular apparatus.

Apart from changes due to anatomic variations, the ocular and skeletal changes may be the result of a common metabolic defect or of defects of unknown origin. The following guideline summarizes the entities to be described:

1. Craniostenoses
   a. Oxycephaly
   b. Apert's syndrome
   c. Crouzon's disease
   d. Carpenter's syndrome
   e. Hypertelorism
2. Mandibulofacial dysostoses
   a. Treacher Collins syndrome
   b. Hallermann-Streiff syndrome
   c. Goldenhar's syndrome
   d. Pierre Robin syndrome
3. Fragile bone diseases
   a. Osteogenesis imperfecta
   b. Fibrous dysplasia
   c. Osteopetrosis
4. Chondroplastic diseases
   a. Achondroplasia
   b. Conradi's disease
   c. Skeletal alterations in the mucopolysaccharidoses
5. Dwarfism
   a. Cockayne's disease
   b. Progeria
   c. Seckel's bird-headed dwarf
   d. Werner's disease
6. "Bull-neck" anomalies
   a. Platybasia
   b. Arnold-Chiari syndrome
   c. Klippel-Feil syndrome
7. Oculoskeletal diseases with skin involvement
8. Miscellaneous syndromes

CRANIOSTENOSES

Craniostenosis refers to the premature closing of the skull sutures. Normally the cranial bones abut each other by approximately one year of age, and interdigitate completely by about eight to ten years of age, only to be closed finally at early adulthood. The brain undergoes significant expansion up to approximately eight years of age. Thus, premature closure causes skull deformity, enlargement of the head (megalocephaly), and mental and motor stunting during these early years of life. This is in response to increased intracranial pressure. However, beyond this prepubertal age the cranium does not permit expansion; therefore, papilledema and possible optic atrophy ensue. If the synostosis particularly affects the orbital region, as in oxycephaly or Crouzon's disease, shallow orbits result, which in turn cause exophthalmos. In the brain's attempt to expand, there results a thinning of the cranial bones that is radiologically manifested by a smooth-edged, beaten-out appearance.

The deformity to which the skull eventuates depends upon which sutures close prematurely. As a rule, brain growth is hindered in a direction perpendicular to the line of the prematurely fused suture (perpendicular here indicates "into the air," not tangential to the closed suture or sutures). For example, plagiocephaly is characterized by a slanted, asymmetrical head with a vertical and lateral bulging on one side. This results from unilateral closure of a coronal suture on the opposite side. That is, the enlarging brain grows in any direction in which it is not severely obstructed.

When more than one suture is fused, growth extends by one of two mechanisms. The brain may protrude in a direction opposite to the fused sutures, which is in the direction of least resistance. This would occur in trigonocephaly, in which the synostitic coronal sutures force the intracranial contents posteriorly. Here, the appearance is of a head whose posterior portion bulges laterally and vertically. Another example of this mechanism is oxycephaly, in which the frontal suture, in addition to the coronal sutures, is prematurely fused. Growth must extend in the opposite direction, namely, superoposteriorly.

In a second mechanism the fused sutures act as an immobile keel which "floats" or elevates. Thus, a prematurely closed sagittal suture extending from the anterior to posterior fontanelles leads to a vertical elevation of this "keel"—called scaphocephaly—and creates a narrow skull on frontal view with a long anterior-posterior diameter. Another example is that of brachycephaly, characterized by a pancake-like, or flat-faced, head with a short anterior-posterior length. This results from fused coronal sutures which "float" ver-

tically instead of forcing posterior growth, as in trigonocephaly.

Oxycephaly (Acrocephaly)

Almost to the exclusion of other craniostenoses, increased pressure tends to occur in oxycephaly. Therefore, oxycephaly is of neurologic and ophthalmologic significance. Other descriptive terms apply for oxycephaly, such as tower skull or dome-shaped, pointed, or bullet-shaped head. There is wide variation in this deformity, and although it is present neonatally, it is rarely recognized in infancy and early childhood. Oxycephaly is essentially an elongation in an anterior-to-superoposterior direction together with a short transverse diameter. There often is a high forehead, or occipital overhang. Acrocephaly is a term often used in place of oxycephaly, but strictly speaking it refers to anterior protrusion such as that seen in Apert's syndrome (high forehead and flat occiput). When the posterior skull protrudes, a flat head is created on the surface of the head sometimes being saddle-shaped, and tends to overhang the cervical spine. This condition is called clinocephaly or platycephaly.

Unlike the other entities, oxycephaly may have hereditary patterns, as evidenced by reports of irregularly dominant pedigrees, a greater incidence in monozygotic twins, its absence in dizygotic twins, its presence in siblings, and occasional cases of consanguinity of parents. Interestingly, oxycephaly is more common in boys than in girls.

Associated skeletal findings are those of malar hypoplasia, a deviated nasal septum, syndactyly, and a heavy lower jaw coupled with a small upper jaw creating prognathism.

Symptomatology depends on the severity of the disease. When severe, headaches, convulsions, and visually crippling eye signs, such as papilledema and optic atrophy, occur. However, minor involvement may exclude neuro-ophthalmic signs. Although there may be no mental retardation, psychosocial cosmetic difficulties may exist.

Over half the cases of oxycephaly have exophthalmos due to shallow orbits. Voluntary protrusion of the globes can occur with crying or coughing. Hypertelorism and exotropia are related to the bony configuration. Ptosis, ectropion, blue sclerae, nystagmus, cataracts, and medullated nerve fibers have been reported in oxycephaly.

Loss of vision is secondary to optic atrophy. The reason for this is not clear, but it may be due to a sharp angulation and stretching of the optic nerve as it enters the optic canal, or secondary to papilledema and increased intracranial pressure.

Diagnosis can be confirmed by x-rays which reveal the absence of suture lines, and a characteristic skull containing digital impressions secondary to brain convolutions.

Apert's Syndrome (Acrocephalosyndactyly)

Apert's syndrome is a craniostenosis characterized by a high forehead, flat occiput, and short anterior-posterior diameter. The head grows laterally and vertically, owing to an incomplete closure of the coronal suture, and is similar to oxycephaly except for its wide transverse diameter. While ocular signs may be similar to those in oxycephaly, the rise in intracranial pressure is minimized because the brain may expand in two directions. It is one of the few diseases associated with an older paternal age, as is observed in achondroplasia and Marfan's syndrome.

Acrocephalosyndactyly may look like Crouzon's disease because of the proptotic eyes, the protruding lower jaw, the mouth which incompletely closes (mordex apertus), choanal atresia, and a saddle-shaped nose. However, the skeletal anomaly of syndactyly, which can vary from partial webbing to complete fusion of the fingers and toes, is present only in Apert's syndrome (Fig. 31–1). Occasionally there are cases that show features of both Crouzon's and Apert's syndromes. Usually there is no mental retardation, but it may exist if sufficient brain damage resulted from craniostenosis.

Crouzon's Disease (Craniofacial Dysostosis)

Maxillary hypoplasia, shallow orbits, exophthalmos, and a prominent jaw create a distinct appearance that characterizes this syndrome (Figs. 31–2, 31–3, and 31–4). The skull is usually of the brachycephalic type (short anterior-posterior length). Because the eyes can be luxated

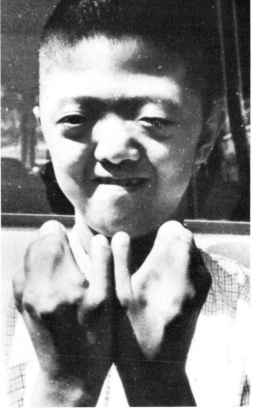

Figure 31–1   Apert's syndrome. (Courtesy of Dr. R. D. Harley.)

spontaneously, these people are often employed in circuses as grotesque anomalies. They have a typical parrot-like beak, and the lower jaw extends beyond the upper teeth, so that the mouth closes posteriorly but occlusion of the front incisor teeth is restricted.

The ocular complications are exotropia due to orbital separation, optic atrophy, and papilledema, possibly related to the bony structures.

Crouzon's disease can be differentiated from oxycephaly by its characteristics of frontal bossing and a large nose, its recognition at birth, and the distinct autosomal dominant transmission.

A special form of Crouzon's has been described by Franceschetti, called pseudo-Crouzon's disease. It is similar to Crouzon's disease in that there are the radiologic convolutions of the skull and the proptotic appearance of the eyes together with frontal bossing. However, in pseudo-

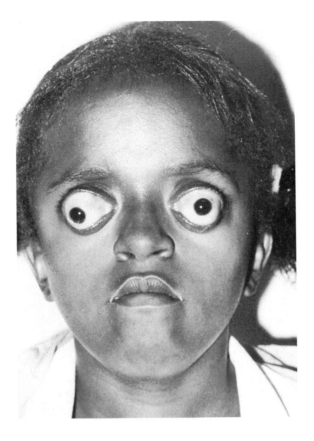

Figure 31–2   Crouzon's disease associated with congenital absence of the superior rectus muscle bilaterally.

Crouzon's disease the large, hooked, parrot-like nose is not present, there is no protrusion of the jaw, and there usually is no exotropia. It is sometimes called "skull of Crouzon," which probably represents an incomplete penetrance and expressivity of a dominant gene.

Carpenter's Syndrome

Carpenter's syndrome is another form of acrocephalosyndactyly along with Apert's and Crouzon's diseases, but it may be an autosomal recessive disease. It has the severe manifestations of Apert's syndrome in addition to hypogenitalism, obesity, and mental retardation and must be differentiated from the Lawrence-Moon-Biedl syndrome.

Hypertelorism

Hypertelorism is an abnormally wide separation of the bony orbits, resulting in an increased interpupillary distance and giving the appearance of wide separation of the eyes (Fig. 31–5). This was described in 1924 by Greig, who speculated that an exuberant bony formation occurred in the lesser wing of the sphenoid bone, leading to a separation of the orbit. Although there are familial cases, no distinct hereditary pattern is established. Hypertelorism is of ocular interest because of its cosmetic effect and the exotropia which may be secondary to the bony anatomy. Hypertelorism is distinguished from telecanthus, which represents a lateralization of the inner canthi, as is seen in Waardenburg's and Down's syndromes. Occasionally a broad nose bridge gives the appearance of hypertelorism.

Hypertelorism is observed in a variety of skeletal syndromes and is frequently seen with nasal and frontal meningoencephaloceles, in Pyle's cranial metaphyseal dysostosis, and in the median cleft face syndrome. Another syndrome was identified by Opitz in which hypospadias is seen in conjunction with hypertelorism and which occurs solely in males without associated ocular difficulties.

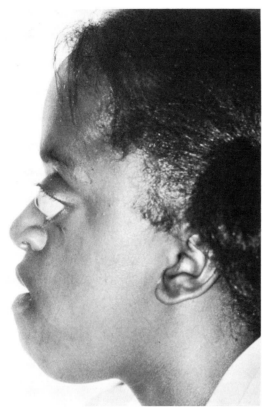

Figure 31–3 Crouzon's disease, profile view of Figure 31–2.

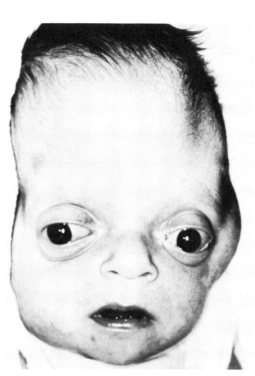

Figure 31–5 Hypertelorism and oxycephaly. (Courtesy of Dr. Harold Falls.)

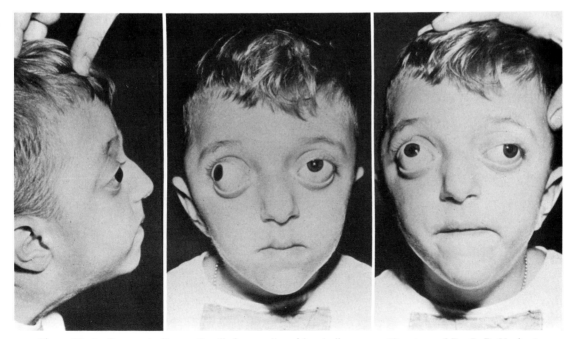

Figure 31–4 Crouzon's disease. Papilledema relieved by skull surgery. (Courtesy of Dr. R. D. Harley.)

MANDIBULOFACIAL DYSOSTOSES

By definition these diseases are bony anomalies of the anterior segment of the head and are categorized together by their similar embryopathic origin from the first and second branchial arches. The early embryo has ventrolateral elevations on the head, consisting of cartilage, connective tissue, muscles, blood vessels, and nerves. They are separated from each other by branchial clefts, otherwise called grooves. The first branchial arch subdivides into two portions: the maxillary and the mandibular. The second branchial arch does not subdivide in this fashion.

The first part of the first branchial arch forms the upper facial structures: the maxilla and zygoma, the lateral portion of the upper lip and cheek (malar bone), the palatine bone, the inferior and anterior aspects of the ear, and the mandibular division of the fifth cranial nerve. The second part of the first branchial arch forms the lower face: the mandible, the lower lip, part of the middle ear, and the temporomandibular joint. The second branchial arch forms the external part of the ear, particularly the posterior portion, part of the middle ear including the seventh cranial nerve, and muscular tissue located inferiorly and posteriorly in the upper part of the neck (submandibular area).

Malformations of the maxillary portion of the first branchial arch lead to the down-slanting fissures, the atypical contour of the lower lids, and the sunken-cheek appearance due to malar hypoplasia. Mandibular abnormalities are usually characterized by a receding chin, which leads to a characteristic profile. With the absence of a nasofrontal angle (Greek nose) and a slanting forehead, there is a snoutlike projection of the face similar to that of a fish. When the nose is prominent, a birdlike appearance is created. Maldevelopment of the second branchial arch causes abnormalities of the external ear, typically, supernumerary auricular appendages, hypoplastic or absent auricles, and blind fistulas between the ear and angle of the mouth. Conduction deafness results from both the mandibular portion of the first arch and the second branchial arch, because both participate in the embryogenesis of the middle ear. Most of these facial dysmorphisms are associated with dental abnormalities.

Although the hereditary pattern is that of irregular autosomal dominance, there is an enormous variability in penetrance and expressivity. Thus, any manifestation among these diseases may be apparent but by itself does not suggest a recognizable pattern or diagnosis. Indeed, with skipped generations there are individuals whose pedigrees cannot be traced and who seem to arise from otherwise "normal" families. As a result of delineating old features and adding "new" findings to a given syndrome, innumerable disease entities have been described, only to be confused further by the myriad eponyms. Occasionally, other skeletal malformations coexist that form no logical pattern with the first and second arch defects.

Treacher Collins Syndrome (Franceschetti's Syndrome)

The prototype mandibulofacial dysostosis is that described at the beginning of the century and labeled in the English literature Treacher Collins syndrome. In 1944 Franceschetti and Klein brought together the numerous associated findings from scattered case reports, and the condition has since been referred to as the Franceschetti syndrome. This eponym tends to appear frequently in the ophthalmic and European literature. The title "first arch syndrome" is somewhat of a misnomer because the second arch also contributes to the malformations.

The characteristic facial appearance of the Treacher Collins syndrome is that of depressed cheek bones; a small jaw; macrostomia; a narrow, beaked nose; malformed ears; and conduction deafness (Fig. 31–6). However, there are certain features that tend to distinguish this entity from the other dysostoses. These include many of the ocular adnexal manifestations: anti-Mongoloid down-slanted fissures, S-shaped colobomas of the outer half of the lower lid, absence of lashes on the inner one third of the lower lid, dystrichiasis, and a tendency toward underdeveloped or aplastic orbicularis oculi muscles, which predisposes to ectropion. Another feature rather unique to the Franceschetti syndrome is a bilateral flame-shaped projection of hair extending

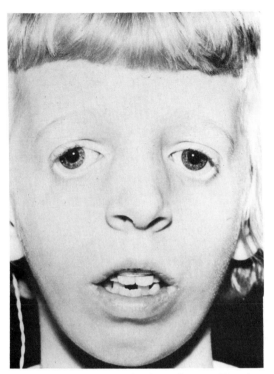

Figure 31–6   Franceschetti syndrome (Treacher Collins). (Courtesy of Dr. R. D. Harley.)

on a line from the ear to the angle of the mouth and lying over the temporal bone. Mental retardation is uncommon, although it is often suspected as a result of the unusual facies and hearing difficulty.

Hallermann-Streiff Syndrome

A severely receded jaw makes a sharp angle with the large parrot-like nose seen in the Hallermann-Streiff syndrome. For this reason the description "bird-face" is often applied to these individuals. The dysplasia lends itself to marked dental abnormalities which at times can result in a complete lack of teeth. The dwarf stature differentiates this condition from other mandibulofacial dysostoses. The head is of proportional size but simulates megalocephaly because of the peculiar facial contour. Hair is sparse, particularly in the axillary and pubic regions, and the skin, especially of the scalp and nose, is thin and atrophic. As a consequence, these people usually appear older than their chronological age. Low-set ears, limitation of mouth opening secondary to maldevelopment of the temporomandibular joint, and hy-

perextensible joints, particularly the knees, represent other distinguishing features of this syndrome. No distinct hereditary pattern has been found.

Ocular complications can be severe in that bilateral microphthalmos and congenital cataracts may accompany this syndrome. Other ocular defects include nystagmus, strabismus, and cataracts with small fine punctate opacities that occasionally reabsorb spontaneously.

Ullrich and Fremerey-Dohna described a similar syndrome but listed more extensive systemic manifestations. For this reason the literature distinguishes between the above syndrome and that labeled the Hallermann-Streiff syndrome. However, François states that all these findings probably constitute one syndrome in which extensive or atypical forms present themselves.

Goldenhar's Syndrome (Oculoauriculovertebral Dysplasia)

Goldenhar's syndrome is characterized by a triad of symptoms: bulbar dermoids or lipodermoids, misshapen or low-set ears, and vertebral skeletal anomalies (Fig. 31–7). Epibulbar dermoids are usually unilateral (but may be bilateral) and located in the lower temporal limbal area or adjacent conjunctiva, whereas lipodermoids tend to be found in the upper quadrant. These dermoids are variable in appearance and on occasion can simulate a pterygium, particularly when conjunctival vessels accompany the lesion. Auricular appendages are usually unilateral, often associated with an ear which is somewhat distorted, smaller in size, and low set. Also, pretragal fistulas to the corner of the mouth may exist. Deafness does not afflict these patients. Various vertebral anomalies coexist but often are undetected unless x-rays are obtained.

Other ocular abnormalities include a unilateral coloboma of the upper lid between the inner third and middle portion. Rarely, there may be microcornea, anophthalmos, colobomas, iris atrophy, cataracts, or strabismus.

Goldenhar's syndrome can be distinguished from Treacher Collins syndrome (Franceschetti's syndrome) on the basis of unilateral involvement. Skull asymmetry, mandibular hypoplasia, palatal asym-

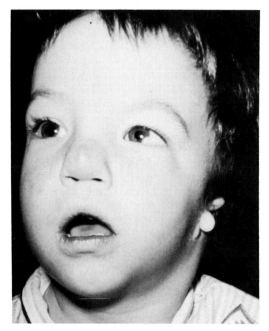

Figure 31–7 Goldenhar's syndrome illustrating corneal dermoid and defective external ear. (Courtesy of Dr. R. D. Harley.)

metry, and malocclusion of the teeth are frequently associated with Goldenhar's syndrome. In Goldenhar's syndrome the lid coloboma is unilateral, involving the upper lid, whereas in Franceschetti's syndrome the colobomas are bilateral and symmetrical, involving the lower lids. Dermoids and vertebral deformities do not exist in the mandibulofacial dysostosis syndrome.

On the other hand, much confusion between these two entities is evidenced by case reports with findings from both syndromes overlapping. In 1958 Weyers and Thier described a mandibulofacial abnormality showing ocular and vertebral involvement and unilateral bony hypoplasia of the face. Other findings included macrostomia, dental malocclusion, and unilateral microphthalmos.

Another unilateral entity was described by François and Haustrate in 1953 but it does not show ocular involvement. This was labeled otomandibular dysostosis and involved hypoplasia of the mandible, malformation of the temporomandibular joint, and auricular distortions.

Pierre Robin Syndrome

Of the first and second arch syndromes the one that may be detected at the earliest age is the Pierre Robin syndrome, because of neonatal respiratory distress and swallowing difficulty that results from severe micrognathia and glossoptosis. The markedly receded jaw predisposes to a posteriorly located but normal-sized tongue which obstructs the breathing and swallowing passages. There may or may not be an associated cleft palate. Occasionally death occurs secondary to aspiration of swallowed material. Low-set ears frequently accompany this syndrome.

Ocular complications are not routinely observed but when they occur they may be severe. Microphthalmos, glaucoma, cataracts, high myopia, a proptotic appearance, and esotropia have been reported. As with most mandibulofacial dysostoses the genetic pattern is not clearly established, although both autosomal recessive and dominant pedigrees have been noted.

FRAGILE BONE DISEASES

Osteogenesis Imperfecta (van der Hoeve's Disease)

The triad of symptoms that characterize osteogenesis imperfecta includes blue sclerae, fragile brittle bones, and conduction deafness. This disease has been described periodically in the past few centuries by Lobstein, Spurway, and Vrolik, each of whom presented some modification of the basic entity. It occurs rarely, by both autosomal dominant and recessive transmission. Two major types are dependent upon the age of onset. The birth onset form is more severe; the second type occurs in childhood and results in fewer fractures. Fractures may occur spontaneously or with minimal trauma, usually affecting the lower limbs, and seem to decrease in incidence with age. Oddly, there is little associated pain.

Other skeletal anomalies include teeth abnormalities, short stature, lax joints that result in dislocations and subluxations, and a characteristic frontal and occipital cranial prominence. Bilateral conduction deafness often occurs later in life and is progressive.

Blue sclerae are more precisely scleral ectasias and are similar to the thin, loose skin common in this disease. Although the blue appearance may be variable in color and affect any part of the globe, the thinness does not progress to staphylomatous stages. Other ocular defects include anterior embryotoxon, cataract, keratoconus, and megalocornea. Cutaneous manifestations consist of a thin, translucent-appearing skin which produces a prematurely aged appearance.

Fibrous Dysplasia of Bone (Albright's Disease)

Fibrous replacement of bone is a disease process of unknown cause which presents itself in a variety of clinical manifestations. This has led to semantic confusion regarding the proper descriptive term and the appropriate eponym. In the mid-1930s McCune and Albright independently described the syndrome of multiple foci of fibrous dysplasia; irregular, brown, patchy skin pigmentation; and sexual precocity. McCune labeled the disease osteitis fibrosa cystica. Albright named the syndrome osteitis fibrosa disseminata. Since that time many more cases have been reported, some not fulfilling all the above criteria, others with additional associated findings. One such descriptive modification is the involvement of one focus, or monostatic fibrous dysplasia, which may or may not show the skin and endocrine manifestations and which is the form that is usually present when the skull is involved. Therefore, ophthalmologists may encounter a unilateral proptosis secondary to fibrous dysplasia without other systemic involvement.

The basic pathologic progression is that of fibrous tissue replacing the medulla of bones in either a densely collagenous or highly cellular fashion. This tissue may contain areas of cartilage, calcification, hyalin, hemorrhage, or cysts. Thus, radiologic widening of bones is seen with thinning of the cortex. The femur and the pelvis are particularly affected. However, facial bones may be involved which include the frontal, sphenoidal, and temporal bones. Its progression is slow and usually begins in childhood, with particular exacerbation during pubertal growth. The weakened bones are predisposed to fractures which in turn cause pain and ultimate deformity.

The brown pigmentary skin changes are usually on the same side of the body as the bony abnormality and may mimic the skin patches in neurofibromatosis. The typical ocular involvement is that of unilateral ex-

ophthalmos which progresses in a downward fashion, secondary to a fibrotic orbital mass. This also predisposes to papilledema and ultimate blindness. Occasionally cranial nerves may be involved, and congenital cataracts have been reported.

Osteopetrosis (Albers-Schönberg's Disease; Marble Bone Disease)

Osteopetrosis is characterized by dense, thick, sclerosing bone which leads to marble-like fragility and replacement of bone marrow. This causes spontaneous fractures and a pancytopenia (particularly a myelophthisic anemia) secondary to marrow obliteration. Although the cause of this very rare disease is unknown, the autosomal dominant type is mild and the autosomal recessive type is potentially severe enough to lead to an anemic or infectious death.

The disease may be evident at birth in the severe form with the possibility of bone marrow destruction in infancy or early childhood. However, the milder forms are usually diagnosed in childhood or early adolescence. Radiologic evidence can be obtained early in life, which unlike the rarefaction of bone in osteogenesis imperfecta demonstrates an increased bone density. Long bones and the base of the skull are especially afflicted. The ossified foramina at the cranial base impinge upon cranial nerves. Therefore, strabismus, optic atrophy, and blindness represent ophthalmologic complications. Also, the orbital and maxillary bones may become misshapen, causing progressive exophthalmos. These usually occur in the more severe form. When there is compression of the foramen magnum, hydrocephalus may occur. When the ocular structures become involved, surgical decompression of the optic canal may be necessary to obviate further progression.

CHONDROPLASTIC DISEASES

Achondroplasia

Achondroplasia, the most common of the chondrodystrophies, is characterized by short stature and a large head. Ophthalmologic interest is based on ocular problems secondary to neurologic complications. Its transmission is autosomal dominant with skipped generations, but it seems to occur sporadically most of the time (90 per cent) as a result of mutation. This is one of the diseases associated with older paternal age, as Apert's and Marfan's syndromes.

By definition, the basic defect is a dysplasia of cartilaginous tissue, and thus long bones are affected primarily. This causes short arms and legs, the femur most usually being involved. All the fingers tend to be similar in length, with short proximal and middle phalanges creating a stubby appearance. Typical of achondroplasia is a divergence of the fingers (trident hand), readily noticeable when the fingers are not in a flexed position. Although the nucleus pulposus of the vertebral column contains cartilage, the trunk is of usual height. However, a marked lumbar lordosis contributes to the characteristic posture.

Neuro-ophthalmologic manifestations are related to cranial malformations which similarly are secondary to cartilage dysplasia. The cranial floor originally is derived from cartilaginous tissue, which in normal neonates is not calcified. In achondroplastic infants there are ossification and fusion of cartilage of the occiput and the two sphenoid bones. Involvement of the occiput by premature calcification narrows the foramen magnum; this contributes to the formation of hydrocephalus and possible eventual bony compression on the spinal cord. While hydrocephalus leads to a relatively larger head, the posterior fossa is relatively smaller.

If the ethmoid and nasal bones prematurely ossify, a flat low nasal bridge results. Optic atrophy and decreased vision have been observed in achondroplasia and may occur when hydrocephalus is not present. Ocular signs of strabismus and optic atrophy are secondary to osseous impingement upon cranial nerves.

Conradi's Disease (Chondrodystrophia Calcificans Congenita; Dysplasia Epiphysealis Punctata)

Conradi's disease is an abnormality in calcium deposition that results in bilateral cataracts, short limbs, and joint stiffness secondary to flexion contractures which may be morphologically suggestive of the mucopolysaccharidoses. The pathologic condition develops before birth as well as neonatally. Most infants die within several years, although a few patients survive, with stigmata of the skeletal and ocular deformities.

Calcium is deposited in the subcutaneous tissues, cardiac valves, and bony epiphyses. X-rays reveal punctate deposits and a ballooning-type widening of these epiphyses. A variety of bony anomalies results, including syndactyly, micrognathia, club foot, dislocated hip, and craniostenosis. Congenital heart defects are a logical consequence of valvular involvement. Because of joint immobility there tend to be muscle wasting and fibrosis.

Ocular manifestations occur in approximately 50 per cent of cases and are typified by complete bilateral cataracts. Rarely, heterochromia iridis and primary optic atrophy have been observed. These also develop prenatally and are therefore present at birth. Similar to Rieger's anomaly, this disease process may result in a prominent Schwalbe's line (posterior embryotoxon), iris-corneal adhesions, and hypoplasia of the iris.

Those children not severely involved who survive to adulthood usually undergo a spontaneous regression of calcium deposition, despite the persistence of the structural disease. Having an autosomal recessive hereditary pattern, the disease is often linked with a history of consanguinity.

Skeletal Alterations in the Mucopolysaccharidoses

Since it is the skeletal deformity which has some similarity to the chondrodystrophies, it will be discussed at this time. The ocular manifestations of this disease are discussed elsewhere.

The skull is noticeably enlarged and bulky, usually of the scaphocephalic type, resulting in a long anterior-posterior diameter with frontal bossing. Occasionally brachycephaly occurs. Also, hydrocephalus may exist, perhaps secondary to meningeal involvement. A depressed nasal bridge, often called "saddle nose," is additive to hypertelorism in creating the appearance of wide-set eyes. Dental defects, particularly malalignment, exist. Because of a short cervical spine the head appears to sit on the shoulders as if no neck exists.

Other syndromes mimic this latter feature, namely, platybasia and Arnold-Chiari and Klippel-Feil syndromes. The thorax has a "humped-back" contour due to cervical kyphosis, and demonstrates flared ribs anteriorly. All the limbs tend to be shortened, which accounts for the short height. Although the fingers are broad and stubby, attention is drawn to the flexion contracture of the fingers ("clawhand"). Joints are relatively immobile to the extent that these patients may walk on their toes.

In general, the above changes can be seen in any of the mucopolysaccharidoses to a greater or lesser degree. Usually the earliest manifestations appear by one to two years of age. These changes are most typical in the prototype, Hurler's disease. Hurler's and Maroteaux-Lamy syndromes include moderately severe limitation of joints. Genu valgum (knock-knee) is seen in Maroteaux-Lamy and Morquio's syndromes. Markedly short stature typifies Morquio's disease. There is only mild joint limitation in Sanfilippo's and Scheie's syndromes (despite severe hand involvement in Scheie's syndrome).

DWARFISM

A variety of dysmorphologic syndromes associated with ocular disease can be characterized as exhibiting unusually small stature, often with premature senility. These include Cockayne's disease, Hutchinson-Gilford's progeria, and Werner's syndrome. Rothmund's poikiloderma congenita is similar to Werner's disease because of the cataractous changes, but it is primarily a dermatologic condition. The Hallermann-Streiff syndrome is similar to progeria in appearance but is not characterized by premature senility. Seckel's bird-headed dwarf is also devoid of senile systemic changes.

Cockayne's Disease

Cockayne described an autosomal recessive disease that begins at approximately two years of age and is characterized by dwarfism and premature senility. Several skeletal and facial anomalies are also present, as well as thin photosensitive skin. Reduced hearing and mental retardation make it difficult to communicate with these patients.

The most typical ocular finding is that of a scattered pigmented and depigmented retinal appearance, sometimes thought to be salt and peppery, suggestive of a degenerative process. Cataracts, nystagmus, decreased tearing and sweating, and optic atrophy are occasionally present. (See p. 878.)

Progeria (Hutchinson-Gilford Disease)

Progeria is a rare form of dwarfism and premature senility with an onset in infancy. These children have a typical emaciated appearance together with hydrocephaly and prominent eyes secondary to subcutaneous tissue atrophy. The broad head and receding jaw create a V-shaped facial contour, and the alopecia may lead to complete baldness. The voice is high pitched. Because of atherosclerotic vascular changes, death from coronary disease usually occurs in the second decade.

Although ocular changes infrequently occur, the presence of a congenital or acquired cataract in these dwarfs with premature senility must be distinguished from Cockayne's, Werner's, and Rothmund's diseases.

Seckel's Bird-Headed Dwarf

These dwarfs described by Seckel do not have the premature senility that typifies Cockayne's or Werner's disease and progeria, but they do have the birdlike facies of the Hallermann-Streiff type of mandibulofacial dysostosis. Malar hypoplasia contributes to this effect. Because of a prenatal growth deficiency there is an infantile onset of dwarfism, and the small head remains nearly bald. The typical frontal appearance includes a large nose together with the low-set ears and a narrow face. In profile, the large nose and mandibular hypoplasia create a birdlike facial contour.

This rare diagnosis is not made by the ocular manifestations. The eyes may appear prominent, and strabismus may be present.

Werner's Disease

Individuals with Werner's disease present themselves during teen age or somewhat beyond the pediatric age group because they experience stunted growth and postpubertal senile changes. Therefore, the dwarfism is not as marked as in Cockayne's disease or progeria. The basic defects in this autosomal recessive entity are a diffuse loss of subcutaneous tissue and a thinning of the skin. This, along with thin gray hair, creates an aged appearance. As with progeria, the high-pitched voice helps to identify this syndrome. It is easiest to conceptualize this process as one of normal childhood development until adolescence, when progressive senile changes replace the usual accelerated growth. A variety of endocrine abnormalities develop, the most important of which is diabetes mellitus.

Accompanying these changes is the onset of cataracts leading to visual impairments. Retinal degenerative changes may also exist. (See p. 871.)

DISEASES OF CERVICO-OCCIPITAL PROXIMITY: "BULL-NECK" ANOMALIES

"Bull-neck" individuals often present with neuro-ophthalmic manifestations that are secondary to skeletal deformity and fusion in the posterior neck region. This "head-on-shoulders" appearance is characteristic of platybasia, the Arnold-Chiari syndrome, and the Klippel-Feil syndrome (congenital brevicollis). Its presence in the following diseases is variable: mucopolysaccharidoses, Paget's disease of bone, osteogenesis imperfecta, rickets, and hyperparathyroidism.

Platybasia (Basilar Impression)

The basic pathologic feature of platybasia is an upward bulge into the posterior fossa of the foramen magnum portion of the occipital cranium, usually associated with partial fusion of the upper cervical vertebrae to each other and to the skull. Thus, mechanical pressure is exerted upon the medulla, cerebellum, and upper spinal cord. Also, the vertebrae do not properly align vertically, resulting in a gradual herniation of the bony processes upon this nervous tissue. This herniation process explains why coughing and straining lead to the periodic neuro-ophthalmologic symptoms and the onset of symptoms in early adulthood.

Pressure upon upper cervical nerves causes numbness of the upper extremities. Cerebellar involvement causes an ataxic and spastic gait, jerky horizontal nystagmus on lateral gaze, and vertical nystagmus on up and down gaze. The affected medulla causes spinal tract pain, numbness, paresthesia, and pyramidal tract spasticity. Increased intracranial pressure secondary to interruption of normal cerebrospinal fluid flow may cause sixth nerve palsy and diplopia and would also account for the occurrence of papilledema and partial optic atrophy. Other cranial nerve disorders are anisocoria, ptosis, and corneal anesthesia. Another mechanism for these signs is that of basilar artery compression.

Because of the age group involved and the variety of neuro-ophthalmologic manifestations, multiple sclerosis must be ruled out. X-ray findings rule out other disease entities in the differential diagnosis. If symptoms are persistent or severe enough, decompression surgery may be of benefit. Platybasia is frequently associated with the Arnold-Chiari syndrome.

Arnold-Chiari Syndrome

Arnold, in 1894, and Chiari, in 1895, described a malformation with symptomatology identical to platybasia. The pathologic process, however, is the reverse of that in platybasia, in that there is central nervous tissue herniating caudally through the foramen magnum, rather than an upward protrusion of cranial bone at the base of the skull. Here there is maldevelopment of the pons, medulla, and cerebellum, almost always associated with hydrocephalus and spina bifida. A wedge or tongue of cerebellar tissue is fused to the posterior surface of the cervical spinal cord, which upon projecting through the foramen magnum obstructs cerebrospinal fluid dynamics. Therefore, hydrocephalus ensues during childhood development, accompanied by cerebellar ataxia and bilateral pyramidal tract signs. However, symptoms usually develop in early adult life, as in platybasia, and are aggravated by sneezing, coughing, and certain head positions. Head and neck pain accompanies both these entities. Differentiation of the Arnold-Chiari syndrome from platybasia may be made by myelography which reveals the nervous tissue herniation. Downbeat nystagmus, slow deviation, and diplopia are additional ocular findings.

Klippel-Feil Syndrome (Congenital Brevicollis)

Congenital brevicollis is a synostosis of the upper cervical vertebrae, always involving the atlas and axis, though occasionally extending caudally to the upper dorsal vertebrae. Cervical rather than cranial nerves are usually involved, despite the occasional deformity of the base of the skull. It sometimes accompanies platybasia, and there is often an upward displacement of the scapula (Sprengel's deformity). Similar to the Arnold-Chiari syndrome, an occult spina bifida in the cervical area periodically occurs. The head appears to emerge from the body, but unlike platybasia and the Arnold-Chiari syndrome there is usually some torticollis. Head movements are somewhat limited owing to webbing of the neck. These findings coupled with the low hairline are suggestive of Turner's disease (pterygium colli).

"Mirror movements" are characteristic of congenital brevicollis; that is, one hand simultaneously moves in a fashion identical to that of the other hand. It is thought that an abnormal decussation of the motor tracts leads to bilateral muscular innervation.

Eye findings associated with congenital brevicollis include congenital strabismus (esotropia), nystagmus, Duane's syndrome, paralysis of conjugate lateral gaze, and external ophthalmoplegia.

OCULOSKELETAL DISEASES WITH SKIN INVOLVEMENT

In the classification of multi-organ syndromes, cumbersome overlap and inadvertent omission may occur when a disease entity is described solely or consistently within one organ system. A group of diseases with significant oculoskeletal involvement might be recognized more readily by their dermatologic lesions. These include Albright's disease, Rothmund's disease, neurofibromatosis, poikiloderma (Goltz's syndrome), incontinentia pigmenti (Bloch-Sulzberger disease), and dyskeratosis congenita. (See Chapter 30.)

Poikiloderma (Goltz's Disease)

Poikiloderma is primarily a dental and dermatologic anomaly. However, syndactyly, strabismus, colobomas, and microphthalmos have been associated. These patients have skeletal asymmetry, a short stature, and joint hypermobility.

Incontinentia Pigmenti (Bloch-Sulzberger Disease)

Incontinentia pigmenti is a well-documented syndrome usually typified by a peculiar bluish truncal skin pigmentation. It tends to appear on the lower back and buttocks and along the dermatomes. Associated dental defects and absence of hair are frequent findings. Approximately 25 per cent of these patients have skeletal involvement including hemivertebrae, additional ribs, syndactyly, and short arms and legs. (See p. 869.)

MISCELLANEOUS SYNDROMES WITH OCULAR AND SKELETAL INVOLVEMENT (See Table)

Syndrome	Skeletal Deformity	Ocular Manifestations
Biemond's	Brachydactyly	Nystagmus
Caffey-Silverman (Infantile cortical hyperostosis)	Idiopathic soft tissue swelling; secondary hyperostosis	Adnexal and orbital misdiagnoses: cellulitis, tumor, edema
Cerebrohepatorenal syndrome	Long narrow head; high forehead; shallow supraorbital ridges; appearance of Down's syndrome	Elevated intraocular pressure; cataract; faulty formation of optic disc; retinal pigmentary scattering
Cryptophthalmos	Multiple defects of ears, nose, teeth, genitals, spinal column; cleft palate; partial syndactyly of fingers and toes	Fused lids, without brows or lashes; microphthalmos with malformed or absent corneas: symblepharon; colobomas

MISCELLANEOUS SYNDROMES WITH OCULAR AND SKELETAL INVOLVEMENT
(See Table) (Continued)

Syndrome	Skeletal Deformity	Ocular Manifestations
Cornelia de Lange	Small, brachycephalic head; micromelia and phocomelia; hand and finger anomalies	Bushy, confluent brows (synophrys); long lashes; down-slant fissures; ptosis; high myopia; disc pallor; anisocoria
Ectodermal dysplasia	Teeth abnormalities with pointlike appearance; full forehead	Thin wrinkled lids; prominent orbital ridges; conjunctivitis
Engelmann's disease (Hereditary diaphyseal dysplasia)	Large head; long limbs; sclerotic, cortical thickening of long bones; progressively painful limbs	Exophthalmos; papilledema; optic atrophy; lagophthalmos; lateral rectus palsy and diplopia; ptosis; cataracts; retinal vascularization
Hereditary Osteo-onychodysplasia, "HOOD" (Nail-patella syndrome)	Hypoplasia and splitting of nails, especially thumb; patella hypoplasia; elbow hypoplasia, iliac horns or spurs	Scalloped iris collarette with darker central area (Lester's line); sclerocornea; heterochromia; keratoconus; microcornea; megalophakia; cataracts; ptosis
Laurence-Moon-Biedl syndrome	Polydactyly; syndactyly; short stature	Retinitis pigmentosa; cataracts, microcornea; nystagmus; strabismus, especially esotropia
Leprechaunism (Donohue's syndrome)	Small stature; stunted growth	Hypertelorism; small but prominent eyes
Marinesco-Sjögren syndrome	Brachydactyly; short stature; hypotonia; ataxia	Cataracts; strabismus; nystagmus
Median cleft face syndrome	Horseshoe-shaped depression in forehead; occult bifidism of cranium; cleft nose, lip, and palate	Hypertelorism; telecanthus
Mieten's syndrome	Thin nose; short forearms; flexion contracture of elbows and wrist; short stature	Corneal opacity
Oculodentodigital syndrome (Lohmann's; Meyer-Schwickerath)	Thin nose with anteverted nostrils; camptodactyly of fifth fingers; dental enamel hypoplasia	Bilateral microphthalmos; iris hypoplasia; anophthalmos; glaucoma; hypertelorism; epicanthal folds
Otopalatodigital syndrome (Taybi's)	Scaphocephaly; broadening at ends of fingers and toes	Hypertelorism
Prader-Willi syndrome	Clinodactyly; syndactyly; joint hyperextensibility; very small hands and feet	Almond-shaped palpebral fissures; strabismus
Pyle's disease (Metaphyseal dysplasia)	Bony elevation at bridge of nose; tall stature; knock-knees; bony compression of skull foramina	Hypertelorism; strabismus; cranial nerve compression upon optic nerve
Rubinstein-Taybi syndrome	Broad, short thumb and toe; narrow nose; short stature	Cataract; coloboma; ptosis; long lashes; down-slant fissures; strabismus; high-arched brows with hypertrichosis
Schwartz-Jampel syndrome	Small stature; limitation of joint movements; myotonia; appearance of Morquio's disease	Blepharophimosis; long irregular lashes; myopia; congenital cataract
Smith-Lemli-Opitz syndrome	Syndactyly of second and third toes; polydactyly; brachydactyly; upturned nostrils	Ptosis; strabismus; epicanthal folds
Stanesco's syndrome (Craniofacial dysostosis with diaphyseal hypoplasia)	Brachycephaly, short upper arms; small stature; mandibular hypoplasia; thickened cortices of long bones	Shallow orbits; prominent eyes
Stickler's syndrome (Progressive arthro-ophthalmopathy)	Painful, stiff joints; subluxation of hip	Progressive, high myopia; secondary retinal detachment and glaucoma

An additional 25 per cent of these patients are afflicted with ocular anomalies and ocular inflammation which can be visually crippling. Retrolental masses have frequently been seen and have been documented as retinal dysplasia, retrolental fibroplasia, or PHPV. Uveitis, keratitis, cataracts, strabismus, nystagmus, papillitis, and myopia have been associated symptoms. Recently, pigmentation of the conjunctiva and retina has been reported.

Dyskeratosis Congenita

Dyskeratosis congenita is characterized by hyperpigmentation of the skin which is recognized in childhood, although it is present at birth. Leukoplakia, nail dystrophy, and pancytopenia contribute to the syndrome. The ocular findings may be the most bothersome because they can consist of blepharitis, ectropion, and nasolacrimal duct impatency. (See p. 862.)

REFERENCES

Bertelsen, T. I.: The premature synostosis of the cranial sutures. Acta Ophthal. (Suppl. 51), 1958.

Coles, W. H.: Ocular manifestations of Cockayne's syndrome. Amer. J. Ophthal., 67:762, 1969.

Duke-Elder, S.: System of Ophthalmology. Vol. III, Part 2. Congenital Deformities. London, Henry Kimpton, 1964.

Falls, H. F., and Schull, W. J.: Hallermann-Streiff syndrome: a dyscephaly with congenital cataracts and hypotrichosis. Arch. Ophthal., 63:409, 1960.

Feingold, M., and Gellis, S. S.: Ocular abnormalities associated with first and second arch syndromes. Survey Ophthal., 14:39, 1969.

Flickinger, R. R., and Spivey, B. E.: Lester's line in hereditary osteo-onychodysplasia. Arch. Ophthal., 82:700, 1969.

Gellis, S., and Feingold, M.: Atlas of Mental Retardation Syndromes. Washington, D. C., U. S. Department of Health, Education and Welfare, 1968.

Hammond, A.: Dysplasia epiphysealis punctata (Conradi's disease). Brit. J. Ophthal., 54:755, 1970.

Ide, C. H., Miller, G. W., and Wollschlaeger, P.B.: Familial facial dysplasia. Arch. Ophthal., 84:427, 1970.

Ide, C. H., and Wollschlaeger, P. B.: Multiple congenital abnormalities associated with cryptophthalmia. Arch. Ophthal., 81:638, 1969.

Jones, S. T.: Retrolental membrane associated with Bloch-Sulzberger syndrome (Incontinentia pigmenti). Amer. J. Ophthal., 62:330, 1966.

Keith, C. G. : Retinal atrophy in osteopetrosis. Arch. Ophthal., 79:234, 1968.

Loh, R. C. K., and Tan, D. S. L.: An unusual case of progeria-like dwarfism with bilateral macular coloboma. Amer. J. Ophthal., 70:968, 1970.

Minton, L. R., and Elliott, J. H.: Ocular manifestations of infantile cortical hyperostosis. Amer. J. Ophthal., 64:902, 1967.

Morse, P. H., Walsh, F. B., and McCormick, J. R.: Ocular findings in hereditary diaphyseal dysplasia (Engelmann's disease). Amer. J. Ophthal., 68:100, 1969.

Nicholson, D. H., and Goldberg, M. F.: Ocular abnormalities in the de Lange syndrome. Arch. Ophthal., 76:214, 1966.

Parks, M. M., and Costenbader, F.: Crouzon's disease. Amer. J. Ophthal., 33:77, 1950.

Punnett, H. H., and Kirkpatrick, J. A.: A syndrome of ocular abnormalities, calcification of cartilage, and failure to thrive. J. Pediat., 73:602, 1968.

Roy, F. H., Sumjitt, R. L., Hiatt, R. L., and Hughes, J. G.: Ocular manifestations of the Rubinstein-Taybi syndrome. Arch. Ophthal., 79:272, 1968.

Schwartz, O., and Jampel, R. S.: Congenital blepharophimosis associated with a unique generalized myotonia. Arch. Ophthal., 68:82, 1962.

Seelenfreund, M., and Gartner, S.: Acrocephalosyndactyly (Apert's syndrome). Arch. Ophthal., 78:8, 1967.

Smith, D. W.: Recognizable Patterns of Human Malformation. Philadelphia, W. B. Saunders Co., 1970.

Smith, J. L., Cavanaugh, J. J. A., and Stowe, F. C.: Ocular manifestations of the Pierre-Robin syndrome. Arch. Ophthal., 63:984, 1960.

Symposium on Congenital Anomalies of the Eye. Trans. New Orleans Acad. Ophthal. St. Louis, The C. V. Mosby Co., 1968.

Walsh, F., and Hoyt, W.: Clinical Neuro-Ophthalmology. Baltimore, Williams & Wilkins Co., 1969.

Sugar, S.: The oculoauriculovertebral dysplasia syndrome of Goldenhar. Amer. J. Ophthal., 62:678, 1966.

CHAPTER 32

OPTICAL AIDS FOR CHILDREN WITH SUBNORMAL VISION

SIDNEY WEISS, M.D.

BLINDNESS

Blindness is defined in the United States as visual acuity for distant vision of 20/200 or less in the better eye with best correction, or visual acuity of more than 20/200 if the widest diameter of the field of vision subtends an angle no greater than 20 degrees, even though central visual acuity is 20/20 (legal blindness).

Total blindness means inability to distinguish light from darkness, or no light perception.

PARTIALLY SIGHTED

Fonda (1965) classifies the partially seeing into four groups:

    I. Light perception to 1/200

    II. Vision ranging from 2/200 to 4/200

    III. Vision ranging from 5/200 to 20/300

    IV. Vision ranging from 20/250 to 20/60

Studies made in the last decade have estimated that there are over 100,000 school children in the United States who function as *partially sighted* (Hatfield, 1966). This amounts to one child out of every 500 children. "For educational purposes a partially seeing child is defined as one who uses his sight as his chief channel of learning. This would include all of the children defined, on the basis of ophthalmic measurements, as partially seeing as well as legally blind children who are able to make use of their remaining vision in the learning situation" (Hatfield, 1966).

CAUSES OF SUBNORMAL VISION IN CHILDREN

Congenital or hereditary diseases are the greatest causes for subnormal vision in children. In a study of 105 children from first grade through high school who were examined for optical aids at the Center for the Blind, the following diseases were found in order of greatest numbers:

1.	Congenital cataract (aphakia)	18
2.	Optic nerve atrophy	17
3.	Retrolental fibroplasia	15
4.	Congenital nystagmus	14
5.	Chorioretinitis	11
6.	High degree myopia	7
7.	Juvenile macular degeneration	5
8.	Albinism	4
9.	Congenital glaucoma	3
10.	Retinal detachment	3
11.	Unilateral amblyopia (other eye blind or enucleated)	2
12.	Retinitis pigmentosa	2
13.	Coloboma of iris and choroid	2
14.	Congenital aniridia	1
15.	High degree hyperopia	1
	Total	105

A child may have a combination of diseases such as congenital cataracts associated with optic atrophy and nystagmus. Children with retrolental fibroplasia frequently have an associated nystagmus. Optic atrophy alone is frequently seen, and children who develop macular degeneration sometimes have an associated pallor of the optic nerves.

Chorioretinitis is frequently central and bilateral and commonly of toxoplasmic origin. The children with congenital aniridia may develop cataracts and glaucoma during their adult life rather than in childhood. The child with amblyopia in one eye and normal vision in the opposite eye is rarely seen in a low vision clinic, except in the presence of injury and impairment of vision in the normal eye.

MANAGEMENT OF THE CHILD WITH SUBNORMAL VISION

The following procedure should be undertaken by the physician attending to a child with subnormal vision:

1. History.

2. Ophthalmological examination, including visual acuity for near and distance, external examination, funduscopic examination (through dilated pupils if possible), slit lamp microscopy, refraction, and muscle balance.

3. Estimation of required magnification.

4. Trial of proposed optical aid and verification of predicted magnification.

5. Ordering of the optical aid, including instructions to optician.

History Taking

In some instances it is advisable to speak to the parent or parents alone before examining the child; however, the presence of the parents may be more advantageous, since it allows the ophthalmologist to observe the interfamily reactions, attitudes of one or both parents toward the child and his problems, as well as the attitude of the child to his parents and to his visual handicap. Behaviour problems of a visually handicapped child may be directly related to the inability of a child to understand the teacher or overprotection on the part of the parents. One should inquire as to the type and grade of class the child is attending. Does the child attend a sight saving class? Or is the child one among many normal sighted children? A very important question is the degree to which the parents help the child with his homework. We have had parents tell us that it is the teacher's job to help the child and not that of the parents. I usually ask older children if they like school. A negative answer will usually be corroborated by the parents that the child is not doing well or that he would rather watch television than study.

Ophthalmological Examination

VISUAL ACUITY. The visual acuity for near and distance is one of the most important parts of the examination of a child with subnormal vision. Preschool children, mentally retarded, and brain-damaged children may pose a problem. However, patience on the part of the examiner and cooperation of the parents are usually rewarding. In such children, the "Flash Card Vision Test for Children" (Faye, 1968) for distance vision is very

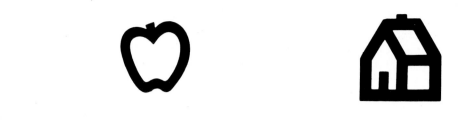

30 ft.   **40 ft.**   **50 ft.**

Figure 32–1   Flash card vision test cards with Snellen notation on each card.

satisfactory. The test cards are a modifica- of the Schering pediatric picture chart.* The cards for distance acuity consist of 12 reversible 4 × 5-inch flash cards with one symbol on each side (Fig. 32–1). Three symbols are used, namely, a house, an umbrella, and an apple. Snellen acuity notation is printed on every card, with three symbols for each acuity level from "200" to "10." The reverse sides of the "200" characters are their "100" counterparts. The "50" and "40" are paired as are the "30" and "20" and the "15" and "10."

Faye found that the three symbols would attract the attention and comprehension from the average child of 27 months, and from the trainable mentally retarded with I.Q.'s ranging from 30 to 70, age range approximately 8 to 12 years. Faye found that a test distance of 10 feet or less (later converted to 20 feet notations) created the greatest degree of interest on the part of the child. If the examiner cannot get the cooperation of the child for this test, the parents are asked to purchase a set of cards and teach the child at home. For older children who know their numbers and for whom visual acuity is 10/200 or less, a standard Snellen numbers chart, illuminated and mounted on a movable stand, can be brought forward and the distance and size of print recorded as Snellen notation, e.g., 5/200, 7/200, and so on (Fig. 32-2).

When vision is tested at less than 20 feet, the fraction can be converted to 20 feet notation by simply multiplying the numerator and denominator of the visual fraction by a number which converts the numerator to 20.

Example: $\dfrac{5}{200} \times \dfrac{4}{4} = \dfrac{20}{800}$

For children who have better than 10/200 (20/400 vision) and who know their numbers or letters, the Project-o-chart is invaluable.

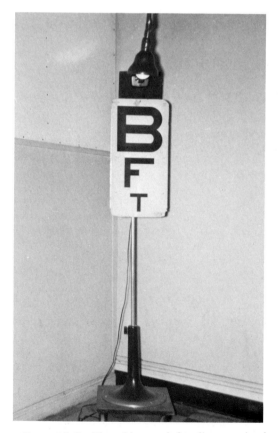

Figure 32–2   Moveable stand for distance visual acuity.

*Schering's Children's Eye Chart, Schering Corporation, Bloomfield, New Jersey, © 1961.

Visual acuity for near. The visual acuity for near is considered to be comparable to the corrected distance visual acuity. The basis for this fact is that all standard reading charts are based on the same optical principle of a letter subtending an angle of 5′ at a given distance, and in which each component is a 1′ angle. In actual practice this does not hold. Kestenbaum and Sturman (1956) stated that near vision of an eye measured with a reading chart and corrected distance vision measured on the Snellen chart corresponded in general, except in the following five conditions:

1. Near vision is better than far vision in irregular astigmatism because the pupil constricts and acts as a pinhole by decreasing the radius of the diffusion circles. Patients with high astigmatism experience proportionately better near vision. Although the smaller pupil is a factor, it is the large blurred retinal image produced by holding the print close to the eyes that improves vision.

2. Near vision is better with peripheral opacities because they are less disturbing when the pupil is narrow.

3. Near vision is better in many patients with pendular nystagmus, which decreases or even disappears with convergence upon the near object.

4. Near vision is poorer than far vision in eyes with central opacities of the cornea or lens, since the normal peripheral parts are covered by the iris in miosis.

5. In incomplete central scotoma or field defects which encroach on the center, near vision measured with a reading chart is often poorer than far vision measured with a Snellen chart.

Visual acuity for near is measured separately for each eye, with and without the child's correction on. For preschool children and illiterates, the near vision test card devised by Faye and Koehler is based on Snellen notation, and consists of a 4 × 5-inch white card using the house, umbrella, and apple from the Schering Eye Chart (Fig. 32–3). Mixed symbols are shown on seven lines diminishing in size from 6.0 meters to 0.5 meter. The print size is shown in Snellen notation and the point size for each line is shown in two separate columns on the right margin.

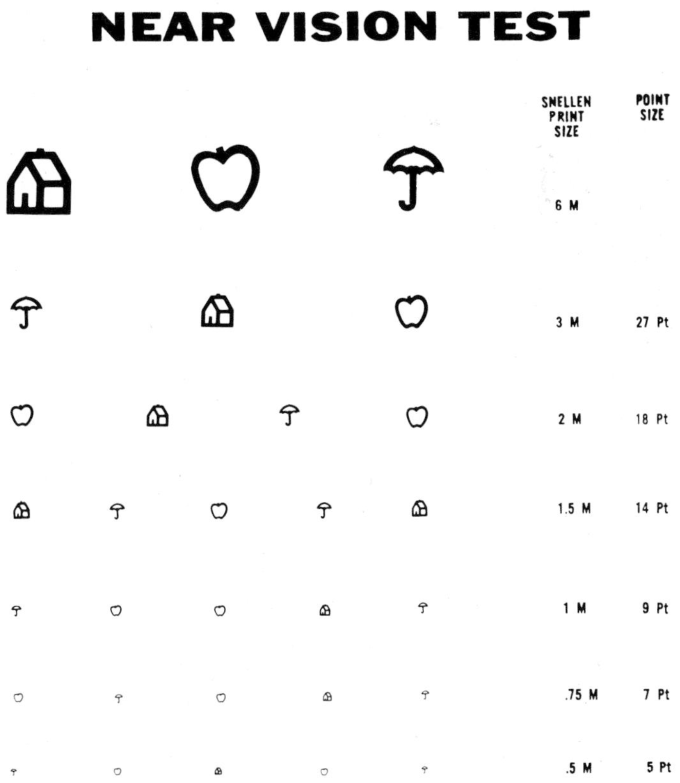

NEAR VISION TEST

Figure 32–3 Near vision test card of Faye and Koehler for illiterate and preschool children, based on Snellen notations. (The Lighthouse Low Vision Services.)

	SNELLEN PRINT SIZE	POINT SIZE
	6 M	
	3 M	27 Pt
	2 M	18 Pt
	1.5 M	14 Pt
	1 M	9 Pt
	.75 M	7 Pt
	.5 M	5 Pt

		NEAR VISION (IN METERS)	DISTANCE VISION (IN FEET)
GAME		6 M	20/360
CRANE		3.5 M	20/200
TOLD	(18 Point)	2 M	20/120
LEFT		1.6 M	20/100
DOT	(12 Point)	1.4 M	20/80
BAKE	(9 Point)	1 M	20/60
CODE		.8 M (800 mm)	20/50
BOTH	(6 Point)	.7 M (700 mm)	20/40
NEAR	(4 Point)	.5 M (500 mm)	20/30
PRINT		.35 M (350 mm)	20/20

Figure 32–4 Near vision test card. Words are substituted for symbols. (The Lighthouse Low Vision Services.)

After the child learns the three symbols, the card may be held at any distance. Acuity is recorded at the distance at which the card is held, for example, 15 cm./1 M. This near acuity is not used to estimate required magnification of the reading addition. The Lighthouse for the Blind has devised a near vision chart in which words are substituted for the symbols (Fig. 32–4). The use of words is valuable because it frequently reveals the word comprehension of the child, the presence of dyslexia, and the presence of scotomas as indicated by the omission of some of the letters in the words. The Rosenbaum pocket screener is useful but has obvious limitations (Fig. 32–5).

FUNDUSCOPY AND SLIT LAMP EXAMINA-TION. May reveal that only one eye can be refracted with any degree of success. The presence of nystagmus or opacities of the lens or cornea may make such determinations difficult. Indirect ophthalmoscopy is valuable in these cases.

KERATOMETRY. When the cornea is irregular, the keratometer is useful in determining the degree and axis of the corneal astigmatism. The keratoscope is valuable in examining the cornea for irregularity.

REFRACTION (SUBJECTIVE TESTING). Having obtained as much information as is possible from previously performed retinoscopy and keratometry, one proceeds with subjective testing. If vision is less than 20/200 the distance chart may be placed at 10 feet or less, since the accuracy of the testing is only slightly affected by the shorter distance. The use of a 1D cross cylinder is frequently helpful. A 1D cross cylinder is equivalent to +1.00D sphere and a −2.00D cylinder or a −1.00D sphere and a +2.00D cylinder.

Estimation of Required Magnification (Reading Addition)

Before attempting to evaluate the near vision needs of a child with subnormal vision, one must determine the child's available accommodation and the size of print he is using and will be using in the coming years. Also, the type of lighting that will be available to him as well as the degree of intelligence of the child are important factors. Field defects are of significance, since in some instances it is

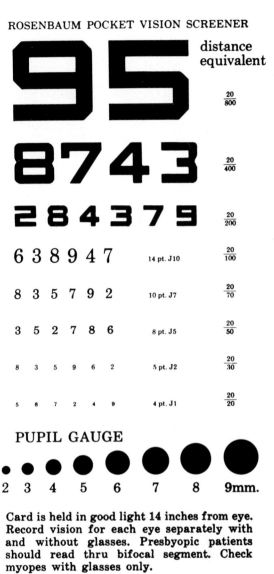

Figure 32–5 Rosenbaum pocket vision screener. (Cooper Laboratories, SMP Division.)

necessary for a child to turn his head in an exaggerated position in order to find the proper and best field of vision.

According to Russell (1963), "One of the most interesting findings in examining children with subnormal vision is the degree of sophistication (know-how) achieved by the children. By the time they come to the low vision center, they have learned to make the most use of the visual acuity and fields of vision available to them. There is very little one can teach them on this score. They are very quick and accurate in comparing performance using the optical aids with the performance using the unaided eye and, indeed, between two different optical aids.

"In evaluating the optical needs of the child, the examining ophthalmologist must be careful not to impose on the child by prescribing an acuity or magnification that is far in excess of his requirements, thus making the optical aid stronger than is necessary, or by prescribing an arbitrary degree of magnification which is insufficient for his needs."*

ESTIMATION BY TRIAL AND ERROR. Have the child bring with him the book or books he is currently using and will be using in the coming years. Place the previously determined distance correction in the trial frame and ask the child to read his book, holding the material at any distance from his eyes that he may choose. Help the child by pushing the printed matter either closer or farther away to determine the clearest point. Some children will naturally hold the print very close to their eyes, especially if they are myopic or have good accommodation. If they appear to have difficulty seeing the print, add plus power in stages of +1.00 or more diopters, until the patient is able to read satisfactorily. Give the least amount of plus necessary.

KESTENBAUM FORMULA. The dioptric power of the addition for reading J-5 type (Jaeger) is equal to the reciprocal of the distant visual acuity. The denominator of the distance visual acuity is divided by the numerator, giving a figure which Kestenbaum calls the RV (reciprocal of vision) (Kestenbaum and Sturman, 1956).

---

*Russell, B. K. (F.A.D.O.): An optician's review of five years' experience with partially sighted and blind children—their difficulties and problems, an analysis of optical aids supplied, together with details of some pathological conditions encountered. Lecture given at the International Optical Congress, Geneva, April, 1963. From Keelen Magazine, April, 1963, p. 6.)

Example: 10/200 = 20
    RV   = +20D for J-5
    For reading J-1 double the reciprocal.

The amount of available accommodation must be subtracted approximately 8D for 10 years.

SLOAN METHOD. Reading additions are selected on the basis of vision measured in M units at 40 cm. and the dioptric power of the reading addition required by the patient to read 1M type (Sloan and Brown, 1963). These reading additions assume that the patient has no accommodation. This value should be decreased by the number of diopters of accommodation the patient is able to sustain. Sloan's special test cards are composed of continuous text in 9 different sizes of type (see Table 32–1) (Fig. 32–6).

Selection of reading additions from measurement of vision at 40 centimeters

Explanation: The smallest type is designated 1M. Ability to read this type requires in Snellen notation 40/100 because the patient reads at 40 cm. what the normal eye can read at 100 cm. One M is equal to newsprint (Jaeger 5). When the patient's reading acuity is measured, he should wear a correction for his refractive error, supplemented by whatever reading addition is required. If accommodation is inadequate, add +2.50D at 40 cm., and +5.00D at 20 cm.

Example: An individual wo can read 4M type at 40 cm. can read 1M type at 10 cm. For this distance, reading addition is 4 × 2.5 or 10 diopters (assuming no accommodation). An emmetropic child

TABLE 32–1   PRINT SIZES USED IN MEASURING READING ACUITY (SLOAN READING CARDS)

Size of Print in M Units	Acuity Required at 40 cm.	Equivalent Distance Acuity	Dioptric Power of Reading Add Required to Read 1 M Print (Assuming Emmetropia and Zero Accommodation)
1.00	40/100	20/50	2.50
1.50	40/150	20/75	3.75
2.00	40/200	20/100	5.00
2.50	40/250	20/125	6.25
3.00	40/300	20/150	7.50
4.00	40/400	20/200	10.00
5.00	40/500	20/250	12.50
7.00	40/700	20/350	15.00
10.00	40/1000	20/500	25.00
14.00	40/1400	20/700	30.00
20.00	40/2000	20/1000	50.00

One day my neighbor asked me if I had met the widow who had just moved into the next block. That night I hobbled down the street and knocked upon her door. I expected to find some sweet, although tottering, lady of 80, but what opened the door was this blonde. I proposed to her immediately. She had a better television set in her house than the one I had in my cottage.

A

Bow ties are of two kinds, those that are ready tied and those that have to be tied. Bow ties that have to be tied are preferred, since the ready tied are too perfect. Imperfections in the tie that has to be tied show that it is not machine-made but hand-wrought. While the tie that has to be tied is imperfect it should not be too imperfect. That is to say, one side should not be longer than the other side, and the tie should sit horizontally and not at an angle of 45 degrees. Tying a bow tie does not come naturally. It has to be learned, like swimming. Written directions may be had, but they are hard to follow. If they cannot be understood a teacher will have to be called in to give practical demonstrations. But since the teacher stands facing the pupil the latter will have to follow the demonstrations in reverse. That is as hard to do as understanding the written directions. Thus many men never learn to tie a bow tie. So they have to do brilliant things, such as graduating in physics, to compensate for not being able to tie a bow tie. Others learn to tie a bow tie after a fashion. But they are mortified when they find themselves at an evening party with many men in bow ties and discover that their bow tie is the worst. One way of solving the bow-tie problem is to look for a girl who can tie a bow tie and request a demonstration. If that is successful the next thing to do is to marry her. Then a man can be assured of having his bow tied by hand. It is an expensive method, but, to a man who has struggled for years with a bow tie, it is worth it.

B

Figure 32–6 *A*, Sloan special test card for near [size 2m/200]. *B*, Sloan special test card for near [size 1m/40/100(20/50)].

<u>Sloan Reading Cards for Patients With Subnormal Vision</u>

(See Amer. J. of Ophth. <u>42</u>, 1956, 863-872)

Cards are to be shown at a distance of 40 cm, preferably in an illuminated reading stand. The patient wears his refractive correction for distance plus a reading add of 2.5 diopters unless accommodation is known to be adequate for this distance.

The reading cards are used to determine the smallest size of print which gives the patient useful reading vision. If the 10M print cannot be read at a distance of 40 cm, larger visual angles may be obtained by viewing the 7M and 10M cards from a distance of 20 cm to give the equivalent of 14M and 20M at 40 cm.

The table below shows for each level of reading acuity the approximate dioptric power of the reading addition needed to permit the patient to read print the size of ordinary newsprint. When a very high dioptric power is needed, a magnifier which rests on the reading page is usually more successful than one worn as a spectacle.

<u>Print Sizes Used In Measuring Reading Acuity</u>

Size of Print in M Units	Acuity Required at 40 cm	Equivalent Distance Acuity	Dioptric Power of Reading Add Required to Read 1M Print (assuming emmetropia and zero accommodation)
1.0	40/100	20/50	2.50
1.5	40/150	20/75	3.75
2.0	40/200	20/100	5.00
2.5	40/250	20/125	6.25
3.0	40/300	20/150	7.50
4.0	40/400	20/200	10.0
5.0	40/500	20/250 or 16/200	12.50
7.0	40/700	20/350 or 11.5/200	15.00
10.0	40/1000	20/500 or 8/200	25.00
14.0 *	40/1400	20/700 or 5.8/200	30.00
20.0 *	40/2000	20/1000 or 4/200	50.00

To obtain the equivalents of 14 and 20M print viewed from a distance of 40 cm, the 7 and 10M sizes are viewed from a distance of 20 cm.

Figure 32–6 *Continued.* *C,* Sloan reading cards for patients with subnormal vision.

with the same reading acuity at 40 cm. can read 1M type by holding the print at 10 cm. without glasses, providing that he has 10D of accommodation.

KEELER NEAR VISION CHART (KEELER "A": SERIES WORD CHART) (FIG. 32–7). This chart is designed for a quick estimation of the magnification required to raise the visual acuity of the partially sighted to read newsprint. It consists of 14 different sizes of print numbered from A-20 [largest size to A-6 (newsprint)]. The assessed magnification to read newsprint is stated in diopters and magnification (X) under each size of print. The chart has been logarithmically calibrated. With the patient's distance correction on, the chart is held at 25 cm. (10 inches) before each eye. If there is no accommodation present, a +4.00-diopter sphere is added to the patient's distance correction to allow reading at 25 cm. The patient is asked to read the smallest print that he is

able, thus giving directly the magnification required to read newsprint. In children, for example, if the child brings the chart to 12.5 cm. (5 inches) in order to read, thus enlarging the image, the assessed magnification would then have to be doubled.

Fonda (1965) states that approximately 70 per cent of children with subnormal vision under 10 years of age require no optical aid but only the correction of their refractive error. These children are able to read without other aids because their available accommodation is great and because many are myopic. Also the type they are required to read (Table 32–2) is large and they normally read at a distance of 10 inches or less.

Verification of Predicted Magnification for Near and Trial of Proposed Aid

The child's predetermined distance correction is placed in the trial frame, and

Ridges could
which is not

A18 = 12X = 48ᴅ

Look down from
on either side of

A17 = 10X = 40ᴅ

The Keeler "A" Series Word-Chart

is designed for a quick estimation of the magnification required
to raise the visual acuity of the partially sighted to read news print.

PLEASE NOTE:

Patient's correction for 25cm. must be worn for this test and each
eye examined separately.

© C. H. KEELER 1958

Figure 32–7   Keeler near vision chart for estimation of required magnification.

over this is placed plus lenses from previously determined estimated magnification. The child is asked to read the material placed before him. He is asked to find the point where the reading material is the clearest. This may or may not be the focal point of the lens combination. Check to see

TABLE 32–2   TABLE COMPARATIVE
NEAR VISION NOTATIONS

Jaeger Notation	Snellen Equivalent	Point Size	Reading Material
J–1	0.50M	4	Small Bible print
J–2	0.60M	5	Want ads (newspaper)
J–3	0.70M	6	Telephone directory
J–4 to J–5	0.80M	8	Newspaper print
J–6	1.00M	9	Magazines
J–9	1.50M	12	Children's books (age 9 to 12) Typewriter print
J–10	1.75M	14	Children's books (age 8 to 9)
J–13	2.00M	18	Children's books (age 7 to 8)
J–14	3.00M	24	Sight saving print

whether or not the cylindrical correction, if any, enhances the reading ability of the child. It has been found that omission of cylinder corrections of 0.50 diopters to 2.00 diopters often does not lessen the efficacy of the optical aid. This may be the case when a full reading lens is to be prescribed. If a bifocal is to be ordered, the cylinder is important for the distance correction.

Prescription for an Optical Aid and Instructions to the Optician

The final decision as to the type of optical aid that a particular child will need depends on several factors:

First, whether or not a simple bifocal type of lens will be better, for example, than just a full reading lens must be determined. The examining ophthalmologist should consider the cosmetic appearance of the aid. If the optical aid is only for home use, the fact that it may have an unusual appearance should not make any difference to the student. Frequently, a special type of lens may be prescribed for home use, and either a full reading glass or bifocals for use at school. Some parents may object to the appearance of the special types of optical aids. Insofar as instructions to the optician are concerned, the ophthalmologist should be specific as to type of frame, bridge, and temples. Also, instead of ordering just "bifocals," he should specify Kryptok, Executive, or Ultex A. The height of the bifocal segments are important. Some opticians will give a child a very low bifocal because the frame size is small, and the child will be looking over the tops of the bifocals instead of through them when looking down to read. A satisfactory height is one-half the height of the lens or possibly 1 mm. below center. When strong reading lenses are ordered, the best vision is obtained through the optical center of the lens.

Single vision lenses can be decentered as much as 3 to 4 mm. When more prismatic effect is needed, prisms should be ordered. This pertains to binocular corrections. When vision is present in only one eye, the eye will find the best spot for reading. Whenever possible, patients should be asked to return with their glasses so that they may be checked. When a child lives too far away to return, the ophthalmologist should insist on a telephone call from the parents.

METHODS OF CORRECTION OF SUBNORMAL VISION

Optical aids improve vision in the partially sighted (1) by eliminating anterior corneal irregularities, (2) by producing a sharper retinal image, and (3) by enlarging the retinal image (Tait, 1951). Vision of more than 97 per cent of patients with subnormal vision is improved by enlarging the retinal image (Fonda, 1961).

Eliminating Anterior Corneal Irregularities

This group is made up chiefly of individuals with keratoconus and those in whom the regularity of the anterior corneal surfaces has been changed by scars resulting from previous corneal ulcers, injuries, and keratitis. In these cases, providing the other media and retina are normal, the vision may be improved by replacing the anterior corneal surface (as far as its optical effect is concerned) by the an-

terior surface of a contact lens. However, contact lenses do not usually help those cases of injury or severe ulceration which result in a dense corneal opacity in the pupillary area of the cornea.

In *keratoconus* the pathological condition causes the substitution of a conic section surface for the nearly spherical or toric one in front of the pupillary aperture of a normal cornea. This results in extensive irregular astigmatism which can only be neutralized by a contact lens.

Producing a Sharper Retinal Image

In those cases in which central retinal function is unimpaired, but in which there are scattered opacities of various sizes and densities with clear areas between them or irregular astigmatism surfaces or areas in the crystalline lens (producing overlapping and irregular retinal blur surfaces), vision can be corrected by limiting the number of refracting systems present—accomplished by the use of pinhole spectacles. By this means, an artifical and smaller pupil is substituted for a normal one, thereby producing a clearer image. However, pinhole spectacles are not practical because they limit the field of vision, require a great deal of light, and one cannot walk with them.

Enlarging the Retinal Image (Magnification)

For Distance Vision. *Nonoptical method.* For distance, the simplest method of enlarging the retinal image is by moving closer to the object of regard. For example, moving from 20 feet to 10 feet from the blackboard increases the magnification by 2X.

Optical method. A second method is by the use of telescopic lenses, through which the object appears larger than it actually is, owing to an increase in the visual angle (Fig. 32–8).

For Near Vision. *Nonoptical methods.* For near vision, the image is enlarged when the object of regard (reading material) is brought closer to the eyes. (Moving a book from 10 inches to 2 inches, increases linear size of the image by 5X.) Uncorrected myopia, available accommodation, and plus lenses all cause enlargement of the retinal image. Another method involves the use of large print books (18- to 24-point print). The principle underlying

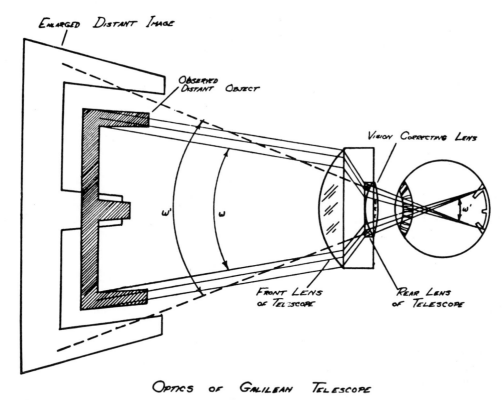

Figure 32–8   Principle of Galilean Telescope: object appears nearer than it actually is due to increase in visual angle. (From IHB Optical Aids Service Survey. The Industrial Home for the Blind, 57 Willoughby Street, Brooklyn, N.Y. September, 1957.)

all visual aids which improve vision by increasing the size of the retinal image can be demonstrated by the following diagram (Fig. 32–9).

Optical methods. In macular and central retinal changes, enlargement of the retinal image is the only way that vision can be improved. The improvement in vision is directly proportional to the degree of macular involvement. Telescopic lenses, when used with a strong reading addition (convex lens), will frequently give good near vision. However, they have the disadvantage of being very critical. In some cases, the use of a plano convex doublet lens (to decrease spherical aberration) is of value for near use (micro-

scopic lens) (Fig. 32–10). This type of lens is of value in individuals with extremely low vision and requires that the individual hold the reading material at the very short focus of the lens.

THE PRINCIPLE OF MAGNIFICATION (IN SUBNORMAL VISION)

The image which falls on the retina is enlarged and the flaws (nonseeing areas of the retina) are therefore smaller in proportion to the image and interfere less with its perception. Or, one may say that any system of lenses that will cause the image to

Figure 32–9   Demonstrates enlargement of the retinal image obtained by moving object of regard closer to the eye, as A to B (20″ to 2″, same size object.) Linear size of retinal image is increased 10 times (10×). (Modified from Fonda, G.: Management of the Patient with Subnormal Vision. St. Louis, The C. V. Mosby Co., 1965.)

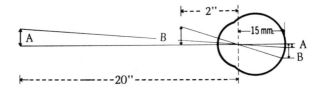

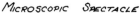

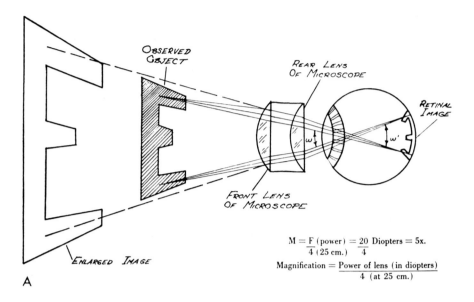

$$M = \frac{F \,(\text{power})}{4\,(25\,\text{cm.})} = \frac{20 \text{ Diopters}}{4} = 5\text{x.}$$

$$\text{Magnification} = \frac{\text{Power of lens (in diopters)}}{4 \,(\text{at } 25 \text{ cm.})}$$

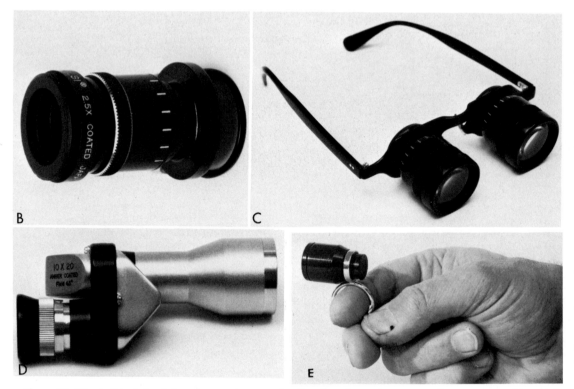

Figure 32–10 *A*, Principle of the microscopic spectacle: Consists of two plano convex lenses separated by an air space. Magnification is achieved by the optical projection of the object to a more distant plane. Upon this distant plane, the image created is magnified and perceived as such by the eye. Permits the viewing of small type at extremely close range at which unaided eye could not possibly perceive it. (From IHB Optical Aids Service Survey. The Industrial Home for the Blind, 57 Willoughby Street, Brooklyn, N.Y. September, 1957.)

    B, Uniocular adjustable telescope (2.5×).

    C, Binocular distance telescope (2.5×) (sports glass).

    D, Prism telescope 10×.

    E, Uniocular distance telescope (1.75×).

spread over more retinal cones will produce magnification. Formula for linear magnification:

$$M = \frac{I}{O} = \frac{\text{image size}}{\text{object size}} = \frac{\text{image distance}}{\text{object distance}}$$

This formula for linear magnification is based on linear distances measured parallel and perpendicular to an optical system.

Angular Magnification

Magnification in association with the eye and the use of ophthalmic instruments involves angular magnification. Angular magnification may be defined as the ratio between the angular size of the image seen through a lens or optical system and the angular size of the object seen without the lens or optical system when the object is at the same distance from the eye in both instances. Angular magnification is dependent upon the angular sizes of the image and object about a reference point. This reference point is usually one of the eye's cardinal points (either entrance pupil of the eye or center of rotation of the eyeball).

Owing to the variability of accommodation, some methods used to compute angular magnification utilize what is commonly called "least distance of distinct vision." As a historical carry-over from the angular magnification of microscopes, this reference viewing distance is usually 25 cm., or 10 inches. Sloan and Habel (1956) use 40 cm. They believe that this distance is more practical and that 25 cm. is too short. Using 40 cm., the magnification required is increased as $20D/2.5 = 8X$, since we are reducing the size of the image by placing the object at a farther distance from the eye.

Formula for magnifiers: $M = \dfrac{\text{diopters}}{4}$

Basis for this formula is that the object is located at the focus of the lens, i.e., u=f, and the image distance is 25 cm. (least distance of distinct vision); therefore

$$M = \frac{v}{u} = \frac{1/4}{1/f} = \frac{D}{4}$$

TABLE 32–3 DIOPTRIC EQUIVALENT OF MAGNIFIERS

Diopters	Magnification	Focus in Centimeters	Focus in Inches
+4D	1X	25.0	10
+8D	2X	12.5	5
+10D	2.5X	10	4.0
+20D	5X	5.0	2.0
+40D	10X	2.5	1.0
+80D	20X	1.25	0.5

u = object distance from lens
f = focal distance of lens
v = least distance of distinct vision

Example: 40-diopter lens has magnification of $\dfrac{40}{4} = 10X$

X = letter denoting magnification as 10 times magnification

CLASSIFICATION OF OPTICAL AIDS (SIMPLIFIED)*

I. Optical Aids to Improve Distance Vision.
  A. Spectacles
    1. Conventional
    2. Telescopic
      a. Uniocular (clip-on) (Fig. 32–10 *A*)
      b. Binocular (sports glass) (Fig. 32–10 *B*)
  B. Nonspectacles
    1. Binocular and uniocular field glasses
    2. Prism telescopes (usually 6X or 10X) (Fig. 32–10*C*)
  C. Contact Lenses
II. Optical Aids to Improve Near Vision
  A. Spectacles
    1. Conventional (full reading lenses)
    2. Bifocals
    3. Half-eye full reading lenses
    4. Special spectacle lenses
      a. Aspheric bifocals (Keeler)
      b. Aspheric full reading lenses
      c. Doublet lens (15X) (bifocal microscopic)
      d. Illuminated spectacle magnifier
  B. Telescopic Spectacles
  C. Nonspectacle Magnifiers
    1. Hand magnifiers (single, double, and triple)
    2. Stand magnifiers
    3. Illuminated nonspectacle magnifier

---

*For a complete list of optical aids, refer to Fonda, G.: Management of the Patient with Sub-Normal Vision. St. Louis, The C. V. Mosby Co., 1965.

III. Auxilliary Optical Aids
  A. Tinted Lenses
  B. Tinted Contact Lenses
  C. Visors

I. OPTICAL AIDS TO IMPROVE DISTANCE VISION

Evaluation of visual acuity needs: In determining the distance visual acuity needs of a school child, one must remember the ease of utilizing nonoptical methods of magnification. For example, moving closer to the object of regard (blackboard) increases the size of the retinal image. A child who walks from 20 feet to within 2 feet of the blackboard increases the magnification 10X. Having the teacher write larger than usual on the blackboard is nonoptical magnification.

A. Spectacle Lenses for Distance Use

1. Conventional Spectacles

Little need be said here about conventional spectacles except that they should be as small as is consistent with the interpupillary distance (P.D.) and facial configuration. They should be as thin as possible to eliminate unsightly thickness of the edges of the lenses. Today there is a law in the United States that all lenses be case-hardened for safety purposes. Plastic lenses may be substituted for glass when desirable. Teen-agers are demanding extra large frames and glasses, which introduces the problem of overdecentration and possibly discomfort on wearing such lenses.

2. Telescopic Spectacles

Telescopic lenses give a small field, approximately 14 degrees for a 2.2X power worn at a vertex distance of 12 mm. In addition, one cannot walk about with telescopic spectacles because they produce motion parallax. We have prescribed uniocular 2.5X adjustable telescopes (Fig. 32–10A) to be clipped on over the patient's distance correction for observing the blackboard. The child may hold the telescope in his hand and place it on the desk when not using it. We have found that a child will enthusiastically welcome this optical aid when it is shown to him in the low vision center. Later, he will discard it when he finds it easier to go up to the blackboard. However, this optical aid has value to the school child for use in the school auditorium for viewing the stage, and also on the street for sighting bus or trolley car numbers. There is also available a binocular clip-on telescope which is light in weight and can be flipped up when not in use.

B. Nonspectacles

These include uniocular and binocular telescopic systems, such as weak field glasses, as well as prism telescopes of 6X to 10X magnification. Such lenses are usually heavy and rather unwieldy to hold (Fig. 32–10C).

C. Contact Lenses

Contact lenses are of value in subnormal vision caused by corneal scars, irregular astigmatism, keratoconus, high myopia, and in congenital or traumatic monocular aphakia. Contact lenses may be tinted for extreme photophobia. Opaque contact lenses have been prescribed for albinism and aniridia, but are of questionable value here. Contact lenses are contraindicated in aphakia with subnormal vision, since they reduce the size of the retinal image. This also applies to high hyperopia with subnormal vision.

II. OPTICAL AIDS TO IMPROVE NEAR VISION

A. Spectacles

1. Conventional Spectacles

School children with subnormal vision who have a degree of hyperopia sufficient to require that they wear their distance correction most of their waking hours will do better in most instances to have plus power added in the form of a bifocal rather than to use reading glasses which they must remove frequently in order to see the blackboard or their surroundings, whereas myopes will raise their spectacles in order to see better for their near reading.

2. Bifocal Spectacles

We have found that bifocals of 2 to 4 diopters or in some cases (6D in a Kryptok or Ultex A) are usually sufficient for their near needs. The Executive type bifocal has been prescribed in some children who tilt their heads to see better, especially seen in nystagmus. If a child has the same or nearly the same vision in both eyes, and bifocals are ordered, proper decentering is necessary. This is more difficult with bifocals than with full reading glasses. The usually narrow P.D. will reduce the amount of decentering required.

3. Half-Eye Full Reading Lenses (Fig. 32–11)

When prisms are needed to produce single binocular vision, these can be more easily added in a half-eye reading lens.

Fonda's rule of thumb for creating base in prism is to decenter each bifocal segment in 1 mm. for each diopter of reading addition for each eye, or in single vision lenses, grind one prism diopter of prism base in for each diopter of reading addition (Fonda, 1965).

Since many children with subnormal vision have useful vision in only one eye, half-eye additions up to 20 diopters may be prescribed. This can be illustrated by a 20-year-old female student about to enter college who had been wearing an optical

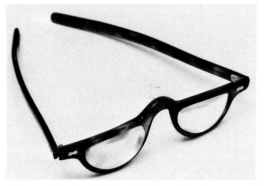

Figure 32–11   Half-eye full reading lenses with prisms.

aid because of retrolental fibroplasia. Vision was present in only one eye. She felt conspicuous with her present optical aid. A 20-diopter lens (5X) in a half-eye full reading lens was prescribed for her seeing eye and a balance lens for the opposite eye.

4. Special Spectacle Lenses

a. ASPHERIC BIFOCALS (KEELER) (Fig. 32–12).   These consist of 22-mm. round plastic aspheric button-like lenses which are threaded for insertion into a plastic distance correction. These lenses vary in power from 2X to 9X (eight different powers of magnification). Because the eyes cannot converge through strong lenses, these are to be used for only one eye. If there is interference from the opposite eye in the form of a "ghost image," a frosted occluder button can be placed in the other lens (Fig. 32–13). Although this lens is made as a bifocal, it

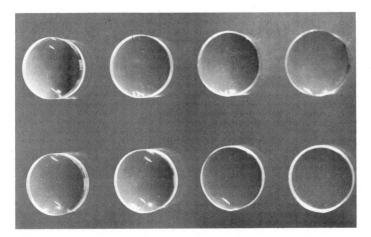

Figure 32–12   Aspheric bifocal lenses (2X to 9X) (Keeler).

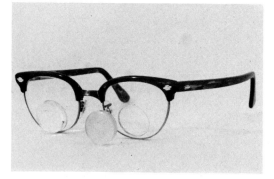

Figure 32–13 Aspheric bifocal in frame with occluder.

is not satisfactory for use when walking, since the bifocal segment is too high. In some instances, however, the bifocal can be placed down low enough so that a person can walk with it. Since there is no correction behind the aspheric button, the power of the distance correction must be incorporated in the bifocal power. A special chart (Table 32–4) is available to supply this figure. One of the former disadvantages of the Keeler bifocal is that the astigmatic correction could not be incorporated. The advanced method of Keeler of grooving out one-half of the thickness of the distance lens and cementing in a sleeve to hold the button has corrected this situation. However, it has been found that the absence of astigmatic corrections in the bifocals of as much as 3 diopters has not lessened the efficacy of the lens.

A special trial set of lenses of similar power is available that allows the examiner to test the patient directly, using the lens power previously determined. An impor-

tant advantage of the Keeler lenses is that the aspheric button can easily be removed and one of a higher power inserted at a later date, should this become necessary because of a decrease in the patient's visual acuity.

b. ASPHERIC FULL READING LENSES. Keeler makes a full width field monocular plastic lens varying from 2X (8D) to 8X (32D). This is also available with a cutaway top for distance vision or a distance telescope of 2.5X (field 7.5 degrees) may be inserted. The opposite lens may be a plano or an occluder lens.

c. DOUBLET LENS. For those individuals who need a high power lens for reading, there is available a 15X (60-diopter) doublet lens that can be used in a manner similar to that for the previously described Keeler aspheric bifocals for individuals with vision of 5/200 or less (Fig. 32–14).

d. ILLUMINATED SPECTACLE MAGNIFIER. Illuminated spectacle magnifier of Keeler 8X to 20X requires close proximity of reading matter to the optical aid (Fig. 32–14A).

e. High add bifocal additions have been successful for surgical aphakia after congenital cataracts. Children have always held the paper close to their eyes to read and therefore adjust readily.

Aolite plastic aspheric high add bifocals are available (American Optical Co.) with reading additions of +6.00, +12.00, and +18.00. These are satisfactory when a reading addition stronger than +4.00 and less than +20.00 is needed. The distance corrections are available from +8.00 to +20.00.

TABLE 32–4 TABLE OF MAGNIFICATION*

Assessed Magnification with Reading or Distance Correction in Use	Patient's Correction (in diopters)								
	−20	−16	−12	−8	−4	+4	+8	+12	+16
X2						X3	X4	X5	X6
X3					2	4	5	6	7
X4				2	3	5	6	7	8
X5			2	3	4	6	7	8	9
X6		2	3	4	5	7	8	9	10
X7	2	3	4	5	6	8	9	10	11

*From Helping the Partially Sighted. Manual by C. H. Keeler.
Magnification adjusted to incorporate the distance or reading correction automatically.

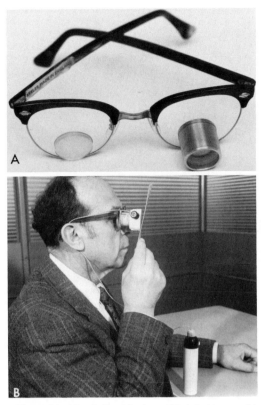

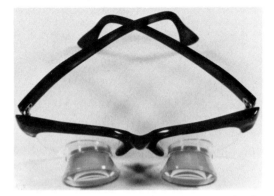

Figure 32–15   Binocular telescopic spectacles for near use (2× to 5× magnification) (Keeler) incorporates the distance correction (all plastic).

Figure 32–14   *A*, Doublet lens (15×) (microscopic). *B*, Illuminated spectacle magnifier (8× to 20× magnification) requires close proximity of reading matter.

The successful use of a Keeler binocular telescopic spectacle can be demonstrated by the following case:

J.W., a female albino, age 17 years, was referred to the low vision center for an optical aid. She was anxious to read the newspaper. Her uncorrected visual acuity was OD 20/260, OS 20/260.

Refraction:
  OD − 100 + 200 cyl. axis 90
  OS − 100 + 200 cyl. axis 90
  corrects to 20/120 each eye

Her assessed magnification to read newsprint was 3X. With a 3X Keeler binocular telescope in front of her spectacle correction, she could read J-5 type. In a follow-up

B. Telescopic Spectacles

We have found the Keeler telescopic binocular spectacles for reading to be the most satisfactory of several on the market. These lenses consist of lightweight, all plastic lenses varying in power from 2X (8D) to 5X (20D) (Fig. 32–15), angulated to the proper P.D., and made to insert into plastic aspheric distance lenses in which part of the distance correction has been reamed out to hold the near lenses. In order to use binocular telescopes satisfactorily, the visual acuity should be the same or near the same in both eyes.

There is also available from Keeler a full width binocular telescope of either 1.6X or 2.0X magnification, which provides a long working distance and is suitable for children (Fig. 32–16).

Telescopic lenses for near have the disadvantage of a small field and are more critical than ordinary lenses.

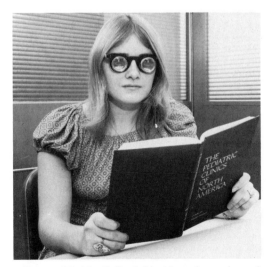

Figure 32–16   Full field binocular telescopic spectacles (1.6× magnification) (Keeler). Note the long working distance.

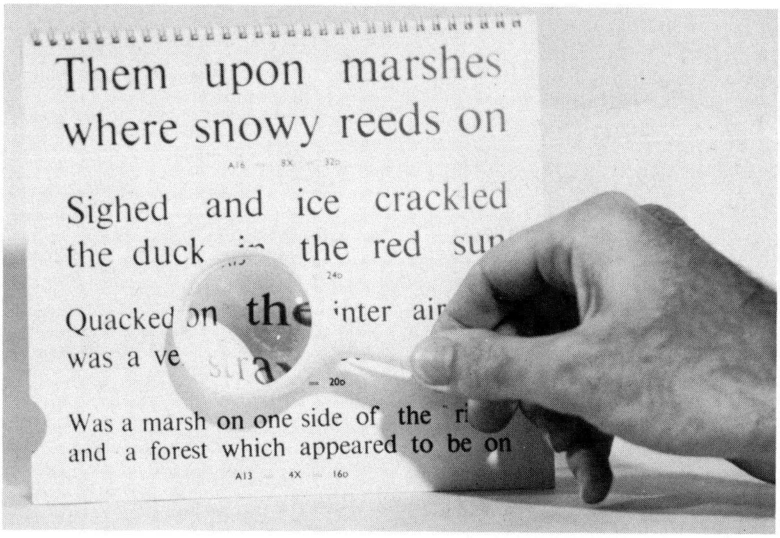

Figure 32-17   Hand magnifier (5× aspheric).

3 years later, she was found to be using her optical aid consistently.

C. Nonspectacle Magnifiers (also known as Loupes)

These magnifiers are convex lenses of powers varying from +8.00 diopters to +80.00 diopters. The most commonly used and least expensive one is the hand magnifier.

1. The Hand Magnifier (Fig. 32-17)

The principle of the hand magnifier is that the image is enlarged if the object lies inside the anterior focal plane of the lens. When so placed, a virtual erect and magnified image is produced (Fig. 32-18). The size of the field varies directly with the diameter of the magnifier and inversely with the distance the loupe is held from the eye. The hand-held magnifier is more valuable in cases in which the field of vision is constricted, since a spectacle magnifier would enlarge the image into a nonseeing area. Hand-held magnifiers are easily carried in the pocket or purse and vary in combinations of from 1 to 3 lenses in a suitable arrangement up to 80 diopters (Fig. 32-19).

2. Stand Magnifiers

These magnifiers have a fixed object-to-lens distance which is less than the focus of the lens, and the virtual image is formed behind the lens. A fair amount of accommodation is needed, depending on the eye-to-lens distance. With such a lens, single binocular vision is obtainable when the reading matter is held at a more or less normal reading distance. We have prescribed this aid for young children just learning to read who need magnification (Fig. 32-20).

3. Illuminated Nonspectacle Magnifier

Where direct light is required on the reading material, the Keeler illuminated nonspectacle magnifier, which varies

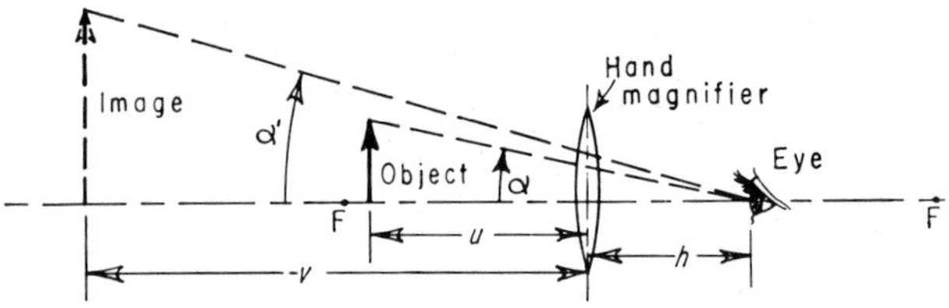

The optical principles of an ordinary hand magnifying lens.

Figure 32-18   Principle of hand magnifier (object placed inside anterior focal plane produces an erect magnified image. (From K. N. Ogle: Optics, An Introduction for Ophthalmologists. Springfield, Ill., Charles C Thomas, 1961.)

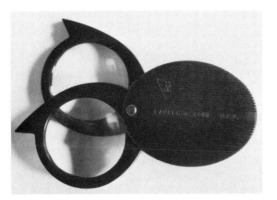

Figure 32–19   Multipower hand magnifier.

from 8X to 20X magnification, is the most practical. (They can be focused by the patient.)

III. AUXILIARY OPTICAL AIDS

A. Tinted Lenses

These lenses are indicated when an individual is bothered by glare from either the sun or from an abnormal intensity of light. Calobar D and G-15 are indicated for strong sunlight. Many colored lenses that are available and are demanded by teenagers are of questionable value except cosmetically. The new Photogray lens on the market changes shade with different light intensities, but it is not intended for strong sunlight. For the latter the Photosun lens is available.

B. Tinted Contact Lenses

It is advisable to tint contact lenses so that the lens may be more easily found if it falls out of the eye or is dropped.

C. Visors

Visors are only indicated if the light source cannot be regulated or adjusted.

INDICATIONS FOR OPTICAL AIDS IN SUBNORMAL VISION

Optical aids function better in those persons with subnormal vision who have depressed macular function (Weiss, 1964). Included in this group are patients with early diabetic retinopathy, high degrees of myopia with central myopic degeneration, healed central choroiditis, and all forms of macular degeneration. In disease processes in which central vision is lost early in life or in which the macula fails to develop, with resultant pendular nystagmus, visual aids are of considerable value. Included in this group are albinism, aniridia, and congenital cataracts.

Optical aids function poorly in persons with field defects such as right homonymous hemianopia, glaucoma, retinitis pigmentosa, advanced optic atrophy, and advanced vascular diseases producing field changes.

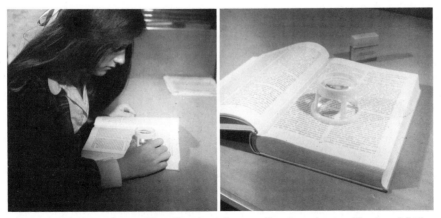

Figure 32–20   Stand magnifier (illuminated or nonilluminated, magnification, 1.8 ✕).

CONTRAINDICATIONS FOR OPTICAL AIDS

Optical aids are contraindicated in acute inflammatory diseases of the eyes, in young diabetics with recurrent hemorrhages, when motivation is poor, or when there is a disinclination to read and when a child's physical state prevents him from holding the reading matter in the necessay position because of muscular weakness or marked tremors (Weiss, 1964).

PSYCHOLOGICAL ASPECTS OF PARTIAL SIGHTEDNESS

When ordering optical aids for partially sighted children, one must consider the psychological aspect of such treatment. I like to use the term "psychological acceptance." By this I mean the realization on the part of the parents that their child has subnormal vision and that because of this he will be required to use some type of optical aid that will make the child conspicuous and appear different from other children in the classroom.

It is also important for the child himself to recognize this fact. This is particularly true today, because the child with subnormal vision (in many instances) is being placed in classes with children who have normal sight. This is the result of desire on the part of the child, demand by parents, and acquiescence by educators. In the majority of cases, we have found that the child's intense desire to learn to read, and thus successfully compete with the fully sighted child, helps him to overcome his reluctance to use the optical aid. This, alone, is usually sufficient to convince the parents and the child that appearances are secondary to his education.

It cannot be stressed too strongly here that the handling of the visually handicapped child in school is a three-way affair, with the child at the apex and parent and teachers at the bases of the triangle. The partially seeing child must be accepted in the schoolroom as a normal human being, without too much emphasis being placed on his visual disabilities. He must be made to feel secure and wanted in the classroom. Normal children in the classroom may be cruel to the child because of his disability, and it is incumbent on the teachers to explain the problem to the rest of the class.

From the parent's standpoint, the child must be made to feel secure at home. Since this type of child is apt to be slow in learning because of his ocular disability, overemphasis on his educational attainment should be avoided. If a child cannot keep up with his class, extra time should be given him by a special teacher. Parents and older children at home must take the time to help the child with his schoolwork, at the same time to do it without making him feel too dependent on them. In other words, the child's confidence must be developed so that he feels he can do the work required of him.

One of the problems which we have found at the Low Vision Center refers to the child who lives in a small town where there are no facilities for the education of partially sighted children, that is, a lack of special teachers properly trained for the handling of the child with subnormal vision. The parents are at a loss as to what should be done. On occasion, I have recommended that parents move to larger cities where special schools or proper facilities are available.

BRAILLE

A frequent question after the examination of a partially sighted child is, "Should my child be taught braille?" In general, one may say that a child who is unable to read 18-point print (Jaeger 13 or Snellen 2M) should be taught braille. The learning of braille requires an intelligent child, one who has good finger sensitivity (Nolan et al., 1965; Crandell et al., 1968) and good motivation.

When the nature of the eye disease or type of congenital eye defects indicates that there is a good possibility for future decrease in vision, the ophthalmologist should consider the necessity for braille. Braille should be taught as a supplement to reading. Fonda (1962), in a study of 161 albinoes, found that 7 per cent of this group had been needlessly taught braille. At the New York State School for the Blind, Faye, Kohler, and Sanborn found that 24 per cent of the students should never have been taught braille. This was confirmed by Jones (1961), who stated that he found that 82 per cent of partially seeing local students and 29 per cent of residential students could read type. In residential schools, almost every child is taught braille.

SCHOOLS FOR THE BLIND

The question frequently arises as to whether or not a child should be sent to a school for the blind. This question requires careful consideration on the part of the ophthalmologist, parent, and educators of the blind. Such schools are widely scattered and may necessitate the child's being sent far away from home. It is a known fact that some children with severe limitations on their sight will often do well in a sighted class, whereas another child less severely limited will not get along well. This may indicate that there are other problems to be considered; a child may feel more secure in a sheltered environment or may not be doing well in a class of sighted pupils.

DYSLEXIA

This chapter would not be complete without some remarks on the subject of dyslexia. The following are excerpts taken from a publication of IDEA (Institute for Development of Educational Activities), entitled "The Role of the Ophthalmologist in Dyslexia."*

"Dyslexia is considered to be a learning disability in a person of normal or even superior intelligence. The term dyslexia takes its origin indirectly from the word alexia or inability to read due to brain damage. Dyslexia in its current usage does not invariably refer to brain damage as a causative factor. Reading disabilities should be considered as one aspect of a total symptom complex of language disturbance (Helveston, 1969).

"The seminar of ophthalmologists generally held 'that the role of the eyes in reading disabilities is limited. That poor vision does not limit reading ability. The child may require larger type or may read slower, but he is certainly not dyslexic. The role of ophthalmology is to help the child attain the most effective, efficient vision possible with corrective lenses or other optical devices, and the treatment of any concurrent eye diseases by the use of drugs, medical, surgical or other means.' It is concluded that not enough objective scientific evidence yet exists to prove that perceptual motor training of the visual system can significantly influence reading disability. Also, that the belief that eye dominance be at the root of so profound and broad a human problem as reading and learning disability is [both] naive, simplistic, and unsupported by scientific data."

Nicholls (1965) classifies reading difficulties in children into three groups:

1. *Congenital Dyslexia* — A specific reading disability in which there is a disturbance of audio-visual perceptions and their interpretations, probably caused by a physiologic disturbance in the parieto-temporal lobe of the dominant cerebral hemisphere.

2. *The Slow Reader* — The child with congenital dyslexia must be differentiated from the slow reader, in whom the retardation is related to low intelligence, to faulty hearing or faulty vision, or to some emotional disturbance, or a combination of these.

3. *The Mixed Type* — A mixture of the previous two types. Goldberg (1959) lists the reading difficulties found most commonly among first grade children having congenital dyslexia as follows:

— inability to work out the pronunciation of a strange word.
— failure to see likenesses and differences in forms of words, i.e., ON-NO PUG-BUD
— failure to hear differences in sounds of letters.
— making reversals u-n stop-tops was-saw
— failure to keep their places while reading.
— failure to read from left to right.
— vocalizing of words.
— failure to read with sufficient understanding.

---

*International Seminar, IDEA publication, 1969.

SOURCES OF INFORMATION FOR OPHTHALMOLOGISTS ON SUBNORMAL VISION

1. National Society for the Prevention of Blindness
   16 E. 40th Street, New York, New York 10016
2. U.S. Department of Health, Education and Welfare
   Division of Handicapped Children and Youth
   Washington, D.C. 20225
3. Social Rehabilitation Service
   Rehabilitation Services Administration, Washington, D.C. 20201
   (Information available on state level relative to special education and rehabilitation.)
4. National Aid to the Visually Handicapped, Inc.
   3201 Balboa Street,
   San Francisco, California 94121
   (Large print textbooks, library materials on request. Sources of information and guidance on resources for the visually handicapped.)
5. Center for the Blind
   Low Vision Lens Service
   3518 Lancaster Avenue,
   Philadelphia, Pennsylvania.
6. Recording for the Blind, Inc.
   215 E. 58th Street,
   New York, New York 10022
   (Recording textbooks and reading materials from elementary through college level.)
7. American Foundation for the Blind, Inc.
   15 W. 16th Street, New York, New York 10011
8. Library of Congress, Division of the Blind
   Washington, D.C. 20225
   [Recorded poetry and literature (talking books).]
9. American Printing House for the Blind
   1839 Frankfort Ave., Louisville, Kentucky 40206
   (Large print text books, tapes, braille books, and tangible aids.)

SOURCES OF LARGE PRINT BOOKS

1. Charles Scribner's Sons
   597 Fifth Avenue, New York, New York 10017
2. Guild for Large Print Books
   211 E. 43rd Street, New York, New York 10017
3. New York Times Large Print Weekly
   229 W. 43rd Street, New York, New York 10036
4. Library for the Blind
   919 Walnut Street, Philadelphia, Pennsylvania
5. Reader's Digest Large Print Edition
   Xerox Corporation, P. O. Box 3300, Grand Central Station, New York, New York 10017

REFERENCES

Crandell, J., Hammill, D., Witkowski, C., and Barkowich, F.: Measuring form discrimination in blind individuals. Internat. J. Educ. Blind, 18:3, 1968.

Faye, E.: A flash card vision test for children. Low Vision Lens Service, The New York Association for the Blind, 111 E. 59th St., New York, N.Y. 10022

Faye, E. E.: A new visual acuity test for partially sighted nonreaders. J. Ophthal., 5:207, 210–212, November, 1968.

Faye, E. E., Koehler, C., and Sanborn, L.: Personal communication, 1960.

Fonda, G.: Evaluation of telescopic spectacles. Amer. J. Opthal., 51:433, 1961.

Fonda, G.: Characteristics of low vision corrections in albinism. Amer. J. Ophthal., 68:754, 1962.

Fonda, G.: Management of the Patient with Sub-Normal Vision. St. Louis, The C. V. Mosby Co., 1965.

Goldberg, H. K.: The ophthalmologist looks at the reading problem. Amer. J. Ophthal., 47:67, 1959.

Hatfield, E. M.: Estimated statistics on blindness and vision problems. National Society for the Prevention of Blindness. New York, N.Y., 1966.

Helveston, E. M.: The role of the ophthalmologist in dyslexia. Institute for the Development of Educational Activities, Inc., Dayton, Ohio, 1969.

Jones, J. W.: The blind child. School Life, 43:7, 1961.

Kestenbaum, A., and Sturman, R. M.: Reading glasses for patients with very poor vision. Arch. Ophthal., 56:451, 1956.

Nicholls, J. V. V.: Reading difficulties in children. Vol. 5, No. 2, pp. 423–440, June, 1965.

Nolan, C. Y., and Morris, J. E.: Development and validation of the roughness discrimination test. Internat. J. Educ. Blind, 15:1, 1965.

Sloan, L., and Brown, D. J.: Reading cards for selection of optical aids for partially sighted. Amer. J. Ophthal., 55:1187, 1963.

Sloan, L., and Habel, A.: Reading aids for the partially blind. Amer. J. Ophthal., 42:863, 1956.

Tait, E. F.: Textbook of Refraction. Philadelphia, W. B. Saunders Company, 1951.

Weiss, S.: Indications for optical aids in sub-normal vision. Eye Ear Nose Throat Monthly, 43:43–47, January, 1964.

CHAPTER 33

TUMORS OF THE EYE, LIDS, AND ORBIT IN CHILDREN

DON H. NICHOLSON, M.D.,*
and W. RICHARD GREEN, M.D.

INTRAOCULAR TUMORS

Retinoblastomas

   rogress in the understanding, diagnosis, and treatment of childhood cancer is nowhere more dramatically exemplified than in the instance of retinoblastoma. Once uniformly fatal, retinoblastoma, the most common intraocular malignant condition of childhood, can now be detected and treated successfully enough to preserve both life and vision. Retinoblastoma occurs with a frequency of 1 case in 17,000 to 34,000 live births and is one of the six most common childhood malignant conditions in the United States (Dargeon, 1960; Ellsworth, 1969). Although the tumor may be present at birth, the diagnosis is most

frequently made between the ages of $1\frac{1}{2}$ and 2 years (Ellsworth, 1969; François and Matton-Van Leuven, 1964).

Pathology

The histogenesis of retinoblastoma has been disputed for over a century, with some authors supporting Virchow's concept of origin from retinal glial elements and others favoring Flexner's theory of origin from retinal sensory receptors. Recent studies from the Armed Forces Institute of Pathology have yielded light and electron microscopic evidence of definite photoreceptor differentiation in 6 per cent of retinoblastomas on file in the Registry of Ophthalmic Pathology, lending support to the latter concept of histogenesis (Ts'o et al., 1970a and 1970b). Albert and Reid have stimulated questions about the possible role of a virus in human retinoblastoma by demonstrating in this tissue an enzyme system similar to that found in certain oncogenic RNA viruses.

*Supported in part by Henry Berol and Heed Ophthalmic Foundation Fellowships in Ophthalmology.

923

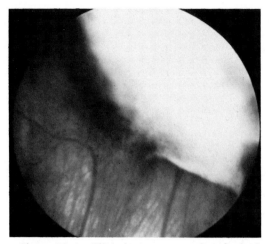

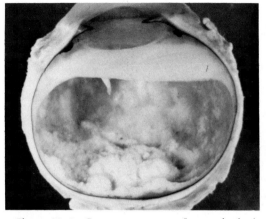

Figure 33–1 Clinical appearance of endophytic retinoblastoma in a 5-year-old boy (5335 Wilmer).

Figure 33–2 Gross appearance of an endophytic retinoblastoma from a 4-year-old girl treated on two occasions with cryotherapy for presumed angiomatosis retinae (E.P. #32066).

The tumor most commonly arises from the inner retinal layers and extends as a fleshy nodular mass into the vitreous cavity, producing the *endophytic* configuration (Figs. 33–1 to 33–4). When it arises and extends primarily externally, producing a secondary retinal detachment but no localized ophthalmoscopically visible vitreous nodule, the gross configuration is termed *exophytic* (Figs. 33–5 to 33–8). Multiple sites of origin in the same and fellow eye are common, and since these do not necessarily arise simultaneously, repeated thorough ophthalmoscopic examinations are mandatory. A diffuse infiltrating type of

retinoblastoma (Figs. 33–9 to 33–11) has been described by Morgan (1971a). This type of retinoblastoma does not form a frank tumor mass but spreads diffusely throughout the retina, breaks into the vitreous, lines the intraocular cavities and infiltrates adjacent structures. This morphologic variant accounted for 1.4 per cent of his total series, was invariably unilateral, and occurred at an older age (average 6.2 years). Anterior involvement with pseudohypopyon (Fig. 33–11) was the presenting sign in 6 of 10 cases. Prognosis appears to be better for diffuse infiltrating retinoblastoma than for exophytic or endophytic

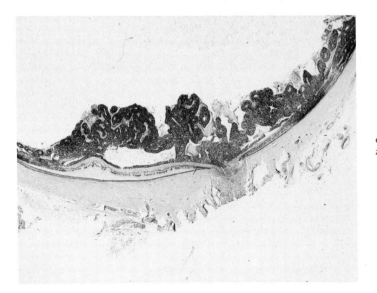

Figure 33–3 Low-power view of endophytic retinoblastoma. (Hematoxylin and eosin ×8.) (E.P. #32066)

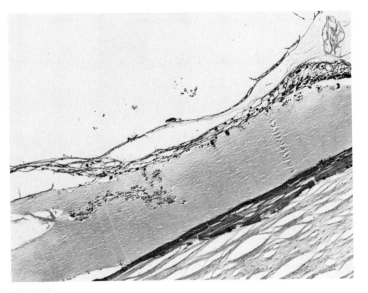

Figure 33–4 Area of retinal atrophy with pigment migration. Site of cryotherapy for suspected retinal angioma in eye with endophytic retinoblastoma. (Hematoxylin and eosin ×65.) (E.P. #32066)

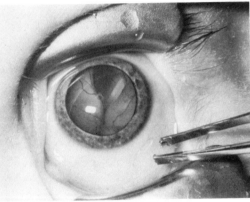

Figure 33–5 Clinical appearance of an exophytic retinoblastoma in a 14-month-old boy. Leukokoria first noted at age 10 months (E.P. #28631).

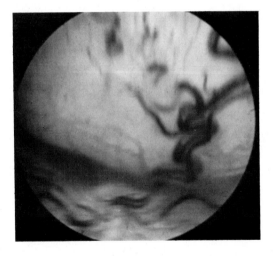

Figure 33–6 Ophthalmoscopic appearance of a single nodule of exophytic retinoblastoma in an 18-month-old child. (Courtesy of the Retina Service, Wills Eye Hospital.)

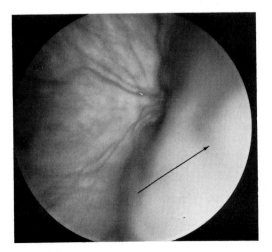

Figure 33–7 Exophytic retinoblastoma with a single nodule of tumor extending through the retina into the vitreous cavity (arrow). This 4-month-old boy had bilateral retinoblastoma with small multifocal tumors in the other eye. (Case of Dr. Harrell Pierce.) (E.P. #33190)

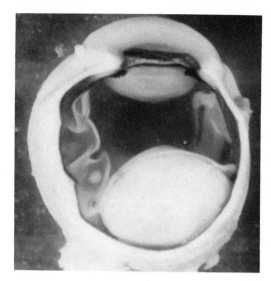

Figure 33–8 Gross appearance of same tumor illustrated in Figure 33–7 after enucleation. (E.P. #33190)

Figure 33–9 Diffuse retinoblastoma in a 5-year-old child whose presenting signs were those of secondary glaucoma. Tumor extends diffusely within the retina, along its inner surface and into the anterior chamber (arrow). (Hematoxylin and eosin, ×4.5.) (E.P. #5580)

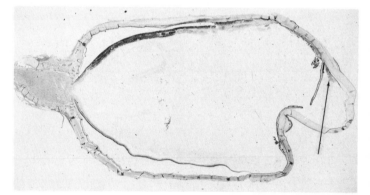

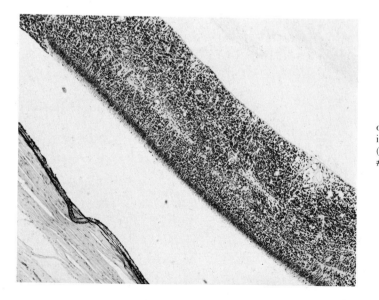

Figure 33–10 Higher magnification demonstrates diffuse nature of intraretinal tumor illustrated in Figure 33–9. (Hematoxylin and eosin, ×65.) (E.P. #5580)

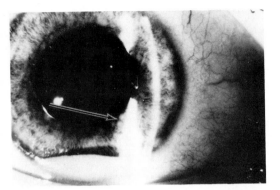

Figure 33–11 Diffuse retinoblastoma with pseudohypopyon and multiple small iris nodules of tumor (arrow). This 8-year-old girl had a two-month history of ocular inflammation. The diagnosis of malignant tumor was confirmed by paracentesis and the diagnosis of retinoblastoma by enucleation. (Courtesy of Dr. F. C. Blodi).

types. All 10 patients were alive and well after enucleation with an average follow-up of 9.3 years.

Microscopically, the bulk of most tumors is composed of undifferentiated, small, round, densely packed cells with hyperchromatic nuclei and scant cytoplasm (Fig. 33–12). Widespread necrosis is often present, with interlacing zones of viable tumor cells surrounding tumor blood vessels (Fig. 33–13). The term "pseudorosettes" which has been applied to these islands of viable tumor cells serves no useful purpose from a histopathologic standpoint but is firmly entrenched in our ter-

minology. The areas of necrotic tumor contain scattered clumps of basophilic material which represents in some instances focal calcium deposition and in other instances clumped nucleic acid breakdown products from necrotic tumor cells (Mullaney, 1969). Generally, the inflammatory response to tumor necrosis is minimal, but on occasion it may be intense enough to produce a clinical picture suggestive of ocular inflammatory disease. In rare instances, tumor necrosis continues to the point of complete spontaneous regression. Boniuk and Zimmerman (1962a) reported the clinical and pathologic findings in 14 patients with spontaneously regressed retinoblastoma. They noted that host immunologic response seemed an unlikely explanation for this phenomenon, since in two cases spontaneous regression was documented in one eye at the same time that tumor extension through the globe into the orbit was noted in the fellow eye. Albert et al. (1970) have observed tumor necrosis in retinoblastoma tissue culture, further suggesting that tumor necrosis occurs independently of host immune mechanisms.

Several degrees of cytodifferentiation have been recognized. *Homer Wright rosettes* (Fig. 33–12) contain no internal limiting membrane, luminal acid mucopolysaccharide, or centrally directed cilia and are morphologically indistinguishable from the rosettes in neuroblastoma and medul-

Figure 33–12 Undifferentiated retinoblastoma with small hyperchromatic cells having no detectable cytoplasm. A Homer Wright rosette is present (arrow). Hematoxylin and eosin. ×530.) (E.P. #6672)

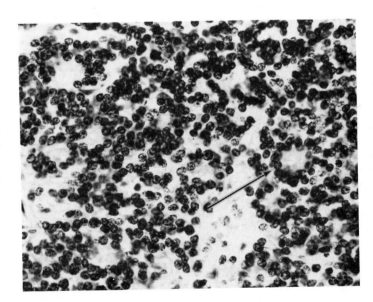

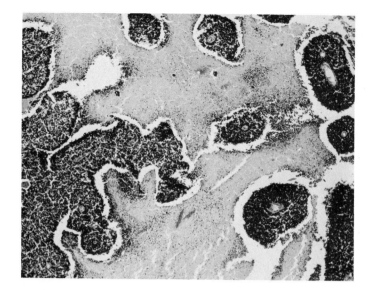

Figure 33–13 Characteristic low-power view of retinoblastoma showing extensive necrosis with collarettes of viable tumor surrounding blood vessels. Small flecks of calcium are present within the necrotic areas. (Hematoxylin and eosin, ×160.) (E.P. #2927)

loblastoma. *Flexner-Wintersteiner rosettes* (Fig. 33–14), on the other hand, are specific for retinoblastoma. These structures consist of a cluster of low columnar cells arranged around a central lumen; the cell nuclei are situated basally, and terminal bars toward the cell apex form a structure analogous to the external limiting membrane. The lumen contains hyaluronidase-resistant acid mucopolysaccharide and filamentous cytoplasmic projections from the surrounding cells (Ts'o et al., 1969). Cells exhibiting even more definite ultrastructural characteristics of photoreceptor differentiation have been recently described by Ts'o et al. (1970a). In 6 per cent of 300 retinoblastomas these authors found small areas of cells with abundant cytoplasm, extensive intercellular matrix into which cytoplasmic processes from tumor cells extended, and uniform mildly hyperchromatic nuclei. Clusters of these cells form "fleurettes" of photoreceptor elements (Figs. 33–15 to 33–17).

Dissemination of retinoblastoma occurs via several routes. Within the globe loosely cohesive cells and nodules of tumor may be exfoliated into the vitreous (Figs. 33–18 and 33–19), onto the adjacent retinal surface, or even into the anterior chamber

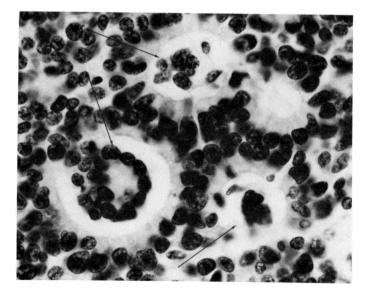

Figure 33–14 Flexner-Wintersteiner rosettes. Occasionally tumor cells are located within the rosette lumen (arrows). (Hematoxylin and eosin, ×750.) (E.P. #6672)

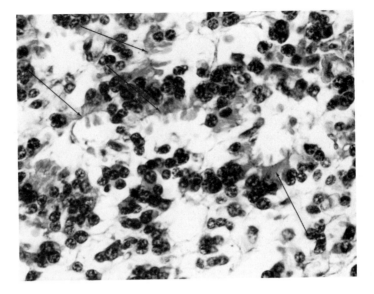

Figure 33–15 Field with numerous retinoblastoma fleurettes (arrows). (Hematoxylin and eosin, ×520.) (E.P. #17882)

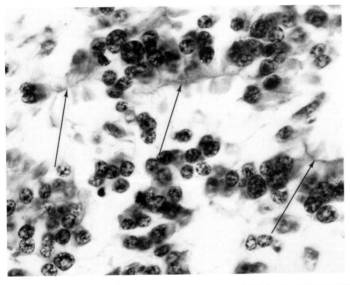

Figure 33–16 Retinoblastoma fleurettes with prominent external limiting membrane-like structure (arrows). (Hematoxylin and eosin, ×800.) (E.P. #17882)

Figure 33–17 Cystic space lined with numerous fleurette-like configurations. (Hematoxylin and eosin, ×450.) (E.P. #17882)

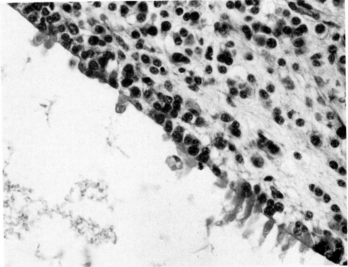

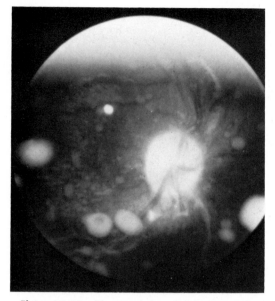

Figure 33–18 Characteristic ophthalmoscopic appearance of retinoblastoma with seeding into the vitreous. (Courtesy of Dr. Morton F. Goldberg.)

(Figs. 33–11 and 33–20) where they may clinically simulate inflammatory cells. The most common route of extraocular extension is along the optic nerve, whereby the tumor gains access to the subarachnoid space and intracranial cavity (Figs. 33–21 to 33–23). Choroidal invasion (Fig. 33–24) provides access to a rich vascular network which serves as a potential route for distant metastases. Finally, in advanced cases

direct extension through the sclera into the orbit may occur (Fig. 33–25).

Approximately 50 per cent of retinoblastoma deaths result from intracranial extension and cerebral involvement, 40 per cent from distant metastasis (bone marrow, liver, and lymph nodes are the most common sites, lung metastases are rare), and 10 per cent from local pharyngeal or tracheal obstruction by massive orbital tumor enlargement (Reese, 1963).

Heredity

Physicians have recorded various details of the hereditary nature of retinoblastoma for over 150 years (Dunphy, 1964). Although we have acquired sufficient understanding to provide guidelines for parents of affected children or for survivors of the malignant disease (see Genetic Counseling), investigation of this area is rendered difficult by the fact that no trait other than retinoblastoma is produced by the genetic alteration. The karyotype is usually normal, although several patients with mental retardation, retinoblastoma, and multiple congenital anomalies have been found to have partial deletion of the long arm of a D-group chromosome (Jensen and Miller, 1971). No clinical or laboratory tests enable us to detect genetic carriers of retinoblastoma at the present time. Brown's preliminary study (1966b) which suggested that urinary vanilmandelic acid and homovanillic acid excretion might be

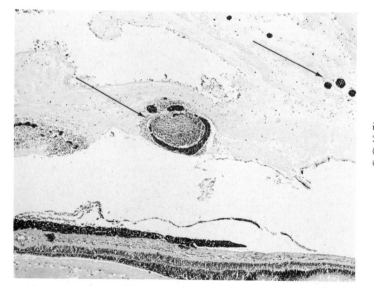

Figure 33–19 Retinoblastoma seedings in the vitreous (arrows). Eye from 2-year-old child with bilateral disease. (Hematoxylin and eosin, ×50.) (E.P. #23694)

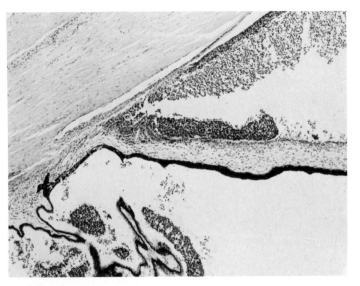

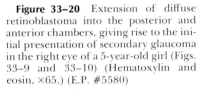

Figure 33–20 Extension of diffuse retinoblastoma into the posterior and anterior chambers, giving rise to the initial presentation of secondary glaucoma in the right eye of a 5-year-old girl (Figs. 33–9 and 33–10) (Hematoxylin and eosin, ×65.) (E.P. #5580)

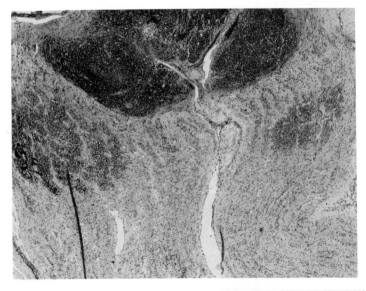

Figure 33–21 Characteristic extension of retinoblastoma into the optic nerve. (Hematoxylin and eosin, ×45.) (E.P. #19822)

Figure 33–22 Extension of retinoblastoma, via the optic nerve, into the subarachnoid space. Tumor is also beginning to invade the fibrovascular pial septa in the periphery of the nerve (arrows). (Hematoxylin and eosin, ×65.) (E.P. #20600)

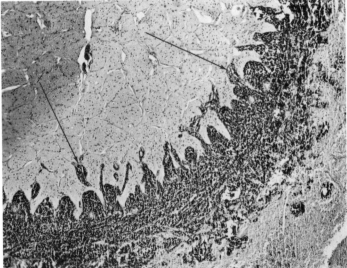

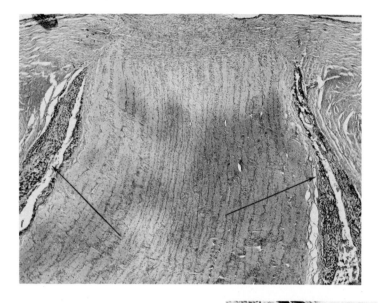

Figure 33–23 Death in this child was due to central nervous system extension via the optic nerve. Retinoblastoma had also extended down the opposite optic nerve (arrows). (Hematoxylin and eosin, ×35.) (E.P. #20600)

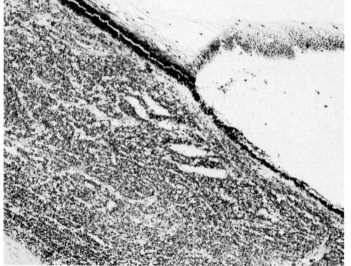

Figure 33–24 Extensive choroidal and ciliary body invasion by retinoblastoma (Hematoxylin and eosin, ×45.) (E.P. #36142)

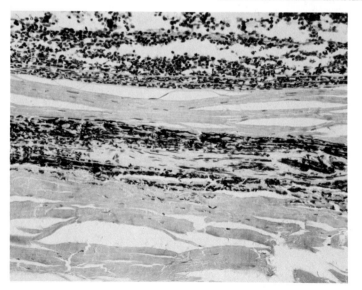

Figure 33–25 Intrascleral extension of retinoblastoma is more apt to be seen with very large tumors. (Hematoxylin and eosin, ×200.) (E.P. #36142)

increased in children with retinoblastoma has not been investigated further (Ellsworth, 1969).

Approximately 6 per cent of retinoblastoma cases are familial, and the mode of inheritance in these cases is that of an autosomal dominant trait. The degree of penetrance (frequency with which the gene becomes manifest in individuals carrying it) varies from 20 to 95 per cent among different reported pedigrees (Ellsworth, 1969; Macklin, 1959), but is most frequently stated to be about 80 per cent (François and Matton-Van Leuven, 1964). This 6 per cent proportion of familial cases should be regarded as a low approximation, since (1) more intensive investigation of families with negative family histories (*sporadic cases*) has revealed affected collateral descendants in 10.5 per cent of cases (Macklin, 1959), (2) long periods of observation of siblings are necessary to exclude familial occurrence after detection of the first case in a family, and (3) exercise of voluntary birth control after one child with retinoblastoma lowers the proportion of detectable familial cases.

In spite of these sources of error, all authorities agree that the great majority of retinoblastoma cases (over 90 per cent) are of the sporadic variety. A number of theories have been proposed to explain the existence of two genetically distinct categories of phenotypically similar patients. The supposition that hereditary cases result from germinal mutations whereas sporadic cases represent somatic mutations is probably incorrect. Follow-up studies of the offspring of "sporadic" unilateral retinoblastoma survivors indicate that from the practical viewpoint of early detection and genetic counseling, sporadic cases should be regarded as germinal mutations with low penetrance in unilateral cases and high penetrance in bilateral cases (Ellsworth, 1969). Although familial and sporadic retinoblastoma are clinically identical in many respects, an important difference is the dissimilar proportion of bilateral tumors in the two categories. The proportion of bilateral retinoblastoma patients is over twice as high among familial cases as among sporadic cases (Table 33–1). Conversely, 50 per cent of offspring of bilateral "sporadic" retinoblastoma survivors develop retinoblastoma, indicating that these

TABLE 33–1   BILATERALITY IN RETINOBLASTOMA

Clinical Category of Patient	Probability of Bilateral Tumor (%)
Sporadic case	18 to 31
Hereditary case	
Parent affected	92 to 95
2 or more siblings affected	83
Distant relative affected	60

After Ellsworth, R. M.: The practical management of retinoblastoma. Trans. Amer. Ophthal. Soc., 67:462, 1969; and François, S., et al.: Recent data on the heredity of retinoblastoma. *In* Boniuk, M. (Ed.): Ocular and Adnexal Tumors; New and Controversial Aspects. St. Louis, The C. V. Mosby Co., 1964, p. 123.

"sporadic" cases are indeed the result of germinal mutations with nearly 100 per cent subsequent penetrance (Ellsworth, 1969).

Genetic Counseling

The probability that *normal parents with 1 affected child* and no prior family history will produce more offspring with retinoblastoma is between 4 and 7 per cent (Ellsworth, 1969; François and Matton-Van Leuven, 1964). The probability of their producing offspring with the carrier state is unknown, since we are unable to identify carriers at present. *Normal parents with 2 or more affected children* will transmit the genetic basis for retinoblastoma to 50 per cent of their children; the proportion of children developing retinoblastoma will be determined by the degree of penetrance in that particular family. Similarly, a *retinoblastoma survivor with established hereditary occurrence* will produce 50 per cent genetically affected offspring. A *survivor of bilateral "sporadic" retinoblastoma* will produce clinically affected offspring in 50 per cent of cases (Ellsworth, 1969). Finally, 10 per cent of *survivors of unilateral sporadic retinoblastoma* produce clinically affected children (Ellsworth, 1969; Nielsen and Goldschmidt, 1968).

Diagnosis

The variety and relative frequencies of initial signs and symptoms in a series of 900 cases of retinoblastoma from the Columbia-Presbyterian Medical Center have

TABLE 32–2 PRESENTING SIGNS OR SYMPTOMS IN RETINOBLASTOMA

Sign or Symptom	Percentages
White reflex or "cat's eye reflex"	56.0
Strabismus	20.0
Esotropia	11.0
Exotropia	9.0
Red, painful eye with glaucoma	7.0
Poor vision	5.0
Routine examination	3.0
Orbital cellulitis	3.0
Unilateral mydriasis	2.0
Heterochromia iridis	1.0
Hyphema	1.0
"Strange facial expression"	0.5
Nystagmus	0.5
White spots on iris	0.5
Anorexia, failure to thrive	0.5

From Ellsworth, R. M.: The practical management of retinoblastoma. Trans. Amer. Ophthal. Soc., *67*:462, 1969.

Figure 33–27 Red, painful, and glaucomatous right eye with yellowish-white reflex. This 3-year-old girl was brought to the clinic with a history of pain in the eye for three months. Examination of the enucleated globe disclosed choroidal and optic nerve invasion by retinoblastoma (E.P. #29104).

been tabulated by Ellsworth (Table 33–2). The initial symptom in the great majority of patients is the familiar white "cat's eye" reflex, usually first noted by the child's mother (Fig. 33–26 and 33–27). The relative frequencies of the numerous causes of *leukokoria* have been studied clinically by Howard and Ellsworth, and their data are recorded in Table 33–3. Most of these conditions are discussed in detail elsewhere in this volume, and Table 33–4 summarizes

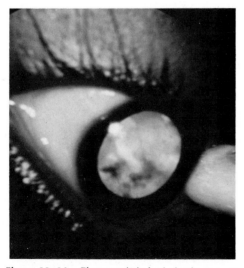

Figure 33–26 Characteristic leukokoria presentation of retinoblastoma in a 13-month-old child. (E.P. #31382)

some of the differential diagnostic features.

The second most frequent initial sign of retinoblastoma is *strabismus*. Exotropia and esotropia are about equally frequent and, together with poor vision, account for the presenting signs in 25 per cent of patients (Table 33–2). Every child with either poor vision or strabismus should receive an adequate fundus examination with mydriasis and, if necessary, under general anesthesia.

Although the remaining presenting signs or symptoms are found in less than 20 per cent of retinoblastoma patients, these are the ones which most frequently lead to misdiagnosis. In a review of 618 histologically proved retinoblastomas Stafford et al. found 92 cases (14.9 per cent) that were initially misdiagnosed. Less than 15 per cent of the misdiagnosed group were examples of "pseudoglioma" which had been followed as benign lesions. On the other hand, over 60 per cent of the misdiagnosed group were thought to represent some form of inflammation or glaucoma (Table 33–5). An average delay of 6.0 months between onset of symptoms and enucleation in the erroneously diagnosed group compared with an average delay of 0.1 month in the correctly diagnosed group. An example of delay in diagnosis because of the impression of ocular

TABLE 33–3 DIAGNOSIS IN 265 PATIENTS WITH LESIONS SIMULATING RETINOBLASTOMA

Diagnosis	Per Cent of Total
Persistent hyperplastic primary vitreous	19.0
Retrolental fibroplasia	13.5
Posterior cataract	13.5
Coloboma of choroid or disc	11.5
Uveitis	10.0
Nematode endophthalmitis	6.5
Congenital retinal fold	5.0
Coats' disease	4.0
Organizing vitreous hemorrhage	3.5
Retinal dysplasia	2.5
Tumor other than retinoblastoma	1.5
White-with-pressure sign	1.0
Juvenile xanthogranuloma	1.0
Retinoschisis	1.0
Tapetoretinal degeneration	1.0
Endophthalmitis	1.0
Persistent tunica vasculosa lentis	1.0
Miscellaneous (Incontinentia pigmenti; cyst in remnant of hyaloid artery; anomalous disc; hematoma under retinal pigment epithelium; myopic chorioretinal degeneration; medullated nerve fibers; traumatic choroiditis; anteriorly dislocated lens with secondary glaucoma; congenital corneal opacity)	<1.0 each

From Howard, G. M., and Ellsworth, R. M.: Differential diagnosis in retinoblastoma. A statistical survey of 500 children. I. Relative frequency of lesions which simulate retinoblastoma. Amer. J. Ophthal., *60*:610, 1965.

inflammation is illustrated in the case of a 14-month-old child treated for two months with two courses of antibiotics (Fig. 33–28). Examination of the fellow eye disclosed retinoblastoma (Fig. 33–29). The tumor depicted in Figures 33–2 and 33–3) masqueraded as an exudative retinal detachment, simulating angiomatosis retinae or Coats' disease closely enough to be treated as such with cryotherapy (Fig. 33–4). Failure to respond to treatment and the development of glaucoma led to enucleation and the correct diagnosis.

Prognosis

The temporal pattern of mortality due to *unilateral retinoblastoma* resembles that of other childhood solid tumors. Essentially all tumor deaths occur within the first two years. The mortality pattern of *bilateral retinoblastoma* is, however, quite different, and this difference should be borne in mind while evaluating published mortality data, which are generally based on 2- or 3-year survival rates. Less than two thirds of tumor deaths occur within 2 years in bilateral cases, and by the end of the third year 76 per cent of tumor deaths have occurred. The remaining 24 per cent of tumor-related deaths occur 5, 10, or even 20 years later (Table 33–6; Brown, 1966a).

Both clinical and histologic criteria have been found helpful in predicting the course of retinoblastoma. As noted in the previous section, the nature of presenting clinical signs or symptoms and the correctness of initial diagnosis may affect prognosis, though present data are inconclusive on these points. Except for the fact that bilateral and unilateral intraocular retinoblastoma have no different survival rates (Boniuk and Zimmerman, 1962a; Brown, 1966a), extent of disease at the time of diagnosis does affect prognosis. If distant metastases can be demonstrated, the disease is invariably fatal in spite of current methods of radio- and chemotherapy (Ellsworth, 1969). If orbital extension is clinically evident, hematogenous dissemination has already occurred in most cases. Ellsworth cites rare instances, however, in which no extraorbital tumor could be demonstrated and the prognosis for life was not so hopeless (see Treatment). In contrast to the situation with gliomas of the optic nerve, roentgenologic evidence of optic canal enlargement by retinoblastoma is virtually diagnostic of intracranial extension, and an orbital surgical approach in such a situation is of no value (Ellsworth, 1969). Extent of disease within the globe at the time of diagnosis also affects prognosis, and the categories which have been found useful in guiding therapy at the Columbia-Presbyterian Medical Center have been tabulated by Ellsworth (Tables 33–7 and 33–8).

The histologic features which provide clues to prognosis are (1) extent of optic nerve invasion, (3) scleral and epibulbar extension, and (4) degree of cytodifferentiation. Mortality data based on these criteria from the AFIP (McKenzie and

TABLE 33–4 LEUKOKORIA: SUMMARY OF DIFFERENTIAL DIAGNOSTIC FEATURES

	Retino-blastoma	Persistent Hyperplastic Primary Vitreous	Retrolental Fibroplasia	Uveitis	Nematode Endophthalmitis	Coats' Disease	Organizing Vitreous Hemorrhage	13–15 Trisomy	Juvenile Retinoschisis	Incontinentia Pigmenti	Norrie's Disease
Sex predilection	-	-	-	-	-	Male	-	-	Male	Female	Male
Familial	(+)	-	-	-	-	-	-	-	+	+	+
Age at onset	Infant	Congenital	Infant	Infant	Juvenile	Juvenile	Congenital (Infant)	Congenital	Congenital (Infant)	Congenital (Infant)	Congenital
Bilateral	(+)	-	+	(+)	-	(+)	-	(+)	+	(-)	+
Microphthalmos	-	+	(-)	-	-	-	-	+	-	(+)	-
Buphthalmos	(-)	(+)	-	-	-	-	-	(-)	-	(+)	(+)
Phthisis	(-)	(+)	(+)	(+)	(+)	-	(+)	-	-	(+)	+
Blindness	(+)	(+)	(+)	(-)	(+)	(+)	+	+	-	+	+
Shallow anterior chamber	-	+	+	-	-	-	-	+	-	+	+
Elongated ciliary processes	-	+	-	+	(-)	-	-	+	-	-	+
Anterior synechia	-	-	-	+	(+)	-	-	+	-	+	+
Posterior synechia	-	+	-	(-)	(-)	-	-	+	-	-	+
Cataract	(+)	(+)	+	(+)	-	+	(-)	(+)	-	+	+
Retinal detachment	+	+	+	(-)	+	+	(+)	(+)	+	+	+
Prematurity	-	-	+	-	-	-	-	-	-	-	-
Systemic abnormalities	-	-	-	-	-	-	-	+	-	+	+

Key:
    + = frequent
    (+) = occasional
    (-) = infrequent
    - = absent or rare

After Warburg, M.: Norrie's disease; a congenital progressive oculo-acoustico-cerebral degeneration. Acta Ophthal. Suppl. 89, 1966.

TABLE 33–5 INITIAL MISDIAGNOSES IN PROVEN CASES OF RETINOBLASTOMA

Erroneous Diagnosis	Number of Cases
Inflammation	
Panophthalmitis	18
Endophthalmitis	14
Uveitis	6
Unspecified	3
Glaucoma	16
Pseudoglioma	13
Blind eye	7
Retinal detachment	5
Retrolental fibroplasia	4
Cataract	3
Trauma	1
Phthisis bulbi	1
von Hippel's disease	1
Total	92

From Stafford, W. R., et al.: Retinoblastomas initially misdiagnosed as primary ocular inflammations. Arch. Ophthal., *82*:771, 1969. Copyright 1969, American Medical Association.

Zimmerman, 1964) and Columbia-Presbyterian Medical Center (Brown, 1966a) are summarized in Table 33–9. The mortality rate among patients with retinoblastoma exhibiting fleurette photoreceptor differentiation is approximately the same as that among children with tumors containing numerous Flexner-Wintersteiner rosettes (T'so et al., 1970b).

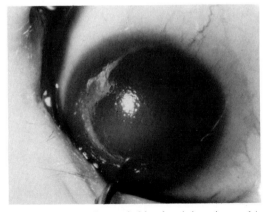

Figure 33–28 Corneal blood-staining in a 14-month-old child who was initially thought to have endophthalmitis in the right eye. No improvement occurred after treatment with systemic antibiotics over a two-month period. Examination under anesthesia disclosed this opaque right cornea and tumor anterior to the equator in the left eye (Fig. 33–29). Retinoblastoma was confirmed by histopathologic study of the right eye (E.P. #35661).

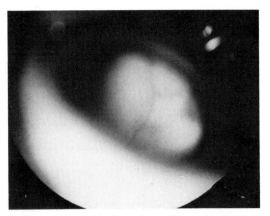

Figure 33–29 Single nodule of retinoblastoma in periphery of left eye of case illustrated in Fig. 33–28 (E.P. #35661).

Treatment

UNILATERAL CASES (Bedford et al., 1971; Ellsworth, 1969). The curative value of early *enucleation* with particular attention to excision of a long optic nerve segment has been the cornerstone of our therapeutic approach to retinoblastoma for over a century. In patients with large unilateral tumors (Groups IV and V, Table 33–7) and no family history of retinoblastoma, prompt enucleation is the treatment of choice. Two groups of patients with unilateral lesions are now being diagnosed at an early enough stage (Groups I to III, Table 33–7) to permit primary treatment with radiotherapy rather than enucleation. These are (1) children with small macular lesions who are brought to medical attention early for evaluation of strabismus or

TABLE 33–6 CUMULATIVE FOLLOW-UP: TIME IN YEARS FROM ENUCLEATION TO FOLLOW-UP

Years	Unilateral		Bilateral	
	Alive	Dead	Alive	Dead
2	59	18	109	27
3	51	18	90	32
5	34	18	68	34
10	18	18	26	38
20			2	41
25			0	42

From Brown, D. H.: The clinicopathology of retinoblastoma. Amer. J. Ophthal., *61*:508, 1966.

TABLE 33–7 PROGNOSIS BASED ON INTRAOCULAR EXTENT OF TUMOR

GROUP I — Very favorable
  a. Solitary tumor, less than 4 disc diameters in size, at or behind the equator;
  b. Multiple tumors, none over 4 disc diameters in size, all at or behind the equator.
GROUP II — Favorable
  a. Solitary tumor, 4 to 10 disc diameters in size, at or behind the equator;
  b. Multiple tumors, 4 to 10 disc diameters in size, behind the equator.
GROUP III — Doubtful
  a. Any lesion anterior to the equator;
  b. Solitary tumors larger than 10 disc diameters behind the equator.
GROUP IV — Unfavorable
  a. Multiple tumors, some larger than 10 disc diameters;
  b. Any lesion extending anterior to the ora serrata.
GROUP V — Very unfavorable
  a. Massive tumors involving over half the retina;
  b. Vitreous seeding.

From Ellsworth, R. M.: The practical management of retinoblastoma. Trans. Amer. Ophthal. Soc., 67: 462, 1969.

poor vision and (2) relatives of retinoblastoma patients whose tumors are detected on routine ophthalmoscopic check. In both these groups external irradiation

TABLE 33–8 3-YEAR CURE RATE BASED ON PROGNOSTIC CATEGORIES IN TABLE 33–7. "CURE-RATE" ENCOMPASSES BOTH PATIENT SURVIVAL AND ERADICATION OF TUMORS NOT TREATED BY ENUCLEATION

	Number of Cases	Cure Rate (%)
GROUP I	20	95
GROUP II	32	87
GROUP III	24	67
GROUP IV	32	69
GROUP V	74	34
ORBIT	10	30

From Ellsworth, R. M.: The practical management of retinoblastoma. Trans. Amer. Ophthal. Soc., 67:462, 1969.

(total dose 3500 R supervoltage, temporal port, over 3 weeks) may be later supplemented by cryotherapy or photocoagulation if necessary. If viable tumor persists nonetheless, the eye should be removed. The ocular complication rate of a second course of external radiotherapy is so high that only about 15 per cent of eyes will retain useful vision. The added risk of radiation-induced malignant disease (see later discussion) is a second argument against a

TABLE 33–9 PROGNOSIS BASED ON HISTOLOGIC CRITERIA

Histologic Criteria		Per Cent Mortality	
		AFIP* (300 Cases)	Columbia-Presbyterian (204 Cases)†
Invasion of Optic Nerve	None	8	28
	To lamina cribrosa	15	16
	Beyond lamina cribrosa, within limits of transection	44	63
	Beyond line of surgical transection	64	82
Invasion of Choroid	None	—	36
	Slight	25	—
	Massive	65	60
Scleral Extension	Absent	—	34
	Present	—	75
Epibulbar Extension	Absent	—	34
	Present	—	70
Degree of Cytodifferentiation	Many Flexner-Wintersteiner rosettes	—	17
	Undifferentiated	—	50

*Armed Forces Institute of Pathology.
†Combines unilateral and bilateral mortality data.

repeated course of irradiation in such cases.

An alternative mode of external irradiation using a direct anterior field has been employed with good results in England and is recommended for large tumors, vitreous seeding, and tumors located near the optic disc (Bedford et al., 1971). These same authors have employed focal modes of treatment (cobalt plaque, photocoagulation, or cryotherapy) as the initial modality in 63 eyes with Group I to III tumors and compared these results with those from a group of 58 eyes treated by whole-eye irradiation (prognostic groups not specified). The recurrence rate was similar in the two groups (46 per cent whole-eye, 42.8 per cent focal) and new primary tumors arose after treatment in 8 per cent of the external irradiation group versus 20 per cent of the focally treated group. All but one of the new primary tumors in the latter group were eradicated with further focal therapy. We are not yet certain whether the obvious ocular dividends of more conservative retinoblastoma therapy will be counterbalanced by an increased mortality risk, and several years must elapse before this uncertainty can be statistically resolved.

BILATERAL CASES (Bedford et al., 1971 Ellsworth, 1969). The majority of bilateral cases are detected at a stage when tumor involvement in one eye is much more advanced than in the other. In such asymmetrical cases, the preferred mode of ·therapy is enucleation of the more involved eye with supervoltage radiotherapy directed to the second eye, with or without chemotherapy. Though several chemotherapeutic agents have been shown effective against retinoblastoma, the one with which most experience has accumulated is *triethylenemelamine* (TEM) administered intramuscularly or by carotid perfusion. Chemotherapy alone is not effective in eradicating retinoblastoma, but it is regarded by Ellsworth as a valuable curative adjuvant to radiotherapy for advanced intraocular cases, orbital recurrences, or residual tumor at the line of surgical transection. The adverse hematologic effects and equivocal benefit in Group I to III cases prompted Ellsworth to suggest that in treatment of intraocular tumor, radiotherapy should be supplemented by TEM

in only Group IV and V cases. In contrast, Bedford et al. have deleted chemotherapy from their attack on retinoblastoma "with no apparent adverse influence on subsequent results." Heyn has recently summarized the available alternative chemotherapeutic regimens for metastatic disease, although all are at present only palliative.

The fortunately rare patients with *bilateral symmetrical* tumors which are advanced (Groups IV and V) are probably best managed by large total tumor doses of external irradiation (e.g., 4500 R supervoltage) to both orbits with concomitant chemotherapy. If response in one of the eyes is good enough to indicate that useful vision might be preserved with supplementary cryotherapy or photocoagulation, the risk to life of retaining the globe would seem justified. If however, tumor regression in neither eye is sufficient to expect salvage of visual function, both eyes should be enucleated. Bilateral symmetrical cases in which small tumor masses are more favorably situated (Groups I to III) may be managed with initial external irradiation and subsequent local treatment if needed.

Several approaches to the treatment of localized areas of residual or new tumor growth have proved effective. Cryotherapy, photocoagulation, radon seed implantation, and cobalt-60 application have all been used with success. The indications and limitations of these modalities are discussed by Ellsworth, Lincoff et al., Stallard, Höpping and Meyer-Schwickerath, and Bedford et al.

RADIATION-INDUCED NEOPLASMS (Forrest, 1962; Soloway, 1966). Enough children treated with radiotherapy now survive retinoblastoma to develop new malignant disease in irradiated tissue as the ironic result of the very treatment which may have been responsible for their survival. Although most of the reported patients were treated with high total doses (8,000 to 16,000 R), 2 of the 25 patients reviewed by Soloway had received a total dose of less than 3,000 R. The latent period between radiotherapy and appearance of secondary tumors ranges from 4 to 30 years. Fifty-two per cent of secondary tumors appear by the tenth postirradiation year. Because the great majority of radiation-induced tumors are sarcomas (Table

TABLE 33–10 HISTOLOGIC CLASSIFICATION OF RADIATION-INDUCED NEOPLASMS FOLLOWING THERAPY FOR RETINOBLASTOMA

Type	Number of Cases
Mesenchymal	
Osteogenic sarcoma	9
Fibrosarcoma	6
Chondrosarcoma	1
Rhabdomyosarcoma	1
Malignant mesenchymoma	2
Sarcoma, not otherwise specified	2
Fibromatosis	1
Epithelial	
Squamous cell carcinoma	1
Basal cell carcinoma	1
Carcinoma, not otherwise specified	1
Total	25

From Soloway, H. B.: Radiation-induced neoplasms following curative therapy for retinoblastoma. Cancer, 19:1984, 1966.

33–10), and because they arise in such close proximity to deep structures of the face and skull, their prognosis is exceptionally poor. Parenthetically, recent epidemiologic evidence suggests that children with retinoblastoma may have an increased risk of developing a second primary malignant condition which is unrelated to prior irradiation (Jensen and Miller, 1971).

Congenital Neuroepithelial Tumors of the Ciliary Body

These rare congenital tumors usually arise from nonpigmented ciliary epithelium and are composed primarily of tissue which resembles primitive embryonal retina prior to differentiation of inner and outer neuroblastic layers (6th week).

The extreme variability of cell type and arrangement which characterizes these tumors may be explained in part by the pluripotential nature of the embryonic medullary epithelium from which they are derived. Differentiation of the medullary epithelium which forms the inner layer of the optic cup eventually produces retinal photoreceptor, glial, and neuronal elements; nonpigmented ciliary epithelium; pigment epithelium of the iris; dilator and sphincter muscles of the iris; and perhaps some of the cellular constituents of the vitreous; in birds the striated muscle of the iris is also derived from this tissue (Zimmerman, 1971).

Zimmerman's classification of congenital tumors of the ciliary body is outlined in Table 33–11. "*Diktyoma,*" a term derived from the histologic appearance of these tumors, is not employed in this classification, but the tumors referred to as diktyomas by other authors would be placed in either the medulloepithelioma or teratoid medulloepithelioma category. The term "embryonal medulloepithelioma," used synonymously with "diktyoma" by others, is regarded by Zimmerman as redundant and is not employed in his classification.

Only two tumors with histologic features which require separation into the *glioneuroma* category have been observed, and the details of these cases may be found in Zimmerman's review.

The basic histologic features of *benign medulloepithelioma* are illustrated in Figure 33–30.

Thin sheets of closely packed tumor cells are folded and rolled to form in cross section a distinctive pattern of juxtaposed membranes, clefts, tubules, and rosettes separated by variable amounts of loose myxoid connective tissue. The usual polarity of cells constituting the sheets suggests that the central lumen, lined by a delicate membrane, is analogous to the cavity of the optic vesicle, whereas the surrounding loose connective tissue is analogous to the primary vitreous (Andersen, 1971). This polarity may be reversed, however, with the luminal tissue instead analo-

TABLE 33–11 CONGENITAL NEUROEPITHELIAL TUMORS OF THE CILIARY BODY

Glioneuroma
Medulloepithelioma
Benign
Malignant
Teratoid medulloepithelioma
Benign
Malignant

From Zimmerman, L. E.: Verhoeff's "teratoneuroma": A critical reappraisal in light of new observations and current concepts of embryonic tumors. Amer. J. Ophthal., 72:1039, 1971.

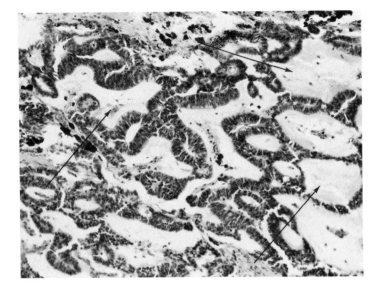

Figure 33–30 Interlacing sheets of medullary epithelium constitute the basic histopathologic feature of benign medulloepithelioma. The cystic cavities (arrows) formed by the neuroepithelium contain a material which is rich in hyaluronidase-sensitive acid mucopolysaccharide. (Colloidal iron, ×160.) (E.P. #34506)

gous to primary vitreous. Other areas of tumor resemble ciliary epithelium rather than embryonic retina, and most tumors contain areas of glial differentiation. Areas of *heteroplastic differentiation* into cell types not found in the normal eye are often identified in addition to the basic medulloepithelioma elements which are analogous to embryonic medullary epithelium, retina, or ciliary body. The presence of such heteroplastic elements—brain tissue (Figs. 33–31 to 33–32), cartilage (Fig. 33–33), or striated muscle—constitutes the criterion for histologic separation of the *tera-toid medulloepithel oma* category. Both medulloepithelioma and teratoid medulloepithelioma may exhibit histologic evidence of malignancy (nuclear pleomorphism; numerous mitoses; areas of densely packed, small undifferentiated cells resembling retinoblastoma; extensive destruction of the internal architecture of the globe). Extension into the orbit, adjacent sinuses, or cranial cavity may occur in the malignant types, and metastasis to cervical lymph nodes has been observed (Zimmerman, 1971). An ultrastructural study of one medulloepithelioma has confirmed

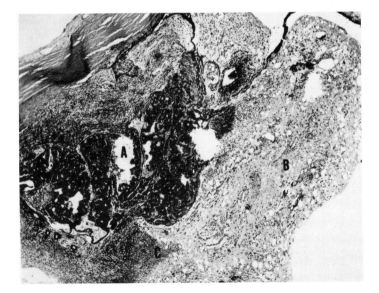

Figure 33–31 Teratoid medulloepithelioma of the ciliary body presented as a white mass (Fig. 33–37) invading the iris and angle in the right eye of a 4½-year-old boy. This tumor has three distinct zones: (*A*) sheets and cords of embryonal medullary type epithelium, (*B*) brainlike tissue with large ganglion cells, and (*C*) a zone of small cells. (Hematoxylin and eosin, ×3.) (E.P. #20059)

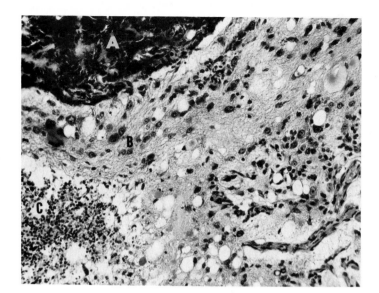

Figure 33–32 Higher power to illustrate the three different areas noted in Figure 33–31 (E.P. #20059).

the existence of cellular elements similar to embryonal retina. No areas of more definite photoreceptor differentiation were identified (Iwamoto et al., 1967).

Clinical Features

The average age at the time of enucleation was 4½ years in Andersen's series of 17 benign medulloepitheliomas, 7 years in his 6 patients with malignant medulloepithelioma, and under 4 years in Reese's series of 13 cases (Reese, 1963). The age of detection ranges from birth through the first decade. The tumor is invariably unilateral, and the presenting signs are generally (1) visible iris tumor (Figs. 33–34 to 33–36) or gross displacement of the iris, (2) signs of secondary glaucoma, (3) a white pupillary reflex (Fig. 33–37), and, rarely, (4) reduced visual acuity or strabismus. The eye harboring a medulloepithelioma may be somewhat microphthalmic, but the fellow eye is completely normal. The tumor arises from the region of ciliary body, but the presenting signs are usually produced by proliferation of cystic or membranous structures over the pupillary margin, behind the lens, or over the anterior iris surface, eventually occupying most of the anterior chamber.

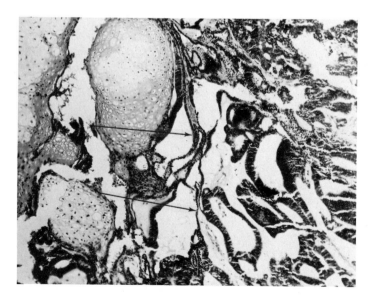

Figure 33–33 Heteroplastic differentiation into cartilage in a teratoid medulloepithelioma. The embryonal epithelium is continuous with adult-type nonpigmented ciliary epithelium in some areas (arrows). (Hematoxylin and eosin, ×100.) (E.P. #34506)

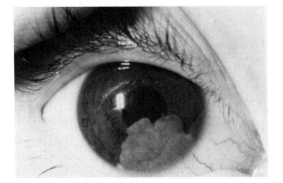

Figure 33–34 This illustrates iris displacement by a medulloepithelioma of the ciliary body in another 4½-year-old child. The initial clinical impression was juvenile xanthogranuloma. Excision of the iris lesion disclosed a medulloepithelioma. Two weeks after this excision, extensive seeding of the vitreous was observed and the eye was enucleated. (Case of Dr. D. E. LaMarche and Dr. P. Horowitz.) (E.P. #32182)

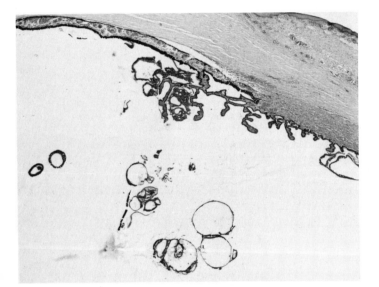

Figure 33–35 Cystic medulloepithelioma with marked seeding into the posterior chamber and vitreous. (Hematoxylin and eosin, ×24.) (E.P. #32182)

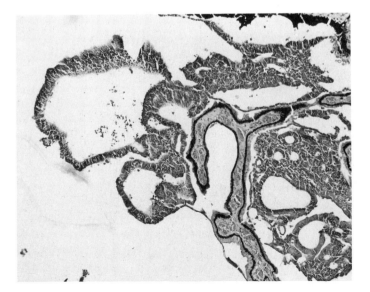

Figure 33–36 Cystic medulloepithelioma in direct continuity with non-pigmented ciliary epithelium. (Hematoxylin and eosin, ×105.) (E.P. #32182)

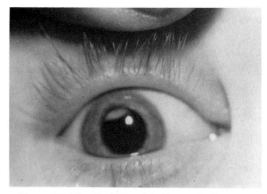

Figure 33-37 Medulloepithelioma of ciliary body presenting as a whitish mass behind the iris and pupil. Lens was tilted posteriorly. The correct clinical diagnosis was made preoperatively. (From Iliff, C. E., and Ossofsky, H. J., Tumors of the Eye and Adnexa in Infancy and Childhood, 1962. Courtesy of Charles C Thomas, Publisher, Springfield, Illinois.) (E.P. #20059)

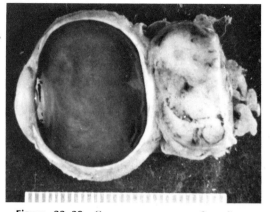

Figure 33-39 Gross appearance of malignant teratoid medulloepithelioma after coronal and vertical sectioning. (E.P. #34506)

Although the most common site of origin of medulloepithelioma is the ciliary body, these tumors may also arise in the retina and optic nerve (Andersen, 1971; Green et al., 1972; Reese, 1957). We have recently observed a malignant teratoid medulloepithelioma of the optic nerve (Figs. 33-38 to 33-40). This 6-year-old girl had a blind, painful, and slightly proptotic right eye when she was first examined. The clinical impression was orbital tumor, possibly a glioma of the optic nerve. She is alive and well two years after orbital exenteration.

Differential Diagnosis

Retinoblastoma is frequently bilateral and multicentric, occurs in normal-size eyes, and may contain areas of calcification on x ray examination. No hereditary cases of medulloepithelioma have been reported. Juvenile xanthogranuloma usually occurs earlier in infancy, rarely exhibits a cystic appearance, and is frequently multicentric, with individual tumors having a fleshy, vascularized appearance. Persistent hyperplastic primary vitreous may closely simulate medulloepithelioma, and this neoplasm should be considered a diagnostic possibility in any child with the clinical diagnosis of persistent hyperplastic primary vitreous, unilateral buphthalmos, anteriorly dislocated lens, or multiple cysts in the anterior chamber (Reese, 1963).

Prognosis and Treatment

If *enucleation* is performed before the tumor has extended into the orbit, the prognosis is excellent. Malignant medulloepitheliomas usually do not metastasize, but tumor deaths may occur as a result of intracranial extension

Malignant Melanomas

Although uveal melanomas are rare in childhood, examples have been recorded at all ages, including the newborn (Chaves and Granville, 1972; Greer, 1966). Generally, however, the frequency of these tumors remains low until puberty, and begins to increase thereafter (Table 33-12). Although some endocrine depend-

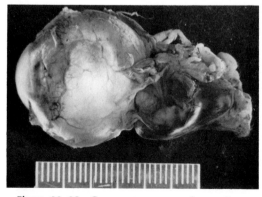

Figure 33-38 Gross appearance of a malignant teratoid medulloepithelioma of optic nerve. The tumor had extended into the optic nerve head, broken through the meninges, and invaded the orbit. (E.P. #34506)

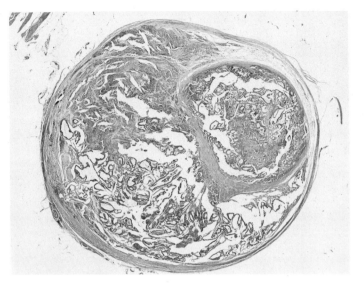

Figure 33–40 Cross-section of proximal end of orbital optic nerve illustrating the characteristic "netlike" appearance of medulloepithelioma. (E.P. #34506)

ence is suggested by this observation, Apt's analysis of 46 uveal melanomas in patients under 20 years of age from the AFIP documents a biological similarity of the prepubertal tumors to their adult counterparts. For example, the proportion of tumor deaths was the same for prepubertal as for pubertal and postpubertal patients. As in the adult, the prognosis was more dependent upon tumor location—iris or posterior uvea—and, among the ciliary body and choroidal tumors, upon the histopathologic appearance. Conditions associated with an increased frequency of uveal melanoma include melanosis oculi (Table 33–20), and possibly oculodermal melanosis (Table 33–20) and neurofibromatosis (p. 1035).

TABLE 33–12 UVEAL MELANOMAS IN CHILDREN AND ADOLESCENTS

Age of Patients (Years)	Location of Tumor	
	Iris (Number of Cases)	Ciliary Body and Choroid (Number of Cases)
0 to 4	2	0
5 to 9	3	5
10 to 14	3	5
15 to 19	11	17
Total	19	27

After Apt, L.: Uveal melanomas in children and adolescents. Int. Ophthal. Clin., 2:403, 1962.

IRIS MELANOMAS*

Iris tumors constitute 41 per cent of uveal melanomas in Apt's series, whereas in adults only 6 to 8 per cent of tumors occur in the iris (Rones and Zimmerman, 1958). Darkening or growth of a pre-existing pigmented iris lesion is the commonest initial clinical sign, although the presence of an iris tumor may also be heralded by heterochromia, glaucoma, distortion of the pupil, or spontaneous hyphema. An illustrative case is that of a 10-year-old patient referred to Dr. C. E. Iliff for evaluation of bilateral congenital ptosis. During the course of the examination, Dr. Iliff noted an extensive iris melanoma superiorly which extended into the chamber angle and a smaller tumor deposit inferiorly (Fig 33–41). Cytopathologic examination of a paracentesis specimen revealed spindle-shaped cells which were consistent with a diagnosis of amelanotic malignant melanoma. The eye was enucleated and a malignant melanoma, mixed cell type, was found arising from the ciliary body temporally with extension into and over the iris both temporally and inferonasally (Figs. 33–42 to 33–44). The patient has remained free of tumor for 13 years.

The prognosis for life is generally good with iris tumors, and histologic classification of these lesions by Callender's criteria

*See Apt, 1962; Lerner, 1970; Verdaguer, 1965.

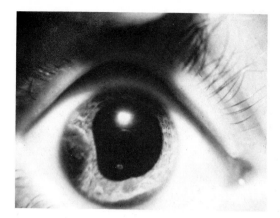

Figure 33–41   Ten-year-old child with malignant melanoma of ciliary body displacing iris in the infero-temporal quadrant. (E.P. #24598)

Figure 33–42 Sections of the temporal area of tumor demonstrating that most of the lesion is in the ciliary body. (Hematoxylin and eosin, ×35.) (E.P. #24598)

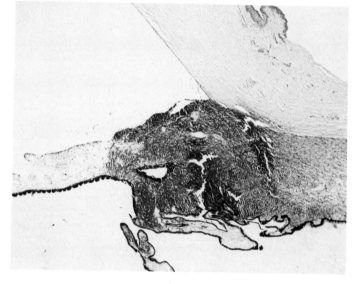

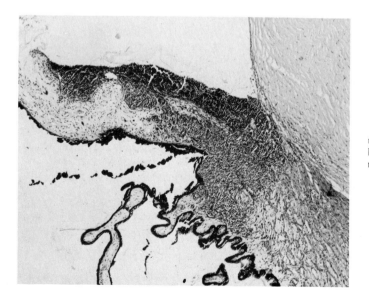

Figure 33–43 Melanoma involves anterior aspect of ciliary body, as well as base and anterior surface of iris. (Hematoxylin and eosin, ×35.) (E.P. #24598)

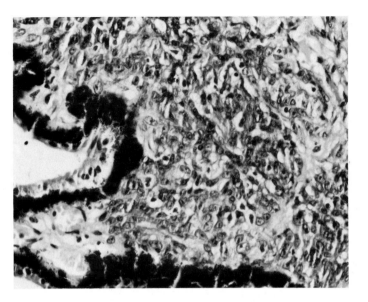

Figure 33–44 Malignant melanoma of ciliary body, mixed cell type. Same case is illustrated in Figures 33–41 to 33–43. (Hematoxylin and eosin, ×390.) (E.P. #24598)

has less prognostic value. Iris melanomas can be classified histopathologically into two groups: those that are composed of spindle-shaped cells which are tightly packed and cohesive (Fig 33–45), and those that are less spindle-shaped, loosely packed, and discohesive (Fig 33–46). Shedding of tumor cells in the discohesive group is more apt to lead to intraocular spread and secondary glaucoma.

Five-year follow-up information was available for 13 of the patients with iris melanoma in Apt's series. Twelve showed no signs of tumor recurrence or metas-

tasis, and one died with metastatic melanoma six years after enucleation.

The iris lesion in Figure 33–47 was present in a 13-year-old girl who was a patient of Dr. Howard Naquin for 17 years thereafter. The lesion was removed by a sector iridectomy and histopathologic examination disclosed a relatively cohesive malignant melanoma (Fig. 33–48). Five years later a pigmented spot was noted beneath the conjunctiva, a few millimeters posterior to the incision site (Fig. 33–49). This lesion enlarged slightly over a period of three years (Fig 33–50) and was ex-

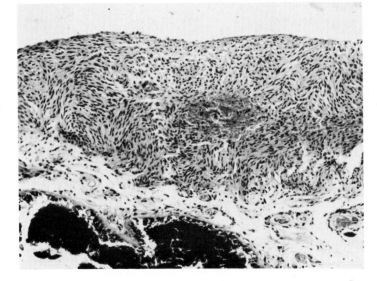

Figure 33–45 Cohesive type of malignant melanoma of the iris. (Hematoxylin and eosin, ×150.) (E.P. #16815)

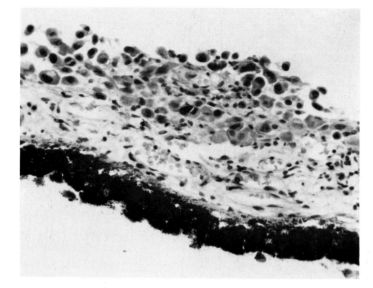

Figure 33–46 Discohesive type of iris melanoma (Hematoxylin and eosin, ×310.) (E.P. #24515)

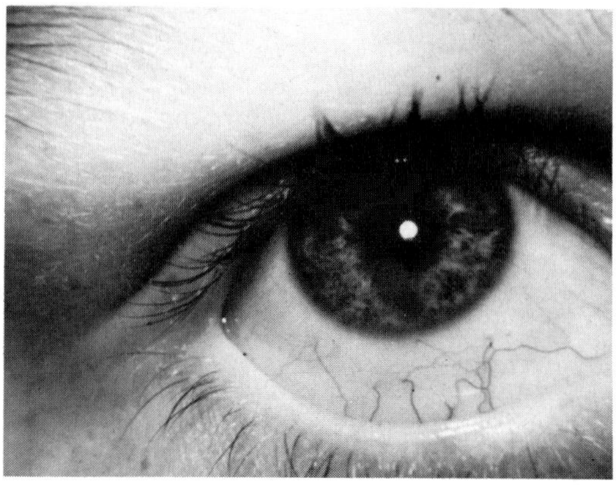

Figure 33–47 Iris melanoma in a 13-year-old girl. (Courtesy of Dr. Richard L. Wolfe.) (E.P. #16815)

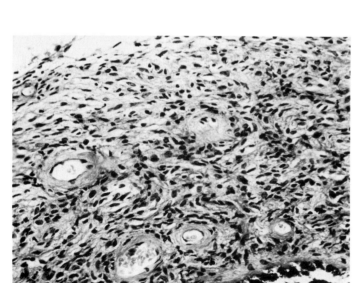

Figure 33–48 Moderately cohesive malignant melanoma of iris clinically illustrated in Fig. 33–47. (Hematoxylin and eosin, ×280.) (E.P. #16815)

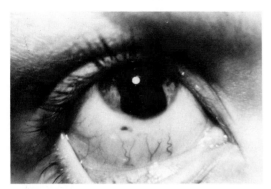

Figure 33–49 Pigmented subconjunctival lesion which appeared 8 years after removal of iris melanoma shown in Figures 33–47 and 33–48. (E.P. #16815)

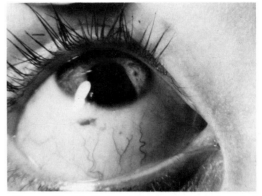

Figure 33–50 Enlargement of subconjunctival pigmented lesion in Figure 33–49 after 5 years' observation. (E.P. #16815)

cised. Histopathologic examination disclosed a malignant melanoma similar to the original iris lesion (Fig 33–51). There was no continuity with the old scar, and this possibly represents seeding at the time of the original surgery. The patient has remained free of tumor for the past nine years.

The principles which have evolved for evaluation and treatment of pigmented iris lesions in adults would seem applicable to children. Serial photographs and gonioscopic examinations are frequently the only means by which definite enlargement of suspicious lesions may be documented. Enlarging lesions localized to one sector of iris should be excised by iridectomy or, with more basally located lesions, by irido-

cyclectomy or corneoscleroiridocyclectomy with graft (Reese et al., 1968; Vail, 1971). Enucleation is indicated when the tumor (1) recurs after more conservative surgery; (2) is too large for excision; or (3) exhibits a diffuse, flat growth pattern or a ring type of growth (Reese et al., 1968).

MELANOMAS OF CILIARY BODY AND CHOROID*

Twenty-seven of the 46 uveal melanomas studied by Apt arose in the ciliary body or choroid. Initial clinical manifestations in this series included decreased visual acuity, field loss, glaucoma, signs of

---

*See Apt, 1962; Verdaguer, 1965.

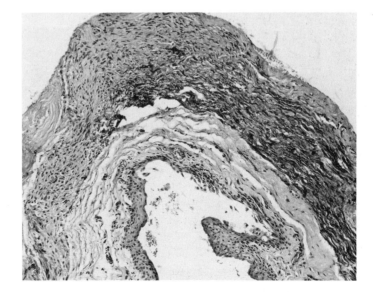

Figure 33–51 Histologic appearance of pigmented subconjunctival mass depicted in Figures 33–49 and 33–50. Moderately cohesive malignant malanoma similar to original iris tumor (Fig. 33–48). (Hematoxyl and eosin, ×135.) (E.P. #25017)

TABLE 33–13   CALLENDER CLASSIFICATION OF CHOROID AND CILIARY BODY MELANOMAS IN CHILDREN AND ADOLESCENTS

Callender Type	Number of Patients	Number of Tumor Deaths
Spindle A	4	0
Spindle B and Fascicular	9	1
Mixed and Necrotic	8	4
Epithelioid	6*	1

*One additional patient in this group had recurrent tumor 6 months after enucleation, but no further information is available.

After Apt, L.: Uveal melanomas in children and adolescents. Int. Ophthal. Clin., 2:403, 1962.

ocular inflammatory disease, pupillary abnormalities, retinal detachment, and one example of acquired esotropia. The subtle early signs of ciliary body melanoma, such as slowly increasing lenticular astigmatism, segmental prominence of episceral vessels, or mild hypotony which are so often missed in adults (Foos et al., 1969), may be virtually impossible to detect in children. Likewise, peripheral field defects associated with small choroidal melanomas will not be noticed even by older children, and medical attention will not be sought until an abnormal pupillary reflex, signs of ocular inflammation or diminished central acuity supervene. When a pigmented fundus lesion is detected at an earlier

stage, comparable to the usual case in adults, the ancillary diagnostic measures of fluorescein angiography (Gass, 1972; Pettit et al., 1970), radioactive phosphorus uptake (Hagler et al., 1970), or, more recently, radioactive chloroquine uptake (Walsh and Packer, 1971) may be of help in the differential diagnosis.

Apt's study confirmed in the pediatric age group the prognostic value of the Callender histologic classification of ciliary body and choroidal melanomas (Table 33–13). Figures 33–52 to 33–56 illustrate the major histologic categories in this classification details of which may be found in standard texts (Hogan and Zimmerman, 1962; Reese, 1963). The survival data recorded in Table 33–13 actually represent a minimum estimate of mortality, since follow-up observations are lacking in some cases or are of insufficient duration to exclude the possibility of later tumor recurrence or metastasis. As is the case with posterior uveal melanomas in adults, the asymptomatic interval between enucleation and the appearance of metastases may be as long as 20 years. Thus, 5-year survival figures are misleadingly optimistic in this group of tumors (Paul et al., 1962).

The generally accepted treatment of posterior uveal melanomas is enucleation. Although conservative treatment of smaller lesions by surface application of *gamma radiation* sources (Newman et al., 1970; Stallard, 1966), or *transcleral diather-*

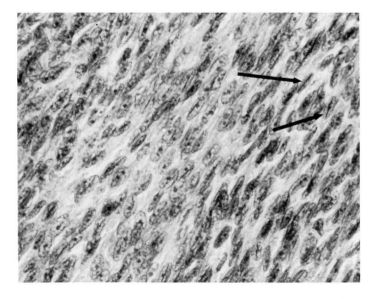

Figure 33–52 This field contains both spindle A and spindle B melanoma cells. The larger spindle cells with prominent nucleoli are the B type and the smaller, more slender, spindle-shaped cells with the central chromatin strip (arrows) are spindle A cells. (Hematoxylin and eosin. ×550.) (E.P. #35303)

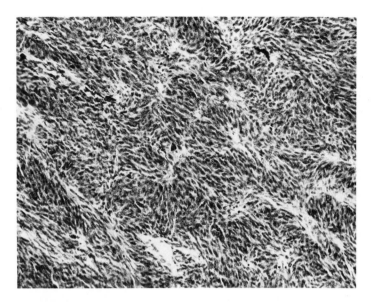

Figure 33–53 The fascicular type of melanoma is composed of spindle-shaped cells (predominantly spindle B) arranged in palisading fascicles and bundles. (Hematoxylin and eosin, ×55.) (E.P. #19660)

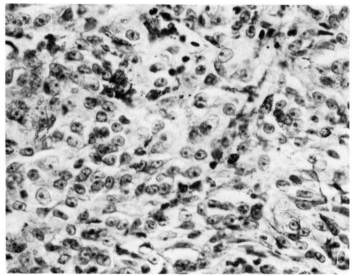

Figure 33–54 Epithelioid type melanoma cells are large, have abundant cytoplasm, and may demonstrate considerable pleomorphism. (Hematoxylin and eosin, ×550.) (E.P. #34384)

Figure 33–55 This large tumor was necrotic except for two small extrascleral nodules (arrows) composed primarily of epithelioid cells (Hematoxylin and eosin, ×45.) (E.P. #34384)

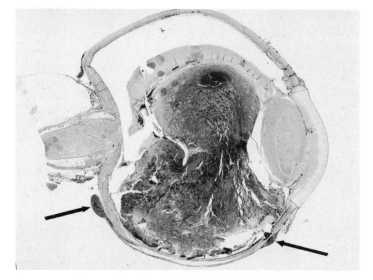

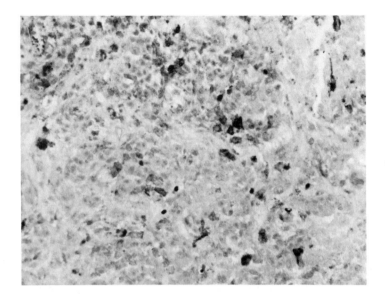

Figure 33–56   Necrotic choroidal melanoma with the globe. Only cell ghosts remain. (Hematoxylin and eosin, ×550.) (E.P. #34384)

my (Davidorf et al., 1970) have been advocated, numbers of patients treated and duration of follow-up periods are insufficient to permit us to recommend such therapy in children or adolescents with good vision in the unaffected eye. Vogel has demonstrated that some choroidal melanomas can be treated successfully by *xenon arc photocoagulation* without increasing the 10-year mortality rate above that reported in other series of patients treated by enucleation. *Cryotherapy* has not proved effective in the treatment of melanoma (Lincoff et al., 1967).

Treatment of metastatic melanoma with currently available chemotherapeutic agents has been generally unsatisfactory (Nathanson et al., 1967) and only further experience wi'l permit conclusions about preliminary reports of remissions induced with newer nitrosurea or colchicine derivatives (Johnson and Jacobs, 1971).

Angiomatosis Retinae

Angiomatosis retinae came to ophthalmoscopic attention less than 20 years after Helmholtz invented his Augenspiegel, and for the succeeding century, ophthalmologists, neurologists, neurosurgeons, endocrinologists, geneticists, pathologists, nephrologists, oncologists, radiologists, hematologists, and urologists have been unraveling the systemic implications of this fascinating fundus finding. Few ocular disorders span a greater breadth of subspecialty interest, both outside and within ophthalmology.

Pathology

The retinal lesions of angiomatosis retinae (von Hippel tumors) are benign vascular neoplasms whose cellular elements bear light microscopic histochemical, and ultrastructural similarity to cerebellar hemangioblastoma. Fluorescein angiographic demonstration of the de novo origin of an angioma (Welch, 1970) and trypsin digestion histopathologic demonstration of a normal vascuature in areas of retina away from the angioma (Goldberg and Duke, 1968; Nicholson et al., in prep.) suggest that the basic lesion may be a neoplasm and not a hamartoma.* Small tumors are usually insinuated between dilated afferent and efferent vessels. The tumor appears in cross section as a fusiform thickening of the entire sensory retina in which normal retinal architecture is replaced by a conglomeration of small blood vessels separated by a cellular matrix of stromal tissue (Fig 33–57). The small vessels within the tumor have normal endo-

---

*Hamartoma: A developmental mass lesion comprising anomalous tissue elements which are normally present at the site where the lesion develops, in contrast to anomalous tissue elements constituting a choristoma.

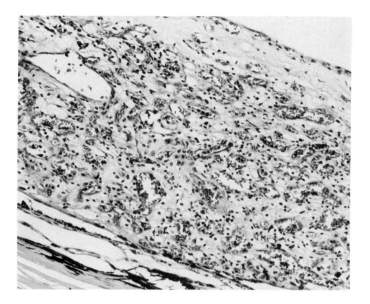

Figure 33–57 One of several retinal angiomas occurring in both eyes of a 48-year-old man who died following removal of a large midline cerebellar hemangioblastoma. (Hematoxylin and eosin, ×180.) (E.P. #33611)

thelium and basement membrane, and each vascular unit in the mass is demarcated by a fine ring of reticulin which extends to a lesser degree out among the adjacent stromal cells (Fig. 33–58). The precise nature of the stromal cells is unknown. They have small, uniform nuclei and abundant clear to vacuolated cytoplasm within which lipid can be demonstrated to accumulate. The adjacent choroid and pigment epithelium are initially normal. As the tumor grows, consequences of repeated hemorrhage into the tumor and vitreous and exudative

retinal detachment dominate the histopathologic picture (Fig. 33–59).

VON HIPPEL-LINDAU DISEASE. The association of cerebellar hemangioblastoma (Lindau tumor) with angiomatosis retinae and cyst or tumor formation throughout the body (Table 33–14) constitutes a dominantly inherited disorder of incomplete penetrance and variable expressivity. Patients who have one or more of the manifestations and who are in a kindred with one documented example of central nervous system hemangioblastoma fulfill the criteria of Melmon and Rosen for the diag-

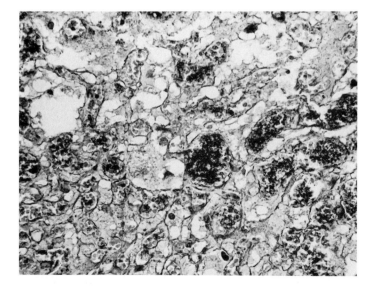

Figure 33–58 Cerebellar hemangioblastoma. A delicate reticulin network outlines each vascular channel. (Gomori's reticulin stain. ×279.) (S.P. 68-8621)

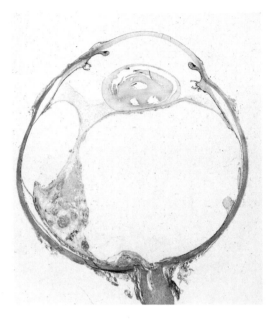

Figure 33–59 Angioma of retina with total retinal detachment and secondary glaucoma. (Hematoxylin and eosin, ×2.5.) (E.P. #4335)

TABLE 33–14 PATHOLOGIC LESIONS DESCRIBED IN VON HIPPEL-LINDAU DISEASE

Structure	Lesion	Structure	Lesion
Cerebellum	Hemangioblastoma Ependymoma	Spleen	Angioma
		Lung	Cyst
Medulla oblongata	Hemangioblastoma	Adrenal cortex	Adenoma Hyperplasia
Spinal cord	Hemangioblastoma Syringomyelia		
		Adrenal medulla	Cyst Pheochromocytoma
Retina	Hemangioma		
Kidney	Cyst Renal cell carcinoma (hypernephroma) Fibroma of medulla Capillary angioma Adenoma Hemangioblastoma	Sympathetic chain	Paraganglioma
		Cerebral cortex	Hemangioblastoma
		Meninges	Meningioma
		Bones	Cysts Anomalies of diploic vessels
Pancreas	Cyst Papillary cystadenoma Hemangioblastoma		
		Bladder	Hemangioblastoma
Epididymis	Cyst Tumor (hypernephroid) Adenoma	Skin and mucosa	Nevus (pigmented or vascular) Café-au-lait spots
Liver	Cyst Adenoma Angioma	Omentum	Cyst
		Mesocolon	Cyst

From Melmon, K. L., and Rosen, S. W.: Lindau's disease; a review of the literature and study of a large kindred. Amer. J. Med., *36*:595, 1964.

nosis of Lindau's disease. The term "von Hippel-Lindau disease" refers to those patients in whom angiomatosis retinae occurs as one of the disease manifestations. According to Lindau, 10 of 47 reported cases of von Hippel's angiomatosis retinae developed intracranial complications, and this observation is perpetuated in the teaching that approximately 20 per cent of patients with angiomatosis retinae are found to have associated systemic abnormalities which place them in the von Hippel-Lindau disease spectrum. This estimate is undoubtedly low, since we now know that intensive medical evaluation of family members on repeated occasions is necessary to detect early or subtle signs of systemic involvement (Melmon and Rosen, 1964). In patients who develop both retinal and cerebellar tumors, the retinal lesion generally becomes symptomatic several years prior to the onset of cerebellar symptoms.

Clinical Features

Our present ideas concerning the age distribution of patients with angiomatosis retinae are derived from Usher's review of 104 patients of known age reported in the literature prior to 1935 whom he considered to have a characteristic fundus appearance and clinical history. His conclusions are recorded in Table 33–15. The contemporary techniques of indirect ophthalmoscopy and fluorescein angiography provide us with much more sensitive methods of detection than were then available, and as more families are studied with Welch's exemplary thoroughness, our present ideas of age distribution will need to be modified. Similarly, Usher's data are

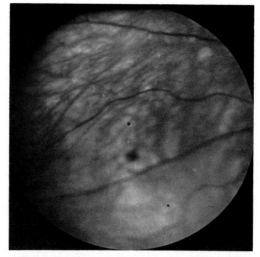

Figure 33–60 Retinal angioma. Small reddish nodule in midperiphery at 8 o'clock (small black dot is an artifact). No demonstrable feeder vessels. (Courtesy of Dr. Robert B. Welch and Trans. Amer. Ophthal. Soc., *68:*367, 1970.)

the source of the generally held concept that about 20 per cent of cases of angiomatosis retinae are genetically determined, whereas 80 per cent occur sporadically. These must therefore be regarded as minimum estimates of familial occurrence and associated systemic disease.

The earliest retinal lesion of angiomatosis retinae was a subject of controversy and some speculation until recently. Welch has photographically documented the origin of a small angioma in retinal tissue which had previously been noted to be normal ophthalmoscopically and by fluorescein angiography. The earliest visible lesion is a small, red-to-gray nubbin of tissue which is *not* associated with abnormal afferent and efferent vessels and which does not fill with fluorescein injected intravenously (Figs. 33–60 and 33–61). At the next stage of development, the lesion may appear either as a small capillary cluster or as a small pink nodule, and both types of angioma stain with fluorescein at this stage (Figs. 33–62 and 33–63). Subsequently, dilation of feeder vessels is observed, and the tumor begins to assume the classic "pink balloon" configuration, tethered to the disc by enormously dilated, tortuous afferent and efferent vessels, both of which may appear to carry oxygenated blood (Figs. 33–64 and 33–65). The

TABLE 33–15 AGES OF 104 PATIENTS WITH ANGIOMATOSIS RETINAE

Age	Number of Patients
1 to 10	8
11 to 20	31
21 to 30	44
31 to 40	13
41 to 50	6
51 to 60	2

From Usher, C. H.: The Bowman lecture: On a few hereditary eye affections. Trans. Ophthal. Soc. U.K., *55:*164, 1935.

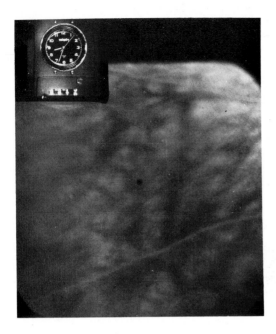

Figure 33–61 Fluorescein angiogram of area shown in Figure 33–60. There is no abnormal fluorescence in this area. (Courtesy of Dr. Robert B. Welch and Trans. Amer. Ophthal. Soc., *68*:367, 1970.)

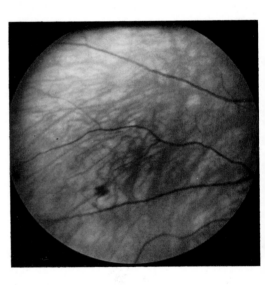

Figure 33–62 Same area illustrated in Figures 33–60 and 33–61, 1½ years later. (Courtesy of Dr. Robert B. Welch and Trans. Amer. Ophthal. Soc., *68*:367, 1970.)

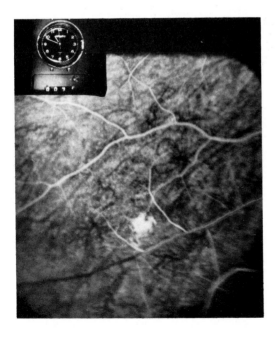

Figure 33–63 Fluorescein angiogram of angioma in Figure 33–62 now shows definite abnormalities. Feeder arteriole and venule as well as the small angioma can be identified. Note that the vein peripheral to exit of efferent venule has not yet filled with fluorescein. This angiogram was obtained 1½ years after the study shown in Figure 33–61. (Courtesy of Dr. Robert B. Welch and Trans. Amer. Ophthal. Soc., *68*:367, 1970.)

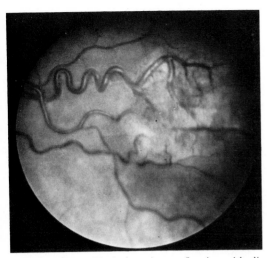

Figure 33–64   Typical angioma of retina with dilated and tortuous vessels leading to and from the lesion. (Courtesy of Dr. Robert B. Welch and Trans. Amer. Ophthal. Soc., *68*:367, 1970.)

angiomas occur most frequently in the temporal periphery, but they have also been described at the optic disc or near the macula (Horowitz, 1971; Landbo, 1972; Welch, 1970). Welch notes that the angiomas are reported to be bilateral in 30 to 50 per cent of cases and that multiple angiomas occur in about one third of involved eyes.

The ophthalmologist should be acquainted with the variety of ways in which peripheral angiomas may reduce visual acuity and thereby first bring the patient to

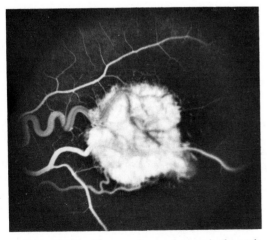

Figure 33–65   Fluorescein appearance in the early venous phase of retinal angioma illustrated in Figure 33–64. (Courtesy of Dr. Robert B. Welch and Trans. Amer. Ophthal. Soc., *68*:367, 1970.)

his attention. The occurrence of lipid maculopathy, vitreous hemorrhage, or exudative retinal detachment should alert the clinician to the possibility of angiomatosis retinae and prompt the meticulous "sensitized" indirect ophthalmoscopic examination which is necessary to discover the tumor in difficult cases (Welch, 1970). Rarely, angiomatosis retinae may be associated with a rhegmatogenous retinal detachment, as we have noted recently in a patient of Dr. J. D. M. Gass (Fig. 33–66).

Treatment

Although rare examples of spontaneous regression of retinal angiomas have been recorded (Welch, 1970), intractable retinal detachment, repeated vitreous and retinal hemorrhage, and secondary glaucoma eventually destroy useful vision in the majority of untreated eyes. If the angiomas can be detected before massive hemorrhage or other late complications have occurred, they can be eradicated successfully with xenon arc photocoagulation or cryotherapy (Figs. 33–67 and 33–68). The indications, technical details, and results of various modes of treatment have been comprehensively reviewed by Welch.

Glial Tumors of the Retina and Optic Disc

Retinal tumors of glial origin, whether neoplastic or hamartomatous, have been described frequently in association with *tuberous sclerosis*, rarely in association with *neurofibromatosis* (Saran and Winter, 1967), and rarely in the absence of identifiable systemic or familial disease (McLean, 1937). These uncommon tumors merit attention because they may clinically mimic retinoblastoma (Cleasby et al., 1967).

Histology

All glial tumors of the retina which have been studied histologically at an early stage appear to arise from the inner retinal layers, usually the nerve fiber and ganglion cell layers, forming a dome-shaped mass (Fig. 33–69). Even in relatively large tumors such as that reported by McLean, the outer retinal layers may be well preserved. The cellular composition of reported tumors varies considerably, rang-

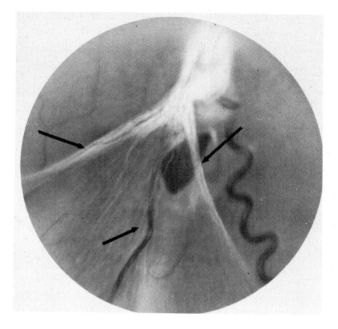

Figure 33–66 Rhegmatogenous retinal detachment associated with angiomatosis retinae. Note vitreous strands (arrows) leading to angioma, which lies just anterior to large retinal break. (Courtesy of Dr. J. D. M. Gass.)

ing from almost pure spindle-shaped astrocytes with prominent glial fibrils (Figs. 33–70 and 33–71) in some cases to large or multinucleated syncytial or ganglion cell-like components in others (Fig. 33–76). The latter tumors resemble the distinctive giant cell astrocytoma of the brain which occurs in tuberous sclerosis, whereas the former type more closely resembles the commoner fibrillary astrocytoma. The core of the tumor frequently contains myriad small calcified concretions (Fig.

33–77) and these are thought to be the histologic counterpart of the golden spherules which are viewed with the ophthalmoscope through the thin transparent overlying layer of tumor cells. Larger areas of calcification and areas of ossification have also been reported. In tuberous sclerosis one may also find *giant drusen of the disc* represented histologically by large calcific concretions embedded in the disc with only moderate surrounding gliosis (Fig. 33–72).

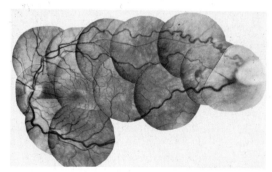

Figure 33–67 Montage demonstrating preoperative appearance of two peripheral angiomas arranged in channel or arcade fashion. Proximal lesion appears to be an angiomatous cluster and peripheral lesion a large tumor (see Figure 33–68). (Courtesy of Dr. Robert B. Welch and Trans. Amer. Ophthal. Soc., *68*:367, 1970.)

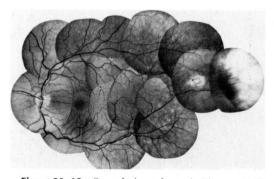

Figure 33–68 Same lesions shown in Figure 33–67 1½ years after treatment of the posterior lesion by photocoagulation and of the larger anterior lesion by cryotherapy. Note the return of vessels to normal size. (Courtesy of Dr. Robert B. Welch and Trans. Amer. Ophthal. Soc., *68*:367, 1970.)

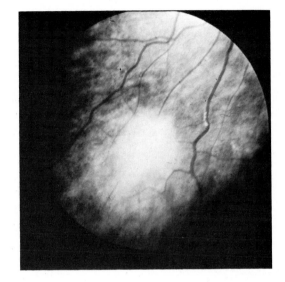

Figure 33–69 Midperipheral retinal glioma in a child with tuberous sclerosis.(Case of Dr. Robison D. Harley.)

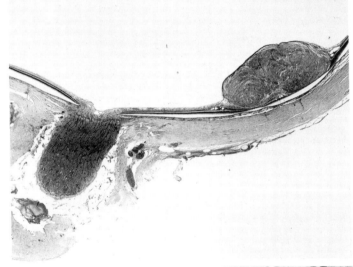

Figure 33–70 Large retinal glioma from adult with tuberous sclerosis. (Hematoxylin and eosin, ×8.) (E.P. #3711)

Figure 33–71 Neurofibrillar appearance of retinal glioma illustrated in Figure 33–70. (Hematoxylin and eosin, ×290.) (E.P. #3711)

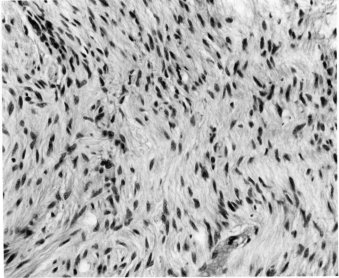

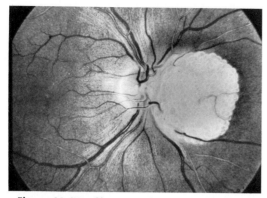

Figure 33–72 Characteristic calcified glioma of optic nerve head in patient with tuberous sclerosis. (Painting by Mrs. Annette Smith Burgess.)

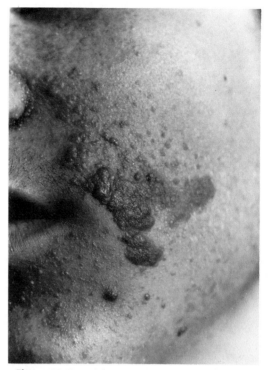

Figure 33–73 Adenoma sebaceum in 15-year-old boy with tuberous sclerosis and astrocytoma of optic nerve head.

Clinical Features

Glial tumors of the retina associated with tuberous sclerosis are frequently multiple, may occur bilaterally, and can arise at the optic disc posterior pole, or peripheral retina. Although many authors regard the tumors as hamartomas, Harley and Grover have observed a new tumor arising from previously normal retina, suggesting that if this lesion was a hamartoma rather than a neoplasm, its original size was subclinical.

An example of *astrocytoma of the optic disc* which occurred in a patient with tuberous sclerosis (Sanderson et al.) is illustrated in

Figures 33–73 to 33–77. Poor vision in the right eye was noted when the patient was 11 years old. Skull x-rays demonstrated multiple areas of intracranial calcification,

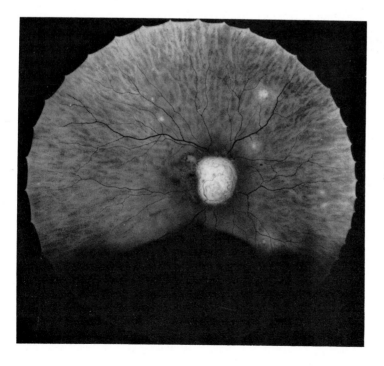

Figure 33–74 Astrocytoma of optic nerve head, vitreous hemorrhage, and multiple gliomas of retina.

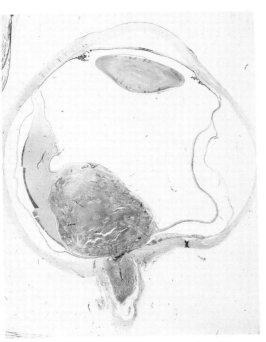

Figure 33–75 Large astrocytoma of optic nerve head in blind glaucomatous eye of a patient with tuberous sclerosis. (Hematoxylin and eosin, ×2.5.) (E.P. #31650)

and typical lesions of adenoma sebaceum of the skin of the face were noted (Fig. 33–73). A large whitish mass was present over the optic nerve head, and several similar but smaller lesions were scattered in the retina (Fig. 33–74). Over a seven-year period the mass of the optic nerve

head grew larger, and the eye became glaucomatous, blind, and painful and was enucleated. Histopathologic examination revealed a large astrocytoma of the optic nerve head (Figs. 33–75 to 33–77).

The earliest lesions are rather flat and translucent and may be confused with medullated nerve fibers. They grow slowly, forming dome-shaped semitranslucent tumors which project internally from the retina (Fig. 33–70). These are the lesions which may be mistaken for *retinoblastoma*. The latter tumors are whiter and more opaque and may have a chalky appearance associated with calcification (Gass, 1965). The characteristic vitreous seeding by retinoblastoma tumor nodules should be carefully looked for, and it is not likely to be confused with release of golden tapioca granules into the vitreous which van der Hoeve reported in his initial observations of advanced tuberous sclerosis lesions. If one or more discrete semitranslucent retinal tumors are present in a child, associated clinical features which should be sought to verify the suspicion of tuberous sclerosis are (1) *mental retardation* (2) *a history of seizures* and (3) the *characteristic skin lesions* in either the patient or family members. Table 33–16 records the frequency of the major clinical signs in a large series of carefully studied patients. *Adenoma sebaceum* (Fig. 33–73) may not develop until later childhood, and its absence does not exclude the diagnosis of tuberous

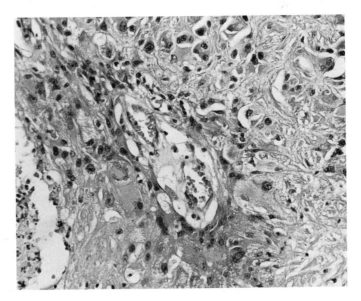

Figure 33–76 Large astrocytes make up much of the tumor. (Hematoxylin and eosin, ×250.) (E.P. #31650)

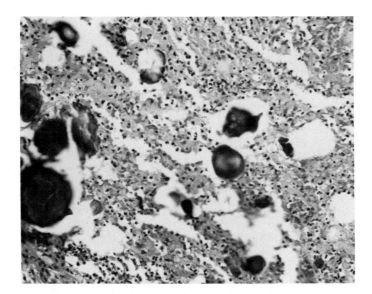

Figure 33–77   Areas of concentric lamellar calcification within an astrocytoma of optic nerve head. (Hematoxylin and eosin, ×220.) (E.P. #31650)

sc'erosis in an infant with retinal tumors. If no additional stigma of tuberous sclerosis or of neurofibromatosis is detected, and if one is in doubt about whether small, discrete tumors are retinoblastomas or glial tumors, enuc'eation should be deferred and the child re-examined weekly. If the lesion is retinoblastoma, growth of the tumor wi l soon be apparent, and appropriate treatment can then be undertaken (Gass, 1965). A glial tumor of the retina grows very slowly, assuming in later childhood or at puberty the classic "gilded mulberry" configuration as much of its bulk is transformed into glistening golden spherules (Fig 33–72).

TABLE 33–16 TUBEROUS SCLEROSIS: CLINICAL FEATURES OF 71 PATIENTS

Abnormality	Per Cent of Patients with Abnormality
Mental Retardation	62
Seizures	93
Retinal phakoma	53
Adenoma sebaceum	83
Other skin lesions	
Shagreen patches	21
Periugual fibromas	17
White macules	15
Intracranial calcification	
by x-ray	51

From Lagos, J. C., and Gomez, M. R.: Tuberous sclerosis: Reappraisal of a clinical entity. Mayo Clin. Proc., *42*:26, 1967.

Prognosis

Glial tumors of the retina do not metastasize or extend outside the globe, and their growth rate is extremely slow. Occasionally a tumor will become large enough to destroy vision in the eye (Wolter and Mertus, 1969).

Hemangioma of the Choroid

Choroidal hemangioma is most commonly thought of in association with facial hemangioma (Milles syndrome) or the facial hemangioma—ipsilateral leptomeningeal angioma syndrome of Sturge-Weber (Figs. 33–78 to 33–82). Histopathologically oriented reviews of reported choroidal hemangiomas indicate that approximately 50 per cent are isolated abnormalities unassociated with facial angioma (Danis, 1952); Jones and Cleasby, 1959).

Pathology

Choroidal hemangiomas generally do not form a localized, well-demarcated choroidal mass, but rather create a diffuse thickening of the choroid which is usually greatest around the optic nerve and gradually tapers into normal thickness choroid peripherally (Fig. 33–83). The closely packed vessels making up the angioma have normal endothelial lining, thin walls, and variable diameters. The overlying

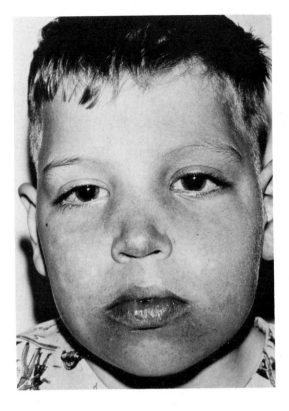

Figure 33–78 Bilateral port-wine stain in 7-year-old patient with Sturge-Weber disease. Facial hemangioma in this patient involves primarily the lower face, sparing the right upper lid and forehead. Bilateral episcleral angiomas are present, and the patient has advanced juvenile glaucoma in both eyes.

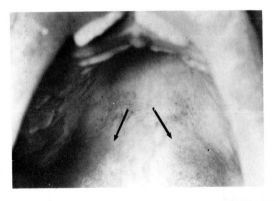

Figure 33–79 Palatal hemangioma (arrows) in patient with Sturge-Weber disease shown in Figure 33–78.

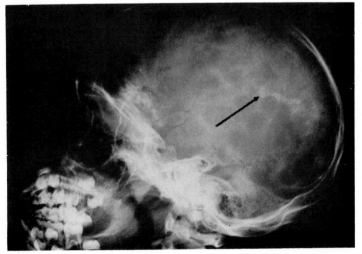

Figure 33–80 Cerebral calcifications in Sturge-Weber disease (arrow). Same patient as in Figure 33–78.

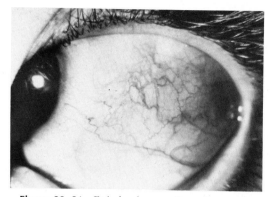

Figure 33–81 Episcleral vascular hamartoma. Same patient as in Figure 33–78.

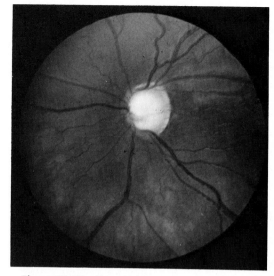

Figure 33–82 Severe glaucomatous optic atrophy, left eye. Same patient as in Figure 33–78.

retinal pigment epithelium may show focal proliferation attenuation or metaplasia, participating in the formation of a connective tissue layer which characteristically separates the angioma from overlying retina (Jones and Cleasby, 1959). The adjacent sensory retina is cystic and frequently detached. Foci of ossification can often be demonstrated in association with long-standing choroidal hemangiomas.

Clinical Features

Of the 25 patients reported by Jones and Cleasby for whom the age of onset of symptoms is known, 13 exhibited symptoms in infancy or childhood. Three of the 13 patients had Sturge-Weber syndrome, and 4 had ipsilateral facial hemangioma

without evidence of intracranial involvement. The predominant signs which they record and which probably reflect the clinical presentation are glaucoma or buphthalmos—6 patients (3 with Sturge-Weber syndrome, 1 with facial hemangioma only); history of "inflammation or infection"—2 patients; history of trauma—2 patients; choroidal hemangioma with secondary cataract and glaucoma—1 patient; and suspected malignant melanoma—1 patient (age 10 years). Other presenting manifestations of choroidal hemangioma

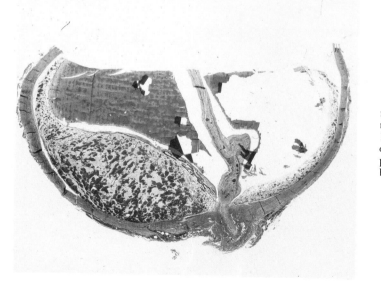

Figure 33–83 Large choroidal hemangioma and secondary detachment of the retina of the left eye of a 14-year-old with Sturge-Weber syndrome. Pain and elevated intraocular pressure prompted enucleation of this blind eye. (E.P. #6596)

include progressive hypermetropia and secondary retinal detachment.

The ophthalmoscopic appearance of the tumor varies with its extent, degree of elevation and associated secondary retinal changes. The flat, diffuse lesions may be detectable only as a darker reddish-orange color than the opposite normal choroid. More elevated lesions have rather indistinct margins, a variable degree of pigment epithelial disturbance, and frequent cystic changes in the overlying retina (Font and Ferry, 1972). Fluorescein angiography demonstrates tumor filling coincident with or prior to retinal arterial filling. In all but the earliest lesions, later phases of the angiogram show extensive pooling of dye in the intraretinal cystoid spaces overlying the tumor (Gass, 1972). Though not pathognomonic of choroidal hemangioma, these angiographic features are characteristic of this tumor and are rarely seen in other lesions.

Treatment

Xenon arc photocoagulation can eliminate the exudative retinal detachment associated with choroidal hemangiomas, although the size of the choroidal tumor itself remains unchanged (Gass, 1972).

Juvenile Xanthogranuloma (JXG)

Juvenile xanthogranuloma (nevoxanthoendothelioma) is a non-neoplastic, self-limited histiocytic proliferation of unknown etiology occurring in infants 2 years of age or younger. The proliferation is most frequently confined to focal areas in the dermis, producing the clinical appearance of yellow or red-brown papular lesions varying in size from a few millimeters to several centimeters in diameter, distributed over the head, neck, and upper trunk (Fig. 33–84). This innocuous and somewhat obscure dermatologic disorder occasionally occurs within the eye, producing a clinical and pathologic picture the distinctive nature of which has been recognized only in the last 15 years. Juvenile xanthogranuloma occurring in the lids or orbit is described elsewhere in this chapter (p. 967).

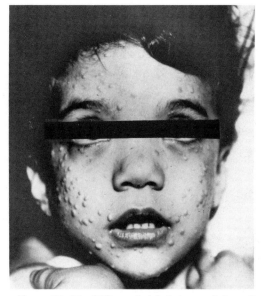

Figure 33–84 Diffuse facial lesions of juvenile xanthogranuloma. (Courtesy of Dr. George W. Hambrick, Jr.)

Pathology*

Intraocular juvenile xanthogranuloma involves the iris and ciliary body in either a focal or a diffuse fashion. Characteristically the lesions are composed of densely packed polyhedral histiocytes with small uniform nuclei and abundant cytoplasm which exhibits varying degrees of vacuolization (Fig. 33–85). Occasional multinucleated giant cells with nuclei distributed regularly around the periphery of the cytoplasm (Touton giant cells, Fig. 33–86) are also present. A prominent network of thin-walled blood vessels is often present on the surface of the tumor (Fig. 33–87), representing the morphologic basis for one of the most frequent presenting signs of JXG—spontaneous hyphema.

In addition to histiocytes, Touton giant cells, and fragile capillaries, a mixed inflammatory infiltrate of variable intensity is often present. Electron microscopic studies of cutaneous JXG lesions show that the histiocytes contain abundant liposomal structures, lipid vacuoles not enclosed by membranes, and single membrane-bound structures resembling altered mitochondria (Esterly et al., 1972; Gonzalez-Crussi

---

*See Zimmerman, 1965.

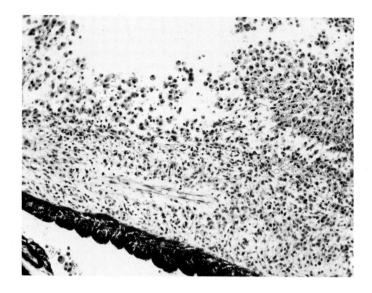

Figure 33–85 Juvenile xanthogranuloma of iris. The infiltrate is primarily composed of histiocytes. (AFIP neg. 60–2781, ×145) (Courtesy of Dr. L. E. Zimmerman and Trans. Amer. Acad. Ophthalmol. Otolaryngol., 69:412, 1965.)

Figure 33–86 Juvenile xanthogranuloma of iris. Numerous Touton giant cells. (AFIP neg. 64–1140), (Courtesy of Dr. L. E. Zimmerman and Trans. Amer. Acad. Ophthalmol. Otolaryngol., 69: 412, 1965.)

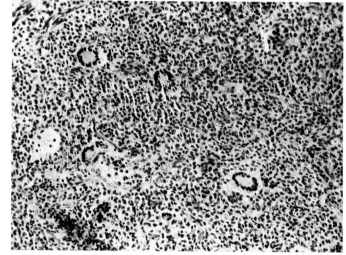

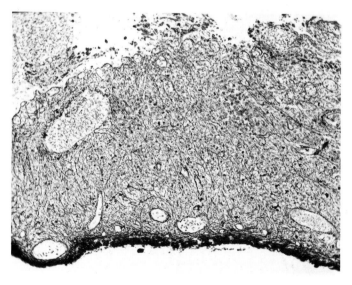

Figure 33–87 Juvenile xanthogranuloma of iris with numerous delicate, thin-walled, and engorged capillaries along anterior surface of diffusely thickened iris (AFIP neg. 60–2783), (Courtesy of Dr. L. E. Zimmerman and Trans. Amer. Acad. Ophthalmol. Otolaryngol., 69:412, 1965.)

and Campbell, 1970). Langerhans' granules, demonstrable by electron microscopy in *histiocytosis X*, are not present in the histiocytes of JXG, supporting the consensus that these processes are unrelated.

Clinical Features

The disorder has no predilection for a particular race or sex, and no hereditary pattern has been recognized. Rare examples of *neurofibromatosis* have been recorded in infants with JXG or their relatives (Okisaka et al., 1970). Eighty-five per cent of ocular cases in Zimmerman's review occurred in infants less than 1 year old, and 64 per cent of the patients were 7 months old or less. Thus, although rare cases have been described in adults (Smith et al., 1969), the disease almost never occurs in a patient over the age of 2 years. Almost all cases are unilateral, though bilateral intraocular involvement has been documented (Smith and Ingram, 1968). The presenting clinical signs, succinctly summarized by Zimmerman, are (1) an *asymptomatic localized* (Fig. 33–88) or *diffuse iris tumor,* usually having a fleshy appearance with prominent surface vessels and stained variably with pigment from previous hemorrhage; (2) *congenital* or *acquired heterochromia of the iris;* (3) *unilateral glaucoma* (Fig. 33–89); (4) *spontaneous hyphema;* and (5) a *red eye with signs of uveitis.* When any of these signs is noted in an infant the ophthalmologist should search thoroughly for the characteristic skin lesions. The lid skin is curiously spared in reported cases of intraocular involvement (Zimmerman,

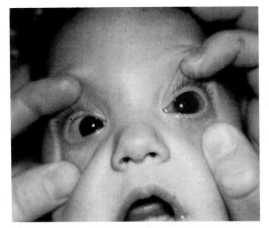

Figure 33–89 Uniocular glaucoma with hyphema due to JXG involvement of iris and ciliary body. (Patient of Dr. M. L. Small.) (From Iliff, C. E., and Ossofsky, H. T., Tumors of the Eye and Adnexa in Infancy and Childhood, 1962. Courtesy of Charles C Thomas, Publisher, Springfield, Illinois.)

1965), but one or more lesions are present elsewhere on the body in the majority of cases in which they have been sought (Sanders, 1966). In some instances typical skin lesions have appeared several months after the iris lesion.

Differential Diagnosis*

Although spontaneous hyphema in infancy is now recognized as the clinical hallmark of JXG, other disorders which may produce this sign include (1) any *intraocular tumor* involving the anterior segment, including retinoblastoma, medulloepithelioma, iris hemangioma, melanoma, leukemia, and lymphoma; (2) diseases associated with formation of *vascular pupillary* or *retrolental membranes,* including retrolental fibroplasia, persistent hyperplastic primary vitreous, and juvenile retinoschisis; (3) unsuspected *trauma* or delayed hemorrhage after trauma; (4) diseases associated with *abnormal bleeding* tendencies such as hemophilia, scurvy, or thrombocytopenic purpura; and (5) *fulminant anterior uveitis,* documented most frequently in adults in association with herpes zoster, herpes simplex, or gonococcal iridocyclitis.

Prognosis and Treatment

The severity of intraocular involvement varies considerably, and the clinical course

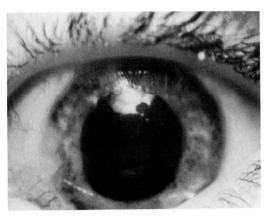

Figure 33–88 Localized iris lesion of juvenile xanthogranuloma (Patient of Dr. A E Maumenee.)

*See Guzak, 1970; Howard, 1962.

of skin lesions might lead one to expect spontaneous resolution of iris lesions in some cases. However, purely expectant management risks the irreversible complications of recurrent uncontrolled bleeding and secondary glaucoma, so that even the smaller lesions should be treated. Topically administered corticosteroids, given in conjunction with oral acetazolamide and topical atropine, may successfully eradicate the tumor and control complications (Clements, 1966; Stern and Arenberg, 1970). More frequently systemically administered steroids have been employed for a period of 4 to 6 weeks (Smith and Ingram, 1968). X-irradiation has also been successful in some cases (Maumenee and Longfellow, 1960), and a schedule of therapy similar to that used by Fonken and Ellis (1966) to eradicate leukemic infiltrates of the iris should provide adequate dosage with minimal risk. Finally, localized iris lesions may be surgically removed, although massive hemorrhage may occur at the time of surgery (Gass, 1964; Smith and Ingram, 1968). The prognosis is good if resolution of the lesion can be secured before secondary glaucoma and hemorrhage have destroyed visual function, since the lesions do not recur. Involvement of the second eye several months after the first has been recorded (Smith and Ingram, 1968), so that continued careful follow-up examinations of both eyes are indicated.

Uncommon Miscellaneous Lesions of the Iris

Uncommon lesions of the iris include *aberrant lacrimal gland tissue* (Bruce, 1952; Christensen and Anderson, 1952). Such lesions are considered to be congenital developmental anomalies, although one has been described in association with an epithelial cyst following intraocular surgery (Fig. 33–90; Green and Zimmerman, 1967).

Hemangiomas of the iris are among the rarest ocular tumors (Ferry, 1972). Histopathologic review of lesions interpreted as iris hemangioma has in some instances resulted in their recognition as *juvenile xanthogranuloma* or in other instances as *melanomas of the iris*. A true iris hemangioma (Figs. 33–91 and 33–92) has

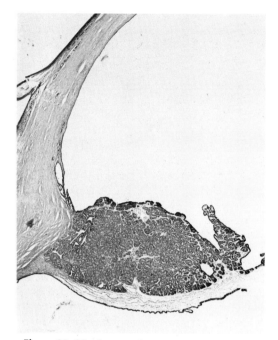

Figure 33–90   Intraocular ectopic lacrimal gland. (AFIP neg. 62–78) (Courtesy of Dr. W. R. Green and Dr. L. E. Zimmerman and Arch. Ophthal., 78:318, Copyright 1967, American Medical Association.)

been observed in a newborn infant with diffuse congenital hemangiomatosis (Naidoff et al, 1971).

Congenital nonpigmented epithelial cysts of the iris (Figs. 33–93 to 33–95) should be considered in the differential diagnosis of iris lesions in infants and children. Such rare lesions can apparently occur as congenital anomalies (Naumann and Green, 1967), but they may also be

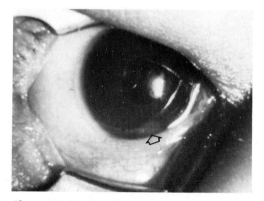

Figure 33–91   Iris hemangioma (arrow) in the right eye of an infant with diffuse congenital hemangiomatosis. (Courtesy of Drs. M. A. Naidoff, K. R. Kenyon, and W. R. Green and Amer. J. Ophthal., 72:633, 1971.) (E.P. #30306)

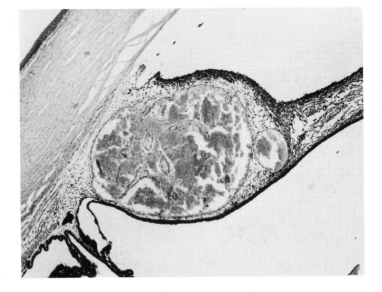

Figure 33–92 Histopathologic section of iris hemangioma illustrated in Figure 33–91. (Hematoxylin and eosin, ×135.) (Courtesy of Drs. M. A. Naidoff, K. R. Kenyon, and W. R. Green and Amer. J. Ophthal., 72: 633, 1971.) (E.P. #30306)

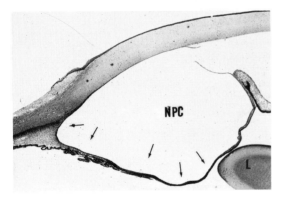

Figure 33–93 Nonpigmented epithelial cyst (NPC) within superonasal iris stroma extends to posterior corneal surface. L indicates lens. (Hematoxylin and eosin, ×19.) (AFIP neg. 66189), (Courtesy of Dr. G. Naumann and Dr. W. R. Green and Arch. Ophthal., 78:496, Copyright 1967, American Medical Association.)

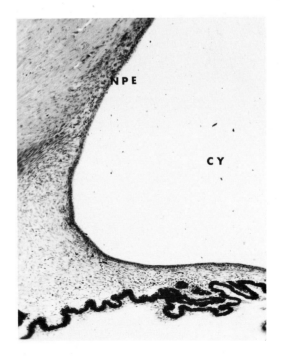

Figure 33–94 Nonpigmented epithelial lining (NPE) of empty cyst (CY) in the region of trabecular meshwork. (Hematoxylin and eosin, ×150.) (AFIP neg. 66–2186.) (Courtesy of Dr. G. Naumann and Dr. W. R. Green and Arch. Ophthal., 78:496, Copyright 1967, American Medical Association.)

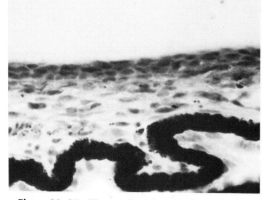

Figure 33–95 Two to three layers of cuboidal non-pigmented epithelium lining cyst of iris. (Hematoxylin and eosin, ×750.) (AFIP neg. 66–13406.) (Courtesy of Dr. G. Naumann and Dr. W. R. Green and Arch. Ophthal., *78*:496, Copyright 1967, American Medical Association.)

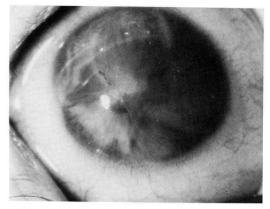

Figure 33–96 Congenital epithelial cysts of the anterior chamber following suspected trauma at the time of amniocentesis. (Case of Dr. H. Cross and Dr. A. E. Maumenee.) (E.P. #33356)

seen following trauma at the time of amniocentesis (Fig. 33–96) (Cross and Maumenee).

EPIBULBAR TUMORS

Table 33–17 summarizes the relative frequencies of various epibulbar tumors among patients under 20 years of age in Ash's review of 1016 specimens from the Armed Forces Institute of Pathology.

The relative frequencies of 298 histopathologically diagnosed epibulbar lesions in children up to the age of 16 years obtained from the files of the Eye Pathology Laboratory of the Johns Hopkins Hospital are listed in Table 33–18. Of course, data based solely on histopathologic diagnosis may not directly reflect the relative clinical frequencies of various epibulbar tumors. In spite of this limitation, the data do provide some numerical reinforcement of the clinical impression that nevi, dermoids, epithelial inclusion cysts, pyogenic granulomas and papillomas are the most frequent epibulbar tumors encountered in children. A more complete differential diagnosis must include a wide variety of inflammatory, neoplastic, congenital, and metabolic lesions which together constitute a significant proportion of epibulbar tumors but which individually are relatively rare (Table 33–19).

TABLE 33–17 RELATIVE FREQUENCIES OF VARIOUS EPIBULBAR LESIONS IN CHILDREN: AFIP DATA

Lesion	Age Group	
	0 to 9 years (Number of Cases)	*10 to 19 years* (Number of Cases)
Nevus	14	38
Dermoid and Teratoma	25	24
Papilloma	9	4
Pterygium and Pinguecula	0	8
Epidermalization	1	3
Carcinoma	0	3
Malignant melanoma	0	3
Miscellaneous benign	10	9
All other	11	12
Total	70	104

From Ash, J. E.: Epibulbar tumors. Amer. J. Ophthal., *33*:1203, 1950.

TABLE 33–18 RELATIVE FREQUENCIES OF VARIOUS EPIBULBAR LESIONS IN CHILDREN: WILMER INSTITUTE DATA

	Number of Cases	Per Cent of Total
Choristomatous tumors	100	34
Dermoids	58	20
Dermolipomas	30	10
Dermis-like choristomas	6	2
Complex choristomas	6	2
Nevi	89	30
Epithelial inclusion cysts	34	11
Granuloma pyogenicum	26	9
Papillomas	22	8
Vascular hamartomas	7	2
Granulomas	6	2
Lipomas	6	2
Squamous cell carcinomas	3	1
Amyloid	1	
Benign hereditary intraepithelial dyskeratosis	1	
Fibrous histiocytoma	1	
Neurofibroma	1	
Rhabdomyosarcoma	1	
Total	298	

From Elsas, F., and Green, W. R.: Epibulbar tumors in children. Presented at the 32nd Wilmer Residents Association Meeting, Baltimore, April, 1973.

Pigmented Epibulbar Lesions

CONJUNCTIVAL NEVI

Nevi are tumors composed of a characteristic cell type, the nevus cell, the precise developmental origin of which is unclear. Many authorities contend that nevus cells stem from epithelial melanocytes which have undergone metaplasia. Others believe that this is a cell type sui generis derived directly from neural crest tissue. Finally, some consider the nevus cell a Schwann cell derivative.

Histopathology*

In a *junctional nevus* circumscribed nests of nevus cells are located entirely within the epithelial layer (Fig. 33–97). Two histo-

---

*See Jay, 1965.

TABLE 33–19 EPIBULBAR TUMORS IN CHILDREN: DIFFERENTIAL DIAGNOSIS

(1) *Congenital Tumors*
Dermoid
Dermolipoma
Lymphangioma
Hemangioma
Epibulbar osseous choristoma
Ectopic lacrimal gland
(2) *Acquired Epithelial Tumors*
Papilloma
Carcinoma in situ
Squamous cell carcinoma
Benign hereditary intraepithelial dyskeratosis
Epithelial inclusion cyst
(3) *Acquired Subepithelial Tumors*
Neurofibroma
Schwannoma
Nodular fasciitis
Xanthoma

Fibrous xanthoma
Juvenile xanthogranuloma
Leukemia
Orbital rhabdomyosarcoma
Lymphoma
(4) *Pigmented Epibulbar Lesions*
Nevus
Epithelial melanosis
Intrascleral nerve loop
Melanosis oculi
Oculodermal melanosis
Malignant melanoma
(5) *Inflammatory and Degenerative Lesions*
Vernal conjunctivitis
Ligneous conjunctivitis
Phlyctenular keratoconjunctivitis
Granuloma pyogenicum
Pterygium and pinguecula

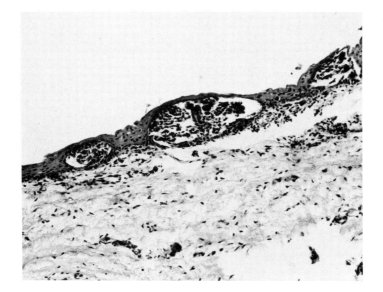

Figure 33–97 Junctional nevus. Nests of nevus cells are located within epithelial layer of conjunctiva. (Hematoxylin and eosin, ×175.) (E.P. #31715)

logic changes are observed at the epithelial-subepithelial interface: (1) formation of nevus cell nests within the basal layers of epithelium and (2) proliferation of nevus cell nests into the underlying subepithelial tissue. These two changes constitute the *junctional activity* of the nevus. A *compound nevus* is composed of both epithelial and subepithelial nevus cell nests (Fig. 33–98). Cysts lined by goblet cell–containing epithelium may be present (Figs. 33–99 and 33–100). Expansion of these cysts can account for clinically evident enlargement of a nevus. A *subepithelial nevus* contains nevus cells which are confined to the subepithelial layer (Fig. 33–101).

The character of the nevus cells themselves varies with the type of nevus. In junctional nevi and the superficial subepithelial layer of active compound nevi, the cells are generally polygonal or epithelioid, with abundant pale-staining cytoplasm and large vacuolated nuclei. The commoner type of nevus cell in most compound nevi is a small cell resembling a lymphocyte, with scanty cytoplasm, indistinct cell borders, and a dense homogeneous nucleus. In the deepest part of com-

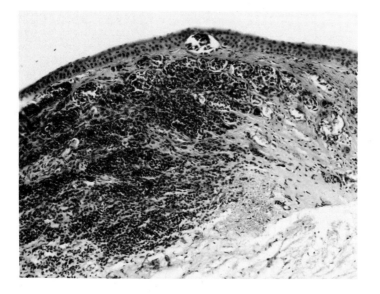

Figure 33–98 This compound conjunctival nevus has a large subepithelial component and a relatively small junctional component. (Hematoxylin and eosin, ×135.) (E.P. #34836)

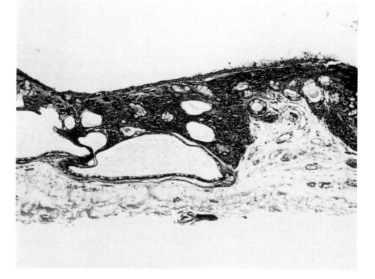

Figure 33–99 Epithelial cysts within a compound conjunctival nevus. (Hematoxylin and eosin, ×70.) (E.P. #30968)

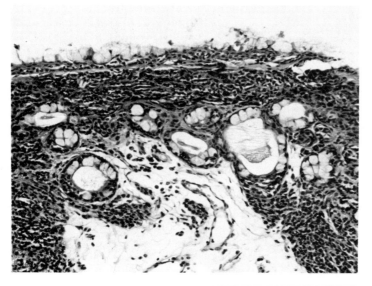

Figure 33–100 Compound conjunctival nevus. Numerous cysts whose epithelial lining contains goblet cells. (Hematoxylin and eosin, ×210.) (E.P. #30968)

Figure 33–101 Subepithelial nevus of the conjunctiva. A narrow zone separates nevus cells from epithelium which exhibits no junctional changes. (Hematoxylin and eosin. ×215.) (E.P.#30369)

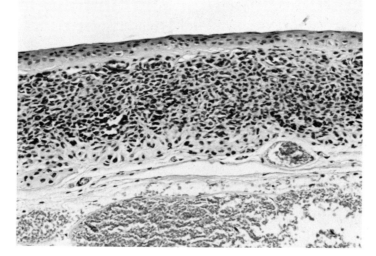

pound or subepithelial nevi, the cells tend to be more fibrillar in form. Solid or cystic downgrowths of surface epithelium into the substance of the nevus are common in compound conjunctival nevi and may also be responsible for the enlargement noted clinically. An inflammatory infiltrate of lymphocytes or plasma cells was present in 24 per cent of the nevi in Jay's series.

The degree of junctional activity varies with the age of the patient. Junctional activity was noted in all conjunctival nevi from patients under 10 years of age in Jay's series, and the proportion progressively decreased to less than 50 per cent of patients by the fifth decade of life. In addition, subepithelial nests of nevus cells in children may contain cells which lack cohesion and exhibit a wide range of pleomorphism. Although these features are indicative of malignant melanoma in an adult, the ophthalmologist and pathologist should be aware that this is not true in children. Malignant melanoma of the conjunctiva is extremely rare in the pediatric age group and the reader is referred to the articles by Jay (1965), Reese (1966), and Zimmerman (1966) for further information about this neoplasm.

Clinical Features

Nevi are the commonest tumors of the conjunctiva. Although some may be evident at birth, Jay found that only 43 per cent become apparent before the age of 10 years and an additional 22 per cent are first noted during the second decade of life.

Most nevi occur at or near the limbus as well-circumscribed pigmented lesions of variable size. Junctional nevi are generally flat (Fig. 33–102) whereas compound nevi (Figs. 33–103 to 33–105) and subepithelial nevi are usually elevated. Clear cysts are more frequently associated with compound nevi (Fig. 33–105). Other sites of predilection of nevi are at the lid margin (Fig. 33–106) and the caruncle (Fig. 33–107).

Many exceptions to these generalizations exist. Approximately 30 per cent of conjunctival nevi are nonpigmented (Fig. 33–103), and many become pigmented only after adolescence. Nonpigmented nevi appear as transparent to pinkish masses which are difficult to

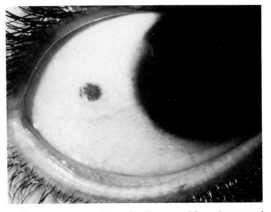

Figure 33–102 Flat, freely movable, pigmented junctional nevus of the conjunctiva in a 12-year-old. It has been present for years but had enlarged recently. (E.P. #31715)

distinguish from other epibulbar lesions such as papillomas, pingueculae, ectopic lacrimal tissue, lymphoid hyperplasia, or juvenile xanthogranuloma. Nevi located on the bulbar conjunctiva may assume a polypoid configuration, in contrast to the generally flat elevation of limbal nevi.

Treatment

Since the risk of malignant change in a conjunctival nevus during childhood is virtually nonexistent, the indication for excision in this age group is cosmetic, and operation can be deferred until an age when local anesthesia can be used. If a large wedge resection for lid margin nevi is necessary, dehiscence of the wound may occur if closure of the wound is inadequate or unaccompanied by a relaxation

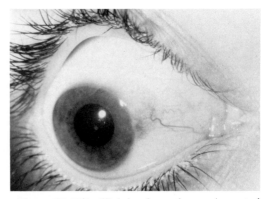

Figure 33–103 Slightly elevated, nonpigmented, freely movable compound nevus of the bulbar conjunctiva of a 13-year-old. (E.P. #13223)

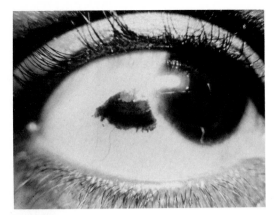

Figure 33–104 Elevated, densely pigmented compound nevus of the bulbar conjunctiva.

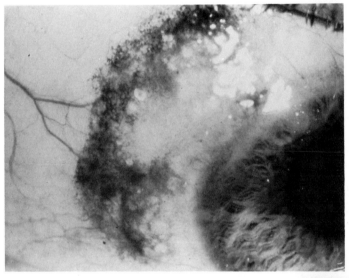

Figure 33–105 Elevated, partially pigmented and cystic compound nevus of the conjunctiva. (Case of Dr. A. E. Maumenee.)

Figure 33–106 Elevated, nonpigmented, fixed compound nevus of the lid margin.

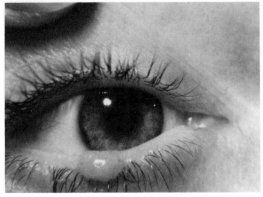

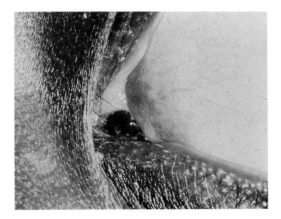

Figure 33–107 Densely pigmented compound nevus of caruncle.

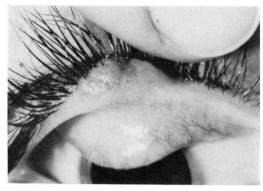

Figure 33–108 Recurrence of a compound nevus of the lid margin 10 years after primary excision had been performed at age 15. (E.P. #33539)

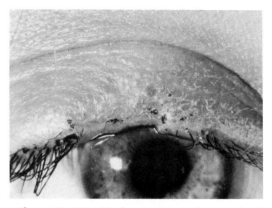

Figure 33–110 Final appearance after repair of lid margin defect depicted in Figure 33–109. (Case of Dr. A. E. Maumenee.) (E.P. #33539)

procedure (Figs. 33–108 to 33–109). Even with subsequent repair, notching and the absence of lashes may yield a less than optimal cosmetic result (Fig. 33–110). In the case of larger nevi of the lid margin, incomplete removal by shaving the lesion off at its base may be the best procedure to obtain a reasonable cosmetic result (Figs. 33–160 to 33–162), as is recommended by Stegmaier for cosmetic management of cutaneous nevi. Nevi are not sensitive to irradiation.

OTHER PIGMENTED LESIONS

Congenital or developmental variations in pigmentation of the eye, lids, and periorbital skin are summarized in Table 33–20). None of these anomalies is a precursor of malignant melanoma of the skin or conjunctiva. However, patients with

melanosis oculi do have an increased incidence of ipsilateral uveal melanoma, and several patients with oculodermal melanosis have developed ipsilateral uveal or orbital melanomas (Font et al., 1967; Henkind and Friedman, 1971; Jay, 1965; Sabates and Yamashita, 1967). Because of these associations and because a type of pigmentary glaucoma has been described in both melanosis oculi and oculodermal melanosis, individuals with either of these congenital pigmentary anomalies should receive periodic ocular examinations (Weiss and Krohn, 1971). The acquired forms of melanosis, benign and cancerous, are generally not pediatric problems, and for a discussion of these lesions, the reader should consult Reese (1966) and Zimmerman (1966).

Dermoids and Dermolipomas

Epibulbar dermoids are choristomas* composed of dense dermis-like collagenous connective tissue containing hair follicles and sebaceous glands and covered by squamous epithelium (Fig. 33–111). They may occur outside the limbus, in conjunctiva, or rarely, on the cornea. The layer of dense connective tissue may contain very few pilosebaceous apparati and overlie a deposit of adipose tissue (Fig. 33–112), in which case the term *dermolipoma* is applied. At the present time, we have no

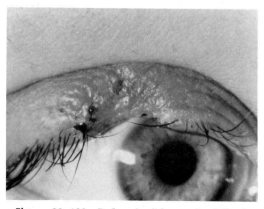

Figure 33–109 Defect in lid margin following wedge resection of recurrent compound nevus of the lid margin. (E.P. #33539)

---

*Choristoma: A developmental anomaly consisting of a mass of tissue which is histologically normal for a part of the body other than the site at which it is located.

TABLE 33–20 PIGMENTED EXTERNAL LESIONS IN CHILDREN

Type	Clinical Appearance and Occurrence	Course	Histopathology	Malignancy Potential
Epithelial Melanosis	Patchy, flat, brownish conjunctival pigmentation mainly on bulbar conjunctiva; pigmented patch movable over sclera.	Present from birth or childhood; stationary.	Increased pigment in cells of basal epithelial layer of conjunctiva.	None
Intrascleral Nerve Loops (Axenfeld)	Single or multiple circumscribed, elevated, pigmented; occasionally tender spots beneath conjunctiva 3 to 4 mm. from limbus.	Present from birth or childhood; stationary.	Uveal melanocytes accompanying external loops of long ciliary nerves.	None
Melanosis Oculi (Congenital Ocular Melanosis)	Unilateral slate-blue mottled episcleral pigmentation; unilateral increase in uveal pigment.	Present from birth; pigmentation may increase at puberty.	Subepithelial aggregates of fusiform melanocytes, increase in uveal melanocytes.	Increased incidence of melanomas of the uveal tract (Reese).
Oculodermal Melanosis (Nevus of Ota)	Varying degree of unilateral slate-blue scleral and conjunctival pigmentation associated with ipsilateral skin pigmentation which may be quite subtle. Predilection for Orientals and Negroes, with involved females outnumbering males 5:1 (Hidano et al.).	Onset most frequent before age 1 yr. or during adolescence (*debut tardif*). Increase in pigmentation during first year of life, then some regression, with seond increase at puberty.	Subepithelial melanocytes in episclera, sclera, and skin; increase in uveal melanocytes.	May develop malignant melanomas of uvea or orbit (more generally in Caucasians).

After Henkind, P.. and Friedman, A. H.: External ocular pigmentation. Int. Ophthal. Clin., *11(3)*:87, 1971.

satisfactory explanation for the origin of these developmental lesions.

Clinical Appearance*

Limbal dermoids appear as cream-colored circular or elliptical elevations (Fig. 33–

*See Duke-Elder, 1964; Haye et al., 1969.

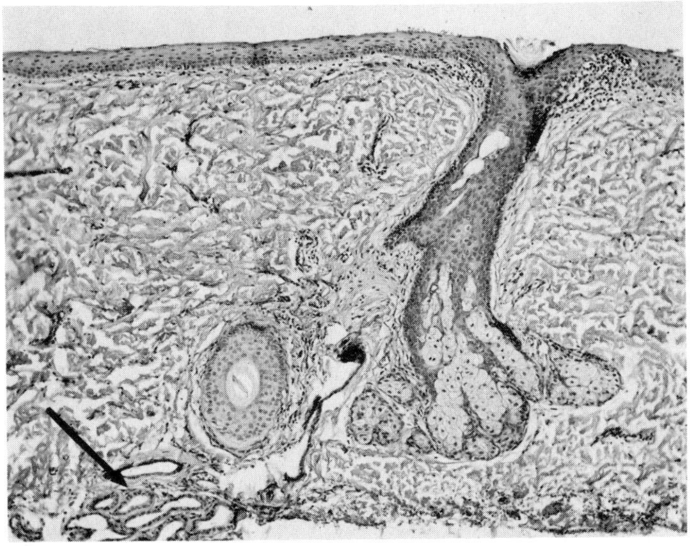

113) varying in size from 1 mm. in diameter to a mass large enough to protrude through the lids. The surface is keratinized and frequently bears fine hairs. The majority of limbal dermoids are single and unilateral (except in association with Goldenhar's syndrome) and they are most frequently located in the lower temporal

Figure 33–111 Limbal dermoid excised from a 3-year-old. The lesion consists of a dense, corium-like connective tissue in which pilosebaceous apparati are present. In addition, apocrine sweat glands are present (arrow). (Hematoxylin and eosin, ×100.) (E.P. #23890)

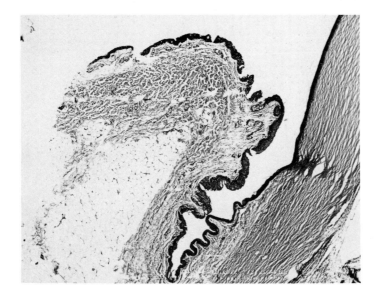

Figure 33–112 Limbal dermolipoma of right eye obtained postmortem from a 10-month-old child with Goldenhar's syndrome. The lesion consists of dense, corium-like connective tissue and adipose tissue. The left eye had a characteristic limbal dermoid. (Hematoxylin and eosin, ×35.) (E.P. #31686)

quadrant (Fig. 33–114). An arc of lipid infiltrate frequently appears along the corneal margin of the dermoid. Purely corneal dermoids are a rare variation of this anomaly (Figs. 33–115 to 33–119). Dermoids are generally evident at birth and may gradually increase in size with time, particularly at puberty (Duke-Elder, 1964).

Conjunctival dermoids (nonlimbal) often are found to be dermolipomas histologically; they are frequently softer and more mobile than limbal dermoids, and surface hair is less frequently seen (Figs. 33–112, 33–120, and 33–121). Duke-Elder indicates that 75 per cent of conjunctival dermoids are located in the upper temporal

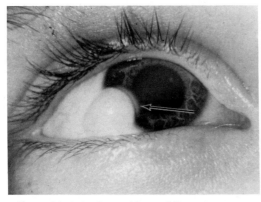

Figure 33–113 Dermoid straddling the limbus. Fine hairs are visible on its surface. An arc of lipid deposit is present in the cornea (arrow.)

quadrant between the insertions of the superior and lateral recti. However, a review of 27 conjunctival dermoids from the files of the Armed Forces Institute of Pathology disclosed that the greatest number, 10, were located temporally, 6 were upper temporal, 3 lower temporal, 4 lower nasal, and none upper nasal (Boniuk and Zimmerman, 1962b).

Associated ocular and systemic anomalies are present in approximately 30 per cent of patients with epibulbar dermoids (Duke-Elder, 1964). Ocular anomalies include lid colobomas (into hiatus of which the dermoid may seem to fit), microphthalmos, aniridia, and coloboma of the various ocular tunics. One case of an associated contralateral retinal vascular anomaly has been reported (Lichter, 1967). Epibulbar dermoids are an integral clinical feature of *oculoauriculovertebral dysplasia* (Goldenhar's syndrome), in which limbal or conjunctival dermoids, frequently bilateral, are associated with unilateral upper lid coloboma (Fig. 33–115), preauricular appendages, aural fistulas, and vertebral anomalies. Baum and Feingold have comprehensively reviewed the ophthalmic findings in Goldenhar's syndrome, and their tabulation of the relative frequencies of major ocular anomalies is presented in Table 33–21. Epibulbar dermoids are not found in the other branchial arch syndromes of Treacher Collins, Pierre Robin, or Hallermann-Streiff (Feingold and Gellis, 1969;

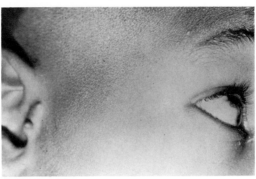

Figure 33–114   Child with Goldenhar's syndrome. Inferotemporal limbal dermoid and auricular appendages are present.

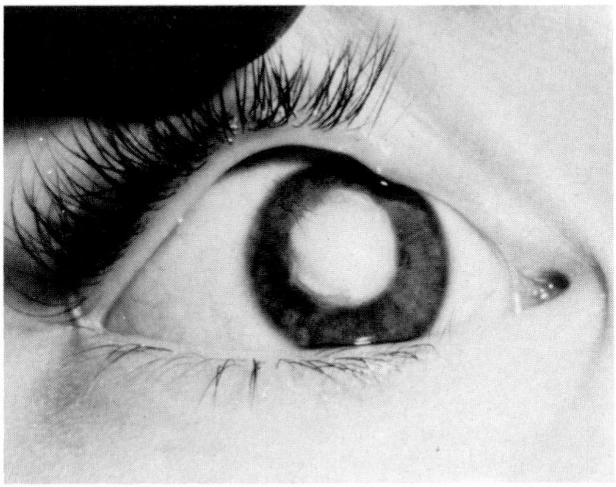

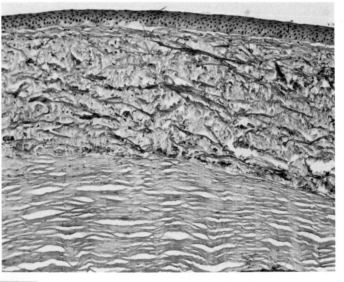

Figure 33–115   Central corneal opacity and coloboma of the upper lid present since birth in a 5½-year-old girl. (Case of Dr. C. E. Iliff.) (E.P. #26936)

Figure 33–116   Examination of the full-thickness keratoplasty specimen disclosed the outer one half of the cornea to be composed of a dense, corium-like choristoma. No skin appendages were observed. (Hematoxylin and eosin, ×110.) (E.P. #26936)

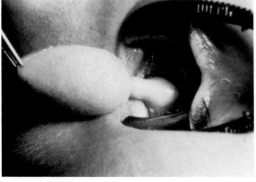

Figure 33–117   Large corneal dermoid with peduncular attachment to a distorted, microphthalmic eye. (Courtesy of Dr. J. D. M. Gass.)

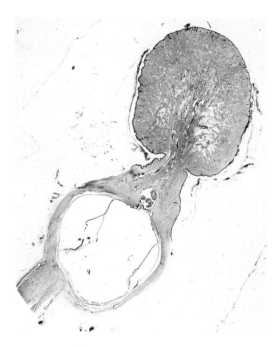

Figure 33–118 Large dermoid and microphthalmic eye illustrated in Figure 33–117. (Hematoxylin and eosin, ×4.)

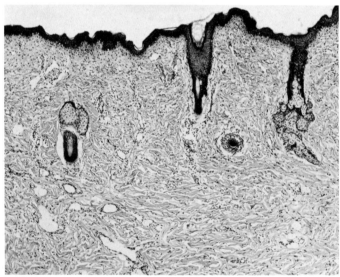

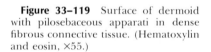

Figure 33–119 Surface of dermoid with pilosebaceous apparati in dense fibrous connective tissue. (Hematoxylin and eosin, ×55.)

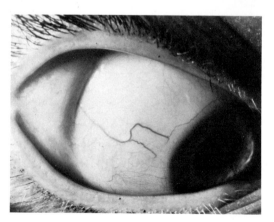

Figure 33–120 Dermolipoma of superotemporal bulbar and palpebral conjunctiva.

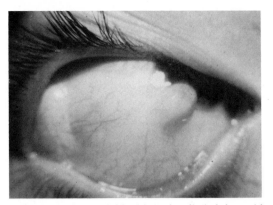

Figure 33-121 Child with both a limbal dermoid and a temporal dermolipoma. (Case of Dr. C. E. Iliff.)

Sugar and Berman, 1968). Epibulbar dermoids have been reported in patients with nevus flammeus (Malik et al., 1967) and oculonasal dysplasia (White, 1969).

Treatment

The usual indication for treatment of *limbal dermoids* is cosmetic, although the chronic irritant effect of hair-bearing elevated limbal lesions may be sufficient to produce a chronic conjunctivitis. Rarely, enlargement of the dermoid or progression of the associated lipid infiltrate may encroach upon the visual axis or cause a progressive astigmatism. The only effective treatment is surgical removal. Opti-

TABLE 33-21 MAJOR OPHTHALMIC ANOMALIES IN 127 REPORTED CASES OF GOLDENHAR'S SYNDROME

Abnormality	Number of Cases	Per Cent
Epibulbar dermoids		
Unilateral	68	53
Bilateral	29	23
No dermoid*	30	24
Dermolipomas		
Unilateral	35	28
Bilateral	24	19
No dermolipoma*	68	53
Coloboma of upper eyelid		
Unilateral	26	21
Bilateral	4	3
No coloboma*	97	76

*Or not mentioned in article.
From Baum, J. L., and Feingold, M.: Ocular aspects of Goldenhar's syndrome. Amer. J. Ophthal., 75:250, 1973.

mism about the efficacy of surgical treatment is tempered by recognition of the potential hazards involved. No definite cleavage plane exists between the dermoid and underlying cornea and sclera, and examples of intraocular extension of limbal dermoids have been recorded, so that careful gonioscopy should be performed prior to surgery (Garner, 1951). Also, the surgeon should bear in mind the occasional association of scleral staphyloma and limbal dermoid (Fig. 33-122). A recent surgical case at the Wilmer Institute (Fig. 33-123) underscores this admonition. During the operation the senior assisting surgeon remarked that one should proceed with caution, since he had previously encountered an extensive staphyloma just posterior to a limbal dermoid. A few moments later, a large lobular staphyloma measuring 16 × 12 mm. was uncovered (Fig. 33-124). A scleral graft was used to support the markedly weakened staphylomatous area (Fig. 33-125). Another interesting finding in this case was the presence of brainlike tissue in the dermoid (Hutchinson et al., 1972).

The exuberant conjunctival reaction following simple excision of a limbal dermoid in an infant may create a pseudopterygium which is as cosmetically objectionable as the original tumor. Dailey and Lubowitz (1962) advocate lamellar keratoplasty to minimize the chance of pseudopterygium formation. Baum and Feingold (1973), on the other hand, find lamellar keratectomy to be sufficient, and they recommend simple shaving of lesions which involve the posterior half of corneal stroma. Beta irradiation has also been used to supplement surgical excision.

Conjunctival dermolipomas (Figs. 33-120 and 33-121) may be intimately related to ocular muscles or the lacrimal secretory apparatus, and they may extend posteriorly into the orbit. Postoperative conjunctival reaction may lead to extensive symblepharon formation with consequent restriction of ocular motility. However, partial excision of the anterior extent of these lesions yields a satisfactory cosmetic result, and the lesion has no tendency to recur (C. E. Iliff, personal observation). Difficulty is primarily encountered when too complete an excision is attempted.

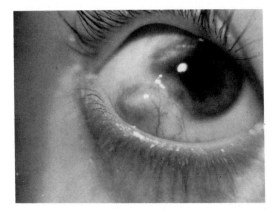

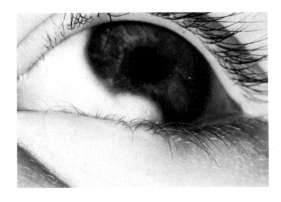

Figure 33–122   Limbal dermoid associated with scleral staphyloma in a 3-year-old girl. (From Iliff, C. E. , and Ossofsky, H. J., Tumors of the Eye and Adnexa in Infancy and Childhood, 1962. Courtesy of Charles C Thomas, Publisher, Springfield, Illinois.)

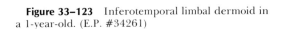

Figure 33–123   Inferotemporal limbal dermoid in a 1-year-old. (E.P. #34261)

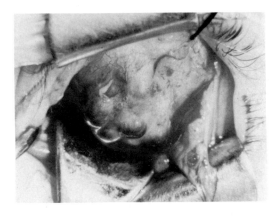

Figure 33–124   Operative appearance of an extensive lobular staphyloma measuring 16 × 12 mm., located posterior to the limbal dermoid illustrated in Figure 33–123. (E.P. #34261)

Figure 33–125   Postoperative appearance following removal of limbal dermoid and scleral patch graft of case illustrated in Figures 33–123 and 33–124. (E.P. #34261)

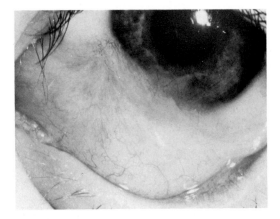

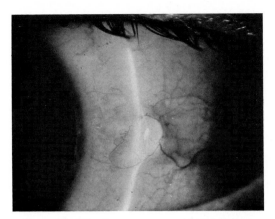

Figure 33–126 Spontaneous epithelial inclusion cyst of the bulbar conjunctiva. (E.P. #34743)

Epithelial Inclusion Cysts

Epithelial inclusion cysts of the bulbar and palpebral conjunctiva (Figs. 33–126 and 33–127) were the third most common childhood epibulbar lesion in the Wilmer Series. These cysts may occur spontaneously or following trauma or surgery. They are lined by conjunctiva-like epithelium and contain a fluid which is generally clear (Figs. 33–128 and 33–129).

Papillomas

Papillomas were fifth in frequency among childhood epibulbar tumors reviewed in the Eye Pathology Laboratory of the Wilmer Institute, constituting 8 per cent of the 298 cases (Elsas and Green,

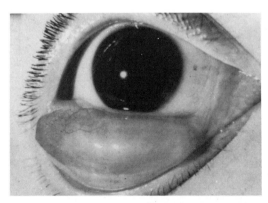

Figure 33–127 Large epithelial inclusion cyst involving bulbar and palpebral conjunctiva. (From Iliff, C. E., and Ossofsky, H. J., Tumors of the Eye and Adnexa in Infancy and Childhood, 1962. Courtesy of Charles C Thomas, Publisher, Springfield, Illinois.)

Table 33–18). These tumors may arise rapidly over a period of a few weeks, and both viral and benign neoplastic etiologies have been postulated.

Clinical Features

Histologically, the lesions consist of a central branching fibrovascular core underlying stratified squamous epithelium which exhibits epidermalization with or without significant keratinization (Fig. 33–130). Papillomas located at the limbus are generally sessile, moderately elevated lesions which range in color from transparent faint yellow to salmon pink. The most characteristic appearance is the speckled pattern of red dots and lines created by the contrast between the core vessel of each transparent microvillous projection and the almost colorless background of adjacent epithelial tissue (Fig. 33–131). In contrast to the low, broad-based limbal lesions, papillomas located in the fornix, in the palpebral conjunctiva, or near the caruncle are often pedunculated and have a fine nodular surface resembling pink caviar (Fig. 33–132). Exceptions to this generalization are frequent (Fig. 33–133).

Treatment

Small papillomas may be excised with cautery of the tumor base and primary closure of the conjunctiva. The large extent of many of these lesions renders simple excision impossible, and in these instances excision with mucous membrane graft or beta irradiation have been recommended. Even after apparently complete surgical excision or treatment with chemical or thermal cautery, the tumor may recur with remarkable rapidity (Fig. 33–134). If *external cryotherapy* of extensive and recurrent conjunctival papillomas proves as successful as preliminary reports suggest, this should probably be the primary mode of treatment, since the difficulties of extensive surgery and the dangers of external irradiation are eliminated (Harkey and Metz, 1968; Omohundro and Elliott, 1970).

Other Epibulbar Tumors

Inflammatory conjunctival and limbal lesions which in children may simulate

(*Text continued on page 986.*)

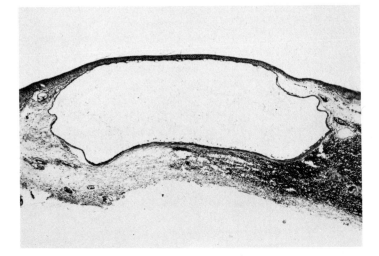

Figure 33–128 Epithelial inclusion cyst of the conjunctiva. (Hematoxylin and eosin, ×40.) (E.P. #34743)

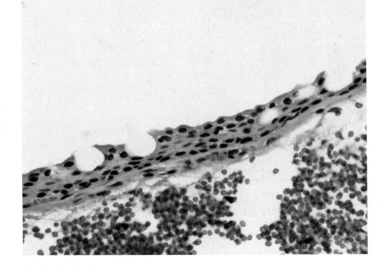

Figure 33–129 The cyst illustrated in Figure 33–126 is lined by goblet cell–containing stratified squamous epithelium. (Hematoxylin and eosin, × 440.) (E.P. #34743)

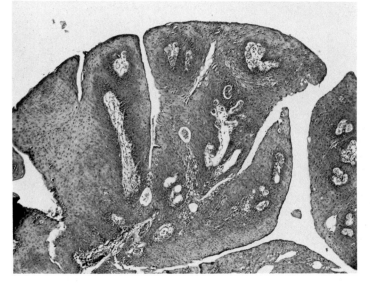

Figure 33–130 Conjunctival papilloma consisting of numerous thin fibrovascular cores covered by normal stratified squamous epithelium. (Hematoxylin and eosin, ×60.) (E.P. #28213)

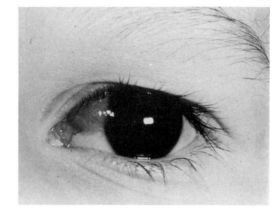

Figure 33–131 Three-year-old girl with a two-week history of rapid growth of conjunctival papilloma. (E.P. #28213)

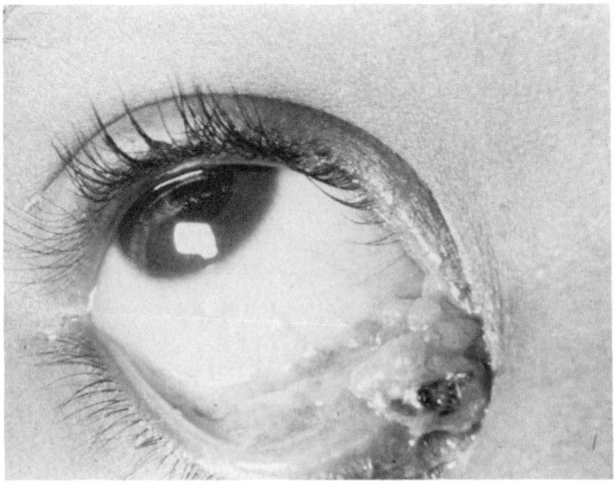

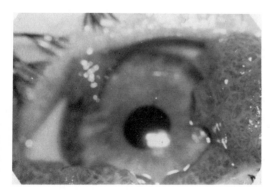

Figure 33–132 Large lobular papilloma of palpebral conjunctiva and caruncle, with involvement of lower lid and punctum in a 2-year-old boy. (E.P. #28891)

Figure 33–133 Sessile papilloma involving the inferior palpebral conjunctiva, lower punctum, and lid margin in a 3-year-old girl. The lesion had been present for five months and was enlarging. (E.P. #35264)

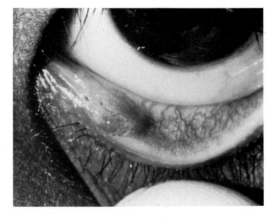

Figure 33–134 Extensive and diffuse recurrence of conjunctival papilloma following initial incomplete excision. (E.P. #31225)

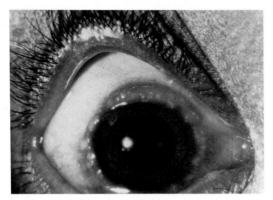

Figure 33–135   Elevated nodular lesions of limbal vernal conjunctivitis in a 6-year-old girl.

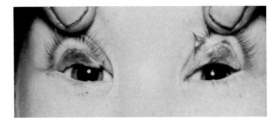

Figure 33–137   Ligneous conjunctivitis. (Courtesy of Dr. A. E. Maumenee.)

neoplasia include *vernal conjunctivitis* (Figs. 33–135 and 33–136), *ligneous conjunctivitis* (Fig. 33–137), and *phlyctenular keratoconjunctivitis.* Similarly, *granuloma pyogenicum* may arise without antecedent trauma or inflammation as a soft, smooth-surfaced, fleshy, pedunculated, rapidly growing conjunctival mass (Friedman and Henkind, 1971). It is more frequently seen in the conjunctiva or skin of the lids in association with chronic inflammatory conditions such as chalazion (Figs. 33–138 and 33–139), pyogenic infection, or suture granuloma (Figs. 33–140 to 33–142). *Nodular fasciitis,* a benign nodular proliferation of connective tissue has in one instance arisen in infancy as a limbal mass indistinguishable from juvenile xanthogranuloma (Font and Zimmerman, 1966).

Although *pterygium* and *pinguecula* are generally considered degenerative changes

found in adults, eight of these lesions were found in the 10 to 19 year age group in Ash's series (Table 33–17).

Malignant epithelial tumors of the conjunctiva are extremely rare in childhood, except in association with a systemic disease such as *xeroderma pigmentosum* (El-Hefnawi and Mortada, 1965). However, both *carcinoma in situ* and frank *squamous cell carcinoma* have been reported in adolescents without any known predisposing disorder (Linwong et al., 1972; Olurin, 1971). In a series of 21 cases of invasive squamous cell carcinoma of the conjunctiva, two occurred in children (ages 4 and 12 years). One of the children (age 12) had xeroderma pigmentosum and one had no associated systemic disease (Iliff et al., 1969). The white elevated plaques of hyperkeratotic conjunctival epithelium associated with vitamin A deficiency (Bitot spots) should not be confused with malignant or premalignant lesions.

In *hereditary benign intraepithelial dyskeratosis* (Fig. 33–143) elevated, semitranslucent granular horseshoe-shaped plaques of tissue associated with prominent conjunctival vessels are present at the temporal and nasal limbus and associated with dyskeratosis of the oral buccal mucosa (Von Sallman and Paton, 1960; Witkop et al., 1960; Yanoff, 1968). The disorder is transmitted as a simple mendelian dominant trait and has been observed in descendants of a triracial group in North Carolina. Histologically the conjunctival lesions consist of localized acanthosis, hyperkeratosis, parakeratosis, mildly disordered maturation, and occasional individual cell premature keratinization (Fig. 33–144).

Conjunctival infiltrates of *leukemia* may produce single or multiple conjunctival nodules, and Schuster et al. calculated that

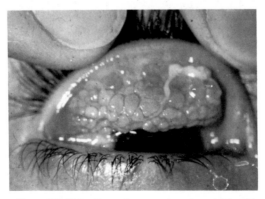

Figure 33–136   Extensive vernal conjunctivitis with papillary formation of the upper tarsal conjunctiva.

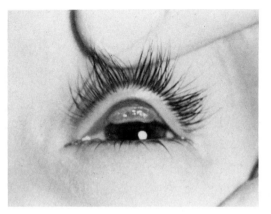

Figure 33–138 Granuloma pyogenicum associated with chalazion. (E.P. #24514)

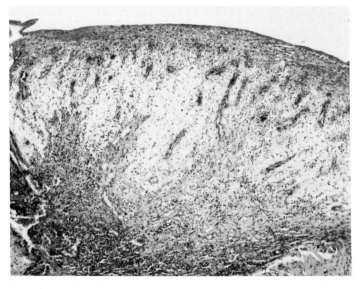

Figure 33–139 Loose connective tissue with fine radial vessels and acute and chronic inflammatory cellular infiltration characterizes granuloma pyogenicum. (Hematoxylin and eosin, ×310.) (E.P. #24514)

Figure 33–140 Six-year-old boy who had strabismus surgery on the right lateral rectus 4 weeks before developing a granuloma pyogenicum. (Case of Dr. S. M. Wolff.) (E.P. #33967)

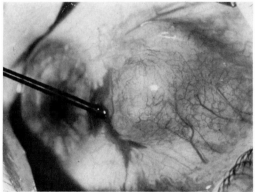

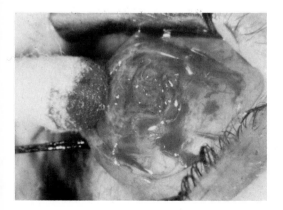

Figure 33–141 Granulation tissue is present over the site of previous muscle surgery. The conjunctiva has been incised and reflected. (E.P. #33967)

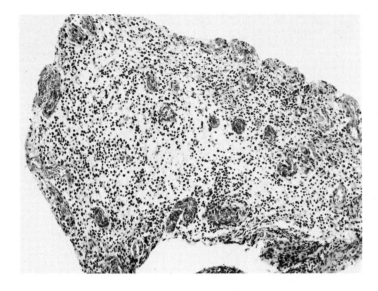

Figure 33–142   Granuloma pyogenicum. Histologic appearance of the tissue excised from case depicted in Figures 33–140 and 33–141. (Hematoxylin and eosin, ×60.) (E.P. #33967)

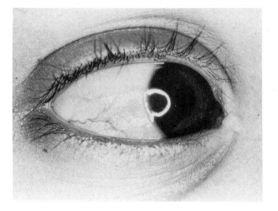

Figure 33–143   Slightly elevated whitish plaque of bulbar conjunctiva in a 5-year-old boy with hereditary benign intraepithelial dyskeratosis of Witkop and Von Sallman. (E.P. #36143)

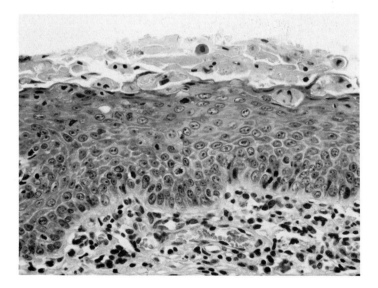

Figure 33–144   The lesions of hereditary benign intraepithelial dyskeratosis show moderate acanthosis, keratinization, some parakeratosis, mildly disordered maturation, and occasional individual cell premature keratinization. (Hematoxylin and eosin, ×380.) (E.P. #36143)

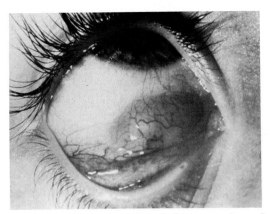

Figure 33-145 Subconjunctival presentation of orbital rhabdomyosarcoma in a 5-year-old. (Case of Dr. David Paton.) (E.P. #23575)

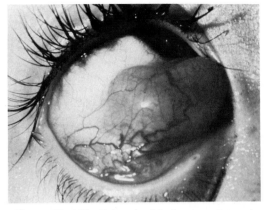

Figure 33-146 Subconjunctival mass shown in Figure 33-145 tripled in size during a one-week period. (E.P. #23475)

7 per cent of reported *orbital rhabdomyosarcomas* have presented as conjunctival masses (Figs. 33–145 to 33–147). *Lymphacytic tumors* of the conjunctiva are rare in children (2 of 12 cases in Ash's series, 0 of 26 cases in Morgan's), but should be considered in the differential diagnosis of childhood epibulbar tumors.

Conjunctival *lymphangiomas* (Fig. 33–148) are benign, slowly progressive tumors which are usually readily recognized by their vermiform or multinodular configuration and water-clear contents, though some of the channels may intermittently fill with blood spontaneously or after minor trauma. These congenital lesions have a tendency to be diffuse and are thus not always easily excised in toto. Although total excision is curative, recurrences after

simple drainage or incomplete excision are frequent. Awdry successfully obliterated isolated ectatic subconjunctival lymphatics with transconjunctival coagulation diathermy in two patients. If the conjunctival lesion is the only visible portion of an extensive lymphangioma of the lid or orbit, successful excision may be impossible. *Conjunctival hemangiomas* are more common vascular tumors than are lymphangiomas, and the diagnosis is generally evident on inspection (Figs. 33–149 and 33–150). Hemangiomas are, in general, more discrete and more easily excised than lymphangiomas. Although these hamartomas (both lymphangioma and hemangioma) may be localized in the lid or epibulbar regions, they frequently extend deeper into the orbit (see Tumors of

Figure 33-147 Exenteration specimen with tumor indenting the globe. (Hematoxylin and eosin, ×2.5.) (E.P. #23475)

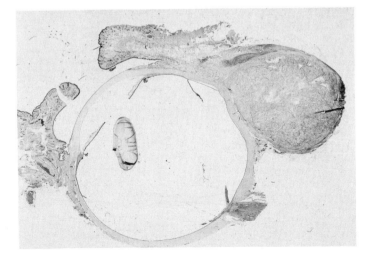

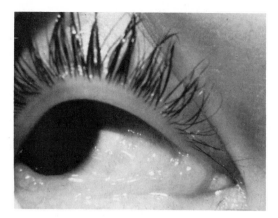

Figure 33–148 Six-year-old boy with lymphangioma involving the conjunctiva, lid, and orbit. (Case of Dr. C. E. Iliff.)

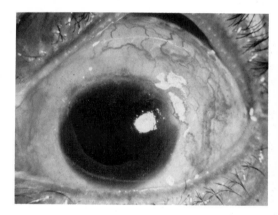

Figure 33–149 Diffuse hemangioma of conjunctiva in an 8-year-old girl. (E.P. #22574)

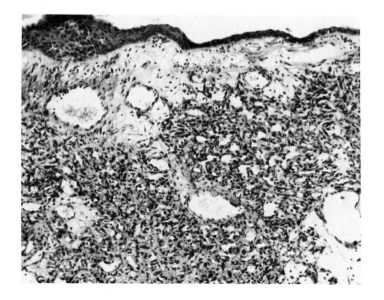

Figure 33–150 Capillary hemangioma illustrated in Figure 33–143. (Hematoxylin and eosin, ×155.) (E.P. #22574)

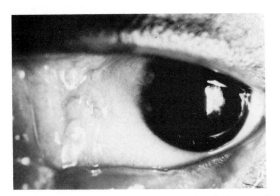

Figure 33–151   Neurofibromatous involvement of conjunctiva in a 9-year-old patient with neurofibromatosis. (E.P. #23783)

Deeper Lid Structures and Orbit, p. 1000.)

Benign peripheral nerve tumors such as *neurofibroma* and *schwannoma* (Figs. 33–151 to 33–153) may arise beneath conjunctiva, in which case they appear as whitish, smooth-surfaced, oval to sausage-shaped lesions (Vincent and Cleasby, 1968).

Epibulbar osseous choristoma (epibulbar osteoma, Fig. 33–154) is a flat, disc-shaped nodule of mature bone, varying from pea- to almond-size, which is located beneath normal conjunctiva characteristically in the superotemporal quadrant of the globe, 5 to 10 mm. from the limbus (Boniuk and Zimmerman, 1962b; Roch and Milauskas, 1968). Ferry and Hein described an example of epibulbar osseous choristoma within

an epibulbar dermoid and called attention to several instances in which these lesions have been closely adherent to the lateral rectus muscle sheath. The clinical diagnosis in most instances has been epibulbar dermoid.

Thirty-seven cases of *ectopic lacrimal gland* have been reviewed by Pfaffenbach and Green. These choristomatous masses are usually noted at birth (72 per cent of cases) and involve the temporal and superotemporal limbal or paralimbal portions of the globe (Fig. 33–155). The preoperative appearance of these vascularized pink-to-yellowish soft conjunctival masses has generally led to a clinical diagnosis of dermolipoma, dermoid, or pterygium. In addition to lacrimal gland tissue (Fig. 33–156) half the reported tumors have contained other choristomatous tissues, such as cartilage, fat (Fig. 33–157), muscle, epidermal structures, and hamartomatous aggregates of nerve or vascular tissue.

Juvenile xanthogranuloma (JXG, pp. 965, 999, and 1054) occurring in epibulbar tissue appears as a yellowish or salmon-pink, somewhat gelatinous mass (Figs. 33–158 and 33–159) clinically similar to dermolipoma, lymphomatous infiltrate of the bulbar conjunctiva, or epibulbar xanthoma (Cogan et al., 1958; Zimmerman, 1965). A careful search for the characteristic skin lesions of JXG may establish the diagnosis, but epibulbar JXG may occur without cutaneous involvement.

(*Text continued on page 994*)

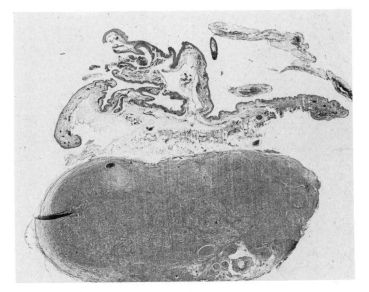

Figure 33–152   Discrete, localized epibulbar schwannoma in an 8-year-old. (Hematoxylin and eosin, ×21.) (E.P. #28751)

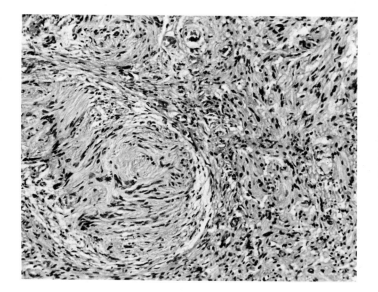

Figure 33–153 Higher power of epibulbar schwannoma in Figure 33–152. The tumor is composed of small spindle-shaped cells and fibrillary processes in swirls, fascicles, and bundles. (Hematoxylin and eosin, ×210.) (E.P. #28751)

Figure 33–154 Epibulbar osseous choristoma from the superior temporal area. It consists of a plaque of compact bone surrounded by a thin fibrous tissue capsule. (Hematoxylin and eosin, ×60.) (E.P. #28812)

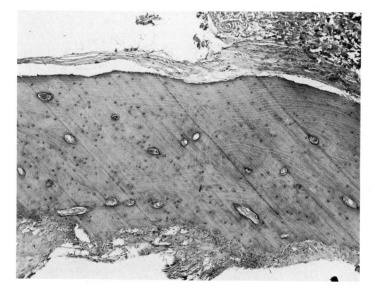

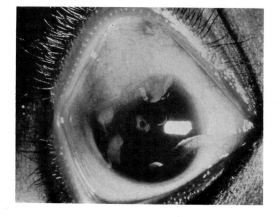

Figure 33–155 Ectopic lacrimal gland of conjunctiva and cornea in a 7-year-old girl. (E.P. #29198)

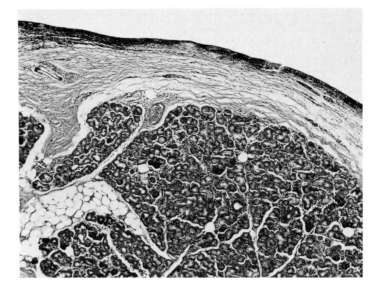

Figure 33–156 Ectopic lacrimal gland illustrated in Figure 33–155. (Hematoxylin and eosin, ×55.) (E.P. #29198)

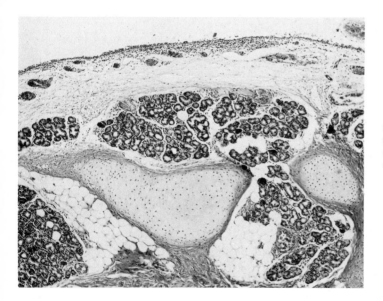

Figure 33–157 Complex choristoma of bulbar conjunctiva with ectopic lacrimal gland, cartilage, and adipose tissue. (Hematoxylin and eosin, ×55.) (E.P. #29321)

Figure 33–158 Juvenile xanthogranuloma with involvement of the bulbar conjunctiva and iris in a 4-year-old boy.

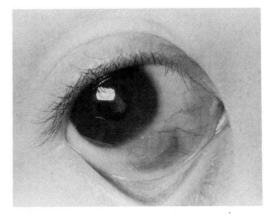

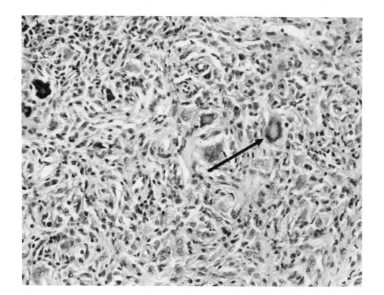

Figure 33–159 Juvenile xanthogranuloma of conjunctiva. The lesion is composed of an infiltrate of histiocytes, lymphocytes, and giant cells, some of which are of the Touton type (arrow). (Hematoxylin and eosin, ×275.) (E.P. #9842)

Xanthomas and *fibrous xanthomas* of the conjunctiva have been described in children with Hand-Schüller-Christian and Letterer-Siwe syndromes, encephalocraniocutaneous lipomatosis, xanthoma disseminatum, and as isolated lesions without any detectable abnormality of lipid metabolism (Albert and Smith, 1968; Grayson and Pieroni, 1970; Haberland and Perou, 1970; Liebman et al., 1966). The conjunctival lesions in these disorders appear as orange or yellowish gelatinous limbal or conjunctival masses which are clinically indistinguishable from each other or from the epibulbar lesions of JXG, and the distinction must be made on the basis of histopathologic and systemic evaluations.

SUPERFICIAL LID TUMORS

In this section we shall consider briefly those lid tumors which arise from surface structures—epithelium and sebaceous glands. Tumors which arise from deeper lid structures—neural, vascular, or connective tissue tumors, for example—merge clinically with orbital lesions of similar origin and will therefore be discussed in the section devoted to orbital tumors.

Nevi

Nevi, the most prevalent of all skin tumors, arise at the epidermal-dermal junction from cells which are probably derived from the neural crest. Only 3 per cent of infants are born with nevi. Most appear in early childhood, usually after the second year of life, and undergo a fairly predictable process of development (Stegmaier, 1967). Nevi in young children are most frequently *junctional nevi* (all nevus cells above basement membrane of epithelium). *Compound nevi*, in which nevus cells are present in dermis and epidermis, are generally first noted during the prepubertal years, and they may darken or enlarge at puberty. At puberty *dermal nevi* first appear. This last histologic pattern—all nevus cells contained within the dermis—predominates in later life. "Kissing nevi" involving adjacent surfaces of upper and lower lids (Figs. 33–160 to 33–

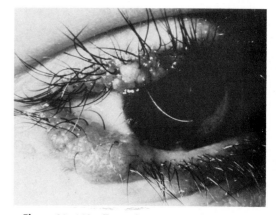

Figure 33–160 Extensive compound nevus (polypoid in areas) involving both upper and lower lids (kissing nevus) in a 10-year-old girl (E.P. #30424)

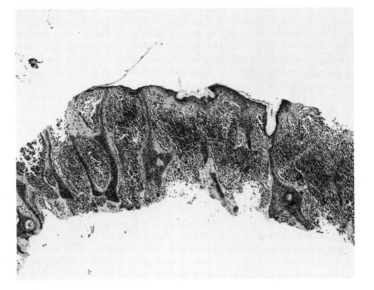

Figure 33–161   Shavings from an extensive compound kissing nevus of the lids. (Hematoxylin and eosin, ×70.) (E.P. #30424)

162) suggest that the cells which are precursors of nevi are already present during the 3rd to 6th months of embryonic development, when the lids are fused. These nevi are histologically of the compound or intradermal type (Ehlers, 1965). The indications for surgical removal of nevi are (1) suspicion of malignancy based on change in size or appearance of the nevus and (2) cosmetic concern. Prophylaxis against possible malignant change is not a valid indication for removal of nevi (Clark and Mihm, 1971; Stegmaier, 1967).

Basal Cell and Squamous Cell Carcinomas

The commonest epithelial malignant conditions of the lids in adults—*basal cell carcinoma* and *squamous cell carcinoma*—are extremely rare in children. Payne et al. had one 9-year-old patient in their series of 256 cases of basal cell carcinoma of the lids, and no other patient in the series was under the age of 20. Several inherited disorders, however, are associated with a skin malignancy diathesis which becomes manifest in childhood. The *basal cell nevus syndrome* is an autosomal dominant disorder characterized by (1) development of multiple basal cell carcinomas early in life, usually after puberty; (2) mandibular cysts, rib and vertebral anomalies, and defective dentition; (3) a variety of neurologic abnormalities including a high incidence of cerebellar medulloblastoma; (4) telecanthus and/or hypertelorism; and (5) anomalies of the reproductive system (Berlin et al., 1966). The skin tumors often appear in childhood. In the case reported by Nover and Korting (1970), multiple skin tumors were present at age 8, though the first lid lesions did not develop until age 14. Chromosomal aberrations have been described in several patients with basal cell nevus syndrome (Happle and Kupferschmid, 1972; Happle et al., 1971). In addition, Happle et al. described one patient with basal cell nevus syndrome who had bilateral retinitis pigmentosa, cataract, and recurrent vitreous hemorrhage.

Xeroderma pigmentosum is an autosomal recessive disorder characterized by sensitivity to ultraviolet light and development of multiple cutaneous malignant condi-

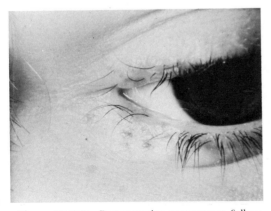

Figure 33–162   Postoperative appearance following incomplete removal of an extensive compound kissing nevus of the lid by shaving. (E.P. #30424)

tions of various types. Squamous cell carcinoma, basal cell carcinoma, malignant melanoma, sarcoma, and keratoacanthoma have all been noted, and death from malignancy usually occurs at an early age (Reed et al., 1969). El-Hefnawi and Mortada (1965) have provided a comprehensive survey of the ocular findings in xeroderma pigmentosum. They examined 46 affected children who ranged in age from 2 months to 12 years. Two patients, each 10 years old, had squamous cell carcinoma of the lid, and one 12-year-old patient had basal cell carcinoma of the lid. Skin fibroblasts from patients with xeroderma pigmentosum lack the genetically determined biochemical mechanism which specifically repairs the normal photochemical damage to DNA pyrimidine bases. However, the connection between this basic defect and carcinogenesis is not clear. A prenatal diagnostic test has recently been developed which should facilitate postconception counseling of families with an affected child (Regan et al., 1971), and treatment with topical application of 5-fluorouracil has been successful in eradicating and suppressing the malignant disease (Reed et al., 1969). Other genetic disorders associated with an increased frequency of early skin cancer are the Rothmund-Thomson syndrome and Fanconi's syndrome with dyskeratosis congenita (Table 33–22).

Sebaceous Carcinoma

Three of 86 cases of sebaceous carcinoma reported from the Armed Forces Institute of Pathology occurred in patients under 20 years of age (Boniuk and Zimmerman, 1968). The youngest patient, age 13, had been treated with x-ray therapy for retinoblastoma 12 years before appearance of the lid tumor which simulated a recurrent chalazion. A nodular brow lesion in a 16-year-old girl was thought to be an epidermal inclusion cyst until excision and histologic study revealed a sebaceous carcinoma.

Metastatic Tumors

Metastatic lid tumors are rare at any age, and recent reviews do not cite any examples in pediatric patients (Brownstein and Helwig, 1972; Riley, 1970). One unusual case of lid metastasis from our laboratory is illustrated in Figure 33–163. This 3-year-old girl developed a rapidly growing mass in the left lower lid that was metastatic from an embryonal sarcoma primary in the buttock area. *Malignant melanoma and neuroblastoma* are two tumors which can also produce cutaneous metastases in early life, so that lid metastasis from one of these tumors in a child is possible.

TABLE 33–22 HEREDOFAMILIAL DISORDERS WITH SKIN TUMOR DIATHESIS

Disorder	Sun Sensitivity	Neurologic Disorders	Dwarfism	Inheritance
Basal Cell Nevus Syndrome	No	Yes	No	Autosomal dominant
Hereditary Adenoid Cystic Epithelioma	No	No	No	Autosomal dominant
Neurofibromatosis	No	Yes	No	Autosomal dominant
Xeroderma Pigmentosum	Yes	Yes	Yes	Autosomal recessive
Ataxia-telangiectasia	No	Yes	Yes	Autosomal recessive
Rothmund-Thomson Syndrome	20 to 40%	Occasional	Yes	Autosomal recessive
Dyskeratosis Congenita with Fanconi's Syndrome	No	Occasional	Occasional	X-linked

After Reed, W. B., et al.: Xeroderma pigmentosum; clinical and laboratory investigation of its basic defect. J.A.M.A., *207*:2073, 1969.

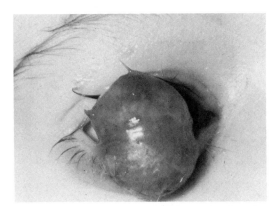

Figure 33–163 This 3-year-old girl developed a chalazion-like lesion which rapidly grew in a three-week period to the large size illustrated. It was interpreted as an embryonal sarcoma, metastatic from the buttock. (E.P. #28392)

Keratoacanthoma

In their histopathologic review of eyelid *keratoacanthoma* from the Armed Forces Institute of Pathology, Boniuk and Zimmerman (1967) reported that the youngest patient in their series of 44 cases was 19 years old. All the lesions in this group of patients were believed to be solitary, localized keratoacanthoma, the common variety which occurs most frequently in the sixth and seventh decades of life. Baer and Kopf note, however, that patients with *multiple keratoacanthomas* frequently note the appearance of lesions in adolescence or early adulthood and may give a family history positive for similar lesions. Although keratoacanthomas are rare in early childhood, Baer and Kopf cite reported examples in infants 5, 16, and 22½ months of age.

Hereditary Adenoid Cystic Epithelioma

An autosomal dominant hereditary disorder in which multiple cutaneous facial tumors begin to develop in childhood is hereditary adenoid cystic epithelioma (Brooke's tumor, multiple trichoepithelioma) (Fig. 33–164). These 0.2 to 0.5 cm. pearly-to-reddish tumors may appear as early as the third year of life but generally become manifest at puberty (Gray and Helwig, 1963; Wolken et al., 1969). Basal cell carcinoma rarely develops in a

Brooke's tumor, in contrast to the lesions of the basal cell nevus syndrome. Skin lesions in these two disorders, however, may appear quite similar (Graham et al., 1965). Histologically, individual Brooke's tumors are indistinguishable from solitary trichoepitheliomas (Figs. 33–165 and 33–166). Islands of basaloid cells and keratin cysts are dispersed in a loose connective tissue stroma which may be infiltrated with a variable number of acute and chronic inflammatory cells.

Adenoma Sebaceum

Adenoma sebaceum (Fig. 33–73) of tuberous sclerosis may also resemble Brooke's tumors clinically. The term "adenoma sebaceum" is a misnomer, since these lesions are in fact vascular fibromas (Fig. 33–167) in skin which is naturally equipped with large sebaceous glands (Graham et al., 1972).

Syringoma

Syringoma often appears at puberty and has a predilection for the eyelids (Fig. 33–168). Individual tumors are flesh-colored to slightly yellowish papules, 1 to 3 mm. in diameter, which clinically resemble trichoepithelioma or Brooke's tumors (Hash-

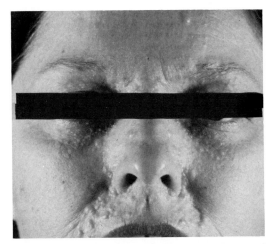

Figure 33–164 Adult female, one of several members of a family with hereditary adenoid cystic epithelioma (Brooke's tumor). (Courtesy of Dr. George W. Hambrick, Jr.)

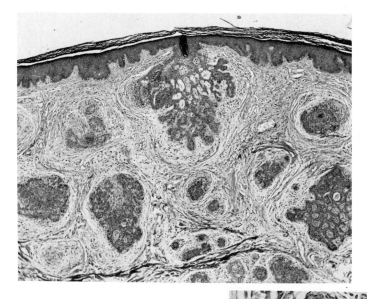

Figure 33–165 Brooke's tumor consisting of islands of basaloid cells with peripheral palisading, prominent stroma, and keratin cysts. (Hematoxylin and eosin, ×50.) (Derm. Path. 72-1543)

Figure 33–166 Brooke's tumor. (Hematoxylin and eosin, ×200.) (Derm. Path. 72-1543)

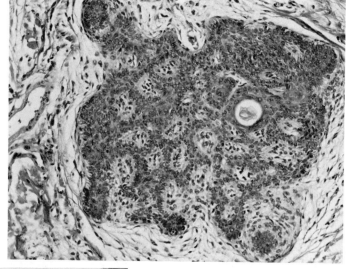

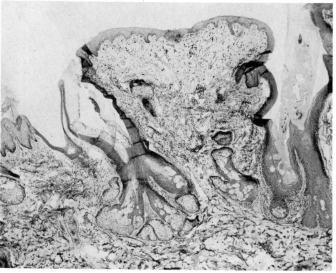

Figure 33–167 Lesion of adenoma sebaceum consists of an elevated nodule of fibrovascular tissue covered by surface epithelium. (Hematoxylin and eosin, ×35.) (Derm. Path. 64-114)

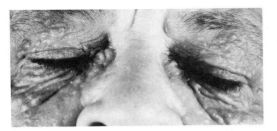

Figure 33–168   Adult with numerous syringomas involving lids of both eyes. (Courtesy of Dr. George W. Hambrick, Jr.)

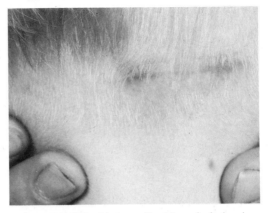

Figure 33–170   Linear yellowish scalp lesion in a 4-year-old with juvenile xanthogranuloma. (Courtesy of Dr. George W. Hambrick, Jr.)

imoto and Lever, 1971). Histologically the tumor is characterized by collections of ductal structures lined by one or two layers of flattened epithelial cells with clear cytoplasm (Fig. 33–169).

Juvenile Xanthogranuloma

Juvenile xanthogranuloma most commonly occurs as an eruption of orange-colored nodular cutaneous granulomas over the scalp, face, trunk, or proximal extremities in otherwise healthy children. The skin xanthomas may occur on the lids with or without other cutaneous lesions (Figs. 33–84, 33–170, and 33–171). They typically appear in the newborn period or first 6 months of life, increase in size and number until 1 to 1½ years of age, and then involute spontaneously. The appearance of the cutaneous lesions is unique and pathognomonic. No other discrete orange nodular skin lesions occur in this age group (Crocker, 1971). This generally innocuous dermatologic disorder acquires systemic significance through its association with neurofibromatosis (Crocker, 1971; Okisaka et al., 1970) and ophthalmic overtones through its occasional occurrence in the orbit or iris (see pp. 965 and 1054).

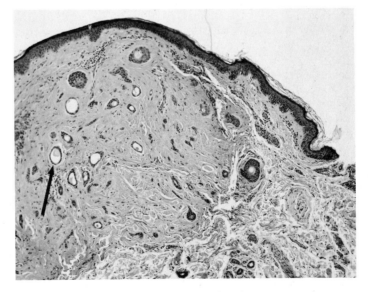

Figure 33–169   Syringoma. One of multiple lesions involving upper and lower lids of both eyes. The clinical diagnosis was xanthoma. The lesion consists of ductal structures surrounded by dense connective tissue, lined by flattened epithelium, and containing an eosinophilic material (arrow). In other areas, only small cords of epithelium are present. (Hematoxylin and eosin, ×100.) (E.P. #31200)

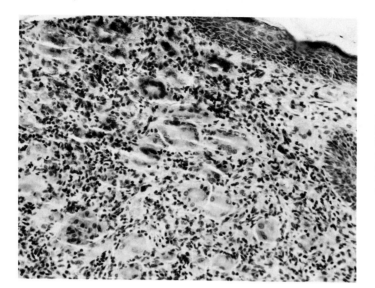

Figure 33–171 Juvenile xanthogranuloma of skin of left upper lid of a 2½-year-old. The lesion consists of an infiltrate of large cells with vacuolated cytoplasm. Numerous Touton giant cells and occasional lymphocytes and eosinophils are present. (Hematoxylin and eosin, ×260.) (E.P. #17525)

TUMORS OF DEEPER LID STRUCTURES AND ORBIT

Differential Diagnosis

The relative frequencies of different orbital tumors in patients 15 years of age and younger are listed in Table 33–23. These data are derived from three clinical centers—Columbia-Presbyterian and Memorial Hospitals in New York (Ingalls, 51 cases), Children's Hospital in Washington, D. C. (Yousseffi, 62 cases), and the Wilmer Institute and Johns Hopkins Hospital in Baltimore (Iliff and Green, 150 cases). The most frequent orbital tumor of childhood in all three series is the *dermoid cyst*, which constitutes 32 per cent of the aggregate total. Fifteen per cent of orbital tumors from the combined series are *hemangiomas*, and again, this tumor is ranked second in frequency in each of the individual tabulations. Thus, these two benign developmental tumors constitute approximately one half the orbital tumors in children. *Rhabdomyosarcoma* is the most common *malignant* orbital tumor in children if one combines the total from the three series, though this lesion was much less frequently encountered in the Washington Children's Hospital files than in those from the other two clinical centers.

Tumors which occur in the orbit secondarily (neuroblastoma, leukemia) are included in the tabulations generally when orbital involvement is the initial clinical manifestation of the primary disease process. However, Yousseffi's series, containing the greatest relative proportion of neuroblastoma, includes 3 cases in which orbital involvement did not antedate the systemic diagnosis. *Neuroblastoma* is the most frequent tumor of this type, constituting 4 per cent of all orbital tumors in the combined series, though its frequency within each of the three series ranges from 1 to 10 per cent of the total.

The commonest intraocular malignant condition of childhood, *retinoblastoma*, may extend into or recur in the orbit. One intuitively considers orbital retinoblastoma a diagnostic problem only in medically underdeveloped countries, and neither Ingalls nor Yousseffi included this tumor in his tabulations. Iliff and Green did review and include 10 examples of orbital retinoblastoma found in their files. In 2 of the 10 cases a primary orbital tumor was the presumptive clinical diagnosis, with a dense congenital cataract obscuring the fundus in one case and multiple associated facial and systemic anomalies in the other, leading clinicians to suspect an intraocular malformation rather than tumor. Thus, these two cases are explicit reminders that one should consider retinoblastoma in the differential diagnosis of childhood orbital tumors and exclude this possibility only after a thorough fundus examination has revealed no suspicious lesions. *Orbital masses arising in the socket after enucleation* for

TABLE 33–23 FREQUENCIES OF VARIOUS ORBITAL TUMORS IN CHILDREN: CLINICAL CENTERS (HISTOLOGIC DIAGNOSIS)

Tumor	Series						Total (263)	
	Ingalls		Yousseffi		Iliff and Green			
	Number of Cases	Per Cent	Number of Cases	Per Cent	Number of Cases	Per Cent	Number of Cases	Per Cent
Dermoid Cyst	15	29.4	29	46.7	39	26.0	83	31.6
Hemangioma	14	27.4	9	14.5	18	12.0	41	15.2
Rhabdomyosarcoma	4	7.8	2	3.2	16	10.7	22	8.4
Neuroblastoma	3	5.9	6	9.7	2	1.3	11	4.2
Neurofibroma	4	7.8	0	0	6	4.0	10	3.8
Pseudotumor	2	3.9	2	3.2	5	3.3	9	3.4
Glioma of optic nerve	1	2.0	1	1.6	7	4.7	9	3.4
Meningioma	1	2.0	0	0	5	3.3	6	2.3
Lymphangioma	0	0	0	0	6	4.0	6	2.3
Leukemia and lymphoma	3	5.9	0	0	2	1.3	5	1.9
Schwannoma	2	3.9	0	0	3	2.0	5	1.9
Lipoma	0	0	0	0	4	2.7	4	1.5
Microphthalmos with cyst	0	0	0	0	4	2.7	4	1.5
Postoperative granulation tissue	0	0	0	0	4	2.7	4	1.5
Retinoblastoma: Extrabulbar extension	—	—	—	—	4	2.7	4	1.5
Orbital recurrence	—	—	—	—	4	2.7	4	1.5
Orbital presentation	—	—	—	—	2	1.3	2	0.8
Teratoma	0	0	0	0	3	2.0	3	1.1
Epithelial or sebaceous cyst	0	0	2	3.2	1	0.7	3	1.1
Prolapsed fat	0	0	0	0	3	2.0	3	1.1
Unexplained proptosis	0	0	3	4.8	0	0	3	1.1
Dermolipoma	0	0	2	3.2	0	0	2	0.8
Fibrous dysplasia	0	0	1	1.6	1	0.7	2	0.8
Organizing hematoma	1	2.0	1	1.6	0	0	2	0.8
Undifferentiated sarcoma	0	0	0	0	2	1.3	2	0.8

Neurosarcoma; sphenoid wing meningioma; ectopic lacrimal gland; thyroid exophthalmos; metastatic embryonal sarcoma; meningo-encephalocele, eosinophilic granuloma; mixed tumor of lacrimal gland; leiomyosarcoma; medulloepithelioma; alveolar soft part sarcoma; metastatic astrocytoma; fibrous histiocytoma; myxosarcoma (one of each)							14	5.3

retinoblastoma may pose diagnostic difficulties. Four of the patients in the series of Iliff and Green had *recurrent orbital retinoblastoma* after enucleation. Two examples of *"postoperative granulation tissue"* (Table 33–23) from Iliff and Green's series were clinically mistaken for orbit recurrences of retinoblastoma. A third possibility in such a situation is *postirradiation sarcoma* (p. 939), though these tumors have in the past appeared several years after irradiation, at a time when recurrent retinoblastoma and orbital granulation tissue are unlikely to become manifest. Finally, *amputation neuroma* may arise as a painful nodular mass in the socket after enucleation (Wolter et al., 1971).

Although the statistically weighted differential diagnosis contained in Table 33–23 is attractive by virtue of the large number of cases analyzed, clinicians should bear in mind its limitations. All three retrospective studies rely primarily on histologic diagnosis. Therefore, lesions in which the diagnosis can be made on the basis of clinical appearance (e.g., hemangioma), radiographic appearance (e.g., mucocele), or therapeutic response (e.g., pseudotumor) will be represented infrequently in such a tabulation. Yousseffi states that he avoids this bias in his series by including cases in which the diagnosis was established clinically; however, we note that 8 of the 9 hemangiomas were obtained from pathologic rather than clinical records. This suggests that the histopathologic bias is still strong in his series, since the great majority of infantile hemangiomas are now managed without surgery (p. 1001). Thus, Table 33–23 provides guidelines to answer the question, "If a child with an orbital mass is operated upon, what are the lesions which may be encountered and what are their relative frequencies?" It does not answer the question, "If a child is seen in my office with exophthalmos, what are the various possible lesions and their relative frequencies?

The pediatric orbital tumors in the Registry of Ophthalmic Pathology at the Armed Forces Institute of Pathology were reviewed by Porterfield in 1962, and his data are summarized in Table 33–24. These figures are a step further removed from clinical relevance than those in Table 33–23, since the previously mentioned his-

TABLE 33–24 FREQUENCIES OF VARIOUS ORBITAL TUMORS IN CHILDREN: AFIP*

Tumor	Number of Cases	Per Cent of Total
Rhabdomyosarcoma	56	26.2
Glioma of optic nerve	36	16.8
Hemangioma	23	10.8
Dermoid cyst	17	7.9
Leukemia, lymphoma	12	5.7
Malignant unclassified	11	5.1
Inflammatory pseudotumor	10	4.5
Postirradiation sarcoma	6	2.8
Lymphangioma	5	2.3
Epithelial tumors of lacrimal gland	4	1.8
Neuroblastoma	3	1.4
Meningioma	3	1.4
Neurofibroma	3	1.4
Malignant schwannoma	3	1.4
Lipoma	3	1.4
Microphthalmos with cyst	3	1.4
Nonchromaffin para-ganglioma	3	1.4
Juvenile xanthogranuloma	2	0.9
Lacrimal duct cyst	2	0.9
Echinococcus cyst	2	0.9
Benign fibromatosis	2	0.9
Teratoma, granular cell myoblastoma, organizing hematoma, complex hamartoma, epithelial implantation cyst (one of each)	5	2.3
Total	214	99.6

*Armed Forces Institute of Pathology.
From Porterfield, J. F.: Orbital tumors in children: A report on 214 cases. Int. Ophthal. Clin., 2:319, 1962.

topathologic bias is compounded by the unique histopathologic referral position of the AFIP. Dermoid cysts are straightforward histopathologically and they are benign, so that a pathologist might well elect not to seek consultation concerning such a lesion, whereas he might be most anxious for a second opinion concerning a rhabdomyosarcoma. The percentages in Table 33–24 thus should be regarded as a statistical catalogue of material on file at the AFIP, and not as probability guidelines in the clinical evaluation of patients. The bias introduced by geographic selection in such tabulations is illustrated by Templeton's histopathologic review of 60 consecutive orbital tumors in African children under the age of 16 (Table 33–25). Burkitt's lymphoma is three times as frequent

TABLE 33–25 FREQUENCIES OF VARIOUS ORBITAL TUMORS IN AFRICAN CHILDREN: HISTOLOGIC DIAGNOSIS

	Number of Cases	Per Cent of Total
Burkitt's tumor	28	47
Chloroma	8	13
Myelocele	6	10
Fibrous dysplasia	6	10
Pseudotumor	3	5
Nasopharyngeal carcinoma	2	3
Rhabdomyosarcoma		
Fibrosarcoma		
Hemangioma		
Retinal anlage tumor		
Aesthesioneuroblastoma		
Neuroblastoma		
Malignant neurilemmoma	1 each	< 2 each
Total	60	

From Templeton, A. C.: Orbital tumors in African children. Brit. J. Ophthal., 55:254, 1971.

as any orbital tumor, whereas no example of the commonest childhood orbital tumor in three series from the United States, orbital dermoid, is recorded by Templeton.

The ophthalmologic staff of the Hospital for Sick Children in Toronto have provided an alternative perspective to the problem of childhood orbital tumors by summarizing the diagnoses in 257 cases of proptosis in children examined at their institution over a 24-year period. Their data are recorded in Table 33–26. They include for completeness a number of known causes of proptosis in children which are not represented in their hospital records. The value of this tabulation is two-fold. First, it is a comprehensive listing which includes the rare causes of proptosis in childhood. Second, it reminds us of common causes which are excluded by the method of ascertainment from studies based on histologic diagnosis. For example, *hyperthyroidism is the most common "cause" of noninfectious proptosis* in the Toronto series. Hyperthyroidism is not rare in children, and the proportion of hyperthyroid patients with exophthalmos is high, ranging from 33 to 82 per cent in different series. Girls outnumber boys 6 to 1, and Graves' disease with exophthalmos may be first noted at birth or any time thereafter (Hayek et al., 1970; Samuel et al., 1971). As is the case in adults, endocrine exophthalmos may occasionally be unilateral.

Dermoid Cysts

These choristomas are the most frequently encountered orbital tumors of childhood, constituting 32 per cent of the 263 cases summarized in Table 33–23.

Pathology

Although the dysembryogenetic basis for their formation is unknown, the essential lesion is an abnormal retention of ectodermal derivatives within the lid, brow, or orbit in the form of a cyst containing desquamated epithelium, cholesterol, fat, hair, and sebaceous secretions. The cyst walls are composed of keratinizing stratified squamous epithelium and pilosebaceous apparati surrounded by a condensation of connective tissue resembling normal dermis (Figs. 33–172 and 33–173).

These cysts are frequently attached to periosteum, particularly in areas adjacent to suture lines. Deep orbital dermoid cysts may in fact arise within the diploë of orbital bones and either expand the bony cortex or extend in hour-glass fashion into the orbit and adjacent intracranial or sinus cavity. The capsule of the dermoid contains a variable number of inflammatory cells, and liberation of cyst contents may elicit a granulomatous inflammatory response in the orbit (Fig. 33–174).

Clinical Features

Although dermoids are congenital tumors, less than 25 per cent are clinically evident at birth. In their review of 44 orbital dermoid cysts, Haye et al. recorded that 10 were noted at birth, 10 became manifest between birth and 12 years of age, 10 were noted between ages 12 and 30 years, and 14 were first noted after the age of 30 years. The delayed appearance of symptoms is presumably the result of gradual postnatal growth, later hemorrhage into the cyst, or orbital inflammation in response to spontaneous or traumatic release of cyst contents within the orbit. The last two mechanisms are invoked to explain the occasional dermoid which presents in later life with the acute onset of orbital mass lesion symptoms.

Many dermoid cysts have an externally visible component (Figs. 33–175 to 33–177). Most can be palpated as nontender, well-circumscribed masses of doughy to

TABLE 33–26 DIAGNOSIS IN 257 CASES OF PROPTOSIS

Lesion	Number of Cases	Lesion	Number of Cases
Developmental		Teratoma	1
Dysostosis of cranial bones	3	Lymphosarcoma	1
Craniostenosis	17	Melanoma	0
Hypertelorism	3	Lacrimal gland tumor	0
		Secondary and metastatic orbital	
Inflammatory		Neuroblastoma	6
Acute ethmoiditis (orbital cellulitis)	57	Chloroma	5
Cavernous sinus thrombosis (orbital cellulitis)	5	Hodgkin's disease	3
		Lymphoma	2
Orbital cellulitis from injury	6	Nasopharyngeal cancer	1
Orbital cellulitis (cause unknown)	6	Sarcoma of ethmoids	1
Subperiosteal orbital abscess	1	Ovarian sarcoma	1
Osteomyelitis of orbital roof	1	Retinoblastoma	1
Ethmoid mucocele	2	Neurofibromatosis	1
Chronic granuloma	1	Osteoma of antrum	1
		Juvenile angiofibroma of nasopharynx	1
Metabolic and systemic disease		Intracranial tumors involving orbit	3
Hyperthyroidism	35		
Histiocytosis X		*Vascular*	
Eosinophilic granuloma	2	Cavernous hemangioma	9
Hand-Schüller-Christian disease	16	Lymphangioma	2
Letterer-Siwe disease	1	Sturge-Weber disease	3
		Carotid-cavernous fistula	1
Diseases involving bone			
Rickets	0	*Orbital hemorrhage*	
Infantile cortical hyperostosis	0	Scurvy	3
Osteopetrosis	0	Leukemia	10
Fibrous dysplasia	0	Hemophilia	0
		Trauma	22
Neoplastic		Hemorrhagic disease of the newborn	0
Primary orbital		Subdural hemorrhage	1
Sarcoma	5	*Unknown*	10
Optic nerve glioma	4		
Dermoid and epidermoid	3		

From Ophthalmic Staff of the Hospital for Sick Children, Toronto: The Eye in Childhood. Chicago, Year Book Medical Publishers, 1967. Copyright 1967 by Year Book Medical Publishers. Used by permission.

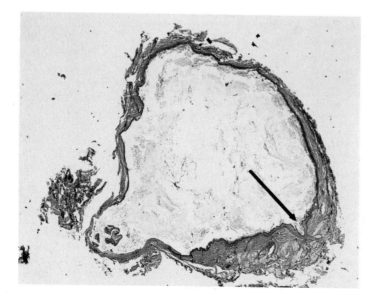

Figure 33–172 Intact dermoid cyst removed from the upper nasal quadrant of the left orbit of a 6-month-old boy. The cyst is filled with keratinous debris and lined by keratinized squamous epithelium. In addition the wall is composed of dense connective tissue in which occasional pilosebaceous apparati are located (arrow). (Hematoxylin and eosin, ×18.) (E.P. #35342)

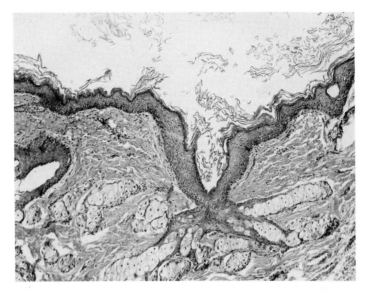

Figure 33–173 Area indicated by arrow in Figure 33–172 showing sebaceous glands opening into the dermoid cyst. (Hematoxylin and eosin, ×100.) (E.P. #35342)

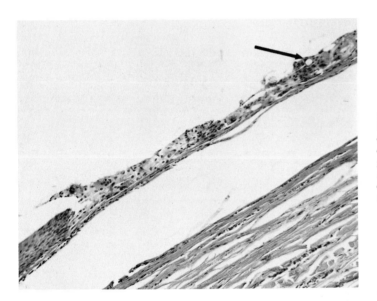

Figure 33–174 This superior temporal orbital dermoid was excised from a 27-year-old man. The lesion had been observed since the age of 5 years. The epithelial lining has been replaced by a granulomatous inflammatory infiltrate. A fine hair shaft is present within a giant cell (arrow). (Hematoxylin and eosin, ×185.) (E.P. #33704)

Figure 33–175 Superior temporal orbital dermoid in an 8-month-old child. (From Iliff, C. E., and Ossofsky, H. J., Tumors of the Eye and Adnexa in Infancy and Childhood, 1962. Courtesy of Charles C Thomas, Publisher, Springfield, Illinois.)

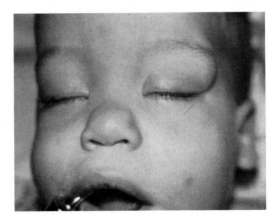

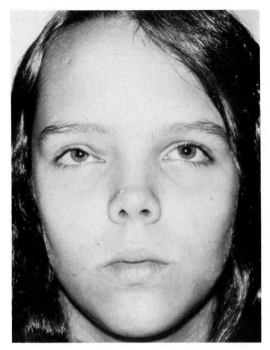

Figure 33–176 Superior nasal orbital dermoid (2 cm. in diameter) in a 15-year-old girl. First noted as a BB-sized lesion at age of 6 years. (E.P. #34104)

TABLE 33–27 LOCATION OF ORBITAL DERMOID CYSTS

Location	Number of Cases	Per Cent of Total
Upper temporal quadrant	61	49
Upper nasal quadrant	29	23
Lower nasal quadrant	14	11
Orbital roof	10	8
Lower temporal quadrant	7	6
Deep within orbit	4	3

After Haye, C., et al.: A propos des kystes dermoïdes de l'orbite. Arch. Ophtal. (Paris), 26:471, 1966.

rubbery consistency. They are frequently attached to bone by a fibrous band which restricts to some degree their passive movement on palpation. Haye et al. (1966a) have tabulated from the literature and their own case material the frequency of location of 125 orbital dermoid cysts, and these data are summarized in Table 33–27. Approximately one half of reported cases have been located in the upper temporal quadrant and approximately one fourth in the upper nasal quadrant. Thus, the latter location is not as rare as roundsmen state. Exophthalmos without palpable mass (Figs. 33–178 and 33–179), passive edema of lids and conjunctiva, ptosis, and restricted motility of the globe are other presenting signs of orbital masses which the dermoid cyst shares. In addition, inflammatory signs of orbital reaction to cyst contents may predominate, and the initial symptoms may simulate orbital cellulitis, abscess, or pseudotumor. Rarely a fistulous tract between the cyst and skin or conjunctival surface may produce intermittent drainage and periodic signs of infection which first prompt the patient to seek medical attention.

Dermoids may also be located on the brow and an example of such a lesion is illustrated in Figures 33–180 and 33–181.

Diagnostic Studies

Pfeiffer and Nicholl emphasize a characteristic *radiographic appearance* of deeply situated dermoids which arise within diploë or suture lines. These tumors produce well-circumscribed defects in the orbital bones, with an increase in density of bone at the tumor margin and a diminished radiographic density within the lesion itself (Fig. 33–182). The x-ray appearance of these lesions can be differentiated from that of *mucocele* (Fig. 33–183) (communication with sinus can be demonstrated, involved sinus relatively opacified, no increased bone density at margin of lesion); *eosinophilic granuloma of bone* (Figs. 33–184 and 33–185) (no increase in bone

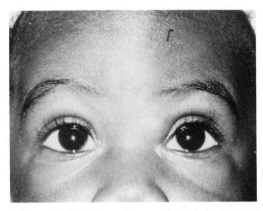

Figure 33–177 Superior nasal orbital dermoid (1.5 cm. in diameter) in a 6-month-old boy. The lesion had gradually enlarged since the age of 2 months. (E.P. #35342)

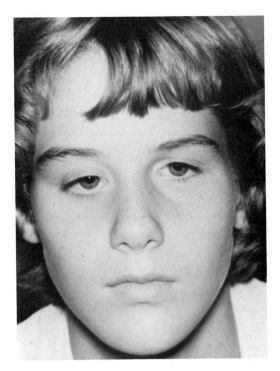

Figure 33–178 Dermoid cyst. This 12-year-old girl had gradually developed 7 mm. proptosis of the right eye over a six-year period. (Patient of Dr. C. E. Iliff.) (E.P. #29214)

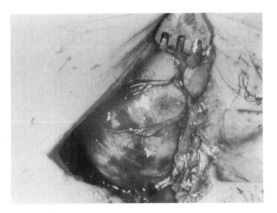

Figure 33–179 Appearance of orbital dermoid in Figure 33–178 at time of surgery. The large dermoid extended posteriorly toward the apex and then medially, measuring 3 × 3 × 2.5 cm. (E.P. #29214)

Figure 33–180 The dermoid in the brow of this 30-year-old woman had been present since birth. The clinical diagnosis was lipoma. At the time of surgery, it was found to be attached to the periosteum. (E.P. #35386)

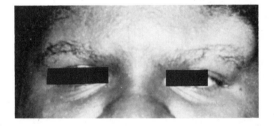

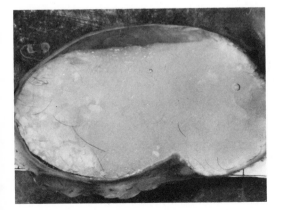

Figure 33–181 Gross appearance of the opened dermoid (measuring 33 × 23 mm.) illustrated in Figure 33–180. The cyst was filled with a yellowish material containing numerous hair shafts. (E.P. #35386)

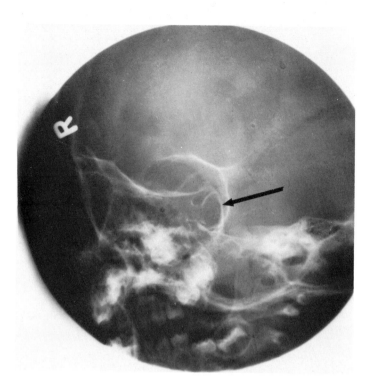

Figure 33–182 Slightly atypical optic foramen view showing an oval radiolucent area with sclerotic margins (arrow) involving the greater wing of the sphenoid in a 2-year-old with an orbital dermoid.

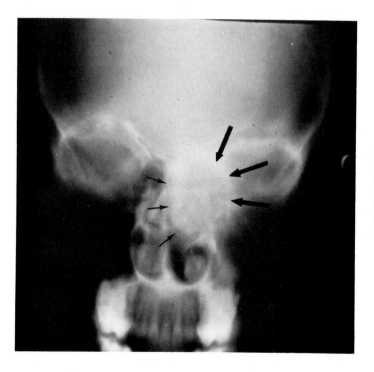

Figure 33–183 Mucocele. Tomogram demonstrates opacification and expansion of the left ethmoid sinus. The lateral wall of the sinus (large arrows) encroaches on the orbit and the medial wall deviates the nasal septum (small arrows). At other levels communication with frontal and maxillary sinuses could also be demonstrated.

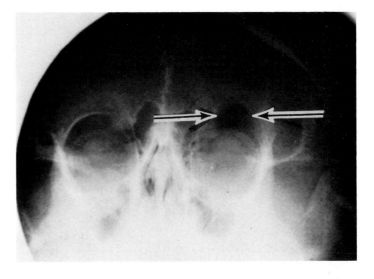

Figure 33–184 X-ray appearance of eosinophilic granuloma involving the frontal bone. Arrows indicate an osteolytic area with no increased bone density at margin. (E.P. #18503)

density at margin of lesion); and *meningocele* or *encephalocele* (Fig. 33–186) (characteristic origin in upper nasal quadrant, communication with cranial cavity on tomograms). Other lesions producing radiographic changes which may be confused with those of the dermoid are meningioma, ossifying fibroma of bone (Fig. 33–249), and orbital wall defects associated with neurofibromatosis (Fig. 33–187). If intracranial extension of the dermoid is suspected, additional neuroradiologic diagnostic procedures should be undertaken to define the extent of intracranial involvement. *Ultrasonography* may be of value in differentiating these cystic orbital lesions from solid tumors.

Prognosis and Treatment

When the cysts are located anteriorly, complete surgical excision can be accomplished without difficulty, and an excellent technique for their removal has been described by Iliff (Iliff and Ossofsky, 1962). A well-defined cleavage plane surrounds the tumor, and its connections to surrounding orbital structures and to periosteum are relatively avascular. If the cyst is ruptured during delivery, postoperative orbital inflammation can be minimized by irrigation

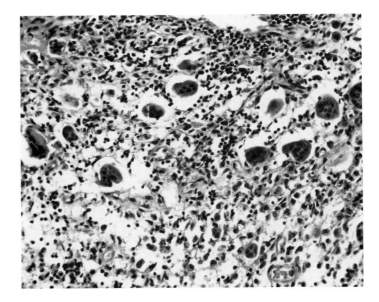

Figure 33–185 Eosinophilic granuloma. Leson consists of eosinophils, mononuclear cells, and multinucleated giant cells, some of which are vacuolated. (E.P. #18503)

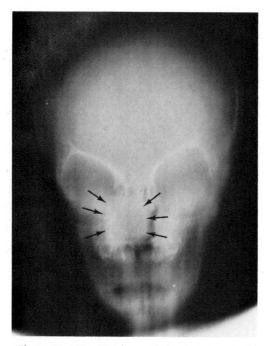

Figure 33–186   Nasal encephalocele (arrows) with right orbital involvement.

curring after previous incomplete surgical excision pose a much more difficult problem in management. Four recurrences were noted among the 45 orbital dermoid cysts reviewed by Haye et al. (1966a), and all could be attributed to incomplete primary excision.

If intracranial involvement is demonstrated radiographically, a neurosurgical approach should be employed as in Carey's series. When a portion of the cyst and its capsule are located posteriorly in the region of the orbital apex, it may be impossible to remove the cyst completely without seriously jeopardizing the function of the eye. In these cases chemical cauterization of the cyst cavity with carbolic acid or trichloroacetic acid has been recommended. Kennedy (1970) recently treated such a patient by marsupialization of the cyst cavity to create a permanently draining cutaneous fistula. External irradiation is of no value in treating surgically inaccessible lesions.

of cyst contents from the orbital tissue, or, if necessary, suppressed by a short postoperative course of systemically administered steroids. Dermoids arising within the orbit, within the bones of the orbit, or re-

Hemangiomas

A small red "beauty mark" on the eyelid of a newborn girl begins in a few months to enlarge rapidly (Fig. 33–188), and the irony of that initial euphemism becomes

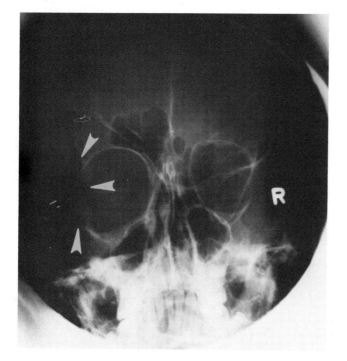

Figure 33–187   Defect in sphenoid bone (arrows) and enlarged orbit in patient with neurofibromatosis.

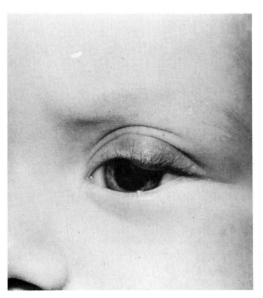

Figure 33–188 Two-year-old girl with a small hemangioma of the left upper lid which was present at birth, grew larger, and then had begun to regress at the time of this photograph. (Courtesy of Dr. A. E. Maumenee.)

increasingly apparent as the disfiguring mass extends over a wider and wider area, periodically bleeds, ulcerates, or becomes inflamed. Dealing with such a patient over a period of several years presents a challenge as demanding as any in pediatric ophthalmology, and the first step toward successful management is a confident, thorough understanding of the natural course of the lesion.

Clinical and Histologic Terminology

The multiplicity of dermatologic and histologic terms for each type of lesion is frequently confusing to the ophthalmologist. The simplified clinical terminology which we prefer stresses the single most important feature of these lesions — that *the great majority of infantile hemangiomas spontaneously regress.* The type of lesions which generally follow a predictable pattern of regression are classified as *involuting hemangiomas* in Table 33–28. Those which do not regress spontaneously and which generally keep pace with the child's growth are termed *noninvoluting hemangiomas.* The relative frequencies of the various types are derived from a series of 347 cutaneous hemangiomas observed over a period of several years by Margileth and Museles.

Since the diagnosis is usually evident clinically, biopsy is not performed in the majority of cases, and the histologic features listed in Table 33–28 are neither as important nor as firmly documented in all cases as the clinical appearance and behavior.

Histogenesis

All of the commonly encountered lesions are hamartomas rather than true neoplasms. If the proliferated capillaries retain the usual appearance of endothelial cells and supporting tissues, the histologic picture of capillary hemangioma (Figs. 33–189 and 33–190) typified by the port-wine stain is produced. Coalescence of these channels or the presence of anastomosing venules produces the histologic picture of cavernous hemangioma (Figs. 33–191 and 33–192). In infants, both capillary and cavernous hemangiomas often exhibit a proliferation of endothelial cells which is not found in adult-type lesions and which, when extensive, produces the histologic picture of benign hemangioendothelioma. Proliferation of the other cellular capillary component — the pericyte — to form a benign hemangiopericytoma is probably not as disproportionately rare in childhood as was previously thought (Backwinkel and Diddams, 1970). An example of hemangiopericytoma arising as a deep lid tumor in a 13-year-old girl has been reported by Oshida et al. (1970). Benign hemangioendothelioma and hemangiopericytoma are probably neoplasms rather than hamartomas, and both may be locally invasive or recur after excision. Further discussion of these rare tumors and of the remaining category of possible vascular neoplasm — Kaposi's sarcoma — may be found in the articles by Kauffman and Stout (1960, 1961), Backwinkel and Diddams (1970), Ortega et al. (1971) and Dutz and Stout (1965).

INVOLUTING HEMANGIOMAS

Natural Course*

The three types of involuting infantile hemangioma (Table 33–28) follow a similar pattern of evolution. Over 80 per cent of the tumors in these three cate-

---

*Bowers et al., 1960; Lampe and Latourette, 1959; Margileth and Museles, 1965; Simpson, 1959.

TABLE 33–28 HEMANGIOMAS IN INFANTS: CLINICAL AND HISTOLOGIC FEATURES

Type	Clinical Characteristics	Histologic Patterns	Relative Proportions (%)
Involuting Hemangiomas			
Capillary hemangioma of infancy (strawberry mark)	Bright or purplish-red with well defined borders; solid mass on palpation, compresses minimally and blanches incompletely with pressure.	Myriad minute capillaries frequently exhibiting endothelial proliferation.	78.0
Mixed cavernous and capillary hemangioma	Cavernous type with overlying capillary component. Spontaneous resolution of capillary component only.	Features of infantile capillary and cavernous hemangioma both present.	9.0
Cavernous hemangioma	Hypodermal tumors are subsurface with poorly defined borders. Dermal lesions are elevated and well circumscribed. Reddish-blue discoloration of overlying skin which may darken with straining or crying. "Bag of worms" on palpation, compresses easily to half original size with pressure.	Larger confluent capillary channels composed of mature vascular elements.	7.0
Noninvoluting Hemangiomas			
Port-wine stain (nevus flammeus)	Pink to deep burgundy color, not elevated, often distributed along the course of trigeminal nerve, bilateral in minority of cases. Does not blanch with pressure.	Thin-walled capillary vessels throughout dermis; areas of cavernous hemangioma may be present.	1.8
Hemangiolymphangioma	Combines features of lymphangioma with one of hemangioma types.	Combines features of lymphangioma and one of hemangioma types.	1.8
Spider nevus (nevus araneus)	Central red spot from which small venules radiate. Fills from center after compression. Occasionally disappears after puberty.	Telangiectatic venous channels with central arteriole.	1.8
Venous angioma	Clinically similar to cavernous hemangioma.	Anastomosing vascular spaces which contain smooth muscle layer characteristic of venous channels.	1.0

After Margileth, A. M., and Museles, M.: Cutaneous hemangiomas in children; diagnosis and conservative management. J.A.M.A., *194*:523, 1965; and Reed, R. J., and O'Quinn, S. E.: Vascular neoplasms. *In* Fitzpatrick, T. B. New York, McGraw-Hill Book Co., 1971, p. 533.

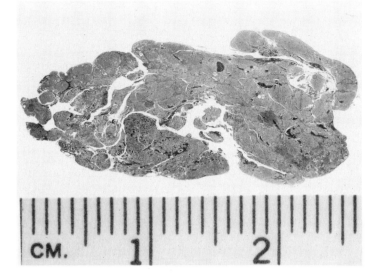

Figure 33–189 Capillary hemangioma of the orbit from a 4-month-old girl. The lesion began to enlarge when the patient was 3 weeks old. The preoperative clinical impression was "probable hemangioma." Complete excision of the mass was attempted even though the lacrimal gland was intimately involved. Fortunately, she did not develop postoperative complications related to the extensive surgery which was required. (Hematoxylin and eosin, ×4.5.) (E.P. #20177)

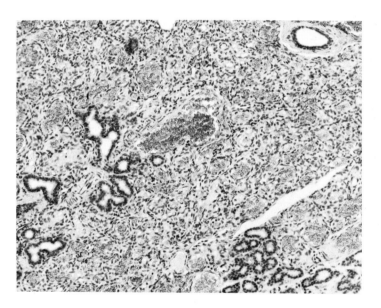

Figure 33–190 Highly cellular capillary hemangioma intermixed with acini and ducts of the lacrimal gland. (Hematoxylin and eosin, ×180.) (E.P. #20177)

Figure 33–191 Small, discrete, and encapsulated cavernous hemangioma of the orbit from an adult. (E.P. #30476)

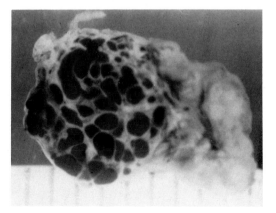

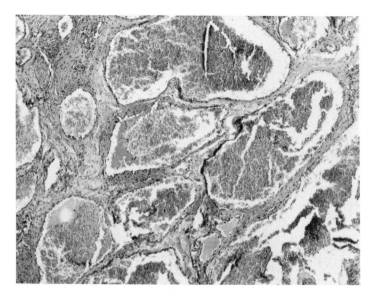

Figure 33–192 Cavernous hemangioma with large vascular spaces lined by normal endothelium and separated by fibrous tissue septa. (Hematoxylin and eosin, ×70.) (E.P. #30476).

gories spontaneously regress (Margileth and Museles, 1965). They occur twice as frequently in girls as in boys and are either present at birth or appear in the first half-year of life. About 15 per cent of the lesions will not increase in size, but the great majority do enlarge over a 6- to 9-month period (Fig. 33–193). After the phase of rapid growth, a stationary or quiescent period ensues which may last from several months to several years. In approximately 80 per cent of the lesions which do eventually regress, early signs of involution are apparent by 12 months of age (Lampe and Latourette, 1959). The phase of spontaneous regression lasts for several years, occasionally through puberty. Margileth and Museles found that involution was maximal by age 3 years in 30 per cent, 4 years in 60 per cent,

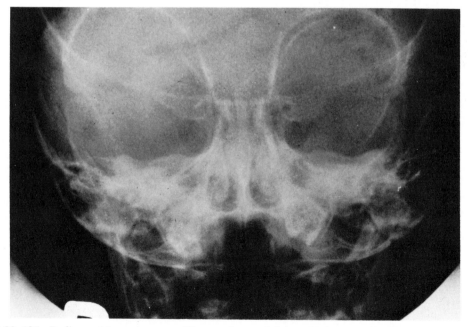

Figure 33–193 Radiographic appearance of hemangioma of right orbit in 4-month-old girl. The right orbit is enlarged and demonstrates increased soft tissue density compared with the left.

and 7 years in 76 per cent of the lesions which they observed.

The initial manifestation of involution is a fading of the bright red color to dull red or pink and finally to gray-white. The color change appears at the center of the lesion first and then gradually extends peripherally. Later, a reduction in volume is first detected as a diminished turgidity of the hemangioma, accompanied by a less tense, even wrinkled, appearance of the overlying skin. The thickness of the lesion then diminishes, and the area of involvement decreases late, if at all (Lampe and Latourette, 1959).

The observations which have been cited thus far are derived from large series of cutaneous angiomas without special reference to those of the lid and orbit. Holland (1968) has presented evidence that our application of this same reasoning to lid lesions is valid. He reported a series of 44 children with lid hemangiomas, 32 of whom were observed without treatment for several years. All 32 of the untreated lesions showed signs of regression, and in 22 (69 per cent) involution was cosmetically complete. Signs of regression were first noted by the age of 2 years in 28 patients and were generally maximal by 4 to 6 years of age.

Local complications during the phase of rapid growth are unusual (less than 5 per cent of lesions) but can include bleeding, ulceration, and local infection. A rare systemic complication associated with large lesions is the development of thrombocytopenia (Kasabach-Merritt syndrome). The ocular complication which is most frequently a source of concern is obstruction of the visual axis by an enlarged lid at an age when amblyopia can develop rapidly and irreversibly.

Treatment

The majority of infantile hemangiomas are best treated by careful observation. Surgery, radiotherapy, cryotherapy, or injection of sclerosing solutions undertaken at an early age for purely cosmetic reasons may produce worse scarring and a higher incidence of complications than would the natural course of spontaneous resolution in the involuting lesions, and these forms of therapy generally fail to improve the appearance of large noninvoluting lesions.

Thus, in the majority of cases management is directed primarily toward enlisting the confidence, cooperation, and patience of the parents. A straightforward explanation of the natural course of the majority of lesions and of the difficulty and possible deleterious effects of more aggressive therapy, plus serial photographs to document the process of gradual involution, help instill a parental attitude which will best minimize psychological trauma while nature is following a course which will best minimize the cosmetic defect.

In those lesions which enlarge at an alarmingly rapid rate or which threaten to obstruct vision, the treatment of choice is systemically administered corticosteroids. Although the mechanism of their action is unknown, these drugs have proved effective in arresting growth of the lesions and in accelerating their regression. A regimen of 20 mg. prednisone or equivalent per day for a period of 2 to 4 weeks with subsequent gradual tapering and discontinuation over a 2- to 4-month period has been effective, though exacerbations may necessitate reinstitution of larger doses during the period of corticosteroid dosage reduction (deVenecia and Lobeck, 1970; Fost and Esterly, 1968; Hiles and Pilchard, 1971). *Treatment should be discontinued in patients whose lesions do not respond after a 3-week trial.* The adverse consequences of exogenous corticosteroid administration in infants are serious enough to demand careful consideration before institution of therapy, meticulous follow-up during the course of therapy, and reduction of drug dosage as soon as improvement is noted with the intention of discontinuing the drug within the shortest period of time possible.

An early example of successful prednisone therapy of lid and orbital hemangioma is illustrated in Figures 33–194 to 33–196 through the courtesy of Dr. Irvin Pollack. When the patient was 6 weeks old, her parents first noted fullness of the right upper lid which progressed gradually until age 3 months, when a more rapid increase in size and bluish discoloration were noted (Figs. 33–194 and 33–195). On July 17, 1967, Dr. Mary Ellen Avery of the Department of Pediatrics began treatment with 20 mg. prednisone per day. Within one week definite improvement was noted, and prednisone

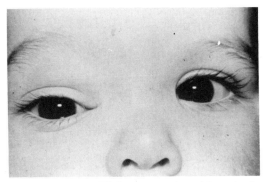

Figure 33–194 Slight proptosis evident in 3-month-old girl with hemangioma of the lid, conjunctiva, and orbit. (Courtesy of Dr. I. P. Pollack.)

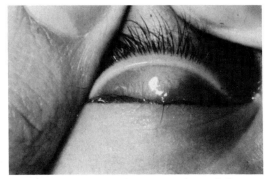

Figure 33–196 Marked regression of hemangioma shown in Figures 33–194 and 33–195 after six-week course of systemically administered prednisone.

dosage was reduced. By the end of the 6-week course of therapy, the hemangioma had regressed dramatically (Fig. 33–196).

Lesions which have become static in size may not improve with corticosteroid therapy (Fost and Esterly, 1968). If a trial of corticosteroid therapy fails to arrest tumor growth or restore an unobstructed visual axis, the alternative modes of therapy which may be considered are irradiation (Figs. 33–197 and 33–198) (Lampe and Latourette, 1959) or surgical excision and primary closure (Simpson, 1959). Cryotherapy by surface application has not been useful in larger lesions, though newer methods of deep tumor cryotherapy may in the future merit consideration. Before undertaking any of these modalities the physician should (1) critically review the reports of their use and (2) assure himself that there is no associated fundus abnor-

mality which might render futile aggressive treatment of a lid hemangioma in an effort to prevent amblyopia.

Although the lesion is generally considered rare in childhood, 2 of the 6 patients with *cavernous hemangioma* of the orbit reported by Kopelow et al. (1971) were under 15 years of age. In patients with this lesion orbital venography and ultrasonography may be of diagnostic value, and the surgical removal of this well-encapsulated tumor is more easily accomplished than is the case with capillary hemangiomas of infancy. A *varix* of the lid or orbit (Fig. 33–199) can generally be clinically differentiated from cavernous hemangioma by its easier compressibility and its engorgement when venous pressure is increased by Valsalva maneuver or lowering the head position.

NONINVOLUTING HEMANGIOMAS: PORT-WINE STAIN (NEVUS FLAMMEUS)

These pink to deep burgundy-colored macular vascular malformations may involve the lids and adjacent face as isolated congenital anomalies or in association with a venous angioma of the leptomeninges of the cerebral cortex in the Sturge-Weber syndrome. In the occasional patient with bilateral angioma the ocular concomitants—glaucoma, episcleral angioma, choroidal angioma—may likewise be bilateral (Figs. 33–78 to 33–82). The facial angioma is best treated with a cosmetic application such as Covermark (Reed and O'Quinn, 1971). The ophthalmologists' primary concern is the detection and treat-

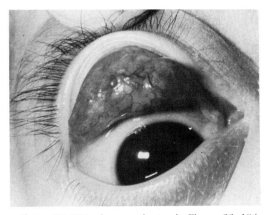

Figure 33–195 Same patient as in Figure 33–194. The upper lid is pulled up, allowing the hemangioma to prolapse.

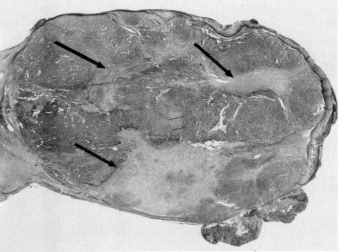

Figure 33–197 This large sclerosing hemangioma was removed from the orbit of a 24-year-old man. It had been present for 10 years and had previously been incompletely excised and treated with irradiation. The lesion is encapsulated and has large areas of fibrous tissue scarring (arrows). (Hematoxylin and eosin, ×7.5.) (E.P. #8766)

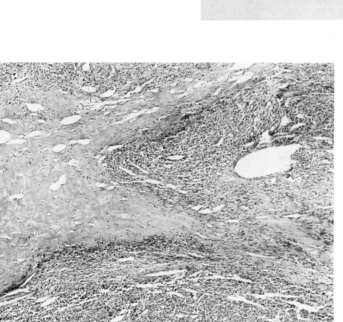

Figure 33–198 Strands of fibrous tissue within a highly cellular capillary hemangioma. (Hematoxylin and eosin, ×75.) (E.P. #8766)

Figure 33–199 Orbital varix in a 3-year-old girl.

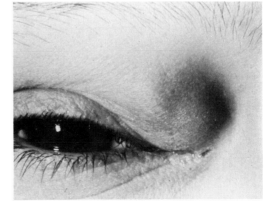

ment of glaucoma, which may not appear until later childhood.

Lymphangiomas

The majority of *lid lymphangiomas* appear as noncompressible firm masses at or soon after birth, involving the upper lid more frequently than the lower. In contrast to the rapid, self-limited growth of infantile hemangiomas, lymphangiomas continue to enlarge slowly during the growing years. If an associated conjunctival extension of the lid lesion is present, the characteristic slit-lamp appearance of the clear, cystic, sinuous conjunctival mass provides a clue to diagnosis. Other features suggestive of lymphangioma are repeated spontaneous ecchymosis, rapid enlargement of the lesion after minor injuries, and secondary cellulitis with or without a concurrent upper respiratory infection. Any of these features may more rarely be seen with hemangiomas, however, and diagnosis usually depends on interpretation of combined clinical and histologic evidence.

Jones' comprehensive study (1959) included 29 patients with *orbital lymphangioma.* In 10 cases the lesion was present at birth and in 11 it appeared between birth and 5 years of age. Sixteen of the patients had associated lid, conjunctival, or facial extension of the orbital tumor. Exophthalmos was present in all patients, and in 6 the exophthalmos was associated with ecchymosis or hemorrhage. In 16 of 22 patients for whom x-ray studies were available, the orbit was radiographically enlarged. The lesion with which orbital lymphangioma is most frequently confused clinically is *hemangioma.* Points of difference are (1) hemangiomas grow at a more rapidly progressive rate, (2) spontaneous regression does not occur in lymphangioma, and (3) associated hemorrhage and cellulitis are more frequent with lymphangioma. Whether response to systemic corticosteroid therapy is a further differential feature is at present uncertain. We have seen an 8-month-old patient in whom a lower lid mass with ecchymosis increased in size after an upper respiratory infection. He was admitted to the hospital with a pre-

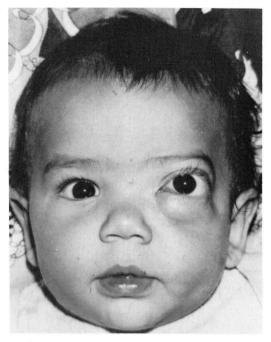

Figure 33–200 Eight-month-old boy with history of rapidly developing proptosis associated with an upper respiratory infection. The lesion was thought to be a lymphangioma both preoperatively and at the time of surgery. Biopsy proved the lesion to be an embryonal rhabdomyosarcoma. (E.P. #35436)

sumptive diagnosis of lymphangioma (Fig. 33–200). Palpation of the mass under general anesthesia gave the impression of a cystic, freely movable lesion, and at operation (Fig. 33–201) a somewhat bluish encapsulated tumor was encountered which was regarded as a perfect clinical and operative example of lymphangioma with ev-

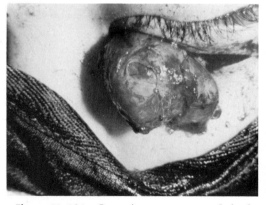

Figure 33–201 Operative appearance of the lesion in Figure 33–200. It had a cystic consistency and bluish color and was thought to be encapsulated. (E.P. #35436)

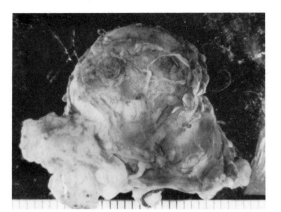

Figure 33-202 Excised pseudolymphangioma, measuring $3 \times 2 \times 2$ cm. (E.P. #35436)

idence of hemorrhage. Histologic sections, however, revealed *embryonal rhabdomyosarcoma* (Figs. 33-202 to 33-205), and exenteration was performed when systemic evaluation showed no evidence of metastasis.

Pathology

These hamartomas are poorly demarcated lesions with variable amounts of connective tissue stroma separating anastomosing channels which contain pale eosinophilic serous fluid. In contrast to infantile hemangiomas, the endothelial cells do not exhibit a proliferative tendency (Fig. 33-206). Nearby blood vessels sev-

ered during excision of the tumor may spill erythrocytes into the lymph channels, and in these instances the clinical history is necessary for interpretation of the histologic appearance. A round-cell inflammatory infiltration of varying intensity (Fig. 33-207), with lymphoid follicles in some instances, may be distributed through the connective tissue stroma. Episodes of spontaneous ecchymosis or rapid enlargement after minor trauma or incomplete excision (Figs. 33-208 and 33-209) may result when hemorrhage into lymph channels causes *blood cyst* formation.

Treatment

Surgical excision, though difficult, is the only reliable method of treatment. It is often impossible to remove completely the poorly encapsulated lesions whose margins are further obscured at surgery by blood from the congested adjacent tissue. Dr. Charles Iliff has observed that some lymphangiomas, on the other hand, have a surprisingly discrete margin which permits fairly easy dissection and total removal (Figs. 33-210 to 33-213). The rare cases which exhibit a partial beneficial response to x-ray therapy are believed to do so as the result of reduction in the stromal inflammatory reaction. Systemically administered corticosteroids should achieve a similar effect in such cases.

(Text continued on page 1023)

Figure 33-203 Embryonal rhabdomyosarcoma with some compact highly cellular zones and other areas of loose spindle-shaped cells. (Hematoxylin and eosin, ×190.) (E.P. #35436)

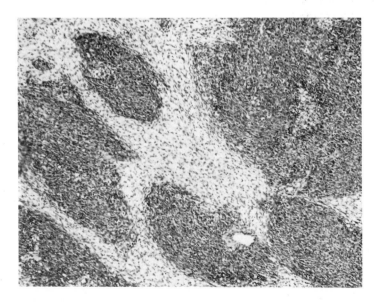

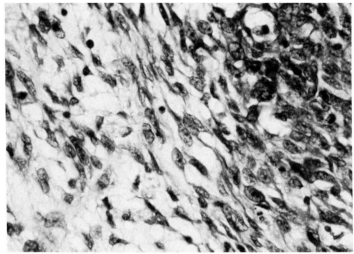

Figure 33–204 Embryonal rhabdomyosarcoma in an area of probable rhabdomyoblastic differentiation with spindle-shaped cells and strap cells. (Hematoxylin and eosin, ×545.) (E.P. #35436)

Figure 33–205 Exenteration of the orbit in case illustrated in Figures 33–200 to 33–204. Even after excision of the apparently encapsulated tumor mass shown in Figure 33–202, a large portion remained in the orbit (arrows). (Hematoxylin and eosin, ×3) (E.P. #35470)

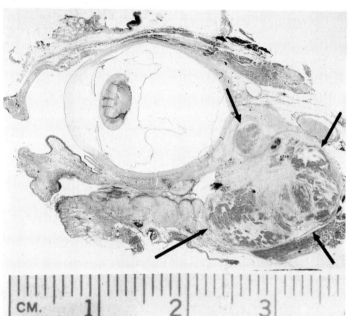

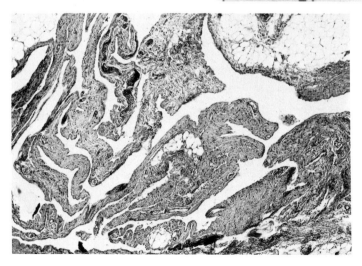

Figure 33–206 Lymphangioma of the orbit in a 2-year-old boy. The right eye had been prominent since birth, but this had increased in the two months prior to admission. The lesion consists of numerous large vascular channels lined with normal endothelium. Very little lymphoid tissue is present. (Hematoxylin and eosin, ×60.) (E.P. #16318)

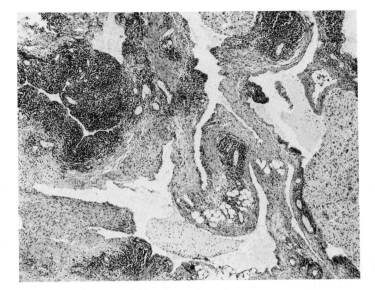

Figure 33–207 Lymphangioma of the orbit of a 10-year-old girl who experienced proptosis of the left eye following a middle ear infection four months before. The proptosis persisted, and the clinical diagnosis was dermoid. The lesion is composed of large endothelially lined vascular spaces filled with lymph. Considerable lymphocytic infiltration is present in surrounding tissues. (Hematoxylin and eosin, ×45.) (E.P. #9894)

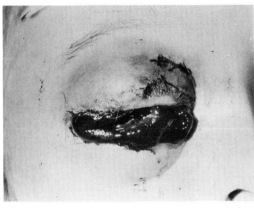

Figure 33–208 Lymphangioma of the orbit. This 7-year-old girl with proptosis of the right eye and mass in the upper lid had a previous excision at the age of 1 year. Severe orbital hemorrhage occurred in the early postoperative period. The tumor gradually increased in size over the ensuing years. At the time of her second excision, lymphangioma was observed in the orbit, lids, and conjunctiva. The result has been satisfactory. (Case of Dr. C. E. Iliff.) (E.P. #34934)

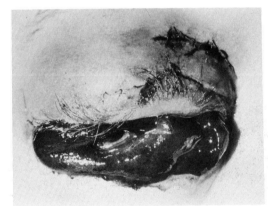

Figure 33–209 Enlargement of Figure 33–208.

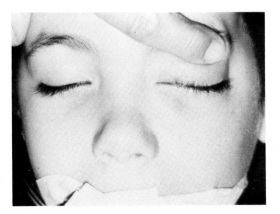

Figure 33–210 Lymphangioma of the orbit. This 6-year-old girl presented with a six-month history of proptosis and a blue, cystic mass in the left lower lid below the eye. (Case of Dr. C. E. Iliff.) (E.P. #34635)

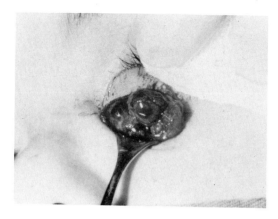

Figure 33–211 At surgery a lobulated grayish-blue, cystic, encapsulated mass was found and was totally excised. (E.P. #34635)

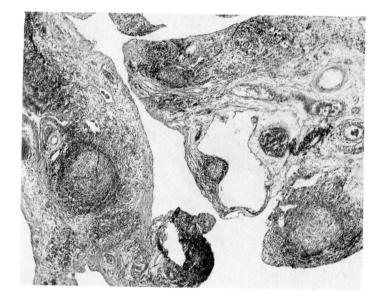

Figure 33–212 Lymphangioma of the orbit. Sections of the 25 × 12 × 12 mm. specimen (Figures 33–210 and 33–211) disclosed large vascular channels containing lymph. The intervening stroma contains a prominent lymphoid infiltrate with follicles. (Hematoxylin and eosin, ×40.) (E.P. #34635)

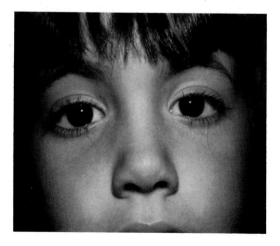

Figure 33–213 One year after excision of lymphangioma shown in Figures 33–210 to 33–212. (E.P. #34635)

Rhabdomyosarcomas

Rhabdomyosarcoma is the most common primary orbital malignant condition in childhood and ranks with Wilms' tumor and neuroblastoma as one of the three most frequent soft tissue malignant conditions in the body in this age group (Porterfield and Zimmerman, 1962; Sutow et al., 1970). Over 90 per cent of orbital rhabdomyosarcomas occur in children under the age of 16 years.

Pathology

Each of the three largest published series of study of orbital rhabdomyosarcoma employs a different histologic classification. Although we shall use the classification of Porterfield and Zimmerman, the reader is advised to expect variations in terminology in other articles on the subject.

Embryonal Type

Seventy-three per cent of orbital rhabdomyosarcomas reviewed by Porterfield and Zimmerman were in this histopathologic category (Table 33–29). The individual cells are generally stellate, round, or spindle-shaped with round or oval nuclei, and they are arranged either in a loose syncytium or in bands of more closely packed cells (Figs. 33–203, 33–204, and 33–214). Cells with ribbon- or straplike eosinophilic cytoplasm are the most likely

TABLE 33–29 ORBITAL RHABDOMYOSARCOMA: FREQUENCY OF HISTOLOGIC TYPES

Histologic Type	Number of Cases	Per Cent of Total
Embryonal	40	73
Alveolar	9	16
Differentiated	6	11

From Porterfield, J. F., and Zimmerman, L. E.: Rhabdomyosarcoma of the orbit; a clinicopathologic study of 55 cases. Virchows Arch. Path. Anat., *335*: 329, 1962.

to contain longitudinal myofibrils or cross striations (Figs. 33–215 and 33–216). The cytoplasm of rhabdomyoblasts stains bright red with Masson's trichrome, a useful adjunct in the search for cells which are most likely to contain myofibrils or cross striations. A second special stain, phosphotungstic acid–hematoxylin (PTAH), is sometimes helpful in the identification of cross striations. Porterfield and Zimmerman were able to identify unequivocal cross striations in 60 per cent of their embryonal rhabdomyosarcomas. These tumors are believed to arise from a primitive mesenchymal nest rather than from formed skeletal muscle, and anaplastic areas in an embryonal rhabdomyosarcoma are morphologically similar to embryonic mesenchyme.

Alveolar rhabdomyosarcoma was second in

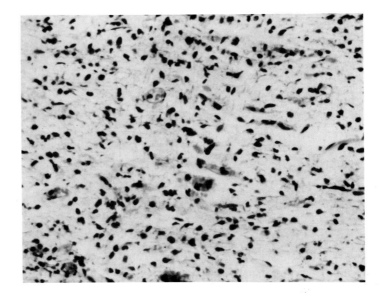

Figure 33–214 Embryonal rhabdomyosarcoma with a loose syncytial arrangement. Cytoplasmic streaming, a possible rudimentary feature of rhabdomyoblastic differentiation, is present in some cells. (Hematoxylin and eosin, ×300.) (E.P. #33136)

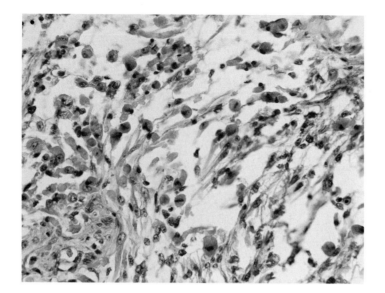

Figure 33–215 Area of differentiated rhabdomyosarcoma with large round cells with abundant cytoplasm (rhabdomyoblasts) and numerous strap cells. (Hematoxylin and eosin, ×260.) (E.P. #23475)

frequency to the embryonal type in Porterfield and Zimmerman's series (Table 33–29). This tumor consists of irregular groups and nests of poorly differentiated cells which exhibit a general loss of cohesion with formation of alveolar spaces (Figs. 33–217 and 33–218). The cell nests are separated and surrounded by a framework of delicate fibrous trabeculae, to which the peripherally located cells may adhere in a manner reminiscent of adenocarcinoma. Neoplastic rhabdomyoblasts could be identified in 77 per cent of the 110 cases of alveolar rhabdomyosarcoma in the AFIP general pathology files,

whereas only 29 per cent exhibited unequivocal cross striation (Enzinger and Shiraki, 1969). In contrast to embryonal rhabdomyosarcoma, 3 of the 9 orbital cases of the alveolar type in Porterfield and Zimmerman's series were thought to have arisen from preformed skeletal muscle.

An unusual case of alveolar rhabdomyosarcoma has been followed by Dr. C. E. Iliff for the past 12 years (Figs. 33–217 to 33–221). The patient was born with a proptotic left eye (Fig. 33–219). When examined at the age of 3 weeks the eye was proptosed 2.5 cm. The orbit was firm but slightly compressible, and a palpable mass

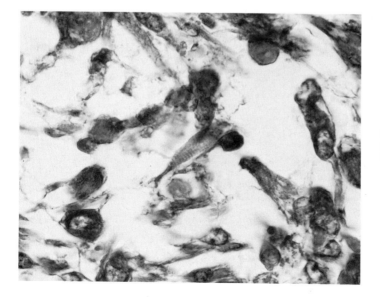

Figure 33–216 Large differentiated cell with well-delineated cross-striations. (Hematoxylin and eosin, ×900.) (E.P. #23475)

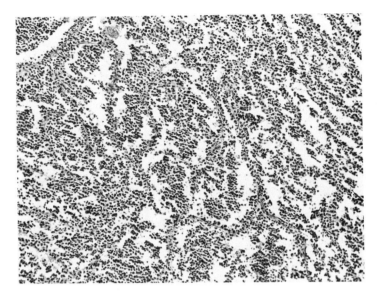

Figure 33–217 Alveolar rhabdomyosarcoma. Fine strands of connective tissue separate the tumor cells into an alveolar pattern. (Hematoxylin and eosin, ×115.) (E.P. #19218)

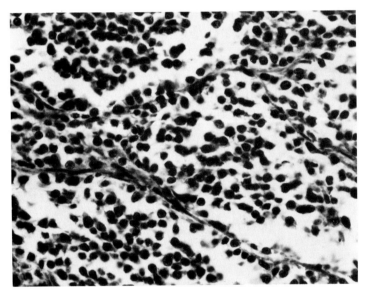

Figure 33–218 Alveolar rhabdomyosarcoma. The delicate strands separate clones of tumor cells, some of which appear to attach to the trabeculae. No cross-striations were observed. (Hematoxylin and eosin, ×470.) E.P. #19218)

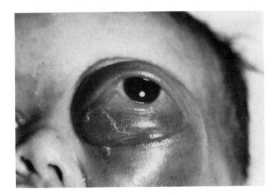

Figure 33–219 Three-week-old child born with proptosis of the left eye. The first clinical impression was orbital teratoma. The lesion grew rapidly and biopsy showed a "malignant sarcoma." (E.P. #19218)

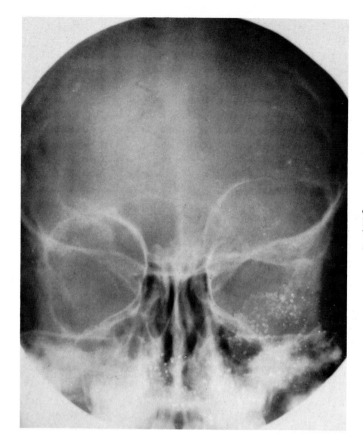

Figure 33–220 Greatly enlarged left orbit due to alveolar rhabdomyosarcoma. No evidence of bony extension of tumor. White stippling over lower portion of orbit and nasal cavity is artifact. (E.P. #19218)

was present in the inferior orbit. On x-ray the orbit was enlarged but showed no evidence of bone invasion (Fig. 33–220). A biopsy was initially interpreted as undifferentiated sarcoma, but later review by Dr. Lorenz E. Zimmerman and others (AFIP 919470) established the diagnosis of alveolar rhabdomyosarcoma. After biopsy Dr. Iliff exenterated the orbit (Fig. 33–221). The patient is alive and well after almost 13 years!

Differentiated rhabdomyosarcoma was the

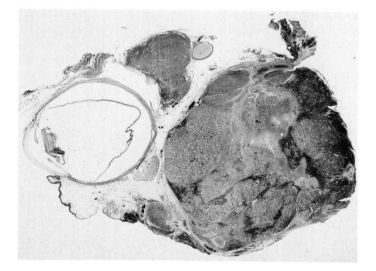

Figure 33–221 Extensive replacement of orbital tissue by the congenital alveolar rhabdomyosarcoma shown in Figures 33–219 and 33–220. (Hematoxylin and eosin, ×2.) (E.P. #19218)

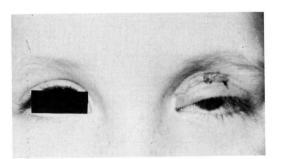

Figure 33–222 This eight-year-old boy initially developed an inflamed nodular lid lesion which the surgeon interpreted as a chalazion. At the time of curettage the surgeon became suspicious and submitted a small piece of tissue to our laboratory. A histologic diagnosis of rhabdomyosarcoma was made, and the patient was referred to the Wilmer Clinic. At this time he had ptosis and limitation of upward gaze but no proptosis. (E.P. #33136)

least frequent histologic type encountered by Porterfield and Zimmerman. Only 6 of their 55 cases were of this variety, and 2 of the 6 were from patients over the age of 20. This category is used for those cases in which virtually every cell has a ribbon of abundant eosinophilic cytoplasm, numerous cells with myofibrils are present, cross striations are found with relative ease, and mitotic figures are less common.

We have recently studied a case in which rhabdomyosarcoma was intimately con-nected with the superior rectus, surrounding this muscle as it extended posteriorly toward the apex of the orbit (Figs. 33–222 to 33–224). In some highly differentiated areas almost every tumor cell was a strap cell (Figs. 33–225 and 33–226). The bulk of the tumor, however, was of the embryonal type (Figs. 33–214 and 33–224).

Several ultrastructural studies of orbital rhabdomyosarcoma (Kroll, 1967; Polack et al., 1971; Schuster et al., 1972) demonstrate the value of electron microscopy in examining poorly differentiated tumors in which cross striations or myofibrils cannot be detected by light microscopy. Electron microscopic studies have also documented rhabdomyoblastic differentiation in an unusual iris tumor (Naumann et al., 1972) and in teratoid cerebellar tumors which resemble medulloblastoma (Misugi and Liss, 1970).

Clinical Features

The average age of onset is between 7 and 8 years. Orbital rhabdomyosarcoma is extremely rare after the age of 20, though instances of its occurrence as late as the eighth decade have been recorded (Polack et al., 1971). In the majority of cases the presenting sign is unilateral proptosis which frequently progresses at an alarming rate. Ptosis accompanies the exoph-

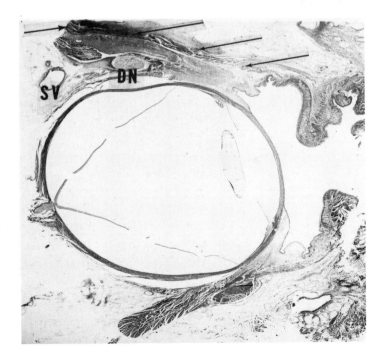

Figure 33–223 Exenteration specimen demonstrated tumor in and around the superior rectus muscle throughout its extent (arrows). Tumor was present in tissue removed separately from the orbital apex. The superior ophthalmic vein (S.V.) is surrounded by a thin rim of tumor which in one area had replaced the wall, giving tumor cells direct access to the vessel lumen. A large nodule of highly differentiated tumor is present (DN) between the tumor and the globe. (E.P. #33136)

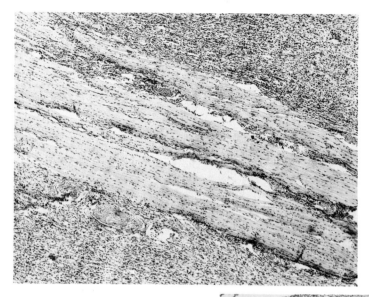

Figure 33–224 Undifferentiated rhabdomyosarcoma within and surrounding the superior rectus muscle along its entire extent. (Hematoxylin and eosin, ×60.) (E.P. #33136)

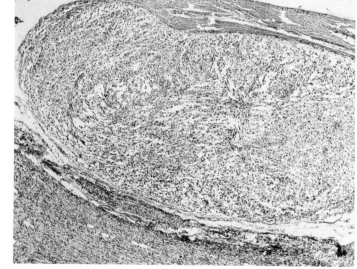

Figure 33–225 Nodule of differentiated rhabdomyosarcoma (see Fig. 33–223). (Hematoxylin and eosin, ×40.) (E.P. #33136)

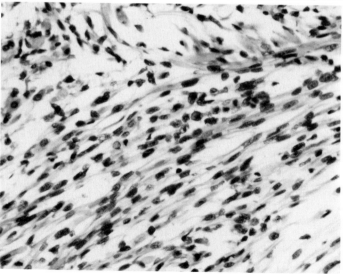

Figure 33–226 Almost all tumor cells in this nodule of differentiated rhabdomyosarcoma have a strap-shaped configuration. (Hematoxylin and eosin, × 300.) (E.P. #33136)

TABLE 33–30 PRESENTING SITE OF RHABDOMYOSARCOMA

Presenting Site	Number of Cases	Per Cent of Total
Orbit	95	71
Lids	29	22
Conjunctiva	10	7

After Schuster, S. A. D., et al.: Alveolar rhabdomyosarcoma of the eyelid; diagnosis by electron microscopy. Arch. Ophthal., *87*:646, 1972.

thalmos in one third of patients, and a palpable orbital or lid mass is present in one fourth (Jones et al., 1965). In one fifth of 134 cases reviewed by Schuster et al. (Table 33–30), orbital rhabdomyosarcoma was initially manifest as a lid mass, and in 7 per cent of cases the conjunctiva was the site of presentation (Fig. 33–145). Porterfield and Zimmerman reported that rhabdomyosarcoma arose most frequently in the upper nasal orbit. However, neither Jones et al. nor Ashton and Morgan confirmed this predilection. The displacement of the proptosed globe inferotemporally by a central retrobulbar mass may give the clinical impression of an upper nasal orbital mass. Radiographic findings are nonspecific, and the diagnosis must be made histologically.

Prognosis

Mortality from orbital rhabdomyosarcoma is highest within the first three years after diagnosis and original treatment (Table 33–31). Recurrences or metastases (most frequent to lungs, brain, and lymph nodes) usually become evident within two years. After the third year the increase in number of tumor deaths or metastases is small enough that the prognosis of children surviving three years without recurrence or metastasis is excellent. The factors which affect prognosis are (1) cell type, (2) extent of disease at diagnosis, and (3) mode of therapy. In addition, a definite tendency for higher survival rate in younger children has been noted for rhabdomyosarcoma in general (Sutow et al., 1970), though this variable has not been studied in orbital rhabdomyosarcoma. The extremely poor prognosis for alveolar rhabdomyosarcoma elsewhere in the body (less than 2 per cent 5-year survival, Enzinger and Shiraki, 1969) is confirmed for orbital tumors by Zimmerman's report that only one of the 9 patients with alveolar rhabdomyosarcoma reported in the 1962 series is now living (written communication, 1971).

Though the number of patients is small, prognosis appeared much better for *differentiated rhabdomyosarcoma* in Porterfield and Zimmerman's series, 3 of 6 patients surviving 5 years or more. The 3-year survival rate for patients with embryonal cell type was 27 per cent (9 of 33 patients). Extent of disease at the time of diagnosis is a second determinant of prognosis. Jones et al. conclude that about 50 per cent of patients with rhabdomyosarcoma confined to the orbit at the time of surgery can be cured by exenteration, whereas those with more extensive disease have a much poorer prognosis, regardless of treatment employed.

Treatment

Two significant therapeutic advances have been made since the reports of Porterfield and Zimmerman, Ashton and Morgan, and Jones et al. First, radiation therapy has proved to be an effective means of treating orbital rhabdomyosarcoma. Sagerman et al. have reported their

TABLE 33–31 ORBITAL RHABDOMYOSARCOMA: PATIENTS SURVIVING WITHOUT DISEASE 3 AND 5 YEARS AFTER DIAGNOSIS

Series	3-Year Follow-Up		5-Year Follow-Up	
	Number of Survivors/ Total Followed	*Per Cent Survival*	*Number of Survivors/ Total Followed*	*Per Cent Survival*
Ashton and Morgan	7/22	32	4/20	20
Jones et al.	20/62	32	18/62	29
Porterfield and Zimmerman	18/45	40	—	—

results in 15 patients who were treated with primary irradiation and without surgery except diagnostic biopsy. Ten of the 15 children are alive without disease at follow-up intervals of 18 to 81 months (average 45.7 months). Three of the 10 survivors received concomitant chemotherapy, but the remaining 7 had no chemotherapy. The 5 children who died with metastatic disease had no evidence of orbital tumor recurrence. These authors employ direct anterior field radiation with cobalt-60 supervoltage beam until 5000 rads tumor dose at 4 cm. depth is achieved over 5 weeks, followed by a lateral booster field of 800 rads to raise the dose in the posterior orbit. This high-dosage therapy is uniformly cataractogenic, but the authors report "useful vision" in 7 of their 10 survivors. These therapeutic results with primary irradiation are encouraging. However, before we can advise abandoning exenteration in favor of radiation, we would like to be certain that (1) all survivors have been followed for a minimum of three years in order to permit comparison with the other series summarized in Table 33–31; (2) other centers are able to apply the methods of Sagerman et al. with similar success; and (3) adequate follow-up studies do not disclose an unacceptably high rate of radiation-induced neoplasms in later life (see p. 939).

The second major recent therapeutic advance is in the field of chemotherapy. Three specific agents have been shown to have definite antitumor effects against rhabdomyosarcoma—*vincristine, actinomycin D,* and *cyclophosphamide.* Each affects tumor cells by a different mechanism, and their major toxic manifestations are not additive. For these reasons two or more of these drugs are frequently administered in combination (Sutow, 1969). Chemotherapy is most effective when the residual tumor cell population has been reduced to a minimum by surgery and/or irradiation. The general experience with combination chemotherapy and surgery or irradiation from the M. D. Anderson Hospital includes 14 patients with rhabdomyosarcoma localized to the orbit at the time of diagnosis (Sutow et al., 1970). As of November, 1972, 10 of the 14 children were living with no evidence of disease, and their survival time ranges from a minimum of 5½ years to a maximum of 12 years (Sutow, written communication). The four tumor deaths occurred 17, 25, 36, and 71 months after diagnosis. Regional perfusion of the orbit with phenylalanine mustard and actinomycin prior to exenteration did not improve survival in a series of 5 patients (Dayton et al., 1969), but the agents were employed when the tumor cell population was maximal, and the orbit was perfused via the external carotid artery, so that the quantity of drug delivered to the posterior orbit is difficult to estimate.

Table 33–32 summarizes a reasonable therapeutic approach to patients with orbi-

TABLE 33–32   THERAPY OF ORBITAL RHABDOMYOSARCOMA

Extent of Tumor	Surgical Therapy	Radiation Therapy	Systemic Chemotherapy*
Localized to orbit	Exenteration	Optional	Begin during surgery, continue course postoperatively
Extension beyond margin of exenteration evident at surgery or on histopathologic study	None	Administer postoperatively	Continue course begun at time of surgery
Extraorbital extension or metastasis evident prior to initial therapy	Exenteration of questionable value	Primary treatment of choice	Begin during course of irradiation
Orbital recurrence or subsequent metastasis	None	To site of recurrence	Repeat course

*Vincristine-actinomycin D-cyclophosphamide regimen (Sutow, 1969) or vincristine-actinomycin D regimen (Heyn, 1971).

tal rhabdomyosarcoma based on our present understanding of its response to surgical, radiation and drug therapy.

Metastatic Orbital Tumors

Albert et al. (1967a) have reviewed the subject of tumor metastasis to the orbit in infants and children. Orbital metastases have been described most frequently in association with neuroblastoma and less frequently with Ewing's sarcoma. Rare instances of metastatic Wilms' tumor (Apple, 1968), testicular embryonal carcinoma (Marcel and Chabrut, 1965), ovarian sarcoma, and renal embryonal sarcoma* have been recorded in children. We shall consider lymphoma, leukemia, and other neoplasms of possible multicentric origin separately. Albert et al. (1967a) retrospectively studied the incidence of orbital metastasis in children with solid tumors from 1950 to 1963 at three Philadelphia hospitals, and from 1963 to 1965 they prospectively studied all children admitted to these hospitals with known disseminated malignant disease. Table 33–33 summarizes their findings.

NEUROBLASTOMAS

Neoplasms derived from neural crest tissue constitute one of the most common childhood malignant conditions, being surpassed in frequency only by leukemia and brain tumors. Approximately half the undifferentiated varieties, neuroblastoma and ganglioneuroblastoma, occur in children under 3 years of age, and most of the remaining cases occur before the age of 10

*See Ophthalmic Staff of the Hospital for Sick Children, Toronto: The Eye in Childhood. Chicago, Year Book Medical Publishers, 1967, p. 358.

(deLorimier et al., 1969; Gross et al., 1959). These tumors arise from cells derived from embryonic sympathetic neuroblasts and thus may originate in the adrenal gland or in the sympathetic ganglia of cervical, mediastinal, retroperitoneal, and abdominal regions. Their neural crest origin is reflected both functionally and histologically. Active catecholamine synthesis and catabolism can be demonstrated in over 90 per cent of neuroblastomas by determination of catecholamine excretory products in the urine (Gitlow et al., 1970). Neural crest tumors are categorized histologically by their degree of differentiation. The least differentiated *neuroblastomas* are composed of masses of small rounded cells devoid of diagnostic arrangement or cellular characteristics. An initial sign of differentiation which permits histopathologic identification is the appearance of rosettes of small cells oriented around a central lumen filled with eosinophilic fibrils which represent developing axons (Fig. 33–227). In more differentiated forms, young ganglion cells become recognizable, and this transitional form is the *ganglioneuroblastoma*. The most highly differentiated neural crest tumors, *ganglioneuromas*, are composed entirely of mature nerve cells and fibers. These latter tumors may grow to a large size, but they remain encapsulated and do not metastasize. Serial biopsies of a neuroblastoma or its metastases may demonstrate a definite tendency toward more mature histologic forms and a less malignant behavior with the passage of time (Greenfield and Shelley, 1965). These observations form a histologic corollary for the clinical observation that spontaneous regression probably occurs more frequently in patients with neuroblastoma than with any other neoplasm (deLorimier et al., 1969). In spite of this characteristic, neuro-

TABLE 33–33 FREQUENCIES OF ORBITAL METASTASES FROM SOLID TUMORS IN CHILDREN

Tumor Type	Total Number of Patients with Tumor	Number of Patients with Orbital Metastasis	Per Cent
Neuroblastoma	108	41 (3)	38
Ewing's sarcoma	12	5 (0)	42
Wilms' tumor	60	0	0

Figures in parentheses indicate number of patients in whom orbital metastasis preceded detection of primary site. From Albert, D. M., et al.: Tumor metastasis to the eye. Part II. Clinical study in infants and children. Amer. J. Ophthal., *63*:727, 1967.

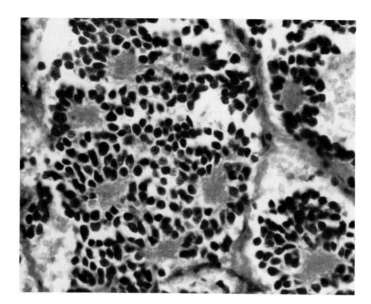

Figure 33–227 Neuroblastoma with rosettes. (Hematoxylin and eosin; ×550.) (E.P. 72-6602)

blastoma remains a lethal but not incurable tumor. As is the case with rhabdomyosarcoma, the great majority of tumor deaths occur within 2 years of diagnosis (96 to 99 per cent) (deLorimier et al., 1969; Gross et al., 1959), so that from a statistical standpoint, 2-year survival is considered equivalent to cure. One of the most important prognostic variables is the age of the patient at the time of diagnosis. D'Angio et al. found that the survival rate was 72 per cent for all infants less than 1 year of age, 28 per cent for those 1 to 2 years old, and 12 per cent for those over the age of 2. The presence of bone metastases is an ominous prognostic sign. Only 2 of 93 patients with demonstrable bone metastases were alive after 2 years in the combined series of Gross et al. and Lingley et al. Conversely, when metastases to liver, spleen, and bone marrow are present but when no radiographic evidence of skeletal metastasis can be demonstrated, the survival rate for all ages is 84 per cent (D'Angio et al., 1971).

Orbital metastasis generally occurs late in the course of neuroblastoma. *Initial orbital involvement* occurs in less than 5 per cent of cases (Table 33–33). Orbital metastasis may, however, precede detection of the primary site of tumor origin by as long as 9 months. Albert el al. (1967a) reported that the orbital and primary tumors were detected simultaneously in 14 of their 41 patients, and that in 24 patients orbital metastasis followed detection of the primary. The metastases were unilateral in 18 of

their cases and bilateral in 23. No tendency for unilateral tumors to occur on the same side of the body as the primary tumor was noted. Neuroblastomas which most frequently metastasize to the orbit arise in the abdomen or pelvis and less frequently in the chest (Albert et al., 1967a). The lesions arising in the neck rarely metastasize to the orbit, although Horner's syndrome is not unusual in these cases (Albert et al., 1967a; Alfano, 1968; Apple, 1969). DeLorimier et al. include one case of neuroblastoma primary in the orbit among their 212 cases, but no further details are given.

Clinical features of metastatic neuroblastoma to the orbit which may be of value in differential diagnosis are (1) frequent occurrence of spontaneous lid ecchymosis which need not be associated with subconjunctival hemorrhage or exophthalmos; (2) associated palpable swelling, often fluctuant, of the adjacent zygomatic bone, indicating bony metastasis to this region; (3) an apparently inflammatory character of the lid or zygomatic swelling, owing to tumor necrosis and hemorrhage; and (4) radiographic evidence of bone destruction (Mortada, 1967). Plain x-ray studies are of particular importance, since metastatic involvement either of orbital bones or of orbital soft tissues above may produce the same clinical picture (e.g., hemorrhagic exophthalmos), although bone metastases are associated with a poorer prognosis.

The influence of various modes of treatment on the course of neuroblastoma is difficult to assess at present, since many of the existing studies do not adequately consider the strong influence on prognosis exerted by age at diagnosis, site of primary origin, and extent of disease at diagnosis. Orbital metastases are generally best treated by irradiation, and one such regimen is outlined in Alfano's study. Although results in older children remain discouraging, the chemotherapeutic agents which have been utilized in a recent large-scale collaborative study are vincristine and cyclophosphamide (Sawitsky et al., 1970).

OTHER TUMORS

In the study of Albert et al. (1967a) 5 of 12 patients with *Ewing's sarcoma* developed orbital metastases. This relatively rare nonosteogenic round cell tumor of bone occurs in young patients and pursues an aggressive, lethal course which is not altered by radical surgical extirpation of the site of origin. Until recently the 5-year mortality rate from Ewing's sarcoma was approximately 90 per cent. However, encouraging preliminary studies are being reported from several centers which rely on intensive adjuvant chemotherapy (cyclophosphamide - vincristine - actinomycin D) and prophylactic whole-brain irradiation without surgery (Johnson and Pomeroy, 1972).

Wilms' tumor occurs almost as frequently as neuroblastoma in children, but reported orbital metastases from this tumor are rare. Apple (1968) reported one such example and reviewed previously reported cases.

Leukemia and Lymphomas

Orbital involvement in *leukemia* may occur as the result of soft tissue infiltration by leukemic cells, orbital extramedullary hematopoiesis, or orbital hemorrhage. Though it is often impossible to differentiate among these mechanisms on clinical grounds alone in a specific patient, the question is not of sufficient practical value to warrant histologic confirmation in patients in whom a diagnosis has previously been established. Although clinical evidence of orbital involvement may be detected in 5 per cent of leukemic patients who are specifically examined for ocular changes (Albert et al., 1967b), proptosis generally occurs late in the course of the disease. Although only 1.9 per cent of orbital tumors in children were leukemic in origin in the three large series which we reviewed (Table 33–23), leukemia may be the leading cause of exophthalmos in some centers of pediatric ophthalmology. Heinrich (1966) reported that leukemia was responsible for 8 of the 11 cases of noninflammatory exophthalmos in children examined at the Universitäts-Augenklinik Innsbruck between 1953 and 1963. Nor is late onset of proptosis in leukemia a universal finding. Heinrich reported that exophthalmos was the initial symptom of leukemia in 6 of these 8 children. Since orbital involvement may occur at a stage when the leukemic process is confined to the bone marrow (aleukemic leukemia), a normal peripheral blood smear does not exclude the diagnosis, and for this reason *bone marrow examination should be considered in the evaluation of any child with proptosis* (Crombie, 1967). The childhood leukemias associated with orbital involvement are most frequently of either the acute stem cell or acute lymphocytic variety, though acute myelocytic leukemia has also been a reported cause (Consul et al., 1967).

The *malignant lymphomas* (lymphocytic, histiocytic, and undifferentiated) and Hodgkin's disease occur much less frequently in children than the leukemias. One clinical, histopathologic, and epidemiologic entity in the lymphoma group which deserves special emphasis because of the frequency of orbital involvement is *Burkitt's lymphoma.* This malignant neoplasm of predominantly undifferentiated lymphoreticular cells was originally thought to occur exclusively in equatorial Africa, though more recent reports have confirmed its endemic occurrence in New Guinea and its sporadic occurrence in England, South America, and the United States (Burkitt and Wright, 1970). The orbit is generally involved by the upward extension of maxillary tumors. Lymphomas other than Burkitt's tumor rarely produce orbital infiltration as an initial symptom. For example, only 3 of 1269 patients with lymphosarcoma reviewed by

Rosenberg et al. presented with orbital tumors. In contrast, 18 per cent of patients from Uganda with Burkitt's lymphoma involving the facial bones had orbital tumors when first examined (Burkitt and Wright, 1970). Although proptosis may be the most conspicuous presenting sign, physical and radiologic examination usually reveals additional sites of infiltration (Olson et al., 1969). Present evidence suggests that in nonendemic areas, including the United States, orbital involvement may be a much less frequent finding (0 of 20 cases reported by Cohen et al., 1969). In both endemic and nonendemic areas the characteristic histologic picture is a "starry-sky" pattern produced by clear histiocytes scattered among a dense sea of uniform, cytologically distinctive immature cells. Several lines of clinical, experimental, and epidemiologic evidence strongly implicate an infectious agent in the etiology of this particular lymphoma, and recent investigations have focused on the striking association of the herpes-type EB virus of infectious mononucleosis with Burkitt's lymphoma (Burkitt and Wright, 1970).

Three children with proptosis secondary to *Hodgkin's disease* were included among the 257 children with proptosis reported from the Hospital for Sick Children in Toronto. The recent report by Strum and Rappaport (1970) is an excellent source of further general information about this lymphoreticular disorder which is relatively uncommon in children.

Prognosis and Treatment

Acute leukemia in children should no longer be regarded as invariably fatal. Collaborative studies have unequivocally documented a 5-year survival rate of 5 to 10 per cent with intensive combination chemotherapy. Projected data further indicate that over half the 5-year survivors will remain free of the disease indefinitely (Burchenal, 1970). In addition to chemotherapy, improved supportive therapy of anemia and infection and judicious use of radiotherapy for reduction of local infiltrations have contributed to the increasing span and improved quality of life for these children. The malignant lymphomas without leukemic transformation, Burkitt's lymphoma, and Hodgkin's disease have

better prognoses than the childhood leukemias, from 10 to 20 per cent in each category surviving 5 years with appropriate chemotherapy and radiotherapy (Carbone et al., 1969; Dargeon, 1960; Strum and Rappaport, 1970). Radiotherapy and chemotherapy remain the treatments of choice for orbital infiltration by lymphoma or leukemia cells. Specific regimens are outlined in the report of the M.D. Anderson Annual Clinical Conference 1970, and guidelines for the radiotherapeutic approach to lymphoma of the orbit in adults have been presented by Foster et al., 1971. With certain chemotherapeutic agents the treatment itself may cause ocular complications such as ocular motor palsies which might be confused with the effects of the underlying disease process (Albert et al., 1967b).

Peripheral Nerve Sheath Tumors

Two types of benign peripheral nerve sheath tumors may occur in the lids or orbit. Both are probably of Schwann cell origin, and both occur with increased frequency in neurofibromatosis. *Schwannoma* (neurinoma, neurilemmoma) is a benign, slow-growing, well-encapsulated neoplasm composed of Schwann cells in a collagenous matrix. Two basic cytoarchitectural patterns are usually present in different areas of the same tumor (Harkin and Reed, 1969). *The Antoni type A* pattern (Fig. 33–153) consists of compactly arranged spindle cells with oval nuclei which frequently have their long axes parallel and which occasionally are aligned in rows, creating a palisade pattern. *The Antoni type B* pattern is much less cellular, consisting of twisting, elongated single-file fascicles of cells widely dispersed in a watery, poorly staining matrix. Examples of schwannoma occurring in the lid and orbit of patients with and without neurofibromatosis have been recorded in children by Sen et al. and Mortada (1968).

The second benign peripheral nerve tumor of schwann cell origin, *neurofibroma*, is, in contrast to schwannoma, poorly encapsulated and less cellular (Figs. 33–228 and 33–229). An abundant mucoid matrix widely separates the fusiform neurofibroma cells and the associated scattered

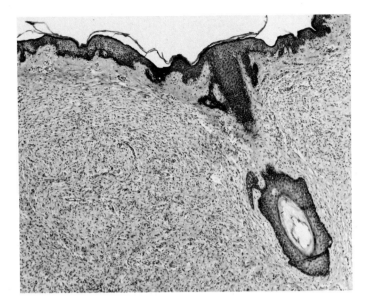

Figure 33–228 Diffuse neurofibroma of skin. (Hematoxylin and eosin, ×60.) (E.P. #18017)

collagen and reticulin fibrils. When most of the fascicles in a segment of peripheral nerve are involved in this process, cylindrical enlargement of the involved nerve segment is observed, and this clinical and gross pathologic configuration is referred to as *plexiform neurofibroma* (Figs. 33–230 and 33–231). In other cases the schwannian proliferation constituting a neurofibroma may diffusely infiltrate the surrounding tissue without respecting the confines of a single peripheral nerve. Stasis and lymphedema contribute to the tissue deformation associated with either plexiform or more diffuse neurofibroma.

Clinical Features

Neurofibromatosis is genetically transmitted as an autosomal dominant trait with variable penetrance. A high rate of genetic mutation has been postulated to explain the fact that a positive family history can be elicited in only about 50 per cent of cases. *Café-au-lait spots* and plexiform neurofibromas, the most common initial clinical manifestations of neurofibromatosis, were

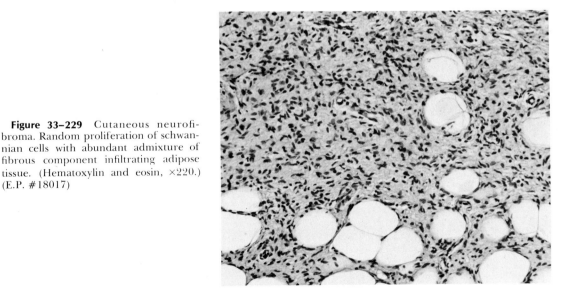

Figure 33–229 Cutaneous neurofibroma. Random proliferation of schwannian cells with abundant admixture of fibrous component infiltrating adipose tissue. (Hematoxylin and eosin, ×220.) (E.P. #18017)

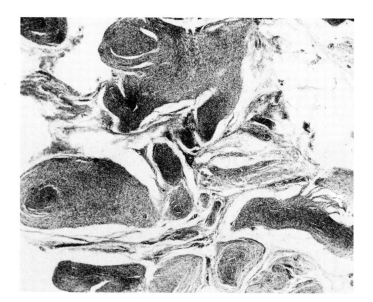

Figure 33–230 Highly cellular plexiform neurofibroma of upper lid in a child with neurofibromatosis. (Hematoxylin and eosin, ×35.) (E.P. #67480)

evident at birth in almost 50 per cent and by the age of 1 year in 63 per cent of the 46 children studied by Fienman and Yakovac. Individual café-au-lait spots, the familiar light-brown macules of neurofibromatosis, are clinically indistinguishable from their counterparts in the normal population. Since café-au-lait spots may be the only external manifestation of neurofibromatosis in childhood (Fienman and Yakovac, 1970) it is critically important for us to know which features distinguish these lesions from café-au-lait spots in normal persons. First, on a statistical basis, if a patient has five or more café-au-lait spots, one may make the diagnosis of neurofibromatosis, whether or not other manifestations of the disease are present. Second, a recent histochemical study has demonstrated that (1) the café-au-lait spots of patients with neurofibromatosis uniformly contain *more* DOPA-positive melanocytes per sq. mm. than does the surrounding skin, whereas café-au-lait spots in patients without neurofibromatosis contain fewer DOPA-positive melanocytes per sq. mm. than does the surrounding skin; and (2) giant pigment granules can be found in melano-

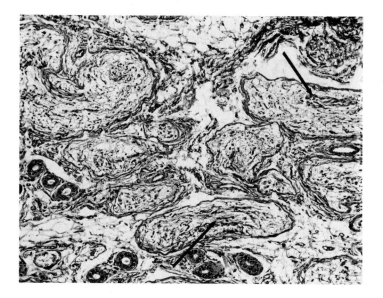

Figure 33–231 Plexiform neurofibroma of the upper lid and orbit with involvement of the lacrimal gland in a 3-year-old boy with neurofibromatosis. Schwann cell proliferation is confined by the sheath of the peripheral nerve. Large pools of acid mucopolysaccharide are present. Residual bundles of nerve fibers are evident (arrows). (Hematoxylin and eosin, ×120.) (E.P. #24840)

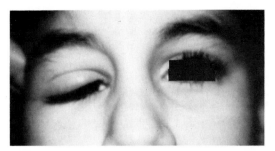

Figure 33–232 Seven-year-old white male with neurofibroma involving the right upper lid and orbit (sine-wave sign).

cytes from café-au-lait spots of the majority of patients with neurofibromatosis, whereas such abnormal granules are not found in patients without neurofibromatosis (Johnson and Charneco, 1970).

Involvement of lids and orbit by plexiform neurofibroma presents a characteristic external appearance (Fig. 33–232). The lid appears thickened and ptotic, and a soft tissue bulge is generally apparent over the adjacent temporal area. Smith and English describe a characteristic configuration of the margin of the ptotic eyelid which arches upward medially and downward temporally, resembling a sine-wave form. The mass feels soft and spongy and con-

tains palpable cords of a more fibrous consistency within its substance. Exophthalmos may be present but does not invariably indicate that the lid mass extends into the orbit (Binet et al., 1969). Rarely, an orbital neurofibroma may be massive enough at birth to simulate teratoma (Moore, 1962). Sarcomas (neurofibrosarcoma; malignant schwannoma) may develop in association with orbital neurofibroma, and a single case of malignant transformation in a benign schwannoma has been recorded (Schatz, 1971).

Roentgenographic Signs*

Neurofibromatosis of the lid may be associated with a congenital defect in the sphenoid bone (Figs. 33–187 and 33–233) which permits expansion of intracranial contents into a portion of the orbit producing pulsatile exophthalmos. Other roentgenologic findings in patients with orbital neurofibromatosis include (1) enlarged optic canal (usually but not always indicative of glioma) (Fig. 33–234), (2) enlarged bony orbit (Fig. 33–233), (3) bulging temporal fossa, and (4) various ab-

---

*See Burrows, 1963.

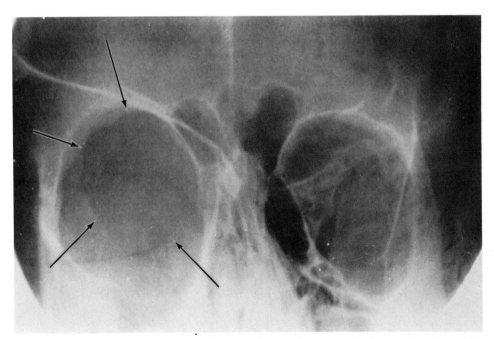

Figure 33–233 Orbital involvement in neurofibromatosis. Thirteen-year-old patient with enlarged right orbit, increased soft tissue density on right, and large defect in roof of right orbit (arrows).

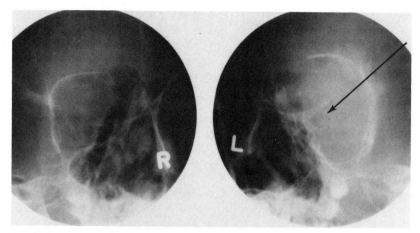

Figure 33–234   Enlargement of optic canals, the left (arrow) greater than the right. The left orbit is also enlarged. Patient had a glioma of the left optic nerve.

normalities of the sella turcica (Fig. 33–235).

ASSOCIATED OCULAR LESIONS (Font and Ferry, 1972).   Several ocular and neurologic associations should be borne in mind by the ophthalmologist examining a child with neurofibromatosis of the lid or orbit. *Congenital glaucoma* may be present in nearly 50 per cent of patients with lid tumors and, conversely, nearly all cases of congenital glaucoma complicating neurofibromatosis occur in patients who have lid involvement (Grant and Walton, 1968). *Gliomas of the optic nerve and chiasm* and primary *meningiomas of the orbit* (p. 1045) probably occur with increased frequency in patients with neurofibromatosis (Walsh, 1970). *Iris nevi* (Fig. 33–236) and *prominent corneal nerves* are familiar anterior segment associations of neurofibromatosis. Other ocular tumors which have been described in patients with neurofibromatosis include *choroidal Schwann cell proliferations* (Font and Ferry, 1972), *uveal malignant melanoma* (Gartner, 1940), and *juvenile xanthogranuloma* (Jensen et al., 1971).

Treatment

Schwannomas and pedunculated neurofibromas may be successfully excised without undue difficulty. Plexiform and diffuse

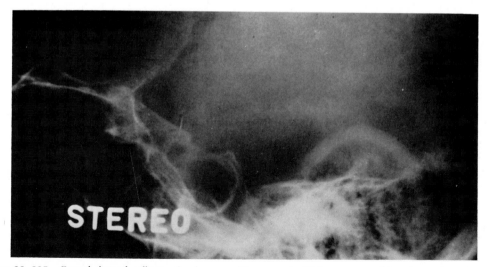

Figure 33–235   Gourd-shaped sella turcica in neurofibromatosis. Thirteen-year-old patient whose anteroposterior projection skull x-ray is reproduced in Figure 33–233 had unilateral exophthalmos and a pale right optic disc.

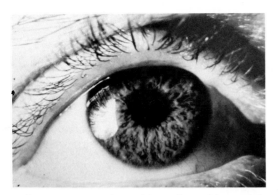

Figure 33–236   Iris nevi in patient with neurofibromatosis.

infiltrating neurofibromas, on the other hand, are highly vascular, poorly circumscribed lesions whose complete excision is a virtual impossibility. The tumors recur slowly after partial excision, and hours of meticulous dissection and hemostasis by a method which minimizes surgical trauma to normal tissue* may occasionally be rewarded by temporary cosmetic improvement. The cosmetic prognosis for reoperations is even more pessimistic.

Gliomas

Gliomas of the optic nerve constitute only 3 per cent of childhood orbital tumors reported from clinical centers summarized

*For example, see Iliff and Ossofsky reference, p. 21.

in Table 33–23, although 16 per cent of orbital tumors on file at the AFIP are of this variety (Table 33–24). Because some chiasmal gliomas may be associated with proptosis and unilateral visual loss, and so may be clinically indistinguishable from optic nerve gliomas (Dodge et al., 1958), we shall consideral all gliomas of the anterior visual pathways in this section.

Pathology and Pathogenesis*

Histologically most gliomas of the anterior visual pathways are benign astrocytomas which possess a more prominent fibrous tissue component and a sparser and less anaplastic cell population than supratentorial astrocytomas in adults (Figs. 33–237 and 33–238). They do not metastasize, and the morbidity and mortality associated with these tumors are due to local enlargement and compression of adjacent neural structures. Gliomas of the nerve and chiasm grow slowly, and their increase in size results from one or more of three processes: (1) active proliferation of tumor cells with extension into adjacent neural and extraneural tissues can be demonstrated *rarely*, and must be an infrequent cause of tumor growth; (2) collateral hyperplasia of adjacent meninges, glial cells, and intraneural septa is a constant finding in the vicinity of these tumors, and the degree of meningeal proliferation may be

*See Anderson and Spencer, 1970; Dodge et al., 1958.

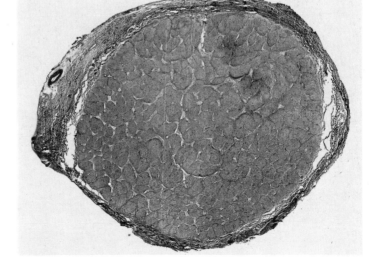

Figure 33–237   Cross-section of glioma of the optic nerve from a 13-year-old boy with neurofibromatosis. The nerve is about three times normal size, and the individual nerve fiber bundles are enlarged by tumor. (Hematoxylin and eosin ×25.) (E.P. #28195)

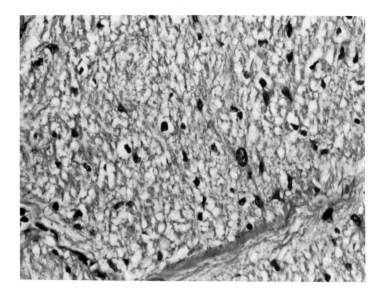

Figure 33–238 Greater magnification of glioma shown in Figure 33–237 reveals occasional larger tumor cells. Early microcystic change (extracellular vacuolization) is present. (Hematoxylin and eosin, ×530.) (E.P. #28195)

great enough to constitute the bulk of the tumor mass (Figs. 33–239 to 33–241); (3) extracellular deposition of hydrophilic mucosubstance (Fig. 33–242) has recently been established as a cause of tumor enlargement by Anderson and Spencer. The occurrence of these tumors in early childhood, their slow and frequently self-limited period of growth, their benign histologic appearance, and the occasional observation of heterotopic, apparently mature ganglion cells within the tumor are cited as features which indicate that these are hamartomas rather than true neoplasms (Dodge et al., 1958; Hoyt and Baghdassarian, 1969).

Clinical Features*

Although certain clinical signs assist in distinguishing gliomas of the optic nerve from those of the chiasm or tract (Table 33–34), in some it is impossible to make this distinction on the basis of clinical and plain radiographic evidence alone. In general, proptosis and concomitant loss of vision dominate the clinical picture in patients with intraorbital optic nerve gliomas, whereas loss of vision with symptoms or

*See Chutorian et al., 1964; Dodge et al., 1958; Fowler and Matson, 1957; Udvarhelyi et al., 1966; Yanoff et al., in prep.

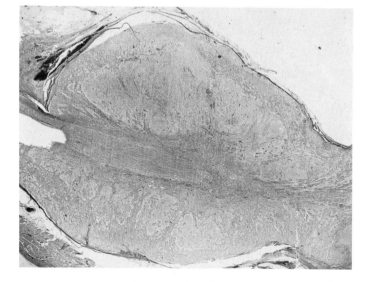

Figure 33–239 Glioma of the optic nerve with extreme degree of arachnoidal proliferation. Over 80 per cent of the lesion consists of this secondary arachnoidal hyperplasia. (Hematoxylin and eosin, ×4.) (E.P. #24840)

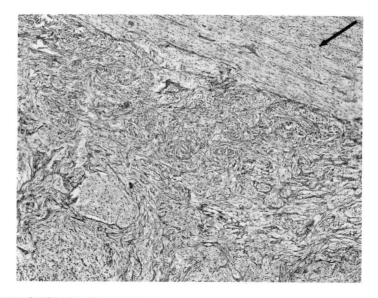

Figure 33–240 Junctional zone between longitudinal section of the glioma (arrow) and arachnoid hyperplasia. (Hematoxylin and eosin, ×55.) (E.P. #24840)

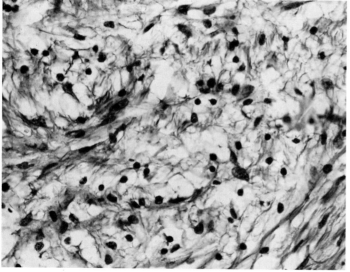

Figure 33–241 Fibrocellular appearance of arachnoid hyperplasia. (Hematoxylin and eosin, ×500.) (E.P. #24840)

Figure 33–242 Deposition of mucopolysaccharide substance in an optic nerve glioma. (Alcian blue, ×175.) (E.P. #24840)

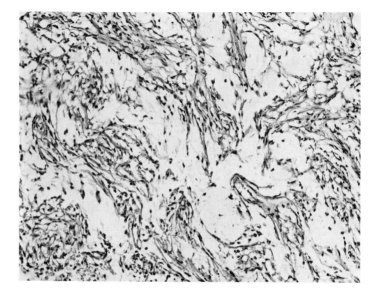

TABLE 33–34 CLINICAL FEATURES OF GLIOMAS OF ANTERIOR VISUAL PATHWAYS

Location of Glioma	Number of Patients	Average Age at Diagnosis	Male/ Female Ratio	Per Cent of Patients with Each Finding								
				Proptosis	Loss of Vision*	Primary Optic Atrophy	Papille-dema	Headache or Eye Pain	Nonpara-lytic Strabismus	Motor Symptoms	Seizures	Endocrine Disorders
I. Optic Nerve	12	9	2/10	100	75	27†	64†	25	58	0	0	0
II. Optic Chiasm or Tract	34	14	19/15	18	97	62	32	47	35	12	9	26

*Four patients in group I and 2 patients in group II were too young for acuity testing and are excluded from this calculation.
†Congenital cataracts prevented visualization of fundus in one patient.
From Dodge, H. W., Jr., et al.: Gliomas of the optic nerves. A.M.A. Arch. Neurol. Psych., 79:607, 1958. Copyright 1958, American Medical Association.

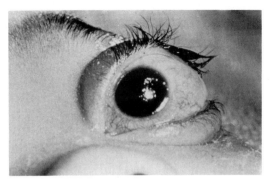

Figure 33–243 Infant with proptosis of left eye due to glioma of optic nerve with massive arachnoid proliferation. (E.P. #24840)

signs of increased intracranial pressure is characteristic of intracranial gliomas of the visual pathway. The tumor may be manifest at birth (Chutorian et al., 1964), but the diagnosis is most frequently made between the ages of 4 and 10, often as a consequence of routine school vision testing.

Because the tumor mass is encapsulated within the muscle cone, the globe is displaced axially or inferotemporally with nerve gliomas (Figs. 33–243 and 33–244). The conspicuous lack of ocular motor palsies is a useful feature in differentiating optic nerve tumors from other orbital neoplasms in children. Nonparalytic strabismus associated with diminished visual acuity may be present, however, as may a searching type of pendular nystagmus.

Diminished visual acuity does not invariably occur, and patients in both the nerve and chiasm-tract categories have been reported with 20/20 acuity bilaterally (Dodge et al., 1958). Conversely, sudden loss of vision may dominate the clinical picture, simulating *acute optic neuritis.* Pfaffenbach et al. reported one such case in which the masquerade was carried a step further when the patient's initial visual loss was rapidly reversed after administration of systemic corticosteroids. *Central retinal artery or vein occlusion* in a child should alert the clinician to the possibility of optic nerve glioma. If retinal vascular occlusion passes unnoticed, subsequent *neovascular glaucoma* may develop and produce the signs or symptoms which first bring the patient to medical attention. Hovland and Ellis (1966) reported an example of hemorrhagic glaucoma in a 6-year-old patient who had chiasmal and optic nerve glioma without exophthalmos. Abnormalities of the disc are noted in over 90 per cent of patients with gliomas of either optic nerve or chiasm. Although these changes are generally described as optic atrophy or papilledema, the latter can be closely simulated by glial proliferation on the nerve head and adjacent retina (Gartner and Feiring, 1966; Verhoeff, 1932). The frequency with which such glial proliferation is responsible for the papilledema observed clinically is difficult to estimate, since the mode of treatment in many cases (radiation or excision of the nerve only) does not

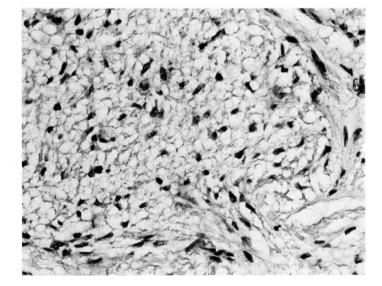

Figure 33–244 Area of optic nerve glioma with moderate degree of deposition of extracellular substance. Same case as in Figure 33–243. (Hematoxylin and eosin, ×550.) (E.P. #24840)

permit histopathologic examination of the optic disc region.

Though the well-known radiographic signs of enlarged optic foramen without erosion (Fig. 33–234) and gourd-shaped sella (Fig. 33–235) are of diagnostic value when clinical findings are suggestive of gliomas of the anterior visual pathways, neither is specific for glioma and neither is as reliable as fractional pneumoencephalography in assessing the intracranial extent of the tumor (Udvarhelyi et al., 1966). Enlarged optic foramina, for example, were noted in 29 per cent of patients in whom the glioma was confined within the orbit, whereas another 29 per cent of patients had normal optic foramina in spite of definite intracranial tumor (Yanoff et al., in prep.). Cutaneous signs of *neurofibromatosis* may be present in approximately 10 per cent of patients with optic gliomas (Reese, 1963; Yanoff et al., in prep.). Since these tumors characteristically occur in early childhood, stigmata of neurofibromatosis may not appear until years after the ocular involvement, however.

Prognosis and Treatment

Uncertainty concerning the histogenesis and natural course of optic gliomas renders evaluation of any treatment modality difficult. After an initial period of growth primarily related to collateral meningeal hyperplasia and extracellular mucosubstance deposition, most gliomas of the anterior visual pathways do not continue to enlarge progressively. Afferent optic nerve axons traversing the tumors may retain good function for many years, though the small-caliber fiber system subserving central visual function does seem more sensitive to pressure effects of gliomas than the large-caliber afferent system (Glaser et al., 1971).

CHIASMAL GLIOMA. Hoyt and Baghdassarian and Glaser et al. (1969) documented a "monotonously static" long-term course in the majority of their 36 patients studied retrospectively at the University of California Medical Center. They were unable to define any difference in visual morbidity between irradiated and nonirradiated patients with chiasmal glioma, and they noted that the principal visual handicap in several patients was the result of attempted surgical excision. These authors conclude that (1) the diagnosis can be conclusively established with neuroradiologic techniques; (2) transcranial operations for excision or biopsy are contraindicated; (3) the only indication for neurosurgical intervention is increased intracranial pressure necessitating shunt procedures; (4) transorbital excision of the tumor should be undertaken only to reduce proptosis in a blind eye, and partial removal of the tumor in such a case has no adverse effect; and (5) radiotherapy is of doubtful efficacy. Whether this very conservative approach will prove the optimal one is uncertain at present. Analysis of 64 AFIP cases by Yanoff et al. confirms the more malignant behavior of intracranial optic gliomas (41 per cent mortality) and the appreciable risk of surgical therapy (2 of 11 deaths were operative). Thus, the role of surgery in the treatment of chiasmal or tract gliomas is questionable. Many authorities would still contend that radiotherapy remains one of the few means by which we might hope to retard the deposition of mucosubstance and proliferation of glial tissue which threaten vision during the actively progressive phase of tumor growth. Finally, some would argue that if radiotherapy is considered, the diagnosis should be confirmed histologically before treatment is begun.

OPTIC NERVE GLIOMA. The generalization of Hoyt and Baghdassarian's recommendations for conservative treatment of chiasmal tumors to gliomas of the intraorbital optic nerve must be questioned. Only 7 patients in the latter category were studied by these authors. Four of these were treated by successful total surgical excision. The treatment in the remaining 3 patients was not specified, but they may have been among the cases treated by subtotal excision. Thus, we do not have enough information about the natural course of untreated glioma confined to the intraorbital optic nerve to justify abandoning primary excision as the preferred mode of treatment. The curative value of total, or often even partial, excision has been repeatedly documented (Chutorian et al., 1964; Dodge et al., 1958; Yanoff et al., in prep.). The realization that meningioma of the optic nerve is not as rare in children as formerly thought (see Meningiomas) is a further important practical reason for requiring histologic confirmation of suspected optic nerve glioma.

Meningiomas

Although intracranial meningiomas are rare in childhood, meningiomas arising in the orbit have a singular predilection for the pediatric age group. Walsh has recently reported 7 children with orbital meningiomas, and Zimmerman states that 8 of the 20 cases of orbital meningiomas on file at the AFIP occurred in patients under the age of 20 (personal communication, 1971).

Histopathology*

The classification of intracranial and spinal meningiomas is complex and variable, with the number of advocated histologic subdivisions ranging from 0 to 22. Most orbital meningiomas arise from the meningothelial arachnoidal tissues and are composed of densely packed clusters and whorls of polygonal cells resembling normal meningothelial cells (Fig. 33–245). Scattered psammoma bodies are often present, and the usual cytologic features of malignancy (mitotic figures, nuclear and cytoplasmic pleomorphism) are absent. Distant metastases and extension into adjacent neural tissue are rare. However,

*See Craig and Gogela, 1949; Walsh, 1970.

many meningiomas do penetrate the dura to invade orbital soft tissue, bone, and, *rarely,* blood vessels (Fig. 33–246).

Diagnosis and Prognosis*

The initial clinical manifestations of meningiomas of the optic nerve—visual loss, proptosis without ophthalmoplegia, and papilledema or optic atrophy—are identical to those associated with *optic glioma.* Both tumors have a definite but unexplained predilection for females. Similarly, the clinical association with neurofibromatosis is at least as frequent with meningiomas as it is with gliomas (Walsh, 1970). Although x-rays of the orbit and optic foramina are helpful in differential diagnosis if the hyperostosis associated with a small percentage of meningiomas is present (Fig. 33–247), normal or enlarged optic foramina without hyperostosis may be seen in either condition. Thus, in most instances, the distinction between these two types of tumor must be made histopathologically. We do not yet know whether newer methods of radioisotope scanning of the orbit will be as helpful with the diagnosis of orbital meningiomas as they have been with intracranial meningiomas.

Ossifying fibroma of bone, a type of fibro-osseous dysplasia, may simulate meningioma clinically and histologically

*See Russell and Rubenstein, 1971; Walsh, 1970.

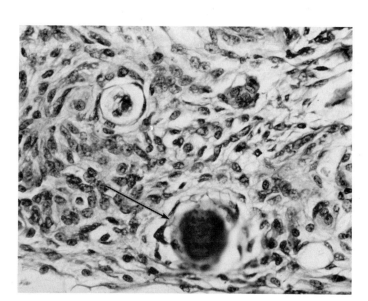

Figure 33–245 Primary orbital meningioma from an 11-year-old girl. Meningothelial cells have a tendency to form swirls (arrow) and psammoma bodies. (Hematoxylin and eosin, ×420.) (E.P. #31652)

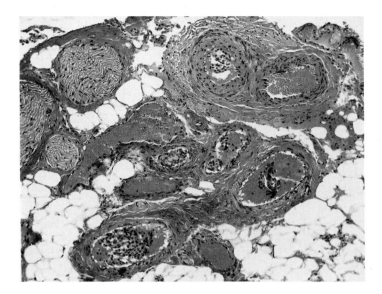

Figure 33–246   Meningioma within ciliary vessels adjacent to tumor and the globe of a 48-year-old woman. (Hematoxylin and eosin, ×120.) (E.P. #3052)

(Lehrer, 1969; Nicholson and Wood, 1972). We recently had a patient who gradually developed proptosis and downward displacement of the globe at about age 13. By the age of 18 (Fig. 33–248) he had 6 mm. proptosis, 20/20 acuity in each eye, 40 prism diopters exophoria-tropia, and a hard, nonpulsatile mass in the upper nasal quadrant of the right orbit. Plain x-rays and tomograms disclosed a monolocular cystic mass surrounded by an intact bony rim (Fig. 33–249). A percutaneous orbital venogram showed downward displacement of the superior ophthalmic vein (Fig. 33–250), and a brachial arteriogram demonstrated no tumor stain. Although the preoperative clinical consensus of ophthalmologists, otolaryngologists, and radiologists in attendance was frontal sinus mucocele, neurosurgeons raised the diag-

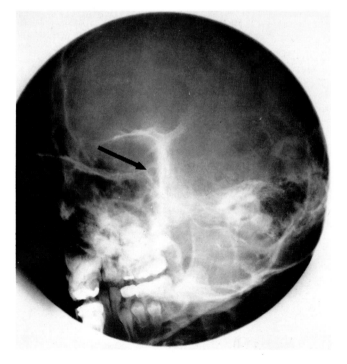

Figure 33–247   Oblique view of right orbit showing hyperostosis of the optic foramen (arrow) of an 8-week-old boy with intracranial middle fossa meningioma.

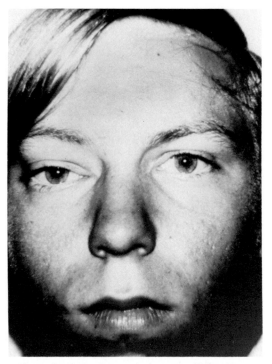

Figure 33–248 Proptosis due to ossifying fibroma of bone involving right orbit in an 18-year-old patient. (E.P. #35065)

nostic possibility of meningioma. Transfrontal craniotomy exposed an extradural mass extending intracranially from the orbital roof, and during its ex-

cision the tumor was noted to have a gritty consistency typical of psammomatous meningioma, though its necrotic center was somewhat unusual. Frozen and permanent histologic sections were reported as meningioma. Several months later, histopathologic review of the tumor disclosed that the "psammoma bodies" were in fact irregular fragments of osteoid embedded in a matrix of highly cellular fibrous tissue (Figs. 33–251 and 33–252). This is ossifying fibroma, not meningioma.

The slow progression of meningiomas plus their clinical similarity to gliomas of the nerve should not lead the clinician to expect a similar excellent prognosis or to adopt a similar conservative therapeutic approach. The fact is that *many meningiomas are locally invasive malignant conditions* which tend to recur repeatedly after incomplete excision. They are insensitive to irradiation or chemotherapy, and *cure depends on adequate surgical removal.* Even when this goal is accomplished subsequent cerebellopontine angle tumors, gliomas, spinal cord tumors, or other central manifestations of neurofibromatosis develop frequently enough to render the ultimate prognosis as uncertain.

The following previously reported case (Walsh, 1970) illustrates the local aggressiveness of primary orbital meningiomas in

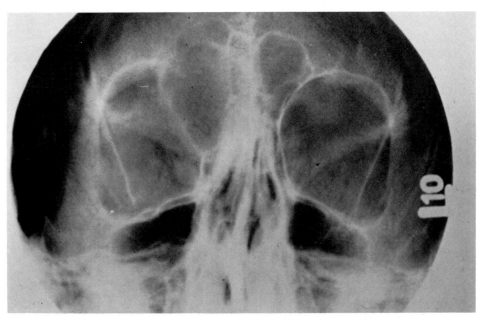

Figure 33–249 Skull x-ray of patient in Figure 33–248. Monolocular cystic mass surrounded by an intact bony rim in upper nasal quadrant of right orbit. (E.P. #35065)

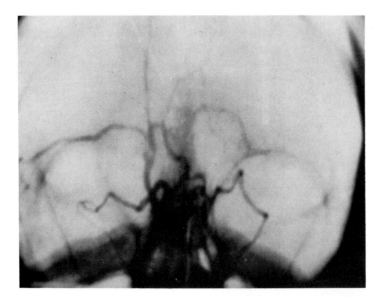

Figure 33–250 Orbital venogram (frontal view). Right superior ophthalmic vein is displaced downward by mass arising in superonasal orbital wall. (E.P. #35065)

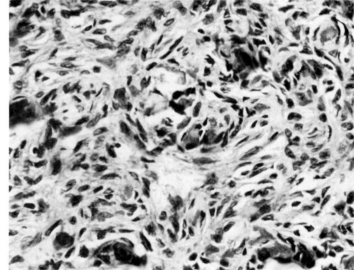

Figure 33–251 Ossifying fibroma of bone. Fibrous tissue proliferation with foci of calcium deposition. (Hematoxylin and eosin, ×550.) (E.P. #35065)

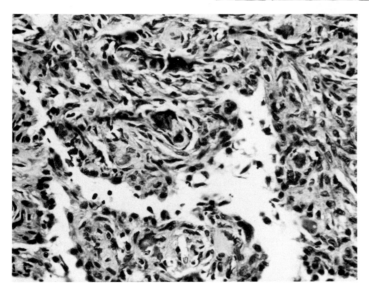

Figure 33–252 Ossifying fibroma of bone. Occasional cystic spaces and inflammatory cells are present. (Hematoxylin and eosin, ×420.) (E.P. #35065)

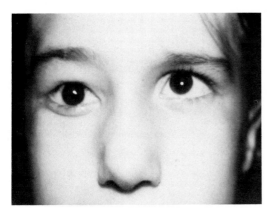

Figure 33–253   Eleven-year-old girl with proptosis due to primary orbital meningioma. (E.P. #31652)

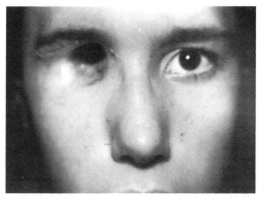

Figure 33–255   Appearance of orbit following exenteration. (Courtesy of Dr. C. E. Iliff.) (E.P. #31652)

children. A 9-year-old girl experienced blurring of vision in her right eye. Examination disclosed no abnormalities. Over the next two years, the right eye became proptotic, and acuity was reduced to light perception (Fig. 33–253). The orbit was explored via a transcranial approach. Biopsy of a mass in the posterior portion of the orbit disclosed meningioma. Subsequently the eye was enucleated and the tumor was thought to have been removed completely in a piecemeal fashion. About one year later there was a recurrence of tumor in the remaining orbital tissue and subconjunctival areas (Fig. 33–254). The orbit was exenterated (Fig. 33–255). Meningioma was found diffusely throughout the specimen (Fig. 33–256), in orbital fat and connective tissue (Fig. 33–257), in tarsal conjunctiva of the upper lid (Fig. 33–258), and along the superior margin and apex of the specimen. She has remained

free of tumor for 19 months after exenteration.

Treatment

In older patients the known slow rate of tumor growth may be relied upon to avoid the risks of surgery. In children, however, even the most slowly growing tumors may have time to produce severe damage. In Walsh's case 1, for example, 17 years after therapeutic enucleation was refused, the meningioma had finally progressed to reach the chiasm, and in spite of subtotal removal of the tumor at this stage, the patient was completely blind within another year. Even when surgery is undertaken early, vision usually cannot be saved, since removal of the tumor without damage to the optic nerve is virtually impossible except with the rare tumors which develop outside the dural sleeve (Walsh, 1970). Therefore, the usual surgical objective is not to preserve vision but to eliminate the possibility of recurrence or spread of the tumor insofar as possible. In many cases this may require orbital exenteration, or transcranial excision followed by exenteration, by the time therapy is undertaken. The rare free-lying orbital meningiomas which are not intimately related to the optic nerve sheath may be treated successfully by simple excision (MacMichael and Cullen, 1969).

Inflammatory Pseudotumors of the Orbit

In his discussion of the paper by Blodi and Gass (1968), Zimmerman divides

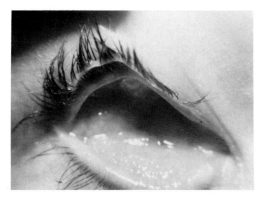

Figure 33–254   Recurrence of primary orbital meningioma one year after enucleation and initial removal of tumor. (E.P. #31652)

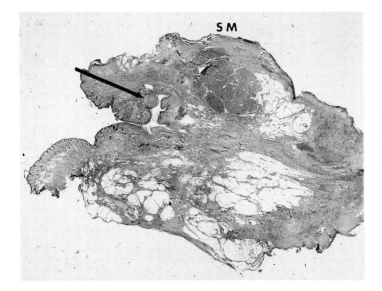

Figure 33–256 Exenteration specimen with recurrent meningioma at the apex, along the superior margin (SM) diffusely invading fat and connective tissue and the tarsal conjunctiva of the upper lid (arrow). (Hematoxylin and eosin, ×4.5.) (E.P. #31652)

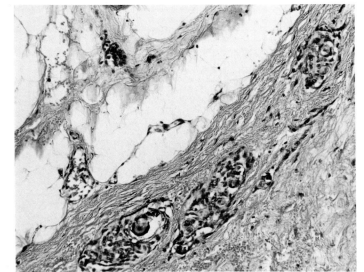

Figure 33–257 Small foci of meningioma diffusely invading orbital fat and connective tissue. (Hematoxylin and eosin, ×180.) (E.P. #31652)

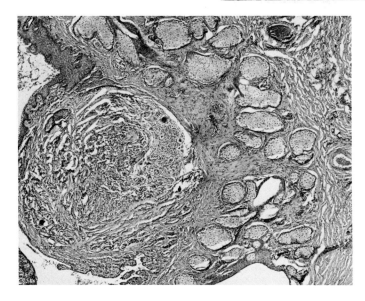

Figure 33–258 Nodule of meningioma in the tarsal conjunctiva of the upper lid. (Hematoxylin and eosin, ×45.) (E.P. #31652)

inflammatory lesions of the orbit which may simulate tumors into three general categories. First, the category of *inflammatory orbital masses associated with systemic disease* includes orbital involvement in Graves' disease, Wegener's granulomatosis, Waldenström's macroglobulinemia, Sjögren's syndrome, polyarteritis nodosa, and sarcoidosis. Weiter and Farkus (1972) reported the case of a 10-year-old girl in whom unilateral pseudotumor of the orbit was the initial clinical manifestation of a limited form of Wegener's granulomatosis. The orbital disease could be suppressed with alternate-day systemic corticosteroid therapy. However, because renal lesions progressed in spite of steroid therapy, azathioprine immunosuppression was substituted for corticosteroid therapy, and she remains in clinical remission 18 months after institution of azathioprine treatment. Blodi's discussion of this paper cites an additional case of an 11-year-old patient in whom orbital pseudotumor was the presenting manifestation of Wegener's granulomatosis. A second category comprises *localized orbital inflammations the cause of which can be determined* by clinical, histologic, or laboratory study. Orbital masses in this group include lesions caused by specific bacteria and fungi, inflammatory reactions around primary tumors such as dermoid cysts or hemangiomas, post-traumatic lesions, and foreign body granulomas. Since in young infants the history of trauma may be either absent or misleadingly trivial, one should carefully examine the lids, brow, and conjunctiva for evidence of previous penetrating injury before excluding retained orbital foreign body as the cause for an inflammatory mass (Heyner and Passmore, 1965). Finally, there is a third category of *inflammatory mass lesions of the orbit for which no cause or pathogenesis can be discovered.* These are the lesions which have been designated inflammatory pseudotumor of the orbit.

Table 33–35 summarizes the age distribution of 19 pediatric patients from the series of 140 histologically documented cases of inflammatory pseudotumor reported by Blodi and Gass (Blodi, written communication, 1972). The youngest patient in their report was 10 months of age. Two examples of orbital pseudotumor in children (ages 4 and 13) are recorded by

TABLE 33–35 AGES OF CHILDREN WITH INFLAMMATORY PSEUDOTUMOR OF THE ORBIT IN SERIES REPORTED BY BLODI AND GASS (1968)

Age (Years)	Number of Patients
Less than 1	1
1 to 5	1
6 to 10	3
11 to 15	9
16 to 17	5

From Blodi, F. C. Personal communication, 1972.

Iliff and Ossofsky.* The 13-year-old patient developed progressive, painful proptosis in the right eye (29 mm. OD, 15 mm. OS), papilledema, impaired motility, and reduced acuity (20/200), all of which resolved completely and spontaneously over a 4-month period. Ten years later, at age 23, the patient developed pain, proptosis, decreased vision, impaired motility, and papilledema in the opposite eye, which resolved completely after systemic administration of corticosteroids. Blodi and Gass reported that patients such as this with bilateral orbital pseudotumor which occurs either simultaneously or consecutively, are statistically more likely to have an associated systemic disease which may become evident long after the orbital involvement.

The most frequent cause of inflammatory proptosis in early childhood is *orbital cellulitis,* and a diagnosis of pseudotumor should be entertained only after excluding acute sinusitis, especially ethmoid sinusitis, and remote foci of infection which may produce metastatic orbital inflammation (Haynes and Cramblett, 1967). Careful exclusion of infectious agents is particularly important, since systemic corticosteroids are the agents most commonly used to treat pseudotumor of the orbit.

Histiocytosis X (Eosinophilic Granuloma of Bone, Hand-Schüller-Christian Disease, Letterer-Siwe Disease)

The proliferative disorders of the reticuloendothelial system cannot be

---

*See Iliff and Ossofsky reference, p. 1063.

TABLE 33–36   PROLIFERATIVE DISORDERS OF THE RETICULOENDOTHELIAL SYSTEM: THE NOSOLOGIC MORASS

Lymphogranulomatosis	Histiocytic medullary reticulosis
Reticulohistiocytosis	Familial reticuloendotheliosis
Paraproteinemic hemoblastosis	Familial erythrophagocytic lymphohistiocytosis
Histiocytosis	Familial lymphohistiocytosis of the nervous system
Malignant histiocytosis	Multicentric reticulohistiocytosis
Malignant hematodermas	
Cutaneous lymphoreticulopathy	Farber's lipogranulomatosis
Atypical cutaneous reticulosis	Reticulohistiocytoma
Malignant reticulopathy	Giant-cell histiocytomatosis
Histiomonocytic reticulosis	Giant-cell reticulohistiocytosis
Histiocytic granuloma	Normocholesterolemic xanthomatosis
Histiocytosis X	Giant-cell histiocytosis
Reticulogranuloma	Reticulohistiocytic granuloma
Systemic reticuloendotheliosis	Giant-cell reticulohistiocytoma
Reticuloblastomatosis	Juvenile xanthogranuloma
Reticuloendotheliosis	Eruptive histiocytoma
Aleukemic reticulosis	Xanthoma disseminatum
Malignant reticulosis	Reticulohistiocytoma cutis
Histiocytic reticulosis	Idiopathic histiocytosis
Leukemic reticuloendotheliosis	Hyperdysplastic granuloxanthomatous histiocytosis
Malignant reticuloendotheliosis	
Malignant leukemic reticulohistiocytosis	
Malignant reticulohistiocytosis	

concisely defined or precisely classified at the present time. Terminology proliferates as rapidly as the most fulminant of the disease processes encompassed, creating for the hapless ophthalmologist a nosologic morass which defies decipherment (Table 33–36). Any concise summary statement about the entire spectrum of diseases would be a misleading oversimplification, and we shall confine our attention in this section to the group of reticuloendothelial proliferative disorders which most frequently produce orbital tumors in childhood—histiocytosis X. In the next section, we shall consider orbital involvement by another of these diseases, juvenile xanthogranuloma.

Definition and Pathology

The common feature of disorders designated histiocytosis X is the proliferation of cytologically benign histiocytes. More variable histologic features include infiltration of eosinophils and, less frequently, foam cells. The histologic similarities among the histiocytoses X are presumed to reflect a common basic disease process, and this is further suggested by ultrastructural demonstration of Langerhans' granule-containing histiocytes in 39 per cent of 54 histiocytosis X specimens of all clinical types reviewed by Basset et al. The Langerhans'

granule organelle is not specific for histiocytosis X, but it is not present in juvenile xanthogranuloma lesions (Gonzalez-Crussi and Campbell, 1970).

Clinical Features

The mechanism of orbital involvement in all forms of histiocytosis X is the same. Proliferating histiocytes in orbital bones form tumors which display a characteristic radiographic appearance and which produce proptosis when they expand sufficiently to reduce orbital volume. The roof and lateral wall of the orbit are most frequently involved, with osteolytic lesions appearing roentgenographically as irregularly marginated radiolucent defects without surrounding sclerosis (Fig. 33–259) (Avery et al., 1957; Nesbit et al., 1970). A less frequently recognized radiographic appearance is thickening and sclerosis of the orbital roof, which apparently occurs as lytic lesions heal in some patients (Nesbit et al., 1970). The sclerotic lesions may resemble those of meningioma, fibrous dysplasia, osteoblastic reaction to lacrimal gland carcinoma or metastatic tumors, osteitis secondary to chronic sinusitis, and Caffey's disease.

Although only one example of probable histiocytosis X is recorded in three series of childhood orbital tumors based on his-

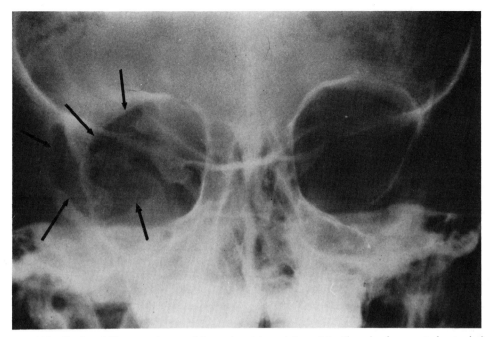

Figure 33–259 Eosinophilic granuloma of bone involving right orbit. Sharply demarcated osteolytic lesion without surrounding sclerosis involves lateral wall and roof of right orbit (arrows).

tologic diagnosis (Table 33–23) 7 per cent of 257 children with proptosis tabulated from clinical records of the Hospital for Sick Children in Toronto are in the histiocytosis X category (Table 33–26).

In reported series of patients with histiocytosis X, exophthalmos occurs most frequently in patients with *simultaneous bone and visceral involvement.* In the series of 29 patients in this category reported by Avery et al. (1957), exophthalmos was present in 10 patients (34 per cent) and was the chief complaint in 4 (14 per cent). Both unilateral and bilateral examples were recorded, and in 2 patients the two eyes were involved at different times. Osteolytic orbital defects were present in 9 patients. Only 1 of the 9 patients with orbital involvement by x-ray did not have exophthalmos. Two patients reported by Avery et al. (1957) and one patient reported by Enriquez et al. (1967) had exophthalmos *without* radiographically demonstrable lesions. Oberman (1968), contrary to the observations of Avery et al., reported that "osseous involvement of the orbit, as noted on x-ray, was far more common than exophthalmos." The frequency of exophthalmos among histiocytosis X patients with initial bone and soft tissue involvement in other series

ranges from 17 to 33 per cent of patients (Lieberman et al., 1969; 1969; Lucaya, 1971; Oberman, 1968). The complete Hand-Schüller-Christian triad-exophthalmos, diabetes insipidus, and multiple lytic osseous lesions—is relatively uncommon in each of the reported series.

In patients with *unifocal eosinophilic granuloma of bone,* orbital involvement and exophthalmos are less common (0 of 50 cases, Lieberman et al.; 7 of 30 patients, Oberman; 0 of 9 cases, Avery et al.; 0 of 12 cases, Lucaya).

Finally, in the most fulminant form of *histiocytosis X, involving multiple soft tissue sites,* exophthalmos is also an infrequent association (1 of 18 patients, Lucaya; 0 of 8 patients, Oberman).

Prognosis and Treatment

All authorities agree that isolated eosinophilic granuloma of bone is a benign disease with excellent prognosis. Treatment of orbital lesions by excision, curettage, systemic corticosteroids, or low doses of external irradiation have been reported effective. More aggressive surgical or irradiation therapy is contraindicated by the basically benign nature of the disease process.

The prognosis for patients with multifocal osseous and/or nonosseous lesions has been elucidated by Lahey (1962). The overall mortality in these patients is about 33 per cent. Age and extent of disease at its onset are the two major prognostic determinants. The mortality rate is inversely related to patient age and directly related to the number of organ systems involved by the disease process. These two factors are not entirely independent, since the majority of children with multiple organ systems affected are in the younger age groups. The specific localization of lesions also influences prognosis: pulmonary, hepatic, splenic, and hematopoietic involvement are associated with a higher mortality rate. Treatment modalities for patients with multifocal forms of histiocytosis X include systemic corticosteroids, external irradiation, and chemotherapy with vinblastine, vincristine, or cyclophosphamide (Avery et al., 1957; Starling et al., 1972).

Juvenile Xanthogranuloma (JXG)

Seven instances of orbital involvement by juvenile xanthogranuloma have been reported (Gaynes and Cohen, 1967; Sanders, 1966; Zimmerman, 1965.). The lesion was first noted when the patient was under 3 months of age in 6 of the 7 cases. Thus, JXG should be included in the differential diagnosis of exophthalmos in the newborn (see Teratoma). A discrete mass near the orbital rim simulated a dermoid cyst in several reported cases. Only 1 of 7 children with orbital JXG had associated skin lesions, in contrast to the high proportion of cutaneous involvement in patients with intraocular JXG (Sanders, 1966). One remarkable patient with histologically confirmed JXG exhibited extensive orbital bone destruction at the time of initial evaluation and surgery and developed a new osteolytic lesion two years later which resolved after x-ray therapy (Sanders, 1966). In a patient reported by Gaynes and Cohen initial JXG was also accompanied by progressive radiographic lucencies in the adjacent malar bone, though in the other 5 cases no bone changes were noted.

Treatment

Sanders recommends surgical excision of as much of the lesion as possible without risking "injury to surrounding structures" and irradiation. Gaynes and Cohen reported a dramatic response to systemic corticosteroid therapy (40 mg. prednisone per day initially, total duration 4 months) after external irradiation had not affected the size of the mass in their 8-month-old patient.

Lacrimal Gland Tumors

Epithelial tumors of the lacrimal gland are extremely rare in children under the age of 10 years, although examples have been recorded (McPherson, 1966). However, a significant proportion of both benign mixed tumors and adenoid cystic carcinomas of the lacrimal gland occur in the 10- to 19-year-old age group. In their review of cases on file at the Armed Forces Institute of Pathology, Zimmerman et al. (1962) found 4 of 68 benign mixed tumors (6 per cent) and 5 of 29 adenoid cystic carcinomas (14 per cent) in this age group. Two additional cases of adenoid cystic carcinoma in 12-year-old girls were recently reported (Ley and Wolter, 1969; Wolter and Henderson, 1969). The prognostic importance of accurate histopathologic classification of these tumors has been emphasized in reviews of AFIP material (Zimmerman et al., 1962) and of the Columbia-Presbyterian Hospital data (Forrest, 1971).

Benign mixed tumors (Figs. 33–260 to 33–262) of the lacrimal gland can be cured if completely excised, although they may recur locally if excision is incomplete, and a small percentage of cases undergo malignant change. Adenoid cystic carcinomas (Fig. 33–263) are the most common malignant lacrimal gland tumors. These are highly invasive, aggressive, relentlessly progressive malignant conditions that are

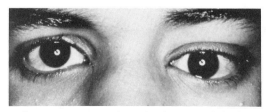

Figure 33–260 Benign mixed tumor of the lacrimal gland in a 15-year-old boy. Painless progressive proptosis of left eye over a nine-month period. (Courtesy of Dr. Kurt A. Gitter.) (E.P. #30696)

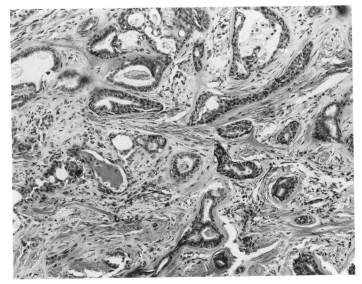

Figure 33–261 Benign mixed tumor of the lacrimal gland with acinar-like structure lined by two layers of low cuboidal epithelium. Spindle and stellate cells stream from the epithelial structures to form a fibrous tissue-like stroma. (Hematoxylin and eosin, ×125.) (E.P. #30696)

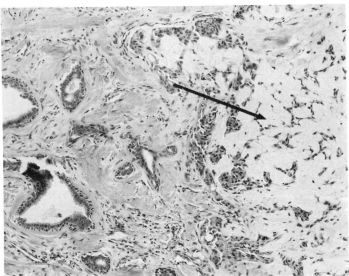

Figure 33–262 Benign mixed tumor of lacrimal gland with an area of chondromatous differentiation (arrow). (Hematoxylin and eosin, ×135.) (E.P. #30696)

Figure 33–263 Adenoid cystic carcinoma of lacrimal gland from a 32-year-old patient whose presenting symptoms were recent retro-orbital pain and diplopia. The tumor is composed of cells with hyperchromic nuclei and scanty cytoplasm. Mucin-containing cystic spaces are present in islands of tumor cells. (Hematoxylin and eosin, ×220.) (E.P. #35092)

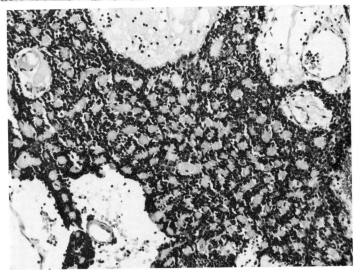

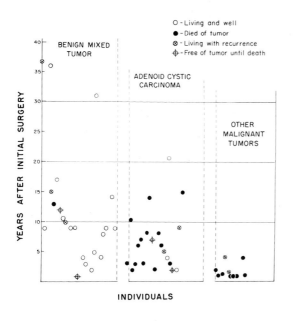

CLINICAL COURSE OF PATIENTS WITH
EPITHELIAL LACRIMAL GLAND TUMORS

Figure 33–264 Graphic illustration of clinical course of patients with epithelial tumors of the lacrimal gland, according to tumor type. (Courtesy of Dr. A. W. Forrest and Amer. J. Ophthal., *71*:178, 1971.)

lethal in a high proportion of patients in spite of radical surgical and modern irradiation therapy. Figure 33–264 depicts this distinct difference in biological behavior based on follow-up data from the Columbia-Presbyterian Hospital. Only 1 of 22 patients with a benign mixed tumor died, whereas 14 of the 20 patients with adenoid cystic carcinoma died as a result of the tumor.

Ectopic Lacrimal Gland

Choristomatous masses of ectopic lacrimal gland tissue may occur within the lid or orbit, producing signs and symptoms of an orbital tumor. Green and Zimmerman (1967) reviewed 8 cases of this type from the files of the Armed Forces Institute of Pathology. Four of their 8 patients were 15 years of age or younger. Proptosis (which was in one instance intermittent), ptosis, limitation of extraocular muscle function, and loss of vision with or without a palpable mass were the presenting signs in these children (Fig. 33–265). An inflammatory reaction of variable intensity was noted in the vicinity of the aberrant lacrimal tissue and was thought to explain the rapid pro-

gression of clinical signs which was observed in some instances (Fig. 33–266). In one 16-year-old patient, adenocarcinoma was found arising from ectopic lacrimal gland deep within the orbit.

Teratomas

By 1969 only 40 of these rare congenital orbital tumors had been reported in the lit-

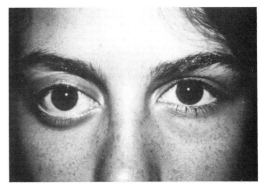

Figure 33–265 Ectopic lacrimal gland in orbit. External appearance of right eye after onset of proptosis in an 11-year-old girl. (AFIP neg. 66-9639-2). (Courtesy of Dr. Marshall Parks and Arch. Ophthal., *78*:318, Copyright 1967, American Medical Association.)

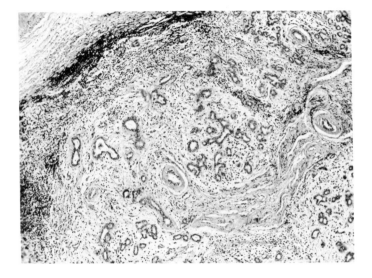

Figure 33–266 Isolated acini of ectopic lacrimal gland surrounded by inflammatory cells and fibrous tissue located within the muscle cone. (AFIP neg. 66-13027). (Arch. Ophthal., 78:315, Copyright 1967, American Medical Association.)

erature (Jensen, 1969). These choristomatous masses contain tissue representative of all three germ layers, though endodermal derivatives such as gut (Fig. 33–267), pancreas, or respiratory epithelium (Fig. 33–268) are generally less conspicuous than ectodermal (Fig. 33–269) or mesodermal elements (Fig. 33–270). The origin of teratomas has been a matter for embryologic speculation for over a hundred years, and current theories stress a primary abnormality which permits development of an aberrant growth center at some distance from the normal growth center near the primitive streak (Haye et al., 1966b;

Hoyt and Joe, 1962). No hereditary predilection has been noted.

Clinical Features

These tumors are evident at birth as grossly visible, cystic orbital masses which are often of grotesque proportions, displacing and destroying the child's globe, distending the lids and conjunctiva, and enlarging the bony orbit. Dr. Kenneth Jaegers provided the clinical photograph reproduced in Figure 33–271. This 10-month-old infant was noted at birth to have a large cystic orbital mass, a small right eye, and a purplish hue of both up-

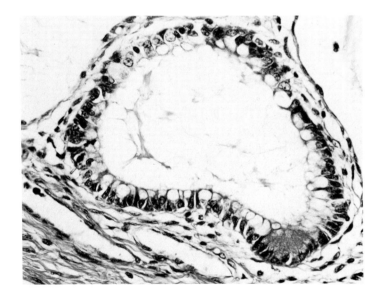

Figure 33–267 Intestinal mucosa. Endodermal component of orbital teratoma. (Hematoxylin and eosin, ×410.) (E.P. #30606)

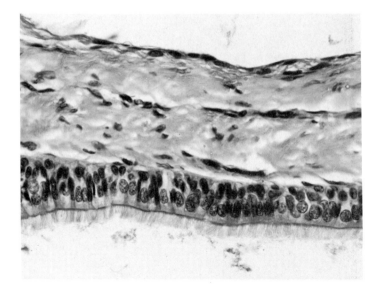

Figure 33–268   Ciliated respiratory epithelium. Endodermal derivative in an orbital teratoma. (Hematoxylin and eosin, ×530.) (E.P. #30606)

Figure 33–269   Cystic cavity lined by keratinized squamous epithelium with pilosebaceous apparati. Ectodermal derivative in orbital teratoma. (Hematoxylin and eosin, ×115.) (E.P. #30606)

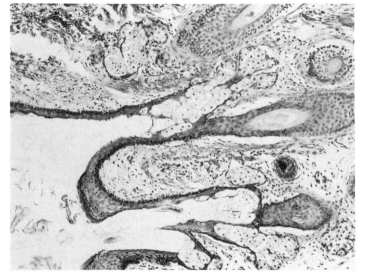

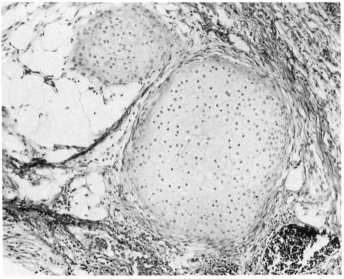

Figure 33–270   Cartilage and fat. Mesodermal derivatives in an orbital teratoma. (Hematoxylin and eosin, ×135.) (E.P. #30606)

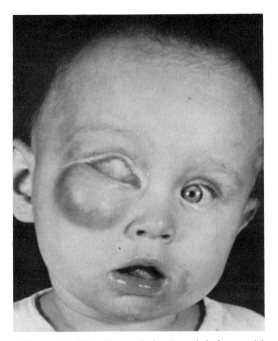

Figure 33–271 Congenital microphthalmos with cystic teratoma of the orbit. This 10-month-old girl was noted at birth to have a microphthalmic eye and a large orbital cyst. The cyst enlarged and was aspirated on two occasions. Enucleation and excision of a multicystic orbital mass were performed at the age of 10 months. (Case of Dr. Kenneth R. Jaegers.) (E.P. #30606)

per and lower lids. Histopathologic study of the exenteration specimen showed that in this instance microphthalmos with cyst and an orbital teratoma were both present! The case was presented in detail elsewhere (Jaegers, 1967; Rones, 1969).

Although malignant change occurs frequently in teratomas located elsewhere in the body, no example of a locally invasive or metastasizing orbital teratoma was encountered in the review of the literature by Hoyt and Joe or by Haye et al. (1966b). Orbital teratomas do enlarge if left untreated, and death may be caused by complications of intracranial erosion or by compression of nasal or oral passages by massive tumor.

Histopathology

Figures 33–267 to 33–270 illustrate the three germ layer derivatives found in the tumor depicted in Figure 33–271. Ectodermal tissues which are frequently found include skin and its appendages (sweat glands, pilosebaceous apparati) and neural tissue; mesodermal tissues include connective tissue, smooth muscle, cartilage, bone, and vessels. Ocular tissue has been described only recently in an orbital teratoma (Jensen, 1969) but has been seen previously in ovarian, testicular, and intracranial teratomas.

Treatment

Early local excision has cured the great majority of orbital teratomas for which follow-up information is available. Though it is not usually possible to preserve the globe, in rare instances useful vision has been salvaged by isolating and excising the tumor.

Microphthalmos With Cyst

The differential diagnosis of teratoma includes other causes of a congenital orbital tumor. Microphthalmos with cyst is one such possibility. This anomaly results when incomplete closure of the embryonic cleft permits herniation of developing ocular

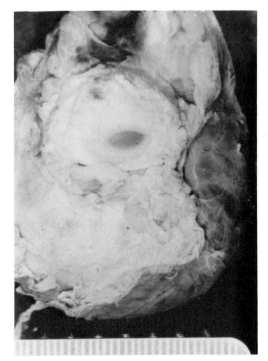

Figure 33–272 Microphthalmos with cyst from a 4-year-old boy who was born with a small right eye. Slowly progressive proptosis started at the age of 2 months. (Case of Dr. R. L. Marback.) (E.P. #34070)

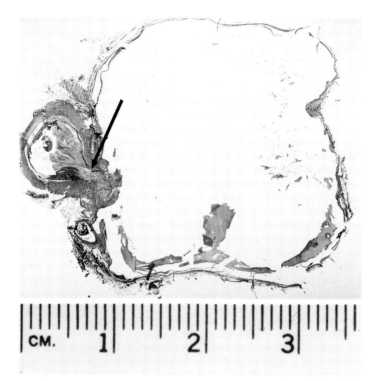

Figure 33–273 Low-power view of microphthalmic eye with scleral defect (arrow) which establishes communication between cyst cavity and globe. (Hematoxylin and eosin, ×3.) (E.P. #34070)

structures into the adjacent orbital tissue. The volume of the cyst cavity may exceed that of the microphthalmic globe (Figs. 33–272 and 33–273), and in extreme cases the tiny globe may be impossible to locate clinically. Large cysts produce taut distention of both upper and lower lids, whereas smaller lesions often project inferiorly, producing an apparent inferior orbital mass. Transillumination is useful to establish the cystic nature of the swelling, and an associated bluish discoloration of the overlying lid skin is an additional diagnostic clue. Other orbital mass lesions which may be present at birth include meningoencephalocele, orbital neurofibroma, dermoid cyst, hemangioma, lymphangioma, rhabdomyosarcoma, and juvenile xanthogranuloma.

ACKNOWLEDGMENTS

The authors gratefully acknowledge the contributions of patient histories and photographs from the resident and senior staff of the Wilmer Institute, Dr. John P. Dorst and Dr. Fred J. Hodges, III, Department of Radiology, and Dr. George W. Hambrick, Jr., Department of Dermatology, Johns Hopkins Hospital, and the technical assistance of Mr. Raymond E. Lund, R.B.P., and Mr. Terry W. George, R.B.P.

REFERENCES

Abele, D. C., and Griffin, T. B.: Histiocytic medullary reticulosis. Report of two cases and review of the literature. Arch. Derm., *106*:319, 1972.

Albert, D. M., Rabson, A. S., and Dalton, A. J.: Tissue culture study of human retinoblastoma. Invest. Ophthal., *9*:64, 1970.

Albert, D. M., and Reid, T. W.: RNA-directed DNA-polymerase activity in retinoblastoma: Report of its presence and possible significance. Trans. Amer. Acad. Ophthalmol. Otolaryngol., *76*:1564, 1972.

Albert, D. M., and Smith, R. S.: Fibrous xanthomas of the conjunctiva. Arch. Ophthal., *80*:474, 1968.

Albert, D. M., Rubenstein, R. A., and Scheie, H. G.: Tumor metastasis to the eye. Part II. Clinical study in infants and children. Amer. J. Ophthal. *63*:727, 1967a.

Albert, D. M., Wong, V. G., and Henderson, E. S.: Ocular complications of vincristine therapy. Arch. Ophthal. *78*:709, 1967b.

Alexander, G. L., and Norman, R. M.: The Sturge-Weber Syndrome. Bristol, John Wright and Sons, Ltd., 1960.

Alfano, J. E.: Ophthalmological aspects of neuroblastomatosis: a study of 53 verified cases. Trans. Amer. Acad. Ophthalmol. Otolaryngol., *72*:830, 1968.

Andersen, S. R.: Medulloepithelioma of the retina. Int. Ophthalmol. Clin., *2*:483, 1962.

Andersen, S. R.: Differentiation features in some retinal tumors and in dysplastic retinal conditions. Amer. J. Ophthal., *71*:231, 1971.

Anderson, D. R., and Spencer, W. H.: Ultrastructural and histochemical observations of optic nerve gliomas. Arch. Ophthal., *83*:324, 1970.

Apple, D. J.: Wilms' tumor metastatic to the orbit. Arch. Ophthal., *80*:480, 1968.

Apple, D. J.: Metastatic orbital neuroblastoma originating in the cervical sympathetic ganglion chain. Amer. J. Ophthal., *68*:1093, 1969.

Apt, L.: Uveal melanomas in children and adolescents. Int. Ophthal. Clin., *2*:430, 1962.

Ash, J. E.: Epibulbar tumors. Amer. J. Ophthal., *33*:1203, 1950.

Ashton, N., and Morgan, G.: Embryonal sarcoma and embryonal rhabdomyosarcoma of the orbit. J. Clin. Path., *18*:699, 1965.

Avery, M. E., McAfee, J. G., and Guild, H. G.: The course and prognosis of reticuloendotheliosis (eosinophilic granuloma, Schüller-Christian disease and Letterer-Siwe disease); a study of forty cases. Amer. J. Med., *22*:636, 1957.

Awdry, P. : Lymphangiectasia haemorrhagica conjunctivae. Brit. J. Ophthal., *53*:274, 1969.

Backwinkel, K. D., and Diddanns, J. A.: Hemangiopericytoma: Report of a case and comprehensive review of the literature. Cancer, *25*:896, 1970.

Baer, R. L., and Kopf, A. W.: Keratoacanthoma. Year Book of Dermatology, 1962–1963 series, p. 7.

Barrow, M. V., and Holubar, K.: Multicentric reticulohistiocytosis; A review of 33 patients. Medicine, *48*:287, 1969.

Barsky, D., and Wolter, J. R.: The retinal lesion of tuberous sclerosis: An angiogliomatous hamartoma? J. Pediat. Ophthal., *8*:261, 1971.

Basset, F., Escaig, J., and LeCrom, M.: A cytoplasmic membranous complex in histiocytosis X. Cancer, *29*:1380, 1972.

Baum, J. L., and Feingold, M.: Ocular aspects of Goldenhar's syndrome. Amer. J. Ophthal., *75*:250, 1973.

Bedford, M. A., Bedotto, C., and MacFaul, P. A.: Retinoblastoma: A study of 139 cases. Brit. J. Ophthal., *55*:19, 1971.

Berlin, N. I., Van Scott, E. J., Clendenning, W. E., Archard, H. O., Block, J. B., Witkop, C. J., and Haynes, H. A.: Basal cell nevus syndrome. Ann. Intern. Med., *64*:403, 1966.

Binet, E. F., Kieffer, S. A., Martin, S. H., and Peterson, H. O.: Orbital dysplasia in neurofibromatosis. Radiology, *93*:829, 1969.

Blodi, F. C., and Gass, J. D. M.: Inflammatory pseudotumour of the orbit. Brit. J. Ophthal., *52*:79, 1968.

Boniuk, M., and Zimmerman, L. E.: Spontaneous regression of retinoblastoma. Int. Ophthal. Clin., *2*:525, 1962a.

Boniuk, M., and Zimmerman, L. E.: Epibulbar osteoma (episcleral osseous choristoma). Amer. J. Ophthal., *53*:290, 1962b.

Boniuk, M., and Zimmerman, L. E.: Eyelid tumors with reference to lesions confused with squamous cell carcinoma. III. Keratoacanthoma. Arch. Ophthal., *77*:29, 1967.

Boniuk, M., and Zimmerman, L. E.: Sebaceous carcinoma of the eyelid, eyebrow, caruncle and orbit. Trans. Amer. Acad. Ophthalmol. Otolaryngol., *72*:619, 1968.

Bowers, R. E., Graham, E. A., and Tomlinson, K. M.: The natural history of the strawberry nevus. Arch. Derm., *82*:667, 1960.

Brown, D. H.: The clinicopathology of retinoblastoma. Amer. J. Ophthal., *60*:508, 1966a.

Brown, D. H.: The urinary excretion of vanilmande-

lic acid (VMA) and homovanillic acid (HVA) in children with retinoblastoma. Amer. J. Ophthal., *62*:239, 1966b.

Brownstein, M. H., and Helwig, E. B.: Patterns of cutaneous metastasis. Arch. Derm., *105*:862, 1972.

Bruce, G. M.: Aberrant glandular tissue in the iris. Trans. Amer. Acad. Ophthalmol. Otolaryngol., *56*:47, 1952.

Burchenal, J. H.: Features suggesting curability in leukemia and lymphoma. *In* M. D. Anderson Hospital and Tumor Institute 14th Annual Clinical Conference on Cancer, 1969: Leukemia-Lymphoma. Chicago, Year Book Medical Publishers, 1970, p. 93.

Burkitt, D. P., and Wright, D. H.: Burkitt's Lymphoma. Edinburgh, E. & S. Livingstone Ltd., 1970.

Burrows, E. H.: Bone changes in orbital neurofibromatosis. Brit. J. Radiol., *36*:549, 1963.

Carbone, P. P., Berard, C. W., Bennett, J. M., Ziegler, J. L., Cohen, M. H., and Gerber, P.: Burkitt's tumor. Ann. Intern. Med., *70*:817, 1969.

Carey, P. C.: Epidermoid and dermoid tumours of the orbit. Brit. J. Ophthal., *42*:225, 1958.

Chaves, E., and Granville, R.: Choroidal malignant melanoma in a two-and-one-half-year-old girl. Amer. J. Ophthal., *74*:20, 1972.

Christensen, L., and Anderson, E. D.: Aberrant intraocular adenomata and epithelization of the anterior chamber. Arch. Ophthal., *48*:19, 1952.

Chutorian, A. M., Schwartz, J. F., Evans, R. A., and Carter, S.: Optic gliomas in children, Neurology, *14*:83, 1964.

Clark, W. H., Jr., and Mihm, M. C., Jr.: Neoplasms of the skin: neoplasms of the melanocyte. *In* Fitzpatrick, T. B., et al. (Eds.): Dermatology in General Medicine. New York, McGraw-Hill Book Co., 1971, p. 491.

Cleasby, G. W., Fung, W. E., and Shekter, W. B.: Astrocytoma of the retina: Report of 2 cases. Amer. J. Ophthal., *64*:633, 1967.

Clements, D. B.: Juvenile xanthogranuloma treated with local steroids. Brit. J. Ophthal., *50*:663, 1966.

Cogan, D. G., Kuwabara, T., and Parke, D.: Epibulbar nevoxanthoendothelioma. Arch. Ophthal., *59*:717, 1958.

Cohen, M. H., Bennett, J. M., Berard, C. W., Ziegler, J. L., Vogel, C. L., Sheagren, J. N., and Carbone, P. P.: Burkitt's tumor in the United States. Cancer, *23*:1259, 1969.

Consul, B. N., Kulshrestha, O. P., and Mehrotra, A. S.: Bilateral proptosis in acute myeloid leukaemia. Brit. J. Ophthal., *51*:65, 1967.

Craig, W. M., and Gogela, L. J.: Intraorbital meningiomas; a clinicopathologic study. Amer. J. Ophthal., *32*: 1663, 1949.

Crocker, A. C.: The histiocytosis syndromes. *In* Fitzpatrick, T. B., et al. (Eds.): Dermatology in General Medicine. New York, McGraw-Hill Book Co., 1971, p. 1328.

Crombie, A. L.: Proptosis in leukaemia. Brit. J. Ophthal., *51*:101, 1967.

Cross, H. W., and Maumenee, A.: Possible ocular trauma during amniocentesis. Arch. Ophthal., *90*:303, 1973.

Cushing, H. W., and Eisenhardt, L.: Meningiomas: Their Classification, Regional Behaviour, Life History and Surgical End Results. Springfield, Illinois, Charles C Thomas, 1938, p. 297.

Dailey, E. G., and Lubowtiz, R. M.: Dermoids of the

limbus and cornea. Amer. J. Ophthal., 53:661, 1962.

D'Angio, G. J., Evans, A. E., and Koop, C. E.: Special pattern of widespread neuroblastoma with a favourable prognosis. Lancet, 1:1046, 1971.

Danis, P.: L'angiome de la choroïde. Arch. Ophtal. (Paris), 12:487, 1952.

Dargeon, H. W.: Tumors of Childhood; a Clinical Treatise. New York, Hoeber, 1960.

Davidorf, F. H., Newman, G. H., Havener, W. H., and Makley, T.: Conservative management of malignant melanoma. II. Transscleral diathermy as a method of treatment for malignant melanomas of the choroid. Arch. Ophthal., 83:273, 1970.

Dayton, G. O., Jr., Langdon, E., and Rochlin, D.: Management of orbital rhabdomyosarcoma. Amer. J. Ophthal., 68:906, 1969.

deLorimier, A. A., Bragg, K. U., and Linden, G.: Neuroblastoma in childhood. Amer. J. Dis. Child., 118:441, 1969.

deVenecia, G., and Lobeck, C. C.: Successful treatment of eyelid hemangioma with prednisone. Arch. Ophthal., 84:98, 1970.

Dodge, H. W., Jr., Love, J. G., Craig, W. M., Dockerty, A. B., Kearns, T. P., Holman, C. B., and Hayles, A. B.: Gliomas of the optic nerves. A.M.A. Arch. Neurol. Psych., 79:607, 1958.

Duke, J. R., and Dunn, S. N.: Primary tumors of the iris. Arch. Ophthal., 59:204, 1958.

Duke-Elder, S.: System of Ophthalmology. Volume III (Congenital Deformities), Part 2. London, Kimpton, 1964, p. 820.

Dunphy, E. B.: The story of retinoblastoma. Trans. Amer. Acad. Ophthalmol. Otolaryngol., 68:249, 1964.

Dutz, W., and Stout, A. P.: Kaposi's sarcoma in infants and children. Cancer, 13:684, 1960.

Ehlers, N.: A case of divided nevus. Arch. Ophthal., 73:664, 1965.

El-Hefnawi, H., and Mortada, A: Ocular manifestations of xeroderma pigmentosum. Brit. J. Derm., 77:261, 1965.

Ellsworth, R. M.: The practical management of retinoblastoma. Trans. Amer. Ophthal. Soc., 67:462, 1969.

Elsas, F., and Green, W. R.: Epibulbar tumors in children. Presented at the 32nd Wilmer Residents Association Meeting, Baltimore, April, 1973.

Enriquez, P., Dahlin, D. C., Hayles, A. B., and Henderson, E. D.: Histiocytosis X: A clinical study. Mayo Clin. Proc., 42:88, 1967.

Enzinger, F. M., and Shiraki, M.: Alveolar rhabdomyosarcoma: an analysis of 110 cases. Cancer, 24:18, 1969.

Esterly, N. B., Sahihi, T., and Medenica, M.: Juvenile xanthogranuloma: An atypical case with study of ultrastructure. Arch. Derm., 105:99, 1972.

Feingold, M., and Gellis, S. S.: Ocular abnormalities associated with first and second arch syndromes. Surv. Ophthal., 14:30, 1969.

Ferry, A. P.: Hemangiomas of the iris and ciliary body. Do they exist? A search for a histologically proven case. Int. Ophthal. Clin., 12 (1):177, 1972.

Ferry, A. P., and Hein, H. F.: Epibulbar osseous choristoma within an epibulbar dermoid. Amer. J. Ophthal., 70:764, 1970.

Fienman, N. L., and Yakovac, W. C.: Neurofibromatosis in childhood. J. Pediat., 76:339, 1970.

Fonken, H. A., and Ellis, P. P.: Leukemic infiltrates in the iris; successful treatment of secondary glaucoma with x-irradiation. Arch. Ophthal., 76:32, 1966.

Font, R. L., and Ferry, A. P.: The phakomatoses. Int. Ophthal. Clin., 12(1):1, 1972.

Font, R. L., Reynolds, A. M., Jr., and Zimmerman, L. E.: Diffuse malignant melanoma of the iris in the nevus of Ota. Arch. Ophthal., 77:513, 1967.

Font, R. L., and Zimmerman, L. E.: Nodular fasciitis of the eye and adnexa. A report of ten cases. Arch. Ophthal., 75:475, 1966.

Foos, R. Y., Hull, S. N., and Straatsma, B. R.: Early diagnosis of ciliary body melanomas. Arch. Ophthal., 81:336, 1969.

Forrest, A. W.: Tumors following irradiation about the eye. Int. Ophthal. Clin., 2:543, 1962.

Forrest, A. W.: Pathologic criteria for effective management of epithelial lacrimal gland tumors. Amer. J. Ophthal., 71:178, 1971.

Fost, N. C., and Esterly, N. B.: Successful treatment of juvenile hemangiomas with prednisone. J. Pediat., 72:351, 1968.

Foster, S. C., Wilson, C. S., and Tretter, P. K.: Radiotherapy of primary lymphoma of the orbit. Amer. J. Roentgen., 3:343, 1971.

Fowler, F. D., and Matson, D. D.: Gliomas of the optic pathways in childhood. J. Neurosurg., 14:515, 1957.

François, J., and Matton-Van Leuven, M. T.: Recent data on the heredity of retinoblastoma. In Boniuk, M. (Ed.): Ocular and Adnexal Tumors; New and Controversial Aspects. St. Louis, The C. V. Mosby, Co., 1964, p. 123.

Friedman, A. H., and Henkind, P.: Granuloma pyogenicum of the palpebral conjunctiva. Amer. J. Ophthal., 71:868, 1971.

Garner, L. L.: Dermoid of the limbus involving the iris angle and lens. Arch. Ophthal., 46:69, 1951.

Gartner, S.: Malignant melanoma of the choroid and von Recklinghausen's disease. Amer. J. Ophthal., 23:73, 1940.

Gartner, S., and Feiring, E. H.: Glioma of the optic nerve and retina. Amer. J. Ophthal., 61:747, 1966.

Gass, J. D. M.: Management of juvenile xanthogranuloma of the iris. Arch. Ophthal., 71:344, 1964.

Gass, J. D. M.: The phakomatoses. In Smith, J. L. (Ed.): Neuro-ophthalmology Symposium of the University of Miami and the Bascom Palmer Eye Institute. Vol. 2. St. Louis, The C. V. Mosby Co., 1965, p. 223.

Gass, J. D. M.: Fluorescein angiography; an aid in the differential diagnosis of intraocular tumors. Int. Ophthal. Clin., 12(1):85, 1972.

Gaynes, P. M., and Cohen, G. S.: Juvenile xanthogranuloma of the orbit. Amer. J. Ophthal., 63:755, 1967.

Gitlow, S. E., Bertani, L. M., Rausen, A., Gribetz, D., and Dziedzic, S. W.: Diagnosis of neuroblastoma by qualitative and quantitative determination of catecholamine metabolites in urine. Cancer, 25:1377, 1970.

Glaser, J. S., Hoyt, W. F., and Corbett, J.: Visual morbidity with chiasmal glioma. Long-term studies of visual fields in untreated and irradiated cases. Arch. Ophthal., 85:3, 1971.

Goldberg, M. F., and Duke, J. R.: von Hippel-Lindau disease; histopathologic findings in a treated and an untreated eye. Amer. J. Ophthal., 66:693, 1968.

Gonzalez-Crussi, F., and Campbell, R. J.: Juvenile

xanthogranuloma; ultrastructural study. Arch. Path., *89*:65, 1970.

Graham, J. H., Johnson, W. C., and Helwig, E. B. (Eds.): Dermal Pathology. Hagerstown, Harper and Row, 1972, p. 17.

Graham, J. H., Mason, J. K., Gray, H. R., and Helwig, E. B.: Differentiation of nevoid basal cell carcinoma from epithelioma adenoides cysticum; a clinico-pathologic and histochemical study. J. Invest. Derm., *44*:197, 1965.

Grant, W. M., and Walton, D. S.: Distinctive gonio-scopic findings in glaucoma due to neurofibroma-tosis. Arch. Ophthal., *79*:127, 1968.

Gray, H. R., and Helwig, E. B.: Epithelioma aden-oides cysticum and solitary trichoepithelioma. Arch. Derm., *87*:102, 1963.

Grayson, M., and Pieroni, D.: Solitary xanthoma of the limbus. Brit. J. Ophthal., *54*:562, 1970.

Green, W. R., Iliff, W. J., and Trotter, R. R.: Malig-nant teratoid medulloepithelioma of the optic nerve. Presented at the 31st Annual Wilmer Resi-dents Association Meeting, Baltimore, April, 1972.

Green, W. R., and Zimmerman, L. E.: Ectopic lacri-mal gland tissue; report of eight cases with orbital involvement. Arch. Ophthal., *78*:318, 1967.

Greenfield, L. J., and Shelley, W. M.: The spectrum of neurogenic tumors of the sympathetic nervous system: Maturation and adrenergic function. J. Natl. Cancer Inst., *35*:215, 1965.

Greer, C. H.: Congenital melanoma of the anterior uvea. Arch. Ophthal., *76*:77, 1966.

Gross, R. E., Farber, S., and Martin, L. W.: Neuro-blastoma sympatheticum; a study and report of 217 cases. Pediatrics, *23*:1179, 1959.

Guzak, S. V., Jr.: Lymphoma as a cause of hyphema. Arch. Ophthal., *84*:229, 1970.

Haberland, C., and Perou, M.: Encephalocraniocu-taneous lipomatosis; a new example of ectomeso-dermal dysgenesis. Arch. Neurol., *22*:144, 1970.

Hagler, W. S., Jarrett, W. H., II, and Humphrey, W. T.: The radioactive phosphorus uptake test in di-agnosis of uveal melanoma. Arch. Ophthal., *83*:548, 1970.

Happle, R., and Kupferschmid, A.: A further case of basal cell nevus syndrome and structural chromo-some abnormalities. Humangenetik, *15*:287, 1972.

Happle, R., Mehrle, G., Sander, L. Z., and Hohn, H.: Basalzellnävus-Syndrom mit Retinopathia pig-mentosa rezidivierender Glaskörperblutung und Chromosomenveränderungen. Arch. Dermatol. Forsch., *241*:96, 1971.

Harkey, M. E., and Metz, H. S.: Cryotherapy of con-junctival papillomata. Amer. J. Ophthal., *66*:872, 1968.

Harkin, J. C., and Reed, R. J.: Tumors of the Periph-eral Nervous System. Washington, D. C., Armed Forces Institute of Pathology, 1969 (Atlas of Tumor Pathology, Second Series, fasc. 3).

Harley, R. D., and Grover, W. D.: Tuberous sclerosis; description and report of 12 cases. Ann. Ophthal., *1*:477, 1970.

Hashimoto, K., and Lever, W. F.: Tumors of the skin appendages. *In* Fitzpatrick, T. B., et al. (Eds.): Dermatology in General Medicine. New York, McGraw-Hill Book Co., 1971, p. 440.

Haye, C., Haut, J., and Romain, M.: A propos des kystes dermoïdes de l'orbite. Arch. Ophtal. (Paris), *26*:471, 1966a.

Haye, C., Haut, J., and Porges, D.: Les tératomes de l'orbite. Arch. Ophtal. (Paris), *26*:569, 1966b.

Haye, C., Haut, J., and Sander, J. -P.: Les dermoïdes épibulbaires. Arch. Ophtal. (Paris), *29*:193, 1969.

Hayek, A., Chapman, E. M., and Crawford, J. D.: Long-term results of treatment of thyrotoxicosis in children and adolescents with radioactive iodine. New Eng. J. Med., *283*:949, 1970.

Haynes, R. E., and Cramblett, H. G.: Acute ethmoi-ditis: its relationship to orbital cellulitis. Amer. J. Dis. Child., *114*:261, 1967.

Heinrich, P.: Exophthalmus bei Leukosen. (2 Kongr. Europ. Ges. Ophth., Wien, 1964). Ophthalmo-logica, *151 (Suppl.)*:775, 1966.

Henkind, P., and Friedman, A. H.: External ocular pigmentation. Int. Ophthal. Clin. *11(3)*:87, 1971.

Heyn, R. M.: Chemotherapy in pediatric orbital tumors. J. Pediat. Ophthal., *8*:141, 1971.

Heyner, F. J., and Passmore, J. W.: Pseudotumor of orbit caused by retained foreign body. Amer. J. Ophthal., *59*:490, 1965.

Hidano, A., Kajima, H., Ikeda, S., Mitzutani, Miya-soto, H., and Niimura, M.: Natural history of nevus of Ota. Arch. Derm., *95*:187, 1967.

Hiles, D. A., and Pilchard, W. A.: Corticosteroid con-trol of neonatal hemangiomas of the orbit and ocu-lar adnexa. Amer. J. Ophthal., *71*:1003, 1971.

Hogan, M. J., and Zimmerman, L. E. (Eds.): Ophthal-mic Pathology; An Atlas and Textbook. 2nd ed. Philadelphia, W. B. Saunders Co., 1962.

Holland, G.: Hämangiome der Lider. Klin. Mbl. Augenheilk., *152*:365, 1968.

Höpping, W., and Meyer-Schwickerath, G.: Light co-agulation treatment in retinoblastoma. *In* Boniuk, M. (Ed): Ocular and Adnexal Tumors; New and Controversial Aspects. St. Louis, The C. V. Mosby Co., 1964, p. 192.

Horowitz, P.: von Hippel-Lindau disease. *In* Tasman, W. (Ed): Retinal Diseases in Children. New York, Harper and Row, 1971, p. 78.

Hovland, K. R., and Ellis, P. P.: Hemorrhagic glau-coma with optic nerve glioma. Arch. Ophthal., *75*:806, 1966.

Howard, G. M.: Spontaneous hyphema in infancy and childhood. Arch. Ophthal., *68*:615, 1962.

Howard, G. M., and Ellsworth, R. M.: Differential diagnosis of retinoblastoma. A statistical survey of 500 children. I. Relative frequency of the lesions which simulate retinoblastoma. Amer. J. Ophthal., *60*:610, 1965.

Hoyt, W. F., and Baghdassarian, S. A.: Optic glioma of childhood. Natural history and rationale for con-servative management. Brit. J. Ophthal., *53*:793, 1969.

Hoyt, W. F., and Joe, S.: Congenital teratoid cyst of the orbit. A case report and review of the literature. Arch. Ophthal., *68*:196, 1962.

Hutchinson, D. S., Green, W. R., and Iliff, C. E.: Lim-bal dermoid with ectopic brain and associated with scleral staphyloma. Presented at the 31st Annual Wilmer Residents Association Meeting, Baltimore, April, 1972.

Iliff, C. E., and Ossofsky, H. J.: Tumors of the Eye and Adnexa in Infancy and Childhood. Spring-field, Ill., Charles C Thomas, 1962.

Iliff, W. J., and Green, W. R.: Orbital tumors in children. Presented at the 31st Annual Wilmer Res-idents Association Meeting, Baltimore, April, 1972.

Iliff, W. J., Marback, R., and Green, W. R.: Invasive squamous cell carcinoma of the conjunctiva. Pre-sented at the 28th Annual Wilmer Residents Asso-ciation Meeting, Baltimore, April, 1969.

Ingalls, R. G.: Tumors of the Orbit and Allied Pseudo Tumors. Springfield, Ill., Charles C Thomas, 1953.

Iwamoto, T., Witmer, R., and Landolt, E.: Diktyoma, a clinical, histological and electron microscopical observation. von Graefe Arch. Ophthal., *172*:293, 1967.

Jaegers, K. R.: Microphthalmos with cyst and orbital teratoma. Presented at the Wills Eye Clinical Conference, February, 1967.

Jay, B.: Naevi and melanomata of the conjunctiva. Brit. J. Ophthal., *49*:169, 1965.

Jensen, N. E., Sabharwal, S., and Walker, A. E.: Naevoxanthoendothelioma and neurofibromatosis. Brit. J. Derm., *85*:326, 1971.

Jensen, O. A.: Teratoma of the orbit. Acta Ophthal., *47*:317, 1969.

Jensen, R. D., and Miller, R. W.: Retinoblastoma: Epidemiologic characteristics. New Eng. J. Med., *285*:307, 1971.

Johnson, B. L., and Charneco, D. R.: Café-au-lait spot in neurofibromatosis and in normal individuals. Arch. Derm., *102*:442, 1970.

Johnson, F. D., and Jacobs, E. M.: Chemotherapy of metastatic malignant melanoma; experience with 73 patients. Cancer, *27*:1306, 1971.

Johnson, R. E., and Pomeroy, T. C.: Integrated therapy for Ewing's sarcoma. Amer. J. Roentgen. Radium Ther. Nucl. Med., *114*:532, 1972.

Jones, I. S.: Lymphangiomas of the ocular adnexa: An analysis of 62 cases. Trans. Amer. Ophthal. Soc., *57*:602, 1959.

Jones, I. S., and Cleasby, G. W.: Hemangioma of the choroid: A clinicopathologic analysis. Amer. J. Ophthal., *48*:612, 1959.

Jones, I. S., Reese, A. B., and Krout, J.: Orbital rhabdomyosarcoma: An analysis of sixty-two cases. Trans. Amer. Ophthal. Soc., *63*:223, 1965.

Kauffman, S. L., and Stout, A. P.: Hemangiopericytoma in children. Cancer, *13*:695, 1960.

Kauffman, S. L., and Stout, A. P.: Malignant hemangioendothelioma in infants and children. Cancer, *14*:1186, 1961.

Kennedy, R. E.: Marsupialization of inoperable orbital dermoids. Trans. Amer. Ophthal. Soc., *68*:146, 1970.

Kogan, L., and Boniuk, M.: Causes for enucleation in childhood with special reference to pseudogliomas and unsuspected retinoblastomas. Int. Ophthal. Clin., *2*:507, 1962.

Kopelow, S. M., Foos, R. Y., Straatsma, B. R., Hepler, R. S., and Pearlman, J. T.: Cavernous hemangioma of the orbit. Int. Ophthal. Clin., *11(3)*:113, 1971.

Kroll, A. J.: Fine-structural classification of orbital rhabdomyosarcoma. Invest. Ophthal., *6*:531, 1967.

Lagos, J. C., and Gomez, M. R.: Tuberous sclerosis: Reappraisal of a clinical entity. Mayo Clin. Proc., *42*:26, 1967.

Lahey, M. E.: Prognosis in reticuloendotheliosis in children. J. Pediat., *60*:664, 1962.

Lampe, I., and Latourette, H. B.: Management of hemangiomas in infants. Pediat. Clin. N. Amer., *6*:511, 1959.

Landbo, K.: A case of optic disc angioma; with a fluorescein angiography. Acta Ophthal., *50*:431, 1972.

Lehrer, H. Z.: Ossifying fibroma of the orbital roof; its distinction from "blistering" or "intra-osseous" meningioma. Arch. Neurol., *20*:536, 1969.

Lerner, H. A.: Malignant melanoma of the iris in children. A report of a case in a 9-year-old girl. Arch. Ophthal., *84*:754, 1970.

Ley, J. A., and Wolter, J. R.: Adenoid cystic carcinoma: as seen in the orbit of a twelve-year-old Vietnamese girl. J. Pediat. Ophthal., *6*:162, 1969.

Lichter, P. R.: Multiple corneal dermoids associated with miliary aneurysms of the retina. J. Pediat. Ophthal., *4*:31, 1967.

Lieberman, P. H., Jones, C. R., Dargeon, H. W. K., and Begg, C. F.: A reappraisal of eosinophilic granuloma of bone, Hand-Schüller-Christian syndrome and Letterer-Siwe syndrome. Medicine, *48*:375, 1969.

Liebman, S. D., Crocker, A. C., and Geiser, C. F.: Corneal xanthomas in childhood. Arch. Ophthal., *76*:221, 1966.

Lincoff, H., McLean, J., and Long, R.: The cryosurgical treatment of intraocular tumors. Amer. J. Ophthal., *63*:389, 1967.

Lindau, A.: Studien über Kleinhirncysten; Bau, Pathogenese und Beziehungen zur Angiomatosis Retinae. Acta Path. Microbiol. Scand., Suppl, 1, 1926, pp. 1–128.

Lingley, J. F., Sagerman, R. H., Santulli, T. V., and Wolff, J. A.: Neuroblastoma; management and survival. New Eng. J. Med., *277*:1227, 1967.

Linwong, M., Hermann, S. J., and Rabb, M. F.: Carcinoma in-situ of the corneal limbus in an adolescent girl. Arch. Ophthal., *87*:48, 1972.

Lucaya, X.: Histiocytosis X. Amer. J. Dis. Child., *121*:289, 1971.

Macklin, M. T.: Inheritance of retinoblastoma in Ohio. Arch. Ophthal., *62*:842, 1959.

MacMichael, I. M., and Cullen, J. F.: Primary intraorbital meningioma. Brit. J. Ophthal., *53*:169, 1969.

Malik, S. R., Sood, G. C., and Gupta, D. K.: Limbal dermoid with naevus flammeus and neurofibromatosis. Eye Ear Nose Throat Mon., *46*:612, 1967.

Marcel, J.-E., and Chabrut, R.: Tumeur du testicule, métastases pulmonaire et orbitaire, sinus pericranii. Arch. Fr. Pediatr., *13*:1111, 1956.

Margileth, A. M., and Museles, M.: Cutaneous hemangiomas in children; diagnosis and conservative management. J.A.M.A., *194*:523, 1965.

Maumenee, A. E., and Longfellow, D. W.: Treatment of intraocular nevoxantho-endothelioma (juvenile xanthogranuloma). Amer. J. Ophthal., *49*:1, 1960.

McKenzie, T. R., and Zimmerman, L. E., cited by Boniuk, M.: Discussion of retinoblastoma. *In* Boniuk, M. (Ed.): Ocular and Adnexal Tumors; New and Controversial Aspects. St. Louis, The C. V. Mosby Co., 1964, p. 198.

McLean, J. M.: Astrocytoma (true glioma) of the retina; report of a case. Arch. Ophthal., *18*:255, 1937.

McPherson, S. D., Jr.: Mixed tumor of the lacrimal gland in a seven-year-old boy. Amer. J. Ophthal., *61*:561, 1966.

M. D. Anderson Hospital and Tumor Institute 14th Annual Clinical Conference on Cancer, 1969; Leukemia-Lymphoma. Chicago, Year Book Medical Publishers, 1970, 392 pp.

Melmon, K. L., and Rosen, S. W.: Lindau's disease; review of the literature and study of a large kindred. Amer. J. Med., *36*:595, 1964.

Mendiratta, S. S., Rosenblum, J. A., and Strobos, R. L.: Congenital meningioma. Neurology, *17*:914, 1967.

Misugi, K., and Liss, L.: Medulloblastoma with cross-striated muscle. Cancer, *25*:1279, 1970.

Moore, J. G. Neonatal neurofibromatosis. Brit. J. Ophthal., 46:682, 1962.

Morgan, G.: Diffuse infiltrating retinoblastoma. Brit. J. Ophthal., 55:600, 1971a.

Morgan, G.: Lymphocytic tumours of the conjunctiva. J. Clin. Path., 24:585, 1971b.

Mortada, A.: Clinical characteristics of early orbital metastatic neuroblastoma. Amer. J. Ophthal., 63:1787, 1967.

Mortada, A.: Orbital neurilemmoma with café-au-lait pigmentation of the skin. Brit. J. Ophthal., 52:262, 1968.

Mullaney, J.: Retinoblastoma with DNA precipitation. Arch. Ophthal., 82:454, 1969.

Naidoff, M. A., Kenyon, K. R., and Green, W. R.: Iris hemangioma and abnormal retinal vasculature in a case of diffuse congenital hemangiomatosis. Amer. J. Ophthal., 72:633, 1971.

Nathanson, L., Hall, T. C., Vawter, G. F., and Farber, S.: Melanoma as a medical problem. Arch. Intern. Med., 119:479, 1967.

Naumann, G., Font, R. L., and Zimmerman, L. E.: Electron microscopic verification of primary rhabdomyosarcoma of the iris. Amer. J. Ophthal., 74:110, 1972.

Naumann, G., and Green, W. R.: Spontaneous nonpigmented iris cysts. Arch. Ophthal., 78:496, 1967.

Nesbit, M. E., Jr., Wolfson, J. J., Kieffer, S. A., and Peterson, H. O.: Orbital sclerosis in histiocytosis X. Amer. J. Roentgen. Rad. Ther. Nuc. Med., 110:123, 1970.

Newman, G. H., Davidorf, F. H., Havener, W. H., and Makley, T. A., Jr.: Conservative management of malignant melanoma. I. Irradiation as a method of treatment for malignant melanoma of the choroid. Arch. Ophthal., 83:21, 1970.

Nicholson, D. H., Green, W. R., and Kenyon, K.: Light and electron microscopic study of angiomatosis retinae. (In preparation.)

Nicholson, D. H., and Wood, W. W.: The meningioma that wasn't. Presented at the 31st Annual Wilmer Residents Association Meeting. Baltimore, April, 1972.

Nielsen, M., and Goldschmidt, E.: Retinoblastoma among offspring of adult survivors in Denmark. Acta Ophthal., 46:736, 1968.

Nover, A., and Korting, G. W.: Zur Kenntnis des familiären Basalzellnävus. Klin. Mbl. Augenheilk., 156:621, 1970.

Oberman, H. A.: Idiopathic histiocytosis. A correlative review of eosinophilic granuloma, Hand-Schüller-Christian disease, and Letterer-Siwe disease. J. Pediat. Ophthal., 5:86, 1968.

Okisaka, S., Ono, H., Asaoka, I., and Uemura, Y.: A case of neurofibromatosis with juvenile xanthogranuloma and congenital glaucoma. Folia Ophthal. Jap., 21:273, 1970.

Olson, C. W., Smith J. H., Testerman, N., Bastin, J.-P., and Frazer, H.: Burkitt's tumor in the Democratic Republic of the Congo. Cancer, 23:740, 1969.

Olurin, O.: Bilateral conjunctival epithelioma in an adolescent. Ann. Ophthal., 3:633, 1971.

Omohundro, J. M., and Elliott, J. H.: Cryotherapy of conjunctival papilloma. Arch. Ophthal., 84:609, 1970.

Ophthalmic Staff of the Hospital for Sick Children, Toronto, Canada: The Eye in Childhood. Chicago, Year Book Medical Publishers, 1967.

Ortega, J. A., Finkelstein, J. Z., Isaacs, H., Jr., Hittle,

R., and Hastings, N.: Chemotherapy of malignant hemangiopericytoma of childhood; report of a case and review of the literature. Cancer, 27:730, 1971.

Oshida, N., Hisatomi, U., Takemura, M., and Kobayashi, Y.: A hemangiopericytoma of the eyelid. Folia Ophthal. Jap., 21:269, 1970,

Paul, E. V., Parnell, B. L., and Fraker, M.: Prognosis of malignant melanomas of the choroid and ciliary body. Int. Ophthal. Clin., 2:387, 1962.

Payne, J. W., Duke, J. R., Butner, R., and Eifrig, D. E.: Basal cell carcinoma of the eyelids; a long-term follow-up study. Arch. Ophthal., 81:553, 1969.

Pettit, T. H., Barton, A., Foos, R. Y., and Christensen, R. E.: Fluorescein angiography of choroidal melanomas. Arch. Ophthal., 83:27, 1970.

Pfaffenbach, D. D., and Green, W. R.: Ectopic lacrimal gland. Int. Ophthal. Clin., 11(3):149, 1971.

Pfaffenbach, D. D., Kearns, T. P., and Hollenhorst, R. W.: An unusual case of optic nerve-chiasmal glioma. Amer. J. Ophthal., 74:523, 1972.

Pfeiffer, R. L., and Nicholl, R. J.: Dermoids and epidermoids of the orbit. Trans. Amer. Ophthal. Soc., 46:218, 1948.

Polack, F. M., Kanai, A., and Hood, C. I.: Light and electron microscopic studies of orbital rhabdomyosarcoma. Amer. J. Ophthal., 71:75, 1971.

Porterfield, J. F.: Orbital tumors in children: A report on 214 cases. Int. Ophthal. Clin., 2:319, 1962.

Porterfield, J. F., and Zimmerman, L. E.: Rhabdomyosarcoma of the orbit; a clinicopathologic study of 55 cases. Virchows Arch. Path. Anat., 335:329, 1962.

Reed, R. J., and O'Quinn, S. E.: Vascular Neoplasms. In Fitzpatrick, T. B., et al. (Eds.): Dermatology in General Medicine. New York, McGraw-Hill Book Co., 1971, p. 533.

Reed, W. B., Landing, B., Sugerman, G., Cleaver, J. E., and Melnyk, J.: Xeroderma pigmentosum; clinical and laboratory investigation of its basic defect. J.A.M.A., 207:2073, 1969.

Reese, A. B.: Medulloepithelioma (dictyoma) of the optic nerve. Amer. J. Ophthal., 44:4, 1957.

Reese, A. B.: Tumors of the Eye. 2nd ed. New York, Harper and Hoeber, 1963.

Reese, A. B.: Precancerous and cancerous melanosis. Amer. J. Ophthal., 61:1272, 1966.

Reese, A. B., Jones, I. S., and Cooper, W. C.: Surgery for tumors of the iris and ciliary body. Amer. J. Ophthal., 66:173, 1968.

Regan, J. D., Setlow, R. B., Kaback, M. M., Howell, R. R., Klein, E., and Burgess, G.: Xeroderma pigmentosum: a rapid sensitive method for prenatal diagnosis. Science, 174:147, 1971.

Riley, F. C.: Metastatic tumors of the eyelids. Amer. J. Ophthal., 69:259, 1970.

Roch, L. M., and Milauskas, A. T.: Epibulbar osteomas. Arch. Ophthal., 79:578, 1968.

Rones, B.: Microphthalmos with cyst and orbital teratoma. Verhoeff Society Meeting, April, 1969.

Rones, B., and Zimmerman, L. E.: The prognosis of primary tumors of the iris treated by iridectomy. Arch. Ophthal., 60:193, 1958.

Rosenberg, S. A., Diamond, H. D., Jaslowitz, B., and Craver, L. F.: Lymphosarcoma: A review of 1269 cases. Medicine, 40:31, 1961.

Russell, D. S., and Rubenstein, L. J.: Pathology of Tumours of the Nervous System. 3rd ed. London, Edward Arnold Publishers, Ltd., 1971, p. 48.

Sabates, F. N., and Yamashita, T.: Congenital melanosis oculi complicated by two independent malignant melanomas of the choroid. Arch. Ophthal., 77:801, 1967.

Sagerman, R. H., Tretter, P., and Ellsworth, R. M.: The treatment of orbital rhabdomyosarcoma of children with primary radiation therapy. Amer. J. Roentgen. Radium Ther. Nucl. Med., 114:31, 1972.

Samuel, S., Pildes, R. S., Lewison, M., and Rosenthal, I. M.: Neonatal hyperthyroidism in an infant born of an euthyroid mother. Amer. J. Dis. Child., 121:440, 1971.

Sanders, T. E.: Infantile xanthogranuloma of the orbit; a report of three cases. Amer. J. Ophthal., 61:1299, 1966.

Sanderson, P., Wong, V. G., and Green, W. R.: Tuberous sclerosis with astrocytoma of optic nerve head: a clinico-pathologic case report. In preparation.

Saran, N., and Winter, F. C.: Bilateral gliomas of the optic discs associated with neurofibromatosis. Amer. J. Ophthal., 64:607, 1967.

Sawitsky, A., Desposito, F., Treat, C., et al.: Vincristine and cyclophosphamide in generalized neuroblastoma. Amer. J. Dis. Child., 119:308, 1970.

Schatz, H.: Benign orbital neurilemmoma; sarcomatous transformation in von Recklinghausen's disease. Arch. Ophthal., 86:268, 1971.

Schuster, S. A. D., Ferguson, E. C., III, and Marshall, R. B.: Alveolar rhabdomyosarcoma of the eyelid; diagnosis by electron microscopy. Arch. Ophthal., 87:646, 1972.

Sen, D. K., Mohan, H., and Chatterjee, P. K.: Neurilemmoma of the lacrimal sac. Eye Ear Nose Throat Mon., 50:179, 1971.

Simpson, J. R.: Natural history of cavernous hemangiomata. Lancet, 2:1057, 1959.

Smith, B., and English, F. P.: Classical eyelid border sign of neurofibromatosis. Brit. J. Ophthal., 54:134, 1970.

Smith, J. L. S., and Ingram, R. M.: Juvenile oculodermal xanthogranuloma. Brit. J. Ophthal., 52:696, 1968.

Smith, M. E., Sanders, T. E., and Bresnick, G. H.: Juvenile xanthogranuloma of the ciliary body in an adult. Arch. Ophthal., 81:813, 1969.

Soloway, H. B.: Radiation-induced neoplasms following curative therapy for retinoblastoma. Cancer, 19:1984, 1966.

Stafford, W. R., Yanoff, M., and Parnell, B. L.: Retinoblastomas initially misdiagnosed as primary ocular inflammations. Arch. Ophthal., 82:771, 1969.

Stallard, H. B.: Radiotherapy for malignant melanoma of the choroid. Brit. J. Ophthal., 50:147, 1966.

Starling, K. A., Donaldson, M. H., Haggard, M. E., Vietti, T. J., and Sutow, W. W.: Therapy of histiocytosis X with vincristine, vinblastine, and cyclophosphamide. The Southwest Cancer Chemotherapy Study Group. Amer. J. Dis. Child., 123:105, 1972.

Stegmaier, O. C.: Cosmetic management of nevi. J.A.M.A., 199:917, 1967.

Stern, S. D., and Arenberg, I. K.: Infantile nevoxanthoendothelioma of the iris treated with topical steroids and antiglaucoma therapy. J. Pediat. Ophthal., 7:100, 1970.

Strum, S. B., and Rappaport, H.: Hodgkin's disease in first decade of life. Pediatrics, 46:748, 1970.

Sugar, H. S., and Berman, M.: Relationship between the mandibulofacial dysostosis syndrome of Franceschetti and the oculo-auriculo-vertebral dysplasia syndrome of Goldenhar. Amer. J. Ophthal., 66:510, 1968.

Sutow, W. W.: Chemotherapeutic management of childhood rhabdomyosarcoma. In M. D. Anderson Hospital and Tumor Institute 12th Annual Clinical Conference on Cancer, 1967: Neoplasia in Childhood. Chicago, Year Book Medical Publishers, 1969, p. 201.

Sutow, W. W., Sullivan, M. P., Ried, H. L., Taylor, H. G., and Griffith, K. M.: Prognosis in childhood rhabdomyosarcoma. Cancer, 25:1384, 1970.

Templeton, A. C.: Orbital tumors in African children. Brit. J. Ophthal., 55:254, 1971.

Ts'o, M. O. M., Fine, B. S., and Zimmerman, L. E.: The Flexner-Wintersteiner rosettes in retinoblastoma. Arch. Path., 88:664, 1969.

Ts'o, M. O. M., Zimmerman, L. E., and Fine, B. S.: The nature of retinoblastoma. I. Photoreceptor differentiation: A clinical and histopathologic study; II. Photoreceptor differentiation: An electron microscopic study. Amer. J. Ophthal., 69:339, 350; 1970a.

Ts'o, M. O. M., Zimmerman, L. E., Fine, B. S., and Ellsworth, R. M.: A cause of radioresistance in retinoblastoma: Photoreceptor differentiation. Trans. Amer. Acad. Ophthalmol. Otolaryngol., 74:959, 1970b.

Udvarhelyi, G. B., Khodadoust, A. A., and Walsh, F. B.: Gliomas of the optic nerve and chiasm in children: An unusual series of cases. Clin. Neurosurg., 13:204, 1965, publ. 1966.

Usher, C. H.: The Bowman Lecture: On a few hereditary eye affections. Trans. Ophthal. Soc. U. K., 55:164, 1935.

Vail, D. T.: Iridocyclectomy. A review; gleanings from the literature. Amer. J. Ophthal., 71:161, 1971.

Verdaguer, J., Jr.: Prepuberal and puberal melanomas in ophthalmology. Amer. J. Ophthal., 60:1002, 1965.

Verhoeff, F. H.: Tumors of the optic nerve. In Penfield, W. (Ed.): Cytology and Cellular Pathology of the Nervous System. Vol. 3. New York, Hoeber, 1932, p. 1027.

Vincent, N. J., and Cleasby, G. W.: Schwannoma of the bulbar conjunctiva. Arch. Ophthal., 80:641, 1968.

Vogel, M. H.: Treatment of malignant choroidal melanomas with photocoagulation; evaluation of 10-year follow-up data. Amer. J. Ophthal., 74:1, 1972.

Von Sallman, L., and Paton, D.: Hereditary benign intraepithelial dyskeratosis. I. Ocular manifestations. Arch. Ophthal., 63:421, 1960.

Walsh, F. B.: Meningiomas, primary within the orbit and optic canal. In Smith, J. L. (Ed.): Neuroophthalmology Symposium of the University of Miami and the Bascom Palmer Eye Institute. Vol. 5, Hallandale, Florida., Huffman Publishing, 1970, p. 240.

Walsh, T. J., and Packer, S.: Radioisotope detection of ocular melanomas. New Eng. J. Med., 284:317, 1971.

Warburg, M.: Norrie's disease; a congenital progressive oculo-acoustico-cerebral degeneration. Acta Ophthal. Suppl. 89, 1966, p. 147.

Weiss, D. I., and Krohn, D. L.: Benign melanocytic glaucoma complicating oculodermal melanocytosis. Ann. Ophthal., *3*:958, 1971.

Weiter, J., and Farkas, T. G.: Pseudotumor of the orbit as a presenting sign in Wegener's granulomatosis. Surv. Ophthal., *17*:106, 1972.

Welch, R. B.: von Hippel-Lindau disease: The recognition and treatment of early angiomatosis retinae and the use of cryosurgery as an adjunct to therapy. Trans. Amer. Ophthal. Soc., *68*:367, 1970.

White, J. H.: Oculo-nasal dysplasia. J. Génét. Human., *17*:107, 1969.

Witkop, C. J., Jr., Shankle, C. H., Graham, J. B., Murray, M. R., Rucknagel, D. L., and Byerly, B. H.: Hereditary benign intraepithelial dyskeratosis. II. Oral manifestations and hereditary transmission. Arch. Path., *70*:696, 1960.

Wolken, S. H., Spivey, B. E., and Blodi, F. C.: Hereditary adenoid cystic epithelioma (Brooke's tumor). Amer. J. Ophthal., *68*:26, 1969.

Wolter, J. R., and Henderson, J. W.: Adenoid cystic carcinoma in the orbit of a child. J. Pediat. Ophthal., *6*:47, 1969.

Wolter, J. R., and Mertus, J. M.: Exophytic retinal as-

trocytoma in tuberous sclerosis. Report of a case. J. Pediat. Ophthal., *6*:186, 1969.

Wolter, J. R., Peterson, N. P., and Barnett, J. M.: Superficial amputation neuroma following enucleation. J. Pediat. Ophthal., *9*:31, 1971.

Yanoff, M.: Hereditary benign intraepithelial dyskeratosis. Arch. Ophthal., *79*:291, 1968.

Yanoff, M., Davis, R., and Zimmerman, L. E.: Glioma of the optic nerve. In preparation.

Yousseffi, B.: Orbital tumors in children. A clinical study of 62 cases. J. Pediat. Ophthal., *6*:177, 1969.

Zimmerman, L. E.: Ocular lesions of juvenile xanthogranuloma; nevoxanthoendothelioma. Trans. Amer. Acad. Ophthalmol. Otolaryngol., *69*:412, 1965.

Zimmerman, L. E.: Criteria for management of melanosis. Arch. Ophthal., *76*:307, 1966.

Zimmerman, L. E.: Verhoeff's "terato-neuroma": A critical reappraisal in light of new observations and current concepts of embryonic tumors. Amer. J. Ophthal., *72*:1039, 1971.

Zimmerman, L. E., Sanders, T. E., and Ackerman, L. V.: Epithelial tumors of the lacrimal gland: Prognostic and therapeutic significance of histologic types. Int. Ophthal. Clin., *2*:337, 1962.

Index